Anatomy & Physiology Essentials

by

Susan J. Hall, PhD, FACSM
Professor of Kinesiology and Applied Physiology
University of Delaware
Newark, Delaware

Michelle A. Provost-Craig, PhD
Associate Professor of Kinesiology and Applied Physiology
University of Delaware
Newark, Delaware

William C. Rose, PhD
Associate Professor of Kinesiology and Applied Physiology
University of Delaware
Newark, Delaware

Publisher
The Goodheart-Willcox Company, Inc.
Tinley Park, IL
www.g-w.com

Manufactured in the United States of America.

ISBN 978-1-63563-574-4

1 2 3 4 5 6 7 8 9 – 20 – 24 23 22 21 20 19 18

Image Credits: Front cover *Foreground*: © Sebastian Kaulitzki/Shutterstock.com; *Background*: zffoto/Shutterstock.com

Library of Congress Cataloging-in-Publication Data

Names: Hall, Susan J. (Susan Jean), 1953- author. | Provost-Craig, Michelle, author. | Rose, William C., author.
Title: Anatomy & physiology essentials / by Susan J. Hall, PhD, Michelle A. Provost-Craig, PhD, William C. Rose, PhD.
Description: Tinley Park, IL : The Goodheart-Willcox Company, Inc., [2020] | Includes index.
Identifiers: LCCN 2018031664 | ISBN 9781635635744
Subjects: LCSH: Human anatomy--Textbooks. | Human physiology--Textbooks. | LCGFT: Textbooks.
Classification: LCC QM23.2 .H338 2020 | DDC 612--dc23 LC record available at https://lccn.loc.gov/2018031664

Brief Contents

Preface

Would you like to live to be 100 years of age? Have you ever wondered why life expectancy varies from country to country across the world? Do you want to stay healthy for your entire life, no matter how long you do live? Can loss of hearing, vision, and mental acuity in later life be prevented? Scientists and physicians have been searching for answers to questions about the body's anatomy and physiology for centuries, and that search continues today. As scientific discoveries increase our knowledge about the human body, the possibilities for living longer and healthier lives are increasing.

No matter what your career aspirations—whether you are destined for a career in a medical field or planning to become an artist or start your own business—knowledge about the human body can be very useful to you in terms of both your health and appearance. Many of the lifestyle choices that you make today will affect your body when you reach age 60 and beyond. And with your own knowledge about the human body, you can help influence the health of your family and friends.

This text will answer numerous questions about the structure and function of the human body that may have crossed your mind. It will spark your curiosity about things you have never thought about. As you discover more and more about the fascinating intricacies of the human body, we believe you will agree with us that the human body is the most interesting topic in all of science.

Susan J. Hall
Michelle A. Provost-Craig
William C. Rose

About the Authors

Susan J. Hall is a professor in the Department of Kinesiology and Applied Physiology at the University of Delaware. She is a fellow of the American College of Sports Medicine and the AAHPERD Research Consortium, and she has served as President of the Biomechanics Academy of AAHPERD, President of the AAHPERD Research Consortium, and Vice President of the American College of Sports Medicine. She is also the author of several successful textbooks and has served on several journal editorial boards. After graduating from Duke University, she began her career as a high school biology teacher. She earned a master's degree from Texas Woman's University and a PhD from Washington State University. She has been teaching at the college level for more than 30 years and served for many years as a department chair and deputy dean.

Michelle A. Provost-Craig is an Associate Professor in the Department of Kinesiology and Applied Physiology at the University of Delaware, where she has taught graduate and undergraduate courses in physiology, clinical exercise physiology, and electrocardiogram interpretation for more than 20 years. She is the recipient of the University's most prestigious awards for Excellence in Teaching and Excellence in Advising and Mentoring. She also received a University grant from the Center for Teaching Effectiveness to develop innovative approaches to teaching anatomy and physiology to college students. At the University of Delaware, she served as the graduate coordinator of the Masters in Exercise Science program and was the founder of their Cardiopulmonary Rehabilitation Program. Dr. Provost-Craig has served in numerous leadership roles for the United States Figure Skating Association (USFSA) and has performed physiological assessments of national and international elite ice figure skaters. She was the Vice President of the Mid-Atlantic Chapter of the Regional American College of Sports Medicine (ACSM) and has participated in several ACSM committees. Dr. Provost-Craig earned a Master's degree from the University of Delaware and a PhD in Exercise Physiology from the University of Maryland.

William C. Rose is an Associate Professor in the Department of Kinesiology and Applied Physiology at the University of Delaware, where he has taught anatomy and physiology for 20 years. He is a member of the American Physiological Society and the American College of Sports Medicine. He is the author of textbook chapters and research articles in the fields of cardiovascular physiology and biomechanics. He has served as a grant proposal reviewer for the National Science Foundation and as a manuscript reviewer for scientific journals such as Circulation and the American Journal of Physiology. After graduating from Harvard University with a degree in physics, Rose earned a PhD in biomedical engineering from Johns Hopkins University. He completed a postdoctoral fellowship in cardiology at Johns Hopkins Hospital, and he worked in research and development for the DuPont Company before joining the University of Delaware.

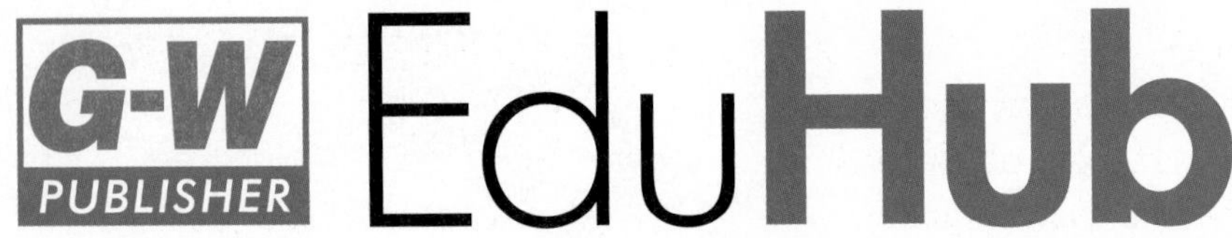

Be Digital Ready on Day One with EduHub

EduHub provides a solid base of knowledge and instruction for digital and blended classrooms. This easy-to-use learning hub delivers the foundation and tools that improve student retention and facilitate instructor efficiency. For the student, EduHub offers an online collection of eBook content, interactive practice, and test preparation. Additionally, students have the ability to view and submit assessments, track personal performance, and view feedback via the Student Report option. For instructors, EduHub provides a turnkey, fully integrated solution with course management tools to deliver content, assessments, and feedback to students quickly and efficiently. The integrated approach results in improved student outcomes and instructor flexibility.

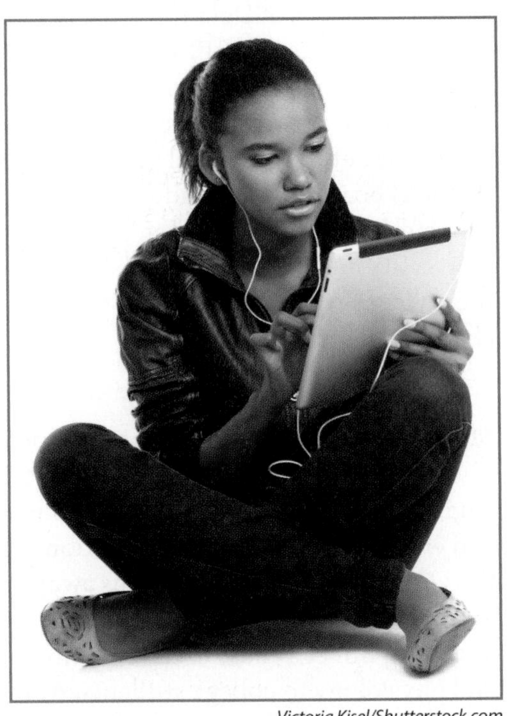

Victoria Kisel/Shutterstock.com

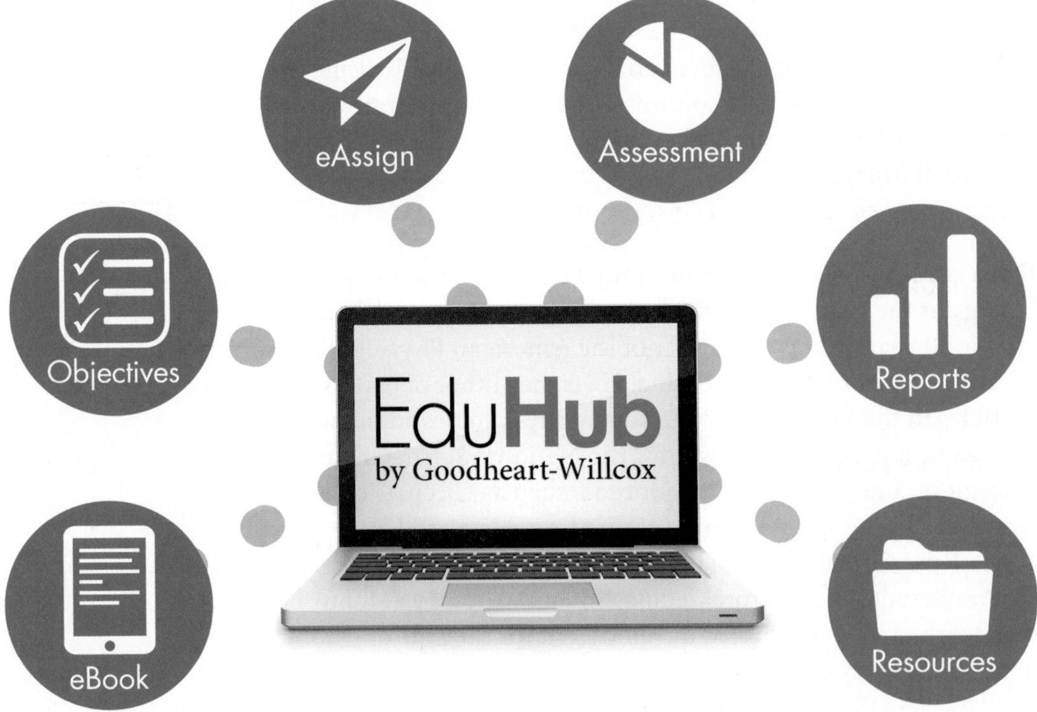

eBook

The EduHub eBook engages students by providing the ability to take notes, access the text-to-speech option to improve comprehension, and highlight key concepts to remember. In addition, the accessibility features enable students to customize font and color schemes for personal viewing, while links to practice activities and animations bring content to life.

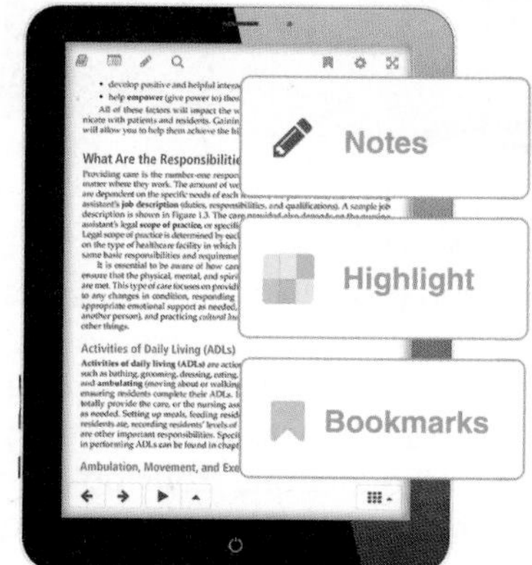

Objectives

Course objectives at the beginning of each eBook chapter help students stay focused and provide benchmarks for instructors to evaluate student progress.

eAssign

eAssign makes it easy for instructors to assign, deliver, and assess student engagement. Coursework can be administered to individual students or the entire class.

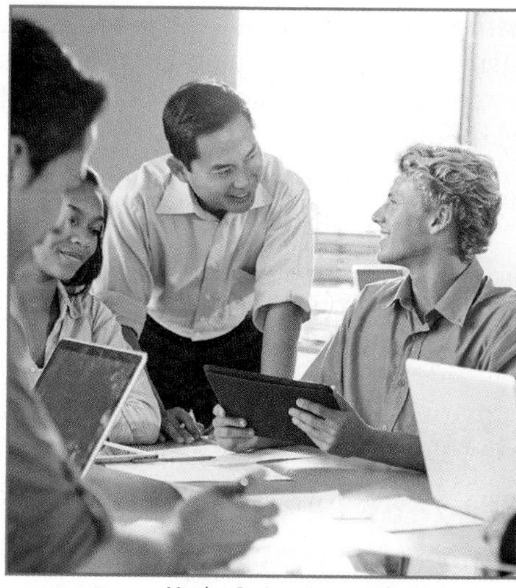

Monkey Business Images/Shutterstock.com

Assessment

Self-assessment opportunities enable students to gauge their understanding as they progress through the course. In addition, formative assessment tools for instructor use provide efficient evaluation of student mastery of content.

Print Export

Score	Items	
100%	●	●
80%	●	●
100%	●	●
80%	●	●
100%	●	●
100%	●	●

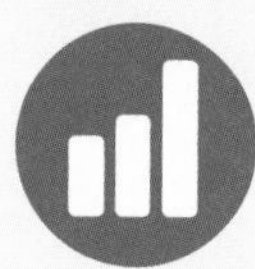

Reports

Reports, for both students and instructors, provide performance results in an instant. Analytics reveal individual student and class achievements for easy monitoring of success.

Instructor Resources

Instructors will find all the support they need to make preparation and classroom instruction more efficient and easier than ever. Lesson plans, answer keys, and PowerPoint® presentations provide an organized, proven approach to classroom management.

Learn more about EduHub at www.g-w.com/eduhub

TOOLS FOR STUDENT AND INSTRUCTOR SUCCESS

EduHub

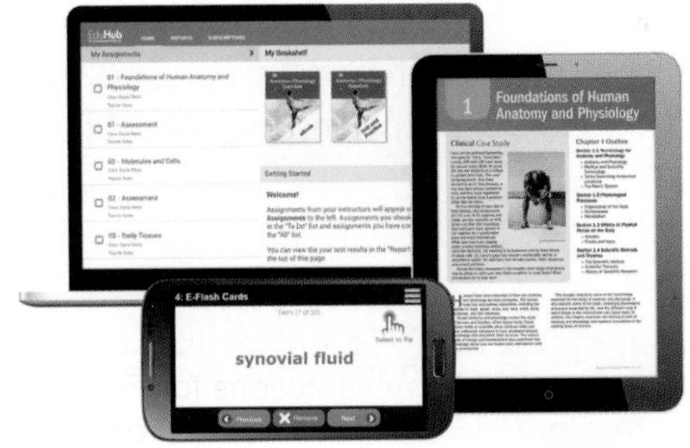

EduHub provides a solid base of knowledge and instruction for digital and blended classrooms. This easy-to-use learning hub provides the foundation and tools that improve student retention and facilitate instructor efficiency.

For the student, EduHub offers an online collection of eBook content, interactive practice, and test preparation. Additionally, students have the ability to view and submit assessments, track personal performance, and view feedback via the Student Report option. For the instructor, EduHub provides a turnkey, fully integrated solution with course management tools to deliver content, assessments, and feedback to students quickly and efficiently. The integrated approach results in improved student outcomes and instructor flexibility. Be digital ready on day one with EduHub!

- **eBook content.** EduHub includes the textbook in an online, reflowable format. The eBook is interactive, with highlighting, magnification, note-taking, and text-to-speech features.
- **eAssign.** In EduHub, students can complete online assignments as specified by their instructor, including text review questions, activities from the Study Guide, and assessments. Many activities are autograded for easy class assessment and management.

Student Tools

Student Text

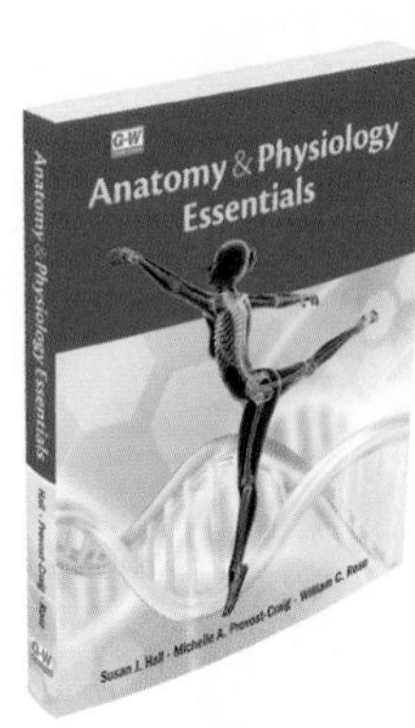

Anatomy & Physiology Essentials provides a solid introduction to human anatomy and physiology. Coverage is broad enough to be useful to students exploring many different career opportunities within the healthcare industry. Starting with the fundamental units from which the human body is built, the content builds to include all of the individual body systems, with an emphasis on terminology as well as structure and function. Attention is also given to diseases, disorders, and conditions that may affect each body system. Clinical scenarios at the beginning of each chapter apply one or more concepts within the chapter, helping to align the topics with realistic cases. Self Checks for each section assess understanding, and review questions at the end of each chapter both assess knowledge and encourage further thinking and research about the topics.

Study Guide

The Study Guide that accompanies *Anatomy & Physiology Essentials* includes instructor-created activities to help students recall, review, and apply concepts introduced in the book.

Instructor Tools

LMS Integration

Integrate Goodheart-Willcox content into your Learning Management System for a seamless user experience for both you and your students. Contact your G-W Educational Consultant for ordering information or visit www.g-w.com/lms-integration.

Instructor Resources

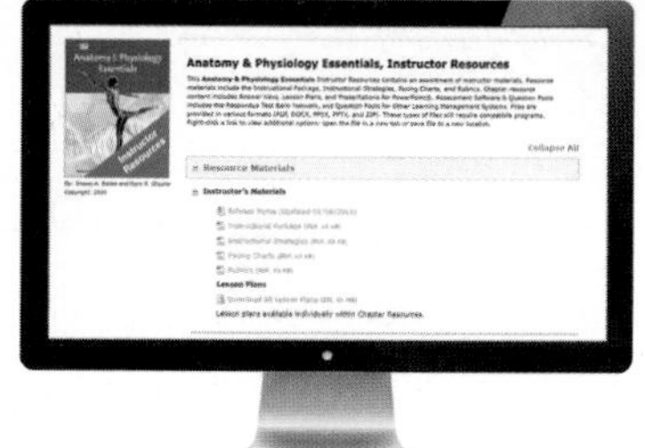

The Instructor Resources provide all the support needed to make preparation and classroom instruction easier than ever. Included are time-saving preparation tools such as answer keys, editable lesson plans, and other teaching aids. In addition, presentations for PowerPoint® and assessment software with question banks are provided for your convenience. These resources can be accessed at school, at home, or on the go.

Instructor's Presentations for PowerPoint® These fully customizable presentations for PowerPoint® provide a useful teaching tool for presenting concepts introduced in the text. Richly illustrated slides help you teach and visually reinforce the key concepts from each chapter.

Assessment Software with Question Banks Administer and manage assessments to meet your classroom needs. The following options are available through the Respondus Test Bank Network.

- A Respondus 4.0 license can be purchased directly from Respondus, which enables you to easily create tests that can be printed on paper or published directly to a variety of Learning Management Systems. Once the question files are published to an LMS, exams can be distributed to students with results reported directly to the LMS gradebook.
- Respondus LE is a limited version of Respondus 4.0 and is free with purchase of the Instructor Resources. It allows you to download question banks and create assessments that can be printed or saved as a paper test.

G-W Integrated Learning Solution

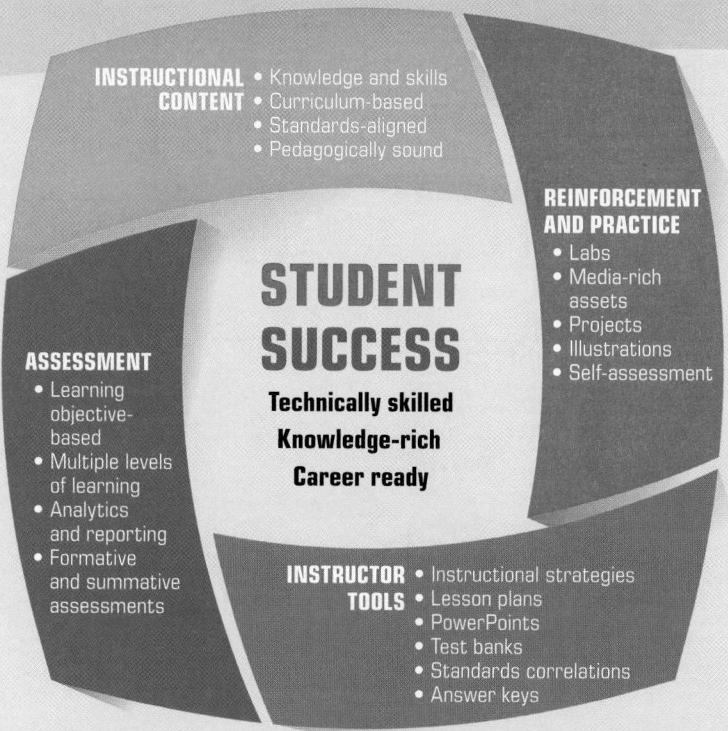

The G-W Integrated Learning Solution offers easy-to-use resources that help students and instructors achieve success.

- **EXPERT AUTHORS**
- **TRUSTED REVIEWERS**
- **100 YEARS OF EXPERIENCE**

EMPLOYABILITY SKILLS · TECHNICAL SKILLS · ACADEMIC KNOWLEDGE · INDUSTRY RECOGNIZED STANDARDS

Guided Tour

Real-World Applications

The *Clinical Case Study* at the beginning of each chapter presents a real-world medical issue related to chapter content. The case study helps prospective healthcare workers understand how the concepts and ideas presented in the chapter are applied in the healthcare field. At the end of the chapter, questions in the Review revisit the case study, asking students to apply chapter content to propose answers to the questions presented in the case study.

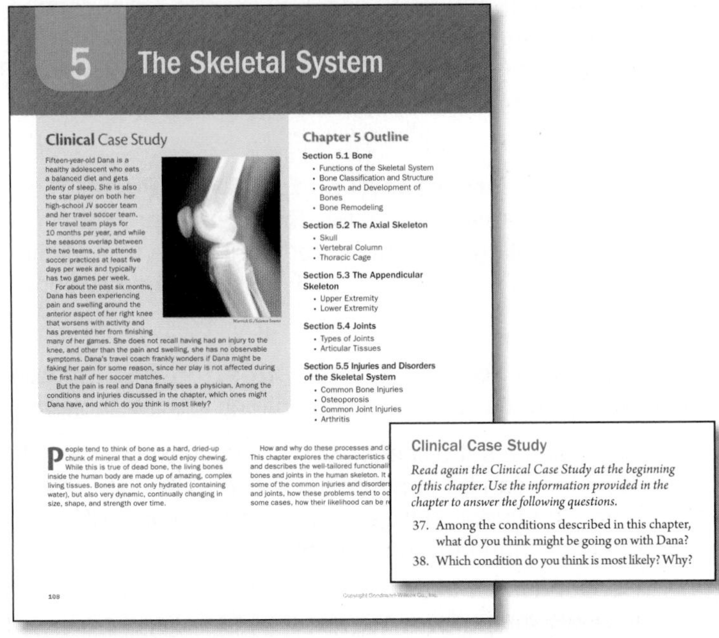

5 The Skeletal System

Clinical Case Study

Fifteen-year-old Dana is a healthy adolescent who eats a balanced diet and gets plenty of sleep. She is also the star player on both her high-school JV soccer team and her travel soccer team. Her travel team plays for 10 months per year, and while the seasons overlap between the two teams, she attends soccer practices at least five days per week and typically has two games per week.

For about the past six months, Dana has been experiencing pain and swelling around the anterior aspect of her right knee that worsens with activity and has prevented her from finishing many of her games. She does not recall having had an injury to the knee, and other than the pain and swelling, she has no observable symptoms. Dana's travel coach frankly wonders if Dana might be faking her pain for some reason, since her play is not affected during the first half of her soccer matches.

But the pain is real and Dana finally sees a physician. Among the conditions and injuries discussed in the chapter, which ones might Dana have, and which do you think is most likely?

Chapter 5 Outline

Section 5.1 Bone
- Functions of the Skeletal System
- Bone Classification and Structure
- Growth and Development of Bones
- Bone Remodeling

Section 5.2 The Axial Skeleton
- Skull
- Vertebral Column
- Thoracic Cage

Section 5.3 The Appendicular Skeleton
- Upper Extremity
- Lower Extremity

Section 5.4 Joints
- Types of Joints
- Articular Tissues

Section 5.5 Injuries and Disorders of the Skeletal System
- Common Bone Injuries
- Osteoporosis
- Common Joint Injuries
- Arthritis

People tend to think of bone as a hard, dried-up chunk of mineral that a dog would enjoy chewing. While this is true of dead bone, the living bones inside the human body are made up of amazing, complex living tissues. Bones are not only hydrated (containing water), but also very dynamic, continually changing in size, shape, and strength over time.

Clinical Case Study

Read again the Clinical Case Study at the beginning of this chapter. Use the information provided in the chapter to answer the following questions.

37. Among the conditions described in this chapter, what do you think might be going on with Dana?
38. Which condition do you think is most likely? Why?

Meaningful Illustrations

Numerous photographs show the effects of various diseases and disorders. Colorful illustrations help students comprehend the complex structure of the human body and how various body systems work together. Well-designed tables provide a concise summary of detailed information.

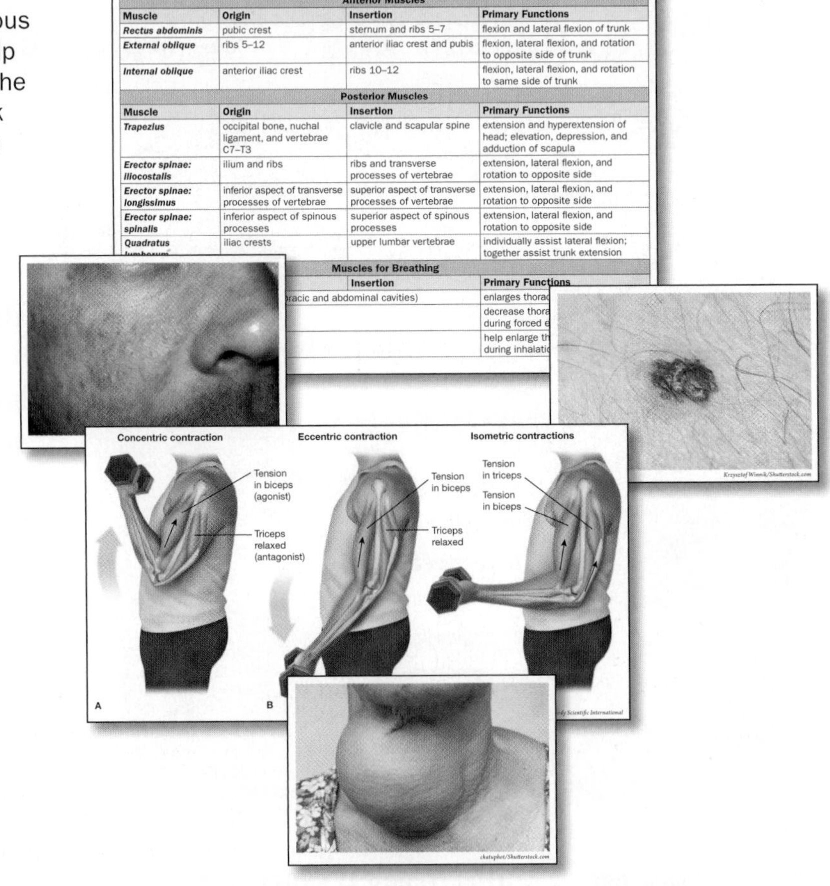

Muscles of the Trunk			
Anterior Muscles			
Muscle	**Origin**	**Insertion**	**Primary Functions**
Rectus abdominis	pubic crest	sternum and ribs 5–7	flexion and lateral flexion of trunk
External oblique	ribs 5–12	anterior iliac crest and pubis	flexion, lateral flexion, and rotation to opposite side of trunk
Internal oblique	anterior iliac crest	ribs 10–12	flexion, lateral flexion, and rotation to same side of trunk
Posterior Muscles			
Muscle	**Origin**	**Insertion**	**Primary Functions**
Trapezius	occipital bone, nuchal ligament, and vertebrae C7–T3	clavicle and scapular spine	extension and hyperextension of head; elevation, depression, and adduction of scapula
Erector spinae: iliocostalis	ilium and ribs	ribs and transverse processes of vertebrae	extension, lateral flexion, and rotation to opposite side
Erector spinae: longissimus	inferior aspect of transverse processes of vertebrae	superior aspect of transverse processes of vertebrae	extension, lateral flexion, and rotation to opposite side
Erector spinae: spinalis	inferior aspect of spinous processes	superior aspect of spinous processes	extension, lateral flexion, and rotation to opposite side
Quadratus	iliac crests	upper lumbar vertebrae	individually assist lateral flexion; together assist trunk extension
Muscles for Breathing			
		Insertion	**Primary Functions**
	racic and abdominal cavities)		enlarges thorac
			decrease thora during forced e
			help enlarge th during inhalatio

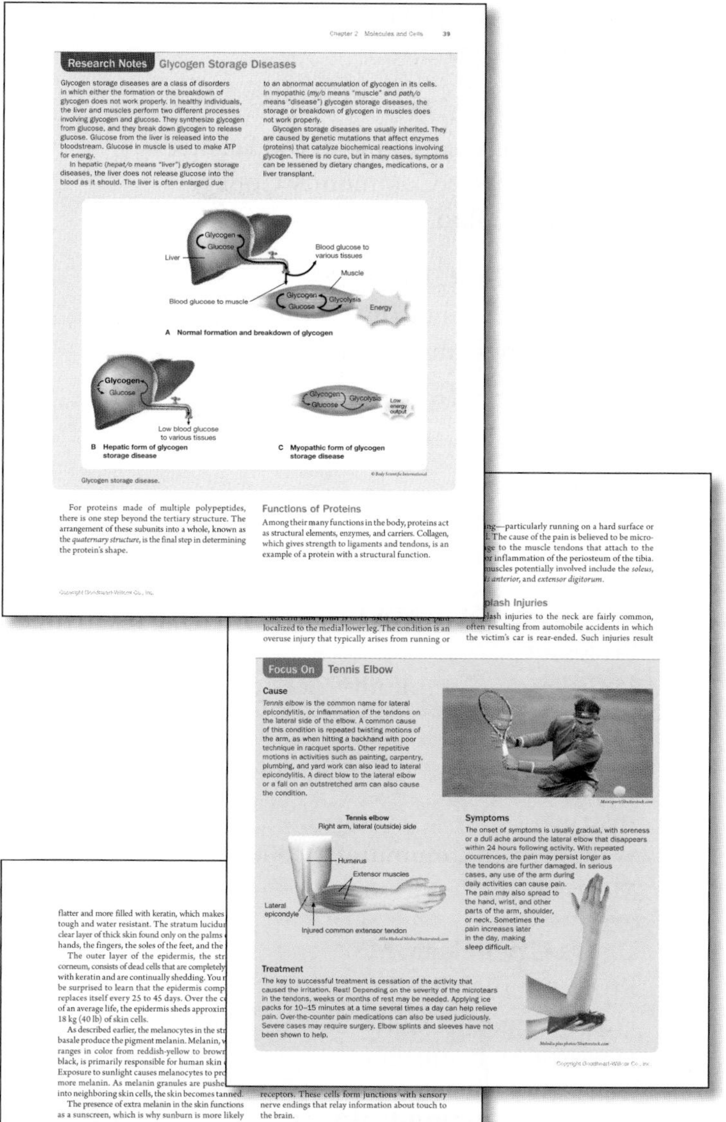

Features

Multiple features address topics of interest to students studying anatomy and physiology. In addition to the *Clinical Case Study* at the beginning of each chapter, *Clinical Applications* throughout the textbook provide insights about how concepts relate to healthcare practices. *Research Notes* highlight recent and ongoing scientific studies related to human anatomy and physiology. *Focus On...* features introduce chapter-related topics of interest to today's students.

Throughout every chapter, *Understanding Medical Terminology* boxes explain the meaning of medical terms, provide insights about why certain structures and medical conditions are named as they are, and provide helpful hints for remembering the terms. In addition, a Medical Terminology section at the end of each chapter helps students practice medical word-building skills.

The Self Check questions at the end of each section help students determine how well they understand the concepts. Review, critical thinking, and research questions at the end of each chapter assess student knowledge and retention, and questions related to the Clinical Case Study help students tie together the chapter concepts in a meaningful way.

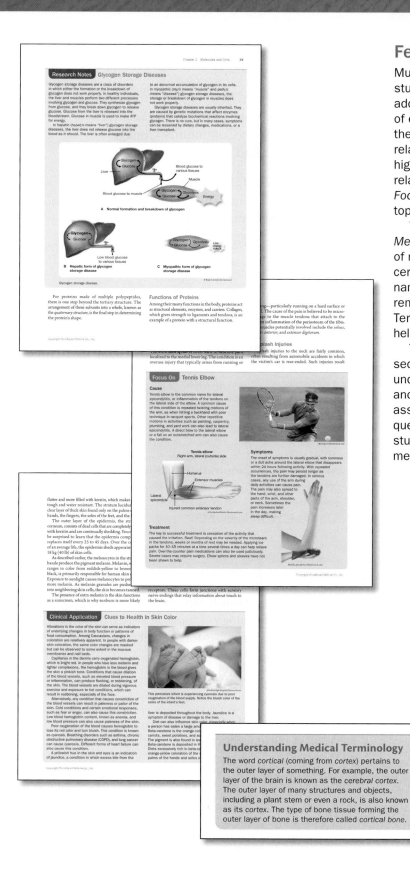

Understanding Medical Terminology

The word *cortical* (coming from *cortex*) pertains to the outer layer of something. For example, the outer layer of the brain is known as the *cerebral cortex.* The outer layer of many structures and objects, including a plant stem or even a rock, is also known as its *cortex.* The type of bone tissue forming the outer layer of bone is therefore called *cortical bone.*

Reviewers

Goodheart-Willcox Publisher would like to thank the following instructors who reviewed selected chapters and provided valuable input into the development of this textbook program.

Gretchen Baumle
Instructor
Sinclair Community College
Dayton, Ohio

Dr. Matthew J. Borcherding
Biology Faculty
Minnesota State Community & Technical College
Fergus Falls, Minnesota

Donna Burge, DVM
Professor of Human Anatomy and Physiology
Lord Fairfax Community College
Warrenton, Virginia

Stephanie M. Burks, MS
Biology Instructor
Hinds Community College
Utica, Mississippi

Tammy Calpin
Instructor
Pennsylvania Highland Community College
Johnstown, Pennsylvania

Kristian Coerper
Anatomy and Physiology Teacher
Kenwood Academy
Chicago, Illinois

George Cornwall
Instructor
Colorado Mountain College
Carbondale, Colorado

Craig Denesha, MS
Academic Director of Science
Spartanburg Community College
Spartanburg, South Carolina

Andrea Dozier
Instructor
Albany Technical College
Albany, Georgia

Miles E. Drake, MD
Adjunct Professor of Biological Sciences
Columbus State Community College
Columbus, Ohio

Lynda DuRant, RN, BSN
Healthcare Science Instructor
South Effingham High School
Savannah, Georgia

Holly Dust
Instructor
Lake Land College
Mattoon, Illinois

Ruby Fogg, MA, MAT
Professor
Manchester Community College
Manchester, New Hampshire

Greg Grass
Instructor
Walters State Community College
Morristown, Tennessee

Debra Grieneisen, MS
Professor, Biology
Harrisburg Area Community College
Harrisburg, Pennsylvania

Kathryn Gronlund, MS
Professor of Biology
Lone Star College—Montgomery
Controe, Texas

Louanne Harto
Instructor
Polk Community College
Winter Haven, Florida

Erin Hattabaugh
Instructor
Cleveland High School
Cleveland, Tennessee

Stephanie Havemann
Instructor
Alvin Community College
Katy, Texas

Ashley Hollern
Instructor
Pennsylvania Highlands Community College
Richland, Pennsylvania

Thomas M. Justice, MS
Professor of Biology
McLennan Community College
Waco, Texas

Tiffany Killblane, MS
Instructor of Biology
Cowley County Community College
Arkansas City, Kansas

Lorin R. King
Professor of Science; Science Department Head
Western Nebraska Community College
Scottsbluff, Nebraska

Phillip Latimer, DC
Assistant Professor of Biology
Andrew College
Cuthbert, Georgia

Dean Lauritzen
Instructor
City College of San Francisco
San Francisco, California

Melinda Lawson, RN, MSN, CNS, OCN
Academy Chair, PLTW Biomedical Teacher
BJHS Medical
Madison, Alabama

Stephen Leadon, PhD
Science Coordinator and Instructor
Durham Technical Community College
Durham, North Carolina

Leontine M. Lowery, MA, RHIA
Instructor, Science
Delaware Technical Community College
Dover, Delaware

Kim McMasters
Instructor
Forsyth Technical Community College
Asheboro, North Carolina

Ann Mills, MS
Biology Instructor
Minnesota West Community
and Technical College
Worthington, Minnesota

Norma Moore
Instructor
Laredo Community College
Laredo, Texas

Laura Ritt
Assistant Professor of Biology
Rowan College at Burlington County
Mount Laurel, New Jersey

James Sciandra
Instructor
Roxbury Community College
Roxbury Crossing, Massachusetts

Jaya Prakash Shah
Instructor
Woodland Community College
Woodland, California

Penelope Wilson
Instructor
Corning Community College
Corning, New York

Erin Windsor
Instructor
Mohave Community College
Bullhead City, Arizona

Contents

Identified features include:
Clinical Application
Focus On
Research Notes

1 Foundations of Human Anatomy and Physiology

Clinical Case Study

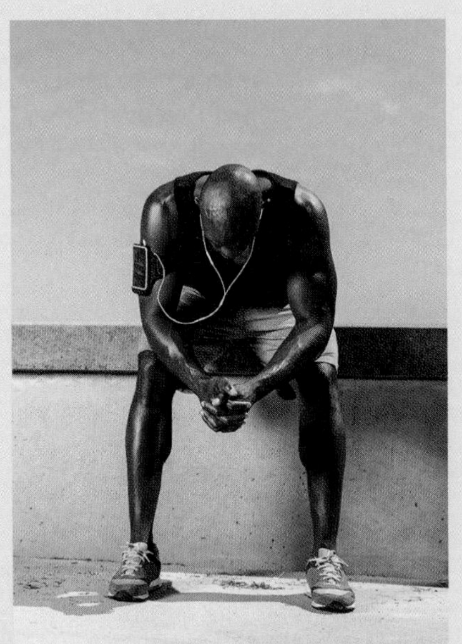
Jacob Lund/Shutterstock.com

Larry and his girlfriend Samantha, who goes by "Sam," have been running 10K and 15K road races for several years. Both 24 years old, they are students at a college in upstate New York. This year for spring break, they have decided to go to New Orleans, a city they have always wanted to visit, and they have registered to run the Mardi Gras marathon while they are there.

On the morning of race day in New Orleans, the temperature at 7:00 a.m. is 82 degrees and rising, and the humidity is 90%. Since it is their first marathon, Sam and Larry have agreed to run together at a comfortable pace and enjoy themselves. While Sam has been sipping water at every hydration station, Larry has declined, not wanting to be bothered until he feels thirsty. At about mile 12, Larry's pace has slowed considerably and he is drenched in sweat. He tells Sam that he has cramps, feels nauseous, and cannot continue.

Among the topics discussed in the chapter, what range of problems may be going on with Larry and which condition is most likely? What should Sam do to help him?

Chapter 1 Outline

Humans have been interested in their own anatomy and physiology for many centuries. The human body has astonishing capabilities, including the abilities to think, speak, move, see, hear, smell, taste, remember, and feel emotions.

Human anatomy and physiology involve the study of the form and function of the human body. These ancient fields of scientific study continue today and have sufficiently advanced to have developed precise terminology that describes what we know. The related fields of biology and biomechanics also contribute new knowledge about how our bodies work and interact with the environment.

This chapter describes some of the terminology essential for the study of anatomy and physiology. It also explains some of the basic, underlying physiological processes essential for life, and the different ways in which forces in the environment can cause injury. In addition, the chapter examines the historical roots of anatomy and physiology and explores innovations in the exciting fields of science.

SECTION 1.1

Terminology for Anatomy and Physiology

Objectives

- Explain the relationship between anatomy and physiology.
- Identify and define the word parts that make up medical terms.
- Use medical terminology to describe locations, planes, and movements of the body.
- Discuss the choice of the metric system as the international system of measurement for all fields of science.

Key Terms

abdominal cavity
abdominopelvic cavity
anatomical position
anatomy
anterior (ventral) cavity
cranial cavity
frontal plane
metric system
middle ear cavities
nasal cavity
oral cavity
orbital cavities
pelvic cavity
physiology
posterior (dorsal) cavity
sagittal plane
spinal cavity
thoracic cavity
transverse plane

Like all fields of science, the related disciplines of anatomy and physiology use a specialized set of terminology to provide accurate descriptions of body structures and functions. This chapter introduces the study of anatomy and physiology, as well as some of the basic terminology that will be used throughout the book.

Anatomy and Physiology

In describing living organisms, the term *anatomy* is often closely followed by the term *physiology*. Although these concepts are closely related in some respects, they are very different in others.

Anatomy is the study of the form or structure of all living things, including both plants and animals. This book focuses on human anatomy. The word *anatomy* is taken from Greek words meaning "to cut apart." The study of the body structures you can see with your eyes is called *gross anatomy*. The study of tiny parts of the body, seen only with a microscope, is termed *microscopic anatomy*.

Physiology is the study of how living things function. This book discusses human physiology. Looking through the table of contents, you will see that most of this book's chapters focus on one of the systems of the human body. The muscular system, skeletal system, and cardiovascular system are familiar examples.

Branches of human physiology exist for all of the different systems of the human body, including muscle physiology, skeletal physiology, and cardiovascular physiology. Each system contributes a unique capability to the human body, and some systems influence other systems.

Why are the studies of anatomy and physiology combined in one book? The answer is that there is a close relationship between how our bodies are structured and how they function.

In a healthy human body, all functions are normal and painless. But when a disease or injury causes a breakdown of even a small part of a body structure, abnormal function and pain can result. An obvious example is the case of a broken femur, which prevents normal leg movement. Another example is a tumor in the digestive tract that prevents the normal passage of materials through the digestive system and rapidly becomes painful and life-threatening. Understanding the normal anatomy and physiology of the human body is the first step in understanding the structures and processes that become dysfunctional with injury and disease.

SELF CHECK

1. What is the difference between anatomy and physiology?
2. What is gross anatomy?

Medical and Scientific Terminology

Most medical and scientific terms are composed of word parts that are combined in certain ways. The four types of word parts are:

- root—the main part of the term that provides its central meaning
- prefix—one or more letters added to the beginning of a root to modify its meaning

- suffix—one or more letters added after the root to modify its meaning
- combining vowel—vowel inserted to link the components of a term and so that the term can be pronounced more easily; usually *o*, but occasionally *a*, *e*, *i*, or *u*

Because the combining vowel is most often used with the root, these two parts are often shown together. For example, the root *cardi* may be written *cardi/o*. Word parts can be combined in many different ways to form medical and scientific terms. Here are some examples using the root *cardi*, meaning "heart":

- prefix, root, suffix: peri/cardi/um (*pericardium*, membrane around the heart)
- root, combining vowel, suffix: cardi/o/gram (*cardiogram*, recording of heart activity)
- root, combining vowel, root: cardi/o/vascular (*cardiovascular*, pertaining to the heart and blood vessels)

Figure 1.1 presents some of the prefixes, roots, and suffixes commonly used in terms related to human anatomy and physiology. Knowledge of these word parts is valuable in understanding specialized medical and scientific terms.

SELF CHECK

1. What is the purpose of a combining vowel?
2. Based on the information in Figure 1.1, what medical term would you expect to be used for "bone disease"?

Terms Describing Anatomical Locations

The body position that serves as a basis for describing positions and directions for the human body is called the ***anatomical position*** (**Figure 1.2**). The anatomical position is a normal standing position, with the feet slightly apart, the head and shoulders facing forward, and the palms of the hands facing forward.

Planes

To describe the human body and its movements, scientists and clinicians refer to three imaginary planes passing through the center of the body (**Figure 1.2**). Collectively, these are referred to as

Word Parts		
Prefixes		
Category	**Prefix**	**Definition**
Related to number	bi-	two, both
	di-	two, double
	quad, quadri-	four
	tri-	three
	uni-	one, single
Related to size	hemi-	half
	hyper-	above normal, excessive
	hypo-	below normal, deficient
	poly-	many, much
Related to position, direction, or location	ab-	away, away from
	ad-	toward
	endo-	in, within
	hypo-	below
	inter-	between
	intra-	within, into
	para-	near, beside
	peri-	around, surrounding
	post-	after, behind
	pre-	before, in front of

(continued)

Goodheart-Willcox Publisher

Figure 1.1

Word Parts *(Continued)*		
Roots and Combining Vowels		
Category	**Root**	**Definition**
General words	bi/o	life
	cyt/o	cell
	electr/o	electricity
	erythr/o	red
	leuk/o	white
	phys/o	function, nature
Related to body parts	arthr/o	joint
	carcin/o	cancer
	cardi/o	heart
	derm/o	skin
	enter/o	intestine
	gastr/o	stomach
	gynec/o	female, woman
	hemat/o	blood
	hepat/o	liver
	neur/o	nerve
	ophthalm/o	eye
	oste/o	bone
	psych/o	mind
	ren/o	kidney
	rhin/o	nose
Suffixes		
Category	**Suffix**	**Definition**
Related to diseases and disorders	-algia	pain
	-cele	hernia, swelling, protrusion
	-edema	swelling, fluid retention
	-emia	blood condition
	-ia	condition
	-itis	inflammation
	-malacia	softening
	-megaly	enlargement
	-oma	tumor, mass
	-osis	abnormal condition
	-pathy	disease
	-penia	deficiency
	-trophy	condition of growth or development
Related to the process of viewing	-gram	record, image
	-graphy	process of recording
	-scope	instrument used to view
Related to surgery	-ectomy	surgical removal
	-lysis	breakdown, separation
	-plasty	surgical repair
	-tomy	process of cutting, incision
Related to careers and research	-ist, -logist	specialist
	-logy	study of

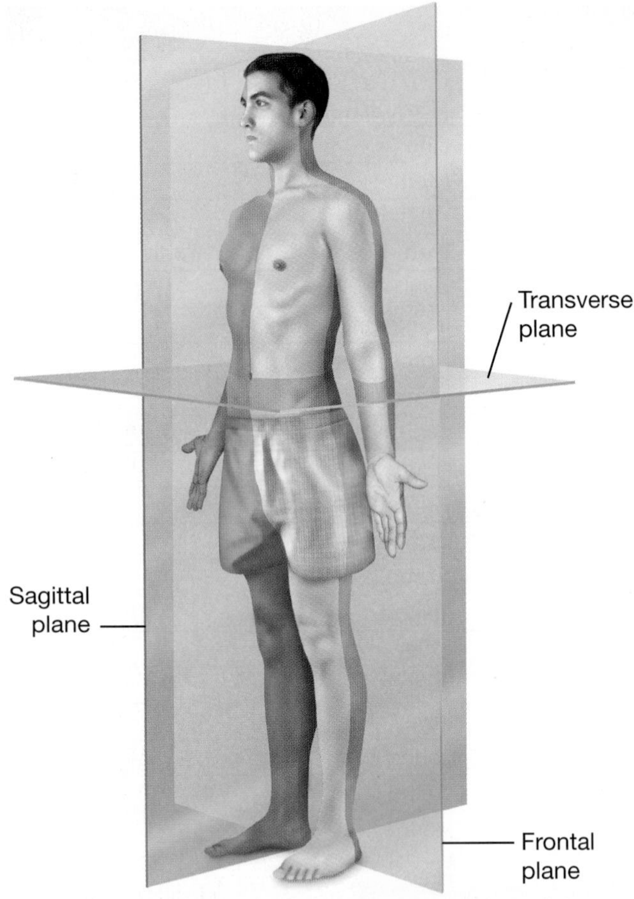

© Body Scientific International

Figure 1.2 The anatomical position is a reference position used when describing locations on a patient's body. Three imaginary planes divide the body into halves in three directions.

the *cardinal planes,* with each plane bisecting the human body into halves.

- The ***sagittal plane*** divides the body into right and left halves—so forward and backward motions of the body or body parts are said to be *sagittal plane movements.*
- The ***frontal plane*** divides the body into front and back halves, with sideways movements considered to be *frontal plane movements.*
- Finally, the ***transverse plane*** divides the body into top and bottom halves, and rotational movements are called *transverse plane movements.*

Of course, many body movements follow a curved path and are not lined up with any one plane. Such movements are described as *nonplanar.*

Directions

Directional terms describe relationships among body parts (**Figure 1.3**). The most commonly used

Common Directional Terms for Anatomy	
Term	**Description**
superior (cranial)	closer to the head
inferior (caudal)	away from the head
anterior (ventral)	toward the front of the body
posterior (dorsal)	toward the back of the body
medial	toward the midline of the body
lateral	away from the midline of the body
proximal	closer to the trunk
distal	away from the trunk
superficial	toward the surface of the body
deep	away from the surface of the body

Figure 1.3 Goodheart-Willcox Publisher

directional terms are paired, describing opposite relationships. For example, the term *superior* means "above" or "over," whereas *inferior* means "below" or "under." So it is correct to state that the chin is superior to the knees. Alternatively, you could say that the knees are inferior to the chin.

Regions

Specific regions of the body are named after the underlying anatomical structures in those regions. For example, the thigh can also be referred to as the *femoral region* after the femur, the major bone of the thigh. The nose is known as the *nasal region of the head* due to the underlying nasal cavity. These regional terms, along with their pronunciations and locations, are listed in **Figure 1.4**.

The abdomen is commonly divided into either four or nine regions. **Figure 1.5** shows the four regions, called *quadrants,* that divide the cavity. The standard terminology for these quadrants is right upper quadrant (RUQ), left upper quadrant (LUQ), right lower quadrant (RLQ), and left lower quadrant (LLQ). Note that "left" and "right" refer to the patient's body as it appears in the anatomical position, not left and right from another person's viewpoint. **Figure 1.6** shows the nine regions that are used when an abdominal area needs to be defined more specifically.

Cavities

The human body contains a number of open chambers called *cavities* (**Figure 1.7**). These cavities hold the internal organs of the body.

Regional Terms for Anatomy

Anterior Term	Pronunciation	Location
abdominal	ab-DAHM-i-nal	anterior trunk, inferior to the ribs
acromial	a-KROH-mee-al	superior, distal shoulder
antebrachial	an-tee-BRAY-kee-al	forearm
antecubital	an-tee-KYOO-bi-tal	anterior to the elbow
axillary	AK-sil-ar-ee	armpit
brachial	BRAY-kee-al	upper arm
buccal	BUCK-al	cheek of the face
carpal	KAR-pal	wrist
cervical	SER-vi-kal	neck
coxal	KAHK-sal	hip
crural	KRU-ral	lower leg
deltoid	DEL-toyd	upper arm
digital	DIJ-i-tal	fingers and toes
femoral	FEHM-oh-ral	thigh
fibular	FIB-yoo-lar	lateral, lower leg
frontal	FRUHN-tal	forehead
inguinal	ING-gwi-nal	groin
mental	MEHN-tal	chin
nasal	NAY-zal	nose
oral	OHR-al	mouth
orbital	OHR-bi-tal	eye
patellar	pa-TEHL-ar	anterior knee
pelvic	PEHL-vik	anterior pelvis
pubic	PYOO-bik	genital area
sternal	STER-nal	breastbone
tarsal	TAR-sal	ankle
thoracic	thoh-RAS-ik	chest
umbilical	uhm-BIL-i-kal	navel

Posterior Term	Pronunciation	Location
calcaneal	kal-KAY-nee-al	heel of the foot
cephalic	seh-FAL-ik	head
femoral	FEHM-oh-ral	thigh
gluteal	GLOO-tee-al	buttock
lumbar	LUHM-bar	lower back
occipital	ahk-SIP-i-tal	posterior head
olecranal	oh-LEK-ra-nal	posterior elbow
popliteal	pahp-LIH-tee-al	posterior knee
plantar	PLAN-tar	sole of the foot
sacral	SAY-kral	between the hips
scapular	SKAP-yoo-lar	shoulder blades
sural	SOO-ral	calf of the leg
vertebral	VER-teh-bral	spinal column

Figure 1.4

Goodheart-Willcox Publisher

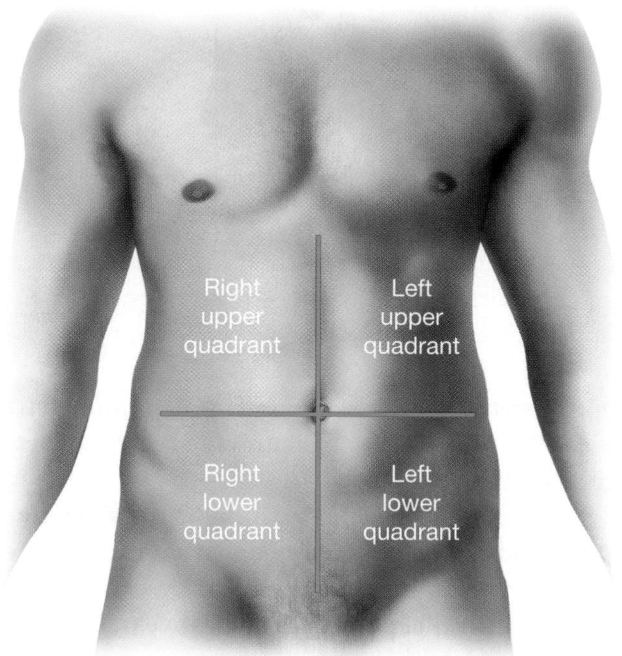

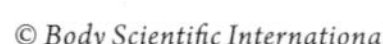

© Body Scientific International

Figure 1.5 The four abdominal quadrants.

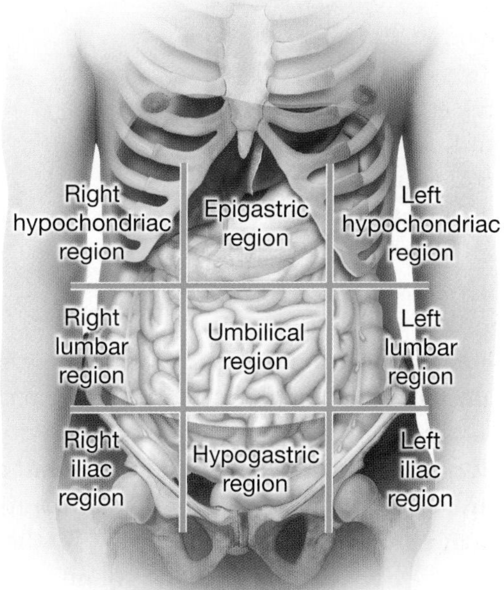

© Body Scientific International

Figure 1.6 The nine abdominal regions.

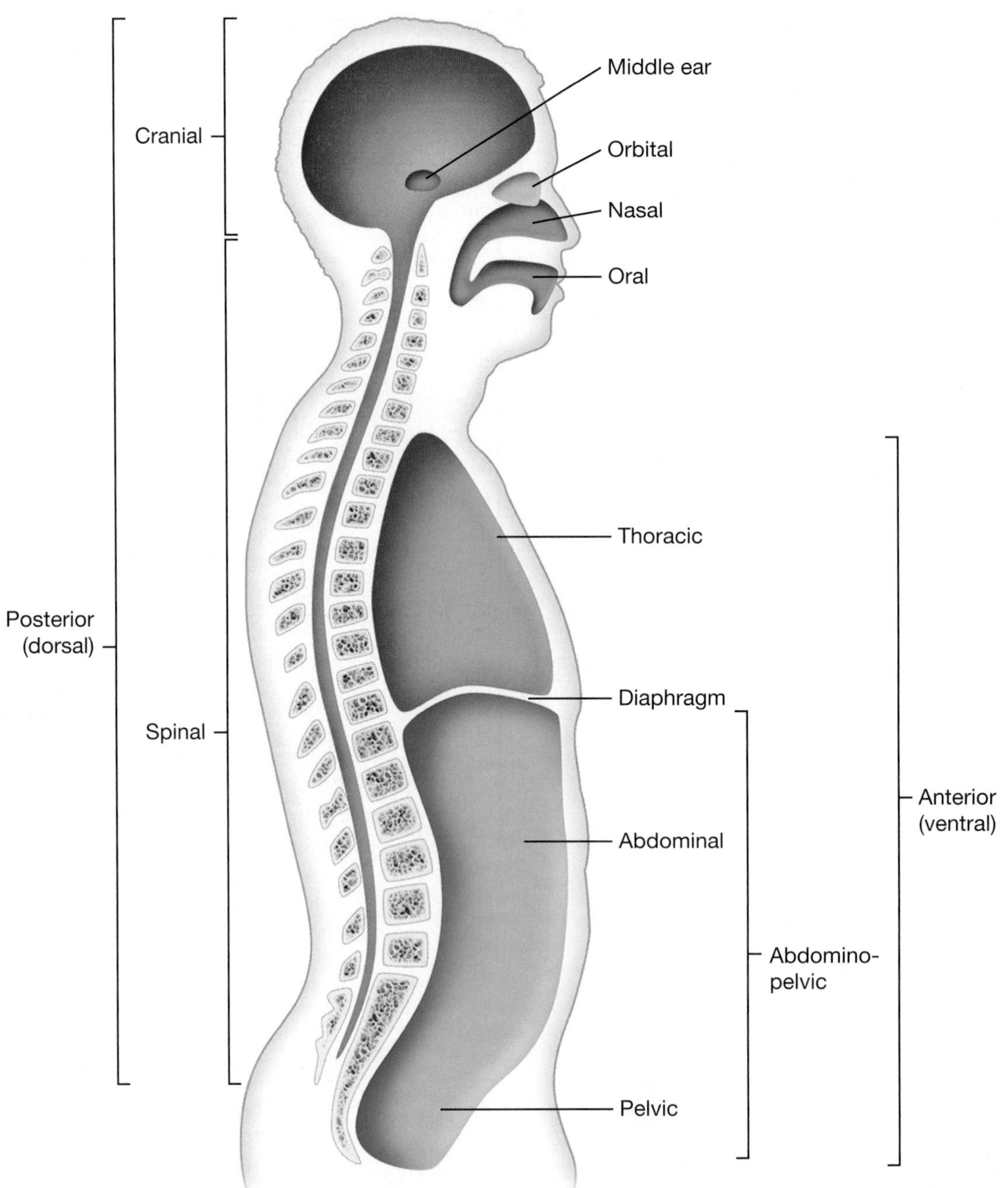

Figure 1.7 The body cavities.

The ***posterior (dorsal) cavity***, located toward the back (posterior side) of the body, includes two named cavities—the cranial cavity and the spinal cavity. The ***cranial cavity*** holds the brain, and the ***spinal cavity*** surrounds the spinal cord. The delicate brain and spinal cord are protected, respectively, by the bony skull and the bones of the vertebral column.

The ***anterior (ventral) cavity***, located at the front (anterior side) of the body, also includes subdivisions. A large, dome-shaped muscle called the *diaphragm* separates the ***thoracic cavity*** and the ***abdominopelvic cavity***. The thoracic cavity houses the heart and lungs, among other organs.

The abdominopelvic cavity includes the ***abdominal cavity*** and the ***pelvic cavity***. No structure separates these cavities. The abdominal cavity contains the stomach and other parts of the digestive tract, as well as the liver and other organs. The pelvic cavity holds the reproductive and excretory organs.

The body also includes several small cavities, including the following:

- ***oral cavity***—within the mouth
- ***nasal cavity***—inside the nose
- ***orbital cavities***—hold the eyes
- ***middle ear cavities***—chambers for transmitting and amplifying sound within the skull

Each of these small cavities is discussed in further detail in Chapter 8.

SELF CHECK

1. What three cardinal planes divide the human body into halves for anatomical purposes?
2. Using the directional terms in Figure 1-3, in what two ways could the relative positions of the nose and ears be described?
3. Which major body cavity contains the thoracic cavity?

The Metric System

The ***metric system*** is used for numerical quantities in all fields of science throughout the world, including the United States. The metric system is also used for everyday measurements by every major country in the world, except the United States. It is popular for several reasons:

- It involves only four base units—the meter (of length); the kilogram (of mass); the second (of time); and the degree Kelvin (of temperature).
- The base units are precisely defined, reproducible quantities that are independent of factors such as gravitational force.
- All units (except those used for time) relate by factors of 10, making conversion between units easy, since only the decimal point needs to move.
- International use of the system facilitates sharing numerical information among countries worldwide.

In the United States, the system of measurement used for nonscientific purposes is called the *English system*. The English system of weights and measures arose over the course of several centuries, mainly for purposes of buying and selling goods and dividing parcels of land. Specific units came largely from royal decrees. For example, a yard was originally defined as the distance from the end of the nose of King Henry I to the thumb of his extended arm. The English system of measurement is not regular, or even logical. There are 12 inches to the foot, 3 feet to the yard, 5,280 feet to the mile, 16 ounces to the pound, and 2,000 pounds to the ton. Metric-English conversion factors are presented in Appendix A.

SECTION 1.1 REVIEW

Mini-Glossary

abdominal cavity the open chamber that contains the stomach, digestive tract, liver, and other organs

abdominopelvic cavity a continuous internal opening that includes the abdominal and pelvic cavities

anatomical position an erect standing position with arms at the sides and palms facing forward

anatomy the study of the form or structure of living things, including plants, animals, and humans

anterior (ventral) body cavity a continuous internal opening that includes the thoracic and abdominopelvic cavities

cranial cavity the open chamber inside the skull that holds the brain

frontal plane an imaginary, vertical flat surface that divides the body into front and back halves

metric system international system of measurement that is used in all fields of science

middle ear cavities openings in the skull that serve as chambers for transmitting and amplifying sound

nasal cavity opening within and behind the nose

oral cavity opening within the mouth

orbital cavities openings that hold the eyes

pelvic cavity internal opening that holds the reproductive and excretory organs

physiology the study of how living things function or work

posterior (dorsal) body cavity continuous internal opening located near the back of the body that includes the cranial and spinal cavities

sagittal plane an imaginary, vertical flat surface that divides the body into right and left halves

spinal cavity the internal opening that houses the spinal cord

thoracic cavity the internal opening that houses the heart and lungs

transverse plane an imaginary, horizontal flat surface that divides the body into top and bottom halves

(continued)

Review Questions

1. Which small cavity is used as a passageway for both air and food?
2. List three reasons the metric system is popular worldwide for both scientific and everyday measurements.
3. Briefly describe the anatomical position.
4. What are the four base units used in the metric system?
5. What two body cavities are named for directional terms?
6. What is the difference between the terms *superior* and *cranial*?
7. Compare and contrast the metric and English systems of measurement.
8. What is the difference between *distal* and *inferior*?

SECTION 1.2 Physiological Processes

Objectives

- Explain how anatomical building blocks, beginning with atoms, combine to comprise organ systems.
- Define *homeostasis* and explain how homeostatic mechanisms help maintain health.
- Explain how the body's metabolism works and describe the factors that can influence metabolic rate.

Key Terms

atoms
cells
control center
effector
homeostasis
homeostatic imbalance
homeostatic mechanisms
metabolic rate
metabolism
molecules
negative feedback
organ
organ system
positive feedback
receptor
tissues

The human body is an elegant biological machine. It is organized into specialized systems that carry out precise functions. Many of these systems interact with and influence the activities of other systems. To appreciate the intricate functions of the body systems, you must first understand how they are constructed (**Figure 1.8**).

Organization of the Body

At the most basic level, tiny particles called ***atoms*** combine in different ways to form larger particles known as ***molecules***. The human body depends on many different kinds of molecules, such as water, proteins, and carbohydrates.

The smallest building blocks of all living beings are ***cells***, which are composed of organized groups of molecules. Groups of similar cells with a common function form ***tissues***. The four basic types of tissues are epithelial, connective, muscular, and neural tissues.

The next level of organization is the ***organ***. An organ is composed of at least two types of tissue that are organized to perform a specific function. The heart, lungs, brain, and liver are all critically important organs. An ***organ system*** includes two or more organs that work together. Each of the human body's organ systems is discussed in a chapter in this book. **Figure 1.9** and **Figure 1.10** provide an overview of these organ systems, which are briefly described here.

The Integumentary System

The integumentary system includes the skin and all of the structures associated with the skin. It serves as a waterproof barrier that cushions and protects the underlying tissues. Receptors in the integumentary system transmit signals for pain, pressure, and temperature at the body's surface. Perspiration through the sweat glands in the skin helps to regulate body temperature.

The Skeletal System

The bones and associated ligaments and cartilage at joints form the skeletal system. The bones provide a rigid framework to which muscles attach, allowing the various motions of which the human body is capable. The bones of the skull, rib cage, and pelvic girdle surround and protect delicate inner organs. The interior of bone is a site at which hematopoiesis, or blood cell formation, takes place.

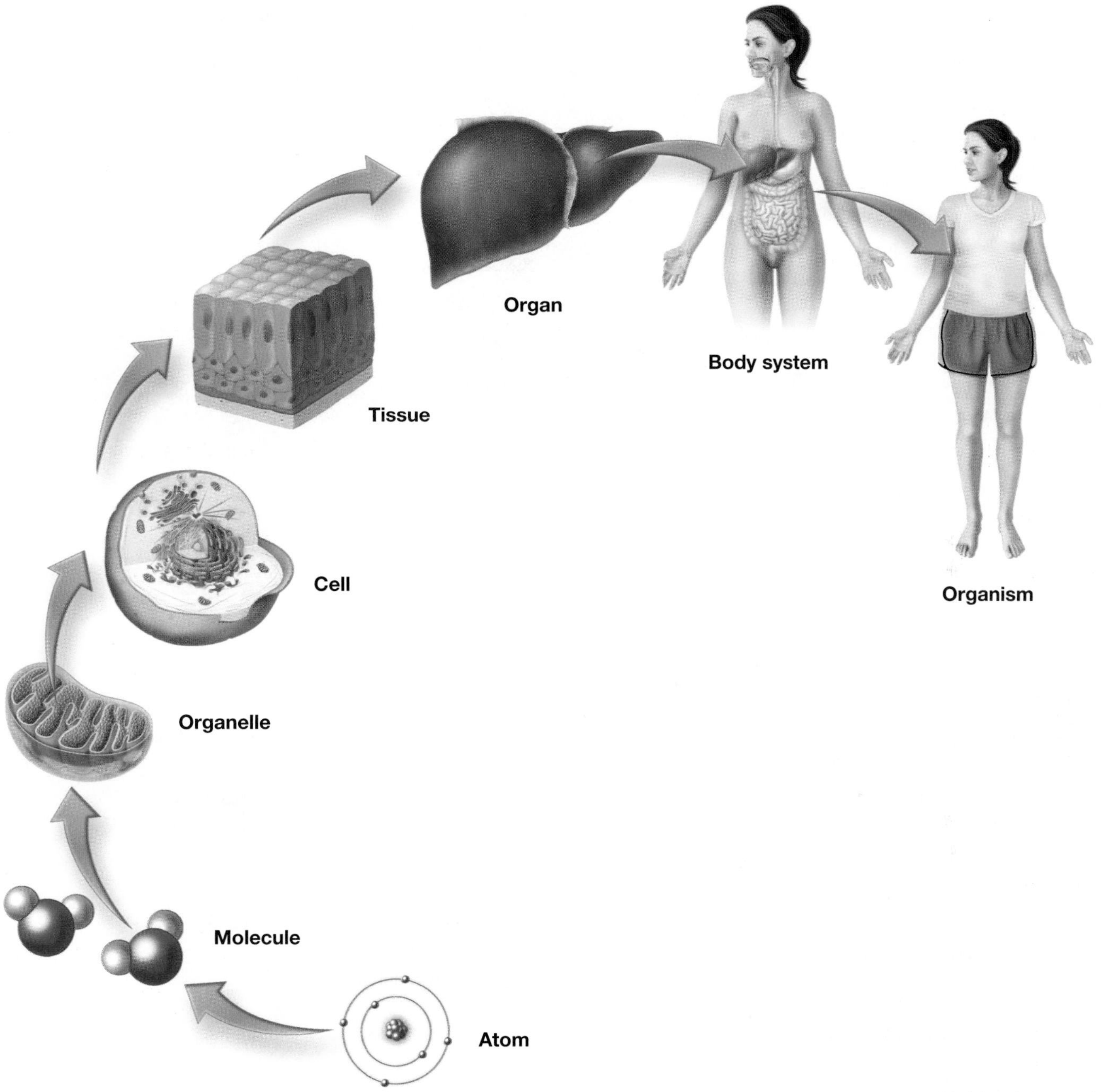

Figure 1.8 Levels of organization within the human body.

The Muscular System

The muscular system includes the skeletal muscles, which contract or shorten to pull on the bones to which they attach. Large, powerful muscles enable walking, running, and vigorous movements of the arms and trunk. Small, fine muscles of the fingers and eyes enable precision movements. This system also includes cardiac muscles, which cause the beating of the heart, and smooth muscles of the inner organs, which help move fluids and other substances through passages inside the body.

The Nervous System

The brain, spinal cord, nerves, and sensory receptors form communication pathways throughout the body that are collectively known as the nervous system. Communication in the nervous system occurs through the transmission of tiny electrical signals called *nerve impulses*. The brain serves as the body's control center, receiving sensory impulses from specialized receptors and sending out impulses to muscles and glands to trigger appropriate actions.

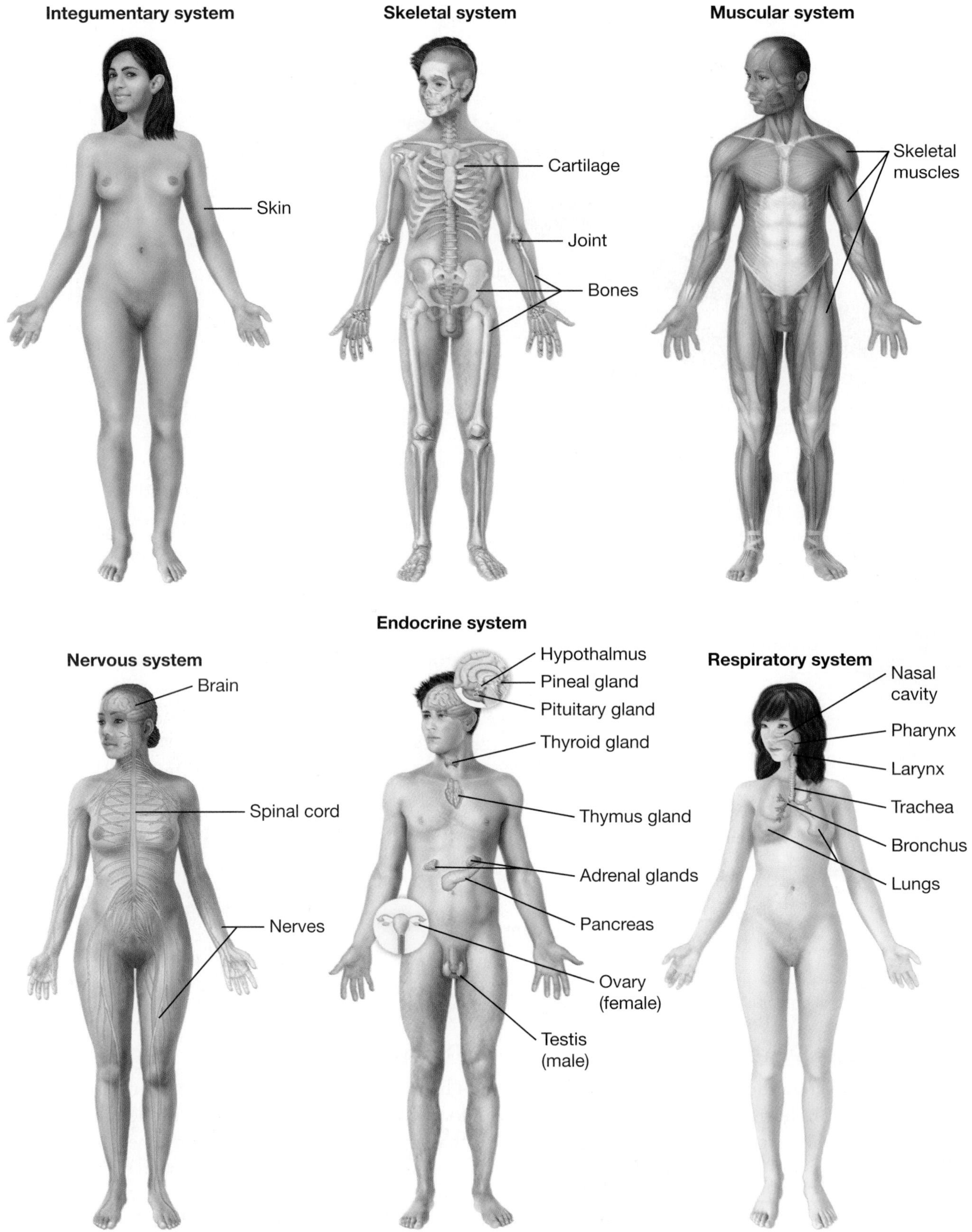

(continued)

Figure 1.9 The organ systems of the body.

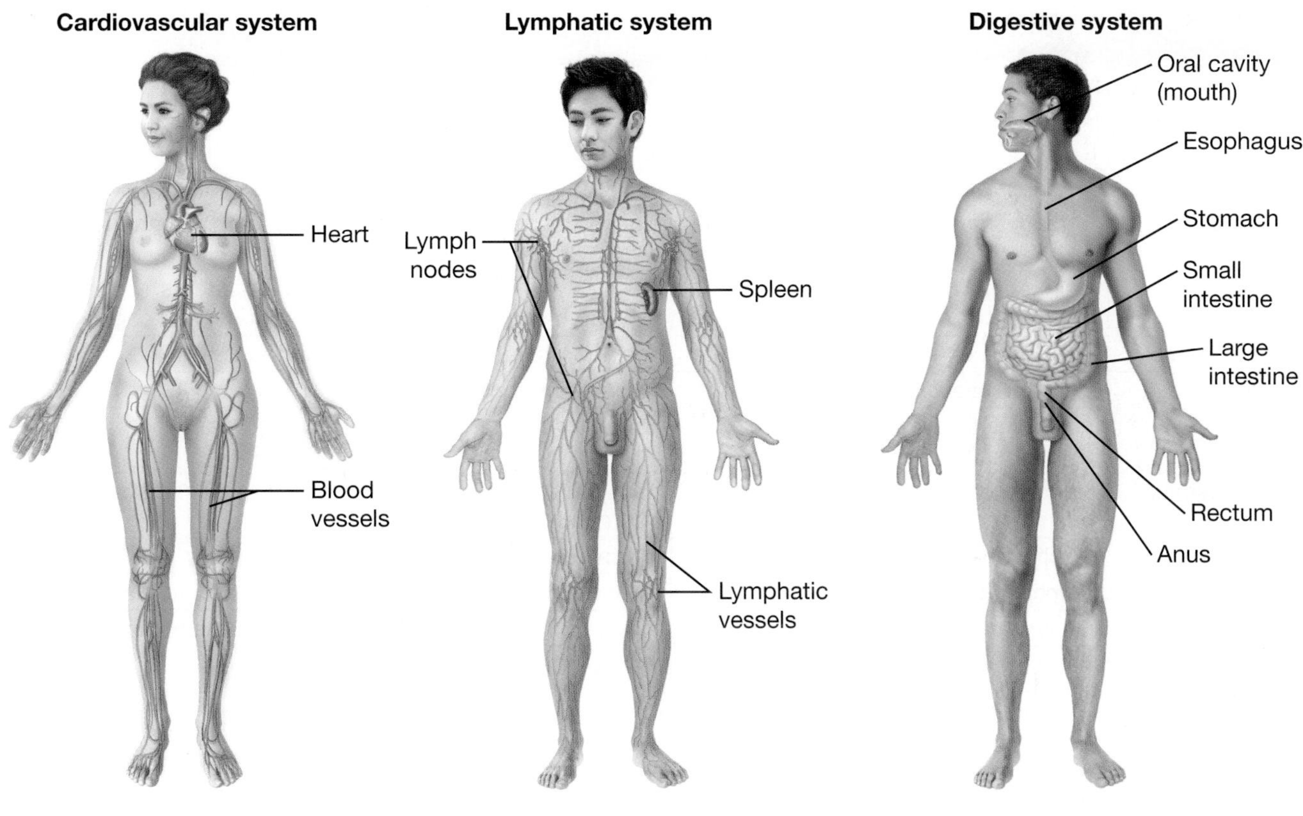
Cardiovascular system
Heart
Blood vessels
Lymphatic system
Lymph nodes
Spleen
Lymphatic vessels
Digestive system
Oral cavity (mouth)
Esophagus
Stomach
Small intestine
Large intestine
Rectum
Anus

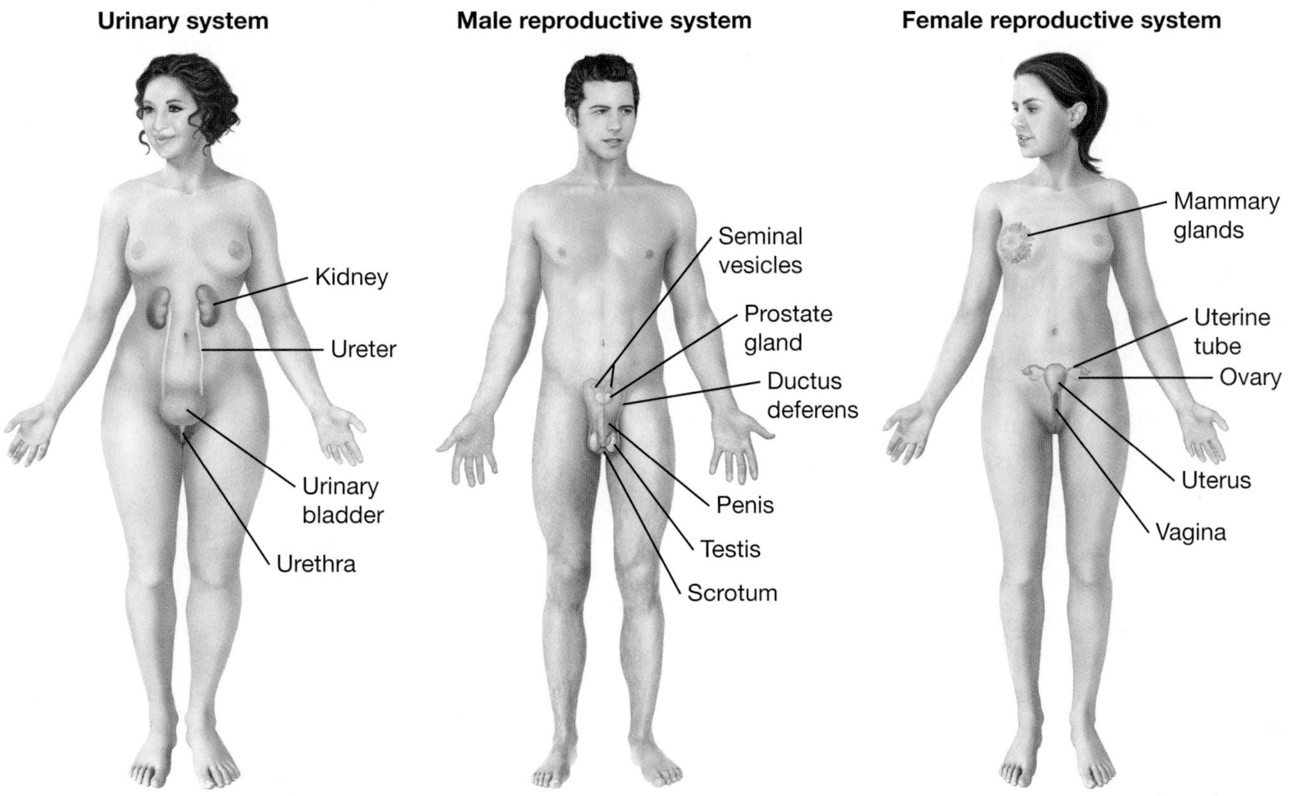
Urinary system
Kidney
Ureter
Urinary bladder
Urethra
Male reproductive system
Seminal vesicles
Prostate gland
Ductus deferens
Penis
Testis
Scrotum
Female reproductive system
Mammary glands
Uterine tube
Ovary
Uterus
Vagina

© Body Scientific International

The Human Organ Systems		
System	**Major Organs**	**Primary Functions**
Integumentary	layers of skin	protects body, eliminates waste, helps regulate body temperature
Skeletal	bones, cartilage, ligaments	supports the body, protects the organs, produces blood cells
Muscular	cardiac, smooth, and skeletal muscle	pumps the heart, helps move materials through the digestive tract, moves the body
Nervous	brain, spinal cord, nerves, sensory receptors	receives and interprets sensory input, directs body movements; includes memory, emotions, and cognition
Special sensory	eyes, ears, organs of smell and taste	enables vision, hearing, smell, and taste
Endocrine	endocrine glands	secretes hormones
Respiratory	lungs, nasal passages, pharynx, larynx, trachea	delivers oxygen to body tissues, removes carbon dioxide from the blood
Cardiovascular	heart, blood vessels	transports oxygen and nutrients to the body's cells, removes waste products
Lymphatic	lymphatic vessels and nodes	returns body fluids to the bloodstream
Digestive	esophagus, stomach, intestines	breaks down foods to allow the body to absorb nutrients
Urinary	kidneys, bladder	removes nitrogen-containing wastes from the blood
Reproductive	male: testes, scrotum, penis female: ovaries, uterus, vagina	enables the production of offspring

Figure 1.10 *Goodheart-Willcox Publisher*

The Sensory Systems

Vision, hearing, and taste are considered the "special senses." Under the control of the nervous system, they provide information to the brain, which in turn processes the information and directs other systems, such as the muscular and skeletal systems, to react appropriately to the environment.

The Endocrine System

The endocrine system also acts to control body functions. Hormones produced by the endocrine system exert powerful influences on reproduction, growth, and metabolism. The glands of the endocrine system include the pituitary, thyroid, parathyroid, pancreas, adrenal, thymus, and pineal glands, as well as ovaries in females and testes in males.

The Respiratory System

The internal pathway responsible for supplying oxygen to the blood and removing carbon dioxide from the body is the respiratory system. Air is inhaled through the nasal passages and travels through the pharynx, larynx, trachea, and bronchi. Oxygen is supplied to very small blood vessels through tiny sacs within the lungs called *alveoli*. Exhalation removes carbon dioxide through a reverse process.

The Cardiovascular System

The cardiovascular system includes the heart and the blood vessels. The heart continually pumps blood through an extensive system of vessels. Blood delivers oxygen, hormones, nutrients, and other substances to body tissues through the capillaries, the smallest of the vessels. White blood cells and other components of the blood protect the body from infections and toxins, and help heal wounds.

The Lymphatic System

Working to support the cardiovascular system, the lymphatic system returns fluid seepage from the blood vessels back to the blood vessels. Lymphatic system components include lymph nodes, lymphatic vessels, the spleen, and the tonsils. The system helps to cleanse the blood, and it plays an important role in the body's immune response to invasion by harmful cells.

The Digestive System

The digestive system takes in foods and liquids, converts them to a form that can be used by the body's tissues for nutrition and hydration, and then expels waste materials. Structurally, this system consists of a long, convoluted tube running from the mouth to the anus. Components include the mouth, esophagus, stomach, and small and large intestines. The salivary glands, liver, pancreas, and other organs all assist with the breakdown and processing of ingested materials.

The Urinary System

Working in conjunction with the digestive system, the urinary system is responsible for extracting waste material from the blood and expelling it from the body in the form of urine. This system includes the kidneys, ureters, bladder, and urethra. The urinary system also plays important roles in maintaining the homeostatic balance of electrolytes and the acid/base composition of the blood.

The Reproductive Systems

The female and male reproductive systems function to produce offspring. The male reproductive system includes the sperm-producing testes, the scrotum, penis, accessory glands, and duct system. The female reproductive system includes the egg-producing ovaries, the uterine tubes, uterus, and vagina.

SELF CHECK

1. List the hierarchy of structure of the human body from the smallest living unit to the largest.
2. What are the four basic types of tissue found in the human body?
3. What part of the body is stimulated by changes in the environment, sending messages to the brain for interpretation and response?

Homeostasis

The organ systems work together to keep factors such as body temperature, blood pressure, blood sugar, water balance, and sodium level within normal boundaries, maintaining a healthy environment inside the body. This state of regulated physiological balance is called ***homeostasis***. The word *homeostasis* comes from Greek words that mean "staying the same."

Organ systems work together to maintain homeostasis through processes called ***homeostatic mechanisms***. The nervous system and endocrine system initiate most homeostatic responses. These systems function through a complex combination of chemical and physical processes. To maintain homeostasis, all of the systems must work together and make adjustments when the body's external and internal environments change.

All homeostatic control mechanisms have three elements in common—a receptor, a control center, and an effector. Changes in the environment stimulate a sensory ***receptor***, a nerve that relays an informational message to a ***control center*** along an afferent pathway. The control center analyzes the information, and when an action is required to maintain homeostasis, the control center sends a command stimulus to an ***effector*** along an efferent pathway. The effector causes an action that helps maintain homeostasis.

Negative Feedback

Most homeostatic mechanisms work on the principle of ***negative feedback***. In a negative feedback loop, conditions exceeding a set limit in one direction trigger a reaction in the opposite (negative) direction. This negative reaction restores the system to the set limit.

A familiar example of a mechanical system that functions on negative feedback is the thermostat on a home heating or cooling system. If the temperature surrounding the thermostat rises or falls outside the set limit, the thermostat triggers either the furnace or air conditioner to turn on. The furnace or air conditioner stays on until the temperature is restored to the set limit.

In the human body, if the temperature begins to rise above the normal 37°C (98.6°F), the hypothalamus of the brain triggers a series of signals to different organs to cause sweating. The evaporation of sweat on the skin cools the body (**Figure 1.11**). Simultaneously, blood vessels that are close to the skin dilate to help release heat.

Alternatively, when the body becomes chilled, the hypothalamus signals the muscles to cause shivering. This increased activity of the muscles produces heat, which helps warm the body. At the same time, blood vessels that are close to the skin constrict to reduce heat loss through the skin.

Positive Feedback

Although most homeostatic mechanisms in the human body operate through negative feedback, positive feedback loops can also occur. In contrast to negative feedback loops, which reduce disruptive influences,

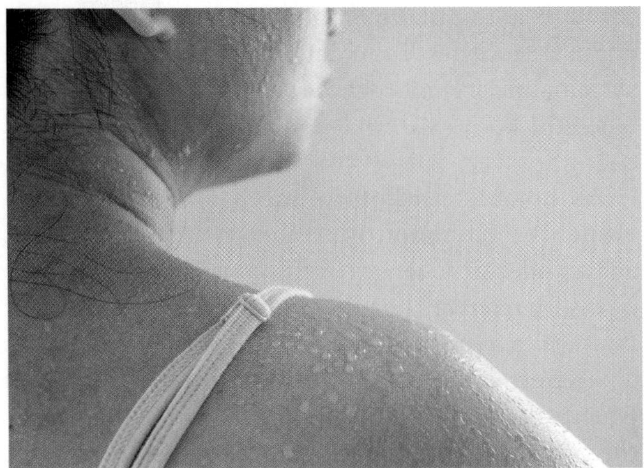

Werayuth Tes/Shutterstock.com

Figure 1.11 Sweating during vigorous exercise helps to cool the body.

positive feedback mechanisms *increase* disruptive influences to restore homeostasis. Positive feedback is involved in accelerating blood clotting, transmitting nerve signals, and stimulating contractions during childbirth.

In the case of body temperature, however, a fever that exceeds 40°C (104°F) can provoke a dangerous positive feedback loop. Body temperature this high increases the body's metabolic rate, which increases body heat still further. This can be fatal if nothing is done to cool the body.

Maintaining Homeostasis

Homeostasis within the human body does not mean that conditions are maintained in a perfectly constant state at all times. Rather, there are routine fluctuations of variables such as blood pressure and body temperature. These normal fluctuations occur in response to a variety of conditions in the external and internal environments. Vigorous exercise, for example, produces a normal elevation in both blood pressure and body temperature. Homeostatic mechanisms work to keep these fluctuations within a normal, healthy range.

Homeostatic Imbalances

A ***homeostatic imbalance*** occurs when the organ systems are unable to keep the body's internal environment within normal ranges. For example, the aging process is accompanied by many homeostatic imbalances. These imbalances can lead to changes, such as the wrinkling and thinning of skin, a reduction of muscle mass and strength, and a decrease in mental acuity.

Disease can also cause homeostatic imbalance. For example, during digestion, food is converted into the simple sugar glucose, which enters the bloodstream and is carried throughout the body to nourish the body cells. The pancreas produces insulin, a hormone that normally controls blood sugar, keeping it in a healthy range. But people with diabetes are unable to move glucose out of the bloodstream because their pancreas does not make enough insulin, or because their cells do not respond normally to insulin. The resulting homeostatic imbalance, if not corrected, can lead to serious problems, such as kidney failure, lower limb amputations, and blindness. Chapter 9 describes diabetes in more detail.

SELF CHECK

1. Explain the difference between positive and negative feedback in maintaining homeostasis. Give an example of each.
2. What is homeostatic imbalance? Include at least one example in your explanation.
3. What are possible consequences of the body's failure to maintain homeostasis?

Metabolism

Metabolism refers to the multitude of chemical reactions constantly going on within the body's cells. The two general types of metabolic activities are anabolism and catabolism. Anabolism is the process through which complex molecules, such as proteins, are constructed from simpler ones. Catabolism is just the opposite: complex molecules such as carbohydrates are broken down into simpler molecules.

Through catabolic processes, the complex molecules in the foods and liquids you consume supply the body with energy in the form of adenosine triphosphate (ATP). ATP, which is further described in Chapter 2, powers activities within the cells. Even while sleeping, the body needs energy for activities, such as breathing, circulating blood, adjusting hormone levels, and growing and repairing cells.

The speed with which the body consumes energy, which is also the rate of ATP production, is a person's ***metabolic rate***. Approximately 60%–75% of the calories that an average person burns is accounted for by the basal metabolic rate, or the energy needed to maintain basic life functions. Another 10% of the calories are burned in digesting and processing the foods and liquids people consume. For this reason, diets that are overly restrictive tend to be counterproductive for losing weight—the body does not burn as many calories because there is not as much to digest.

The remainder of the calories burned depends on the amount of physical activity in which a person engages. Because muscle maintenance requires more energy than maintenance of other tissues, even at rest, muscular individuals burn more calories and have higher metabolic rates than others.

Research Notes Homeostatic Mechanisms during Distance Running

The number one danger associated with marathons, triathlons, and other long-distance running events is overheating. Overheating is a condition in which the body's homeostatic mechanisms for temperature control are overwhelmed. Overheating begins with heat cramps, which can progress to heat exhaustion, eventually leading to heat stroke and death. How does overheating happen, and what steps can runners take to avoid it?

Researchers have recognized that long-distance running poses a severe challenge to the body's homeostatic processes. One reason is that some runners do not drink sufficient fluids during long-distance events. Inadequate water intake impedes the body's ability to sweat—a process that has a cooling effect on the body. An inability to sweat leads to hyperthermia, or dangerously high body temperature. Hyperthermia encompasses both elevated core temperature and elevated skin temperature.

Inadequate water intake can also cause dehydration, which reduces total body blood volume. This limits blood supply to the working muscles, skin, and brain. As a result, the muscles fatigue, the skin is less able to release heat, and judgment may be impaired. Research has shown that losing 3% or more of total body water causes increased strain on the cardiovascular system and a marked decline in aerobic performance. This makes it more difficult to sustain exercise at a steady pace and increases the perception of effort. Hyperthermia may also directly affect the central nervous system, causing it to contribute to total body fatigue.

Overheating can lead to heat exhaustion. The symptoms of heat exhaustion may include profuse sweating, weakness, nausea, vomiting, headache, lightheadedness, and muscle cramps. Individuals experiencing any of these symptoms due to overheating should immediately be placed in a cool environment and adequately hydrated. If nausea or vomiting prevents the person from drinking enough water, intravenous fluids may be required.

In some cases, heat exhaustion progresses to heat stroke. A body temperature of 41°C (106°F) and the absence of sweating are signs that the normal homeostatic processes have been overwhelmed. Under these conditions, individuals become confused and lethargic and may have a seizure. These symptoms represent a life-threatening emergency, and immediate medical attention is needed.

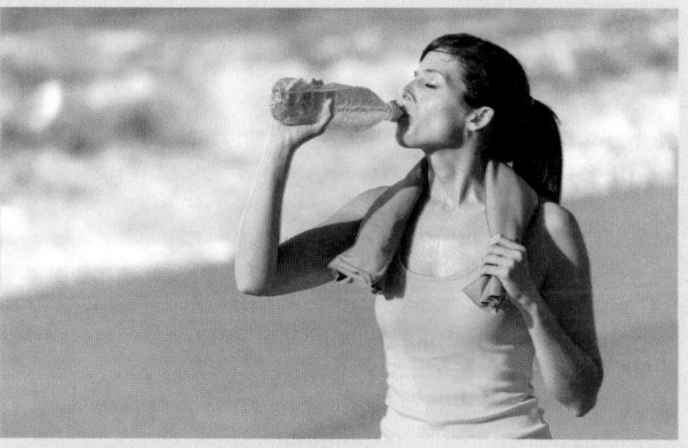

Dirima/Shutterstock.com

It is important to maintain a proper level of hydration during exercise.

Ironically, a related danger during long-distance running can be drinking too much water. Runners in the Boston, Chicago, and Big Sur marathons have died from consuming too much water during the race. The problem is that an excessive amount of water dilutes the blood. This causes the sodium concentration in the blood to fall too low, resulting in swelling of the brain, which can be fatal.

Under normal conditions, the body expels extra water in the form of urine. However, research has shown that an inflammatory response occurs during long-distance endurance events, altering hormone levels and reducing the body's ability to produce urine.

Running experts suggest weighing yourself before and after a long training run. If you have gained weight after running, you have consumed too much water, but if you have lost weight, you need to drink more. It is recommended that you consume 3 to 6 ounces of liquid for every 20 minutes of vigorous exercise. You must take into account, however, that your sweating rate and the environment may necessitate drinking more or less.

SECTION 1.2

REVIEW

Mini-Glossary

atoms tiny particles of matter

cells the smallest building blocks of all living beings

control center a system that receives and analyzes information from sensory receptors, and then sends a command stimulus to an effector to maintain homeostasis

effector a unit that receives a command stimulus from the control center and causes an action to help maintain homeostasis

homeostasis a state of regulated physiological balance

homeostatic imbalance a state in which the organ systems are unable to keep the body's internal environment within normal ranges

homeostatic mechanisms the processes that maintain homeostasis

metabolic rate the speed at which the body consumes energy

metabolism all of the chemical reactions that occur within an organism to maintain life

molecules particles that contain two or more atoms

negative feedback a mechanism that restores homeostasis by reversing a condition that has exceeded the normal homeostatic range

organ a body part organized to perform a specific function

organ system two or more organs working together to perform specific functions

positive feedback a mechanism that restores homeostasis by further increasing a condition that has exceeded the normal homeostatic range

receptor a transmitter that senses environmental changes

tissues organized groups of similar cells

Review Questions

1. What is an organ?
2. Name the two types of homeostatic mechanisms.
3. What happens to homeostasis when a person ages?
4. How might the transmission of nerve signals be an example of a positive feedback system?
5. Compare and contrast the signs and symptoms of dehydration with hyponatremia, which is a condition in which the concentration of sodium ions (Na^+) in cells is too high.
6. Using a hot stove as an example, describe how the afferent and efferent nerves in the body protect a person from being burned.

SECTION 1.3

Effects of Physical Forces on the Body

Objectives

- Explain the kinetic concepts of force, mass, weight, pressure, and torque.
- Identify the external forces that can act on the human body, and explain their effects, including the factors that determine whether an external force causes bodily injury.

Key Terms

bending
combined loading
compression
elastic
force
kinetics
mass
net force
plastic
pressure
shear
stress
tension
torque
torsion
weight

The human body both generates and resists forces during daily activities. The internal forces produced by your muscles enable body movements, whereas external forces such as air resistance and friction slow you down. Sports activities involve applying forces to balls, bats, racquets, or clubs, as well as absorbing forces from impacts with balls, the ground or floor, and opponents (in contact sports). This section introduces key concepts to help you understand the effects that these activities have on the human body.

Kinetics

The field of ***kinetics*** analyzes the actions of forces. The field of human biomechanics is based on analysis of the forces, both internal and external, that act on the human body. A basic knowledge of kinetic concepts will help you understand the movements of the body and the effects of forces that can potentially cause injury.

Force

Force is a push or pull acting on a structure. It is described in terms of its size or magnitude, its direction, and the point at which it acts on a structure. Body weight, friction, and air or water resistance are all forces that commonly act on the human body.

Because a force rarely acts alone, it is important to recognize that what we see and feel are the effects of ***net force***. Net force is the single force resulting from the summation of all forces acting on a structure at a given time (**Figure 1.12**). Thus, net force represents the size and direction of all acting forces.

The size and direction of net force determines the overall effect of the forces acting on a structure. When the forces acting on a structure are balanced, or cancel each other out, there is no net force and no resulting motion. For example, if two people simultaneously apply equal and opposite forces on the two sides of a swinging door, the door will not move. However, if a net force is present—if one person pushes harder than the other—the door will move in the direction of the net force.

Mass and Weight

Mass is the quantity of matter contained in an object. The action of a force causes an object's mass to accelerate, either increasing or decreasing in speed. ***Weight*** is a force equal to the gravitational acceleration exerted on an object's mass. As the mass of an object increases, its weight increases proportionally. If you were to travel to the moon or another planet with a different gravitational acceleration than on Earth, your weight would be different, but your mass would remain the same.

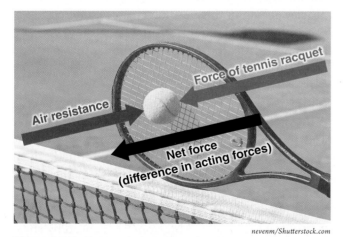

nevenm/Shutterstock.com

Figure 1.12 The net force acting on a tennis ball at the moment of impact with a racquet is the difference between the force exerted by the racquet and the opposing force of air resistance.

Pressure

Pressure is defined as the amount of force distributed over a given area. For example, how much pressure is exerted on the floor beneath you if you shift your weight to one foot? To find out, divide your body weight by the surface area of the sole of your shoe. Thinking about this, would you prefer to have your foot stepped on by a woman wearing athletic shoes or a woman wearing stilettos (shoes with a thin, spiked heel)? The woman's weight would be distributed over a much smaller area in the stilettos, resulting in a much larger pressure against your unfortunate foot.

Torque

When a force causes a structure to rotate, the rotary effect of the force is called ***torque***. Pulling or pushing a suspended bicycle tire causes the wheel to begin spinning. The harder the wheel is pulled or pushed, the faster it spins. From a mechanical perspective, torque is being created on the bicycle wheel.

Torque can be quantified as the size of the force multiplied by the perpendicular distance from the line of force application to the center of rotation. In the case of a spinning bicycle wheel, perpendicular distance is the distance from the outside of the tire to the axis of the wheel. The greater the amount of torque acting at the center of rotation, the greater the tendency for rotation to occur.

When a muscle in the human body contracts, it applies a pulling force on a bone. A sufficiently large force causes movement of the bone, with the bone rotating at the nearby joint center. The amount of torque generated at the joint center is the size of the muscle force multiplied by the distance between the muscle attachment and the joint center. You will learn more about how to measure and calculate forces in Chapter 6, *The Muscular System*.

SELF CHECK

1. What term describes the process of analyzing actions of forces?
2. Name and define two forces that commonly act on the body.
3. What causes an object to rotate?

Forces and Injury

What factors determine whether forces acting on the human body result in injury? The effect of a given force depends not only on its size, direction, and application point, but also on the duration of force application.

Stress and Directional Force Distribution

The way in which a force is distributed affects the outcome of the force acting on the human body and affects the potential for injury. While pressure represents the distribution of external force on a body, ***stress*** represents the resulting force distribution inside a body. Stress is quantified in the same way as pressure, by dividing the size of the force by the area over which the force acts. As **Figure 1.13** shows, a force acting on a small surface produces greater stress than the same force acting over a larger surface.

When the human body sustains a blow, the likelihood of injury to body tissue is related to the magnitude and direction of the stress created by the blow. *Compressive stress, tensile stress,* and *shear stress* are terms that indicate the direction of the acting stress. The protective pads and helmets worn in many sports are designed to distribute forces over a large area, minimizing the stress sustained by the underlying body parts.

Compression

Compressive force, or ***compression***, can be thought of as a squeezing force (**Figure 1.14**). An effective way to press wildflowers is to place them inside the pages of a book and stack other books on top of that book. The weight of the books creates a compressive force on the flowers. Similarly, when a person lands from a jump, the weight of the body plus the force of landing inflict a compressive force on the bones of the skeleton.

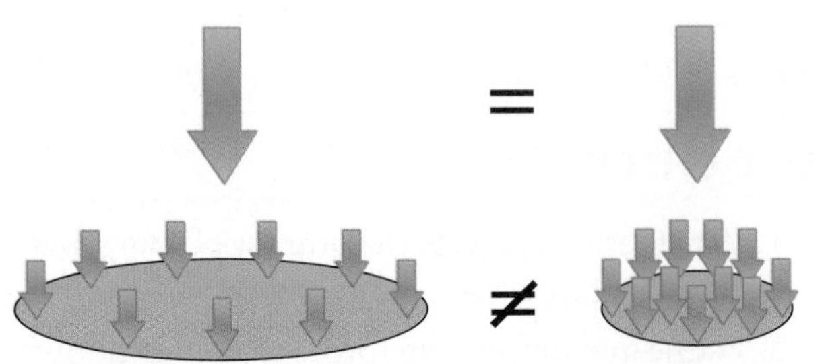

© Body Scientific International

Figure 1.13 When a force of a given size is distributed over an area, the amount of stress generated depends on the size of the area.

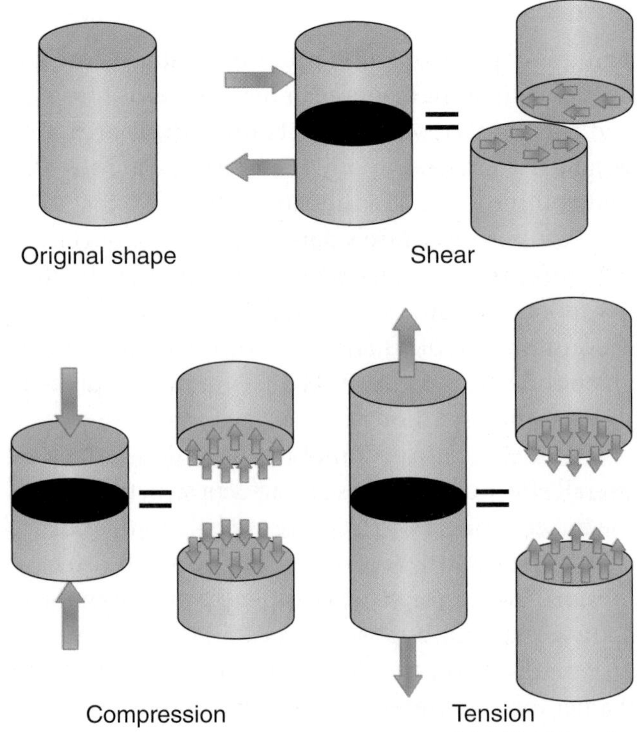

© Body Scientific International

Figure 1.14 Compression, tension, and shear represent three directions of stress distribution within a body.

Tension

The opposite of compressive force is tensile force, or ***tension*** (**Figure 1.14**). Tensile force is a pulling force on the object to which it is applied. When a person hangs from a pull-up bar, tension is created in the arms as they support the weight of the body. A heavier person in this position creates more tension in the arms than a lighter person. When they contract, the muscles also produce tensile force that pulls on attached bones.

Shear

A third direction of force is ***shear***. While compressive and tensile forces act along the length of a bone or other object to which they are applied, shear force acts perpendicular to the length of the object (**Figure 1.14**). Shear force tends to cause a portion of the object to slide, or shear, with respect to another portion of the object. Abrasions are caused by shear force acting on the skin. When a baseball player slides into a base, for example, the shear force created by the ground against any exposed skin can cause an abrasion.

Combined Loads

When multiple forces act at the same time, more complicated force distribution patterns are set up within the body. A combination of off-center forces can create a loading pattern known as ***bending*** (**Figure 1.15**).

Torsion occurs when a structure is made to twist about its length, typically when one end of the structure is fixed (**Figure 1.15**). Torsional fractures of the tibia can occur in football and skiing accidents when the foot is held in a fixed position and the rest of the body twists.

The simultaneous action of two or more types of forces is known as ***combined loading***. Because of the variety of forces people encounter during daily activities, combined loading patterns are relatively common. Fortunately, these patterns do not usually result in injury.

The Effects of Force Application

When a force acts on an object, there are two potential effects: acceleration and deformation. Acceleration is a change in the velocity of the object to which the force is applied. The more massive or heavy the object, the smaller the acceleration will be.

The second effect is deformation, or a change in shape. When a racquetball is struck by a racquet, the ball is both accelerated (put in motion in the direction of the racquet swing) and deformed (flattened on the side that is struck). The amount of deformation that occurs in response to a given force depends on the stiffness of the object acted on.

When an external force is applied to the human body, several factors influence whether an injury occurs. Among these are the size and direction of the force, as well as the area over which the force is distributed. The material properties of the body tissues to which the force is applied are also important.

With relatively small forces, deformation of the softer tissues occurs, but the response is ***elastic***, meaning that when the force is removed, the tissue returns to its original size and shape. Stiffer materials, such as bone, display less deformation in response to a given force. Sometimes the force causes the deformation to exceed the tissue's elastic limit. When this occurs, the response is ***plastic***, meaning that some amount of deformation is permanent. Within the human body, a plastic response translates to injury.

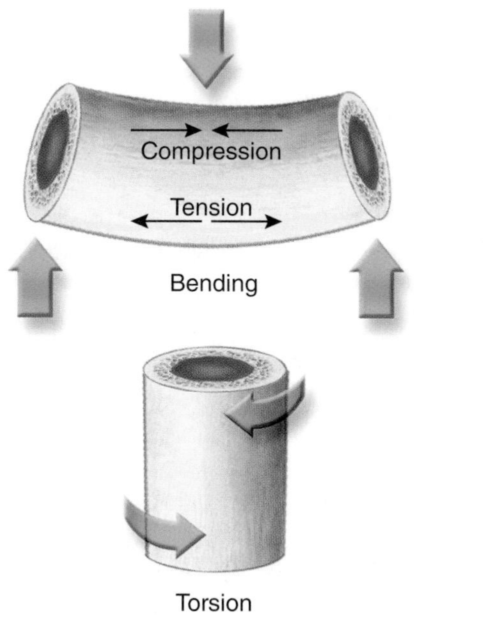

Figure 1.15 Bending and torsion are forms of combined loading.

Repetitive vs. Acute Loads

Yet another factor that influences the likelihood of injury is whether the forces sustained by the body are repetitive or acute. When a single force acts on the body and causes an injury, the force is said to be *acute*, and the result is an acute injury. For example, the force produced by a check in ice hockey or the force resulting from an automobile accident may cause an acute injury, such as a bone fracture.

Injury can also result from relatively small forces sustained on a repeated basis. For example, each time a person's foot hits the ground while running, a force of approximately two to three times the person's body weight is sustained. Although a single force of this magnitude is not likely to result in a fracture to healthy bone, many repetitions of such a force may cause a fracture in an otherwise healthy bone of the foot or lower leg. Injuries caused by repetitive forces are called *chronic injuries* or *stress injuries*.

SECTION 1.3

REVIEW

Mini-Glossary

bending a loading pattern created by a combination of off-center forces
combined loading the simultaneous action of two or more types of forces
compression a squeezing force that creates compression in the structure to which it is applied
elastic a response in which a structure returns to its original size and shape after the application of force
force a push or pull acting on a structure
kinetics a field of study that analyzes the actions of forces
mass the quantity of matter contained in an object
net force the single force resulting from the summation of all forces acting on a structure at a given time
plastic a response in which a structure retains some permanent deformation after a force is applied
pressure the force distributed over a given area
shear a force that acts along a surface and perpendicular to the length of a structure
stress the force distribution inside a structure
tension a pulling force on a structure
torque the rotary effect of a force
torsion a loading pattern that can cause a structure to twist about its length
weight the force equal to the gravitational acceleration exerted on the mass of an object

Review Questions

1. Compare mass and weight.
2. What is net force?
3. Name the three types of directional forces that can act on the human body.
4. What type of load pattern occurs when a long object, such as an arm bone is made to twist along its length?
5. What is the difference between an elastic response to a force and a plastic response?
6. A player gets hit by a lacrosse ball. What is the predominant type of force generated by the ball on the player?
7. Explain how a torn ligament is an example of a plastic response.
8. A linebacker and running back are running toward each other. The linebacker is hit and knocked over by the running back. Using net force as the basis for your answer, explain why the linebacker was knocked over.
9. Every morning, a woman jogs three miles before breakfast. One morning, she stumbles over a curb and falls, breaking her ankle. Is this an acute or chronic injury? Explain your answer.

SECTION 1.4

Scientific Methods and Theories

Objectives

- Describe the scientific method and explain why it is important.
- Discuss the role of data in scientific research.
- Explain what a scientific theory is and how it is derived.
- Identify the important early anatomists and physiologists, and discuss the impact of their work.

Key Terms

data
hypothesis
research question
science
scientific method
scientific theory
statistical inference
statistical significance

To many, the word *science* creates a mental image of a person wearing safety glasses and a white lab coat, swirling solutions in test tubes, and scribbling down equations. But only some scientists wear lab coats and work in laboratories. Others work in a variety of settings as they study plants, animals, birds, insects, volcanoes, ocean currents, weather patterns, Earth's solar system, distant galaxies, food safety, human behavior…and human anatomy and physiology.

The word *science* comes from the Latin word *scientia*, which means "knowledge." Thus, ***science*** is a systematic process that creates new knowledge and organizes that knowledge in the form of testable explanations and predictions about some aspect of the universe. Of course, *testable* is a key word in that definition. Some questions are outside the realm of science because they deal with phenomena that are not scientifically testable.

The Scientific Method

A systematic process called the ***scientific method*** is used to answer questions or find solutions to problems in many fields. The scientific method includes seven steps.

Step 1: Identifying a Research Question

All research begins with the identification of a specific ***research question*** for which someone seeks an answer, or a problem that someone would like to have solved. The research question or problem is the reason for conducting the research.

Almost all scientists today work in teams. Team research is expensive, so investing time and money in an investigation is a substantial commitment. The research question should therefore be important enough to warrant the time and cost required to answer it.

A sound research question must be sufficiently specific that it can be tested adequately using available resources. It should also be testable through the use of various tools. These tools are used to collect, organize, analyze, and interpret data.

Data are systematically collected and recorded observations. They may be observations about any topic imaginable. Sometimes the data are quantitative, consisting of numbers. In other cases, they are qualitative, consisting of recorded comments. Sometimes they are a combination of the two (**Figure 1.16**).

Step 2: Formulating One or More Hypotheses

In scientific research, a ***hypothesis*** is an *educated guess* about the outcome of a research study. It is not merely a hunch or a feeling, but an intelligent expectation based on a thorough understanding of the research topic. Researchers usually base their hypotheses on related information discovered by scientists in the same field and published in research journals. Scientists are constantly communicating their research findings and the information they have extracted from various sources to other scientists.

An example of a research hypothesis might be, "We hypothesize that reaction time will be significantly longer following 24 hours of sleep deprivation." Notice that this hypothesis, like all legitimate research hypotheses, can be confirmed (accepted) or not confirmed (rejected) based on the results of the study. Thus, all hypotheses are tentative, testable statements.

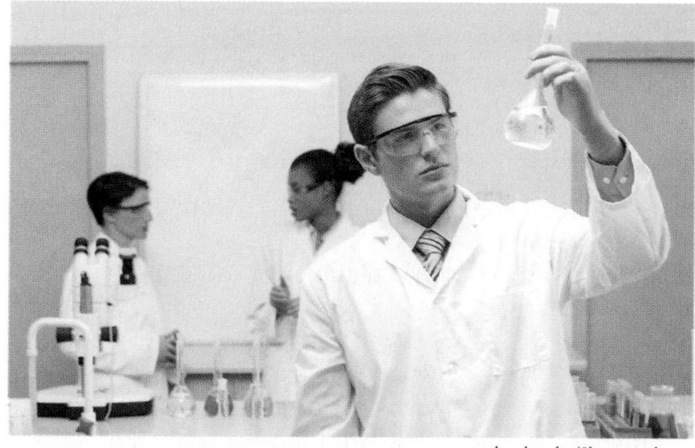

wavebreakmedia/Shutterstock.com

Figure 1.16 This scientist may make both qualitative and quantitative observations about the precipitate in the flask. Qualitatively, he may record that the precipitate is white and appears crystalline. Quantitatively, he may separate and strain the precipitate, weigh it, and record its mass and volume.

Step 3: Planning the Organization of the Study

The organizational aspects of a study involve determining how, where, when, and by whom the data will be collected. In studies involving human participants, organizing the study includes determining

- the criteria to be used for selection of participants;
- the number of participants needed;
- what each participant will be expected to do;
- the equipment or surveys to be used in data collection; and
- the statistical tests that will be used to analyze the data.

Step 4: Collecting the Data

Empirical research involves the recording of observations, or data. Scientists collect data in many different ways. For example, they can use various tools to take precise, accurate measurements. They can use a computer-linked laboratory apparatus to record data values (**Figure 1.17**). They can distribute questionnaires or conduct interviews. Scientists use tools as varied as incubators, meter sticks, and calculators.

No matter what the type of data or medium for collection, scientists must collect all data objectively, using the same procedures. One of the hallmarks of good research is that if other competent researchers were to repeat the study using the same procedures, they would get the same results. For this to be possible, the data collection procedures must be well controlled, and they must be accurately and fully described in the research report.

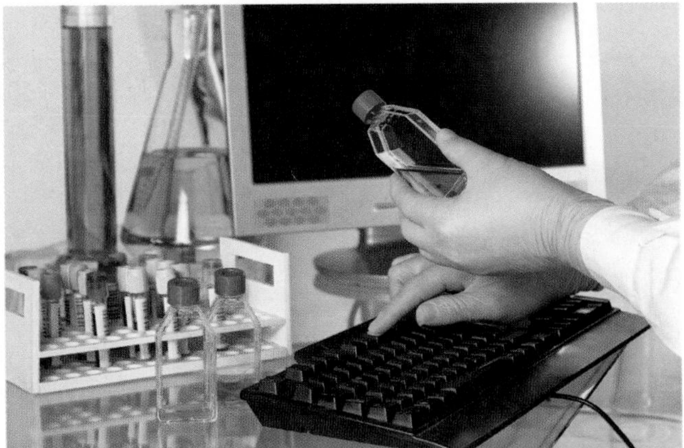
angellodeco/Shutterstock.com

Figure 1.17 Many research laboratories have computerized scales and other equipment that can automatically record data into the lab's computer system. Other labs provide keyboards and input devices that allow researchers to input their data into the computer.

Step 5: Analyzing and Evaluating the Data with Statistical Tools

The analysis and evaluation of data using statistical tools is a vitally important step in the research process. Researchers use statistical tests to determine whether the findings of a study have ***statistical significance***.

When the results of a research study are statistically significant, it suggests that what has been observed from the data collected in the study is also true in general. When data are collected on human participants, statistically significant findings suggest that what is true of the participants in the study is also true of the larger population they represent. The practice of translating the findings of a research study from a small pool of participants to a large population is known as ***statistical inference***.

The ability to accurately predict the characteristics of a very large group based on measurements from a small subset of the large group is a powerful tool. Suppose you would like to know what percentage of US college students take a course in human anatomy and physiology. You could survey students at every college in the country and compile the information, but this would be quite tedious and time-consuming. A more efficient method would be to take data from a number of representative colleges, and then generalize your findings to the entire United States. By looking at such data over a period of years, you could even predict trends in anatomy and physiology course enrollment.

In order to legitimately generalize conclusions from your findings, you must make sure that your sample of representative colleges is truly representative. This might entail collecting data from all of the colleges in a small state, such as Delaware, which has been shown to have a population that is representative of the entire population of the United States in terms of key demographic variables such as rural/urban living distribution and ratios of racial and ethnic groups. Due to its representative nature, findings from a state such as Delaware could be generalized to the entire United States. This could be done with other representative areas as well.

Step 6: Interpreting and Discussing the Results

Interpreting and discussing the results of a study are usually the most interesting and challenging components of the scientific research process. Unfortunately, there is no formula for discussing the results of a study. Researchers typically discuss whether the results support the original hypothesis and compare the findings of the study to the findings of similar studies. Depending on the nature of the study, researchers may also discuss the reasons the findings are important and point out practical or clinical applications that may logically follow from the results.

Step 7: Deriving Conclusions from the Results

The conclusions of a study are composed of one or more concise statements that communicate the key findings of the study. Legitimate, valid conclusions are directly related to the original hypothesis of the study and explain whether the hypothesis is supported by the data collected.

When scientists read the conclusions of a study, they may or may not agree with or accept the conclusions. Scientists are trained to carefully analyze, evaluate, and critique scientific explanations. They do this by considering the empirical evidence (data) presented as the result of the experimental or observational testing. They also consider the logical reasoning behind the interpretation of the study results. A knowledgeable scientist also examines all sides of the scientific evidence presented in the study by considering whether the results are in agreement or conflict with the published results of other similar studies.

SELF CHECK

1. How does an educated guess differ from a hunch or feeling?
2. What elements must be present in a research population to allow researchers to extend the results legitimately to a larger population?
3. How are statistical significance and statistical inference related?
4. The conclusion of a research project needs to be related back to which part of the study?

Scientific Theories

Many people use the word *theory* when they really mean a guess or a hunch. For example, "My theory is that our teacher will give us a pop quiz tomorrow if his football team loses this evening." Sometimes the word *theory* is also used when the speaker really means an educated guess, or hypothesis. In science and medicine, the word *theory* has a much more specific meaning. A ***scientific theory*** is an explanation of some aspect of the natural world that is based on rigorously tested, repeatedly confirmed research. When a hypothesis has been thoroughly tested under a variety of conditions, and it is found to accurately explain a natural or physical phenomenon, it becomes a theory.

The strength of a scientific theory is based on the extent to which it explains a diverse set of circumstances. Theories can be improved and refined as more research is conducted and new technologies and areas of science are developed. Scientists use theories to advance scientific knowledge, create new inventions, and treat diseases.

SELF CHECK

1. What is a scientific theory?
2. What is the relationship between scientific theories and hypotheses?

History of Scientific Research

To appreciate the development of science, consider a brief historical perspective. The history of scientific research dates back to the dawn of civilization. One of the earliest topics of interest was the anatomy and physiology of humans.

Early Greek and Roman Anatomists

One of the first people to systematically study topics related to anatomy was the early Greek philosopher, Aristotle (384–322 BCE). Aristotle studied and wrote about more than 540 species of animals in his anatomy book, *On the Parts of Animals*.

Another early anatomist and physiologist was the Roman physician, surgeon, and philosopher Galen (129–c.200 CE). While serving as the personal physician to several Roman emperors, Galen compiled numerous anatomical reports from his dissections of pigs and monkeys. During Galen's life, dissection of human cadavers was prohibited, so many of his assumptions about human anatomy were based on animal anatomy.

Based on his experiments, Galen was the first to advance the idea that the brain controls the muscles through signals from nerves. Galen also, however, believed that arteries carry the purest blood to the brain and lungs from the left ventricle of the heart, while veins carry blood to the other organs from the right ventricle. This is, of course, incorrect. For his belief to be true, some openings were needed in the walls of the ventricles, which Galen incorrectly claimed to have found.

Anatomists in the Renaissance

Spanning the mid-fourteenth to the mid-seventeenth centuries, the Renaissance was a period of significant cultural and scientific developments. Interest in science increased during this era, leading to new and exciting discoveries. This section lists some of the key anatomists of the Renaissance and describes the contributions they made to the study of anatomy and physiology.

Leonardo da Vinci

During the Renaissance period, the renowned artist Leonardo da Vinci (1452–1519) also distinguished himself as a scientist, engineer, and inventor. Among his many contributions was advancing knowledge of human anatomy and physiology.

To better understand the human body for his paintings, da Vinci was given permission to dissect human corpses at hospitals in Rome, Florence, and Milan. He was known to have dissected at least 30 corpses, including males and females of different ages. From his studies, he prepared a theoretical work on human anatomy with more than 200 drawings,

Research Notes Research

If you pursue a career in the health professions, you might become involved in research projects, even if you do not work in a setting where research is usually done. Scientific investigations happen in laboratories, but research also happens in many other places. For example, a company that makes dentistry tools may want to get feedback from dental hygienists who have used the tools.

Safety and Resources

Whether the research takes place in the lab or in the field, healthcare professionals must be aware of the many safety and resource issues that can arise during research. They must consider how the research could affect their own health, their patients' health, and the environment.

Your Own Health

If the research requires you to change your work routine, are the usual steps that you take to ensure workplace safety compromised? Is a new piece of equipment a potential tripping hazard? Are you exposed to potentially hazardous body fluids? Do you have the right personal protective equipment (PPE), such as safety glasses, gloves, and lab coat? If you are working with needles or blades, do you have a safe place (sharps container) to dispose of them? The questions you ask yourself will depend on your situation, but it is important to anticipate the unexpected when thinking about safety. Note that in some situations, items such as PPE and sharps containers are required by federal Occupational Safety and Health Administration (OSHA) regulations.

Your Patient's Health

If a research project involves people or animals, the research review process involves extensive consideration of the potential risks to the subjects. Even a research project that has been reviewed and approved could present risks that did not occur to the reviewers. Never hesitate to tell your supervisor if you have a concern about patient safety, and be sure you understand federal safety regulations before beginning your research.

The Environment

Always try to find ways to minimize the resources needed for your research and the waste created by it. Also look for ways to recycle resources. Be sure to follow proper procedures for disposing of waste materials. For more information about requirements for disposing of wastes, look up the specific wastes on the website of the Environmental Protection Agency (EPA.gov).

Types of Research

Just as research occurs in many different settings, it takes many forms. For example, research projects may be classified as *descriptive*, *comparative*, or *experimental*.

Descriptive research entails accurately measuring "what is out there." This could mean measuring the height, weight, oral temperature, and age of each child who comes into a clinic. It could also mean testing saliva samples from adults at a senior center for the presence of a newly discovered virus.

Comparative research involves making comparisons between one group and another. For example, you might want to compare the fitness of the students who drive to school to the fitness of those who walk or ride their bicycles to school.

Experimental research is more "active" than descriptive or comparative research. It involves doing something and observing the results. For example, you might ask subjects to complete a math test 15 minutes after drinking coffee, and then have them do a similar math test without the coffee a week later. You might do an experiment to see whether putting people on a program of regular exercise for two weeks improves their performance on tests of short-term memory.

including individual bones, muscles, tendons, ligaments, veins, and arteries.

The Vitruvian Man by da Vinci is one of the best-known drawings in the world (**Figure 1.18**). This drawing represents da Vinci's concept of the ideal proportions of man, and illustrates the blending of science and art that was an important trend during the Renaissance.

Andreas Vesalius

A Flemish physician, Andreas Vesalius (1514–1564), is regarded as the founder of modern human anatomy. Vesalius authored a comprehensive and influential work on human anatomy entitled *De Humani Corporis Fabrica (On the Structure of the Human Body).*

In the course of his work, Vesalius proved that some views of human anatomy proposed by Aristotle and Galen were incorrect. Vesalius correctly observed, for example, that the human heart has four chambers, the liver has two lobes, and the blood vessels originate in the heart, not the liver. These findings were all in contrast to the assertions of Aristotle and Galen.

Vesalius did, however, support Galen's views on bloodletting, which was the standard treatment of the day for most illnesses. The classical Greek procedure, advocated by Galen, was to drain blood from a site

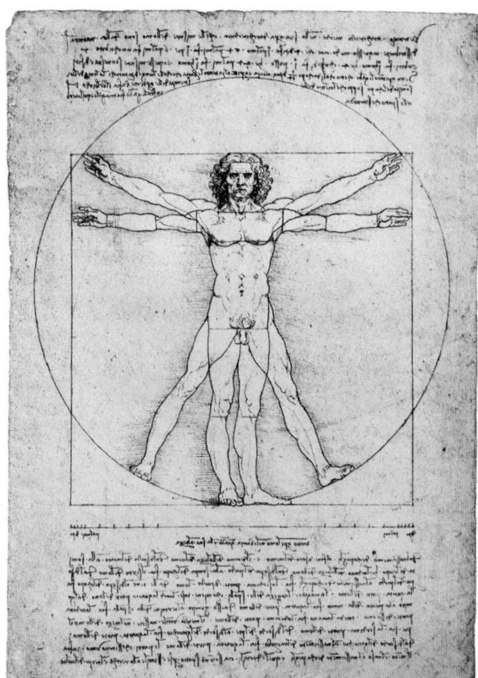

Jakub Krechowicz/Shutterstock.com

Figure 1.18 Leonardo da Vinci's famous anatomical drawing, *The Vitruvian Man*.

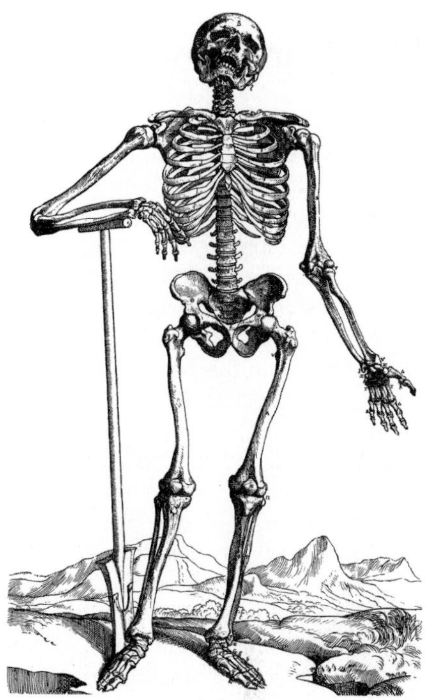

Suzan Oschmann/Shutterstock.com

Figure 1.19 An early anatomical drawing from Vesalius' 1543 text, *De Humani Corporis Fabrica*.

near the part of the body believed to be associated with an illness.

Using knowledge gained from dissecting human cadavers, Vesalius was able to construct anatomical drawings of the human body that were more detailed than other medical illustrations of the day. One of Vesalius' anatomical drawings is shown in **Figure 1.19**.

William Harvey

One of the first accurate descriptions of human physiology was provided by William Harvey (1578–1657), a physician to two kings of England. Harvey and Michael Servetus (1511–1553) were the first to understand that blood circulates continuously through the body, with the heart serving as the pump.

Robert Hooke and Antonie van Leeuwenhoek

Science took another large step forward thanks to the work of the Englishman Robert Hooke (1635–1703) and a Dutch textile merchant named Antonie van Leeuwenhoek (1632–1723). Hooke made a number of improvements to the microscopes of the day, which magnified only about 30 times (as opposed to modern microscopes, some of which can magnify up to 10 million times). Using his improved microscope, Hooke was the first to view and name cells. He published a book about microscopy called *Micrographia* in 1665.

Leeuwenhoek further advanced the quality of the microscope, designing an instrument with a magnification of about 200 times for the purpose of close examination of the weave of fabrics. With the new power of his microscope, however, he was soon examining drops of water, as well as specimens of blood, sperm, muscle tissue, and bacteria. Through his investigations, Leeuwenhoek confirmed that many biological materials are made of cells.

Looking Ahead

Scientists have come a long way in advancing scientific knowledge since the discovery of cells. As is clear from reading about some of these early scientists, the prevailing views of human anatomy and physiology have changed greatly over time. This is true of all fields of science, and change continues today. As new discoveries are made and current assumptions are challenged, scientists continue to advance our knowledge of many phenomena.

The scientific discoveries being made today dramatically impact our lives and improve our environment. Recent scientific breakthroughs, as a result of research sponsored by the National Aeronautics and Space Administration (NASA), have contributed to the development of many products related to human anatomy and physiology. Examples include memory

Focus On Anatomical Fugitive Sheets

During the Renaissance period, physicians and artists engaged in the study of the human body. These perspectives were combined in the form of anatomical fugitive sheets. An anatomical fugitive sheet is an illustration of the human body constructed to display a three-dimensional approximation of the internal organs and structures. This was achieved with several different layers of paper, with each successive layer displaying organs located deeper in the body. The layers were hinged, so that they could be lifted to create views of various stages of dissection.

The earliest anatomical fugitive sheets date back to the 1530s. The original purpose of these sheets is unknown, although some have speculated that they were used as labeled instructional aids for aspiring physicians and surgeons. The first sheets were labeled in Latin, but they were printed in languages of the day over time.

The German engraver and printer Heinrich Vogtherr was among the earliest to publish anatomical sheets in 1538. Jean Ruelle, a French physician and botanist, published anatomical sheets he personally constructed in 1539. However, Andreas Vesalius is believed to have produced the first anatomically accurate drawings in his comprehensive *De Humani Corporis Fabrica*, published in 1543.

Anatomical fugitive sheets, which were popularly distributed from the 1530s through the late seventeenth century, were typically printed as a single sheet rather than as part of a volume. For this reason, very few sheets from these centuries have survived, leading to their "fugitive" designation.

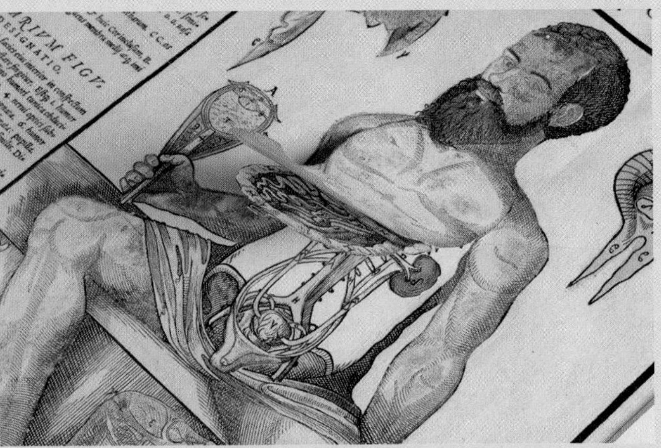

Example of an anatomical fugitive sheet from the 16th century.

A few of the anatomical fugitive sheets dating back to the Renaissance can be found today in library collections focused on the history of medicine. They serve as beautiful examples of Renaissance art, as well as interesting historical documents.

The concept of layering views of the internal human organs has re-emerged periodically in recent times. In fact, a 1983 pop-up book by Jonathan Miller, entitled *The Human Body*, uses this same principle.

foam for comfortable seating, scratch-resistant lenses, cochlear implants, software for viewing partial blockages of the carotid artery, and insulin pumps. Research by NASA scientists has also improved our environment. They have made discoveries leading to technology for superior water filters and a compound called *emulsified zero-valent iron* that can be injected into groundwater to neutralize toxic chemicals. Their research has also led to solar-powered appliances, improved insulation materials for residential and commercial buildings, and better fertilizer for plants.

SECTION 1.4 REVIEW

Mini-Glossary

data systematically collected and recorded observations

hypothesis an educated guess about the outcome of a study

research question the question to be answered or problem to be solved in a research study

science a systematic process that creates new knowledge and organizes it into a form of testable explanations and predictions about an aspect of our universe

scientific method a systematic process that can be used to answer questions or find solutions to problems

scientific theory an explanation of some aspect of the natural world that is based on rigorously tested, repeatedly confirmed research

statistical inference the practice of generalizing the findings of a research study to a large population

statistical significance an interpretation of statistical data indicating that the results of a study can legitimately be generalized to the population represented in the study sample

(continued)

Review Questions

1. Which famous artist was also a preeminent anatomist?
2. The improvement of which scientific tool produced significant advancements in the study of anatomy and physiology?
3. List, in order, the steps of the scientific method.
4. What is the difference between a hypothesis and a scientific theory?
5. Working with the definition of *science* and the information about science provided in this lesson, explain the limitations, if any, of science.
6. Give an example of a scientific theory that has been refined or improved since it was first established as a theory.
7. If Aristotle and Galen had been able to dissect cadavers, how might advancements in the study of anatomy have been different?
8. Explain how da Vinci's study of anatomy influenced the future of anatomical science and art.
9. How would you evaluate the impact of scientific research on a society and the environment in your city, state, or region of the country?

Medical Terminology

As explained in this chapter, medical words are made up of four basic word parts: roots, prefixes, suffixes, and combining vowels. Understanding the meaning of common word parts can help you determine the meaning of words you have not encountered before. Review the word parts in ***Figure 1.1*** *to be sure you understand their meanings. Then use word parts from the figure to form valid medical words that fit the following definitions. When you finish, use a medical dictionary to check your work.*

1. surgical removal of the stomach
2. nerve pain
3. heart specialist
4. inflammation of the intestine
5. above-normal growth and development
6. cancerous mass or tumor
7. specialist in the function of living organisms
8. joint inflammation
9. blood specialist
10. softening of the bone

Chapter 1 Summary

- Anatomy and physiology are studied together because the structure of a cell, tissue, organ, or organism is closely related to its function.
- Scientists use universal terminology for anatomical positions, planes, and directions to accurately describe body positions and movements.
- The metric system is used in science throughout the world to measure numerical quantities.
- The human body is composed of a hierarchy of structures, from atoms as the most basic unit to organ systems at the highest level.
- Although the human body is in a constant state of flux, it is kept healthy and in balance by maintaining homeostasis.
- Metabolism is the constant breaking down and building up of molecules to provide energy, create cells, and perform bodily functions needed to sustain life.
- Kinetics is the study of forces applied to the human body. These forces include pressure, compression, torque, shearing, and stress.
- Forces can cause tissues to experience acceleration and deformation. Deformation may be either elastic or plastic.
- Scientific knowledge is increased via research conducted using the scientific method to ensure uniformity in experimentation.
- A scientific theory emerges from a hypothesis that has been rigorously and repeatedly researched and tested and all evidence points to the accuracy of the theory in explaining a natural occurrence.
- Scientific knowledge continues to grow with advancements in research methods and tools.

Chapter 1 Review

Understanding Key Concepts

1. The ______ cavity contains the skull and brain.
2. The universal starting point for describing positions and movements of the human body is the ______.
3. ______ is the study of the functions of the human body.
4. Which of these organs is found in the thoracic cavity?
   A. heart
   B. stomach
   C. liver
   D. kidneys
5. The knee is ______ to the ankle.
   A. lateral
   B. posterior
   C. distal
   D. proximal
6. The dorsal surface of a person or object is the ______ surface.
   A. superior surface
   B. inferior surface
   C. posterior surface
   D. anterior surface
7. The smallest living structure is the ______.
8. The body maintains a stable internal environment via ______.
9. ______ nerves carry a signal from the external environment to the control center.
10. The lungs are part of the ______.
    A. circulatory system
    B. integumentary system
    C. endocrine system
    D. respiratory system
11. The next most complex level of organization after the cellular level in organisms is the ______.
    A. organ
    B. tissue
    C. body system
    D. chemical
12. Which of the following is *not* one of the four main types of tissue in the body?
    A. muscle tissue
    B. connective tissue
    C. alveolar tissue
    D. nerve tissue
13. Specialized cell parts that perform specific functions within the cell are called ______.
    A. tissues
    B. organs
    C. molecules
    D. organelles
14. ______ is a force that pulls or stretches the tissue.
15. ______ is a force that, with enough energy, crushes tissue.
16. ______ is a force that moves parallel with tissue.
17. ______ is caused by a combination of off-center forces.
18. A bruise is caused by ______.
    A. compression
    B. tension
    C. shearing
    D. torque
19. ______ is the single force resulting from the summation of all forces acting on an object at a given time.
    A. Net mass
    B. Net force
    C. Net torque
    D. Net weight
20. Tissue displacement is said to be ______ when a force is removed and the object returns to its original shape.
    A. plastic
    B. torqued
    C. efferent
    D. elastic
21. All research begins with the identification of a(n) ______.
22. Early anatomists studied ______ because of religious or political influences prohibiting the dissection of ______.

23. Step 2 of the scientific method is ______.
    A. formulating a hypothesis
    B. planning the organization of the study
    C. identifying a research question
    D. collecting the data
24. When a hypothesis has been thoroughly investigated and found to accurately explain a natural or physical phenomenon, it is ______.
    A. a hunch
    B. a preliminary guess
    C. an educated guess
    D. a theory

Thinking Critically

25. What plane(s) can the shoulder move in? Explain your answer.
26. Using the common directional terms for anatomy that you learned in this chapter, provide a written description for the location of the index finger of the left hand.
27. It is a hot, dry day, and you are going to be running a race in the middle of the afternoon. What challenges does your body face in trying to maintain homeostasis while you run?
28. A football player's foot is planted, and he is in the process of turning when his knee is hit from the side, resulting in a serious injury to the ligaments of the knee. Which two forces acted on the knee to produce this injury?
29. Assume that your body is struck by a baseball and a basketball of the same weight traveling at the same speed. Which will exert more pressure on your body—the baseball or the basketball? Why?
30. Is skin or bone more elastic? Why?
31. Suppose that a hypothesis is proven incorrect. Does this mean that the research was a waste of time? Defend your answer.

Clinical Case Study

Read again the Clinical Case Study at the beginning of this chapter. Use the information provided in the chapter to answer the following questions.

32. Among the topics discussed in the chapter, what condition(s) may Larry be experiencing?
33. Which condition is most likely?
34. What should Sam do to help Larry?

Analyzing and Evaluating Data

The graph below shows the average number of steps (foot contacts) resulting in chronic injury, as they occur in groups of people in different weight categories. Use the graph to answer the following questions.

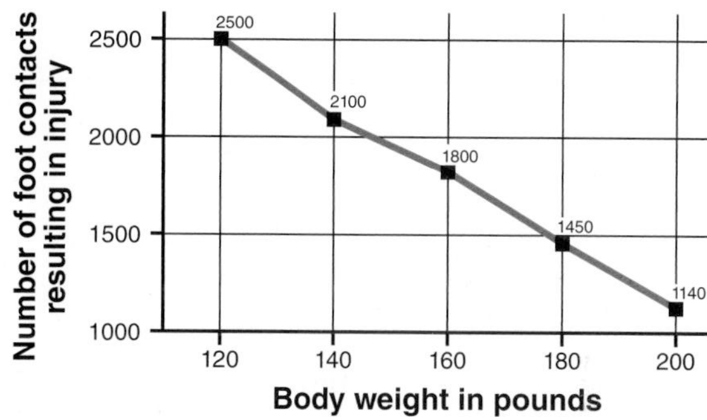

35. How many foot contacts is the group with a body weight of 160 pounds able to make before an injury occurs?
36. Which group is generating the most pressure per foot contact?
37. What prediction would you make about the number of foot contacts leading to injury for people in the 170- to 175-pound range?
38. Based on the data provided in the graph, write a hypothesis about body weight and foot contacts resulting in chronic injuries.

Investigating Further

39. Create a measurable hypothesis about study time and its relationship to success on exams. Make precise, accurate measurements of both time and grades. What can you infer from your data? What trends can you predict?
40. With the students in your anatomy and physiology class as the participants, research the impact of exercise on the homeostatic state of the respiratory system. Collect, organize, analyze, and evaluate both quantitative and qualitative data using appropriate tools. Will this population sample be considered statistically significant? How could you improve this experiment?

2 Molecules and Cells

Clinical Case Study

Stan is a 55-year-old online customer support representative. He is married with one child in college. He exercises by walking about one mile, three times a week. Stan is slightly overweight and does not smoke. He is generally healthy. He had his appendix removed at age 26. He takes a statin drug to control his blood cholesterol.

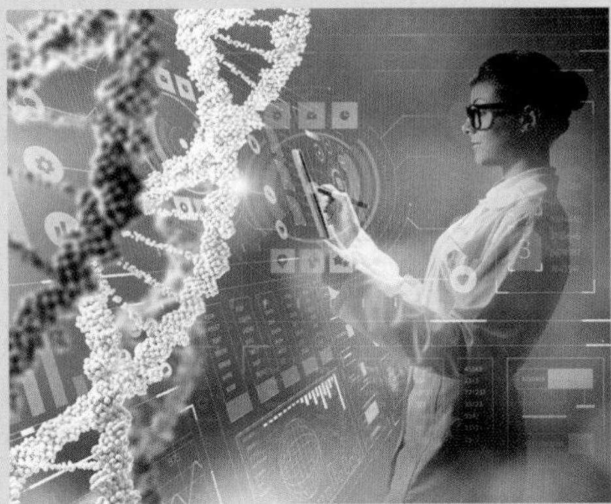

Sergey Nivens/Shutterstock.com

Stan goes to the local urgent care center because he has significant pain in the upper-left side of his abdomen. He tells the nurse practitioner that he has felt unusually tired for the last couple of months. He has lost five pounds because he does not need as much food as usual to feel full.

Stan's temperature is normal. His spleen can be felt below the edge of his left ribs, which indicates that it is enlarged. Microscopic examination of a blood sample reveals an unusually high number of white blood cells, as well as many immature white blood cells, which are not usually seen. His red blood cells have the normal shape and color, but are slightly less abundant than normal. The nurse practitioner suspects that Stan may have cancer. If he does have cancer, she hopes that it is a particular type of cancer, for which there is now a highly effective drug therapy. A definitive diagnosis will require advanced testing of the blood sample.

Chapter 2 Outline

The human body is made of trillions of cells. Although scientists do not agree on exactly how to define life, they all agree that our individual cells are alive. These cells cannot survive independently; they need one another to stay alive. They reproduce through the process of mitosis. They evolve and transmit information from one generation of cells to the next through DNA. They transform energy from one form to another, and they use energy to maintain their internal environment in the face of outside influences.

Each cell is a specialist with its own job to do. Certain tasks, such as maintaining an internal environment different from that of the surrounding fluid, are performed by all cells. Other tasks, such as making ATP, are done by most cells. Some tasks, such as making antibodies, are done by only one type of cell.

You must understand how cells work, and how they work together, to understand anatomy and physiology. An understanding of cells and the molecules they are made of is also necessary for understanding diseases and their treatment. This is even truer now than it was a generation ago, because modern medicine relies more than ever on therapies targeted at molecular and cellular processes.

This chapter reviews the fundamental principles of chemistry. It describes the parts of a cell and how those parts cooperate to keep the cells alive, allow them to reproduce, and help them accomplish specialized tasks.

SECTION 2.1

Atoms and Forces

Objectives

- Describe the relationships among the fundamental particles of an atom.
- Discuss the three basic types of atomic bonds.
- Understand the importance of isotopes in human physiology and medicine.

Key Terms

anion
atom
atomic number
cation
covalent bond
electron
element
hydrogen bond
ion
ionic bond
isotope
molecule
neutron
proton

The cells that make up the human body, as well as the drugs people sometimes take, are made of molecules. Molecules are made of atoms. An ***atom*** is considered the fundamental building block of matter and is made of one or more protons, neutrons, and electrons.

Fundamental Particles

A ***proton*** is a positively charged fundamental particle found in the nucleus, or center, of an atom. Atoms are classified by their ***atomic number***, or the number of protons they have in their nuclei. An ***element*** is a substance composed of atoms that all have the same atomic number. Hydrogen, carbon, nitrogen, and oxygen are the four most abundant elements in the human body. Every hydrogen atom has one proton in its nucleus. Every carbon atom has six protons in its nucleus, every nitrogen atom has seven, and every oxygen atom has eight.

Neutrons are another type of particle found in the nucleus. Neutrons get their name from the fact that they are electrically neutral: they have no electric charge. Most hydrogen atoms do not have any neutrons. Most carbon, nitrogen, and oxygen atoms have six, seven, and eight neutrons, respectively.

Atoms also have ***electrons***, which are negatively charged particles that occupy a space around the nucleus. Atoms in their pure form (not linked to other atoms of different types) have as many electrons as they have protons. Since the negative charge on an electron is equal but opposite to the positive charge on a proton, an atom in its pure form has an electric charge of zero (**Figure 2.1**).

Atomic Bonds

An atom can interact with a nearby atom by exerting a force on it. Attractive forces between certain atoms allow them to link up, or bond, to one another to form a ***molecule*** (**Figure 2.2**). An electron can lower its energy by "sharing" an orbital (a region of space near an atomic nucleus) with another electron. A state of lower energy is more stable.

Covalent Bonds

When two atoms lower their combined energy by sharing a pair of electrons, they have formed a ***covalent bond***. Covalent bonds are strong and not easily pulled apart. The simplest covalent molecule consists of two hydrogen atoms, which share their electrons to form a hydrogen molecule, which is written H_2. The subscript "2" shows how many hydrogen atoms make up the hydrogen molecule. Water, or H_2O, is

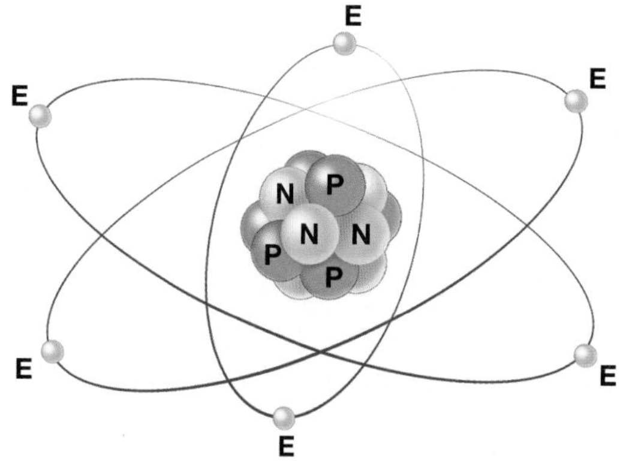

© Body Scientific International

Figure 2.1 A simplified representation of a carbon atom. Carbon atoms have an atomic number of 6.

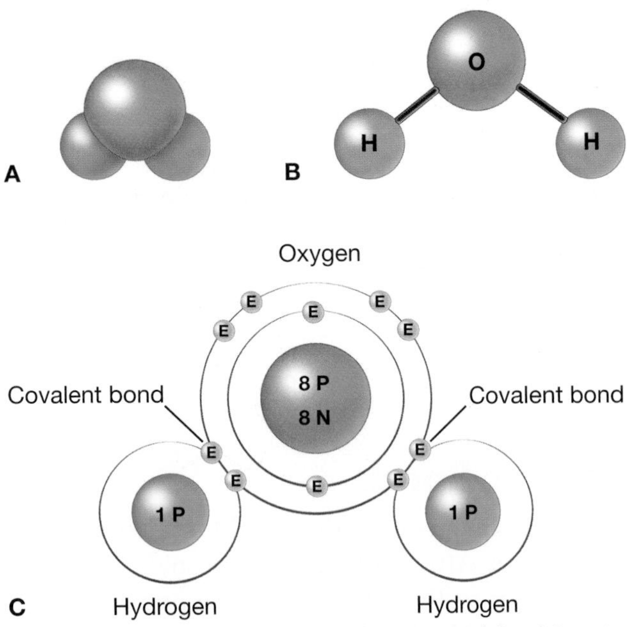

Figure 2.2 Three views of the atoms that make up a water (H_2O) molecule. A—The three-dimensional structure of a water molecule. B—The atoms and the bonds connecting them. C—Covalent bonds form when electrons are shared by two nuclei.

formed when an oxygen atom forms covalent bonds with two separate hydrogen atoms. The bonds in a water molecule are covalent because each involves an electron of oxygen and an electron of hydrogen sharing an orbital.

Amino acids, sugars, and fats are examples of molecules formed by covalently linked atoms. Almost all of the molecules in biology are formed by covalent bonds. Large molecules, such as proteins, may have hundreds or thousands of atoms, and therefore hundreds or thousands of covalent bonds. Chromosomes, the largest biological molecules, have billions of atoms and billions of covalent bonds.

Ionic Bonds

Some atoms, such as chloride, can lower their total energy by "picking up" an extra electron, if one is available. Other atoms, such as sodium, can lower their energy by losing an electron. When two such atoms come near each other, an electron may move from one to the other. The chloride becomes negatively charged when it picks up an electron from the sodium. Similarly, the sodium becomes positively charged when it loses the electron.

Atoms and molecules that are charged are called ***ions***. An ion with a positive charge is a ***cation***, and an ion with a negative charge is an ***anion***. When atoms are oppositely charged, like the sodium and chloride ions in the previous example, they are electrically attracted to one another. A bond between atoms due to this simple electric attraction is called an ***ionic bond***. A crystal of table salt (sodium chloride or NaCl) is held together by ionic bonds between the sodium and chloride ions. Ionic bonds are also present in the human body. Bone is hard because it contains a complex combination of charged subunits linked by ionic bonds.

Hydrogen Bonds

Molecules can also interact with each other through ***hydrogen bonds***, which are a type of van der Waals force. Van der Waals forces are forces that attract molecules to each other.

Because hydrogen bonds are weaker than covalent bonds, they are more easily broken. Molecules linked by these forces can, and often do, become "unstuck" from one another. Many important biological processes take advantage of the reversible nature of these bonds.

A molecule of DNA is an excellent example of the difference between covalent and hydrogen bonds and the importance of both. DNA looks like a twisted ladder and is often called a *double helix.* As seen in **Figure 2.3**, the "sides" of the ladder consist of atoms joined by strong covalent bonds. Each side has "half-rungs," which connect with the other side's half-rungs through hydrogen bonds. The relative weakness of the hydrogen bonds means that DNA can "unzip" down the middle. However, due to their stronger covalent bonds, the two sides do not break. The relatively weak hydrogen bonds *between* the sides, and the strong covalent bonds *along* the sides, are essential for the proper and efficient function of DNA. You will learn more about DNA later in this chapter.

Most proteins that interact with each other do so through hydrogen bonds and other types of van der Waals forces. For example, as described in Chapter 6, every move the body makes is due to the repeated attaching and detaching of actin and myosin proteins in muscle cells. These connections can be made and unmade quickly due to the reversible nature of the bonds that join them.

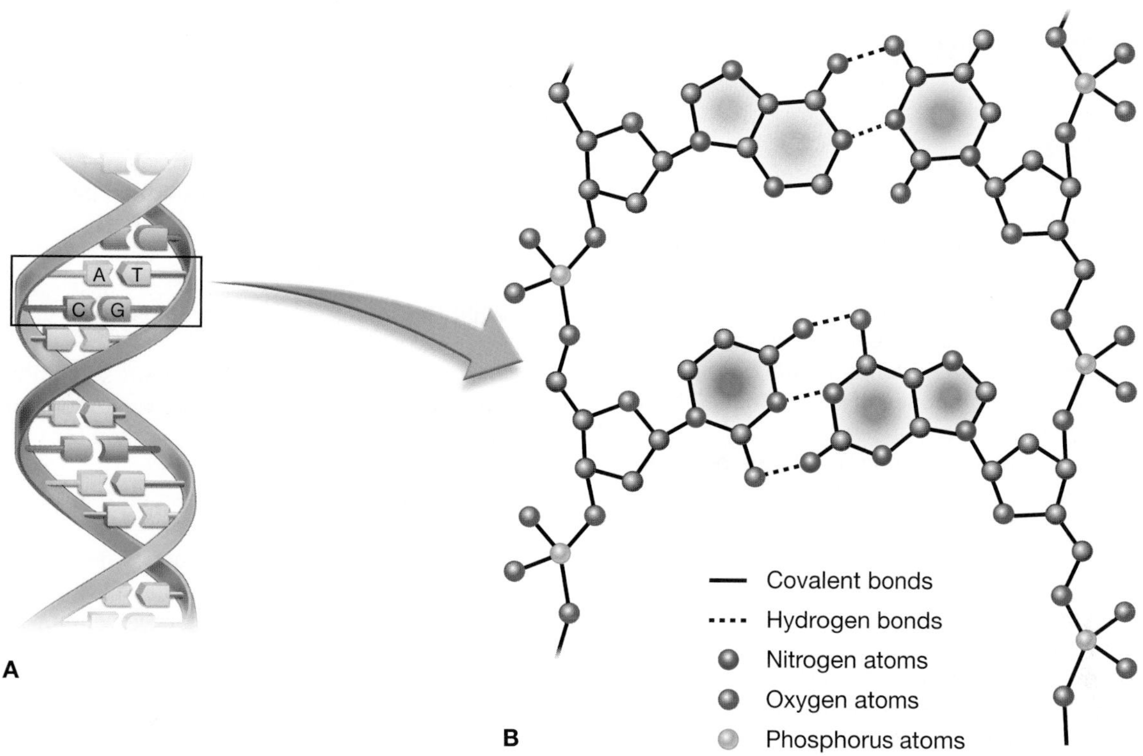

Figure 2.3 A—A segment of a DNA molecule, showing the two strands of the double helix, joined by base pairs. B—The atoms and bonds of a DNA molecule, including two "rungs" formed with hydrogen bonds. Hydrogen atoms that are not involved in base pair bonding are omitted for clarity.

SELF CHECK

1. In practical terms, what is the difference between a proton and a neutron?
2. What is a covalent bond?
3. What type of atomic bond is responsible for most interactions among proteins?

Isotopes

Each type of atom ordinarily has a particular number of neutrons in its nucleus. Atoms that have the same number of protons, but different numbers of neutrons, are called ***isotopes*** of the same element. Carbon-12, an isotope that has six protons and six neutrons, makes up 99% of the carbon in the atmosphere. The remaining 1% is almost all carbon-13, which has six protons and seven neutrons. About one carbon out of every trillion carbons is carbon-14, which has eight neutrons.

Isotopes can be either stable or unstable. Stable isotopes of an element are almost identical in their ability to form bonds with other atoms. Therefore, the presence of stable isotopes in the body's molecules is usually unimportant.

Some isotopes are unstable, meaning that they tend to lose particles over time. This is called *radioactive decay*, and the unstable isotopes are called *radioisotopes*. When an atom undergoes radioactive decay, energy is released. If a radioactive substance enters the body, the energy it releases through radioactive decay may damage cells and cause illness. For example, radioactive iodine was released by the Chernobyl nuclear reactor accident in 1986, and it is believed to have caused several thousand cases of thyroid cancer among nearby residents.

Although they may cause damage, radioactive molecules can also be put to good use in medicine. A drug containing radioactive molecules can be given to a person, and then its location in the body can be tracked with sensors that detect the source of radiation. Cancer scans and positron emission tomography (PET) scans use this technique.

SECTION 2.1

REVIEW

Mini-Glossary

anion a negatively charged ion
atom a basic building block of matter
atomic number the number of protons in an atom's nucleus
cation a positively charged ion
covalent bond a strong connection formed between two atoms when they share a pair of electrons
electron a negatively charged fundamental particle
element a substance composed of atoms that all have the same atomic number
hydrogen bond a weak connection that forms between two molecules through an electrostatic (van der Waals) attraction
ion an atom or molecule that has a positive or negative charge
ionic bond a connection that forms between atoms due to electric attraction
isotope a form of an element that contains an equal number of protons but a different number of neutrons than other forms, or isotopes, of the element
molecule a group of atoms bonded together
neutron a fundamental particle that has no electric charge
proton a positively charged fundamental particle

Review Questions

1. What three fundamental particles make up most atoms?
2. The atomic number of the element sodium is 11. How many protons does an atom of sodium have?
3. Why is a covalent bond stronger than ionic and hydrogen bonds?
4. What is the difference between carbon-12 and carbon-14?
5. Explain the principle of radioactive decay.
6. The notation for a water molecule is H_2O. Given that the symbol for carbon is C, how many of which types of atoms make up a CO_2 molecule?
7. Explain how carbon-14 can be used in some cases to identify the age of carbon-containing materials that have been on Earth for centuries.

SECTION 2.2

Molecules

Objectives

- Explain the types and functions of carbohydrates.
- Describe the structure and functions of amino acids and proteins.
- List the types and properties of lipids, including fatty acids, glycerides, phospholipids, and steroids.
- Discuss the structure and purpose of the two major types of nucleic acids.
- Describe the polarity of water and its contribution to pH balance.

Key Terms

amino acids
base pairs
chromosome
deoxyribonucleic acid (DNA)
enzyme
fatty acid
glucose
glycogen
human genome
lipids
nucleic acids
nucleotides
peptide bond
pH
phospholipids
polymer
polypeptide
ribonucleic acid (RNA)
steroids
triglycerides

The human body contains an almost countless number of different types of molecules. Biochemistry is the study of the molecules of life, how they are made, how they interact, and how they are broken down. This section describes the molecules that are most important in anatomy and physiology.

Most of the chemicals important for life are organic molecules. Organic molecules are those that contain carbon and hydrogen. They usually contain oxygen, and they sometimes contain nitrogen, phosphorous, sulfur, and other elements. Major classes of organic molecules in the body include carbohydrates, proteins, lipids, nucleic acids, and ATP. Important inorganic molecules and elements include sodium, potassium, chloride, calcium, phosphate, and, of course, water.

Carbohydrates

Carbohydrates, also known as *saccharides,* are sugar and starch molecules. Carbohydrates made of just one or two simple subunits are called *simple carbohydrates,* or *sugars.* ***Glucose*** ($C_6H_{12}O_6$) is a monosaccharide—a simple sugar with one subunit (*mono-*). It is the main form of sugar that circulates in the blood

(**Figure 2.4**). Sucrose ($C_{12}H_{22}O_{11}$), (table sugar) is a disaccharide made of two monosaccharides: glucose and fructose.

Simple sugars can join together to form long chains known as *complex carbohydrates.* A molecule made of many similar subunits (several simple sugars, for example) is called a ***polymer. Glycogen*** is a polymer of glucose that is found in animals (**Figure 2.5**). Starch is a polymer of simple sugars that is found in plants.

Understanding Medical Terminology

The term *polymer* comes from the combining forms *poly*, meaning "many," and *mer*, meaning "unit." Monomers (*mono* means "one") are the building blocks from which polymers are made. Other "-mers" include *dimers* (two subunits), *trimers* (three subunits), and *tetramers* (four subunits).

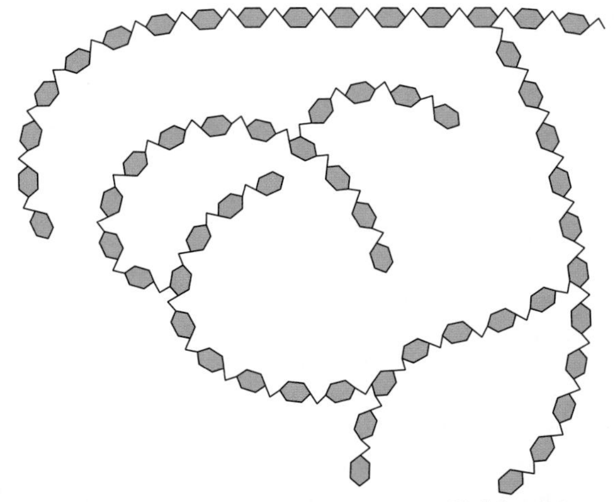

© Body Scientific International

Figure 2.5 Glycogen is a polysaccharide made of glucose monomers, which are shown here as hexagons. Notice the many branches in the monomer chains.

Liver and muscle cells make glycogen molecules from glucose. A single glycogen molecule may contain hundreds of thousands of glucose subunits. The glycogen serves as a form of stored fuel. When a muscle cell needs fuel, it can break glucose molecules off the glycogen and use the glucose for energy. If blood sugar becomes too low, liver cells can break glucose molecules off the glycogen and release the glucose into the blood.

The main function of carbohydrates in the body is to serve as a source of chemical energy, or fuel. The body can quickly utilize this fuel to make ATP, which you will learn about later in this chapter.

Understanding Medical Terminology

The term *carbohydrate* is derived from the elements that combine to make up a carbohydrate. The term also provides a clue to the atomic formula for carbohydrates. All carbohydrates are made of carbon, hydrogen, and oxygen atoms. The hydrogen and oxygen are usually present in a two-to-one ratio; for example, water has two hydrogen molecules and one oxygen molecule: H_2O. *Hydrate* is a chemical term for water. Therefore, carbohydrate means "carbon and water."

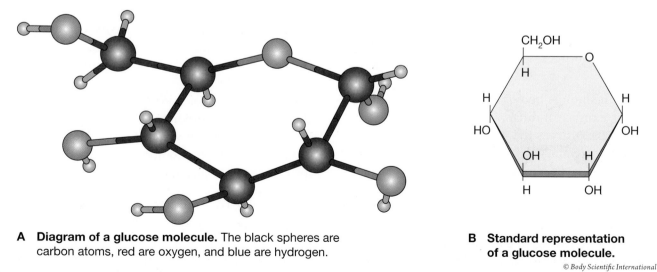

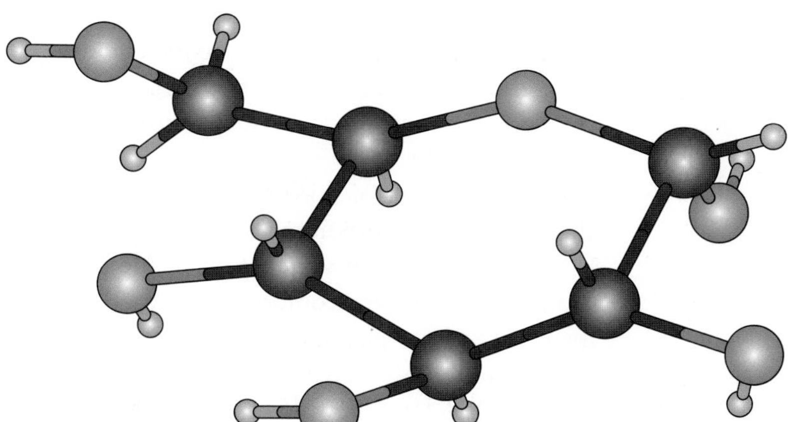

A Diagram of a glucose molecule. The black spheres are carbon atoms, red are oxygen, and blue are hydrogen.

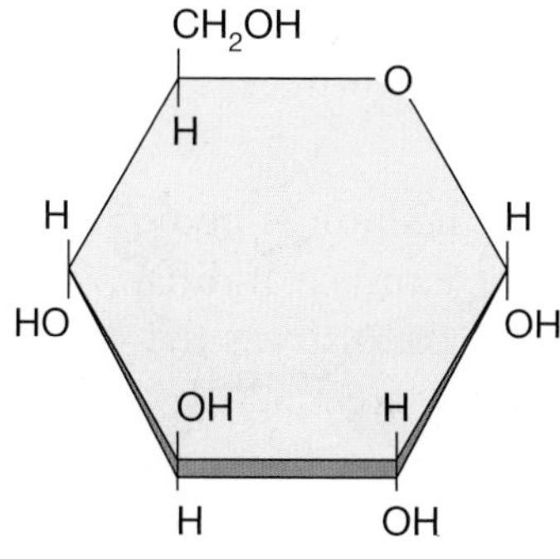

B Standard representation of a glucose molecule.

© Body Scientific International

Figure 2.4 Glucose is an organic molecule. Notice the difference in the number of carbon atoms in A as opposed to B. The reason for this difference is that, in the standard method of representing the molecular structure of glucose (B), a carbon atom is assumed to be present at each unlabeled "corner" where two or more lines (bonds) meet.

SELF CHECK

1. What does the word *carbohydrate* mean?
2. What term describes simple sugars that join together in long chains?
3. Where in the body are glycogen molecules made from glucose?

Proteins

Proteins are large molecules made of chains of ***amino acids***. These chains include anywhere from dozens to hundreds of amino acids. Some proteins help form the structure of cells. Other proteins, called *enzymes*, catalyze (speed up) specific biological reactions. Still others (notably hemoglobin) act as carriers. (Hemoglobin carries oxygen in red blood cells.)

Amino Acids

Twenty common amino acids serve as the building blocks of proteins. All 20 amino acids share a common design: each has an identical "backbone" consisting of an amino group (-NH_2), an acid group (-COOH), and a central carbon between them (**Figure 2.6**). The central carbon has a hydrogen and a variable group of atoms attached to it. The variable group differs from one amino acid to another. Biochemists call this group the *residual group*, so an *R* indicates this group in **Figure 2.6**.

In glycine, the simplest amino acid, the residual group consists of a single hydrogen atom. Tryptophan has the largest residual group (C_9H_4N). Some amino acids have residual groups that are acidic, some have residual groups that are basic, and two amino acids have residual groups that contain sulfur. The sulfur residual group is important because disulfide bonds, which connect sulfurs of different amino acids, are essential to the structure of some proteins.

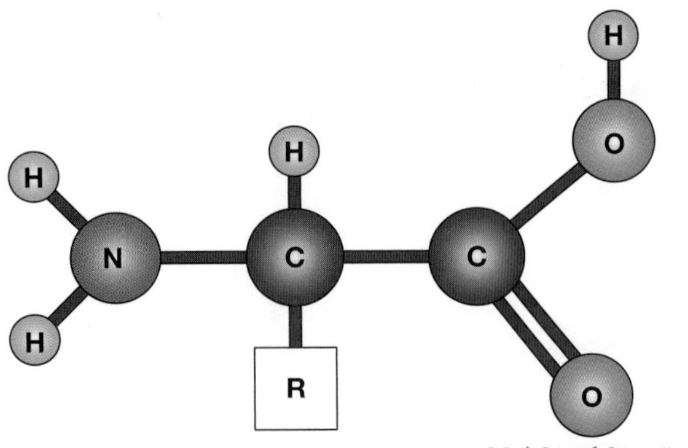

© Body Scientific International

Figure 2.6 The backbone of an amino acid includes an amino group (to the left in the drawing), a carboxylic acid group (to the right), and a central carbon. A residual group (R) is attached to the central carbon. The residual group varies from one amino acid to another.

Peptide Bonds

Amino acids join together by forming a ***peptide bond***, which links the amino group of one amino acid to the acid group of another. Short chains of amino acids (fewer than 50) are often referred to as *peptides*. Examples include the octapeptide (8 amino acids) oxytocin, a hormone that is important in childbirth; and enkephalin (ehn-KEHF-a-lin), a pentapeptide (5 amino acids) that acts in the brain to inhibit the perception of pain.

A longer chain of amino acids is called a ***polypeptide***. Many proteins, such as actin (275 amino acids) and titin (more than 33,000 amino acids), consist of a single polypeptide chain. Both actin and titin are found in muscle tissue. Other proteins include multiple polypeptide chains. The oxygen-carrying protein hemoglobin is made of four polypeptide chains, each between 140 and 150 amino acids long.

Structure of Proteins

The structure, or shape, of a protein is determined by the sequence of amino acids it contains (**Figure 2.7**). The amino acid sequence is known as the *primary structure* of a protein. Polypeptide chains folds up into specific shapes that are determined by their primary structure. This folding process reduces the potential energy of the protein. Just as a marble "wants" to roll downhill, a polypeptide "wants" to fold. Folding allows energetically favorable interactions among amino acid residual groups and with surrounding molecules, including water.

The first level of folding is called the *secondary structure*. One common form of secondary structure is the alpha helix, in which part of the polypeptide chain assumes a spiral conformation. Another common form is the beta-pleated sheet, in which part of the chain assumes a "flat with slight folds" conformation.

The next level of folding is called the *tertiary structure*. At this level, helical sections, pleated sheet sections, and other sections fold together into a three-dimensional whole. If the protein consists of a single polypeptide, the tertiary structure is the final level of protein structure.

Research Notes Glycogen Storage Diseases

Glycogen storage diseases are a class of disorders in which either the formation or the breakdown of glycogen does not work properly. In healthy individuals, the liver and muscles perform two different processes involving glycogen and glucose. They synthesize glycogen from glucose, and they break down glycogen to release glucose. Glucose from the liver is released into the bloodstream. Glucose in muscle is used to make ATP for energy.

In hepatic (*hepat/o* means "liver") glycogen storage diseases, the liver does not release glucose into the blood as it should. The liver is often enlarged due to an abnormal accumulation of glycogen in its cells. In myopathic (*my/o* means "muscle" and *path/o* means "disease") glycogen storage diseases, the storage or breakdown of glycogen in muscles does not work properly.

Glycogen storage diseases are usually inherited. They are caused by genetic mutations that affect enzymes (proteins) that catalyze biochemical reactions involving glycogen. There is no cure, but in many cases, symptoms can be lessened by dietary changes, medications, or a liver transplant.

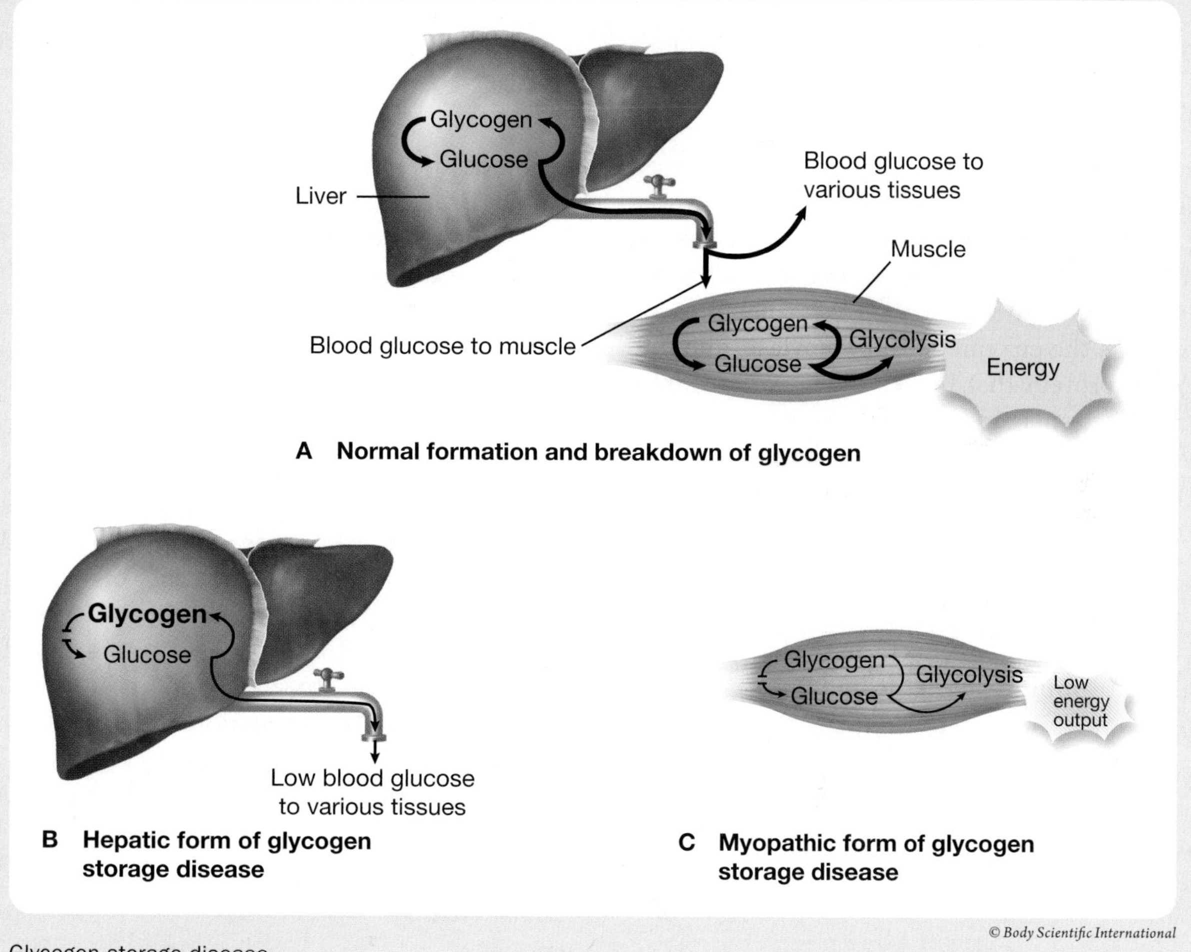

Glycogen storage disease.

For proteins made of multiple polypeptides, there is one step beyond the tertiary structure. The arrangement of these subunits into a whole, known as the *quaternary structure,* is the final step in determining the protein's shape.

Functions of Proteins

Among their many functions in the body, proteins act as structural elements, enzymes, and carriers. Collagen, which gives strength to ligaments and tendons, is an example of a protein with a structural function.

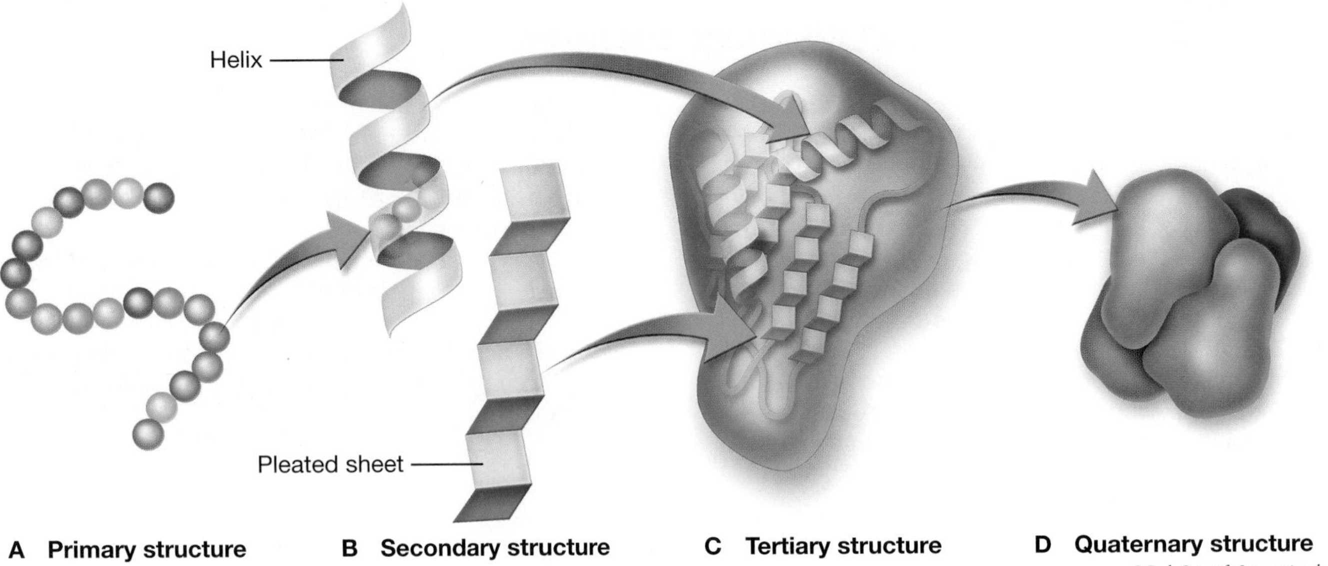

Figure 2.7 Levels of protein structure.

An ***enzyme*** is a protein that participates in a chemical reaction without being consumed or destroyed in the reaction. Enzymes act as molecular facilitators, which allow specific reactions to occur much faster than they would if the enzyme were not present. For example, the enzyme salivary amylase, found in saliva, is a protein that breaks down carbohydrate molecules into smaller sugar molecules.

Myoglobin and hemoglobin are proteins that act as carriers. Myoglobin carries oxygen in muscle; hemoglobin carries oxygen in blood.

SELF CHECK

1. What three components form the backbone of all 20 amino acids in the body?
2. What are the functions of proteins in the body?
3. What is the difference between a peptide and a polypeptide?
4. What is an enzyme?

Lipids

Lipids are fats and oils, as well as related molecules, such as glycerides, phospholipids, and steroids. Lipids are rich in carbon and hydrogen, usually with a ratio of about two hydrogen atoms for every carbon atom. They also contain oxygen atoms and sometimes other types of atoms.

Lipids do not dissolve well in water or blood, although there are special proteins that help carry lipids in the blood. Lipid molecules do not get as big as large proteins and carbohydrates, but they have a wide range of structures and functions.

Fatty Acids

A ***fatty acid*** is a hydrocarbon chain with a carboxylic acid group (COOH) at one end. Fatty acids may consist entirely of single bonds, in which case they are called *saturated*. Fatty acids with one or more double bonds are *unsaturated*. The presence of double bonds in a fatty acid often puts a "kink" in the molecule. Stearic acid ($C_{18}H_{36}O_2$) and oleic acid ($C_{18}H_{34}O_2$) are examples of saturated and unsaturated fatty acids, respectively. Stand-alone fatty acids are not very common in the body, but they are key building blocks for other lipids, particularly glycerides and phospholipids.

Glycerides

Glycerides are composed of a glycerol molecule (a simple sugar) with one, two, or three fatty acids attached to make mono-, di-, and ***triglycerides*** (**Figure 2.8**). Glycerides are important energy storage molecules in the body. Triglycerides make up most of the fat in fat cells.

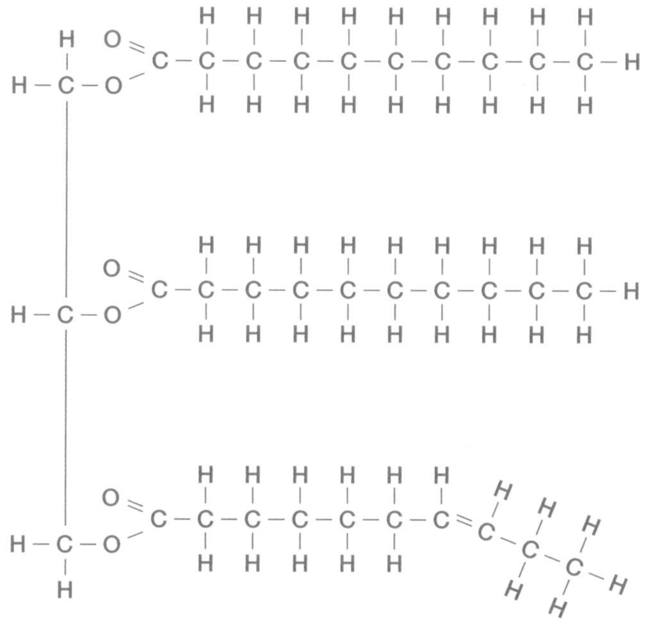

© *Body Scientific International*

Figure 2.8 A triglyceride has a glycerol head (blue) and three fatty acid chains (red). The triglyceride shown here has two saturated fatty acids (top two chains) and one unsaturated fatty acid (bottom chain), which is a result of the double bond.

Phospholipids

Phospholipids are similar to glycerides. The phosphate-bearing head of the phospholipid is hydrophilic, which means that it can form hydrogen bonds with water molecules. The fatty acid tails of the phospholipid are hydrophobic; they cannot form hydrogen bonds with water. As a result, phospholipids in a watery environment tend to form bilayers, liposomes, or micelles ("little spheres"). In these arrangements, the heads of the phospholipids face toward the water and line up the tails adjacent to one another (**Figure 2.9**).

Understanding Medical Terminology

Molecules, and parts of molecules, differ in how well they bond with water. Molecules that bond easily with water are *hydrophilic*, which means "water-loving." Molecules that do not bond well with water are called *hydrophobic*, or "water-fearing." Most lipids, including fatty acids, triglycerides, and steroids, are significantly hydrophobic. That is why oil and water do not mix. Phospholipids are different: they have hydrophilic heads and hydrophobic tails. This makes them ideally suited for making cell membranes, as shown in **Figure 2.9**.

Steroids

Steroids are a class of lipids whose structure is very different from that of other lipids. Three well-known steroid molecules—cholesterol, testosterone, and estrogen—are shown in **Figure 2.10**. All steroids have the same four-ring backbone, but their attached side groups differ. Cholesterol is a component of cell membranes. Testosterone and estrogen are hormones that help regulate the reproductive system.

Focus On Energy Storage

The ability to carry a reserve fuel supply has a survival benefit if food becomes scarce. The body stores chemical energy for future use in the form of carbohydrates (especially glycogen) and fats (especially triglycerides). Which is the better way to store energy?

Each form of stored chemical energy has advantages and disadvantages. For example, glycogen can be turned into usable chemical energy more quickly than triglycerides because glycogen provides glucose directly to cells. This glucose can then be used rapidly by virtually all body cells to make ATP (discussed later in this chapter). By contrast, the breakdown of triglycerides yields fatty acids, which cannot be used by as many cells and, in addition, cannot be used as quickly as glucose.

Glycogen, but not triglycerides, can provide energy fast enough to sustain prolonged rigorous exercise—at least until the glycogen stores run out. It should be noted, however, that fat is also used to some extent during exercise, causing unwanted fat to be consumed. Fat is also used during recovery from exercise to restock the body's storehouse of glycogen.

The big advantage of fat over glycogen is that it stores about twice as much energy per kilogram (or pound) as glycogen or other carbohydrates. One gram of glycogen stores about four to five kilocalories of chemical energy. One gram of fat stores about nine kilocalories of energy. There is obviously a benefit to carrying the same amount of energy reserves with fewer pounds. That is why, if one consumes more calories than are needed to meet the demands of living, the body stores the excess energy as fat rather than as glycogen.

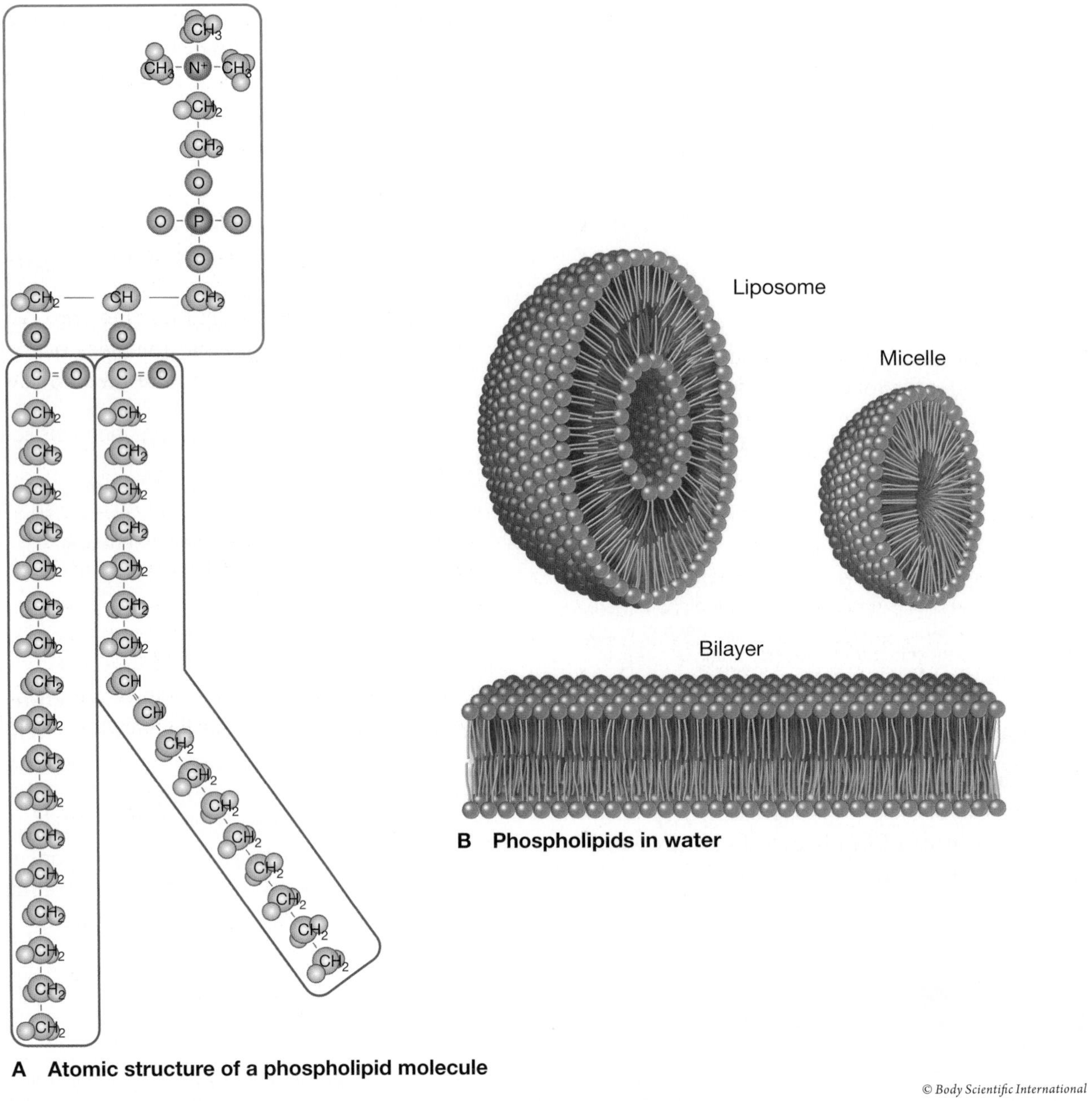

Liposome

Micelle

Bilayer

B Phospholipids in water

A Atomic structure of a phospholipid molecule

Figure 2.9 A—The atomic structure of a phospholipid includes a "head" (outlined in red) and two fatty acid tails (outlined in blue). The head is hydrophilic and the tails are hydrophobic. B—Phospholipids in water can form a bilayer, a liposome, or a micelle. In each of these arrangements, the hydrophilic phosphate heads face outward, toward water, and the hydrophobic tails "hide" themselves by facing inward.

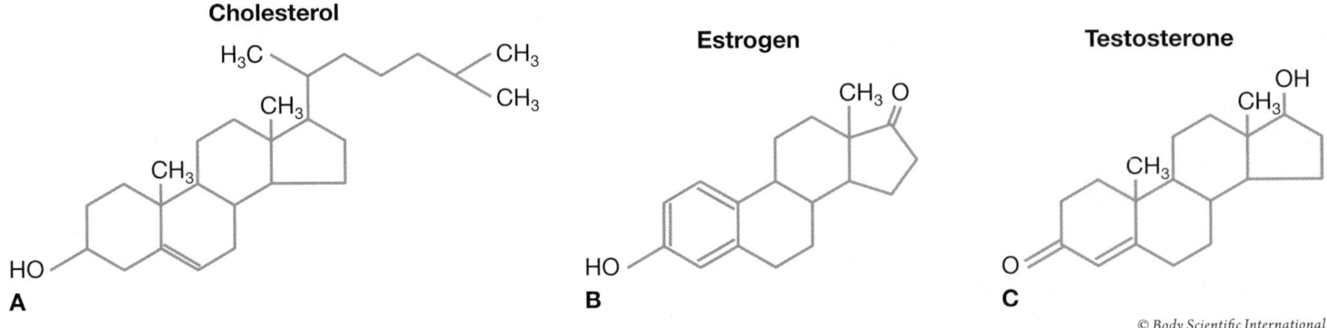

Figure 2.10 Steroid molecules: cholesterol, estrogen, and testosterone.

SELF CHECK

1. Identify the four types of lipids.
2. What are the two classes of fatty acids?
3. What does it mean when a molecule is hydrophilic?
4. Name three well-known steroids.

Nucleic Acids

Nucleic acids are key information-carrying molecules found in cells. Ribonucleic acid (RNA) and deoxyribonucleic acid (DNA) are the two kinds of nucleic acids found in cells. Some nucleic acids also function as enzymes. Like proteins and complex carbohydrates, nucleic acids are polymers, which means they are made of many similar subunits.

The subunits that make up nucleic acids are called ***nucleotides***. Each nucleotide consists of a phosphate group (PO_4), a sugar group, and a nitrogenous (nitrogen-containing) base (**Figure 2.11**). Two nucleotides can join together by forming a bond between the phosphate of one nucleotide and the sugar of another, with the bases "hanging off" to the side. In the process of forming this bond, a water molecule is produced and released.

Just as different variable groups distinguish the different amino acids, different bases distinguish the nucleotides. However, there are only five kinds of nucleotides in the human body, as opposed to 21 different amino acids. The five bases are adenine (A), guanine (G), cytosine (C), thymine (T), and uracil (U). DNA is made of nucleotides containing A, G, C, and T. RNA is made of nucleotides containing A, G, C, and U.

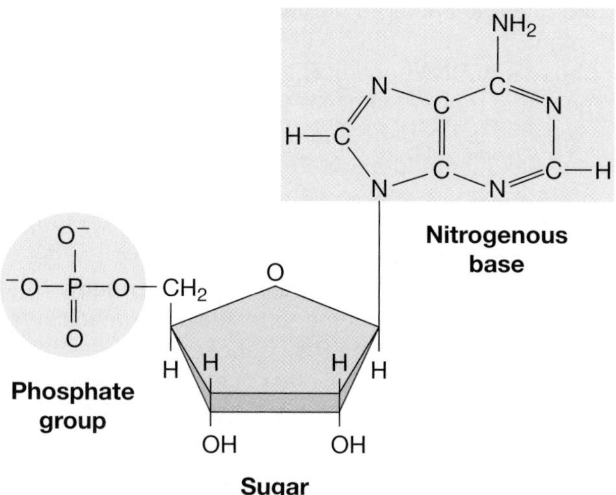

Figure 2.11 A nucleotide is made up of a phosphate group, a sugar group, and a nitrogenous base. Adenine is the base shown here, and the entire molecule—base plus sugar plus phosphate—is called *adenosine monophosphate*.

DNA

Deoxyribonucleic acid (DNA) is a polymer composed of two nucleotide chains, or strands, coiled around each other to form a double helix, which is similar in structure to a twisted ladder (**Figure 2.12**). Sugar and phosphate groups form the sides of the ladder. The bases attached to each side meet in the middle to form the rungs.

Each base can join with only one other base to form a rung, or ***base pair***: A and T form base pairs, and C and G form base pairs. Thus, if you know the base sequence of one strand, you can predict the base sequence of the complementary strand.

As described earlier in this chapter, base pairs are joined in the middle by hydrogen bonds, but the sugar-phosphate sides are held together by covalent bonds. Because hydrogen bonds are weaker than covalent bonds, a DNA molecule can "unzip" down

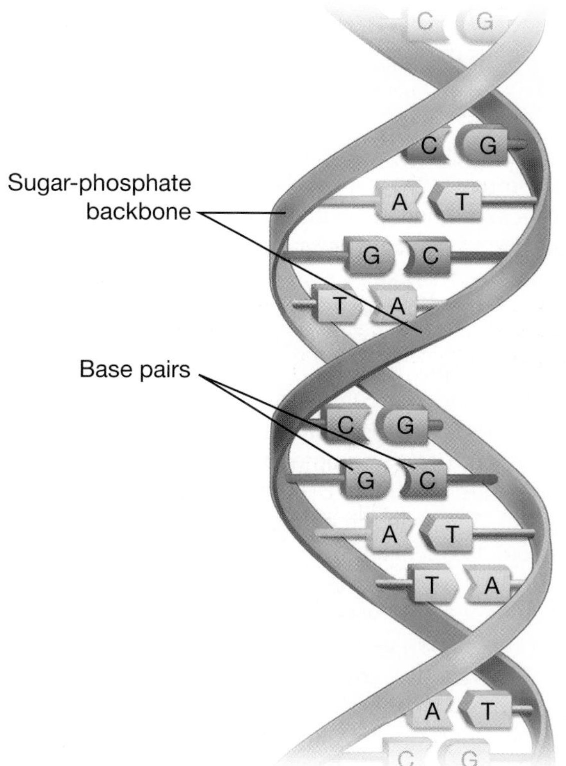

Figure 2.12 The parts of a DNA molecule.

the middle with relative ease, while the sides remain intact. The ability of DNA to unzip is crucial for two processes: copying the DNA before a cell divides, and transcribing short segments of the DNA.

Chromosomes

A ***chromosome*** is a structure that contains the genes, or genetic code, for an individual. It consists of a DNA molecule and the associated proteins that help it coil. Almost every human cell contains 46 chromosomes—23 from each parent. These include 22 pairs of similar chromosomes (numbered 1 through 22), plus one X and one Y chromosome (in males) or two X chromosomes (in females).

Exceptions to the "46-chromosomes-per-cell" rule include sperm cells and egg cells, each of which has just 23 chromosomes. Another exception is red blood cells, which have neither nuclei nor chromosomes.

Glycogen is a very large molecule, with a molecular weight in the tens of millions, but DNA is much bigger. Chromosome 1, with about 250 million base pairs, has a molecular weight of about 150 billion atomic units, which does not include the proteins that bind to it and help it coil.

If laid out straight, the 46 DNA molecules in a single cell would be about 2 meters long. The extreme thinness of DNA allows it to fit in a nucleus with a diameter of 10 micrometers or less. This is similar to the ability of a fisherman to keep a quarter mile or more of fine fishing line in a small tackle box.

Human Genome

A genome is the complete DNA complement of an organism. The DNA of a human is referred to as the ***human genome***. Although the sequence of base pairs along the DNA strand is very similar in all humans, it is not exactly the same except in identical twins. On average, about one base in every thousand bases is variable. The DNA sequences of identical twins are essentially the same.

Certain base locations are much more likely to differ among individuals than other base locations. The base locations that tend to vary are called *single nucleotide polymorphisms*, or SNPs (pronounced "snips"). SNPs are the subject of much study because they account for the genetic differences among individuals, including innate differences in athletic ability, disease susceptibility, and other inherited tendencies.

DNA Blueprints

It is interesting to note that cells can be very different even though they all contain the same DNA. For example, the bone cells, muscle cells, skin cells, and

Research Notes DNA Sequencing

When scientists discovered the basic structure and role of DNA in the 1950s, they realized that the inherited differences among individuals and among species were largely due to differences in the sequence of bases in their DNA. This led to continuing efforts to develop methods and machines that could determine the DNA sequence. This process is typically referred to as *sequencing DNA*.

In 1995, the first complete DNA sequence of a bacterium (*Haemophilus influenzae*, with about 1.8 million base pairs of DNA) was determined and published. In 2000, the first complete DNA sequence of an animal was published. This was the sequence for the fruit fly, which has about 120 million base pairs of DNA in its genome.

In 2003, the human genome sequence, with about 3 billion base pairs, was completed and published. The map of the human genome took hundreds of scientists about 13 years and several billion dollars to complete. The speed and accuracy of DNA sequencing has increased since then, and the cost and amount of raw material required has decreased greatly. These improvements are the result of engineers and scientists developing new chemical methods and better hardware and software. The process of DNA sequencing will become still more affordable and easier to perform as more advances are made.

The use of DNA sequencing has become practical in more and more healthcare situations. For example, the process is used in tests that determine whether a person has inherited a mutated version of the BRCA1 or BRCA2 gene. A woman with a mutated version of this gene has a significantly higher risk of developing breast and ovarian cancer. As a result, she is advised to get frequent and thorough tests to catch cancer early. This test also allows women time to take certain medicines or have surgery to reduce their cancer risk.

DNA "fingerprinting" is another use for DNA sequencing technology. This technique is used to identify or rule out individuals in criminal and other situations. As the technology has improved, DNA fingerprinting has been done successfully with smaller and poorer-quality samples than were previously required. The accuracy of DNA identification continues to be a subject of scientific and legal debate.

nerve cells in one person all contain complete and identical genetic blueprints, yet the cells are very different in structure and function.

DNA provides the blueprint for making proteins. The sequence of bases along DNA molecules specifies which amino acids should be arranged in a particular order to make the proteins needed for life. It takes three bases of DNA to specify one amino acid in a protein. This set of three bases is called a *codon*. A segment of DNA containing all the codons to make one polypeptide chain is called a *gene*.

RNA

Ribonucleic acid (RNA), like DNA, is a polymer of nucleotides. Its bases are adenosine, guanine, cytosine, and—instead of thymine, which is found in DNA—uracil. An RNA molecule is a single chain of nucleotides with a sugar-phosphate backbone (**Figure 2.13**). In some RNA molecules, part of the chain forms a "hairpin" that doubles back on itself. When this occurs, the bases form pairs analogous to the pairs seen in the DNA double helix: C and G form pairs, and A and U form pairs.

There are several forms of RNA: messenger RNA (mRNA), transfer RNA (tRNA), ribosomal RNA (rRNA), and the most recently discovered and least well understood—regulatory RNA. Each type of RNA has its own unique function:

- Messenger RNA carries information related to the manufacture of proteins.
- Transfer RNA assists in the manufacture of proteins.
- Ribosomal RNA forms *ribosomes*, large enzymes that act as catalysts for protein synthesis.
- Regulatory RNAs (actually several individual types of RNA) help regulate which proteins are produced.

The ability of RNA to function as both an information carrier (mRNA) and an enzyme (rRNA) has led biologists to speculate that RNA may have been the first self-replicating molecule and, thus, a key molecule in the development of life.

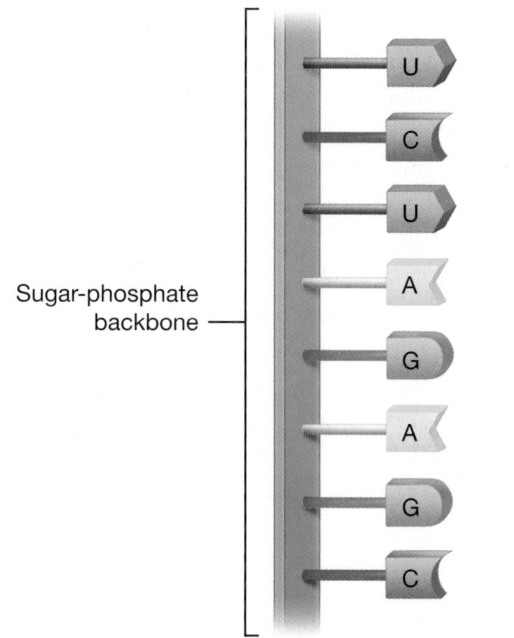

© Body Scientific International

Figure 2.13 An RNA molecule is a chain of nucleotides. The four nucleotides—abbreviated A, C, G, and U—can occur in varying order. The chain can "fold up" in many possible ways, depending on the molecule's function.

SELF CHECK

1. Identify the three components of a nucleotide.
2. How many chromosomes does each parent contribute to its offspring?
3. What is the human genome?
4. Name the four major forms of RNA.

Water and pH

Another molecule essential to life is dihydrogen oxide, more commonly known as *water*. All life as we know it is water-based. Water makes up about two-thirds of the mass of the human body.

Polarity of Water

Water is a polar molecule, which means that it consists of a negatively charged region (the end of the oxygen atom that is situated away from the hydrogen atoms) and positively charged regions (at the far ends of the hydrogen atoms). The molecular configuration of water is shown in **Figure 2.14A**.

Hydrogen Bonding

The polarity of water molecules allows them to form hydrogen bonds with one another or with other polar molecules. Water molecules also form short-lived hydrogen bonds with one another, as shown in **Figure 2.14B**. Hydrogen bonds in water quickly form, break, and then reform as the molecules move around in a solution.

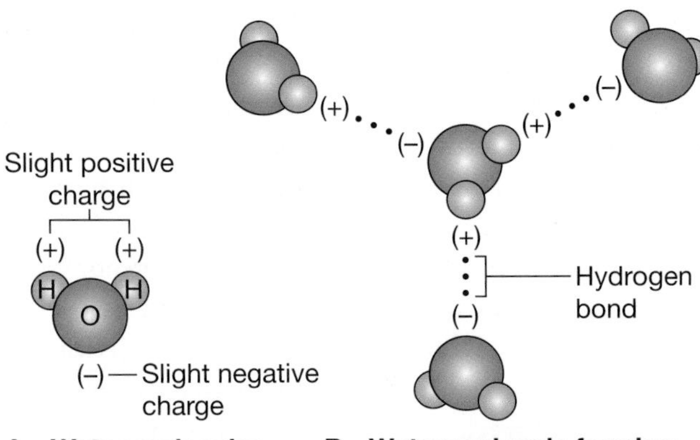

Figure 2.14 A—A water molecule is polar: one side is positively charged and the other side is negatively charged. B—A water molecule can form hydrogen bonds with other water molecules by orienting oppositely charged regions toward each other. In this diagram, the central water molecule is forming hydrogen bonds with surrounding water molecules.

Hydrogen bonds are relatively weak chemical bonds, but they are responsible for several biologically important properties of water. These properties include high heat capacity, relatively high boiling point, and ability to act as a solvent.

Hydrogen bonding gives water the ability to absorb or release a great deal of energy without much of a change in temperature. It is this ability that creates the high heat capacity of water. Water's high heat capacity, coupled with the fact that the human body consists mostly of water, means that body temperature does not change much when people gain or lose heat energy.

Water cannot form hydrogen bonds in a gaseous state, so it is energetically difficult for a water molecule to leave the liquid environment. This means that water has a high heat of vaporization (it takes a lot of energy to boil water) and a high boiling point. Water's high heat of vaporization means that we can rid ourselves of heat when water evaporates from our skin, which occurs when we sweat.

Water as a Solvent

A solvent is a liquid in which another substance, known as a *solute*, is dissolved to form a solution. The polar nature of water makes it a good solvent for many compounds. For example, ionic compounds, such as sodium chloride, dissolve well in water. This is because the positively charged sodium ions are attracted to the negative parts of water molecules, and the negatively charged chloride ions are attracted to the positive parts of water molecules.

Other hydrophilic but uncharged compounds, such as glucose, have positive and negative regions. This means that they can also interact with the oppositely charged parts of water molecules.

Acids and Bases

A very small fraction of the H_2O molecules in a container of water will always break apart, or *dissociate*. When a molecule of H_2O dissociates, it forms a hydrogen ion (H^+) and a hydroxide ion (OH^-). Therefore, pure water contains a small concentration of hydrogen ions and hydroxide ions. A substance that, when added to water, increases its hydrogen ion (H^+) concentration is called an *acid*. An acidic solution has more hydrogen ions than pure water. A substance that reduces the hydrogen ion concentration of a solution is called a *base*. A basic solution has fewer hydrogen ions than pure water.

If you add both an acid and a base to a container of water, the acid and base tend to cancel each other out, or neutralize one another. The same result occurs if you add an acid and a base to a cell, which is essentially a very small container of water and other chemicals.

pH is a measure of the acidity of a solution. Pure water has a pH of seven. An acidic solution has a pH less than seven, and a basic solution has a pH greater than seven. *Alkalinity* is a measure of a solution's ability to neutralize acid. A basic solution (that is, a solution with a high pH) is often called an *alkaline solution*. While this is usually true, remember that pH and alkalinity refer to different aspects of the chemistry of solutions. pH is a measure of the number of hydrogen ions in a solution, whereas alkalinity refers to the ability of a solution to absorb or "mop up" hydrogen ions.

Carbonic acid (H_2CO_3) is an important acid in the body because it dissociates to form H^+ and bicarbonate (HCO_3^-), which helps regulate body pH. It is considered a weak acid because, when added to water, not all of it dissociates. You may have the sodium salt of bicarbonate ($NaHCO_3$) in your kitchen. It is the white powder in the box labeled *baking soda*.

pH Regulation

Several mechanisms keep the pH of body fluids within a narrow range. This physiological regulation of pH is important because the enzymes in the body cells, which trigger biochemical reactions, work best at a certain pH level. Abnormal pH is often a sign of illness. The normal pH of arterial blood ranges from 7.35 to 7.45. An arterial blood pH value lower than 7.35 means the patient has *acidosis* (too much acidity). A value higher than 7.45 means the patient has *alkalosis* (too much alkalinity, not enough acidity).

The body has three overlapping systems that help keep pH within the normal range. These systems are the chemical buffers in blood, the respiratory system, and the kidneys. The fastest-acting mechanisms are the chemical buffers in the blood. The kidneys are the slowest-acting mechanisms, but they can most effectively resist changes in pH.

Chemical buffers react with acids or bases to "soak up" excess H^+ ions or provide H^+ ions if they are in short supply. There are several chemical buffers present in the blood and in the body cells. The carbonic acid/bicarbonate buffer system is the most abundant buffer system in blood plasma. Hemoglobin, which is found in red blood cells, and other proteins also act as buffers. The phosphate buffer system is an important pH buffer inside the cells.

The respiratory system also plays a role in the regulation of pH. The carbonic acid/bicarbonate buffer system creates a connection between breathing and pH. By pushing carbon dioxide (CO_2) out of the body, breathing changes the level of CO_2 in the blood, as will be explained more in Chapter 10. CO_2 reacts with water (H_2O) to make carbonic acid (H_2CO_3), which dissociates into bicarbonate (HCO_3^-) and hydrogen ions (H^+). When the level of CO_2 in the body changes, the pH level also changes. As you breathe more, the level of CO_2 decreases, and the pH level goes up. If the chemical buffers in blood cannot keep the pH in the desired range, the body can adjust its breathing to help control its pH.

Over the long term, the kidneys have the greatest capacity to correct excess acidity or alkalinity. If the blood pH is too low, the kidneys excrete urine that is more acidic. If the blood pH is too high, the kidneys excrete urine that is more alkaline. Through these processes, the kidneys push the appropriate amount of acid out of the body to bring the blood pH back to the optimal level.

Patients with lung or kidney disease often have abnormal pH levels. Caregivers who work with such patients, and those who work in emergency rooms and settings in which a patient's breathing is externally controlled (such as an operating room or intensive care unit), must pay careful attention to blood pH. They must also have a good understanding of the physiological regulation of pH.

SECTION 2.2 REVIEW

Mini-Glossary

amino acids the building blocks of proteins

base pairs pairs of complementary nucleic acid bases; A and T or C and G

chromosome a structure that contains the genes, or genetic code, for an individual; consists of a DNA molecule and the associated proteins that help it coil

DNA a polymer of nucleotides with the bases adenosine, guanine, cytosine, and thymine; deoxyribonucleic acid

enzymes proteins that speed up specific biological reactions

fatty acid a molecule that consists of a hydrocarbon chain with a carboxylic acid group at one end

glucose the main form of sugar that circulates in the blood; a monosaccharide

glycogen a polymer of glucose that is found in animals; the stored form of glucose

human genome the complete DNA sequence of a human

lipids fatty molecules that dissolve poorly in water but dissolve well in a nonpolar solvent; fats and oils

nucleic acids key information-carrying molecules in cells

nucleotides subunits that make up nucleic acids

peptide bond the chemical bond that links two amino acids by connecting the amino group of one to the acid group of another

pH a measure of the acidity of a solution

phospholipids lipids that contain phosphate groups

polymer a molecule made of many similar subunits

polypeptide a long chain of amino acids

RNA a polymer of nucleotides with the bases adenine, guanine, cytosine, and uracil; ribonucleic acid

steroids lipids with a structure that is different from other lipids; includes cholesterol, testosterone, and estrogen, among others

triglycerides compounds composed of a glycerol molecule with three fatty acids attached

(continued)

Review Questions

1. Organic chemicals always include ____ and ____ atoms.
2. The main purpose of carbohydrates in the body is to provide a source of ____.
3. A long chain of amino acids is called a(n) ____.
4. Amino acids join together by forming a(n) ____ bond.
5. What does an enzyme do, and what happens to it in a chemical reaction?
6. Fats and oils in the body are known as ____.
7. Phospholipids are ideally suited for making ____.
8. List the three nucleotides found in both DNA and RNA. Then identify the nucleotide found only in DNA and the one found only in RNA.
9. What property of a water molecule allows it to form hydrogen bonds?
10. Describe the way ATP is used to create energy in the body.
11. What property does pH measure?
12. Is life possible without water? Why or why not?
13. Why is DNA essential for multicellular life?

SECTION 2.3 Cellular Anatomy and Physiology

Objectives

- Identify the major parts of a typical cell, including the plasma membrane, cytoskeleton, mitochondria, Golgi apparatus, ribosomes, endoplasmic reticulum, and nucleus.
- Explain the relationship among DNA, RNA, and proteins.
- Identify the phases and subphases of interphase and mitotic cell division.

Key Terms

active transport
adenosine triphosphate (ATP)
anticodon
centrioles
channel proteins
cilia
codon
cytokinesis
cytoplasm
cytoskeleton
endoplasmic reticulum (ER)
extracellular fluid
extracellular matrix
glycoproteins
Golgi apparatus
messenger RNA (mRNA)
microvilli
mitochondria
mitosis
nucleus
passive transport
plasma membrane
ribosomes
RNA polymerase
transcription
transfer RNA (tRNA)

You can learn a lot by looking at the outside of the body, as healthcare providers do with every patient they see. The clinical value of observing of the "unopened" body with unaided eyes should not be underestimated. However, a great amount can be learned only by opening up the body and looking inside—either through surgery in life or dissection after death. Artists such as Michelangelo and Leonardo da Vinci, who was also a scientist, are among those who have used human dissection to increase knowledge of the body's inner workings.

The invention of the microscope around 1600 A.D. allowed scientists to observe the body with a tool that extended the capability of the human eye. Cells were discovered soon thereafter. As microscopes improved, scientists learned that cells had nuclei and other internal structures. Healthcare providers found microscopes useful in diagnosing disease, especially when examining samples of blood or urine. However, many cellular structures were still too small to see, even with good conventional microscopes.

Electron microscopes were invented in the 1930s (**Figure 2.15**). These microscopes use electrons instead of visible light to make images, so they can magnify much more than conventional (light) microscopes. Many of the structures discussed in this chapter are only "visible" through an electron microscope.

In 1895, X-rays were discovered, opening up yet another avenue of observation—seeing inside the living body without surgery. CT (computed tomography) scans, PET (positron emission tomography) scans, MRIs (magnetic resonance images), and ultrasound images extend the ability to see inside the body without surgery.

Enhancements to these technologies have been essential in the study of anatomy and physiology, and in the diagnosis and treatment of illness. Biomedical imaging will continue to evolve and improve for years to come.

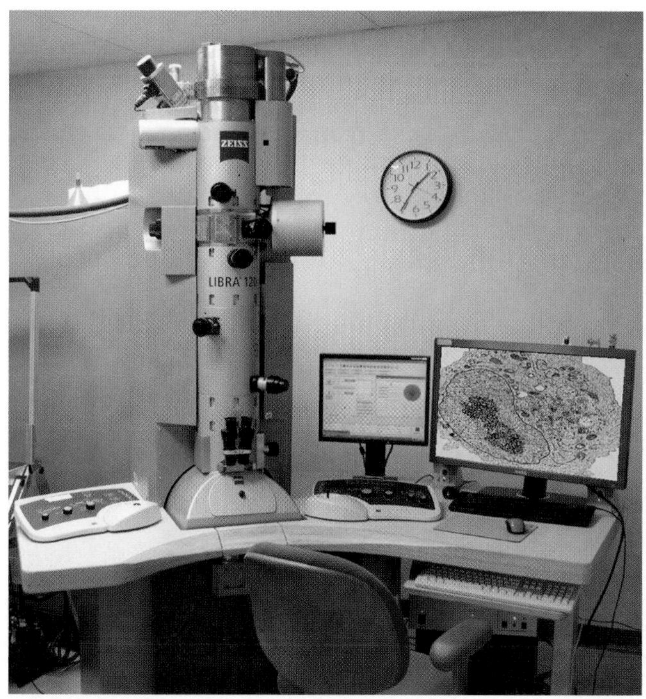

Richard Wisk

Figure 2.15 Some electron microscopes can resolve objects as small as 0.5 nanometers, which is about 10 times smaller than a single hemoglobin protein and 4 times smaller than the diameter of a DNA molecule.

Parts of a Cell

The cells of the human body are surrounded by ***extracellular fluid***, which is mostly water, and an ***extracellular matrix***. The extracellular matrix may be solid or gel-like, depending on the type of tissue. The ***plasma membrane*** is the outer shell of a cell. Inside the membrane are the ***nucleus*** and the ***cytoplasm***, which contains various organelles, or "little organs." (**Figure 2.16**). The type and number of organelles in a cell vary with the type of cell, but most cells contain the organelles described in this chapter.

Plasma Membrane

The plasma membrane keeps the inside of the cell in and the outside of the cell out. It also controls what passes through the cell (**Figure 2.17**). The plasma membrane is a phospholipid bilayer (refer again to **Figure 2.9**). In addition to phospholipids, the membrane contains cholesterol and a variety of proteins. These proteins include structural proteins, ion and water channels, and glycoproteins.

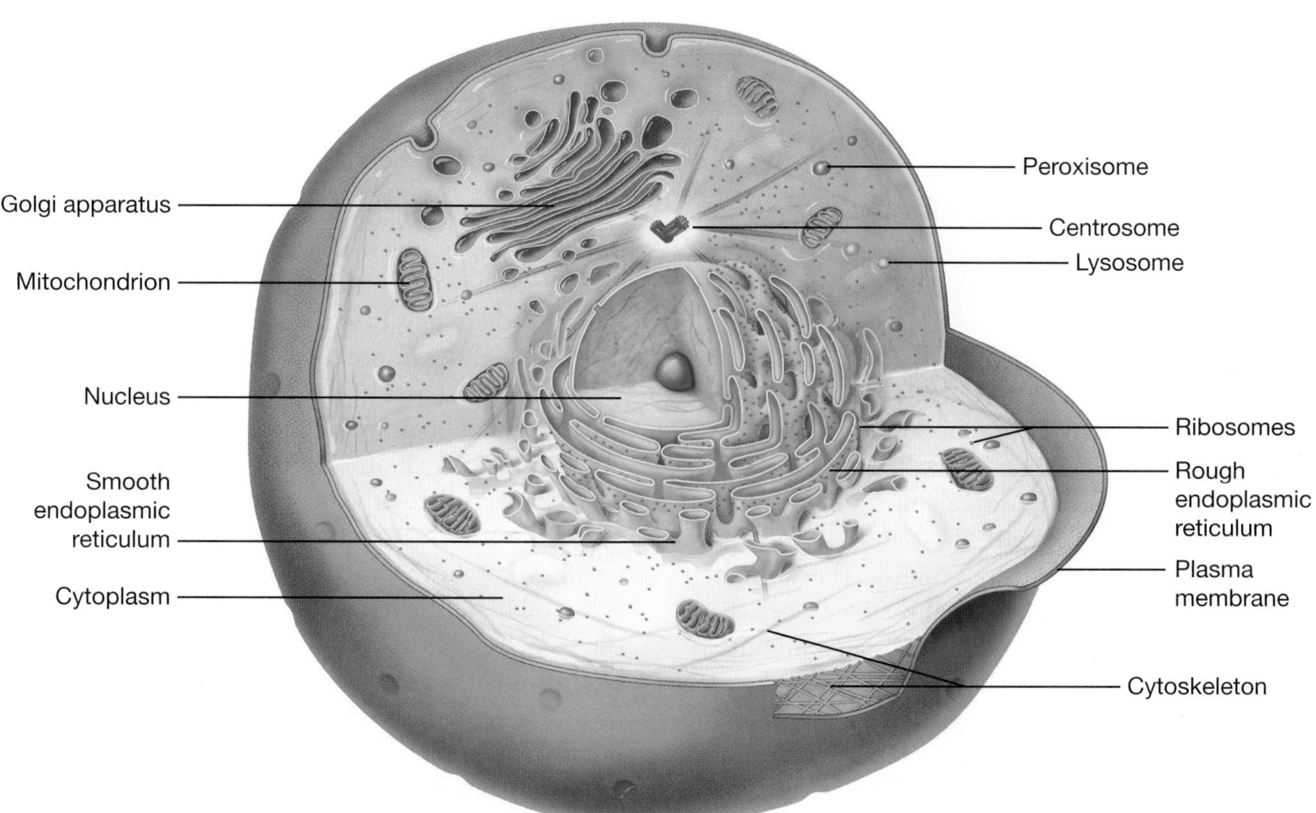

© Body Scientific International

Figure 2.16 A typical cell.

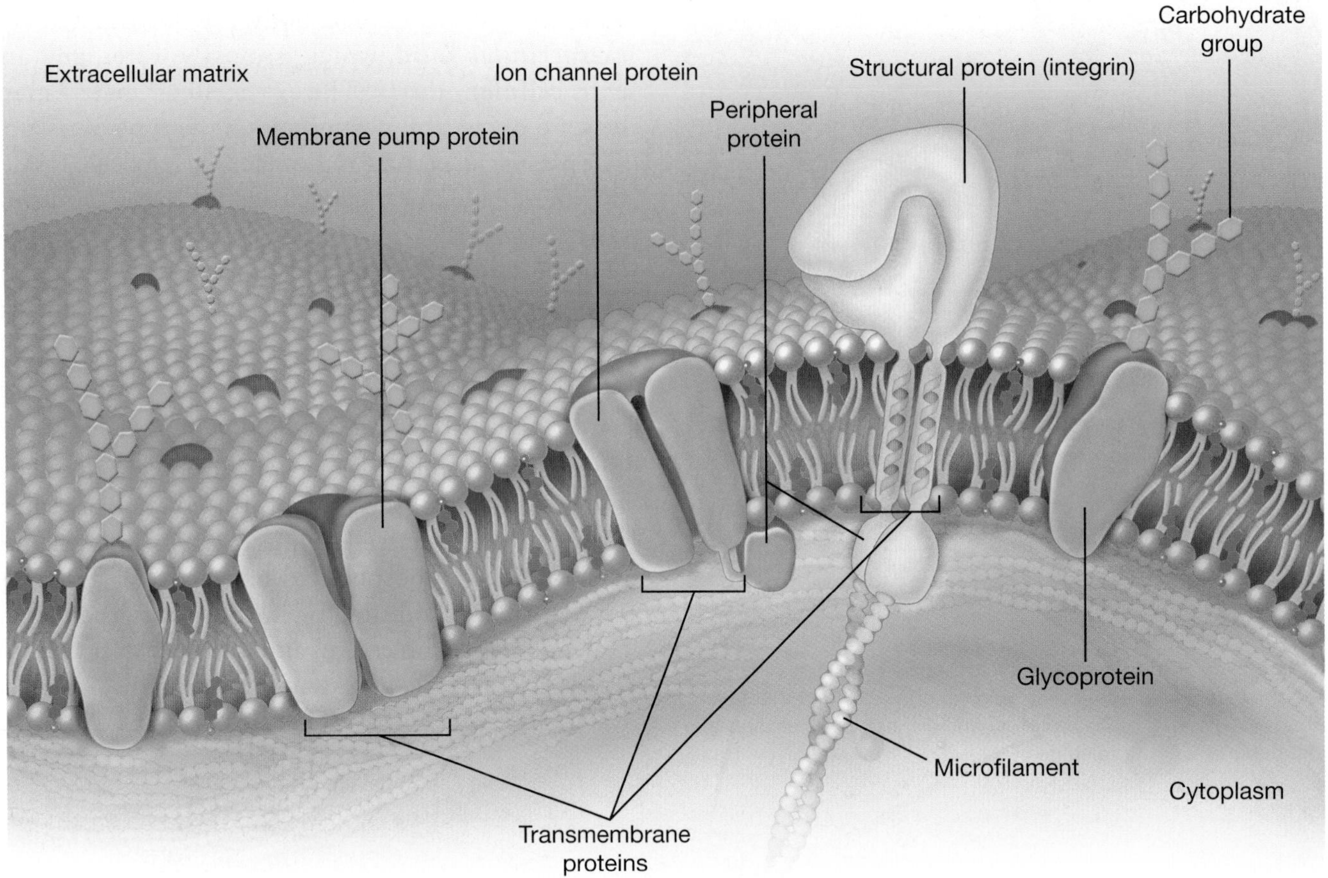

© Body Scientific International

Figure 2.17 The plasma membrane.

Proteins in the Plasma Membrane

Structural proteins such as cadherin, integrin, and spectrin connect the cell to neighboring cells, the extracellular matrix, and the cytoskeleton inside the cell. In this way, these structural proteins form a link between the inside and the outside of the cell.

Channel proteins have a hollow central pore, or channel, that allows water or small, charged particles such as sodium, potassium, calcium, and chloride to pass into or out of the cell. These substances cannot enter or leave the cell without channels because their polarity, or charge, makes them unable to penetrate the phospholipid bilayer of the plasma membrane.

Channels can be extremely selective about which substances they allow to cross the membrane, and when they can cross. For example, water channels, known as *aquaporins*, allow H_2O to cross, but do not allow H^+ or OH^- to cross, even though these two substances are smaller than H_2O. This important selective property helps the cell control its pH.

Potassium channels are another interesting example of channel selectivity. They allow potassium ions to cross, but they do not let sodium ions through, even though sodium ions have the same charge as potassium ions (+1) and are smaller. Imagine using a wire screen to sort coarse gravel from sand. The sand goes through small holes in the screen, and the gravel does not. Potassium channels do the opposite: they let the large ions through (the gravel), but not the small ones (the sand). Scientists have studied potassium channels carefully for many years to understand their remarkable selectivity. These studies have shown that the structure of the channel protein creates a micro-environment within the channel that is energetically favorable for potassium-sized ions to pass through, but not for larger or smaller ions.

Glycoproteins are proteins with carbohydrate groups attached. These proteins are usually found in the plasma membrane, with the carbohydrate group projecting into the extracellular fluid. The layer of carbohydrate groups surrounding a cell is called the *glycocalyx* (gligh-koh-KAY-liks). The glycocalyx helps cells interact with other cells and substances.

The cells that line the blood vessels are called *endothelial cells*. The glycocalyx of endothelial cells plays a key role in regulating the movement of cells and other material from inside the blood vessels to the surrounding tissue. The glycocalyx also allows the endothelial cells to sense how much blood is flowing past. When the blood flow is higher, it exerts more drag force on the glycocalyx.

Membrane Transport

Living cells take in some substances (such as oxygen and glucose) and move out others (such as carbon dioxide and other metabolic wastes). Membrane transport is the mechanism of movement of these substances across the cell's plasma membrane. Membrane transport can occur in one of two basic ways: by passive transport or active transport.

Passive transport does not require the expenditure of any extra energy. It usually involves diffusion: the movement of material from a place where it is concentrated to a place where it is less concentrated. For example, if you drop food coloring into a pot of water, the coloring is initially concentrated at the point where it hits the water. Gradually, however, the food coloring spreads and evens out as a result of diffusion.

Channel proteins provide pathways across a cell membrane for specific substances to diffuse into or out of the cell. Aquaporin channels, for example, allow water to enter and leave cells by passive transport. Dissolved gases such as oxygen and carbon dioxide also enter and leave cells by passive transport, but they do not need a channel pathway. In some cells, glucose enters by passive transport.

Active transport requires energy because it involves making a substance go where it "does not want to go." It is natural for substances to want to move to areas

Research Notes Integrating Physical and Chemical Processes

Various processes and control systems in the body interact with one another to maintain homeostasis—ongoing balance within the body's internal environment. This happens even when the body faces extreme challenges.

Active and Passive Transport

Active and passive transport are inherently stable processes. Small disturbances to the body's internal environment naturally tend to be corrected because of the way in which these processes work. The movement of potassium into and out of a muscle cell illustrates this point.

Research has shown that during exercise a small amount of potassium leaves a muscle cell with each muscle twitch. During intense exercise, the amount of potassium inside the cell may start to drop slightly, and the amount outside the cell may start to rise. This change in potassium balance across the cell membrane causes more potassium to enter the cell by passive transport. There is more potassium outside the cell and less inside the cell than usual, so diffusion occurs. The passive transport process tends to bring the cell back to its normal, steady state.

The lower levels of potassium inside the cell also cause the sodium-potassium pump, which actively transports sodium out of the cell and potassium into the cell, to run slightly faster. This active transport process also helps to correct the potassium imbalance.

You might think that pushing sodium out of the cell would disrupt its sodium balance. This is not the case, however, because exercise also causes excess sodium accumulation inside the cell. Thus, speeding up the pump helps to fix the sodium imbalance as well as the potassium imbalance. In short, the active and passive transport processes, working together, naturally tend to correct temporary imbalances.

Equilibrium vs. Homeostasis

A cell maintaining homeostasis is in a steady state, but it is not at equilibrium. The difference between a steady state and equilibrium is important. In fact, it is a matter of life and death.

Life is a nonequilibrium state of affairs. A living organism is not in equilibrium with its surroundings. However, an organism that is no longer living is, or soon will be, in a state of equilibrium.

Body temperature is a good example of this concept. Humans and other mammals are warm-blooded. The scientific term for this is *homeothermic* (from the Greek word for "same temperature"). The nervous and endocrine systems help the body maintain a constant internal body temperature, which is in a steady state but not at equilibrium with its surroundings. If core body temperature starts to deviate from the norm, the nervous system and the endocrine system initiate responses that bring the temperature back to normal.

of lower concentration—this is the passive process of diffusion. By contrast, active transport involves movement of substances from areas of lower concentration to areas of higher concentration. The most important and widespread examples of active transport are the movement of sodium *out* of a cell and the movement of potassium *into* a cell.

A resting cell contains much less sodium than the surrounding extracellular fluid, so energy is required to move the sodium out. Similarly, a resting cell contains more potassium than the surrounding fluid, so it needs energy to move potassium in. To accomplish this movement of substances, the cell membrane has a sodium-potassium pump protein. This pump breaks down the high-energy ATP molecule and uses the resulting energy to pump sodium out of the cell and potassium into the cell.

SELF CHECK

1. Where are glycoproteins usually found?
2. What is the difference between active and passive transport?

Cytoskeleton

The ***cytoskeleton*** is a network of proteins that defines the shape of a cell and gives it mechanical strength (**Figure 2.18A**). The cytoskeleton rearranges itself as necessary to change the shape of the cell or to allow the cell to move to a new location.

The cytoskeleton contains three types of long fibers, or struts:

- Microfilaments, the thinnest of these fibers, are made of actin subunits. They are found in most cells and are especially prominent in muscle cells.
- Intermediate filaments are made of keratin. They extend across a cell and give the cell strength to resist external pulling forces.
- Microtubules, composed of tubulin subunits, are the cytoskeletal fibers with the largest diameters. They help to separate and organize chromosomes during cell division. Motor proteins, such as kinesin and dynein, move along microtubules as they transport vesicles and other structures inside the cell (**Figure 2.18B**).

Some cells have ***microvilli***, which are finger-like extensions that increase the surface area of the cell. Microfilaments, stringy proteins inside the microvilli, provide structural support.

Other cells have hair-like projections called ***cilia***, which are longer than microvilli. Cilia actively flex back and forth to move fluid or mucus across the outside of the cell. The active movement of cilia is caused by microtubules inside them.

Most cells have a pair of ***centrioles*** in their centrosome, an area near the nucleus. Each centriole is a short cylinder made of nine triplets of parallel microtubules. The centrioles help guide the movement and separation of chromosomes during cell division.

Mitochondria and ATP Production

Organelles ("little organs") are specialized structures that reside in the cytoplasm of cells. ***Mitochondria***, one type of organelle, are tube-shaped structures responsible for making ATP, the universal carrier of energy within cells. For this reason, mitochondria are often called the "powerhouses" of the cell. Cardiac muscle cells have abundant mitochondria to meet their large and unending demand for energy to drive muscular contraction. Cells with minimal energy needs have fewer mitochondria. A mitochondrion has a smooth outer membrane and an inner membrane with many cristae (folds) that increase its surface area (**Figure 2.19**).

The Role of ATP

Adenosine triphosphate (ATP) is a nucleotide composed of an adenine base, a sugar, and three phosphate groups. A significant amount of chemical potential energy is stored in the bonds between the phosphates in ATP. The energy in the bond between the last and middle phosphates can be released by splitting off the last phosphate. This process yields adenosine diphosphate (ADP) and inorganic phosphate (Pi), so named because it contains no carbon. This reaction is shown in **Figure 2.20** by the arrow on the left. ATP can be resynthesized by combining ADP, Pi, and energy. This process is shown by the arrow on the right side of **Figure 2.20**.

To understand the role that ATP plays in cells, consider the role that money plays in the economy. If there were no money, people would have to trade to get the items they needed and wanted. For example, if Alice raises goats, she can trade goat's milk to get bread from Bob the bread maker. In an economy without money, Alice would have a hard time getting bread if Bob did not like goat's milk because that would be all she had to trade. But in an economy with money, Alice can convert her goat's milk into money

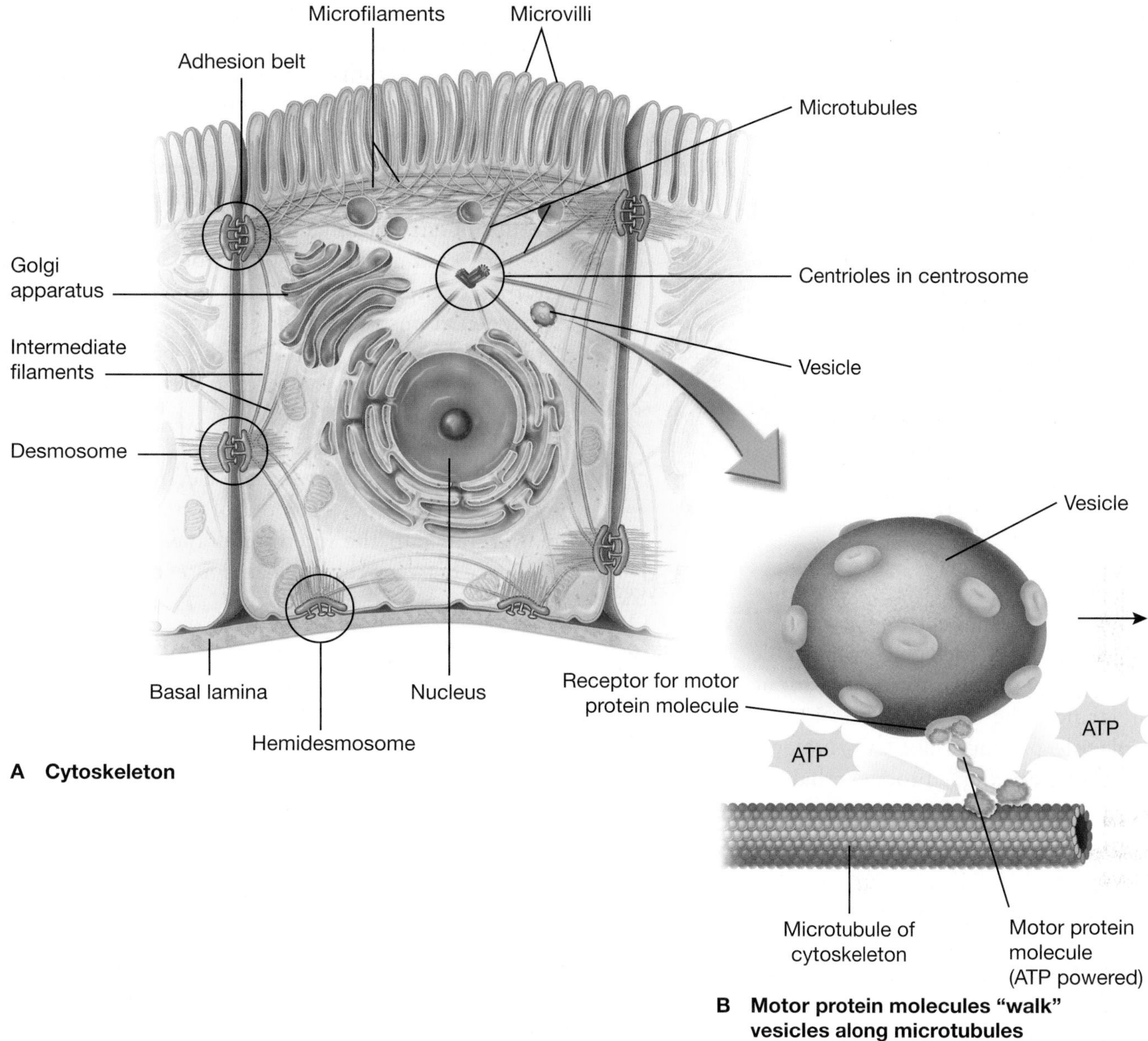

Figure 2.18 A—The cytoskeleton. B—The role of microtubules in cell division.

(by selling it) and use that money to get something that she wants. Money carries value and is accepted by everyone.

ATP plays a similar role in the energy economy of cells. Cells take chemical potential energy that is stored in molecules (such as glucose, glycogen, or triglycerides) and exchange it for ATP. They do this by breaking down the energy-containing chemical (glucose, for example) and using the energy to make ATP. ATP is an energy carrier that is accepted by all kinds of enzymes that need a source of energy. Those enzymes work by breaking down ATP into ADP plus Pi, and then using the energy obtained to accomplish some other energy-requiring process.

ATP Synthesis

The synthesis of ATP begins with glycolysis (gligh-KAHL-i-sis), the breakdown of a glucose molecule into two pyruvate molecules. Glycolysis occurs in the cytoplasm, outside the mitochondrion. The pyruvates pass from the cytoplasm into the mitochondrial matrix, which is the space inside the mitochondrion's inner membrane. Enzymes in this space catalyze the reactions of the citric acid cycle (also known as the *Krebs cycle* or the *tricarboxylic acid cycle*).

The citric acid cycle uses the energy in the pyruvates to make molecules of NADH (nicotinamide adenine dinucleotide with hydrogen) and $FADH_2$ (flavin adenine dinucleotide with hydrogens). The three

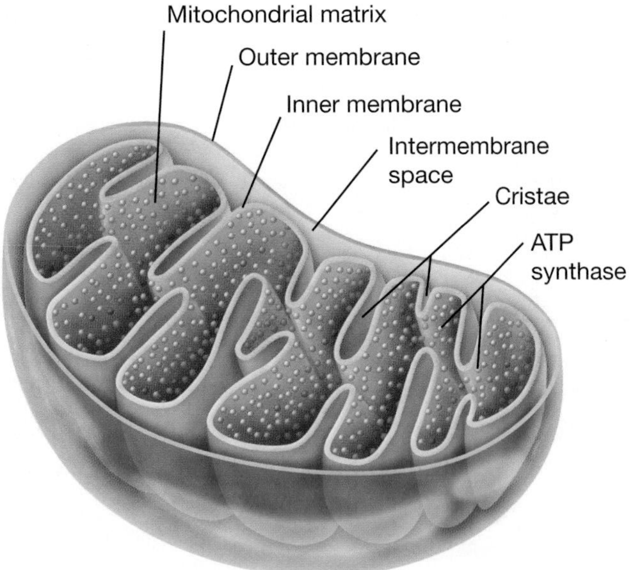

Figure 2.19 A mitochondrion.

carbon atoms in each pyruvate combine with oxygen molecules to make three carbon dioxide (CO_2) molecules. Since each glucose molecule produces two pyruvates, and each pyruvate produces three CO_2 molecules, the complete breakdown of a glucose molecule produces six CO_2 molecules. The CO_2 molecules are waste products that are generated all the time, in the manner just described, by cells throughout the body. Like any waste product, the CO_2 must be removed from the body. The major method for disposing of CO_2 is by breathing it out, as described in Chapter 10.

NADH and $FADH_2$ contain electrons that are bound to hydrogen and have relatively high energy. Groups of enzymes that are embedded in the inner membrane of each mitochondrion are called the *electron transport chain*. These enzymes take the hydrogen atoms, with their electrons, from NADH and $FADH_2$ and pass them along the chain. Eventually these hydrogen atoms and electrons bind to oxygen atoms to make water (H_2O).

As enzymes in the electron transport chain pass the electrons along, they use the electrons' energy to pump hydrogen ions (H^+) out of the mitochondrial matrix and into the intermembrane space. This is the space between the inner and outer mitochondrial membranes.

The hydrogen ions in the intermembrane space are all positively charged, so they repel one another. This mutual repulsion means the hydrogen ions in the intermembrane space can lose energy by going somewhere else.

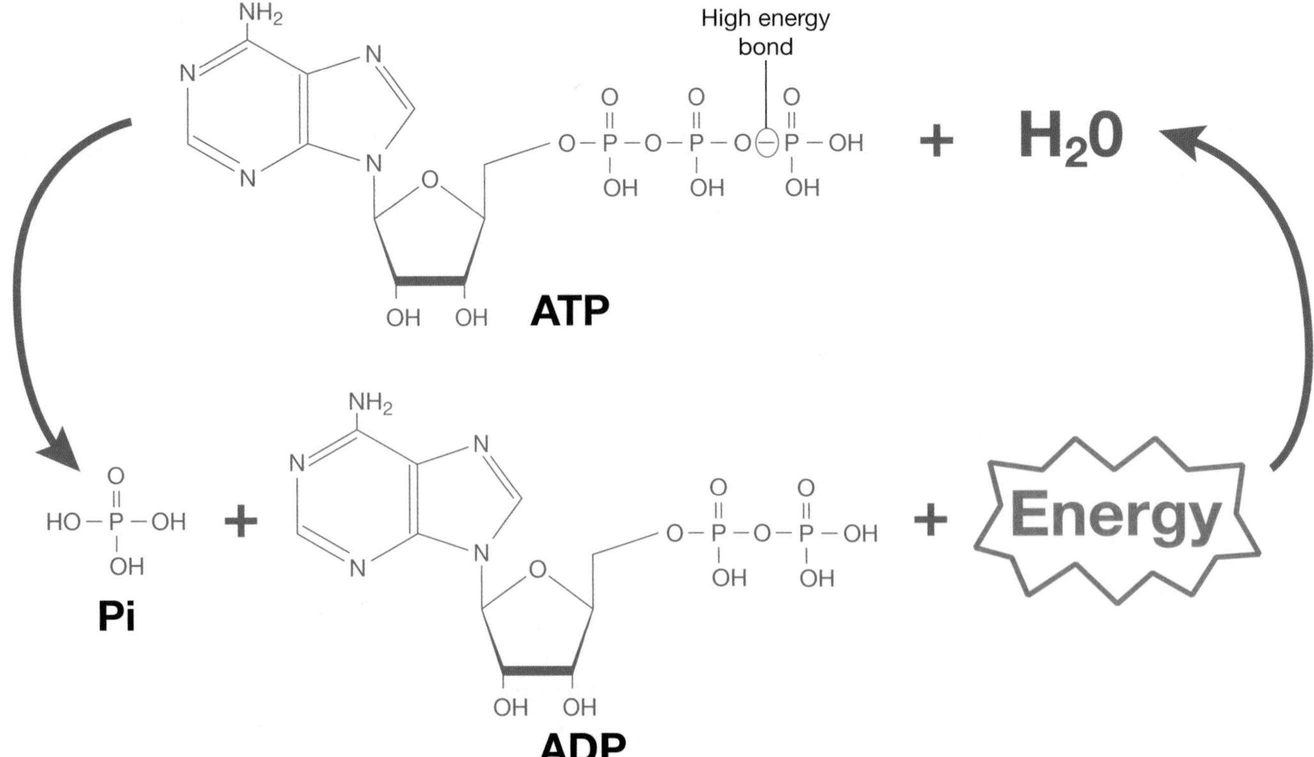

Figure 2.20 Breakdown and formation of ATP. ATP (top) can be broken down to yield ADP plus phosphate plus energy (bottom).

As the hydrogen ions escape from the intermembrane space, ATP synthase, an enzyme present in large numbers in the inner membrane, captures their energy. It then uses that energy to add inorganic phosphate (Pi) to ADP, thus completing the synthesis of ATP. The newly formed ATP leaves the mitochondrion and enters the cytoplasm, where it can be used as an energy source for many different processes.

Golgi Apparatus

The ***Golgi*** (GOHL-jee) ***apparatus***, or Golgi, is an organelle that consists of a set of membranous discs. It is usually located between the endoplasmic reticulum and the plasma membrane of the cell (**Figure 2.18**). The Golgi apparatus produces small, membranous spheres called *vesicles*.

Some vesicles deliver new membrane, perhaps with newly embedded proteins, to the cell's plasma membrane. Some vesicles are packed with proteins or glycoproteins that are destined for secretion from the cell. Other vesicles are *lysosomes*—compartments in which reactions involving potentially dangerous enzymes and reactants can be conducted in isolation from the rest of the cytoplasm.

All the vesicles may need proteins, which are received at the inner side of the Golgi (the forming face) as transport vesicles from the endoplasmic reticulum. The proteins may be modified or sorted in the Golgi before they are released in vesicles from the outer side of the Golgi (the maturing face).

Ribosomes and Endoplasmic Reticulum

Ribosomes, another type of organelle, are very large enzymes that make polypeptides. A ribosome is made up of a small and a large subunit. Each subunit includes ribosomal RNA and protein subunits. Even a ribosome's small subunit is large by molecular standards, containing thousands of bases of RNA and dozens of protein subunits.

The small and large subunits are assembled separately in the nucleolus (part of the nucleus). They then move out to the cytoplasm, where they join to form a functional ribosome. Some ribosomes are found free in the cytoplasm; others are attached to the rough endoplasmic reticulum.

The ***endoplasmic reticulum (ER)***, shown in **Figure 2.21**, is an organelle made up of a network of membranes in the cytoplasm. The ER is located near, and connected to, the nuclear envelope (the membrane that defines the boundary of the cell nucleus). The ER can be either rough or smooth. Rough ER, when viewed through an electron microscope, looks rough (as the name implies) because it has ribosomes attached to it. It often contains flattened, sheet-like chambers known as *cisternae* (sis-TER-nee). Smooth ER does not have ribosomes attached to it, and it often has tubular cisternae.

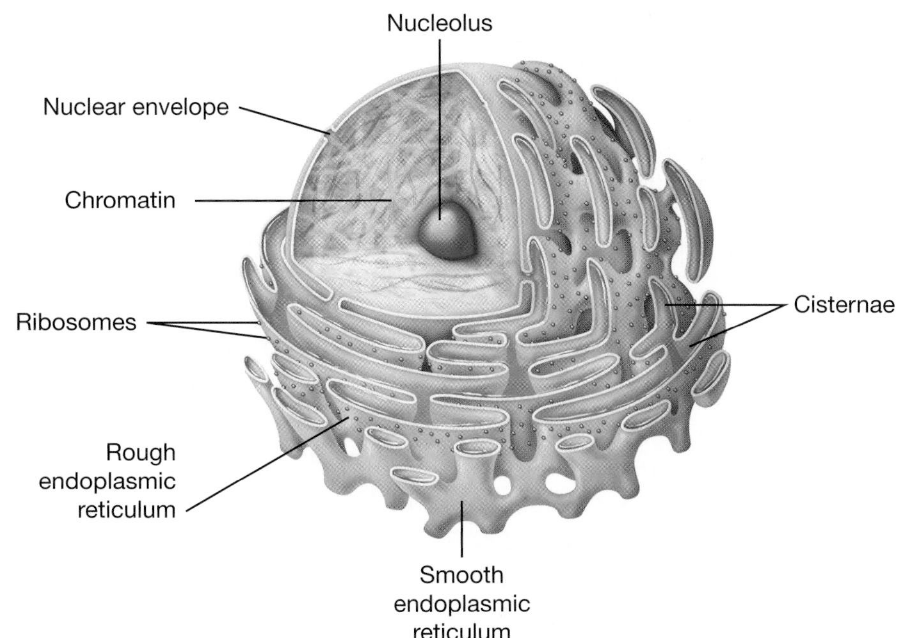

Figure 2.21 The nucleus and associated endoplasmic reticulum.

A cistern is a chamber or tank for holding water. The corresponding Latin words are *cisterna* (singular) and *cisternae* (plural). Besides referring to the interior of the endoplasmic reticulum, these words refer to the interior of the Golgi apparatus membrane compartments and to the interior of the sarcoplasmic reticulum in muscle.

Protein production and modification takes place in the rough endoplasmic reticulum. Ribosomes on rough ER make polypeptides and secrete them into the cisternae. There, the polypeptides may join with other polypeptides to form a multi-subunit protein, or they may be modified by chemical reactions that alter their size or shape. Not all proteins are made on the rough ER, however. Free ribosomes in the cytoplasm also make many proteins.

Smooth endoplasmic reticulum is a site for production of "replacement" membrane for membranous structures in the cell, including the plasma membrane, nuclear envelope, mitochondria, ER, and Golgi. It is also a site of steroid hormone production in cells of the reproductive organs and a site of triglyceride formation in adipocytes, or fat cells, and hepatocytes, or liver cells.

The Nucleus

The cell nucleus, shown in **Figure 2.21**, contains the cell's genetic information—its DNA. It also contains RNA (but not all RNA) and many proteins that are involved with coiling, uncoiling, copying, and maintaining DNA.

The nuclear envelope is a lipid bilayer folded over to form a double membrane. It contains protein-lined pores that allow small molecules to pass in and out of the nucleus. The nucleolus is an area in the nucleus where ribosomal RNA is made and packaged with protein subunits to make the small and large ribosomal subunits. Nucleoli are not present in all cells all the time.

All of a cell's DNA resides in the nucleus. When a cell is neither dividing nor about to divide, the DNA is spread throughout the nucleus. It wraps around small proteins called *histones*. The mixture of DNA and associated protein is called *chromatin*.

When cell division is about to begin, the DNA becomes much more organized. It coils into tight bundles called *chromosomes*. Each chromosome contains one DNA molecule plus the many proteins that enable it to coil.

SELF CHECK

1. What are two functions that a cytoskeleton performs for a cell?
2. What is the function of the mitochondria?
3. What does *ATP* stand for and what are its components?
4. What are lysosomes?
5. Where are ribosomes located?

Roles of the Nucleic Acids and Proteins

Three biological polymers—DNA, RNA, and proteins—are made of similar but not identical subunits that must be present in a specific order to work correctly. DNA and RNA are each made of four different types of nucleotides. Proteins are made of 21 types of amino acids. The order, or sequence, of subunits is a form of information. The use, modification, and passing on of this information are hallmarks of living things.

The DNA sequence is used to determine the RNA sequence, and the RNA sequence is used to determine the protein sequence. The DNA sequence is also used to make new DNA. Another way of stating this is that information flows from DNA to RNA to protein. Francis Crick, who shared with James Watson the Nobel Prize for determining the structure and function of DNA, called this fundamentally important concept "the central dogma of molecular biology."

Making RNA from DNA

The sequence of bases in DNA contains the information essential for making the proteins and RNA needed for life. The production of RNA from DNA is shown in **Figure 2.22**. This process is called ***transcription***.

RNA polymerase is the enzyme that makes an RNA molecule that is complementary to a gene on DNA. RNA polymerase binds to a region of DNA at the starting point of a gene. The DNA "unzips," or opens up, in the region where the RNA polymerase binds to it. The RNA polymerase then starts moving along the DNA, one base at a time. As it moves, it generates an RNA strand whose nucleotides are complementary to the DNA nucleotides. RNA uses

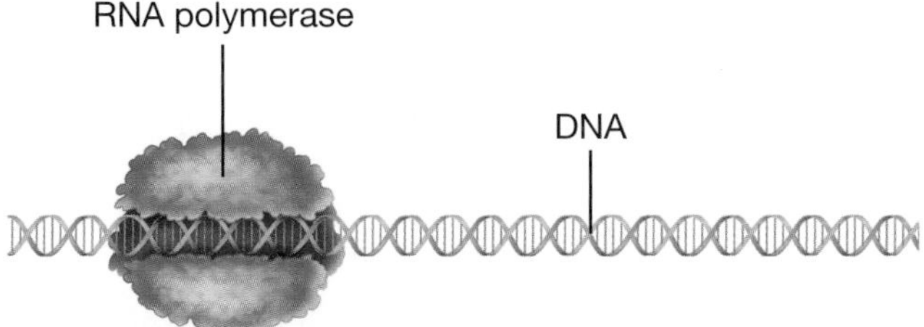

A RNA polymerase binds to DNA

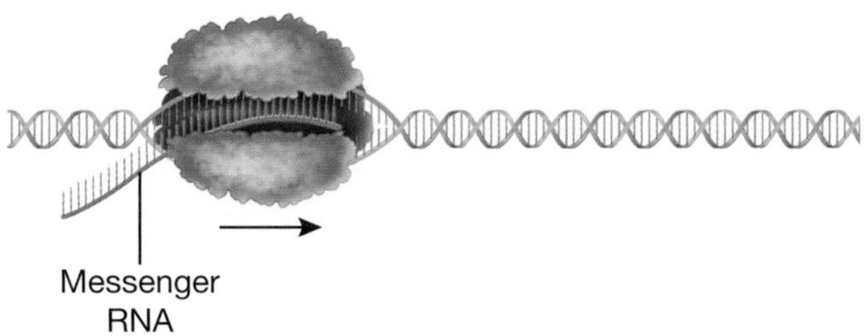

B RNA polymerase "unzips" the DNA and begins forming mRNA

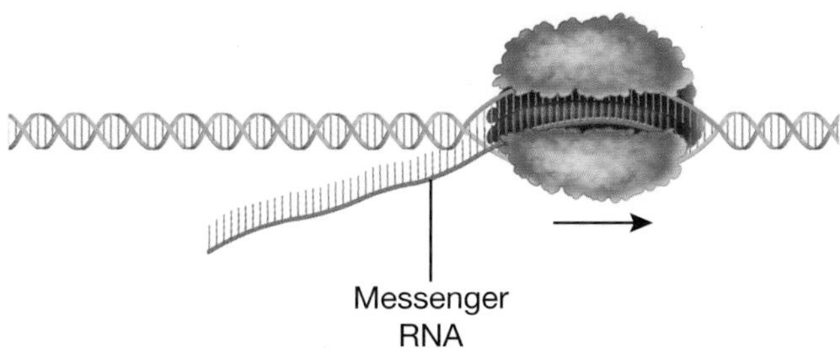

C RNA polymerase continues to form mRNA as it moves along the DNA

Figure 2.22 A—Transcription, which occurs in the nucleus, is the creation of a new RNA molecule. 1. The enzyme RNA polymerase binds to DNA. 2. RNA polymerase partially unwinds the DNA double helix and begins to form a molecule of messenger RNA (mRNA). The arrow shows the direction of RNA polymerase movement. 3. RNA polymerase continues along the DNA, adding new bases to the growing mRNA molecule. B—Translation is the process of interpreting the information in mRNA to create proteins from amino acids.

uracil (U) as the base complementary to adenine (A). In DNA, thymine (T) is the base complementary to A.

As the RNA polymerase moves along, the DNA strands reclose behind it. When the RNA polymerase encounters the end of the gene, it detaches from the DNA and releases the RNA strand. The RNA strand is called ***messenger RNA (mRNA)*** because it carries a message: the base sequence information that will be used to make a polypeptide. (Remember that a protein consists of one or several polypeptides.) The mRNA leaves the nucleus through a nuclear pore.

Understanding Medical Terminology

Transcription and translation—which comes first, and what does each accomplish? It helps to remember that "DNA makes RNA makes protein," and to think of the everyday meaning of *transcribing* and *translating*.

Transcribing means copying information from one place to another, without changing it. Someone taking precise notes in class is transcribing the teacher's words. If you copy a line from a book into an e-mail, you are transcribing. When a cell makes RNA from DNA, it is simply copying, or transcribing, the information from one nucleic acid molecule to another.

Translating involves converting information from one language to another. When we translate, the meaning is the same, but the words are not exactly the same. When a cell makes protein from RNA, it is converting from the language of nucleotides to the language of amino acids.

So, in physiology, what is the difference between transcription and translation? Transcription is making RNA from DNA, and translation is making protein from RNA.

Making a Polypeptide from mRNA

In an mRNA molecule, every set of three bases is called a ***codon*** because it specifies, or codes for, one amino acid in the polypeptide. It takes a 300-base (100-codon) mRNA molecule to code for a protein that is 100 amino acids long.

The mRNA molecule acts as a blueprint for making a polypeptide. **Figure 2.22** shows the molecules and steps involved in making polypeptides. In the cell's cytoplasm, a small ribosomal subunit attaches to the beginning of the mRNA strand. A ***transfer RNA (tRNA)*** molecule binds to the mRNA-ribosome complex. Each tRNA molecule, which can bind to only one kind of amino acid, has a specific ***anticodon***, a set of three bases that are complementary to those in a codon on the mRNA strand. The tRNA, with its attached amino acid, binds to the ribosome and mRNA.

With the help of the ribosome, the tRNA aligns its three-base anticodon with the complementary three-base codon of the mRNA. The large ribosomal subunit then binds, and a second tRNA molecule arrives with an anticodon complementary to the next codon on the mRNA strand. The result is a complex that includes mRNA, two tRNA molecules (each with an amino acid attached), and rRNA (in the ribosome).

The ribosome catalyzes the formation of a peptide bond between the amino acids attached to the two tRNA molecules. It also catalyzes the breaking of the bond that connects the first amino acid to its tRNA. The first tRNA molecule detaches from the mRNA-ribosome complex, and the ribosome moves to the next codon on the mRNA strand.

A third tRNA molecule, which is complementary to the third codon of the mRNA strand, arrives at the complex. This tRNA molecule, with its attached amino acid, aligns its anticodon with the third codon of the mRNA strand. The ribosome catalyzes the attachment of the amino acid on the third tRNA molecule to the two amino acids that are already present. It also catalyzes the breaking of the bond between that third amino acid and its tRNA molecule.

Then the process repeats: the ribosome moves along the mRNA strand, one codon at a time, attaching a new amino acid to the growing chain of amino acids with each move. This continues until the ribosome reaches the end of the mRNA strand. At that point, the large and small ribosomal subunits detach from one another and from the mRNA strand, and the complete polypeptide is released.

SELF CHECK

1. What is transcription?
2. Which type of RNA provides a blueprint for making a polypeptide?

Cell Division

It is perhaps surprising to learn that most cells in the human body have a life span that is considerably shorter than that of humans. For example, the cells lining the intestines have a life span of just 2 to 7 days. Red blood cells live for about 120 days. Many of the nerve cells in the brain, on the other hand, live for an individual's entire lifetime.

Because most cells have shorter lives than people do, they must regularly divide to make new cells for the body. The life cycle of a cell has two major phases: interphase and the mitotic phase. During interphase,

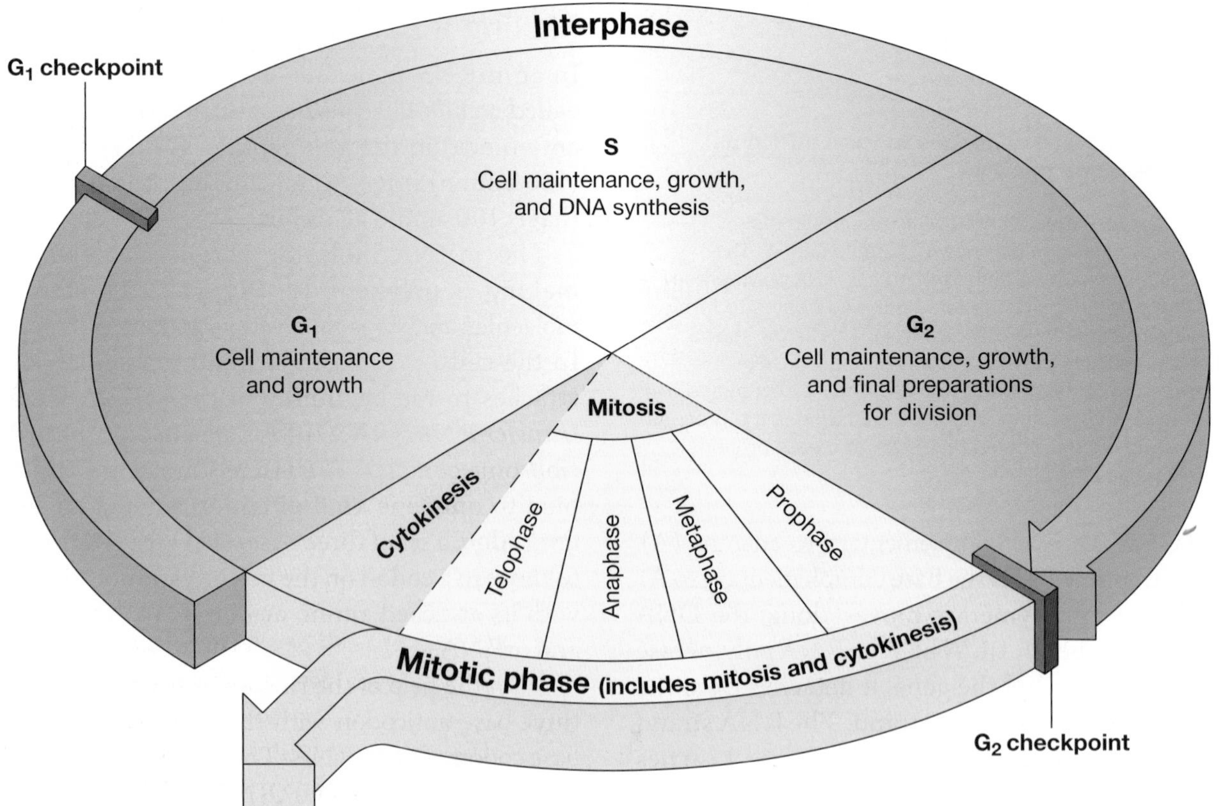

Figure 2.23 The two phases in the life cycle of a cell are interphase, when it is not dividing, and the mitotic phase, when it is dividing. Each of these phases is divided into subphases.

Focus On Cancer

When the cell division process just described does not work properly, serious problems, such as cancer, occur. Cancer is the uncontrolled division and growth of abnormal cells. Normal cells divide just enough to allow us to grow when we are young, and just enough to replace dead or injured cells when we are mature. This is not true of cancer cells.

Normal cells grow only where they are supposed to grow. This means that muscle cells do not grow in our brain, nor do brain cells grow in our muscles. A normal cell will notice if its DNA is damaged, and it will try to repair the damage. If the cell cannot repair the DNA, it will, in a sense, "commit suicide" through a process called *apoptosis*. In general, cancer cells grow more than they should, grow in places where they do not belong, and do not self-destroy when they should.

Cancer is caused by damage to a cell's DNA molecules. A mutation is damage to DNA that changes the genetic code—the pattern of As, Ts, Cs, and Gs. A mutation does not always, or even usually, cause cancer.

Certain mutations, however, can put a cell on the pathway to cancer. Mutations in genes that govern DNA repair, cell cycle checkpoints, and apoptosis have all been implicated in cancer development. For example, if a cell's DNA repair mechanism is damaged, more and more mutations begin to accumulate in the cell.

Cancer is caused by damage to DNA, but what causes damage to DNA? Some mutations seem to occur by random chance or for reasons that are unknown. We do know that various chemicals, cigarette smoke, alcohol, sunlight, X-rays, and viruses can cause mutations. This means that we can reduce our risk of cancer by not smoking, limiting alcohol intake, wearing sunscreen, and being vaccinated for human papillomavirus.

Some chemicals that disrupt the cytoskeleton are useful in cancer treatment because they interfere with mitosis. For example, *paclitaxel* interferes with microtubules and, therefore, prevents cells from segregating their chromosomes during mitosis. Paclitaxel is used as a chemotherapy drug for cancers of the lung, breast, and other organs.

You will learn more about various types of cancer in chapters throughout this text.

the cell performs its usual functions and prepares for cell division. It is during the mitotic phase that the cell actually divides. The diagram in **Figure 2.23** illustrates the phases and subphases in the life cycle of a cell.

Interphase

Interphase is divided into three subphases. It includes two "gap" phases, G_1 and G_2. Between the gap phases is a synthetic (S) phase. Of these three phases, the duration of G_1 varies the most among cell types. G_1 is long—sometimes years long—in cells that have a long life span, and short in cells that have a brief life span. The other two phases of the cycle—G_2 and S—are usually short (just minutes or hours).

Each of the 46 chromosomes in a typical human cell is duplicated in the S phase. The synthesis of new DNA is what gives this phase its name. After the S phase, the cell enters the second gap phase (G_2). During G_2, the cell completes its preparations for cell division.

Multiple "checkpoints" occur during interphase. At a checkpoint, a cell verifies that it has successfully completed the appropriate steps for that phase of the cycle and is ready to progress to the next phase. This verification process often involves checking for DNA damage and repairing any damage, if found, before clearing the checkpoint.

It should be noted that some cells never divide. Examples include red blood cells and most nerve cells in the brain. Cells such as these are said to be in phase G_0.

Mitotic Phase

The mitotic phase includes two types of division: mitosis and cytokinesis. ***Mitosis*** is the division of a cell nucleus and chromosomes into two nuclei, each with its own set of identical chromosomes. ***Cytokinesis*** is the division of the cytoplasm. Mitosis followed by cytokinesis results in the formation of two identical daughter cells.

Mitotic cell division is the process by which a single fertilized egg cell develops into an adult made of trillions of cells. Meiosis, a different kind of nuclear division, will be discussed in Chapter 16. This section takes a closer look at mitosis—divided into prophase, metaphase, anaphase, and telophase—and cytokinesis (**Figure 2.24**). Keep in mind that the DNA has already been duplicated when mitosis begins.

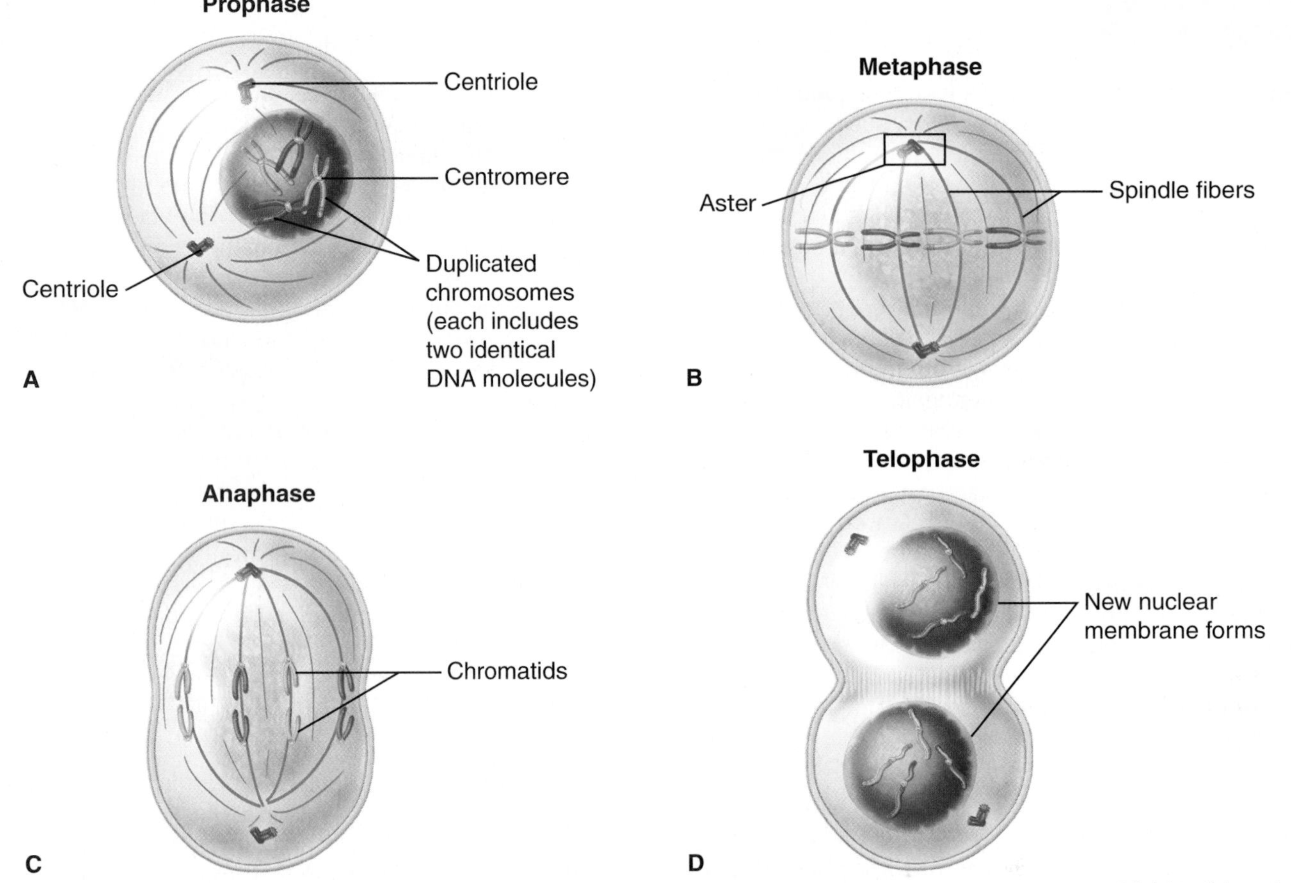

Figure 2.24 Mitosis. Another process—cytokinesis—begins during telophase.

Prophase

In prophase, the chromatin (DNA plus associated proteins) "condenses" to form chromosomes, which are visible in a light microscope. Each chromosome is made of two identical DNA molecules, called *sister chromatids,* which are joined to each other at the centromere. As a result, each chromosome resembles a narrow X, with the centromere at the center of the X.

While the chromosomes are forming, the nuclear membrane is breaking down, and the centrioles are migrating to opposite sides of the cell. Microtubules start to grow away from the centrioles, forming spindle fibers. The spindle fibers form asters (from the Latin term for "star").

Metaphase

In metaphase, some spindle fibers lock onto the centromeres of the chromosomes. At least one spindle fiber from each of the two centrioles attaches to each centromere. Then the spindle fibers pull in a balanced way on each chromosome, positioning the chromosomes along the midline of the cell.

Anaphase

In anaphase, the enzyme separase, which functions like a molecular scissor, cuts each centromere in half so that the sister chromatids are free to move apart. Each chromatid pulls itself along the spindle toward the centriole. As a result, 46 chromatids go to one side, and the other 46 chromatids go to the other side.

Telophase

In telophase, the chromosomes gather around each centriole, where they spread out and are no longer visible using a light microscope. The spindles disappear, and a new nuclear membrane forms around the DNA. Mitosis is now complete. One nucleus has become two, and the DNA has been equally divided.

Cytokinesis

During telophase, cytokinesis begins. Cytokinesis is the final step in cell division. A ring of actin microfilaments forms a circle around the cell. Myosin proteins pull on the actin filaments, making them shorten. As a result of this pulling process, a cleavage furrow, or deepening groove, forms around the middle of the cell. The cleavage furrow gets tighter and tighter, until the cell splits into two daughter cells. This completes the process of cell division.

SECTION 2.3 REVIEW

Mini-Glossary

active transport movement across a cell membrane that requires energy to move a substance against the gradient of concentration

adenosine triphosphate (ATP) a nucleotide composed of an adenine base, a sugar, and three phosphate groups; adenosine triphosphate

anticodon a set of three bases in transfer RNA that are complementary to those in a codon on messenger RNA

centrioles short cylinders that help guide the movement and separation of chromosomes during cell division

channel proteins molecules with a hollow central pore that allows water or small, charged particles of certain substances to pass into or out of cells

cilia hair-like projections that actively flex back and forth to move fluid or mucus across the outside of a cell

codon a set of three bases in DNA or RNA that codes for one amino acid

cytokinesis division of the cytoplasm in a cell, which begins during the telophase portion of mitosis.

cytoplasm the part of a cell that contains everything inside the cell membrane except the nucleus

cytoskeleton a network of proteins that defines the shape of a cell and gives it mechanical strength

endoplasmic reticulum (ER) an organelle that consists of a network of membranes in the cytoplasm

extracellular fluid the liquid—consisting of mostly water—that surrounds a typical cell

extracellular matrix the solid or gel-like substance that surrounds a typical cell

glycoproteins proteins with carbohydrate groups attached

Golgi apparatus an organelle that produces vesicles; consists of membranous discs

messenger RNA (mRNA) a single-strand RNA molecule whose base sequence carries the information needed by a ribosome to make a protein

microvilli finger-like extensions that increase the surface area of a cell

mitochondria organelles in the cytoplasm that make ATP

mitosis the division of a cell nucleus and chromosomes into two nuclei, each with its own set of identical chromosomes

nucleus a rounded or oval mass of protoplasm within the cytoplasm of a cell that contains the cell's DNA and is bounded by a membrane

passive transport movement across a cell membrane that does not require energy because the substance is moving from an area of greater concentration to one of lower concentration

plasma membrane the membrane that defines the outer boundary of a cell

ribosomes very large enzymes that make polypeptides

RNA polymerase the enzyme that makes an RNA molecule complementary to a gene on DNA

transcription the production of RNA from DNA

transfer RNA (tRNA) a molecule that binds to the mRNA-ribosome complex and helps assemble amino acids into polypeptides

Review Questions

1. The liquid outside of and between cells is called _____.
2. What is the glycocalyx?
3. In what part of the cell can you find mitochondria?
4. Vesicles are produced in the _____.
5. DNA is contained in the _____ of a cell.
6. How does mRNA leave the nucleus?
7. How might the human body be different if body cells had walls instead of membranes?
8. Explain the relationship between sodium and potassium in active transport.

Medical Terminology: Molecules and Cells

By understanding the word parts that make up medical words, you can extend your medical vocabulary. This chapter includes many of the word parts listed below. Review these word parts to be sure you understand their meanings.

adip/o	fat, fatty
an-	negative, minus
carcin/o	cancer
cyt/o	cell
de-	without, lack of
-gen	substance that produces something
gluc/o	glucose, sugar
glyc/o	glucose, sugar
-ic	pertaining to
-meter	instrument
neutr/o	neutral
-oid	derived from, resembling
oxy-	oxygenated, containing oxygen
phosph/o	phosphorus
pro-	for, plus
som/o	body
tri-	three

Now use these word parts to form valid medical words that fit the following definitions. Some of the words are included in this chapter. Others are not. When you finish, use a medical dictionary to check your work.

1. containing three glycerides
2. RNA without oxygen
3. cancer-producing substance
4. atomic element with a positive charge
5. atomic element with a net charge of 0
6. ion with a negative charge
7. derived from a solid structure
8. fat cell
9. instrument for measuring cells
10. body that contains pigment or color

Chapter 2 Summary

- The fundamental particles that form atoms include protons, neutrons, and electrons.
- The attractive forces that form links between atoms include covalent, ionic, and hydrogen bonds.
- The isotope of an atom is determined by the number of neutrons in its nucleus.
- Carbohydrates, which always contain carbon and hydrogen, are the sugar and starch molecules that provide fuel for the body's work.
- Proteins, which help form the structure of cells or speed up biological processes, are made up of long chains of amino acids.
- Lipids are fats and oils in the body, and they store energy or regulate the reproductive system.
- DNA and RNA are nucleic acids that contain the body's genetic information or carry it from cell to cell.
- Water is essential to life, and it comprises about two-thirds of body mass.
- Cell parts include the plasma membrane; the cytoskeleton; various organelles, including mitochondria, Golgi apparatus, ribosomes, and endoplasmic reticulum; and the nucleus.
- The base sequence in DNA is used to determine the base sequence in RNA, and RNA directs the manufacture of the various polypeptides and proteins.
- The nucleus of a cell contains the cell's DNA that makes it possible for the cell to transmit information to new cells.
- The life cycle of a cell consists of two major phases—interphase and the mitotic phase—both of which can be divided into several subphases. Cell division occurs in the mitotic phase.

Chapter 2 Review

Understanding Key Concepts

1. What unit is considered the building block of all matter?
2. A substance that is composed of atoms that all have the same atomic number are called ______.
   A. protons
   B. neutrons
   C. elements
   D. electrons

3. The strongest type of atomic bond is the ______ bond.
   A. hydrogen
   B. covalent
   C. cohesive
   D. ionic
4. What three atoms make up a water molecule?
5. What is the difference between an anion and a cation?
6. Explain the difference between carbon-12 and carbon-14.
7. Define *radioactive decay*.
8. Glucose is the main form of ______ that circulates in the blood.
9. A molecule made up of many similar subunits, such as simple sugars, is called a(n) ______.
10. Adenosine triphosphate (ATP) provides ______ for many cellular processes.
11. Fatty acids are key building blocks for certain lipids, especially ______ and ______.
12. The type of bond that links the amino group of one amino acid to the acid group of another is a(n) ______.
    A. acid bond
    B. amino bond
    C. peptide bond
    D. residual bond
13. Name the three types of glycerides and explain the relationship between fatty acids and the different types of glycerides.
14. DNA is formed in the shape of a(n) ______.
    A. double pleat
    B. double helix
    C. triple helix
    D. pleated helix
15. What characteristics do the amino acids glycine and tryptophan have in common? What is one key difference between them?
16. Identify and describe the four levels of protein structure.
17. Charged particles can only enter or leave a cell via ______.
18. Glycoproteins are proteins with ______ groups attached.
19. Located in the centrosome, the ______ help guide the movement and separation of chromosomes during cell division.
20. Because of their great need for energy to power muscle contractions, cardiac muscle cells contain a high number of ______.
21. The breakdown of a glucose molecule into two pyruvate molecules is called ______.
22. The type of RNA that carries the basic information that will be used to make a protein is ______.
    A. tRNA
    B. rRNA
    C. mRNA
    D. pRNA
23. The cytoskeleton does *not* include ______.
    A. cytofilaments
    B. intermediate filaments
    C. microfilaments
    D. microtubules
24. Which of the following organelles consists of a set of membranous discs in the cytoplasm?
    A. mitochondria
    B. endoplasmic reticulum
    C. Golgi apparatus
    D. ribosomes
25. Which of the following statements does *not* describe a ribosome?
    A. It is a very large enzyme.
    B. It is found in the nucleus.
    C. It makes polypeptides.
    D. It includes a large and a small subunit.
26. The enzyme that unzips DNA to produce an RNA molecule is called ______.
    A. adenine
    B. transfer RNA
    C. lipase
    D. RNA polymerase
27. Describe the functions of rough and smooth endoplasmic reticulum.

Instructions: *Identify the parts of a cell by indicating the* **letter** *that corresponds to the name of the cell structure.*

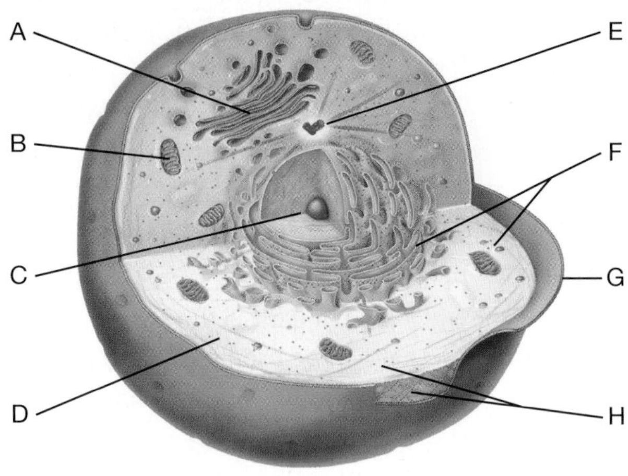

28. mitochondrion
29. ribosomes
30. Golgi apparatus
31. cytoskeleton
32. centrosome
33. nucleus
34. plasma membrane
35. cytoplasm

Thinking Critically

36. Which bodily functions might *not* be possible in the absence of the enzymes discussed in this chapter?
37. Using the information and figures in this chapter, describe at least two different types of chemical reactions that provide the body with energy.
38. What might be the consequences of DNA damage in a person's cells?
39. Compare and contrast microvilli and cilia.
40. Investigate the physical and chemical processes that contribute to homeostasis, including equilibrium, temperature, pH balance, chemical reactions, active and passive transport, and biofeedback. Describe how these processes are integrated.

Clinical Case Study

Read again the Clinical Case Study at the beginning of this chapter. Use the information provided in the chapter to answer the following questions.

41. What diagnoses are possible? Explain your reasoning for each possibility.
42. Evaluate the possible diagnoses in this case. Which seems the most likely in Stan's case?

Analyzing and Evaluating Data

The chart below lists 12 elements in order of their percentage of total body weight. Use the chart to answer the following questions.

Element	Percentage of total body weight
Oxygen	65%
Carbon	18%
Hydrogen	10%
Nitrogen	3%
Calcium	1.5%
Phosphorus	1%
Sulfur	0.25%
Potassium	0.20%
Sodium	0.15%
Chlorine	0.15%
Magnesium	0.05%
Iron	0.006%

43. Elements not shown in this chart that play a role in human physiology and contribute to total body weight are called *trace elements.* What percentage of body weight is made up of these trace elements? Round your answer to the nearest hundredth of a percent.
44. How much more nitrogen than potassium does your body contain? Give your answer as a percentage.

Investigating Further

45. The usefulness of radioisotopes in research depends on their half-life. Investigate what *half-life* means and find the half-life of at least three of the radioisotopes you listed in the previous question. Why is half-life an important consideration in choosing isotopes for a research study?

3 Body Tissues

Clinical Case Study

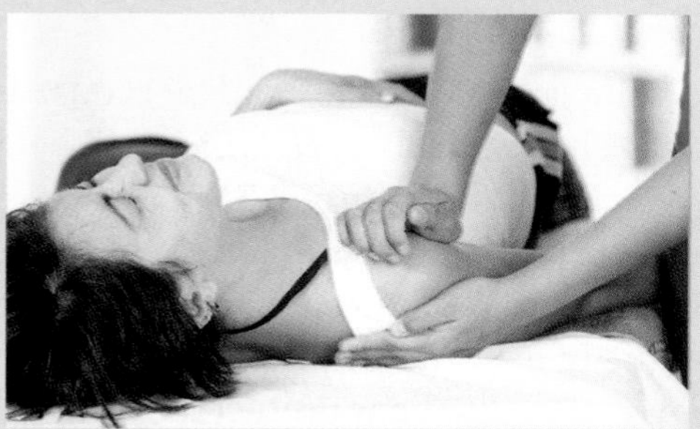
Fotos593/Shutterstock.com

Sara is a 20-year-old college student, 61 inches tall and 101 pounds. A friend brings Sara to the emergency department when Sara hurts her right shoulder. Forty-five minutes earlier, Sara had been walking up a flight of stairs when she tripped. She grabbed the stair railing with her right hand, and as she held on to stop her fall, she felt something pop in her shoulder. Now it hurts a great deal.

The physical examination suggests that Sara has dislocated her shoulder. X-rays confirm the diagnosis. Sara reports that she sprained her ankles and wrists multiple times while growing up, and she says her joints and muscles are frequently painful. Sara says she gets bruises and cuts more easily than her friends, and is not very strong. Her skin has a scarred appearance in many locations, and it is unusually stretchy when gently pinched and pulled.

After giving Sara medication to relax the shoulder and control her pain, the medical team reduces the shoulder dislocation; in other words, they pop the shoulder back to its normal position. Her shoulder feels much better after that. Sara is advised to follow up with a rheumatologist—a physician who specializes in diseases affecting the skeletal system.

Chapter 3 Outline

The previous chapter described the fundamental units of life—cells. This chapter will build on the information about cells to help you understand tissues.

A tissue is a collection of similar cells that have a shared function. Different types of tissues combine in various ways to make organs and organ systems. The four basic types of tissues—epithelial, connective, muscle, and nervous tissues—appear throughout the body. Epithelial tissues cover the body and line the body tracts that connect to the outside world, such as the gastrointestinal tract. Cartilage is an example of connective tissue. Muscle tissue enables movement. Nerve tissue is concentrated in the brain and spinal cord.

This chapter also discusses the specific ways in which injuries and diseases affect the structure and function of tissues. The diagnosis of illness frequently requires examination of tissue samples under a microscope. Healthcare providers must have working knowledge of normal tissues to recognize and classify abnormal tissue, and to assess the progression of recovery from injury or illness.

SECTION 3.1

Tissues

Objectives

- Identify the four main types of body tissue.
- Describe the embryological origin of each type of body tissue.

Key Terms

connective tissue
ectoderm
endoderm
epithelial tissue
extracellular matrix
histology
mesoderm
muscle tissue
nerve tissue

A tissue is created when cells that have a similar structure join together to accomplish a common function. Tissues also include the material between the cells, which is called the ***extracellular matrix***. In some cases, the extracellular matrix makes up most of the mass and volume of a tissue. The study of tissues is called ***histology***.

Types of Tissues

The different tissues in the body have been classified into four main types: epithelial, connective, muscle, and nervous. Each of these has its own subtypes, which will be discussed in the next section (**Figure 3.1**).

Epithelial tissues act as barriers between the body and its surroundings. The structure of epithelial tissues allows them to accomplish several functions. They protect the body from physical damage, control which substances enter and leave the body, provide sensory information, and secrete various substances.

Connective tissue is found throughout the body. It includes the rigid skeleton and the flexible ligaments and tendons, all of which are necessary for movement.

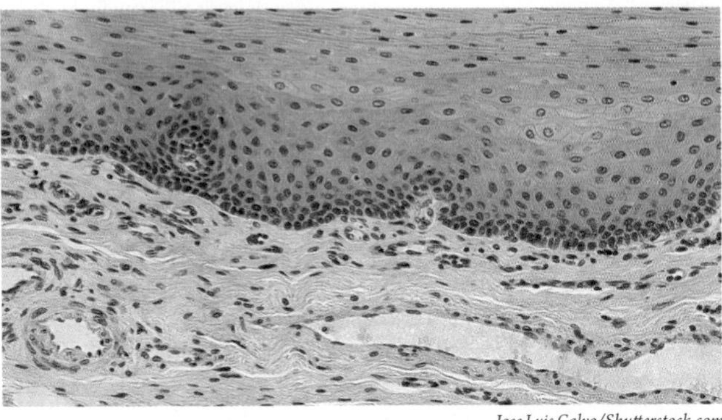

A *Jose Luis Calvo/Shutterstock.com*

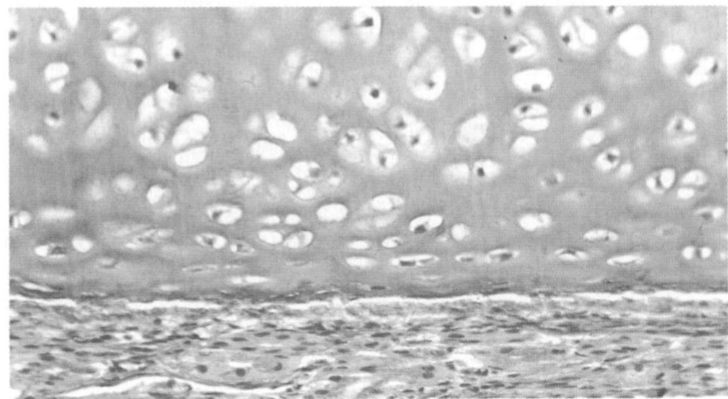

B *Anna Jurkovska/Shutterstock.com*

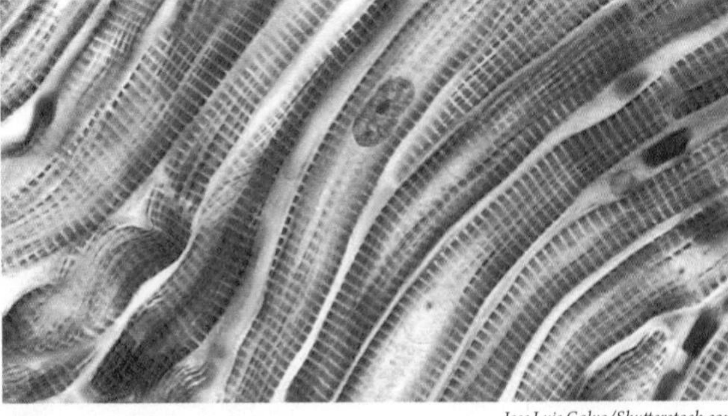

C *Jose Luis Calvo/Shutterstock.com*

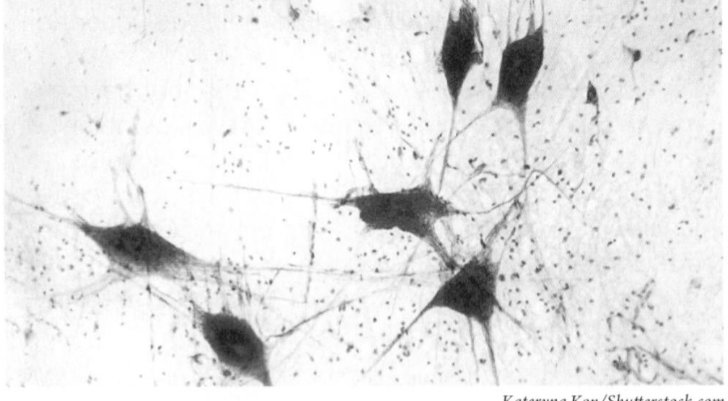

D *Kateryna Kon/Shutterstock.com*

Figure 3.1 A—Epithelial tissue. This is a low-magnification micrograph of a non-keratinized stratified squamous epithelium from the superior surface of the epiglottis. B—Connective tissue. This micrograph shows elastic cartilage. The upper two-thirds of the image shows the extracellular matrix of the cartilage (pink), with spaces (lacunae) occupied by cartilage cells (chondrocytes). The lower third of the image is a fibrous layer (perichondrium) that covers the cartilage. C—Striated muscle. This is a medium-magnification image of cardiac muscle cells. D—Neurons and glial cells in human brain tissue.

Connective tissue gives the body the strength to resist external forces such as gravity, protects internal organs, and helps maintain the proper shape of organs.

Muscle tissue allows the body to move. The three kinds of muscle tissue are skeletal, cardiac, and smooth muscle. Skeletal muscle, the most common type, pulls on bones to create movement. Cardiac muscle, which makes up most of the mass of the heart, propels the blood by contracting. Smooth muscle is found in the walls of hollow organs, including the blood vessels, airways, gastrointestinal tract, bladder, and uterus.

Nerve tissue has the unique ability to convey information through electrical signals. Nerve tissue is found throughout the body, and it is most abundant in the brain and spinal cord.

SELF CHECK

1. What is the purpose of epithelial tissue?
2. List two examples of connective tissue.
3. What are the three types of muscle tissue?
4. Where in the body is nerve tissue most abundant?

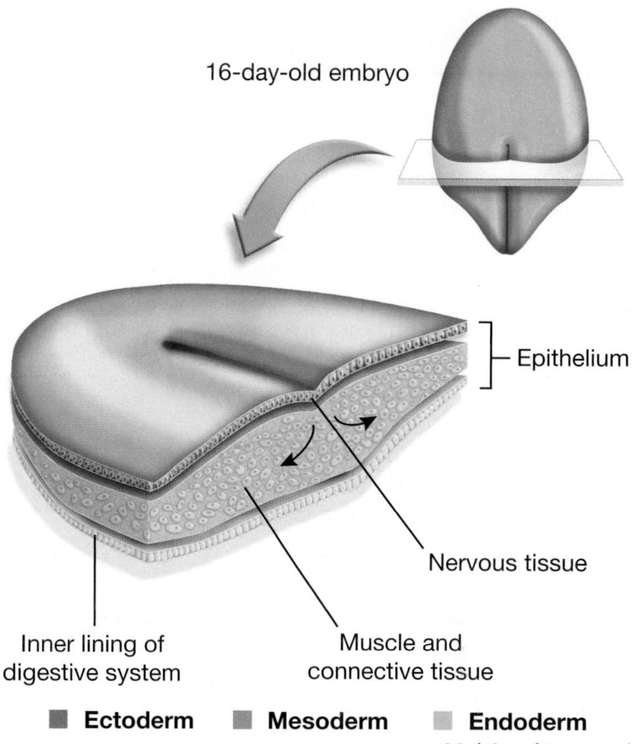

Figure 3.2 The three cell layers in the early embryo give rise to the four major types of tissues.

Origin of Tissues

When a human embryo is about 16 days old, the bundle of cells that will become the body is a flat disk about 0.5 mm long. This disk consists of three layers of cells, as shown in **Figure 3.2**. From outermost to innermost, these layers are the ***ectoderm***, the ***mesoderm***, and the ***endoderm***. Cells from these layers create the four major types of tissues in the body.

Epithelial tissues, including glands and the outer layers of the skin, are derived from cells in all three layers. The linings of the lungs and the gastrointestinal tract, which are epithelial tissues, are specifically derived from cells of the endoderm. Most connective tissues and muscle tissues are derived from cells of the mesoderm. Nervous tissue is derived from cells of the ectoderm.

Normal embryonic development requires cells to divide, move to new locations, and differentiate. Differentiation is the process by which cells change from one type to another, usually becoming more "specialized" as they divide and develop. For example, some embryonic cells of the ectoderm divide and become one of many different types of neurons, each expressing a distinct set of genes and having its own distinct appearance. As the cells differentiate, they migrate to new locations. If cells do not migrate to the correct places, abnormalities are likely.

Spina bifida, a congenital disorder of the nervous system, is one of the most common birth defects. It is an example of a disorder caused by the failure of embryonic cells to go to their correct positions. In normal development of neural tissue, ectodermal cells in the midline of the embryo fold inward toward the mesoderm and pinch off to form the "neural tube." In spina bifida, the neural tube does not pinch off completely, so part of it is left open to the back of the embryo. Spina bifida ranges from mild to severe, depending on how much of the neural tube fails to close.

The study of tissues is essential for understanding health and disease. More than two hundred types of cells make up the different tissues of an adult human. When the right types of cells are present in the right locations at the right times, good health is very likely to occur.

Clinical Application Pathology, Tissues, and Forensic Science

Pathology is the study of injury and disease. All physicians study pathology in medical school. A physician who specializes in pathology is called a *pathologist*. The practice of pathology involves identifying and diagnosing abnormal anatomy by carefully observing tissue samples taken from living or dead patients. The observation of tissue is done with the naked eye (gross anatomy) and with a microscope (microscopic anatomy). Pathologists diagnose disease and determine whether treatment, such as chemotherapy for cancer, is working. This requires pathologists to be extremely familiar with the wide range of "normal" appearances of tissues, as well as the abnormal appearance associated with various diseases, infections, and injuries.

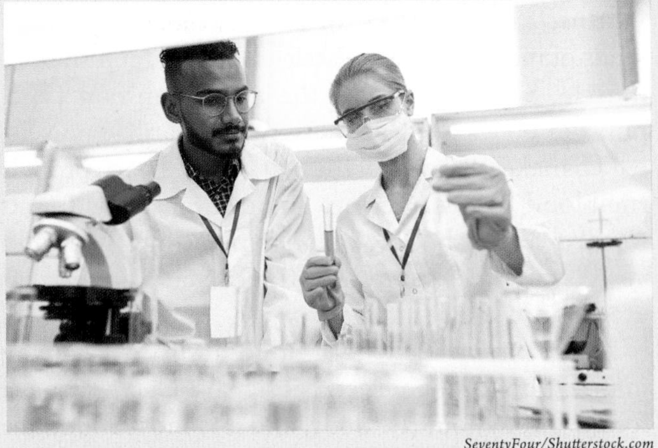

SeventyFour/Shutterstock.com

Tissue Acquisition and Preparation

In a living patient, the samples of tissue used for pathological examination may be obtained by surgery or by scraping off or withdrawing cells, such as blood cells, with a syringe. Tissue samples may be obtained from a deceased subject by autopsy, the surgical examination of a dead body.

After a tissue sample is obtained, it must be prepared for examination. The preparation usually includes four processes: fixation, embedding, sectioning, and staining. Fixation is the chemical treatment of the tissue to preserve it and prevent decay. Embedding is the conversion of the tissue to a fairly solid form so that it can be sliced. Sectioning is the slicing of the embedded tissue into very thin slices, as is required for examination under the microscope. Staining is the treatment of the sample with chemicals, or stains, that make certain features stand out more clearly under the microscope. The most common stains used most commonly in pathology are hematoxylin and eosin (H&E). A tissue sample stained with H&E has purple or blue cell nuclei and pink cytoplasm.

Forensics

Forensic pathologists apply their understanding of anatomy and of body tissues to aid the legal process. Forensic pathology is the application of pathology to legal issues, and in particular to the understanding of deaths that are sudden, unexpected, or violent. Anatomical examination of the body with the naked eye is very important in forensic pathology, since it may reveal injections, bruises, foreign material on the body surface, and other features that can clarify the cause of death. Microscopic examination of tissue is also important; it may reveal signs of injury or disease that could have contributed to death.

SECTION 3.1 REVIEW

Mini-Glossary

connective tissue a class of tissue that connects, supports, binds, or separates other tissues or organs

ectoderm the outermost layer of cells or tissue of an embryo in early development

endoderm the innermost layer of cells or tissue of an embryo in early development

epithelial tissue membranous tissue that covers internal organs and other internal surfaces of the body

extracellular matrix the material between the cells in tissues

histology the study of tissues

mesoderm the middle layer of an embryo in early development

muscle tissue a type of tissue that generates force and allows the body to move

nerve tissue a type of tissue that conveys information through electric signals

(continued)

Review Questions

1. What are the four main types of body tissue?
2. What functions does connective tissue perform?
3. What characteristic of nerve tissue sets it apart from other types of tissues?
4. From what three embryonic layers do body cells originate?
5. Define *differentiation* and explain why it is necessary in human development.
6. What is the probable result if embryonic cells do not differentiate correctly or move to the appropriate place in the developing embryo?
7. How many types of cells are present in the adult human body?

SECTION 3.2 Human Tissues

Objectives

- Describe the various types and functions of epithelia.
- Explain the properties and functions of different types of connective tissue.
- Identify the major types of muscle tissue.
- Describe the basic types and functions of nerve tissue.

Key Terms

cardiac muscle
cartilage
chondroblasts
compressive strength
elasticity
endocrine gland
exocrine gland
glands
lumen
neurons
osseous tissue
simple epithelia
skeletal muscle
smooth muscle
stratified epithelia
tensile strength

This section examines the four main types of tissue: epithelial, connective, nerve, and muscle tissues. It focuses on the different cell types, structures, and functions of each different tissue.

Epithelial Tissue

Epithelial tissue includes epithelia and glands. Epithelia (singular: *epithelium*) are tissues that cover the body and line the cavities within the body. Glands secrete chemicals, either to the outside world (exocrine glands) or within the body (endocrine glands). Epithelial tissues form the interface between the body and its surroundings.

Epithelial Surfaces

One feature that distinguishes an epithelium from other types of tissues is that it has an "inside" and an "outside." The outside is the apical surface (think *apex*, or *top*). The inside is the basal surface (think *base*). The skin is an example of an epithelium. Its apical surface faces the outside world, and the basal surface faces the internal body cells. It forms a barrier that separates the inside of the body from the external environment.

The cells that line the gastrointestinal tract (GI tract), the airways, and the reproductive and urinary tracts also separate the outside from the inside, so they are considered epithelial cells. In these cases, the definition of "inside" and "outside" is less obvious.

Figure 3.3 illustrates this concept of inside and outside. The figure shows the body as a rectangle with tubes in it and through it. The GI tract is a tube that runs through the body, from mouth to anus. The center of the tube is called the ***lumen***, from the Latin word meaning "light." The lumen connects to the outside world, and it could be considered "outside." The respiratory system, urinary system, and reproductive system also have hollow structures with lumens that connect to the outside world. The side of the GI tract's epithelium that faces the lumen is the apical side. The same is true of the epithelia that line structures in the respiratory system, urinary tract, and reproductive tract.

The only epithelial tissues that do not separate the outside from the inside are located in the lining of the cardiovascular system, and in endocrine glands (which are not shown in **Figure 3.3**).

Epithelial Cell Layers and Shapes

Epithelia are classified according to number of cell layers and cell shape, as shown in **Figure 3.4**. ***Simple epithelia*** have a single layer of cells, and ***stratified epithelia*** have multiple layers of cells. Cell shapes in both simple and stratified epithelia include squamous (almost flat), cuboidal (height about equal to width), and columnar (tall and narrow). If an epithelium has

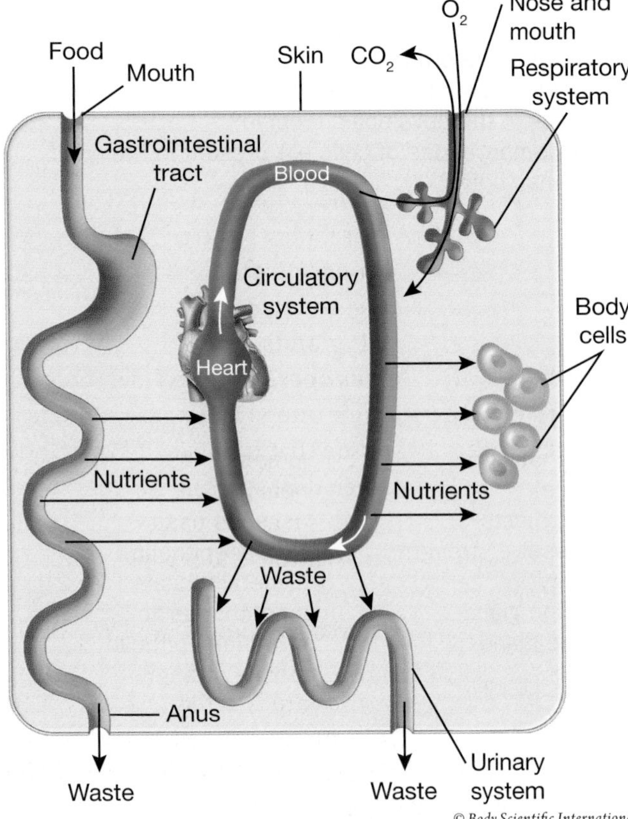

© Body Scientific International

Figure 3.3 Most forms of epithelia separate inside from outside, in the sense that "outside" means a place connected to the external world, without any intervening tissues.

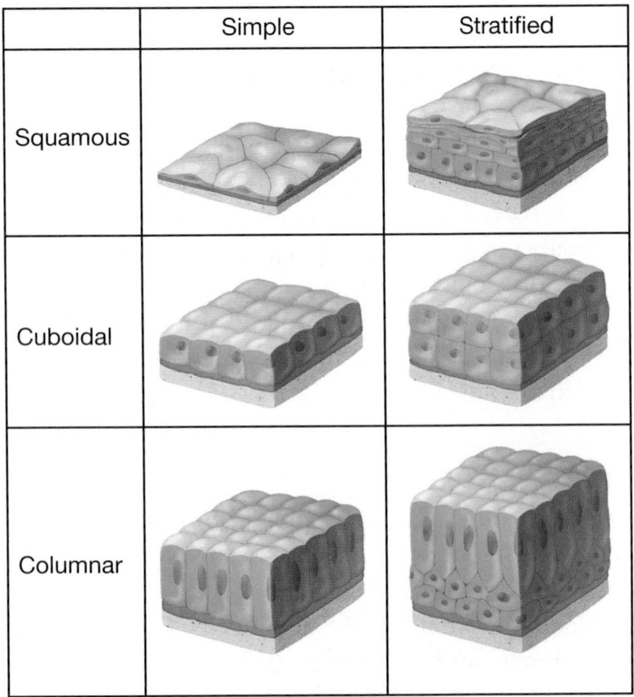

© Body Scientific International

Figure 3.4 Types of epithelia. Transitional epithelium and pseudo-stratified columnar epithelium are not shown.

multiple layers of cells that are not all the same shape, it is classified according to the shape of the most apical cells.

Simple Epithelia

A simple squamous epithelium has a single layer of flattened cells. The thinness of simple squamous epithelia allows rapid diffusion of substances. Examples of simple squamous epithelia in the body include the:

- gas-exchanging cavities (alveoli) of the lungs
- lining of the abdominal cavity
- endothelium, a single layer of cells that lines the blood vessels and the inside of the heart

Simple cuboidal epithelia have a single layer of cuboidal cells. They surround tubules in the kidneys and are present in various secretory glands. These epithelia are typically involved with secretion or absorption.

Simple columnar epithelia have a single layer of columnar cells. They are found in the lining of some ducts in the kidneys, in the stomach, and in the intestines. These epithelia sometimes have microvilli on their apical surfaces to increase their surface area.

Figure 3.5 shows the simple columnar epithelium in the small intestine. Like simple cuboidal epithelia, these epithelia have secretory and absorptive functions.

Stratified Epithelia

Stratified squamous epithelia are found where chemical and mechanical protection are most needed. The most familiar stratified squamous epithelium is the surface of the skin. Stratified squamous epithelia are also found in areas that are closely connected to

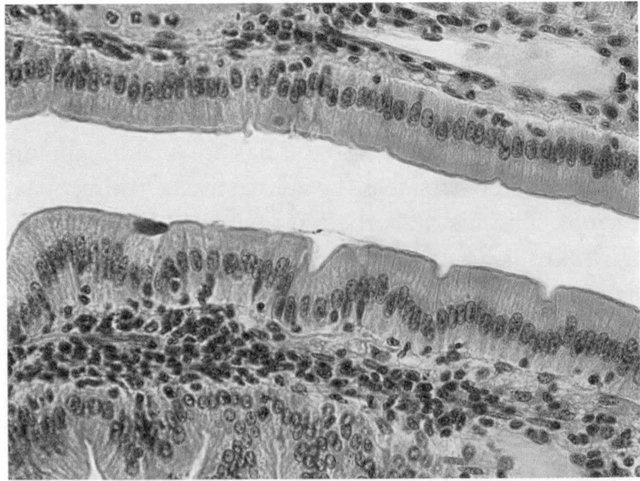

Science Stock Photography/Science Source

Figure 3.5 Light micrograph of a simple columnar epithelium in the small intestine. The purple ovals are cell nuclei.

the outside of the body, including the mouth and throat, as well as the anus and rectum. **Figure 3.6** shows the stratified epithelium of the esophagus.

The most apical cells in the epithelium of the skin are actually dead and dying skin cells filled with keratin (a protein that is also a key component of hair and fingernails). The layer of keratinized cells helps prevent water loss through the skin and provides additional protection.

Stratified cuboidal and stratified columnar epithelia are relatively rare, but they do occur in some areas of the body. Stratified cuboidal epithelia are found in the ducts of some exocrine glands, including sweat glands. Stratified columnar epithelia line the ducts of the pancreas and the salivary glands.

Other Epithelia

Some epithelia do not fit easily into a tidy classification system. Transitional epithelia are stratified epithelia found in the linings of hollow organs that can stretch, such as the bladder. When the bladder is empty, it is relaxed, and the cells near the surface are rounded, or cuboidal. When the bladder is full, however, the apical cells are stretched and have a more squamous appearance.

Pseudostratified columnar epithelia are epithelial tissues composed of a single layer of columnar cells. The cells vary in height and in the position of their nuclei. As a result, they may appear to have more than one layer when observed under a microscope. Pseudostratified columnar epithelia are found in the lining of the trachea and in certain parts of the male and female reproductive organs.

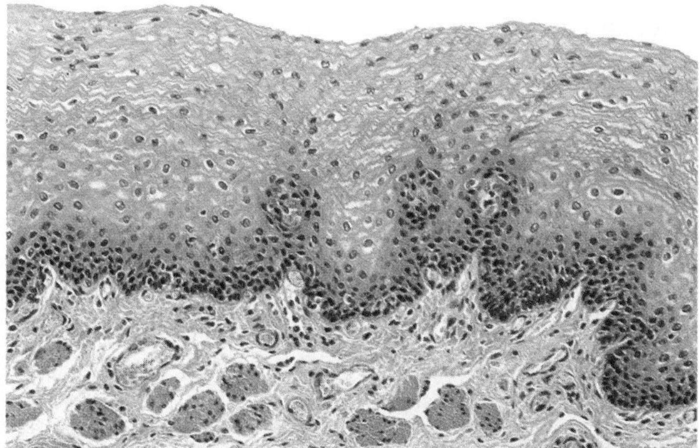

Biophoto Associates/Science Source

Figure 3.6 Light micrograph of stratified squamous epithelium from the esophagus. Here the epithelium extends from the surface, at the bottom, up to the basal cells, whose tightly packed nuclei form a dark layer. A lighter-staining layer of connective tissue lies above the epithelium. The dark circles are cell nuclei.

Glands

Epithelial cells that are organized to produce and secrete substances are called ***glands***. A gland may have just a handful of cells, or it may be large and complex, with blood vessels and connective tissue. Large, complex glands are considered glandular organs.

The two types of glands are endocrine and exocrine glands. An ***endocrine gland*** secretes its product into the tissue's interstitial space, which is the space within the tissue that is outside of the blood vessels. The secretion then diffuses from the interstitial space into the blood and is carried to the rest of the body. Chapter 9 discusses the endocrine glands in more detail.

An ***exocrine gland*** secretes its product to the outside world. Exocrine glands are classified by their structure. Unicellular exocrine glands are isolated secretory cells in an epithelium. In humans, unicellular exocrine glands are found in portions of the linings of the respiratory and digestive tracts. These cells are called *goblet cells* due to their shape. A goblet cell secretes mucus from its apical end—that is, the end that faces the "outside world." The mucus forms a protective layer over the epithelial surface.

Multicellular exocrine glands have two basic parts. One part is a secretory unit composed of cells that make and secrete a glandular product. The other part is a duct that connects the secretory unit to the surface of the epithelium.

An exocrine gland is considered simple if it has a single, unbranched duct, or compound if the duct branches off to multiple secretory units. The secretory units of a gland may be tubular or alveolar (spherical). Some secretory units have both shapes and are therefore called *tubuloalveolar* (too-byool-oh-al-VEE-oh-lar) glands. **Figure 3.7** shows examples of different types of exocrine glands.

SELF CHECK

1. Where in the body are epithelial tissues found?
2. What are the two surfaces of an epithelium?
3. Describe the characteristics of a stratified squamous epithelium.
4. What is the difference between an exocrine gland and an endocrine gland?

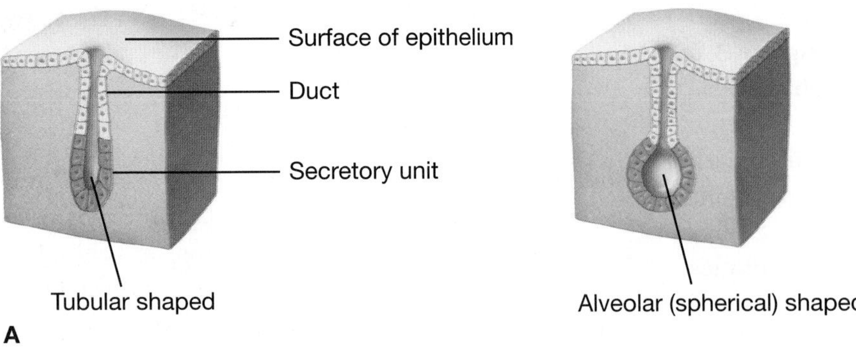

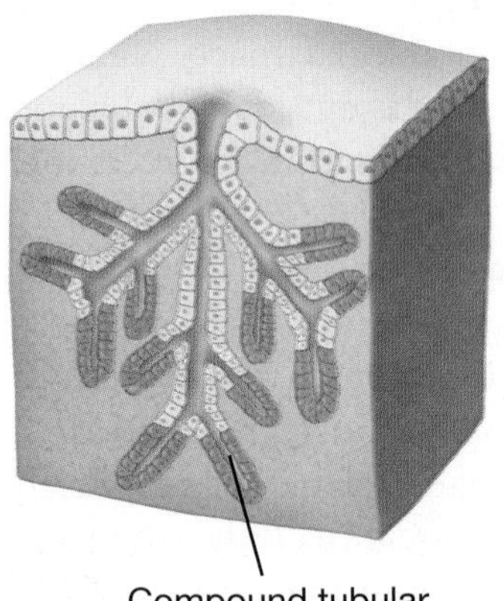

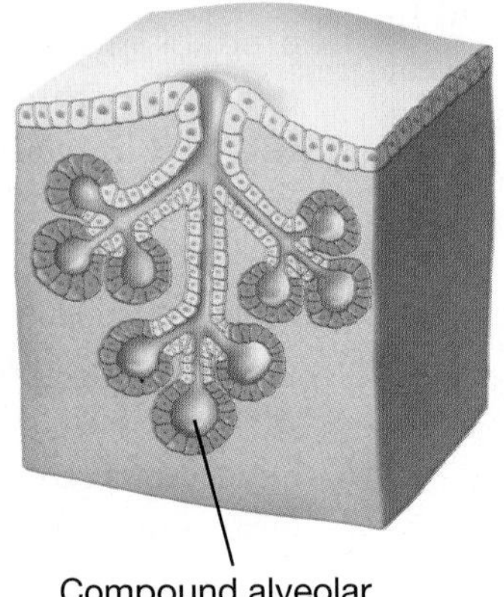

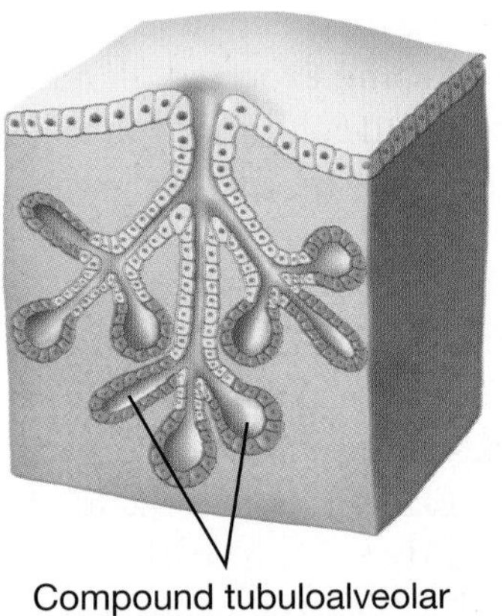

Figure 3.7 The basic structures of multicellular exocrine glands. A—A simple duct structure has a single duct to the secretory unit. B—A compound duct structure has a duct that branches before reaching the secretory units.

Connective Tissue

Connective tissue is found throughout the body, and it comprises several major classes: connective tissue proper, cartilage, bone, and blood. Blood connects distant areas of the body by circulating to all regions and carrying substances from place to place. Chapter 11 describes the blood in more detail.

All forms of connective tissue include both cells and the material in between cells, called the *extracellular matrix*. Each major class of connective tissue has distinctive cells and a different extracellular matrix (**Figure 3.8**).

The extracellular matrix of any connective tissue includes fibers that play an important role in determining the strength and elasticity of the tissue. Three types of fibers are found in connective tissue, although not all connective tissue contains all types of fibers.

Collagen fibers are formed from tropocollagen proteins that link together. Collagen fibers are strong and resistant to stretch. They give tensile strength to tissue.

Reticular fibers are thinner and weaker than collagen fibers. They help to provide a structural framework that keeps cells in place.

Elastic fibers can lengthen considerably when stretched, and then spring back to their original length when the stretching force is removed. Elastic fibers give springiness, or elasticity, to tissues.

Tension, Compression, and Elasticity

The word *tension* is often used to describe a state of mental or emotional stress or anxiety. Tension also has an older meaning, which is still used by physiologists and engineers: a force that pulls something apart. ***Tensile strength*** is the ability to withstand a pulling force. The opposite of tension is *compression*: a force that pushes in. ***Compressive strength*** is the ability to withstand compression.

A rope illustrates the difference between tensile and compressive strength: it has tensile strength, as is evident during a tug-of-war, but no compressive strength. If you try to push the ends of a rope together, it does not resist.

Major Classes of Connective Tissue					
Class	**Subclasses**	**Cells**	**Extracellular Matrix**	**Extracellular Fibers**	**General Features**
Connective tissue proper	loose • areolar • reticular • adipose	fibroblasts adipocytes mast cells macrophages lymphocytes	loose includes fibers; areolar is gel-like; adipose has very little	all three subclasses: • collagen • reticular • elastic	variety of locations and functions; loose tissue provides support, strength, and elasticity; plays a role in immune defenses
	dense • regular • irregular • elastic		dense is mainly fibers; little else		dense fibers provide tensile strength and elasticity; resist stretching
Cartilage	hyaline elastic fibrocartilage	chondroblasts chondrocytes	secreted by chondroblasts; contains proteoglycan molecules, which blend to immobilize water molecules	collagen in all; elastic in some	provides support and flexibility; minimizes friction
Bone (osseous) tissue	cortical (compact) trabecular (spongy)	osteoblasts osteocytes (see Chapter 5 for more information)	secreted by osteoblasts	collagen	provides framework; protects organs; supports body
Blood	no major classes; see cell types in Chapter 11	red blood cells (erythrocytes); white blood cells (leukocytes); platelets	plasma	none	provides transportation, regulation, and protection; carries oxygen and nutrients to cells; carries away wastes and carbon dioxide

Figure 3.8

Goodheart-Willcox Publisher

Elasticity is the ability to stretch when tension is applied, and then spring back to the original length when tension is withdrawn. Elastic fibers give elasticity to skin. Unfortunately, elastic fibers in skin, like the elastic fibers in clothes, tend to lose their elasticity as they get older. As a result, skin and clothes tend to become more baggy and wrinkly with age.

Connective Tissue Proper

Connective tissue proper is often subdivided into two categories: loose and dense. Loose connective tissue includes cells and an extracellular matrix that has fibers running through it. Dense connective tissue includes relatively few cells and an extracellular matrix that is composed mainly of fibers.

Loose Connective Tissue

Loose connective tissue includes areolar, reticular, and adipose tissue. Areolar connective tissue is found throughout the body, typically as a layer beneath epithelial tissues (**Figure 3.9**). It has collagen fibers, reticular fibers, and elastic fibers in its gel-like extracellular matrix, which can hold water. It provides support, strength, and elasticity to overlying epithelia. Areolar connective tissue also plays a role in inflammation and immune system defenses because it contains most of the key cell types involved in these processes, including mast cells, macrophages, and lymphocytes.

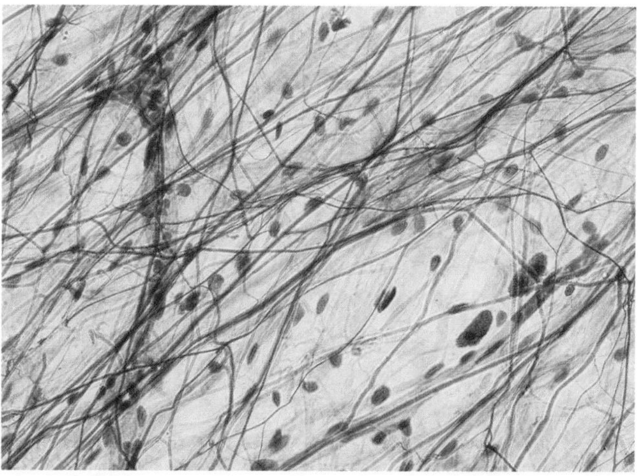

Science Stock Photography/Science Source

Figure 3.9 Light micrograph of areolar connective tissue.

Reticular connective tissue, which contains mostly reticular fibers in its extracellular matrix, is found in lymph nodes, bone marrow, and the spleen. Reticular connective tissue provides a loose framework for blood cell formation in bone marrow, and for immune system defenses in the spleen and lymph nodes. Since it has few collagen fibers, reticular connective tissue is not very strong. This is not a problem for bone marrow, which is surrounded by protective bone. However, this lack of strength can be problematic for the spleen, which can be torn or ruptured by a sharp blow to the abdomen.

Adipose connective tissue consists almost entirely of fat cells (adipocytes), with very little extracellular matrix (**Figure 3.10**). This tissue provides a reservoir of metabolic fuel and generates hormones that regulate metabolism. It also provides thermal insulation and cushioning for organs. Adipose tissue located just under the skin is called *subcutaneous fat*, and adipose tissue in the abdomen or thorax is called *visceral fat*. A small fraction of adipose tissue is relatively rich in mitochondria, the intracellular organelles that produce ATP (described in Chapter 2). This gives the tissue a brown color, so it is called *brown adipose tissue*, or *brown fat*. However, most adipose tissue has few mitochondria, so it is called *white adipose tissue* or *white fat*. The tissue shown in Figure 3.10 is white adipose tissue. Brown fat is metabolically more active than white fat, and it plays a key role in body temperature regulation and cold adaptation.

Dense Connective Tissue

As mentioned earlier, dense connective tissue contains few cells, and its extracellular matrix is made up primarily of fibers. The three types of dense connective tissue are regular, irregular, and elastic tissue.

Dense regular connective tissue consists of collagen fibers that are mostly parallel to one another (**Figure 3.11**). It contains occasional fibroblasts, which secrete collagen. Dense regular connective tissue is found in tendons and ligaments. Its abundant collagen fibers give it high tensile strength, particularly when pulled parallel to the fiber direction.

Dense irregular connective tissue is also composed primarily of collagen fibers. However, unlike those in dense regular connective tissue, the fibers are not all parallel; they run in all directions. As a result, dense irregular connective tissue is good at resisting stretching forces from a variety of directions. It is found in the dermis (the deep layer of the skin) and in the fibrous capsules around joints, among other places.

Dense elastic connective tissue has an extracellular matrix full of elastic fibers (**Figure 3.12**). Not surprisingly, it is highly elastic. This tissue is found in the walls of the airways and large arteries.

Cartilage

Cartilage is part of the skeleton, and it provides support and cushioning where bones join. It also minimizes friction when bones move relative to one another. Cartilage is found between bones and on the ends of bones.

Chondroblasts secrete the extracellular matrix of cartilage. This matrix contains collagen fibers and proteoglycan (proh-tee-oh-GLIGH-kan) molecules (proteins with carbohydrates added), including hyaluronic acid and chondroitin. These large molecules bind to and immobilize many water molecules.

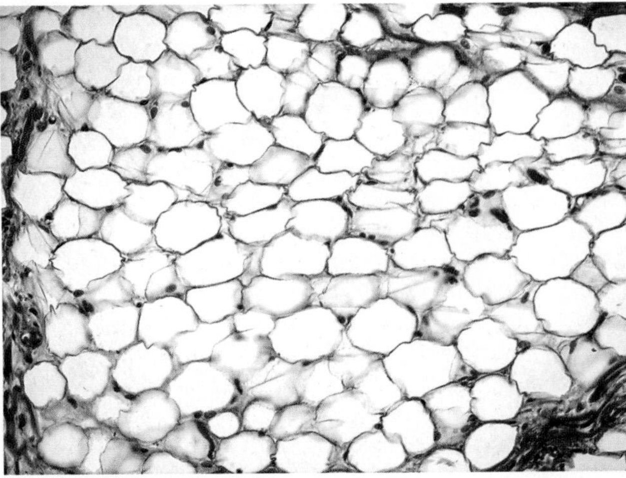

Alvin Telser/Science Source

Figure 3.10 Light micrograph of adipose connective tissue.

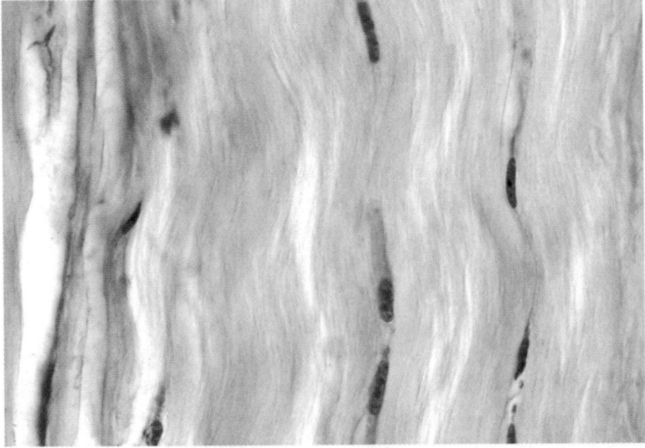

Alvin Telser/Science Source

Figure 3.11 Light micrograph of dense regular connective tissue (human tendon).

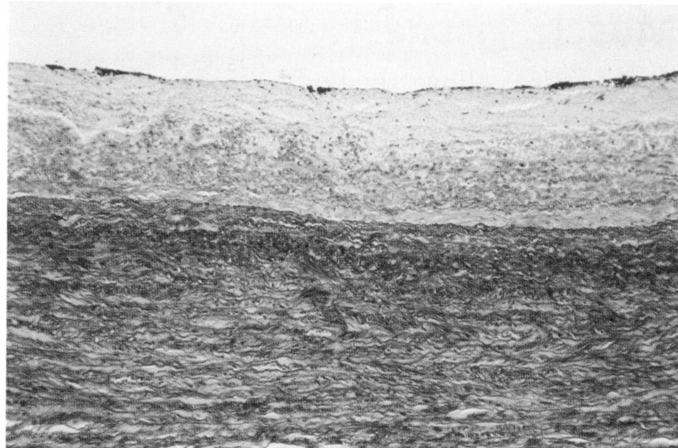

Astrid & Hanns-Frieder Michler / Science Source

Figure 3.12 Light micrograph of dense elastic connective tissue.

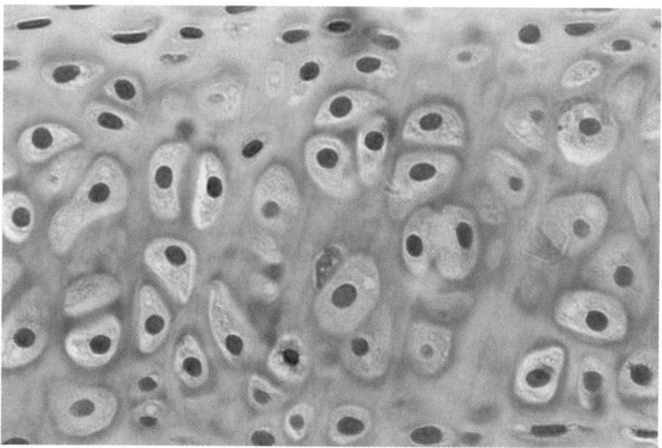

Chuck Brown/Science Source

Figure 3.13 Light micrograph of hyaline cartilage, showing lacunae and chondrocytes.

The large amount of "bound water" in cartilage, and the fact that water is incompressible, explains why cartilage is highly resistant to compression. The high water content also helps make cartilage a low-friction surface, which can make cartilage feel slippery.

The most common form of cartilage is hyaline cartilage, shown in **Figure 3.13**. The smooth, shiny substance at the end of a chicken or turkey leg bone is hyaline cartilage. Hyaline cartilage acts as a smooth covering on the ends of long bones, and it covers the ends of the ribs where they connect to the sternum, or breastbone. It is also found in the nose, trachea (windpipe), and larynx (voice box).

Elastic cartilage is similar to hyaline cartilage, but it contains more elastic fibers, which allow it to bend and spring back to its original shape. Elastic cartilage is found in the external ear and in the epiglottis, a flap of tissue in the throat that prevents food and water from entering the lungs.

Fibrocartilage has more collagen fibers than hyaline or elastic cartilage, so it has more tensile strength. Fibrocartilage is found in the discs between vertebrae and in the discs in the knee joint.

Bone

Bone, also known as ***osseous tissue***, protects organs and supports the body, providing a rigid framework on which muscles can pull (**Figure 3.14**). Osteoblasts secrete the extracellular matrix of bone. This matrix contains collagen fibers, which give bone its tensile strength, and calcium salts, which make bone hard and give it compressive strength. The structure and function of bone is discussed in more detail in Chapter 5.

Understanding Medical Terminology

The combining forms *blast/o* and *cyt/o* are used in many cell names. *Blast/o* is derived from the Greek word for "bud," and it has traditionally been used to denote a cell that can give rise to (precede) a variety of daughter cells. The words *blastula* and *blastocyst*, which refer to early stages in embryo development, are based on this combining form.

Blast cells are sometimes called *stem cells*, which seems reasonable given the close relationship between buds and stems. The descendant cells of stem cells can branch out and develop into various subtypes of specialized mature cells.

The combining form *blast/o* is now also used for cells that actively secrete components of the extracellular matrix, especially with regard to connective tissue. For example, fibroblasts secrete collagen (which is used to make fibers, hence the combining form *fibr/o*). Chondroblasts secrete proteoglycans in cartilage, and osteoblasts secrete osteoid, which hardens into bone.

The combining form *cyt/o* comes from the Greek word for "container," and it is used to refer to cells in general. *Cytology* is the study of cells. When compared to the traditional use of *blast/o* to denote a stem cell, *cyt/o* usually denotes a mature cell that, unlike a blast cell, can only produce descendants that are identical to the parent, or that cannot divide at all. For example, lymphoblasts give rise to lymphocytes, and erythroblasts give rise to erythrocytes. In connective tissue, *cyt/o* is also used to denote a cell that is quiescent—that is, it does not actively secrete extracellular matrix components. Thus the terms *osteocyte*, *fibrocyte* (rare), and *chondrocyte*.

SELF CHECK

1. Identify the four classes of connective tissue.
2. Explain the difference between tensile strength and compressive strength.
3. What is the difference between loose connective tissue and dense connective tissue?
4. What is the function of chondroblasts?
5. Which type of cells is responsible for producing the extracellular matrix of bone?

Muscle Tissue

Muscle tissue allows the body to move. The distinguishing property of muscle is its ability to generate force on command. All muscle cells use intracellular filaments made of actin and myosin proteins to generate force, and they all require ATP as fuel for contraction.

The three kinds of muscle tissue are skeletal, cardiac, and smooth muscle. Skeletal and cardiac muscle are both called *striated muscle* because striations, or stripes, can be seen on them when viewed through a light microscope.

Research Notes Artificial Tissues

There is no substitute for the tissues of a healthy human body. However, when tissue is lost due to illness or accident, artificial tissues can play an important role, either temporarily or permanently. The development of artificial tissues requires the collaboration of cell biologists, chemists, engineers, and physicians, among others. A successful artificial tissue recreates key physiological functions and anatomical features of the real tissue. In addition, artificial tissue must be *biocompatible*, which means it will not provoke an attack from the recipient's immune system.

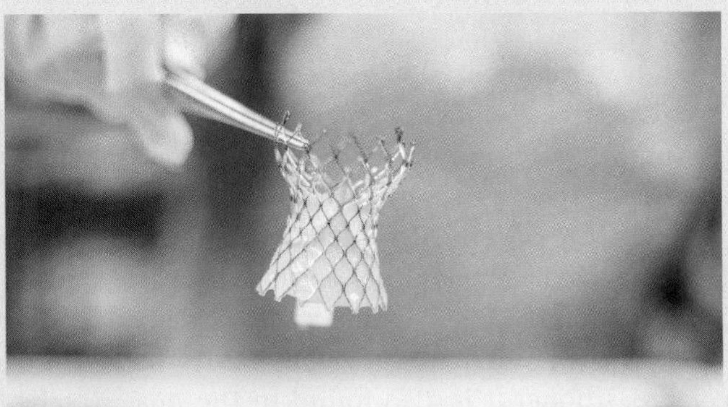

Pan Xunbin/Science Source

Heart Valves

A heart valve can be replaced if it has become damaged and nonfunctional due to disease. An ideal replacement heart valve allows blood to flow easily and without disruption in the right direction at the right times, stops blood flow when it should be stopped, lasts a lifetime, and does not trigger the formation of blood clots. Although an ideal replacement heart valve does not exist, replacement options do exist.

Approximately half of the hundreds of thousands of heart valves replaced annually are artificial. The other half are bioprosthetic, which means they are derived from cow or pig heart valves and tissues. Both artificial and bioprosthetic heart valves have advantages and disadvantages. Artificial heart valves made of carbon fiber, plastic, Dacron®, or similar materials are more durable than bioprosthetic valves, but they are more likely to cause blood clots.

A new type of replacement heart valve includes both artificial and bioprosthetic components, and it is arranged in a tightly folded configuration. This replacement valve is inserted through the femoral artery in the leg and guided up to its final position in the heart. This allows replacement of the aortic heart valve in patients who, for medical reasons, cannot undergo traditional valve replacement surgery.

Blood Substitutes

A blood substitute would be of great value for trauma victims and some surgical patients. Donated blood saves many lives, but it has a limited shelf life and must be matched to the recipient. Donated blood can also carry disease, although it very rarely does, due to extremely rigorous screening. For these reasons, scientists have been trying for decades to develop "artificial blood."

Blood has many functions, but perhaps the most important is the delivery of oxygen to tissues. Solutions of saline and polymers such as dextran are valuable for replacing lost blood volume and restoring blood pressure, but they do not have the oxygen-carrying ability of blood.

Bioengineered versions of hemoglobin, and chemicals known as *fluorocarbons*, have been investigated as potential oxygen carriers for artificial blood. Scientists continue to investigate possible oxygen carriers. One approach currently in development is to modify the genes of stem cells so that they can efficiently produce daughter red blood cells in a laboratory setting. The fact that scientists have not yet developed a good substitute for blood, despite decades of effort, demonstrates the complexity of tissue engineering.

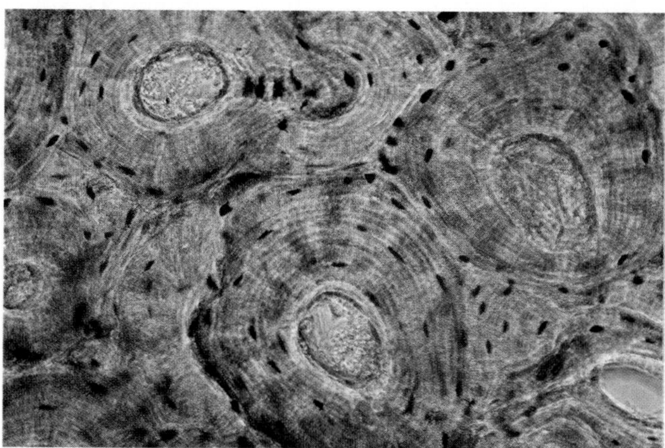

Science Stock Photography/Science Source

Figure 3.14 Light micrograph of human bone.

Skeletal muscle, by far the most common type of muscle, pulls on bones to make the body move (**Figure 3.15**). Skeletal muscle cells are long and thin. They have multiple nuclei because they are formed when multiple embryonic cells merge. The striations in skeletal muscle are at right angles to the long axis of the cells.

Cardiac muscle is the major tissue of the heart. It is similar to skeletal muscle, but its cells are much shorter. Because the heart never stops working, cardiac muscle must generate ATP continuously. As a result, cardiac muscle cells have many mitochondria.

Smooth muscle is found in the walls of hollow organs, including the bladder, uterus, GI tract, airways, and blood vessels. As the name implies, the cytoplasm of smooth muscle cells appears uniform, or smooth, under a light microscope.

SELF CHECK

1. Identify the three types of muscle tissue.
2. Which types of muscle tissue are striated?

Nerve Tissue

Nerve tissue is found in all parts of the body. It is most concentrated in the brain and spinal cord, which comprise the central nervous system.

The nerves outside the brain and spinal cord comprise the peripheral nervous system. The peripheral nervous system has separate nerve fibers for sending out signals (motor commands to the muscles and glands) and for receiving incoming signals (sensory signals from the eyes, ears, skin, and other sensory organs).

Nerve tissue includes supporting cells, called *glial* (GLIGH-al) *cells* (from the root word for "glue"), and ***neurons***, which are the cells in the nervous system that generate, transmit, and receive electrical signals. **Figure 3.16** shows neurons in the brain. An individual neuron has a compact cell body and extensions that carry electrical signals to its targets (muscles, glands, or other neurons) and receive input from other neurons. Chapter 7 describes nerve tissue in more detail.

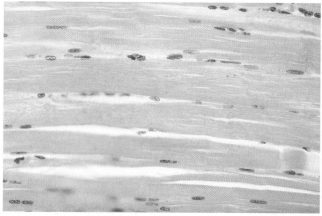

Science Photo Library

Figure 3.15 Skeletal muscle.

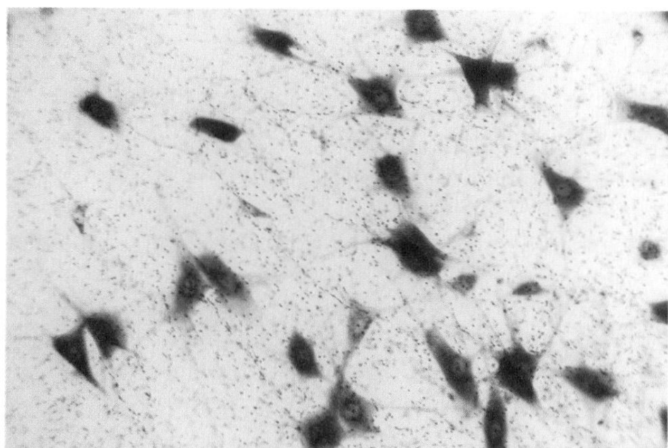

Manfred Kage/Science Source

Figure 3.16 Light micrograph of a neuron. The dark-staining *soma*, or cell body, has dendrites and an axon extending from it.

SECTION 3.2

REVIEW

Mini-Glossary

cardiac muscle the major muscle tissue of the heart
cartilage a class of connective tissue that provides support and flexibility to parts of the skeleton
chondroblasts cells that secrete the extracellular matrix of cartilage
compressive strength the ability of a material to withstand compression (inward-pressing force) without buckling
elasticity the ability of a material to stretch when tension is applied, and spring back to its original shape when the tension is removed
endocrine gland a gland that secretes its product into the interstitial space
exocrine gland a gland that secretes its product to the outside world
glands epithelial cells that are organized to produce and secrete substances
lumen the hollow, inner portion of a body cavity or tube
neurons cells that generate, transmit, and receive electrical signals
osseous tissue bone tissue
simple epithelia epithelia that have a single layer of cells
skeletal muscle the most common type of muscle tissue; usually attached to bone and helps the body move
smooth muscle the muscle tissue found in the walls of hollow organs
stratified epithelia epithelia that have multiple layers of cells
tensile strength the ability of a material to withstand tension (outward-pulling force) without tearing or breaking

Review Questions

1. What is the difference between simple and stratified epithelia?
2. What are the two types of glands and how do they differ?
3. What type of strength do collagen fibers provide to tissues?
4. The most common type of cartilage is ____.
5. Bone is also known as ____ tissue.
6. Identify the two types of protein that make up the intracellular filaments in muscle.
7. Compare and contrast skeletal and cardiac muscles. What do they have in common? How are they different?
8. What would be the consequences if the human body lacked internal epithelial tissues?
9. Assume that you are looking at cell cultures from the lining of the stomach, the wall of the heart, and a leg muscle, but the slides are not labeled. How can you identify the location of each culture?

SECTION 3.3

Disorders of the Body Tissues

Objectives

- Identify and describe major disorders that affect epithelial tissue.
- Describe the disorders that selectively affect connective tissue.
- Explain the histological classifications for carcinomas.

Key Terms

biopsy
carcinoma
cystic fibrosis
eczema
leukemia
lymphoma
Marfan syndrome
sarcoma
systemic lupus erythematosus

One of the best ways to understand a disease is to learn how it affects the body at the cellular and tissue levels. The cause and progression of a disease, the symptoms that patients experience, and the effects of treatment all make more sense when you know what a disease does to particular tissues.

Pathology, the study of the causes of disease, requires the microscopic examination of tissue specimens, often obtained through a biopsy. A ***biopsy*** is the removal of a tissue sample for microscopic examination to diagnose disease.

Epithelial Tissue Disorders

In addition to separating the inside of the body from the external environment, epithelial tissues comprise glands that make and secrete various substances. Disorders of epithelial tissue disrupt these key functions.

Cancer often originates in epithelial tissue. Other relatively common diseases affecting epithelial tissue include eczema and cystic fibrosis. Burns are injuries to epithelial tissue that will be discussed in Chapter 4.

Eczema

Eczema, also known as *atopic dermatitis*, is the most common skin condition. The hallmark symptom of eczema is unrelenting itchiness in affected areas of skin. This condition usually begins within the first year of life. In eczema, the barrier function of the skin's epithelial layer is disrupted due to a combination of genetic and environmental factors. These factors seem to interfere with the physical connections between neighboring epithelial cells. As a result, the skin dries out and becomes itchy. Inflammation and scratching further disrupt the integrity of the epithelium and increase the likelihood of infection (**Figure 3.17**).

Most patients experience periods of remission, when the condition improves, and periods of exacerbation, when the condition worsens. There is no cure for eczema, but it often spontaneously resolves itself around the time of puberty. As they get older, children with eczema have a higher than normal likelihood of developing allergic conditions that involve epithelial tissues, such as nasal allergies, food allergies, and asthma.

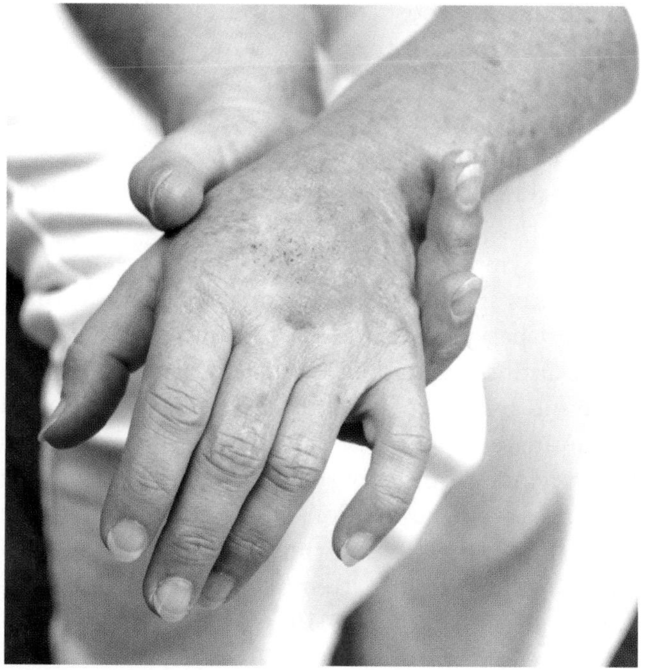

AJPhoto/Science Source

Figure 3.17 Eczema results in dry, itchy, inflamed skin. Scratching the site should be avoided because it may lead to infection.

Treatment for eczema includes the use of skin creams or ointments that have a high lipid content. These products prevent drying of the skin by partially correcting the loss of barrier integrity. Patients may reduce the severity of exacerbations by avoiding triggers such as wool clothing. Drugs that block activation of immune cells can also help treat eczema.

Cystic Fibrosis

Cystic fibrosis is one of the most common inherited diseases. The condition is caused by mutations in a gene known as the cystic fibrosis transmembrane conductance regulator (CFTR). The CFTR gene regulates the movement of chloride ions across cell membranes, so mutations in this gene disrupt the flow of chloride ions. Cystic fibrosis shows an autosomal recessive pattern of inheritance: A person with one good CFTR gene and one bad CFTR gene has no symptoms, but a person with two bad CFTR genes will have cystic fibrosis.

Exocrine glands, which are a form of epithelial tissue, are affected by defective CFTR genes. The altered transport of chloride that results from a CFTR mutation causes the fluid secretions of exocrine glands to be abnormally salty and abnormally thick, creating buildup in many areas of the body.

The thick secretions of the pancreas plug up the organ's ducts. This means the digestive enzymes made in the pancreas cannot reach the small intestine, causing nutritional deficits. It also results in the formation of cysts and scar tissue (fibrosis) in the pancreas, giving the condition its name. Mucus that coats the epithelium of the airways is so thick that it plugs up the airways, resulting in recurrent infections that cause cumulative lung damage, which is the usual cause of death in cystic fibrosis patients. Other secretory glands are also affected.

There is no cure for cystic fibrosis. However, improved treatment of symptoms has increased the life expectancy of cystic fibrosis patients in the United States to over 40 years of age.

SELF CHECK

1. When does eczema typically first appear?
2. Which epithelial tissue disorder affects exocrine glands?
3. Which gene is defective in cystic fibrosis patients?

Connective Tissue Disorders

There are many disorders that selectively affect connective tissue. Some connective tissue disorders occur due to changes in certain genes that are inherited from one or both parents. Others are autoimmune diseases. This means the disease symptoms occur because the immune system makes antibodies that target the body's own tissues. The root cause of autoimmune illness is unclear in many cases. This section discusses two connective tissue disorders: Marfan syndrome and systemic lupus erythematosus. Marfan syndrome is an inherited disorder, and systemic lupus erythematosus is autoimmune.

Marfan Syndrome

Marfan syndrome is an inherited connective tissue disease. It is caused by mutation in the FBN1 gene, which provides instructions for making the protein fibrillin-1. Fibrillin-1 is a glycoprotein (a protein-carbohydrate complex) that is present in the extracellular matrix of connective tissues throughout the body. Fibrillin-1 helps make connective tissue strong. A mutation in the FBN1 gene can reduce the amount of available fibrillin-1. The symptoms and severity of Marfan syndrome differ depending on the specific mutation in the fibrillin-1 gene. Symptoms may be present at birth; others may not become apparent until later in life.

The skeletal system, the cardiovascular system, and the eyes are most often affected by Marfan syndrome. Skeletal abnormalities are the most obvious effects of this condition. Patients with Marfan syndrome are tall and thin. Their fingers, toes, arms, and legs are unusually long in comparison to their height (**Figure 3.18**). They may develop scoliosis, an abnormal curvature of the spine. Their sternum (breastbone) may be sunken, or it may stick out more than normal. Patients with Marfan syndrome also have unusually flexible joints.

The ocular, or eye-related, symptoms of Marfan syndrome include significant nearsightedness, as well as heightened risk of a detached retina or a dislocated lens. The cardiovascular symptoms of Marfan syndrome are the most serious because they can be life threatening. These symptoms include an increased risk of bulging or tearing of the aorta, the largest artery in the body. Patients may also have an unusually floppy and ineffective mitral valve. The mitral valve is a tissue flap that prevents blood from traveling "backward" through the heart.

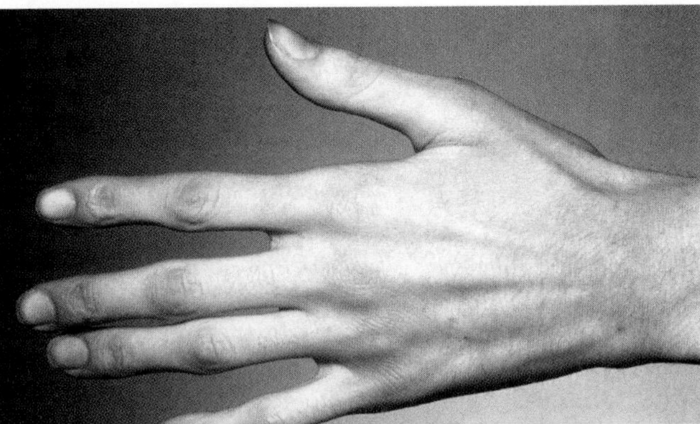

Tim Joyce and The Marfan Foundation, marfan.org

Figure 3.18 A patient with Marfan syndrome is tall, thin, and has unusually long arms, fingers, legs, and toes. Notice the long fingers on this patient's hand.

There is no cure for Marfan syndrome. When Marfan syndrome has been diagnosed, the patient can have regular check-ups to identify and treat problems as soon as they occur.

Systemic Lupus Erythematosus

Systemic lupus erythematosus, also known as *lupus* or *SLE*, is an autoimmune disease in which cells of the immune system attack the body's own connective tissue. Because all organs include connective tissue, almost any organ system may be affected by this condition. The most commonly affected organs and structures include the skin, kidneys, joints, nerve tissue, and blood cells. Lupus has a strong genetic component, and many different genes can be involved in the condition's development.

The severity of SLE, and the organ systems affected by it, varies greatly. Over 90% of SLE cases occur in women. Symptoms usually first appear between 20 and 40 years of age, but the disease may begin at any time.

Most patients with SLE have immune cells that make antibodies to their own DNA. This causes the immune system to attack body tissues, resulting in inflammation and tissue damage. Specific symptoms may include a butterfly-shaped rash across the nose and cheeks, inflammation of the connective tissue coverings of the lungs or the heart, inflammation of the joints (arthritis), extreme sensitivity to light, and kidney disease (**Figure 3.19**).

There is no cure for lupus. However, certain drugs can reduce the likelihood of flare-ups and manage specific symptoms. Researchers continue to seek

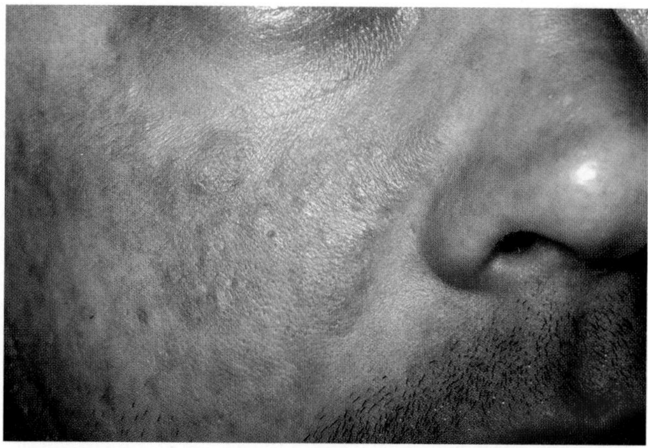

Dr P. Marazzi / Science Source

Figure 3.19 A lupus skin rash is often referred to as a butterfly rash because of the shape of the affected area on the face, along both cheeks and over the nose.

better drug treatments and a better understanding of what causes the immune system to attack the body's own tissues.

SELF CHECK

1. Which gene's mutation causes Marfan syndrome?
2. What are the most obvious effects of Marfan syndrome?
3. Which organs and structures are commonly affected by lupus?

Cancer Classifications

Cancer is a condition characterized by the uncontrolled growth and spread of abnormal cells. Cancers can be classified by the type of tissue in which they originate (the histological classification), or by the location in the body where they originate (lung, breast, and so on). The histological classifications for cancers include carcinoma, sarcoma, lymphoma, leukemia, and others.

Carcinomas originate in epithelial tissue, including glands. ***Sarcomas*** originate in connective tissue, including bone and muscle. ***Lymphomas*** are solid tumors that originate in lymph nodes and other lymphatic tissues (see Chapter 13). ***Leukemias*** are "liquid cancers" of the white blood cells that cause the bone marrow to produce abnormal white blood cells.

About 80–90% of cancers are carcinomas, including most of the top four types of cancer in the United States: lung, breast, prostate, and colorectal (colon and rectum). Most carcinomas originate in glandular epithelial tissues, including the breast (mammary gland) and the prostate gland. Although the lungs, colon, and rectum are not glands, they contain unicellular exocrine glands, which secrete mucus. Almost half of lung cancers, and most colorectal cancers, originate from these mucus-secreting cells. Other lung cancers arise from squamous epithelial cells and other sources.

Understanding Medical Terminology

The ancient Greek physician Hippocrates thought that tumors looked like crabs, with a solid central body and arms that extended into surrounding tissue. Therefore, he gave the disease the name *karkinos*, the ancient Greek word for "crab." From this word, we get the term *carcinoma*, a cancer that originates in epithelial tissue. When people say *cancer* or *carcinoma*, they are really saying *crab*.

SECTION 3.3 REVIEW

Mini-Glossary

biopsy removal of a tissue sample for microscopic examination to diagnose disease

carcinoma cancer that originates in the epithelial tissue

cystic fibrosis a common inherited disease that causes exocrine gland secretions to become abnormally thick, creating buildup

eczema a common skin condition that is characterized by unrelenting itchiness in affected areas of skin; also known as *atopic dermatitis*

leukemia cancer that affects the bone marrow, causing production of abnormal white blood cells

lymphoma cancer that originates in lymph nodes and other lymphatic tissues

Marfan syndrome an inherited connective tissue disease that causes skeletal, ocular, and cardiovascular symptoms

sarcoma cancer that originates in connective tissue

systemic lupus erythematosus an autoimmune disease in which the immune system attacks the body's own connective tissue; also known as *lupus* or *SLE*

(continued)

Review Questions

1. What is the scientific name for eczema?
2. Describe the most common treatments for eczema.
3. What are the physiological effects of the gene mutation that causes cystic fibrosis?
4. Which type of tissue is affected when the body's supply of fibrillin-1 is decreased?
5. What is an autoimmune disease?
6. Into which cancer classification do colon, breast, and prostate cancer fall?
7. In what way are leukemias different from all other classifications of cancer?

Medical Terminology: Body Tissues

By understanding the word parts that make up medical words, you can extend your medical vocabulary. This chapter includes many of the word parts listed below. Review these word parts to be sure you understand their meanings.

-ar	pertaining to
blast/o	embryonic or immature cell
cellul/o	cell
chondr/o	cartilage
derm/o	skin
ecto-	outer, outside
endo-	inner, within
exo-	out, away from
extra-	outside
meso-	middle
-meter	equipment, device
neur/o	nerve
-oma	tumor
ophthalm/o	eye
osse/o	bone, bony
tens/o	stretched
uni-	one

Now use these word parts to form valid medical words that fit the following definitions. Some of the words are included in this chapter. Others are not. When you finish, use a medical dictionary to check your work.

1. inner layer of the skin
2. pertaining to outside a cell
3. inflammation of the middle of a nerve
4. within the larynx
5. the outer layer of a cyst
6. pertaining to bone
7. machine for measuring tension
8. protrusion of the eyeball
9. consisting of one cell
10. embryonic cartilage cell
11. relating to both bone and cartilage
12. tumor of embryonic cells

Chapter 3 Summary

- The four main types of body tissues are epithelial, connective, muscle, and nerve tissue.
- The bundle of cells that make up a 16-day-old embryo contains three layers: the ectoderm, mesoderm, and endoderm—from which all body tissues originate.
- Epithelial tissues include epithelia—the skin and linings of internal body cavities—and glands, which secrete chemicals.
- Connective tissue comprises several major classes: connective tissue proper, cartilage, bone, and blood.
- Muscle tissues generate force to move the body.
- Nerve tissue conveys information through the body via electrical signals.
- Common epithelial tissue disorders include atopic dermatitis (eczema) and cystic fibrosis.
- Marfan syndrome and systemic lupus erythematosus are disorders that specifically affect connective tissue.
- The histological classifications for cancer include carcinoma, sarcoma, lymphoma, and leukemia.

Chapter 3 Review

Understanding Key Concepts

1. The study of tissues is called ______.
2. The type of tissue that acts as a barrier between the body and the outside world is ______.
   A. nerve tissue
   B. muscle tissue
   C. connective tissue
   D. epithelial tissue

3. One purpose of connective tissue is to ______.
   A. convey information throughout the body
   B. help maintain the proper shape of organs
   C. provide sensory information
   D. create body movement
4. Tissues derived from the ______ include the gastrointestinal tract and the lining of the lungs.
5. The process by which cells change from one type to another, more specialized type is known as ______.
6. One of the most common birth defects is a congenital disorder of the nervous system called ______.
7. Epithelial tissues have two different surfaces: an apical surface and a ______ surface.
8. Which of the following functions is *not* accomplished by the epithelial tissues?
   A. providing support and strength to connective tissues
   B. protecting the body from physical damage
   C. providing sensory information
   D. determining which substances enter and leave the body
9. The hollow inside part of a body cavity or tube is called the ______.
10. What is the difference between simple and stratified epithelia?
11. The lining of the abdominal cavity is an example of a simple ______ epithelia.
12. Stratified epithelia that change their shape depending on whether the tissue is stretched are known as ______ epithelia.
13. A(n) ______ gland is one that secretes a product into the interstitial space of a tissue.
14. The two parts of a multicellular exocrine gland are the secretory unit and the ______.
15. *True or False?* Blood is a type of connective tissue.
16. *True or False?* Collagen fibers are very elastic.
17. The type of fibers in connective tissue that help keep cells in place are ______ fibers.
18. Which of the following is *not* a connective tissue?
   A. cartilage
   B. epithelia
   C. blood
   D. bone
19. What kind of epithelia make up alveoli?
20. Which of the following is *not* a form of loose connective tissue?
   A. adipose
   B. areolar
   C. columnar
   D. reticular
21. Explain why cartilage is resistant to compression.
22. Identify three types of cartilage.
23. What type of cells secrete the extracellular matrix of cartilage?
24. One of the functions of osseous tissue is to provide a rigid ______ on which muscles can pull.
25. Where in the body is smooth muscle found?
26. Which of the following is typically not the target of a neuron's electrical signals?
   A. muscles
   B. bones
   C. glands
   D. other neurons
27. The study of the causes of disease is ______.
   A. histology
   B. biopsy
   C. biology
   D. pathology
28. A tissue sample for microscopic examination and disease diagnosis is obtained by performing a(n) ______.
29. The major symptom of eczema is ______.
30. Fluid secretions from the exocrine glands of a person who has cystic fibrosis are ______.
   A. frothy
   B. pinkish in color
   C. thick and salty
   D. highly infectious
31. The most common cause of death in cystic fibrosis patients is ______.
   A. cumulative lung damage
   B. chronic heart disease
   C. pancreatitis
   D. nutritional deficiency
32. Diseases in which the body's immune cells make antibodies that target the body's own tissues are known as ______ diseases.

33. A mutation in the FBN1 gene causes ______.
    A. cystic fibrosis
    B. Marfan syndrome
    C. systemic lupus erythematosus
    D. sarcoma
34. The ______ symptoms of Marfan syndrome can be life-threatening, including a heightened risk of tearing of the aorta.

Thinking Critically

35. Why is it important to avoid scratching the skin during episodes of eczema?
36. Why do people with only one mutated CFTR gene show no sign of disease?
37. Review the general properties of epithelial tissue and connective tissue. Then explain why connective tissue is better suited than epithelial tissue for constructing cartilage.
38. Evaluate the cause and effect of cancer on the structure and function of cells, tissues, organs, and systems.

Clinical Case Study

Read again the Clinical Case Study at the beginning of this chapter. Use the information provided in the chapter to answer the following questions.

39. What is a possible common thread connecting Sara's shoulder injury, physical presentation, and past medical history?
40. What connective tissue disorders might Sara have?

Analyzing and Evaluating Data

The chart below summarizes the percentage of children under the age of 18 diagnosed with eczema or a related skin allergy from 2000 to 2010. Use the chart to answer the following questions.

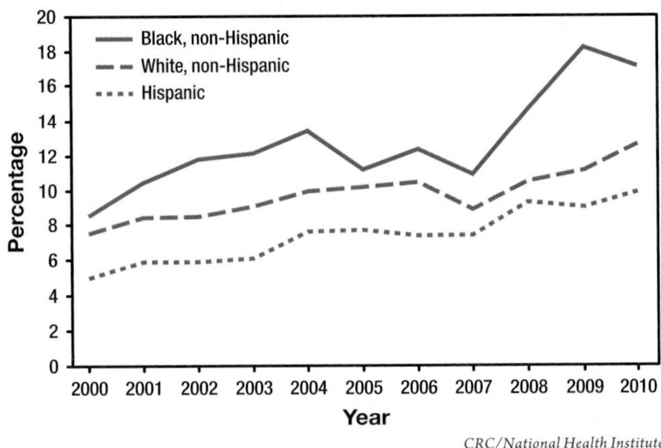

CRC/National Health Institute

41. In which group did the percentage of children decrease between 2004 and 2005?
42. What is the overall trend for all of the racial/ethnic groups included in the study for the first decade of the 21st century?
43. By what percentage did the incidence of eczema increase in Hispanics between the year 2000 and the year 2004?

Investigating Further

44. Investigate and describe current research in therapeutic measures for cystic fibrosis.
45. Systemic lupus erythematosus is not the only type of lupus. Conduct research to find out more about other types of lupus. List and describe at least three types.

4 Membranes and the Integumentary System

Clinical Case Study

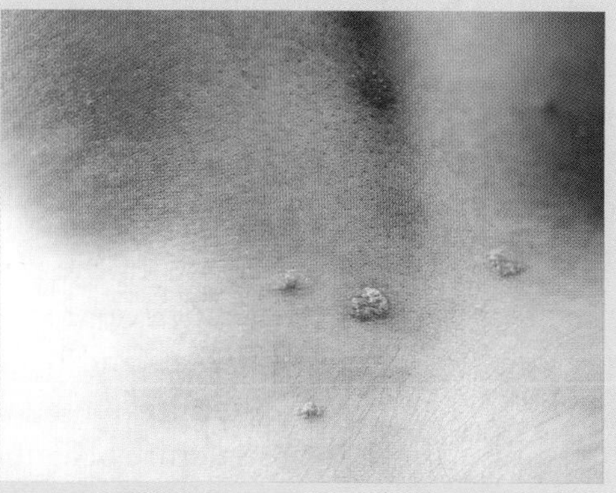
komokvm/Shutterstock.com

Judy is a 20-year-old college student. As a child, she had all of the usual childhood diseases—measles, chickenpox, and mumps—when they affected other children in her elementary school. Today, though, she is healthy and typically runs a three-mile circuit several mornings each week with a group of friends. A couple of years ago she had persuaded her father to join her in following one of the popular healthy weight loss/maintenance diets, which they both continue today.

For the past two weeks, however, Judy has not exercised and has felt a significant amount of stress as she studied for final exams in three courses that she must do well in for her major. Understandably, Judy was surprised and concerned when she awoke one morning with an itchy and somewhat painful rash on her lower back. When she positioned a mirror to see her back, she noticed that the skin in the affected area was raised and appeared scaly. Trying to think what this might be, she recalled that her grandmother once had a painful rash on her back which was diagnosed as shingles and that her father had recently battled psoriasis, with outbreaks on his elbows and back.

Judy makes an appointment to see a caregiver at her student health service. Based on the description of her situation and symptoms, what diagnoses are possible and which seems most likely? Why?

Chapter 4 Outline

People tend to think about their skin mainly when they are interested in getting a tan or avoiding sunburn, but the skin is actually a body organ like the heart or lungs. In fact, this organ called *skin* makes up approximately 15% of total body weight!

The skin is quite a remarkable organ. It is far more than just an outer layer or covering for the body. The skin contains glands and sensory receptors that perform specialized functions; it also grows hair and nails. For these reasons, the skin and its contents are considered a body system—the integumentary system.

This chapter describes the anatomy and functions of the integumentary system, including its associated structures and membranes. The chapter also discusses some of the common injuries and disorders of the skin and membranes, along with their symptoms and current treatments.

SECTION 4.1

Membranes

Objectives

- Identify the types of epithelial membranes and explain their functions.
- Describe the structure and functions of synovial membranes.

Key Terms

cutaneous membrane
epithelial membranes
membranes
mucous membranes
pericardium
peritoneum
pleura
serous fluid
serous membranes
synovial fluid
synovial membrane

The body ***membranes*** surround and help protect the body's surfaces. These surfaces include cavities that open to the outside world, internal cavities that house body organs, capsules that surround ball-and-socket synovial joints, and the skin. This section explores the similarities and differences among the membranes that cover the different body surfaces.

Epithelial Membranes

The ***epithelial membranes*** provide linings for the internal and external surfaces of the body. These membranes include a sheet of epithelial cells and an underlying layer of connective tissue. The three main types of epithelial membranes are the mucous, serous, and cutaneous membranes.

Mucous Membranes

The ***mucous membranes*** line the body cavities that open to the outside world (**Figure 4.1**), including the hollow organs of the respiratory, digestive, urinary, and reproductive tracts. The mouth, nose, lungs, digestive tract, and bladder are examples of hollow organs lined with mucous membranes.

The structure of a mucous membrane comprises a layer of epithelium on top of loose connective tissue called *lamina propria*. All mucous membranes are moist: the membranes of the digestive and respiratory tracts secrete mucus, and glands in the urinary tract add mucus there. Mucus is a slippery solution that protects the mucous membranes and aids in transporting substances.

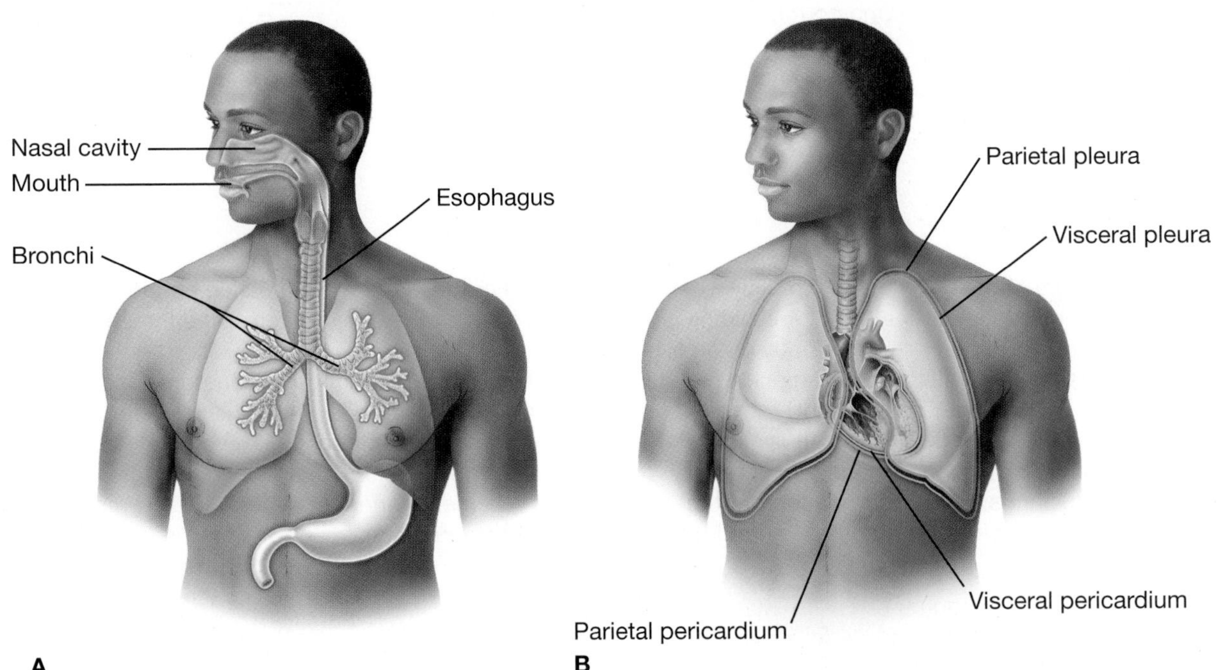

Figure 4.1 Two classes of epithelial membranes. A—Mucous membranes line body cavities that open to the outside world. B—Serous membranes line body cavities that are closed to the outside world.

Serous Membranes

Serous membranes line body cavities that are closed to the outside world (**Figure 4.1**). Examples include the ***pleura***, which encloses the lungs; the ***pericardium***, which surrounds the heart; and the ***peritoneum*** (per-i-toh-NEE-um), which lines the abdominal cavity.

The structure of serous membranes includes an outer layer of simple squamous (flattened) epithelium on a thin layer of loose connective tissue. Each serous membrane forms a double lining, providing both an outer lining and an inner lining for body cavities. The outer lining of each body cavity is called the *parietal layer.* The inner lining, which covers each organ in the cavity, is called the *visceral layer.*

Serous membranes secrete a thin, clear liquid called ***serous fluid***. This fluid serves as a lubricant between the parietal and visceral layers to minimize friction and "wear and tear" on organs that move within the linings, such as the beating heart.

Cutaneous Membrane

The ***cutaneous membrane*** is the skin. The basic structure of skin is a stratified (layered) squamous epithelium over dense, fibrous connective tissue. Although the skin contains sweat glands, it is a dry membrane when sweat is not present.

SELF CHECK

1. Where are epithelial membranes located? Name at least three locations for mucous membranes and three for serous membranes.
2. What is the difference between mucous membranes and serous membranes?
3. What two components make up epithelial membranes?

Synovial Membranes

Only one type of membrane in the body is composed solely of connective tissue and includes no epithelial cells: the ***synovial*** (si-NOH-vee-al) ***membrane***. Synovial membranes line the capsules that surround synovial joints, such as the shoulder and the knee (**Figure 4.2**). These membranes also line tendon sheaths (the connective tissue that surrounds tendons), as well as bursae, the small sacs of connective tissue that serve as cushions for tendons and ligaments surrounding the joints. Synovial membranes in all of these locations secrete a clear substance called ***synovial fluid***, which provides cushioning and reduces friction and wear on moving structures.

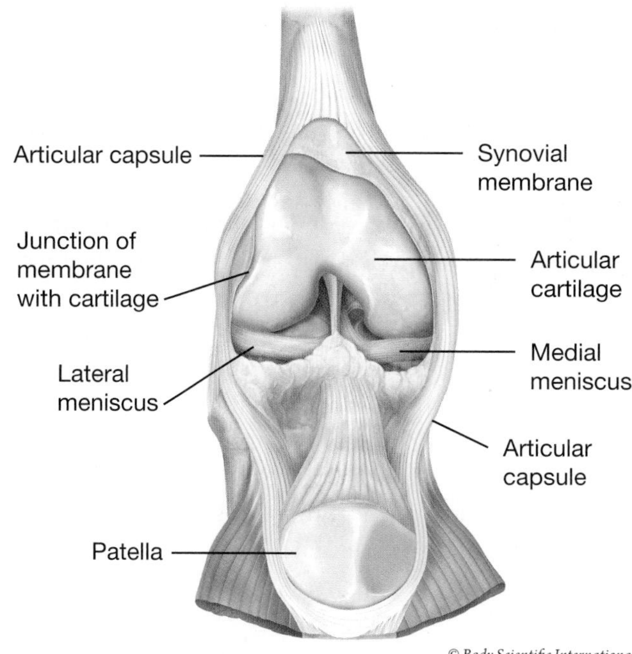

Figure 4.2 Synovial joint—anterior view.

SECTION 4.1 **REVIEW**

Mini-Glossary

cutaneous membrane another name for skin
epithelial membranes thin sheets of tissue lining the internal and external surfaces of the body
membranes thin sheets or layers of pliable tissue
mucous membranes thin sheets of tissue lining the body cavities that open to the outside world
pericardium the membrane that surrounds the heart
peritoneum the membrane that lines the abdominal cavity
pleura the membrane that encases the lungs
serous fluid a thin, clear liquid that serves as a lubricant between parietal and visceral membranes
serous membranes thin sheets of tissue that line body cavities that are closed to the outside world

(continued)

synovial fluid a clear liquid secreted by synovial membranes that provides cushioning for and reduces friction in synovial joints

synovial membrane thin sheet of tissue that lines the synovial joint cavity and produces synovial fluid

Review Questions

1. List the two main categories of body membranes.
2. List the three main types of epithelial membranes.
3. Describe the basic structure of skin.
4. In what way is the structure of synovial membranes different from that of epithelial membranes?
5. Name three examples of serous membranes.
6. List the areas of the body in which mucous membranes are found.
7. What is the primary purpose of the fluid that is produced by serous membranes?
8. If synovial fluid were not present, what would happen to the joints in the body?

SECTION 4.2

The Integumentary System

Objectives

- Explain the functions of the integumentary system.
- Describe the layers of the skin and their functions.
- Identify the appendages that support the skin.

Key Terms

dermis
epidermal dendritic cells
epidermis
hypodermis
integumentary system
keratin
keratinocytes
melanin
melanocytes
Merkel cells
papillary layer
reticular layer
sebaceous glands
sebum
stratum basale
stratum corneum
stratum granulosum
stratum lucidum
stratum spinosum
sudoriferous glands

The skin is the major organ of the ***integumentary*** (in-teg-yoo-MEHN-ta-ree) ***system***. The term *integumentary* comes from the Latin word *integumentum*, which means "covering," but the skin is not simply a membranous covering like those discussed in the previous section. It is an entire system that includes a cutaneous membrane, sweat and oil glands, and nails and hair. Working together, these structures perform critical functions that are not only convenient but also essential for life.

Functions of the Integumentary System

The skin forms a protective cover for the body that serves a variety of purposes. When you sustain a cut or an abrasion, your skin acts as the first line of defense in protecting the underlying tissues. The skin's outermost layer contains ***keratin*** (KER-a-tin), a tough protein also found in hair and nails that adds structural strength. Keratin also helps protect the skin against damage from harmful chemicals.

Keratin and naturally occurring oils serve as a barrier that ensures that water does not escape or enter the body through the skin. The skin substantially lessens the evaporation of water, and the essential molecules the water contains, from inside the body. Furthermore, keratin prevents water from entering the body during bathing or swimming.

The skin is also critically important in regulating body temperature, due to the extensive array of tiny capillaries and sweat glands that lie near the surface of the skin. The capillaries contain blood, which circulates throughout the body. When the body is overheated, the capillaries dilate (expand), bringing more blood near the surface of the skin. The blood cools as it nears the skin's surface, dissipating body heat. Likewise, during hot conditions, the sweat glands become active, producing sweat that evaporates and has a cooling effect on the skin. When the environment is cold, the capillaries constrict (tighten), and blood flow moves to deeper vessels away from the skin to minimize heat loss.

Skin is also involved in certain chemical processes in the body. Specialized cells in the skin called ***melanocytes*** (MEHL-a-noh-sights) produce ***melanin***, a pigment that protects the body against the harmful effects of ultraviolet rays from the sun. Exposure to ultraviolet-B (UVB) rays causes the skin's modified cholesterol molecules, called *provitamin* D_3, to convert into vitamin D. Vitamin D is essential for bone health.

In addition, during the process of sweating the body eliminates chemical waste products, including urea, uric acid, and salts. Because the fluid secreted by the sweat glands is acidic, it also helps protect the body against bacterial infections.

Finally, the skin contains cutaneous sensory receptors that are part of the nervous system. These receptors transmit nerve signals that contain information about the environment, including touch, pressure, vibration, pain, and temperature.

The table in **Figure 4.3** summarizes the functions of the integumentary system.

SELF CHECK

1. In what two ways does the skin help regulate body temperature?
2. What waste products are eliminated from the body through sweat?

Anatomy and Physiology of the Skin

The skin has two layers—an outer ***epidermis*** (EHP-i-DERM-is) and an underlying ***dermis*** (**Figure 4.4**). A blister is produced when friction or a burn causes these two layers to separate, forming a fluid-filled pocket. The epidermis and dermis are thick in certain areas, such as the soles of the feet, and thin in delicate areas, such as the eyelids.

Understanding Medical Terminology

The word *dermis* means "true skin." The prefix *epi-* means "upon" or "over." The prefix *hypo-* means "below," or "under." Thus, the epidermis lies above the dermis, and the hypodermis lies below the dermis.

Beneath the dermis is the ***hypodermis***, or subcutaneous fascia, which serves as a storage repository for fat. The hypodermis is not part of the skin, but it connects the skin to the underlying tissues. It also provides cushioning and insulation against extreme external temperatures.

Epidermis

The epidermis is the outermost layer of skin, which contains five layers of tissue (**Figure 4.5**). From superficial to deep (from the outside going inward), these include the ***stratum corneum, stratum lucidum, stratum granulosum, stratum spinosum***, and ***stratum basale***.

All epidermal layers consist of cells, but none of them includes a blood supply to provide nutrients to the skin. The innermost layer, the stratum basale, absorbs nutrients from the adjacent, underlying dermis. The cells in the stratum basale are constantly producing new skin cells. As new cells germinate, they are pushed toward the surface and away from nutrients. Eventually, these cells die.

Most of the cells within the epidermis are ***keratinocytes*** (keh-RAT-i-noh-sights), which produce keratin. Moving up through the stratum spinosum and stratum granulosum, cells become progressively

Functions of the Integumentary System	
Function	**Mechanisms**
Protection	Tough keratin protects against mechanical injury and chemical damage. Melanocytes produce melanin to protect against UV ray damage. Acidic sweat protects against bacterial infections.
Water barrier	Keratin and oils in the skin reduce loss of water through evaporation and form a barrier against water infusion.
Temperature regulation	Capillaries dilate to dissipate heat and constrict to conserve heat. Sweat evaporation provides a cooling effect.
Vitamin D production	Sunlight converts modified cholesterol molecules to vitamin D, which is essential for bone health.
Waste elimination	Urea and uric acid are eliminated in sweat.
Sensory perception	Receptor cells transmit information about touch, pressure, vibration, pain, and temperature to the central nervous system.

Figure 4.3 Goodheart-Willcox Publisher

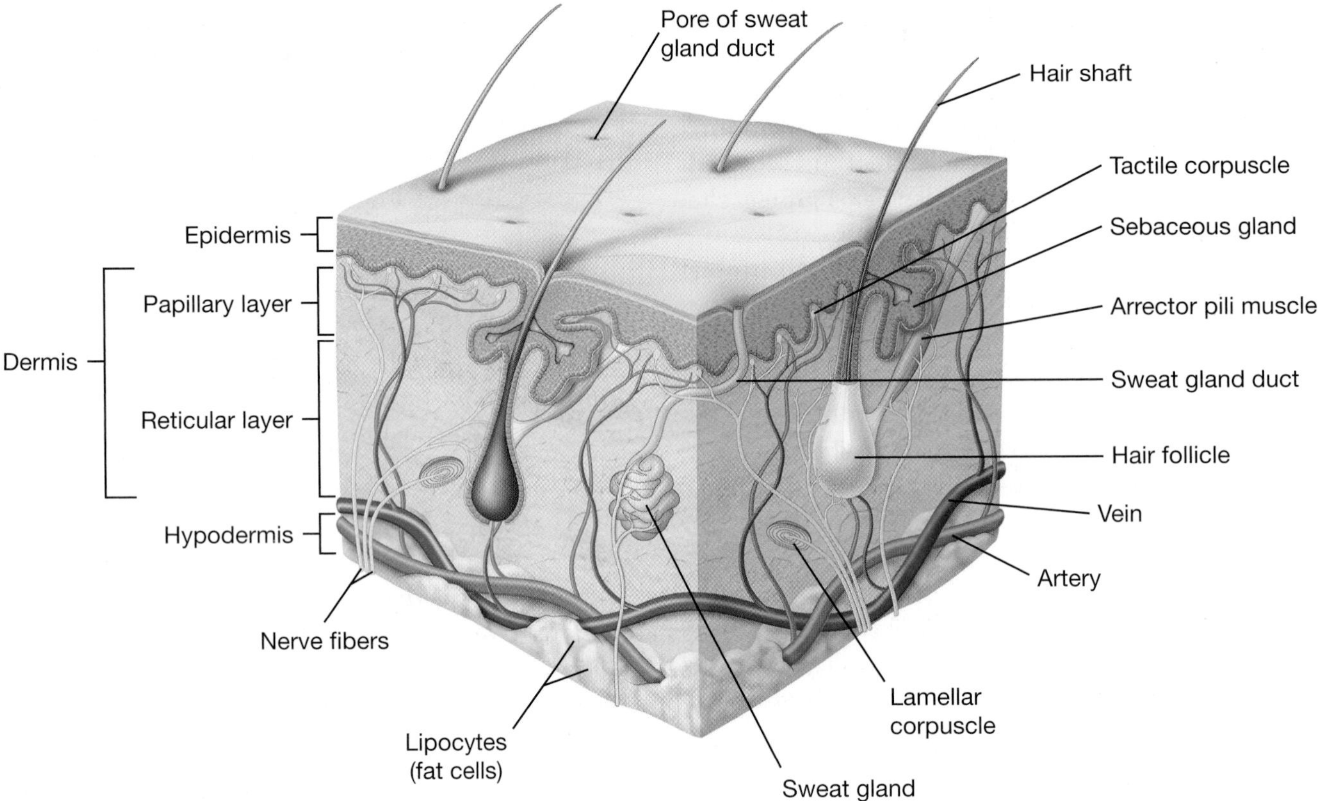

Figure 4.4 The integumentary system, as represented by a section of skin.

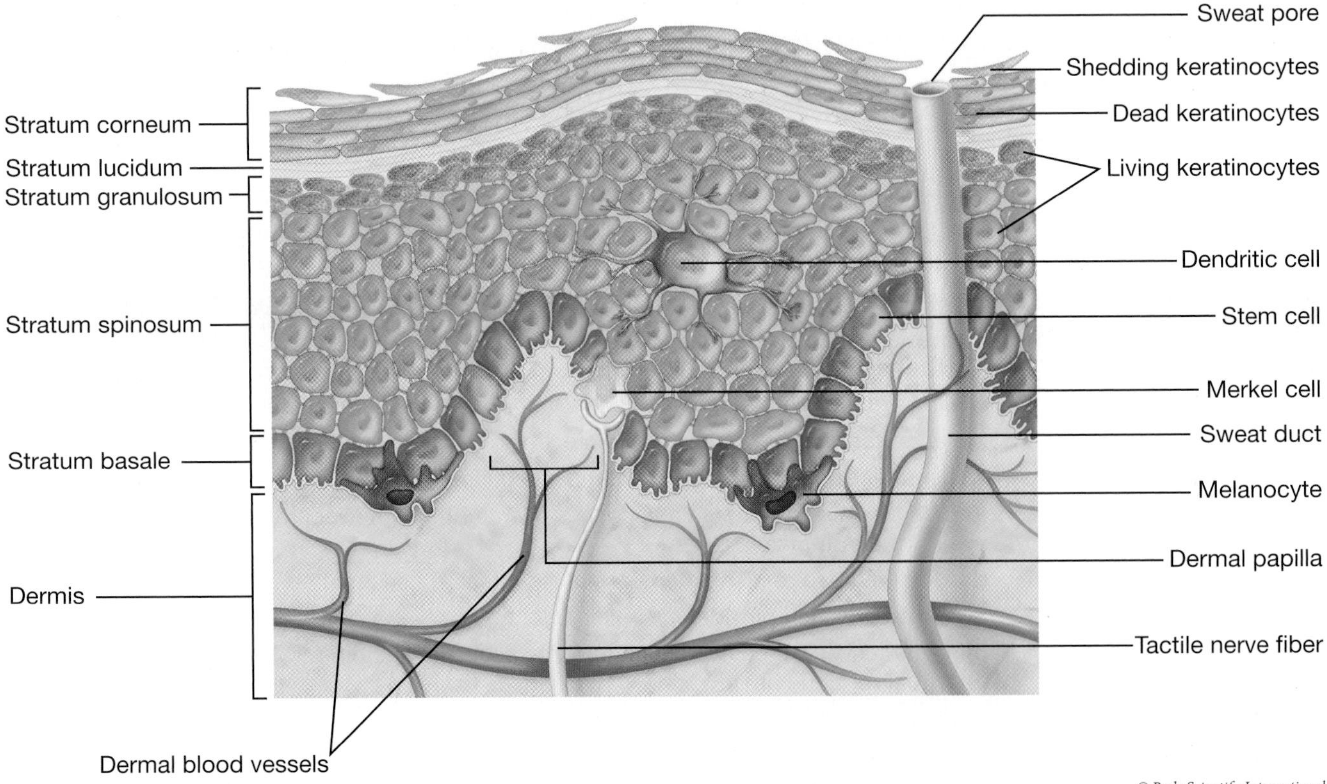

Figure 4.5 The layers of the epidermis.

flatter and more filled with keratin, which makes them tough and water resistant. The stratum lucidum is a clear layer of thick skin found only on the palms of the hands, the fingers, the soles of the feet, and the toes.

The outer layer of the epidermis, the stratum corneum, consists of dead cells that are completely filled with keratin and are continually shedding. You might be surprised to learn that the epidermis completely replaces itself every 25 to 45 days. Over the course of an average life, the epidermis sheds approximately 18 kg (40 lb) of skin cells.

As described earlier, the melanocytes in the stratum basale produce the pigment melanin. Melanin, which ranges in color from reddish-yellow to brown and black, is primarily responsible for human skin color. Exposure to sunlight causes melanocytes to produce more melanin. As melanin granules are pushed out into neighboring skin cells, the skin becomes tanned.

The presence of extra melanin in the skin functions as a sunscreen, which is why sunburn is more likely to affect individuals with light skin. Sunburn is also less likely once a light-skinned person has a tan.

An inherited condition called *albinism* (AL-bi-nizm) prevents the normal production of melanin. Albinism is characterized by very little pigment in the skin, hair, and eyes. Individuals with albinism have extremely pale skin and white hair.

The epidermis also contains specialized cells associated with the immune and nervous systems. ***Epidermal dendritic cells*** respond to the presence of foreign bacteria or viruses by initiating an immune system response, which brings in other cells to attack the foreign invaders. The skin contains as many as 800 dendritic cells per square millimeter to help ward off infections.

Merkel cells (also called *Merkel-Ranvier cells*), located in the stratum basale, function as touch receptors. These cells form junctions with sensory nerve endings that relay information about touch to the brain.

Clinical Application Clues to Health in Skin Color

Alterations in the color of the skin can serve as indicators of underlying changes in body function or patterns of food consumption. Among Caucasians, changes in coloration are relatively apparent. In people with darker skin coloration, the same color changes are masked but can be observed to some extent in the mucous membranes and nail beds.

Capillaries in the dermis carry oxygenated hemoglobin, which is bright red. In people who have less melanin and lighter complexions, the hemoglobin in the blood gives the skin a pinkish tone. Conditions that cause dilation of the blood vessels, such as elevated blood pressure or inflammation, can produce flushing, or reddening, of the skin. The blood vessels are dilated during vigorous exercise and exposure to hot conditions, which can result in reddening, especially of the face.

Alternatively, any condition that causes constriction of the blood vessels can result in paleness or pallor of the skin. Cold conditions and certain emotional responses, such as fear or anger, can also cause this constriction. Low blood hemoglobin content, known as *anemia*, and low blood pressure can also cause paleness of the skin.

Poor oxygenation of the blood causes hemoglobin to lose its red color and turn bluish. This condition is known as *cyanosis*. Breathing disorders such as asthma, chronic obstructive pulmonary disease (COPD), and lung cancer can cause cyanosis. Different forms of heart failure can also cause this condition.

A yellowish hue in the skin and eyes is an indication of jaundice, a condition in which excess bile from the liver is deposited throughout the body. Jaundice is a symptom of disease or damage to the liver.

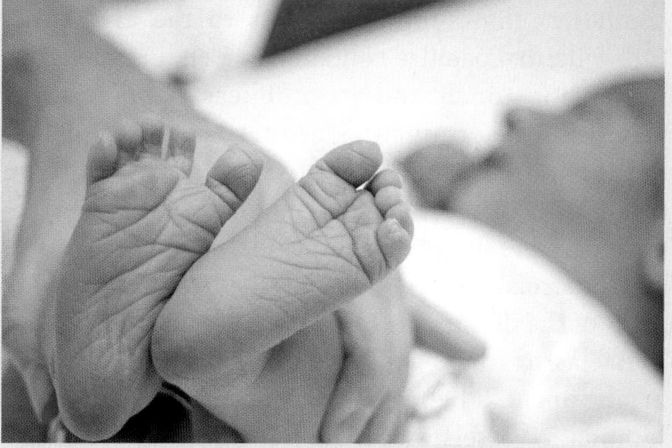

John Radcliffe Hospital/Science Source

This premature infant is experiencing cyanosis due to poor oxygenation of the blood supply. Notice the bluish color of the soles of the infant's feet.

Diet can also influence skin color, especially when a person has eaten a large amount of beta-carotene. Beta-carotene is the orange-colored pigment that gives carrots, sweet potatoes, and acorn squash their color. The pigment is also found in leafy green vegetables. Beta-carotene is deposited in the stratum corneum. Diets excessively rich in beta-carotene can produce an orange-yellow coloration of the skin, especially in the palms of the hands and soles of the feet.

Dermis

The dermis, or "true skin," is a dense, fibrous connective tissue composed of collagen and elastic fibers. The collagen fibers provide toughness and also bind with water molecules to help keep the inner skin moist. The elastic fibers keep the skin looking young, without wrinkles or sagging. During the normal course of aging, the number of collagen and elastic fibers in the dermis decrease.

The dermis has a rich supply of blood vessels, which dilate to help dissipate body heat or constrict to help retain body heat. A variety of sensory receptors for touch, vibration, pain, and temperature are also present throughout the dermis. These receptors communicate with nerve endings to transmit information about what the body is sensing to the brain. White blood cells called *phagocytes* (FAG-oh-sights), which are distributed throughout the dermis, are responsible for ingesting foreign material, including bacteria and dead cells.

The outer layer of the dermis is the ***papillary*** (PAP-i-lar-ee) ***layer***, named after the dermal papillae (pa-PIL-ee) that protrude up into the epidermis (**Figure 4.6**). Some of the dermal papillae contain capillaries that supply nutrients to the epidermis. Other dermal papillae contain nerve endings involved in sensing touch and pain. These papillae form genetically determined, ridged patterns on the palms of the hands, the fingers, the toes, and the soles of the feet. It is the papillae patterns on the fingers that create each person's unique fingerprints.

Underneath the papillary layer lies the ***reticular layer*** of the dermis. As **Figure 4.6** shows, the collagen and elastic fibers in this layer have an irregular arrangement. The reticular layer includes blood and lymphatic vessels, sweat and oil glands, involuntary muscles, hair follicles, and nerve endings.

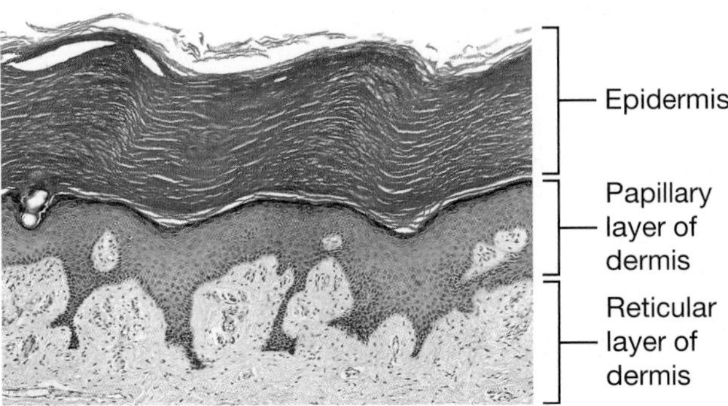

Jose Luis Calvo/Shutterstock.com

Figure 4.6 Light micrograph showing the two regions of the dermis below the epidermis.

Hypodermis

The hypodermis, or subcutaneous fascia, includes fibrous connective tissue and adipose (fatty) tissue. The lipocytes (LIP-oh-sights), or fat cells, reside within the hypodermis. Some amount of body fat is important for padding and insulating the interior of the body. Fat also serves as a source of energy.

SELF CHECK

1. What are the two main layers of skin?
2. Where does the body store fat?
3. How does the epidermis receive nutrients?
4. Which cells are responsible for human skin color?

Supporting Appendages

Structures considered to be appendages of the skin include the sudoriferous (sweat) glands, sebaceous (oil) glands, hair, and nails. In this case, appendages are the related structures that support the functions of the skin.

Sudoriferous (Sweat) Glands

Sweat glands, or ***sudoriferous*** (soo-doh-RIF-er-us) ***glands***, are distributed in the dermis over the entire body, with larger concentrations in the axilla (under the arms), on the palms of the hands and soles of the feet, and on the forehead. Each person has approximately 2 to 3 million sweat glands.

Sweat glands contain nerve endings that cause sweat to form when body temperature or external temperature is elevated. Evaporation of sweat from the skin's surface is very effective in dissipating body heat. During periods of physical activity in a hot environment, you can lose as much as a liter of liquid per hour in the process of sweating. In such circumstances, it is important to drink appropriate amounts of fluids to avoid serious, potentially life-threatening conditions.

There are two types of sweat glands: eccrine glands and apocrine glands (**Figure 4.7**). The eccrine (EK-rin) glands are the major sweat glands of the body. They cover most of the body and open directly onto the external surface of the skin. The sweat secreted by eccrine glands is a clear, acidic fluid that consists of approximately 99% water but also contains waste products such as urea, uric acid, salts, and vitamin C.

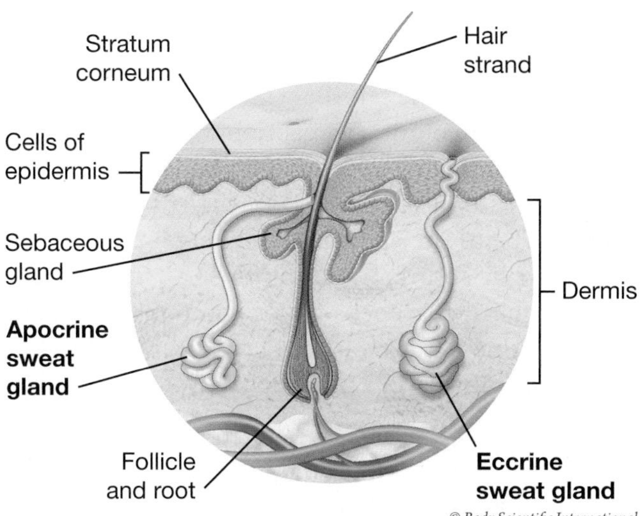

Figure 4.7 The eccrine and apocrine sweat glands.

Sweat is odorless, but if it is left on the skin, bacteria can chemically change it to produce an unpleasant odor.

The apocrine (AP-oh-krin) glands, which begin to function during puberty, are located in the genital and axilla (armpit) areas. The apocrine glands are larger than the eccrine glands, and they secrete a milky fluid consisting of sweat, fatty acids, and proteins. Unlike the eccrine gland ducts, which open directly onto the skin, the apocrine gland ducts empty into hair follicles.

Sebaceous Glands

Sebaceous (seh-BAY-shus) ***glands*** are located all over the body except for the palms of the hands and soles of the feet. These glands produce an oily substance called ***sebum*** (SEE-bum). Most sebaceous glands empty into a hair follicle, though some secrete directly to the skin. Sebum helps to keep the skin and hair soft, and it also contains chemicals that kill bacteria. Because the sebaceous glands are particularly active during adolescence, teenagers' skin tends to be oily.

Hair

Hair follicles are bulb-shaped structures within the dermis that produce hair (**Figure 4.8**). The base of the follicle is "invaded" by a papilla of connective tissue containing a rich capillary supply, which provides nourishment for hair cell formation. The matrix, or growth zone, within the base of the follicle contains specialized cells that divide and generate living hair cells. Like the epithelial cells generated in the stratum basale, as these cells are pushed up toward the scalp, they become filled with keratin and die. Most of a shaft of hair is, therefore, nonliving material composed mainly of protein.

Focus On Tattoos

In his travels around the Tahitian islands in the 1700s, Captain James Cook documented the natives' practice of etching permanent markings on their bodies using bone needles and a stain derived from an oily nut. The word *tattoo* is derived from the Tahitian term *tatua*, meaning "to mark." During the 1800s, tattoos were considered fashionable among the English upper class. In fact, Winston Churchill's mother, Lady Randolph Churchill, had a snake tattoo around her wrist.

In western cultures today, decorative tattoos are popular as a form of self-expression, but they are also used for cosmetic purposes. For example, tattoos are used to help normalize the skin color of patients with vitiligo, a condition in which the melanocytes fail to produce normal color, causing white blotches in the skin. Tattoos may also be used to cover unsightly birthmarks or burn marks.

People who are interested in getting a tattoo should take care to select a tattoo parlor that conforms to the standards of the Association of Professional Tattooists (APT). The client selects the tattoo design, called the *flash*, which is then converted to a stencil, or inked color copy of the flash that can be applied to the client's skin.

The tattoo machine consists of a handheld needle gun that moves up and down like the needle on a sewing machine, penetrating the skin to inject ink into the dermis at 50 to 30,000 times per minute.

The finished tattoo site needs to be cared for, especially during the first two weeks. Similar to a minor burn, the site is likely to become crusted or scabbed and should be kept clean and moist. Complications that may arise include:

- allergic reactions that cause an itchy rash
- skin infections
- overgrowth of scar tissue
- bloodborne diseases such as hepatitis and HIV, if the tattoo needles have not been properly sterilized
- complications during subsequent magnetic resonance imaging (MRI) exams due to the metal content of the ink

Removal of a tattoo is possible through dermabrasion, excision, and laser surgery, but all of these procedures are difficult, expensive, and usually not successful in fully removing the tattoo. The affected area may also lose the ability to produce normal pigmentation, resulting in white blotches in the skin.

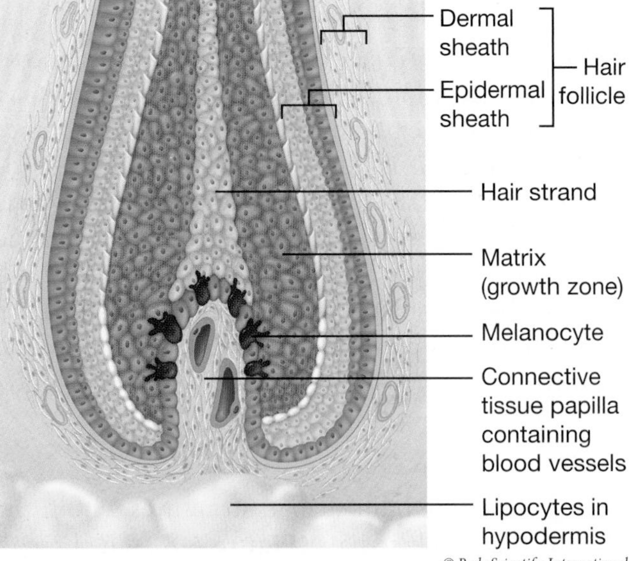

Figure 4.8 The base of a hair follicle—longitudinal section view. If you were to ask a stylist or barber to trim all the "dead ends" from your hair, you would be practically bald.

What gives a person's hair a particular color and texture (straight, wavy, or curly)? Melanocytes within the follicle produce the pigment that gives hair its color. As a person ages, the melanocytes produce less pigment, resulting in gray or white hair. The shape of the hair follicle is genetically determined. A round hair follicle produces straight hair, an oval follicle causes hair to be wavy, and a flat follicle produces curly hair.

What causes the familiar "goose bumps" that are part of an involuntary reaction when people are cold or frightened? Tiny muscles called *arrector pili* (ah-REHK-tor PIGH-lee) connect either side of a hair follicle to the epidermis. When stimulated, the arrector pili contract, pulling the hair upright and causing the appearance of goose bumps on the skin. The erect hair traps a layer of air close to the skin, which adds insulation and helps to warm the body.

Nails

Underlying each nail is a specialized region of the stratum basale known as the *nail bed*. The proximal end of the nail bed is a thickened region called the *nail matrix*. As with hair, nail growth occurs in the matrix, with new cells rapidly becoming keratinized and dying.

Nails are transparent, but they appear pinkish in color because of the capillary supply beneath the stratum basale. The white, crescent moon-shaped region at the base of the nail, which is positioned over the thickened nail matrix, is called the *lunule* (LOO-nyool). The word *lunule* gets its name from the Latin word *luna*, which means "moon."

SECTION 4.2 REVIEW

Mini-Glossary

dermis the layer of skin between the epidermis and hypodermis; includes nerve endings, glands, and hair follicles

epidermal dendritic cells skin cells that initiate an immune system response to the presence of foreign bacteria or viruses

epidermis the outer layer of skin

hypodermis the layer of skin beneath the dermis; serves as a storage repository for fat

integumentary system term for the skin and its appendages; includes the epidermis, dermis, sudoriferous and sebaceous glands, nails, and hair

keratin a tough protein found in the skin, hair, and nails

keratinocytes cells within the epidermis that produce keratin

melanin a pigment that protects the body against the harmful effects of ultraviolet rays from the sun

melanocytes specialized cells in the skin that produce melanin

Merkel cells touch receptors in the skin; also known as *Merkel-Ranvier cells*

papillary layer the outer layer of the dermis

reticular layer the inner layer of the dermis; includes blood and lymphatic vessels, sweat and oil glands, involuntary muscles, hair follicles, and nerve endings

sebaceous glands that produce sebum and are located all over the body

sebum an oily substance that helps to keep the skin and hair soft

stratum basale the deepest layer of the epidermis

stratum corneum the outer layer of the epidermis

stratum granulosum the layer of somewhat flattened cells just superficial to the stratum spinosum and inferior to the stratum lucidum

stratum lucidum the clear layer of thick skin found only on the palms of the hands, the fingers, the soles of the feet, and the toes

stratum spinosum the layer of cells in the epidermis superior to the stratum basale and inferior to the stratum granulosum

sudoriferous glands sweat glands that are distributed in the dermis over the entire body

(continued)

Review Questions

1. List the important features of the epidermal dendritic cells and Merkel cells of the epidermis.
2. Describe collagen fibers.
3. What is the purpose of the elastic fibers in the dermis?
4. Describe two ways in which skin helps to protect the body.
5. What is the other name for sweat glands?
6. Describe the two types of sweat glands.
7. Where does hair and nail growth occur?
8. The epidermis completely replaces itself every 25 to 45 days. Describe the process of skin shedding and how the body constantly supplies nutrients to the outer layers of the skin.
9. In the summer months, exposure to extreme temperatures can be life threatening, but glands close to the surface of the skin help to keep the body cool. What are these glands and how do they help to regulate body temperature?
10. The skin is involved in chemical processes. Which vitamin is essential to bone health, and what role does the skin play in producing that vitamin?

SECTION 4.3 Disorders of the Integumentary System

Objectives

- Describe common injuries to the skin, including decubitus ulcers and burns.
- Explain the characteristics of common viruses, fungi, and bacteria that may cause infections in the integumentary system.
- List disorders that may cause inflammation in the integumentary system.
- Describe the three types of skin cancer.

Key Terms

basal cell carcinoma
cellulitis
common warts
first-degree burns
fourth-degree burns
herpes simplex virus type 1 (HSV-1)
herpes simplex virus type 2 (HSV-2)
herpes varicella (chickenpox)
herpes zoster (shingles)
impetigo
malignant melanoma
peritonitis
plantar warts
pleurisy
psoriasis
rule of nines
second-degree burns
squamous cell carcinoma
third-degree burns
tinea

As the first line of defense in protecting the body from the external environment, the skin is routinely subject to minor injuries and is exposed to a variety of common infections. Fortunately, the skin is a multilayered system with a remarkable capacity for self-healing.

Injuries

The skin commonly sustains minor cuts, abrasions, and blisters that tend to heal quickly. This healing is aided immensely by the skin's normal self-renewal process.

Infection is a major concern with all minor skin injuries. Injuries to the skin that penetrate to the underlying tissues are more complicated, and infection is still the most significant concern.

Decubitus Ulcers

A decubitus (deh-KYOO-bi-tus) ulcer, commonly known as a bedsore, is a skin injury caused by an area of localized pressure that restricts blood flow to an area of the body. Without the normal blood supply to provide nutrients and oxygen, the skin cells die. These skin injuries typically occur in people who undergo prolonged bed rest. When a bedridden patient is not turned often enough, sustained pressure over a particular area can result in a decubitus ulcer. These ulcers can occur anywhere on the body, but most form over bony areas such as the lower back, coccyx (tailbone), hips, elbows, and ankles.

A decubitus ulcer begins as an area of reddened skin, but as cells start to die, small cracks or openings in the skin appear. As the condition progresses, the tissue continues to degenerate and an open ulcer forms (**Figure 4.9**). If not treated, tissue degeneration can progress all the way to the bone and eventually can be fatal.

Although the common term *bedsore* suggests that these injuries affect only bedridden individuals, decubitus ulcers can develop in any situation in which the blood supply to tissues is restricted. People who use wheelchairs, for example, can develop ulcers over pressure points. Individuals who experience numbness in parts of the body from a spinal injury or diabetes

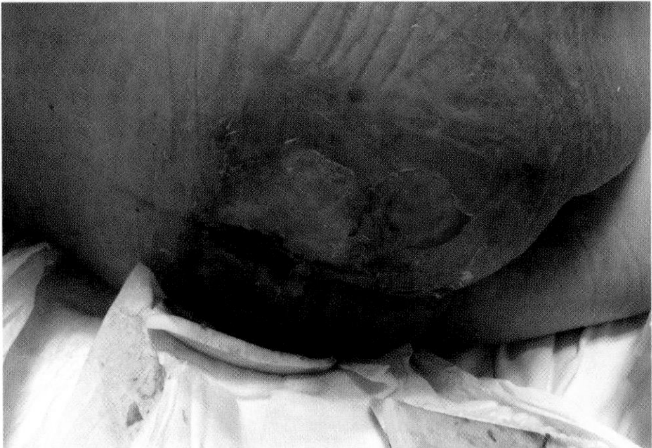

Duangnapa Kanchanasakun/Shutterstock.com

Figure 4.9 A decubitus ulcer is caused by continuous pressure on the skin.

mellitus must be particularly careful to avoid remaining in the same position for prolonged periods.

Treatment for decubitus ulcers includes prescription of oral antibiotics to address or prevent infection. Removal of damaged tissues is another component of treatment. Because dead tissue prevents healing, it must be removed for proper healing to occur.

There are two approaches to removing ulcer-damaged tissues—debridement and vacuum-assisted closure. Debridement is the removal of dead tissue using a surgical or chemical procedure. In vacuum-assisted closure, a vacuum tube is attached to the wound. The vacuum draws moisture from the ulcer, thereby shortening the healing process and reducing the risk of infection.

Proper nutrition is an important factor in both the prevention and healing of decubitus ulcers. Vitamins A, B, C, and E and the minerals magnesium, manganese, selenium, and zinc all contribute to skin health. Sufficient amounts of dietary protein are also important.

Burns

Burns are injuries that can arise from exposure to excessive heat, corrosive chemicals, electricity, or ultraviolet radiation (from sunburn, for example). Burns, which vary considerably in severity, cause tissue damage and cell death.

First-degree burns affect only the epidermal layer of skin (**Figure 4.10A**). These burns involve reddening of the skin and mild pain, and they tend to heal in less than a week. Most types of sunburn are first-degree burns.

Second-degree burns involve damage to both the epidermis and the upper portion of the underlying dermis (**Figure 4.10B**). Second-degree burns are characterized by blisters, which are fluid-filled pockets that form between the epidermal and dermal layers of skin. Second-degree burns are painful and take longer to heal than first-degree burns. Larger blisters require a longer period of healing.

Third-degree burns are a more serious type of skin burn (**Figure 4.10C**). Because these burns destroy the entire thickness of the skin, they are also called *full-thickness burns*. First- and second-degree burns are called *partial-thickness burns*.

The area affected by a third-degree burn appears grayish-white or blackened. Although a third-degree burn is a serious injury, it is initially not painful because the nerve endings in the skin have been destroyed. Later, scarring and pain will occur. A third-degree burn cannot heal on its own because the stratum basale, which generates new skin cells, has been destroyed. Treatment involves grafting skin over the damaged area.

Fourth-degree burns are the most severe type of burn. These burns involve destruction of all layers of skin, as well as nerve endings and some of the underlying tissues such as muscle, tendon, ligament, and bone (**Figure 4.10D**). Because the nerve endings are destroyed in a fourth-degree burn, this burn may result in little to no pain. Like third-degree burns, these injuries require grafting of new skin, but also sometimes necessitate artificial reconstruction of the underlying tissues.

When a large region of skin has been burned, clinicians use the ***rule of nines*** to estimate the extent of burned tissue. **Figure 4.11** illustrates the rule of nines. According to the rule of nines, the percentage of total body surface area covered by burns is approximated as follows:

- 9% for both the anterior and posterior of the head and neck
- 18% for the anterior of the torso
- 18% for the posterior of the torso
- 9% for both the anterior and posterior of each arm
- 18% for both the anterior and posterior of each leg
- 1% for the genital region

Using this approach, clinicians can approximate the affected surface area in the case of a burn. For example, if the anterior of the torso and the anterior of one arm were burned, the affected surface area would be approximately 23% (4.5% for the anterior of the arm and 18% for the anterior of the torso).

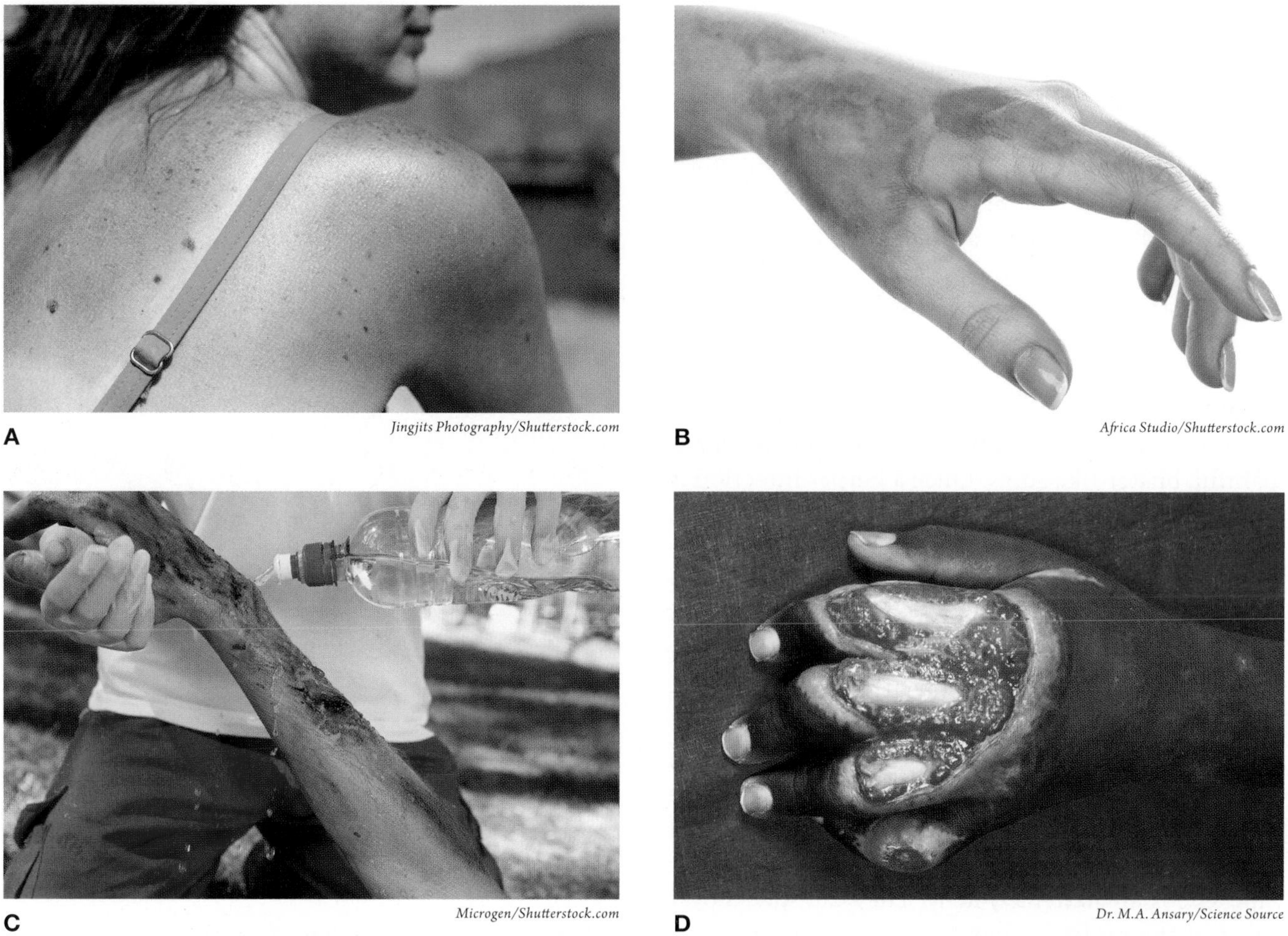

A
Jingjits Photography/Shutterstock.com
B
Africa Studio/Shutterstock.com
C
Microgen/Shutterstock.com
D
Dr. M.A. Ansary/Science Source

Figure 4.10 Different types of burns. A—First-degree burn. B—Second-degree burn. C—Third-degree burn. D—Fourth-degree burn.

SELF CHECK

1. What causes decubitus ulcers?
2. Where on the body do decubitus ulcers commonly occur?
3. Describe two types of treatment for removal of ulcer-damaged skin tissue.
4. What would the affected surface area be if a patient has burns that extend down the back of both legs?

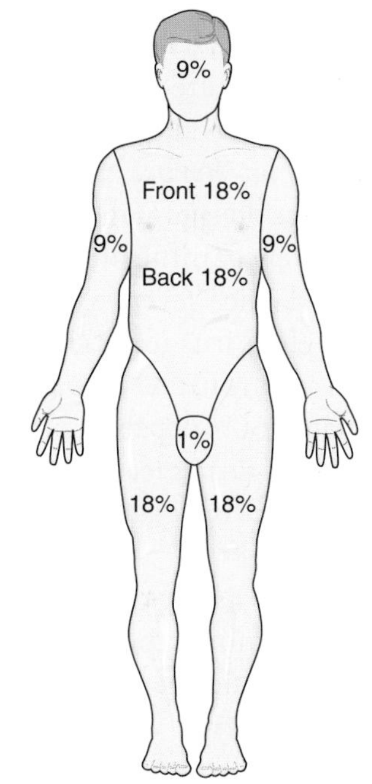

9%
Front 18%
9%
9%
Back 18%
1%
18%
18%
Blamb/Shutterstock.com

Figure 4.11 The rule of nines.

Infections

Skin infections can be caused by contact with an infectious agent that is present on another person or a surface. Infections can also be caused by airborne particles such as viruses or bacteria, or by contamination introduced by a foreign object into a penetrating wound.

Viral Infections

Viruses are extremely small infective agents; most are 100 times smaller than bacterial cells. They consist of a DNA or RNA molecule covered with a protein coat, without any internal mechanism for multiplying. They can reproduce only by invading a living cell and using the cell's reproductive system. Two types of viruses that commonly affect humans are the various strains of herpes viruses and the human papillomavirus.

Herpes

Herpes is a viral infection that produces small, painful, blister-like sores. Once a herpes infection is present, it lasts for the rest of a person's life. Fortunately, herpes infections tend to stay dormant most of the time, with no noticeable sign of infection. Occasional flare-ups do occur, however, and the resurgence of symptoms usually accompanies periods of stress or sickness. Several strains or variations of the herpes virus are known to exist.

Herpes varicella (VAIR-i-SEHL-a), better known as *chickenpox*, is a common childhood disease. Because chickenpox is highly contagious, it tends to spread quickly and widely. The fluid-filled blisters caused by chickenpox are extremely itchy. They can spread over most of the body, or they can be limited in scope. A vaccine for chickenpox is available. The vaccine decreases the chances of infection or reduces the seriousness of the illness if infection does occur.

Once a person infected with chickenpox has recovered, the virus lies dormant. In an adult, the illness can recur as ***herpes zoster*** (ZAHS-ter), commonly known as *shingles* (**Figure 4.12A**). Shingles involves an extremely painful, blistering rash accompanied by a headache, fever, and general unwell feeling. The shingles virus may trigger more serious symptoms, such as chronic nerve pain. In the United States, approximately 50% of people older than 80 years of age have had shingles at least once. A vaccine for shingles is recommended for adults older than 60 years of age.

Herpes simplex virus type 1 (HSV-1), sometimes associated with the common cold, generates "cold sores" or "fever blisters" around the mouth (**Figure 4.12B**). ***Herpes simplex virus type 2 (HSV-2)*** is the genital form of herpes. Both types of the herpes simplex virus are highly contagious and can be transmitted to the mouth or genital area. In the United States, about one in six people has genital herpes.

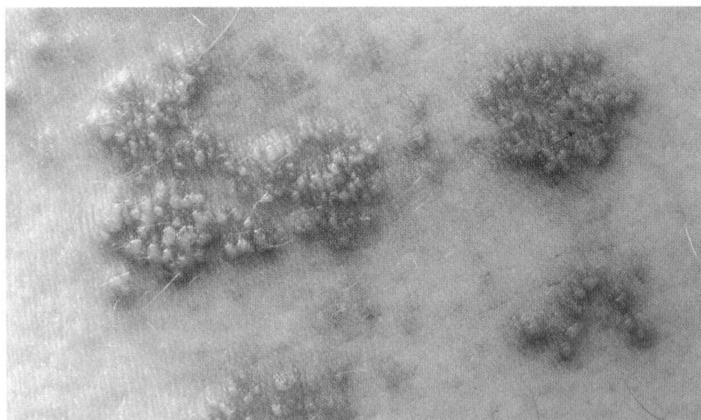

A

CLS Digital Arts/Shutterstock.com

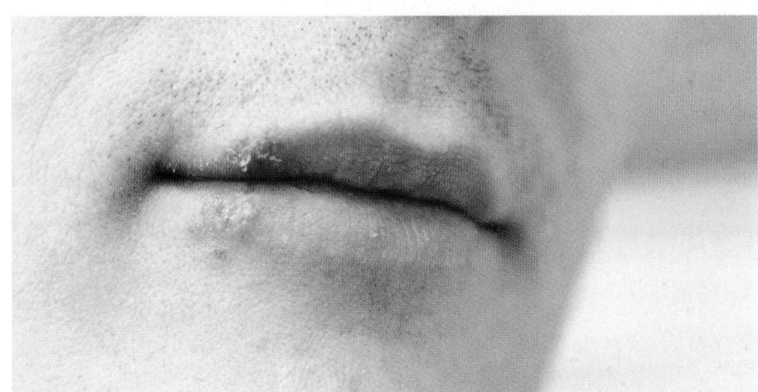

B

vita pakhai/Shutterstock.com

Figure 4.12 Two different types of herpes infections. A—Herpes zoster (shingles) infection. B—Herpes simplex (cold sore) infection.

Transmission of the herpes simplex virus from an infected male to a female partner occurs with greater ease than from an infected female to a male partner. Thus, more women than men are infected with the virus.

During the first outbreak of genital herpes, a person may experience flu-like symptoms such as fever, body aches, and swollen glands. Repeat outbreaks are common, particularly during the first year of infection. Symptoms during repeat outbreaks are usually shorter in duration and less severe than those in the first outbreak. As with all herpes infections, once a person has been infected by a herpes simplex virus, it remains dormant, with the potential to reactivate throughout the remainder of the person's life, although the number of outbreaks tends to decrease over time.

Human Papillomavirus

Warts are raised, typically painless growths on the skin that vary in shape and size. Warts can spread from one part of the body to another. Less commonly, warts can spread from one person to another. All types of warts are caused by the human papillomavirus (HPV).

HPVs are a group of more than 150 related viruses. ***Common warts*** typically appear on the hands or fingers and tend to disappear without treatment (**Figure 4.13**). ***Plantar warts***, which develop on the soles of the feet, grow inward and can become painful. When warranted, warts can be removed by surgery, cryotherapy (freezing), and topical medications such as salicylic acids. Warts can easily be ignored, but it is important to ensure that a wart-like growth on an adult is not a form of skin cancer.

Genital warts caused by HPV infections are the most common sexually transmitted infections in the United States. More than 40 of the HPVs can be easily spread through direct, skin-to-skin contact during vaginal, anal, and oral sex. More than 50% of all sexually active people are infected with an HPV at some point during their life.

There are two major categories of HPVs: low risk and high risk. HPVs are identified by number, and a physician can explain whether a possible HPV infection is categorized as low risk or high risk.

Low-risk HPVs can cause warts on the skin around the genital area and anus but are not known to cause cancer. High-risk HPV infections, however, cause nearly all cervical cancers. This is why some healthcare professionals advocate the papillomavirus vaccine for teenage girls and boys. High-risk HPV infections also cause most anal cancers and about 50% of all vaginal, vulvar, and penile cancers. In addition, HPV infections cause cancer of the soft palate, the base of the tongue, and the tonsils. High-risk HPVs account for about 5% of all cancers.

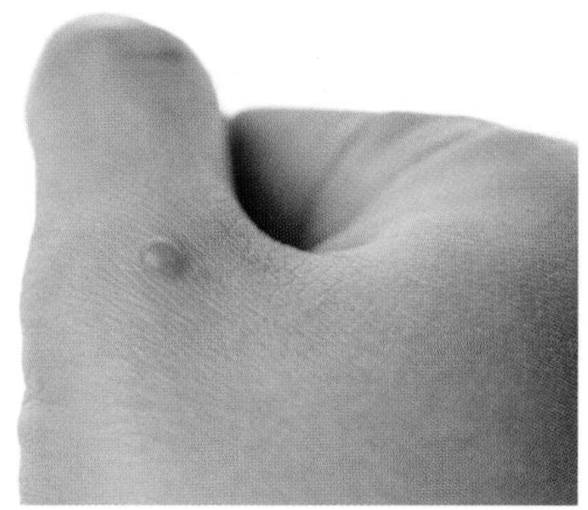

Sakuoka/Shutterstock.com

Figure 4.13 Common warts.

Fungal Infections

Fungal infections, or ***tinea*** (TIN-ee-a), tend to occur in areas of the body that are moist. Therefore, these infections tend to be more prevalent during warm weather, and they are more common in individuals whose work or sporting activities involve frequent periods of sweating.

Tinea Pedis

Tinea pedis (athlete's foot) is the most common fungal infection. It is characterized by cracked, flaky skin between the toes or on the side of the foot. The skin may also be red and itchy. Because tinea pedis is highly contagious, it spreads rapidly on locker room and shower floors. Treatment and prevention includes keeping the feet clean and dry, especially between the toes, and using over-the-counter antifungal powder or cream that contains clotrimazole, miconazole, or tolnaftate.

Research Notes High-Risk HPVs and Cancer

The human papillomavirus (HPV) infects epithelial cells on the skin and in the membranes that line areas such as the genital tract and anus. When an HPV enters an epithelial cell, it begins making specialized proteins. Two of these proteins initiate cancer by interfering with the cell's normal functions, enabling the cell to grow in an uncontrolled manner and resist cell death.

When the immune system recognizes HPV-infected cells, it attacks and attempts to destroy them. When the immune system fails, however, these infected cells continue to grow, and infection takes root. As the cells multiply, they can develop mutations that further promote cell growth, sometimes leading to tumor development.

Researchers believe that 10 to 20 years can pass between the initial HPV infection and tumor formation. They estimate, however, that less than 50% of high-risk HPV infections lead to cancer. Fortunately, HPVs do not enter the bloodstream, so an HPV infection in one part of the body should not spread to other parts of the body.

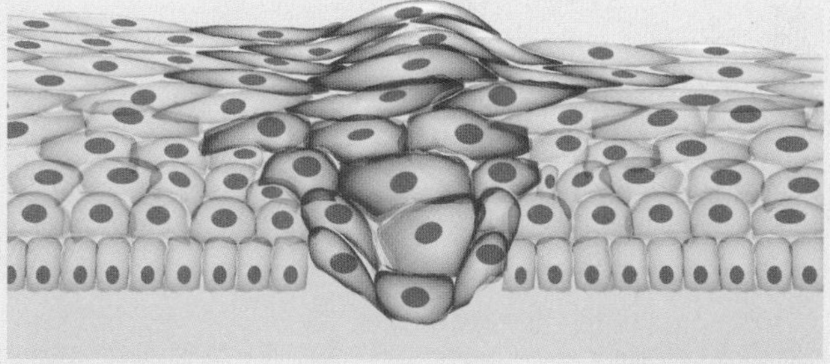

inbevel/Shutterstock.com

Development of cancer cells. Explain how HPV-infected cells can develop into a tumor.

Tinea Cruris

Tinea cruris, or jock itch, primarily affects males in the area around the groin and scrotum. It is caused by the combination of prolonged sweating and friction from clothes. It can be spread through direct contact with infected skin or unwashed clothing. Tinea cruris is typically treated by keeping the skin clean and dry, wearing loose clothing, and applying a topical antifungal or drying powder that contains clotrimazole, miconazole, or tolnaftate.

Tinea Corporis

Tinea corporis, more commonly known as *ringworm*, does not actually involve any type of worm. The common name refers to the characteristically red, ring-shaped rash with a pale center, which somewhat resembles the shape of a worm.

Tinea corporis, which is usually caused by prolonged sweating and poor hygiene, is especially common in children. It is highly contagious and can be spread through direct contact with the infection on someone's body or through contaminated areas such as pool surfaces. Treatment involves keeping the skin clean and dry and applying an over-the-counter antifungal cream that contains clotrimazole, miconazole, ketoconazole, or oxiconazole.

Tinea Unguium

Tinea unguium is a fungal infection under the nails of the fingers or toes (**Figure 4.14**). It causes discoloration and thickening of the infected nail. In general, over-the-counter antifungal creams do not help this condition. Instead, a prescription antifungal medication must be taken orally for several weeks.

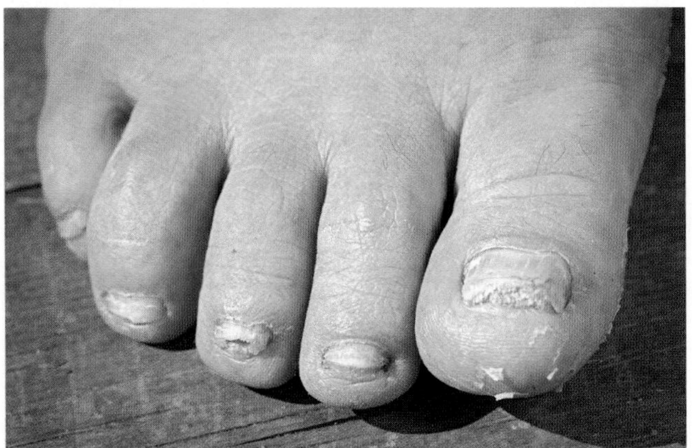

Elena11/Shutterstock.com

Figure 4.14 Tinea unguium, or toenail fungus.

Bacterial Infections

Impetigo (im-peh-TIGH-goh) is a highly contagious infection caused by staphylococcus bacteria that is common in elementary school children. Its symptoms are pink, blister-like bumps, usually around the mouth and nose, which develop a yellowish crust before they rupture.

Cellulitis (SEHL-yoo-LIGH-tis), another staphylococcus infection, is characterized by an area of skin that is red, swollen, and painful. The origin of cellulitis is often an open wound or ulceration. Cellulitis is a serious condition that can become life threatening if not treated with antibiotics.

SELF CHECK

1. What is the difference between a first-degree burn and a second-degree burn?
2. Explain why third- and fourth-degree burns are usually not painful.
3. Why are some HPV viruses considered "high-risk"?
4. What causes warts?
5. What are the most common sexually transmitted infections in the United States?
6. What is impetigo?

Inflammatory Conditions

Inflammation is a general response of body tissue to any injury or disease that damages cells. It is a protective response that involves increased blood flow to the distressed area, along with assembling of specialized cells that attack infectious agents and destroy dead tissue. The increased blood flow causes redness; major inflammation also causes pain and swelling.

Most infections and disorders of the skin and membranes provoke an inflammatory response. This section describes a few inflammatory conditions that have one or more specific causes.

Pleurisy

Pleurisy (PLOOR-i-see) is an inflammation of the pleura, which is the membrane that lines the thoracic (chest) cavity and lungs. Pleurisy can be caused by an infection, such as pneumonia or tuberculosis. It can also be caused by cancer, rheumatoid arthritis, lupus, an injury to the chest, a blockage in the blood supply to the lungs, or the harmful presence of inhaled asbestos.

Pleurisy causes the normally smooth surfaces of the pleura to become rough. With each breath, the pleura lining the chest cavity and the pleura lining the lungs rub against each other, producing a grating sound called a *friction rub*, which can readily be heard with a stethoscope (**Figure 4.15**).

The primary symptom of pleurisy is chest pain that sharpens with inhalation or coughing. The pain may radiate to one or both shoulders. Pleurisy can cause an accumulation of fluid in the thoracic cavity. This fluid accumulation can make breathing difficult and may cause cyanosis, shortness of breath, rapid breathing, and coughing.

The course of treatment for pleurisy depends on the cause. Bacterial infections are treated with antibiotics. When fluid has accumulated in the chest cavity, it can be drained through a surgical procedure. Anti-inflammatory drugs can help control the pain caused by pleurisy.

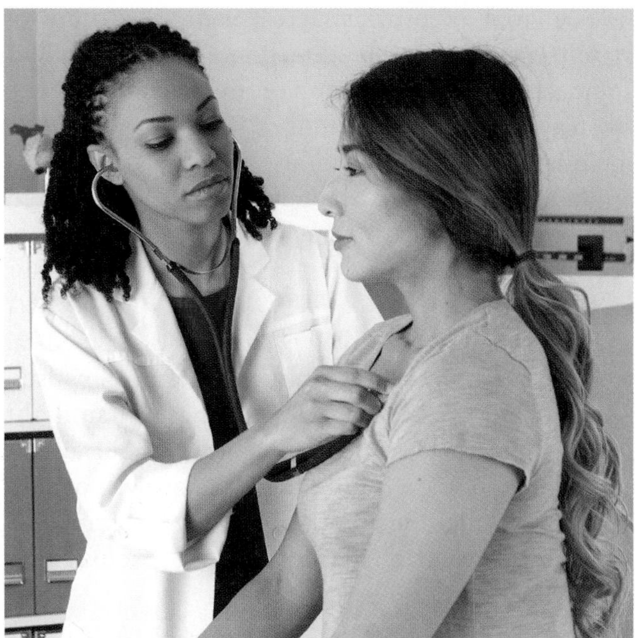

Rocketclips, Inc./Shutterstock.com

Figure 4.15 Doctor examining patient.

Peritonitis

Peritonitis is an inflammation of the peritoneum, or the membrane that lines the inner wall of the abdomen and covers the abdominal organs. Peritonitis is caused by the accumulation of blood, body fluids, or pus in the abdomen. Symptoms include abdominal pain and tenderness that may worsen with movement or touch. The abdomen may also be swollen. Other symptoms may include fever and chills, nausea and vomiting, fatigue, shortness of breath, rapid heartbeat, and decreased urine and stool output.

Peritonitis is a serious, potentially life-threatening condition. Medical treatment typically involves surgery to repair the internal damage that caused the condition, along with a course of strong antibiotics.

Psoriasis

Psoriasis (soh-RIGH-a-sis) is a common skin disorder that involves redness and irritation. The condition is characterized by regions of thick, red skin with flaky, silver-white patches called *scales* that itch, burn, crack, and sometimes bleed (**Figure 4.16**).

According to a prevailing hypothesis, psoriasis has its roots in an autoimmune disorder, which involves an inappropriate immune response to a substance or tissue that is present in the body. In the case of psoriasis, the body's immune system causes skin cells to be produced too quickly. This overproduction of skin cells yields raised patches of skin, or scales.

Psoriasis is not contagious and may be hereditary. It typically develops between 15 and 35 years of age and can progress quickly or slowly. It may disappear and return, or it may persist indefinitely. Outbreaks of psoriasis most commonly affect the elbows, knees, and trunk region, although they can occur anywhere on the body.

A variety of conditions can trigger or exacerbate psoriasis. These conditions include bacterial or viral infections, minor injuries to the skin, dry skin, stress, too little or too much sunlight, excessive alcohol consumption, and certain medications. Psoriasis is also worsened by a weakened immune system due to AIDS, chemotherapy, or autoimmune disorders such as rheumatoid arthritis.

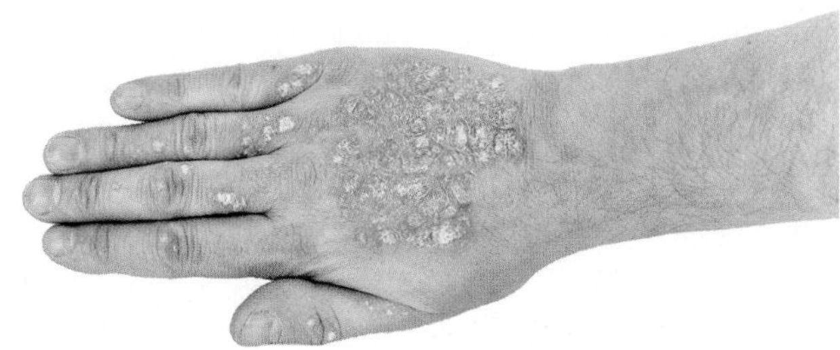

2Ban/Shutterstock.com

Figure 4.16 Psoriasis.

The goal of psoriasis treatment is to control symptoms and prevent infection. Three treatment approaches are available: topical treatments, systemic treatments, and light therapy. Topical treatments include special skin lotions, ointments, creams, and shampoos that are applied to the affected area. Systemic treatments, which treat the whole body, include medications that can be injected or taken orally.

Light therapy, also called *phototherapy,* is a medical treatment in which the skin is carefully exposed to ultraviolet light. The UVB in natural sunlight is an effective treatment for psoriasis because it penetrates the skin and hinders the growth of skin cells affected by the condition. In light therapy, the skin is exposed at regular intervals to a source that delivers artificial UVB.

SELF CHECK

1. What causes the redness associated with inflammation?
2. What is pleurisy?
3. Which skin disorder is characterized by regions of thick, red skin with flaky, silver-white patches?

Skin Cancers

Many skin conditions involve bumps or small, noncancerous lesions. Common warts are an example. Thus far, this chapter has described conditions that involve benign growths—that is, they do not metastasize, or spread, to other regions of the body.

When a tumor is malignant, or cancerous, it tends to metastasize to body parts other than the one in which it originated. Skin cancer is the most common type of cancer in the United States; at some point in their lives, about one-fifth of the population experiences skin cancer. Overexposure to the sun is a major risk factor in skin cancer's prevalence.

Basal cell carcinoma (KAR-si-NOH-ma) is the most common form of skin cancer and, fortunately, it is also the least malignant (**Figure 4.17**). It is caused by overproduction of cells in the stratum basale that push upward, forming dome-shaped bumps. These bumps appear most often on areas of the face that have been exposed to the sun. Slow-growing basal cell carcinomas are usually noticed and surgically removed before they can spread and become dangerous.

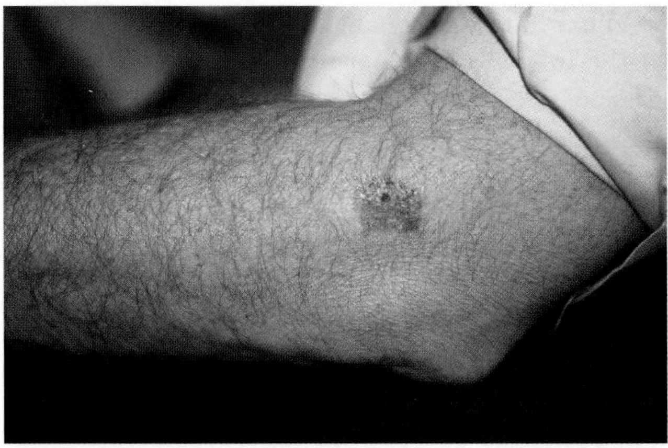

DermPics/Science Source

Figure 4.17 Basal cell carcinoma. Although this common form of skin cancer is less likely than other forms to be malignant, it should not be ignored.

Squamous cell carcinoma is caused by overproduction of cells in the stratum spinosum layer of the epidermis. These cancers appear as a scaly, reddened patch that progresses to an ulcer-like mass with a raised border (**Figure 4.18**). Among fair-skinned people, the most commonly affected locations are the scalp, ears, lower lip, and backs of the hands. Dark-skinned people, however, typically develop this condition in areas not exposed to the sun, such as the legs or feet. Squamous cell carcinomas grow rapidly and can easily spread to nearby lymph nodes. These cancers can be completely cured through early removal by surgery or radiation treatment.

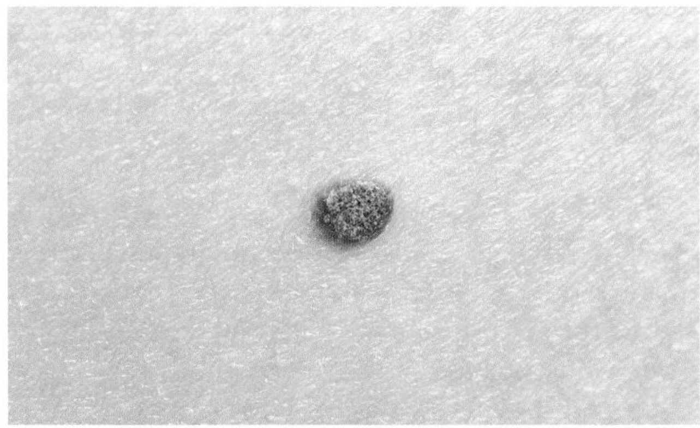

DermPics/Science Source

Figure 4.18 Squamous cell carcinoma.

The most serious form of skin cancer is ***malignant melanoma*** (MEHL-a-NOH-ma), or cancer of the melanocytes (**Figure 4.19**). Although typically dark colored and irregular in shape, a malignant melanoma can appear pink, red, or "fleshy." Changes in the size, shape, color, or elevation of a mole are typical warning signs of a malignant melanoma.

The American Cancer Society advocates the ABCD rule for determining the presence of melanoma:

A. **Asymmetry**: The shape of the mole is irregular.

B. **Border irregularity**: The outside borders of the mole are not smooth.

C. **Color**: More than one color is present in the mole. Melanomas may contain different shades of black and brown, blues, reds, or pinks.

D. **Diameter**: The mole is larger than about one-quarter of an inch in diameter, or larger than the diameter of a pencil.

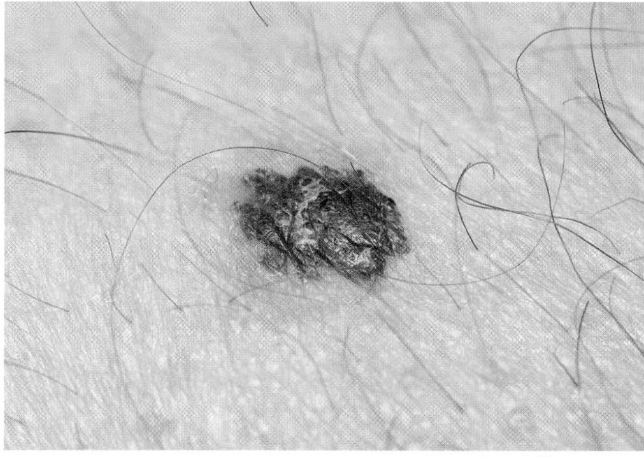

Krzysztof Winnik/Shutterstock.com

Figure 4.19 Malignant melanoma.

It is important for people who suspect that they may have a malignant melanoma to see a health-care provider immediately. Although these cancers comprise only about 5% of all skin cancers, they can be deadly.

Focus On Indoor Tanning

Indoor tanning through the use of a bed, booth, or sunlamp has been popular in the United States since the 1980s. Indoor tanning devices deliver high levels of UV radiation, including both UVA and UVB rays, in a short time. Although most of these devices operate on a timer, the amount of UV radiation delivered varies based on the type and age of the light bulbs. Studies have shown that newer tanning beds are not safer than older models.

Several federal and international agencies and organizations have issued warnings about the negative effects of indoor tanning on health. The US Food and Drug Administration has declared that the UV radiation in tanning devices poses serious health risks. A recent report by the International Agency for Research on Cancer (IARC), part of the World Health Organization, also warns that indoor tanning is dangerous. The Healthy People 2020 initiative, which provides science-based, 10-year national objectives for improving the health of all Americans, includes goals for dramatically reducing the use of indoor tanning devices.

Exposure to UV radiation, whether from the sun or indoor tanning devices, can contribute to the development of skin cancer, skin burns, wrinkles, lax skin, brown spots, cataracts, and cancers of the eyes. Cancers caused by indoor tanning include melanoma, basal cell carcinoma, squamous cell carcinoma, and ocular melanoma. Numerous research studies have shown that the incidence of melanoma and other skin cancers is increased among indoor tanning users, with risk increasing as the number of tanning sessions increases.

You may have heard or read that exposure to UV rays is beneficial in elevating levels of vitamin D within the body. However, indoor tanning is *not* a safe way to get vitamin D. In fact, the best way to get adequate vitamin D is to eat nutritious foods that contain it, such as milk, eggs, mushrooms, and many types of fish.

Because of the known dangers associated with indoor tanning, the practice has been banned or restricted in many regions. The states of California, Delaware, Hawaii, Illinois, Louisiana, Minnesota, Nevada, Oregon, Texas, Vermont, and Washington, as well as some cities and counties in other states, prohibit indoor tanning by children and adolescents younger than 18 years of age. Internationally, Austria, Belgium, Finland, France, Germany, Iceland, Italy, Norway, Portugal, Spain, and the United Kingdom have also banned indoor tanning for people younger than 18 years of age. Brazil and five out of six states in Australia have made indoor tanning illegal altogether.

SECTION 4.3

REVIEW

Mini-Glossary

basal cell carcinoma the most common and least malignant form of skin cancer

cellulitis a bacterial infection characterized by a red, swollen, and painful area of skin

common warts warts that typically appear on the hands or fingers and disappear without treatment

first-degree burns burns that affect only the epidermal layer of skin

fourth-degree burns burns that involve destruction of all layers of skin, as well as nerve endings and some of the underlying tissues such as muscle, tendon, ligament, and bone

herpes simplex virus type 1 the form of herpes that generates cold sores or fever blisters around the mouth

herpes simplex virus type 2 the genital form of herpes

herpes varicella (chickenpox) a highly contagious, common childhood disease that is characterized by extremely itchy, fluid-filled blisters

herpes zoster (shingles) a disease that involves a painful, blistering rash accompanied by headache, fever, and a general unwell feeling

impetigo a bacterial infection common in elementary school children that is characterized by pink, blister-like bumps, usually on the face

malignant melanoma cancer of the melanocytes; the most serious form of skin cancer

peritonitis inflammation of the peritoneum

plantar warts warts that develop on the soles of the foot, grow inward, and can become painful

pleurisy inflammation of the pleura

psoriasis a common skin disorder that involves redness, irritation, and scales (flaky, silver-white patches) that itch, burn, crack, and sometimes bleed

rule of nines a method used to calculate body surface area affected by burns

second-degree burns burns that involve damage to both the epidermis and the upper portion of the underlying dermis; characterized by blisters

squamous cell carcinoma a type of rapidly growing cancer that appears as a scaly, reddened patch of skin

third-degree burns burns that destroy the entire thickness of the skin

tinea a fungal infection that tends to occur in areas of the body that are moist

Review Questions

1. Describe how the skin regenerates.
2. Name two interventions that can help to reduce a bedridden patient's risk for developing decubitus ulcers.
3. Describe the four types of skin burns.
4. List two types of skin infections common in school-age children.
5. Identify three types of medical treatments for warts.
6. List and briefly describe four common fungal infections.
7. Why are third- and fourth-degree burns unable to heal on their own?
8. What is the connection between herpes varicella (chickenpox) and herpes zoster (shingles)?
9. Imagine that you are a physician, and one of your elderly patients has decubitus ulcers in the coccyx area of her body. When you inform the patient that she has bedsores, she seems confused, saying that she sleeps fewer hours per night than most people she knows, and so spends less time in bed. What explanation would you give your patient so that she could better understand her condition?

Medical Terminology: The Integumentary System

By understanding the word parts that make up medical words, you can extend your medical vocabulary. This chapter includes many of the word parts listed below. Review these word parts to be sure you understand their meanings.

-al	relating or pertaining to
-ar	pertaining to
bronchi/o	bronchial tube
cutane/o	skin
cyt/o	cell
derm/o	skin
epi-	above
epitheli/o	epithelium
gastr/o	stomach
hypo-	below
-ic	pertaining to
-ium	structure or tissue
-logy	study of
melan/o	black; pigmented
-meter	instrument
muc/o	mucus
-ous	pertaining to
-pathy	disease
peri-	around, surrounding
reticul/o	network
ser/o	serum
sub-	below, under
sud/o, sudor/o	sweat

Now use these word parts to form valid medical words that fit the following definitions. Some of the words are included in this chapter. Others are not. When you finish, use a medical dictionary to check your work.

1. pertaining to the skin
2. pertaining to mucus
3. pertaining to around the heart
4. pertaining to serum
5. pertaining to under the skin
6. relating to a mucous membrane
7. pertaining to surrounding a bronchus
8. disease of the epithelium
9. layer of skin below the dermis
10. keratin-producing cells
11. pigment-producing cells
12. pertaining to (a layer) containing a network of blood and lymphatic vessels
13. pertaining to under the dermis
14. pertaining to above the stomach
15. study of cells
16. instrument that measures the amount of sweat produced

Chapter 4 Summary

- Three types of epithelial membranes line or cover the internal and external surfaces of the body: mucous, serous, and cutaneous membranes.
- Synovial membranes, which are composed entirely of connective tissue, cushion the tendons and ligaments surrounding joints.
- The integumentary system protects the body against damage from harmful chemicals and ultraviolet rays from sunlight, serves as a water barrier, and helps to regulate body temperature.
- The two layers of the skin are the epidermis (outer layer) and the dermis (underlying layer).
- The appendages that support the skin include the sweat glands, sebaceous glands, hair, and nails.
- Common skin injuries include decubitus ulcers, which are caused by an area of localized pressure that restricts blood flow to one or more areas of the body, and burns.
- Skin infections may be caused by viruses (herpes, human papillomavirus), fungi (tinea), or bacteria (staphylococcus).
- Conditions that may cause inflammation of the skin include pleurisy, peritonitis, and psoriasis.
- The three types of skin cancer are basal cell carcinoma, squamous cell carcinoma, and malignant melanoma.

Chapter 4 Review

Understanding Key Concepts

1. Synovial membranes surround and protect which of the following surfaces?
   A. ball-and-socket joints
   B. internal cavities housing organs
   C. cavities open to the outside world
   D. the nails and hair follicles
2. _____ line or cover the internal and external surfaces of the body.

3. The ______ line the body cavities that open to the outside of the body.
4. Which of the following are lined with mucous membranes?
   A. blood vessels
   B. nerve networks
   C. respiratory tract
   D. the brain
5. *True or False?* Mucous membranes tend to be dry.
6. Which type of membrane is composed only of connective tissue and includes no epithelial cells?
7. Which type of membrane makes up the pleura, pericardium, and peritoneum?
8. *True or False? Cutaneous membrane* is the name for skin.
9. *True or False?* The visceral layer is the outer lining of each serous membrane.
10. *True or False?* The epithelial membranes line or cover the internal surfaces of the body only.
11. *True or False?* The body membranes surround and help to protect the body's surfaces.
12. Which type of protein, found in the outermost layer of the skin, adds structural strength to the skin?
13. What is the name of the receptors that transmit nerve signals containing information about the environment, including touch, pressure, vibration, pain, and temperature?
14. Which two layers make up the skin?
    A. epidermis and hypodermis
    B. epidermis and dermis
    C. hypodermis and dermis
    D. dermis and underlying tissues
15. Which of the following are considered appendages of the skin?
    A. bone
    B. teeth
    C. hair
    D. muscle
16. Collagen and elastic fibers make up the dense, fibrous connective tissue called ______.
17. *True or False?* Keratin is primarily responsible for human skin color.
18. *True or False?* The epidermis completely replaces itself every 25 to 45 days.
19. *True or False?* The skin has two layers, the outer epidermis and the underlying dermis.

Instructions: *Identify each structure in the integumentary system by indicating the* ***letter*** *that corresponds to the name of the structure.*

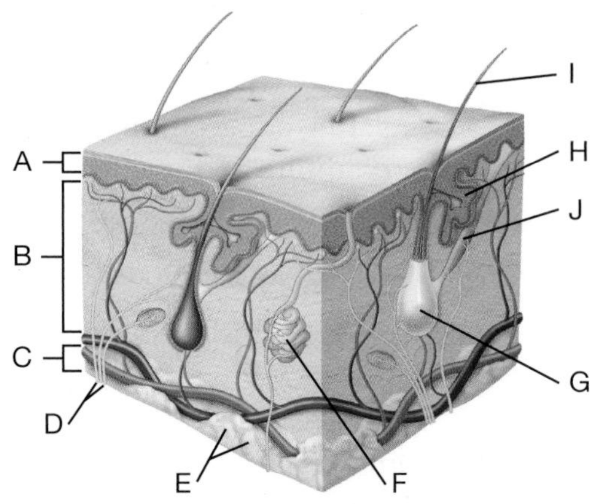

20. lipocytes
21. hypodermis
22. sebaceous gland
23. arrector pili muscle
24. dermis
25. hair follicle
26. epidermis
27. sweat gland
28. hair shaft
29. nerve fibers
30. Which type of burn, referred to as a full-thickness burn, destroys the entire skin but not the underlying structures?
31. Which of the following is *not* a type of viral infection?
    A. herpes
    B. psoriasis
    C. plantar warts
    D. genital warts
32. *True or False?* Psoriasis is a highly contagious disease characterized by scaly skin patches that itch, burn, crack, and sometimes bleed.
33. ______ is a highly contagious staphylococcus infection that is common in elementary school children.

34. ______ is a common skin disorder characterized by regions of thick, red skin with flaky, silver-white patches.

35. The most serious form of skin cancer is ______.
    A. basal cell carcinoma
    B. squamous cell carcinoma
    C. malignant melanoma
    D. lymphoma

36. *True or False?* Burns can be caused by exposure to electricity.

37. *True or False?* First-degree burns damage the epidermis and parts of the underlying dermis.

Thinking Critically

38. Explain the main difference between a mucous membrane and a serous membrane. Discuss examples of both membrane types in your explanation.

39. Explain the skin's function in regulating body temperature. Compare and contrast the ways in which the skin helps the body cool to the way it helps the body warm.

40. Explain to an imaginary person why his or her hair color and texture (straight, wavy, or curly) have developed as they have.

41. The skin can be described as stratified squamous epithelial tissue. Describe what this description means in relation to the structure and function of the skin.

42. Name the two major categories of HPVs and explain how they differ.

43. Which form of skin cancer is the most serious? What are some of its typical characteristics?

44. Describe the effects of decubitus ulcers on the body.

Clinical Case Study

Read again the Clinical Case Study at the beginning of this chapter. Use the information provided in the chapter to answer the following questions.

45. What diagnoses are possible?

46. Which diagnosis is most likely, given the description? Why?

Analyzing and Evaluating Data

Using the information in this chapter about skin burns and the rule of nines, examine the figure below to answer the following questions.

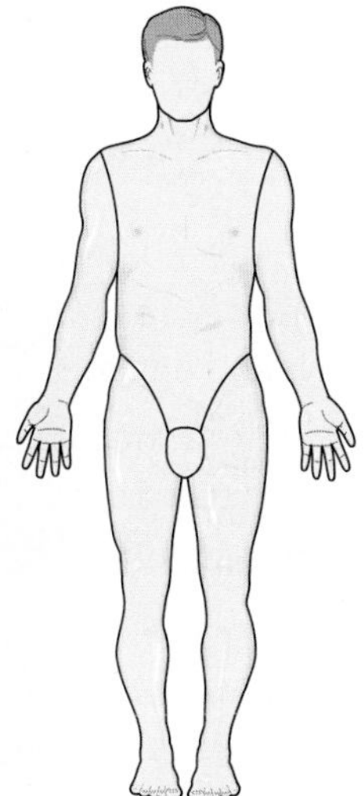

47. What percentage of burned tissue would you assign to a patient who suffered burns to the anterior and posterior portions of the head and the anterior portion of both arms?

48. What percentage would you assign to a patient who suffered burns to the anterior portion of the left leg and the anterior portion of the torso?

49. What percentage would you assign to a patient who suffered burns to the anterior and posterior right leg, the anterior portion of the torso, and the posterior portion of the right arm?

Investigating Further

50. Research skin injuries and disorders that commonly occur in the work environment and develop a written plan to prevent possible dermal exposure in the workplace.

51. Phenol is a chemical that is commonly used in medications such as sore throat sprays and lozenges. Investigate the potential hazard incurred by topical exposure to phenol by workers in medical manufacturing companies that produce medications containing phenol. Write a report describing your findings.

5 The Skeletal System

Clinical Case Study

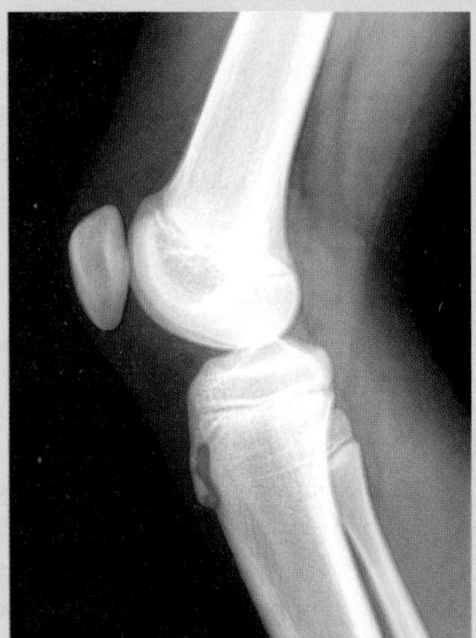
Warrick G./Science Source

Fifteen-year-old Dana is a healthy adolescent who eats a balanced diet and gets plenty of sleep. She is also the star player on both her high-school JV soccer team and her travel soccer team. Her travel team plays for 10 months per year, and while the seasons overlap between the two teams, she attends soccer practices at least five days per week and typically has two games per week.

For about the past six months, Dana has been experiencing pain and swelling around the anterior aspect of her right knee that worsens with activity and has prevented her from finishing many of her games. She does not recall having had an injury to the knee, and other than the pain and swelling, she has no observable symptoms. Dana's travel coach frankly wonders if Dana might be faking her pain for some reason, since her play is not affected during the first half of her soccer matches.

But the pain is real and Dana finally sees a physician. Among the conditions and injuries discussed in the chapter, which ones might Dana have, and which do you think is most likely?

Chapter 5 Outline

Section 5.1 Bone

- Functions of the Skeletal System
- Bone Classification and Structure
- Growth and Development of Bones
- Bone Remodeling

Section 5.2 The Axial Skeleton

- Skull
- Vertebral Column
- Thoracic Cage

Section 5.3 The Appendicular Skeleton

- Upper Extremity
- Lower Extremity

Section 5.4 Joints

- Types of Joints
- Articular Tissues

Section 5.5 Injuries and Disorders of the Skeletal System

- Common Bone Injuries
- Osteoporosis
- Common Joint Injuries
- Arthritis

People tend to think of bone as a hard, dried-up chunk of mineral that a dog would enjoy chewing. While this is true of dead bone, the living bones inside the human body are made up of amazing, complex living tissues. Bones are not only hydrated (containing water), but also very dynamic, continually changing in size, shape, and strength over time.

How and why do these processes and changes occur? This chapter explores the characteristics of living bone and describes the well-tailored functionality of the major bones and joints in the human skeleton. It also discusses some of the common injuries and disorders of the bones and joints, how these problems tend to occur, and in some cases, how their likelihood can be reduced.

SECTION 5.1

Bone

Objectives

- Describe the functions of the skeletal system.
- Classify various types of bones and describe the structure of each.
- Explain the processes through which bones grow in length and diameter during normal human development.
- Discuss bone remodeling, including the cells responsible for this process and the practices and environments that can influence it.

Key Terms

appositional growth
articular cartilage
bone marrow
cortical bone
diaphysis
epiphyseal plate
epiphysis
Haversian canals
Haversian system
hematopoiesis
medullary cavity
ossification
osteoblasts
osteoclasts
osteocytes
osteon
perforating (Volkmann's) canals
periosteum
remodeling
Sharpey's fibers
trabecular bone

Human bones are remarkably adaptive. They grow and change throughout a person's life and play several major anatomical and physiological roles.

Functions of the Skeletal System

The approximately 206 individual bones comprising the human skeleton come in many different sizes and shapes, each uniquely well designed to serve a particular function. The skeletal system, in general, performs the following important functions.

Support

It is hard to imagine humans without bones because, like the framework of a house, human bones form the internal support system that provides shape and support to the trunk and limbs. The bones in your legs enable you to stand upright, while your ribs support your chest cavity.

Protection

Bones surround and support the body's delicate internal organs. For example, the ribs serve as bony protectors of critical organs nestled in the thoracic cavity, such as the heart and lungs. Equally important, the skull provides protection for the brain, and the vertebral column surrounds and protects the delicate spinal cord.

Movement

What produces human movement? Although gravity and other external forces can cause movement, the internal forces produced by muscles cause purposeful movements. When muscles contract or shorten, they pull on the bones they are attached to, thereby causing movement.

The design of the skeletal system, with bones that are able to rotate or glide in certain ways around joints, is extraordinarily functional. Each joint, where two or more bones articulate, is designed to enable specific movements while preventing others. For example, the shoulder joint allows movement in multiple directions, while movement at the knee is largely constrained to one direction. This amazing design enables walking, running, jumping, pushing, pulling, and throwing, as well as all of the routine activities that we take for granted every day. You will learn more about the muscles and how they work in the next chapter.

Storage

Bones also serve as a storage repository for minerals, notably phosphorus and calcium. Phosphorus (P) plays a vital role in the development and maintenance of healthy bones and teeth, as well as the chemical reactions that release energy in the body. Calcium (Ca^{2+}) is essential for normal functioning of the neuromuscular system, contractions of the heart, and blood clotting. Through a chemical balancing procedure known as *homeostasis*, discussed in Chapter 1, the body can draw upon the stored phosphorus or calcium in bone if the levels of these minerals in the bloodstream should fall below normal.

Another storage site within the skeletal system is the ***medullary cavity***, which is a central hollow space inside most of the long bones, such as those of the arms and legs. The medullary cavity is also known as the *marrow cavity* because it stores **bone marrow**, a specialized flexible tissue found inside bones.

There are two types of bone marrow: yellow and red. Both types contain a rich blood supply. Yellow marrow, found in the medullary cavity, is a major storehouse for fat within the body. Red marrow is found in the cavities of many bones, including flat and short bones; bodies of the vertebrae, sternum, and ribs; and the articulating ends of long bones.

Blood Cell Formation

It is in the red marrow that the critically important function of ***hematopoiesis*** (hee-ma-toh-poy-EE-sis), or blood cell formation, occurs. Red blood cells deliver oxygen to tissues throughout the body and transport waste in the form of carbon dioxide to the lungs, where it can be exhaled. Because red blood cells have a life span of only about 120 days, it is important for the red bone marrow to constantly produce new red blood cells.

SELF CHECK

1. List the five functions of the skeletal system.
2. What are two functions of bone marrow?

Bone Classification and Structure

The composition and structure of bone make it remarkably strong and resilient given its relatively light weight. The shapes of bones vary according to their specific functions.

Composition of Bones

Cells are the structural building blocks of bone, as they are in other body tissues. Mature bone cells are called ***osteocytes***.

One factor that distinguishes bone from other tissues is that 60% to 70% of a bone's weight comes from its mineral content—primarily calcium carbonate and calcium phosphate. These mineral salts make bone hard and resistant to compression. The remaining 30% to 40% of a bone's weight comes from collagen—a protein that provides bone's flexibility and resistance to tension (being stretched)—and water. Both the minerals and the water content contribute to bone strength. The bones of children tend to be more flexible than the bones of adults due to higher collagen and water content.

Types of Bone Tissue

Bone includes two different types of tissue: cortical bone and trabecular bone. Whereas ***cortical bone*** tissue is relatively dense, ***trabecular bone*** tissue, also known as *spongy bone* or *cancellous bone*, is relatively porous, with a honeycomb structure (**Figure 5.1**). Cortical (compact) bone is stiffer due to its higher mineral content, so it is generally stronger than trabecular bone. Trabecular bone, with its spongy structure, is more flexible than cortical bone.

Most bones contain both cortical and trabecular tissue. The function of a given bone determines whether it is composed mostly of cortical or trabecular bone. For example, the long bones in the arms and legs are primarily composed of strong cortical bone tissue, although there is trabecular bone inside the ends of these bones. The bones in the spinal column contain a large amount of trabecular bone inside their cortical shells, giving them a certain amount of shock-absorbing capability. However, in all bones, the outer layer is always composed of hard, protective cortical bone, with spongy trabecular bone present to varying degrees inside. **Figure 5.2** compares the properties of these two types of bone tissue.

Understanding Medical Terminology

The word *cortical* (coming from *cortex*) pertains to the outer layer of something. For example, the outer layer of the brain is known as the *cerebral cortex*. The outer layer of many structures and objects, including a plant stem or even a rock, is also known as its *cortex*. The type of bone tissue forming the outer layer of bone is therefore called *cortical bone*.

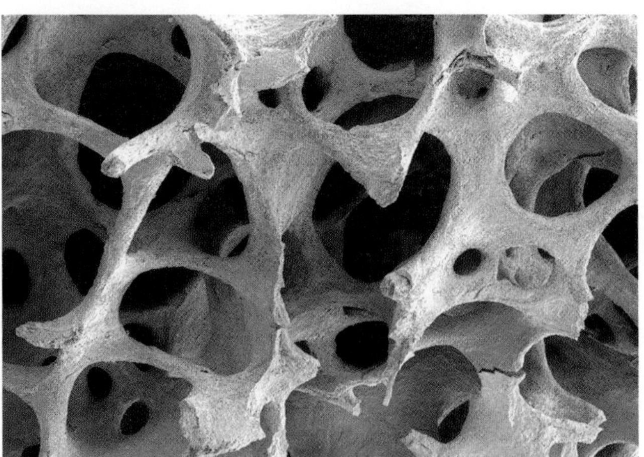

Steve Gschmeissner/Science Source

Figure 5.1 A scanning electron micrograph of trabecular bone tissue.

Properties of Bone Tissue		
	Cortical Bone	**Trabecular Bone**
Structure	dense	porous (honeycomb structure)
Mineral content	relatively high	relatively low
Strength	relatively high	low
Flexibility	low	relatively more
Shock-absorbing ability	low	relatively more
Primary locations	outer surface of all bones, long bones of limbs	interior of vertebrae, femoral neck, wrist, and ankle bones

Figure 5.2

Goodheart-Willcox Publisher

Shapes of Bones

Because of the large variety of sizes and shapes of the bones in the human skeleton, bones are traditionally divided into five categories for the purpose of discussion (**Figure 5.3**):

- Long bones have a long, somewhat cylindrical shaft made of cortical bone, with bulbous knobs of trabecular bone encased in cortical bone at both ends. The shaft encloses the central hollow medullary cavity or canal. The major bones of the arms and legs are long bones.

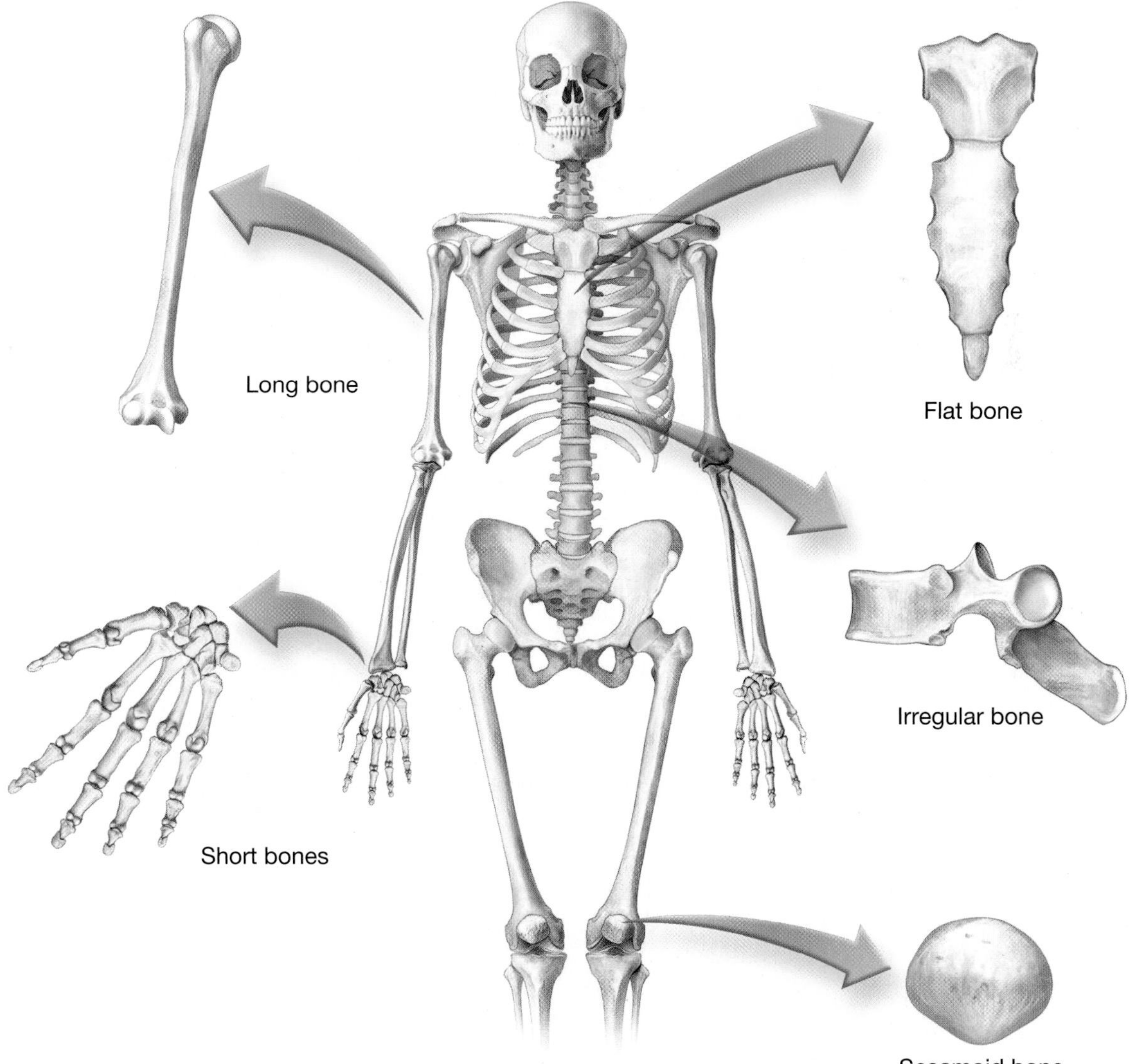

Figure 5.3 The five shape categories of bones.

- Short bones are shaped roughly like a cube and are composed mainly of trabecular bone. The bones of the wrists and ankles are short bones.
- Flat bones are thin, relatively large in surface area, and generally curved to some extent. Structurally, they consist of two thin layers of cortical bone with a layer of trabecular bone in between. These bones function to protect underlying organs and provide large areas for muscle attachments. The scapula, ribs, and the bones of the skull are considered flat bones.
- Sesamoid bones are formed within tendons. The most prominent example of a sesamoid bone is the patella.
- Irregular bones are all those bones that do not fit into one of the preceding categories. They have individualized shapes to fulfill specific functions. The bones of the spinal column and hip girdle are in this category.

Surface Anatomy of Bones

The external surfaces of bones are somewhat like the surface of the moon, scored with crater-like cavities, lined with ridges, and supporting hill-like bulbs. Though they may seem random, the locations of these various irregularities and markings on any given bone are consistent from person to person (**Figure 5.4**).

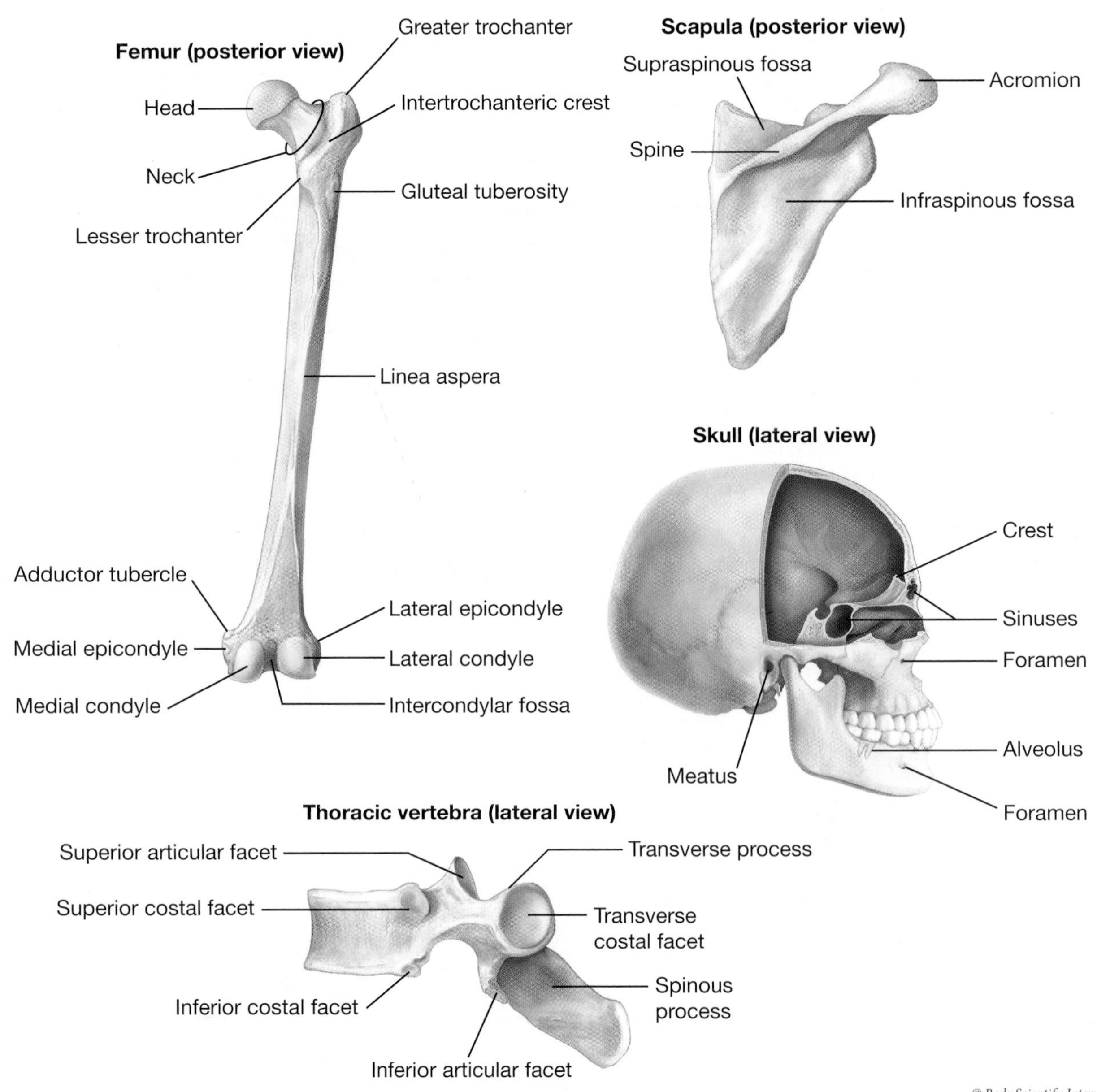

Figure 5.4 Examples of bone markings and irregularities.

This is because the surface features are functional, having been formed by the attachments of tendons and ligaments, or providing reciprocally shaped articulations for blood vessels and nerves at joints or channels. The names of many of these surface features identify the locations of muscle attachments and other points of interest. **Figure 5.5** lists and describes the general names of the anatomical surface features of bones.

Anatomical Structure of Long Bones

The ***diaphysis*** of a long bone is the hollow shaft composed of cortical bone (**Figure 5.6**). A fibrous connective tissue membrane called the ***periosteum*** surrounds and protects the diaphysis. Mats of tiny fibers composed primarily of collagen, known as ***Sharpey's fibers***, firmly bind the periosteum to the underlying cortical bone. The periosteum contains blood and lymph vessels, as well as nerves. It is involved in bone growth, repair, and nutrition.

The hollow center of the diaphysis is the medullary canal, or cavity. Beginning when a person is about 5 years old, this cavity is filled with yellow bone marrow, which has a rich supply of blood vessels and acts as a storehouse for fat. The medullary cavity is lined by a membrane known as the *endosteum*.

The bulbous ends of long bones are known as ***epiphyses***. These regions are composed of trabecular tissue that contains red marrow, which participates in the formation of red blood cells (erythrocytes) and some white blood cells (leukocytes). Although all bone marrow is red at birth, only about half of the marrow is red by adulthood; the other half is yellow. Epiphyses are also the sites of bone growth in long bones and continue to enlarge as a person ages, adding length to the bone. Each epiphysis is surrounded by a protective covering of ***articular cartilage***. You may have noticed the shining white covering of articular cartilage over the ends of the bone in a chicken drumstick.

Surface Anatomy of Bones		
Components of Joints		
Feature	**Description**	**Example**
facet	small, smooth articular surface	facet joints of a vertebra
condyle	knob-like articular surface	femoral condyles
head	prominent, expanded end of a bone	head of a femur
Projections		
Feature	**Description**	**Example**
process	any bony prominence	transverse process of a vertebra
trochanter	process on the proximal femur	greater trochanter of femur
crest	prominent, narrow bony ridge	intertrochanteric crest of femur
line	slightly elevated, long, narrow ridge	linea aspera of femur
spine	sharp, slender process	spine of scapula
tubercle	small, rounded process	adductor tubercle of femur
tuberosity	rough, elevated surface	gluteal tuberosity of femur
epicondyle	elevation superior to a condyle	femoral epicondyles
neck	column supporting a head	femoral neck
Depressions and Openings		
Feature	**Description**	**Example**
fossa	shallow depression	supraspinous fossa of scapula
sinus	cavity or hollow filled with air	sinuses of skull
alveolus	small hollow	tooth socket
foramen	rounded opening	foramen of the skull
meatus	opening into a canal	external acoustic meatus (ear)
canal	tube-like passageway	auditory canal in skull

Figure 5.5 *Goodheart-Willcox Publisher*

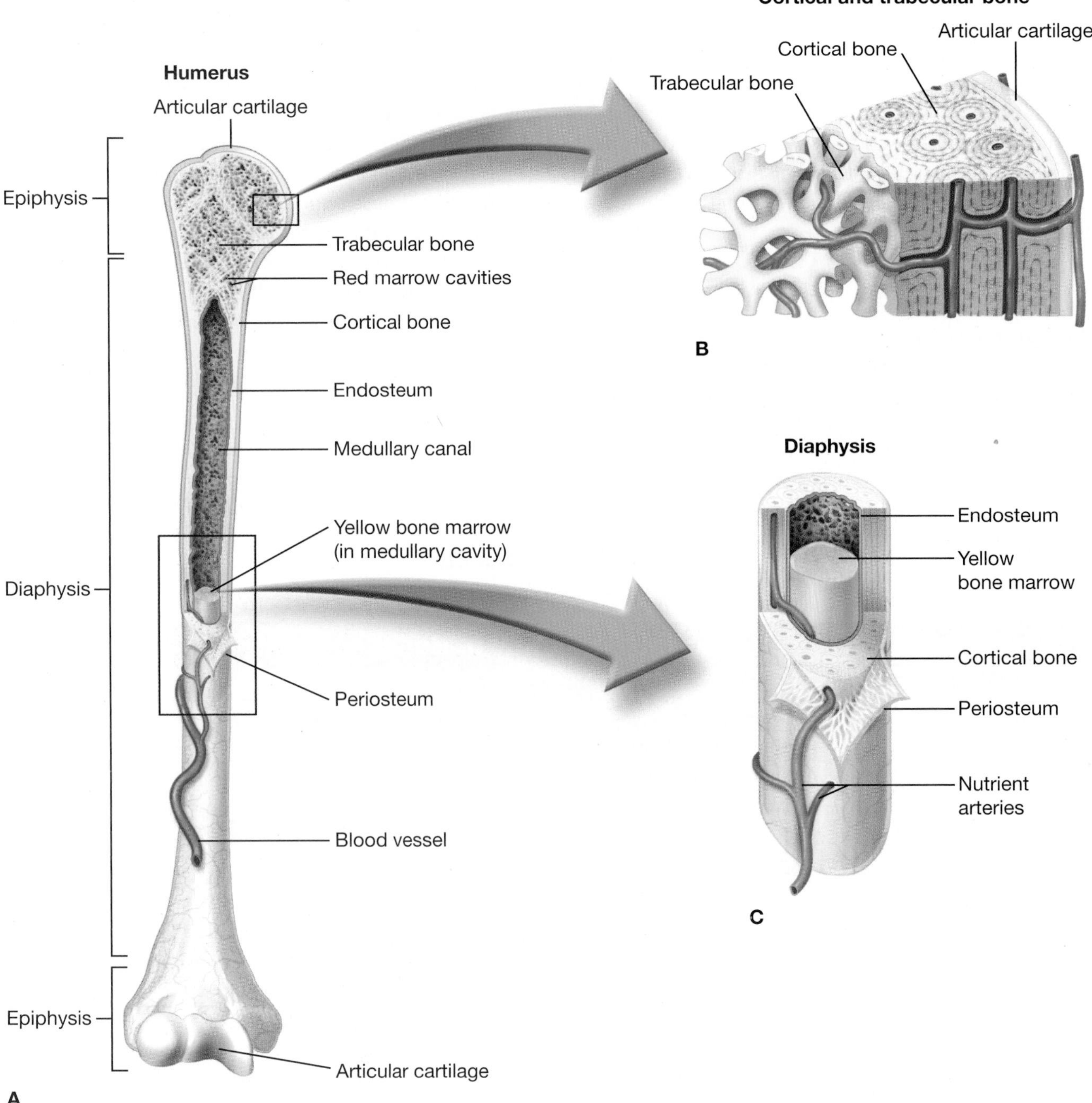

Figure 5.6 The anatomical structure of a long bone. A—Anterior view of the humerus with the interior of the top half exposed. B—Cortical and trabecular bone of the epiphysis. C—Enlargement of the diaphysis.

How does living bone receive nourishment and get rid of waste products? Bone has what you might think of as its own subway system. An intricate array of passageways exists at a microscopic level inside the mineralized part of bone. Blood vessels and nerves course through these tiny tunnels (**Figure 5.7**). Major passageways running in a lengthwise direction through the bone are called ***Haversian canals***. Tiny cavities called *lacunae* (la-KOO-nee) are laid out in concentric circles called *lamellae* (la-MEHL-ee) around the Haversian canals. Osteocytes are housed in the lacunae, which act as protective islands for these cells.

Each Haversian canal, with its surrounding layers of lacunae, forms a structural unit called an ***osteon***, or ***Haversian system***. Within the system, there are tiny sideways canals called *canaliculi* (kan-a-LIK-yoo-ligh). The canaliculi connect with the lacunae, forming a comprehensive transportation matrix for the supply of

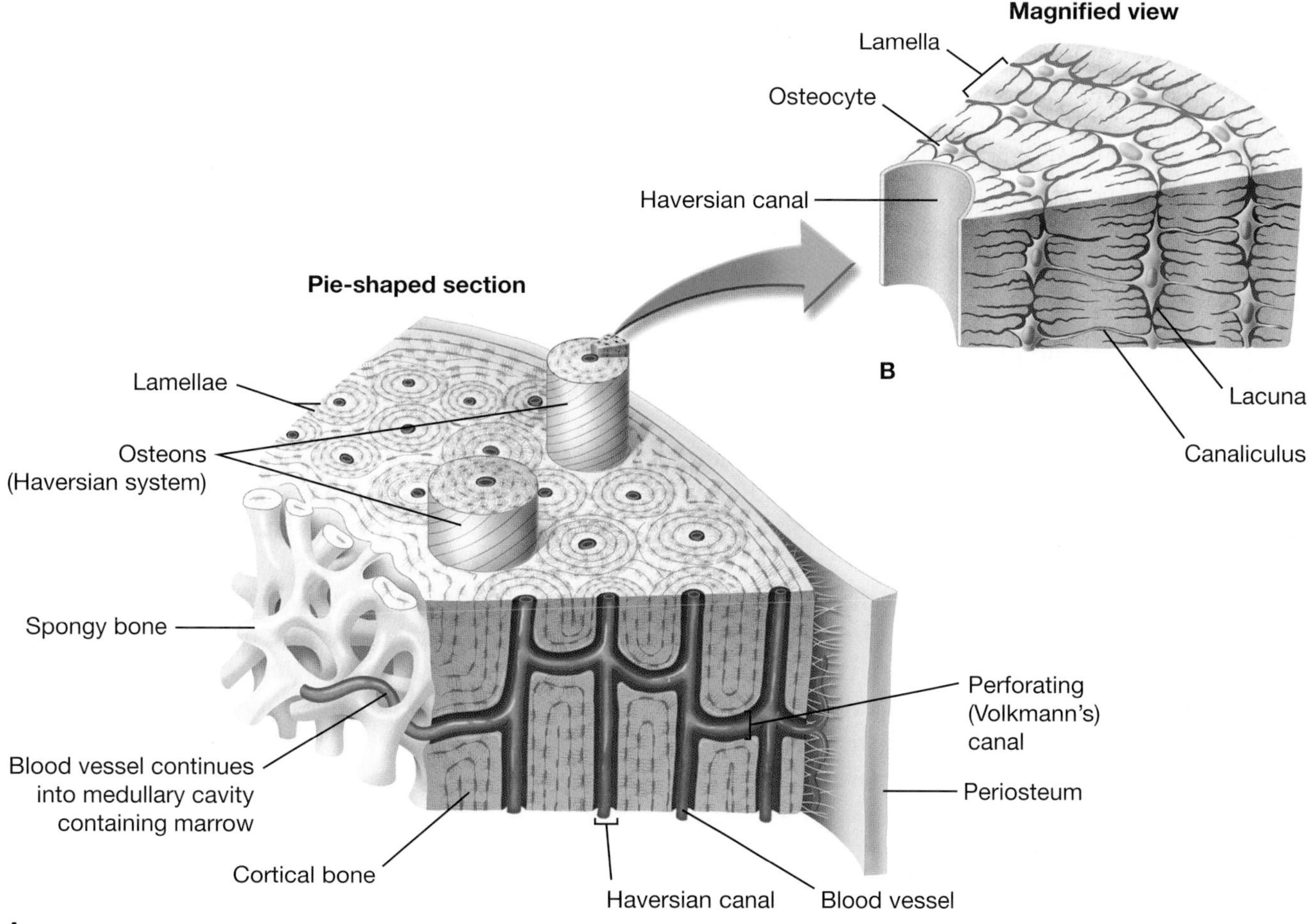

© Body Scientific International

Figure 5.7 A—A microscopic view of the inside of bone tissue. B—An even more magnified view of the diaphysis.

nutrients and removal of waste products throughout the Haversian system. The multiple Haversian systems are joined by ***perforating (Volkmann's) canals***, also running sideways.

SELF CHECK

1. What percentage of bone weight comes from its mineral content?
2. What is collagen?
3. Where is cortical bone typically found?
4. Where is trabecular bone typically found?
5. What is the purpose of a Haversian system?

Growth and Development of Bones

Over the course of the life span from birth through old age, some parts of the body grow, while others tend to shrink. Knowledge of the processes by which bones grow and develop is the key to understanding why these phenomena occur.

Osteoblasts and Osteoclasts

Specialized bone cells called ***osteoblasts*** carry out the work of building new bone tissue. Other specialized cells called ***osteoclasts*** resorb, or eliminate, weakened or damaged bone tissue.

Understanding Medical Terminology

Osteoblast and *osteoclast* are similar-sounding names for these specialized bone cells. An easy way to avoid confusing them is to remember the "b" in *osteoblast* is the same as the "b" in *build*. Similarly, the "cl" in *osteoclast* is the same as the "cl" in *clear*. Osteoblasts *b*uild bone and osteoclasts *cl*ear away old or damaged bone.

Bone growth involves more osteoblast activity than osteoclast activity. However, both osteoblasts and osteoclasts remain extremely busy over the course of a normal person's life. In healthy adult bone, the activity of osteoblasts and osteoclasts is balanced. As a result of this balance, the bones stay strong and optimally designed for their various functions.

Bone Formation

Bone modeling is the process in which new bone is created through osteoblast activity. The skeleton of early-developing embryos is composed mainly of a flexible tissue called *hyaline cartilage*. Although cartilage forms parts of the adult nose, ribs, and some joints, cartilage is rapidly replaced with bone even within the developing fetus.

The process of bone formation is called ***ossification***. Before birth, ossification occurs in two phases. During the first phase, a bone matrix shell covers the hyaline cartilage through the activity of osteoblasts. Next, osteoclasts resorb the enclosed hyaline cartilage, creating a medullary cavity within the bony superstructure.

Longitudinal Growth

Bones grow in length at the ***epiphyseal plates***, which are located close to the ends of long bones (**Figure 5.8**). During childhood growth, osteoblasts on the central side of the epiphyseal plate produce new bone cells, resulting in an increase in bone length. At the end of the growth period, occurring during or shortly after adolescence, the plate dissolves and the bone on either side of the plate fuses, effectively ending the longitudinal growth of the bone.

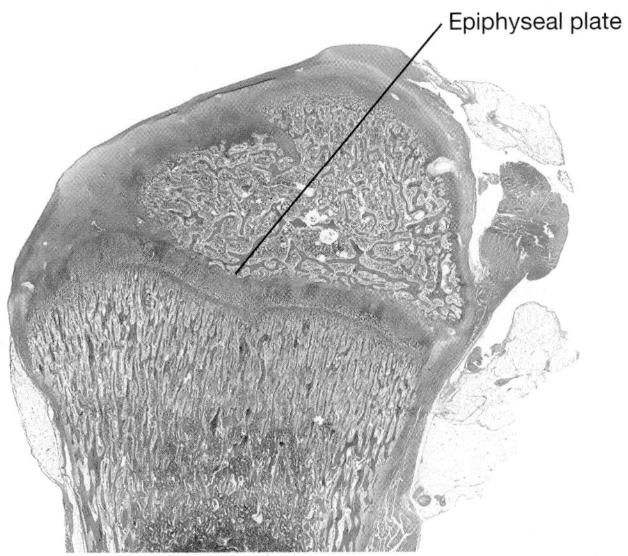

Jose Luis Calvo/Shutterstock.com

Figure 5.8 Bones grow in length at the epiphyseal plates (the dark pink area).

Circumferential Growth

Although most bone growth occurs during childhood, bones actually grow in diameter, or width, throughout the life span (**Figure 5.9**). Osteoblasts in the internal layer of the periosteum build concentric layers of new bone on top of existing ones. To understand the process, you might visualize the way in which the rings on a cross-cut tree stump reveal the tree's growth.

At the same time that the osteoblasts are doing their work, the osteoclasts resorb layers of bone inside the medullary cavity, causing the diameter of the cavity to be progressively enlarged. This beautifully engineered process, known as ***appositional growth***, occurs in such a way that a healthy bone remains optimally functional, lightweight, and strong enough to resist daily stresses.

Adult Bone Development

While osteoblast and osteoclast activity tends to maintain bones at functional sizes and shapes throughout life, age-related changes in the proportion of mineralized to nonmineralized bone do occur. As people age, there is a progressive loss of collagen (which provides elasticity) and an increase in bone brittleness. This means that children are often able to sustain falls and other accidents without harm, while older adults tend to be increasingly vulnerable to bone fractures.

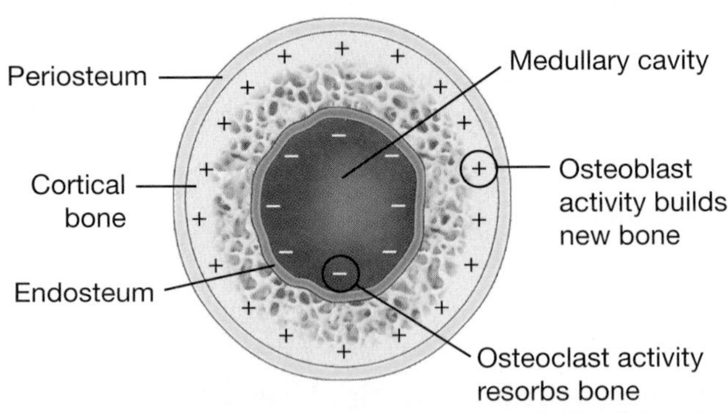

© Body Scientific International

Figure 5.9 Cross section of a long bone showing normal bone throughout life.

Bone mineral content normally peaks in women at about 25 to 28 years of age and in men at about 30 to 35 years of age. Thereafter, bone mass is progressively lost. Because women tend to have smaller bones than men, the loss of bone mass and bone mineral density is generally more problematic for women.

SELF CHECK

1. What is the periosteum? Name at least three functions of the periosteum.
2. Where is the endosteum found?
3. What covers the ends of long bones?
4. Describe the functions of osteoblasts and osteoclasts.
5. Describe and analyze the effects of less elasticity on the body as people age.

Bone Remodeling

Although bones grow and change dramatically during childhood and adolescence, living adult bone is also a very active tissue. It is always changing at a microscopic level in bone mineral content (and thereby strength) and sometimes in size or shape. This occurs through osteoblast and osteoclast activity during a process called ***remodeling***.

Forces such as gravitational force, muscle forces, forces sustained when people push or pull on something, and impact forces created when people bump into something all influence the bones. The remodeling process converts the size and direction of the forces acting on bone into changes in bone mineral density. In some circumstances, the remodeling process also causes changes in the size or shape of bone.

Research Notes Physical Activity and Bones

There are many documented examples of bone remodeling and hypertrophy in response to regular physical activity. Sports that required repeated, forceful use of a certain limb promote not only muscle hypertrophy, but also bone hypertrophy, in the stressed area. For example, clinical case studies have shown increased bone mass, circumference, and mineralization in the dominant forearm of professional tennis players and in the dominant upper arm of baseball players.

It also appears that the larger the forces habitually encountered, the more dramatic the effect. In one interesting study, researchers measured the density of the femur among 64 nationally ranked athletes from different sports. The densest femurs were those of the weight lifters, followed by hammer and discus throwers, runners, soccer players, and swimmers. As you might expect from this research, the size of the regularly acting forces on the body is one factor that appears to be related directly to bone mass.

The other important factor contributing to bone mineral density is absorption of repeated impacts, such as those routinely encountered during running and landings from jumps. In an investigation involving collegiate female athletes, those participating in high-impact sports (basketball and volleyball) were found to have much higher bone mineral densities than the swimmers, with soccer and track athletes having intermediate values. Another study compared the bone mineral densities of trained runners and cyclists to those of sedentary individuals of the same age. Not surprisingly, the runners were found to have increased bone density, but the cyclists did not.

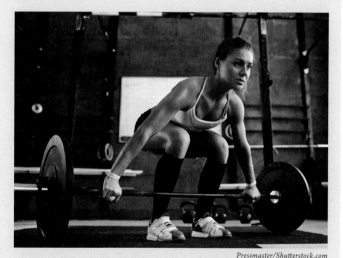

Pressmaster/Shutterstock.com

Repeated, forceful use of the arms or legs during exercise can result in both muscle and bone hypertrophy.

On the whole, the evidence suggests that physical activity involving impact forces is necessary for maintaining or increasing bone mass. One need not be an athlete, however, to exercise for bone health—even vigorous walking generates bone-building impact forces.

Competitive swimmers, who spend a lot of time in the water where the buoyant force counteracts gravity, may have even less bone mineral density than that of sedentary individuals. It is important for competitive swimmers to also participate in activities such as weight training and running to maintain normal bone density.

Blood calcium level can also influence bone density. If blood calcium is too low, the parathyroid glands (discussed in Chapter 9) release parathyroid hormone (PTH) into the bloodstream. PTH, in turn, activates osteoclasts to resorb bone matrix and release calcium into the bloodstream. If blood calcium is elevated above a balanced, homeostatic level, calcium is deposited in the bone matrix through the release of another hormone, called *calcitonin*, from the thyroid gland. These two hormones chiefly focus on homeostasis of blood calcium but indirectly affect the density of bones.

Hypertrophy

Generally, when bone is subjected to larger (stronger) forces it tends to hypertrophy (high-PER-troh-fee), with increases in density and growth at the sites of force applications (often muscle attachments). As a result, the bones of people who are physically active are usually denser and stronger than the bones of people who are sedentary. Dynamic activities such as running and jumping involve landing impacts, which cause motion of fluid within the bone matrix. This motion is particularly effective at triggering osteoblasts to build bone.

Research Notes Bones in Space

Maintaining good bone health and strength requires forces that act on the skeletal system to create the right balance between resorption of older, existing bone and formation of new bone. The single most important force acting to help maintain normal bone metabolism is the powerful force of gravity. When astronauts spend time in space, where they are deprived of gravitational force, "Houston, we have a problem!"

Scientists studying the effects of space flight on humans have long recognized that bone density and total body calcium are diminished during time spent outside of Earth's gravitational field. Generally, the longer the mission, the greater the amount of bone and calcium lost. This seems to occur due to increased bone resorption combined with largely unchanged bone formation. Bone microarchitecture is also weakened, with disruptions created in the trabecular structure.

A number of strategies have been employed to counteract these changes. Research has shown that heavy resistance exercise, coupled with appropriate nutritional and vitamin D intake, can effectively reduce the loss of bone mineral density on long-duration International Space Station missions. While in orbit, every US astronaut is scheduled for an hour of exercise, either treadmill or cycle ergometer, and an hour of resistive exercise (cable ergometer).

Remember that lifting weights in space is not exactly exercise, given that the weights are weightless! The exercise and nutritional intake that may be optimal for preventing bone loss are unknown and still under study. It is also unclear whether the bone loss that occurs while in space is fully reversible after time back on Earth.

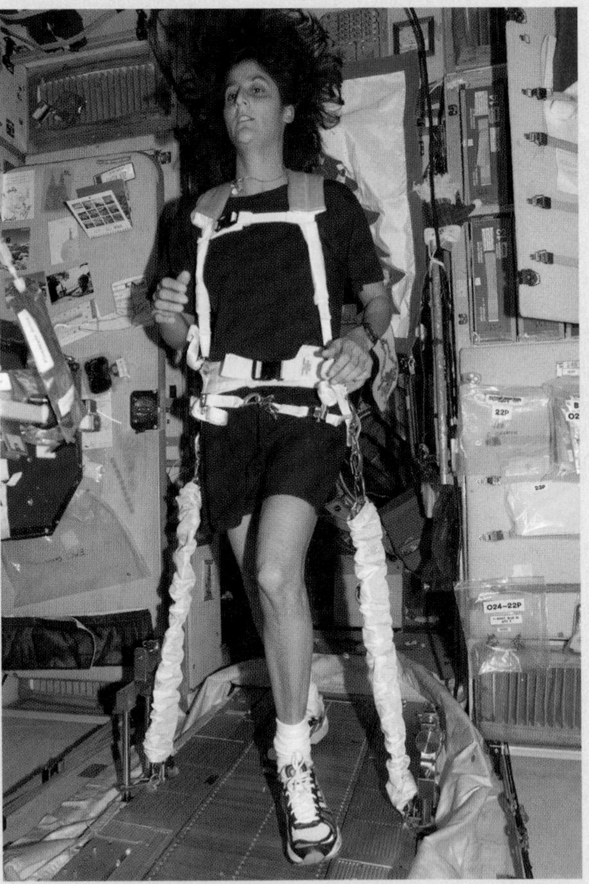

NASA

Astronaut Sunni Williams exercising on a treadmill in the International Space Station.

NASA's Orion program currently projects a manned mission to Mars to occur around the year 2035. Using current technology, robotic missions to Mars take about eight months from launch on Earth to landing on Mars. Today more than 500 people have spent up to a year in space and have maintained remarkably good health. However, for a manned mission to and from Mars to be successful, we will likely need a better understanding of ways to address bone loss, as well as other health-related consequences of long-term space flight.

Because gravity is also a force that continuously acts on bones, people who are heavier tend to have greater bone mass and density than people who are lightweight for their heights. Bone accounts for only about 15% of a person's body weight. This tends to be true whether a person is underweight, of average weight, or overweight. No one is overweight because of heavy bones. Being overweight is almost always the result of carrying excess body fat.

Atrophy

People who are subject to reduced forces are prone to bone atrophy, or loss of bone mineral density and strength. This has been observed, for example, in individuals who are bedridden for long periods of time.

Somewhat surprisingly, bone atrophy has also been observed in elite swimmers who spend hours a day training in a swimming pool. Swimming involves a large amount of muscle activity, but the buoyancy of the water counteracts much of the force of gravity. So, while swimmers are in the water, their bones are subjected to greatly reduced stresses.

Loss of bone mass and strength is an even more significant problem for astronauts, who spend time completely out of Earth's gravitational field. The loss of bone in astronauts in space is so rapid that it is currently one of the major factors preventing a manned space mission to Mars.

SECTION 5.1 REVIEW

Mini-Glossary

appositional growth growth accomplished by the addition of new layers to those previously formed

articular cartilage dense, white connective tissue that covers the articulating surfaces of bones at joints

bone marrow material with a rich blood supply found within the medullary cavity of long bones; yellow marrow stores fat, and red marrow is active in producing blood cells

cortical bone dense, solid bone that covers the outer surface of all bones and is the main form of bone tissue in the long bones

diaphysis the shaft of a long bone

epiphyseal plate growth plate near the ends of long bones where osteoblast activity increases bone length

epiphysis the bulbous end of a long bone

Haversian canals major passageways running in the direction of the length of long bones, providing paths for blood vessels

Haversian system structural unit that includes a single Haversian canal along with its multiple canaliculi, which branch out to join with lacunae, forming a comprehensive transportation matrix for supplying nutrients and removing waste products; also known as an *osteon*

hematopoiesis process of blood cell formation

medullary cavity central hollow area found in long bones

ossification process of bone formation

osteoblasts specialized bone cells that build new bone tissue

osteoclasts specialized bone cells that resorb bone tissue

osteocytes mature bone cells

osteon a Haversian system

perforating (Volkmann's) canals large canals that connect the Haversian canals; oriented across bones and perpendicular to Haversian canals

periosteum fibrous connective tissue membrane that surrounds and protects the shaft (diaphysis) of long bones

remodeling process through which adult bone can change in density, strength, and sometimes shape

Sharpey's fibers tiny connective tissue fibers that join together to firmly bind the periosteum to the underlying cortical bone

trabecular bone interior, spongy bone with a porous, honeycomb structure

Review Questions

1. List each of the five functions of the skeletal system and describe how they benefit the body.
2. Explain the differences between cortical bone and trabecular bone.
3. Describe where the diaphysis of a long bone is in relation to the epiphysis, and where the periosteum is in relation to the endosteum.
4. Compare and contrast osteoblasts and osteoclasts and explain how they work together to reshape and remodel bones.
5. Explain why a physician would be worried about a child who broke a long bone close to the epiphyseal plate.

SECTION 5.2

The Axial Skeleton

Objectives

- Explain the ways in which the skull of an infant is similar to and different from an adult skull.
- Describe the regions of the spine and the shapes and sizes of the vertebrae in each region.
- Explain the structures and functions of the thoracic cage.

Key Terms

atlas
axial skeleton
axis
cervical region
coccyx
cranium
facial bones
fontanel
intervertebral discs
lumbar region
mandible
maxillary bones
median sacral crest
sacral canal
sacral hiatus
sacrum
skull
sternum
sutures
thoracic cage
thoracic region
vertebra

Anatomists divide the body into the axis—the head and trunk—and the appendages—the arms and legs (**Figure 5.10**). Consequently, the major bones of the axis are known as the ***axial skeleton***, which includes three major parts—the skull, vertebral (spinal) column, and thoracic cage. The axial skeleton is designed to provide stability to the core of the body.

Skull

The 22 bones of the ***skull*** are divided into two groups: the cranial bones and the facial bones (**Figure 5.11**). The thin, curved bones of the ***cranium*** surround and protect the delicate brain. The round shape of the cranium is structurally strong. It resists impact forces and tends to absorb less force than if it were composed of flat surfaces. The ***facial bones*** protect the front of the head, give the face its individual shape, protect and orient the eyes, and allow chewing of food.

Most of the bones of the skull and face are joined together by irregularly shaped, interlocking, immovable joints called ***sutures***. A suture is a joint in which bones are bound together by strong, tiny fibers. The sutures permit a very small amount of movement, which contributes to the compliance (ability to change size and shape in response to force) and elasticity of the skull. The one exception is the mandible, or jaw bone, which is attached to the skull by a movable joint.

The skull of a newborn infant is quite different from an adult skull. Compared to adults, babies have big heads relative to the size of their bodies. While the skull of an adult accounts for about one-eighth of total body height, the skull of a newborn represents about one-fourth of body height.

As previously discussed, the skeletal system of a child includes regions of hyaline cartilage. In an infant, the sutures of the skull are composed of this soft connective tissue, which ossifies (turns to bone) in early childhood. In regions of the infant skull where several bones join together, there are openings connected only by pockets of fibrous membranes. Because the baby's pulse can be felt through these "soft spots," they are called ***fontanels***, based on the French word for "little fountains."

The soft sutures and fontanels serve two important functions. They enable some compression of the skull (the largest part of the body) during birth. Equally important, they enable brain growth during late pregnancy and early infancy. The fontanels ossify to bone by 22 to 24 months following birth.

Cranium

The cranium includes eight bones. There are two sets of paired (left and right side) bones; the rest are single bones. Following is a list of the bones that make up the cranium:

- The frontal bone forms the forehead and the superior portions of the eye sockets.
- The two paired parietal bones form the majority of the top and sides of the skull, joining together at the sagittal suture and connecting with the frontal bone at the coronal suture.
- The two paired temporal bones surround the ears, interfacing with the parietal bones at the squamous sutures.

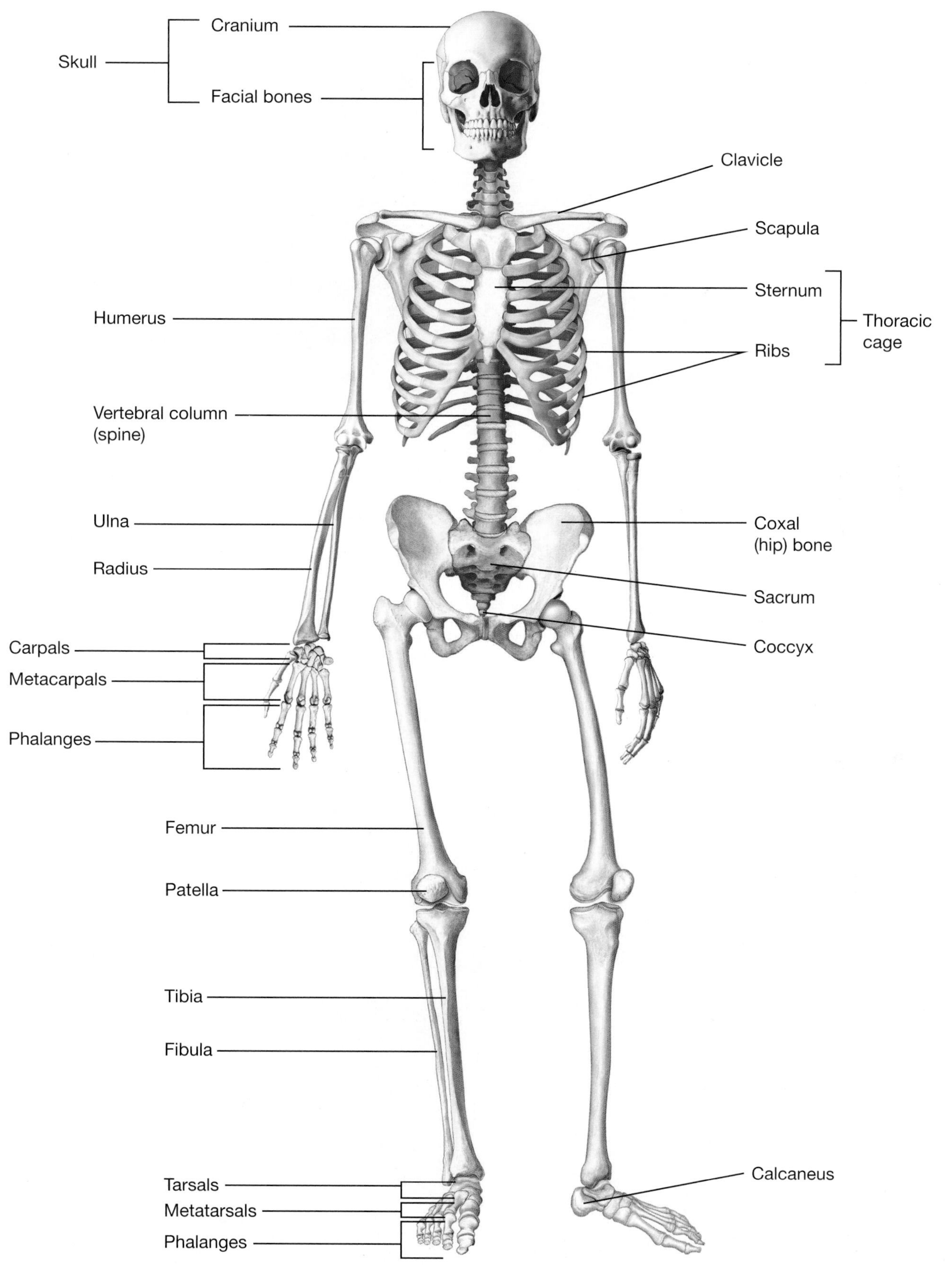

Figure 5.10 The axial skeleton (shown in a reddish color) and the appendicular skeleton.

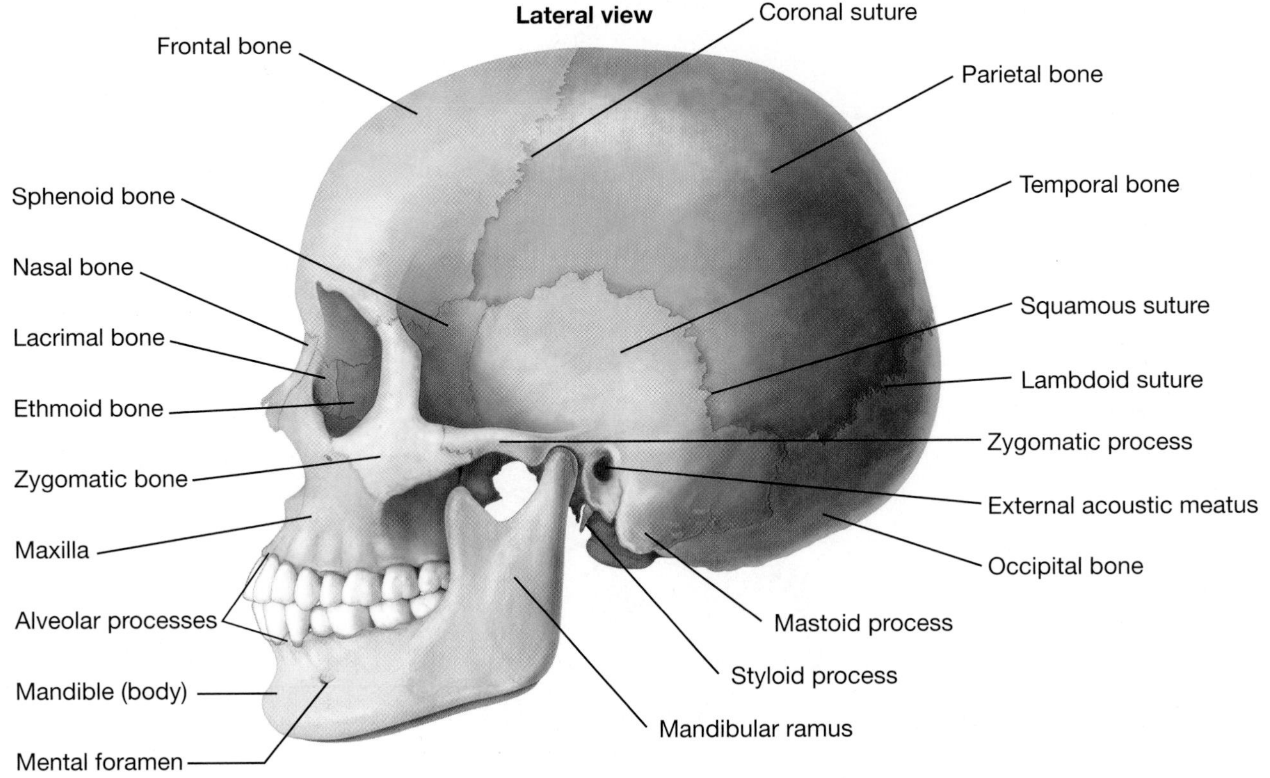
Lateral view
Frontal bone
Coronal suture
Parietal bone
Temporal bone
Sphenoid bone
Nasal bone
Squamous suture
Lacrimal bone
Lambdoid suture
Ethmoid bone
Zygomatic process
Zygomatic bone
External acoustic meatus
Maxilla
Occipital bone
Alveolar processes
Mastoid process
Styloid process
Mandible (body)
Mandibular ramus
Mental foramen

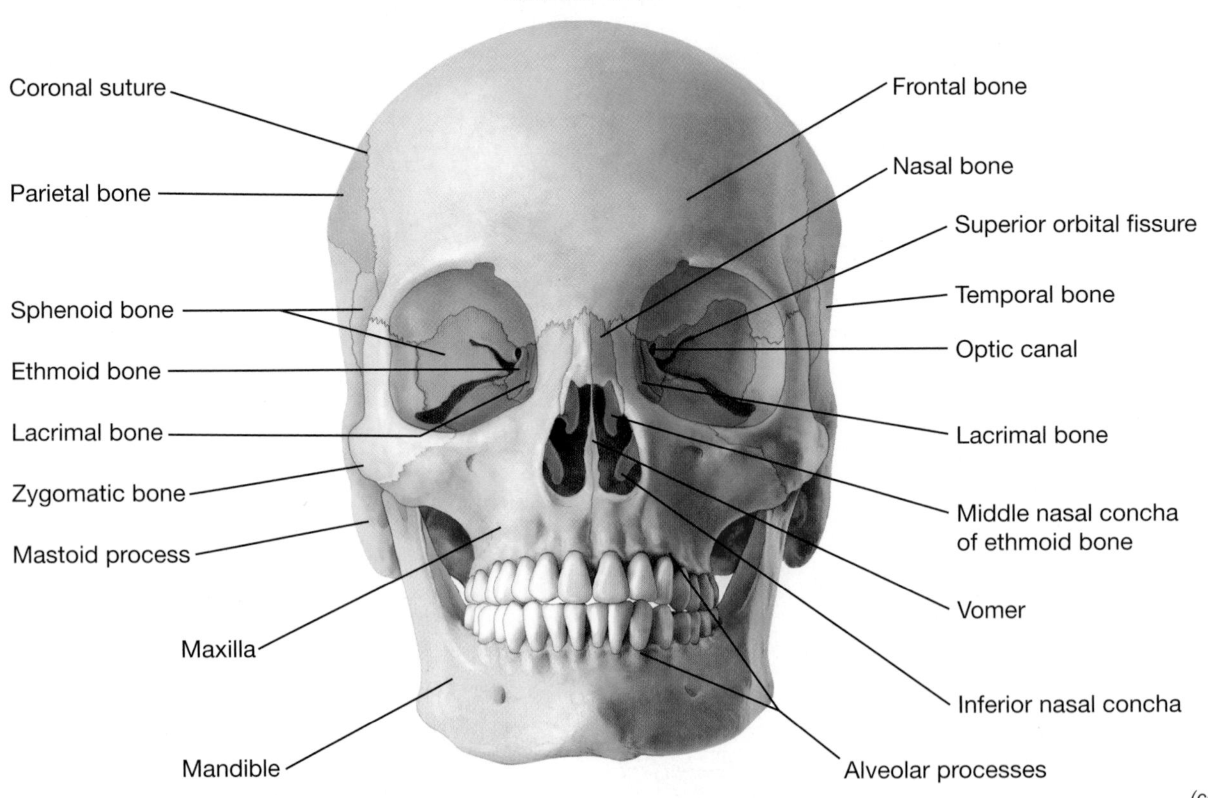
Anterior view
Coronal suture
Frontal bone
Nasal bone
Parietal bone
Superior orbital fissure
Sphenoid bone
Temporal bone
Optic canal
Ethmoid bone
Lacrimal bone
Lacrimal bone
Zygomatic bone
Middle nasal concha of ethmoid bone
Mastoid process
Vomer
Maxilla
Inferior nasal concha
Mandible
Alveolar processes

(continued)

Figure 5.11 Bones of the skull.

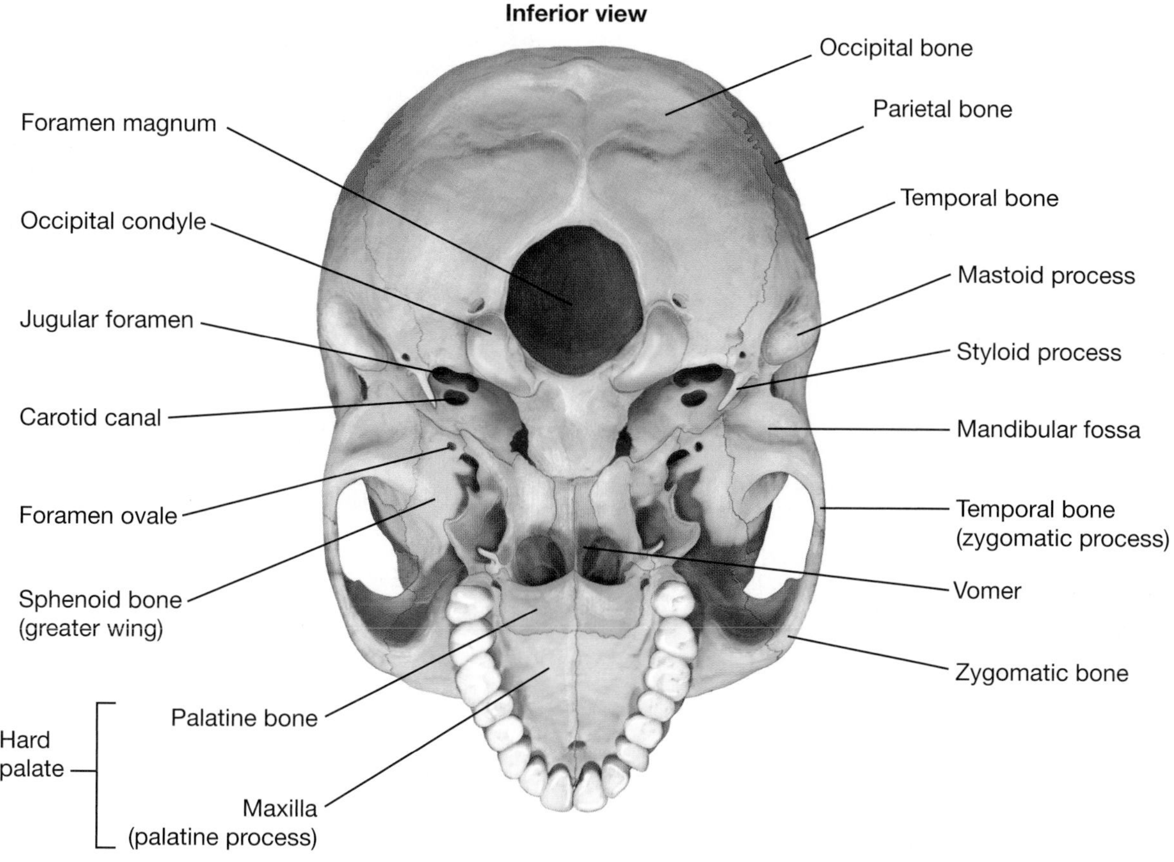
Inferior view
Occipital bone
Parietal bone
Foramen magnum
Temporal bone
Occipital condyle
Mastoid process
Jugular foramen
Styloid process
Carotid canal
Mandibular fossa
Foramen ovale
Temporal bone (zygomatic process)
Sphenoid bone (greater wing)
Vomer
Zygomatic bone
Hard palate
Palatine bone
Maxilla (palatine process)

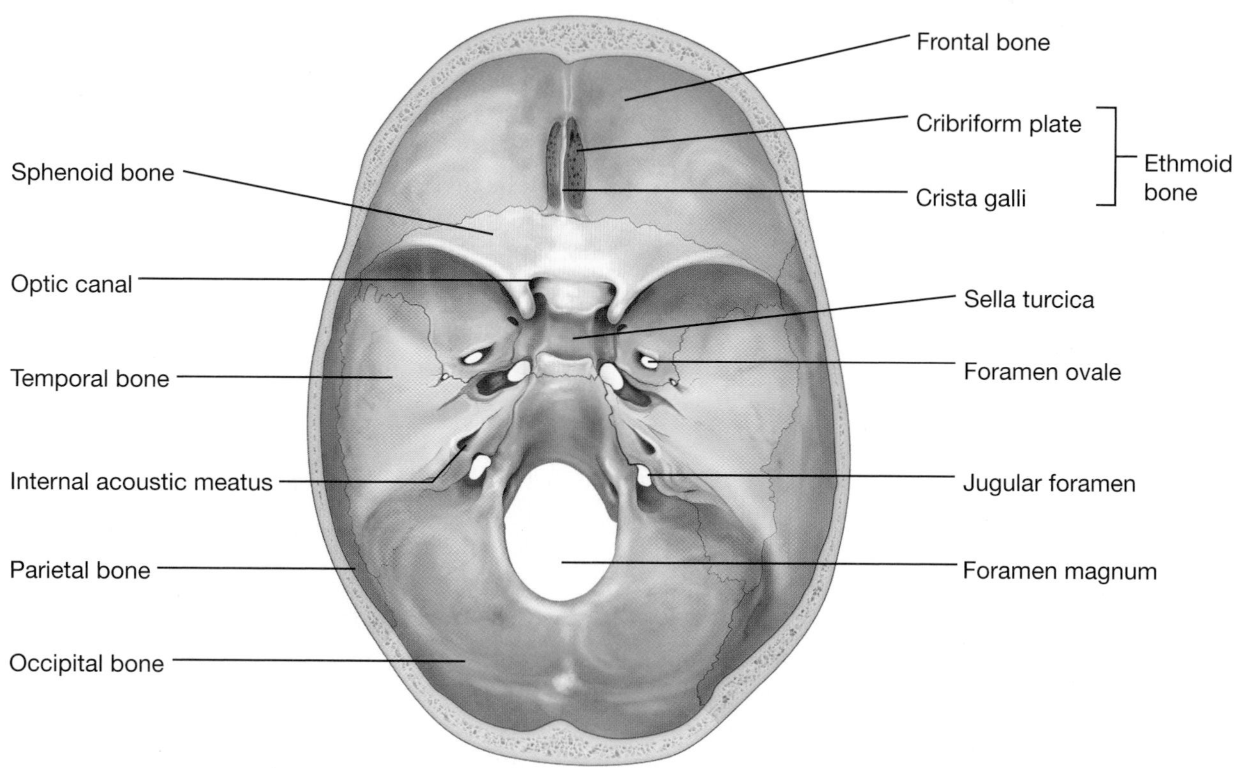
Superior view (top of cranium removed)
Frontal bone
Cribriform plate
Ethmoid bone
Sphenoid bone
Crista galli
Optic canal
Sella turcica
Temporal bone
Foramen ovale
Internal acoustic meatus
Jugular foramen
Parietal bone
Foramen magnum
Occipital bone

© Body Scientific International

- The occipital bone forms the base and lower back portions of the skull. It joins to the parietal bones at the lambdoid suture and includes the foramen magnum ("large hole"), through which the spinal cord connects with the brain.
- The irregularly shaped ethmoid bone forms part of the nasal septum and includes the crista galli, ("cock's comb"), a superior projection to which the outer covering of the brain attaches. The ethmoid bone is surrounded by the cribriform plate, a porous region through which the olfactory (smell) nerves pass. The bone also includes the superior and middle nasal conchae, projections that increase the turbulence of airflow through the nasal passages.
- The sphenoid bone is butterfly shaped and centrally located within the skull. The sphenoid bone supports part of the base of the brain, forms part of the orbits of the eyes, and is connected to all of the other bones of the skull. It includes a small cavity called the *sella turcica,* ("Turk's saddle"), which encases the pituitary gland. The foramen ovale is a large opening in the sella turcica through which the trigeminal nerve passes. Other openings in the sphenoid bone include the optic canal, a passageway for the optic nerve, and the superior orbital fissure, through which cranial nerves III, IV, and V, which control eye movements, pass. The central portion of the sphenoid bone is filled with small cavities known as the *sphenoid sinuses* (**Figure 5.12**).

The temporal bones include the following important features:

- zygomatic process—a raised ridge that joins to the zygomatic bone (cheek bone)
- styloid process—a thin, needle-like projection that serves as an attachment site for several neck muscles
- mastoid process—a neck muscle attachment site that includes cavities known as the mastoid sinuses
- external acoustic meatus—a canal that includes the eardrum and connects to the middle ear
- jugular foramen—a passageway for the jugular vein, the largest vein leading from the brain
- internal acoustic meatus—an opening for the facial and vestibulocochlear nerves

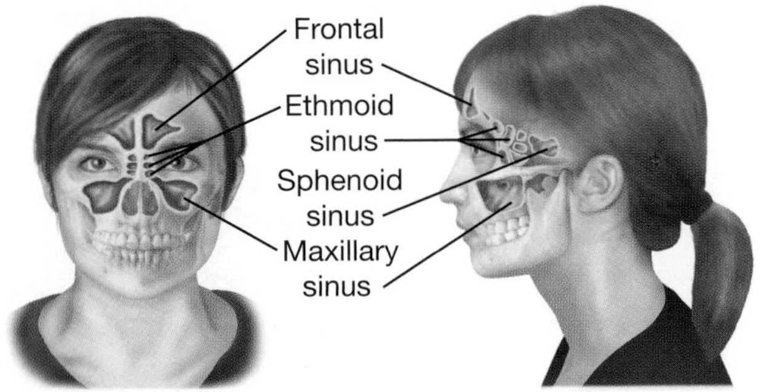

Figure 5.12 The sinuses of the skull.

- carotid canal—a tunnel through which the internal carotid artery, (the major source of blood to the brain), passes

Facial Bones

A total of fourteen bones form the face, including the mandible, vomer, and six pairs (left and right) of bones.

- The two fused ***maxillary bones***, which form the upper jaw, house the upper teeth in the alveolar process, and connect to all other bones of the face, with the exception of the mandible.
- The two palatine bones form the posterior part of the hard palate, or roof of the mouth, and include the paranasal sinuses, which amplify sounds from the vocal chords and reduce the weight of the head.
- The two zygomatic bones, or cheekbones, also form much of the sides of the orbits, or eye sockets.
- The two lacrimal bones are tiny bones connecting to the orbits and surrounding the tear ducts.
- The two nasal bones form the bridge of the nose.
- The vomer (plow-shaped) bone comprises most of the bony nasal septum.
- The two inferior concha bones form the sides of the nasal cavity.
- The ***mandible***, or lower jaw bone, is the largest facial bone, as well as the only movable facial bone, housing the lower teeth within the alveolar process.
- The *hyoid bone,* which is located in the mid-neck just above the larynx, is linked by ligaments to the styloid process of the temporal bones, and forms a moving base for the tongue as well as an attachment site for the muscles that raise and lower the larynx when a person swallows.

SELF CHECK

1. Scientists often divide the human skeleton into two parts. What are these parts called?
2. Which bones make up the axial skeleton?
3. What holds the bones of the skull together? Is movement possible at these joints? Why is this important?
4. List the two functions of the fontanels in a baby's skull.
5. List the eight cranial bones and tell where each is found.
6. List the fourteen facial bones and tell where each is found.

Vertebral Column

Although the word *spine* suggests a straight, rigid bar, the human spine, or vertebral column, is anything but straight and rigid. The human spinal column is well designed to perform its functions of protecting the extremely delicate spinal cord, while supporting the weight of the trunk and allowing flexibility in multiple directions.

Thirty-three stacked, individual bones called ***vertebrae*** comprise the spine. The vertebrae differ in size and shape in the different regions of the spine to best fulfill their respective functions (**Figure 5.13**).

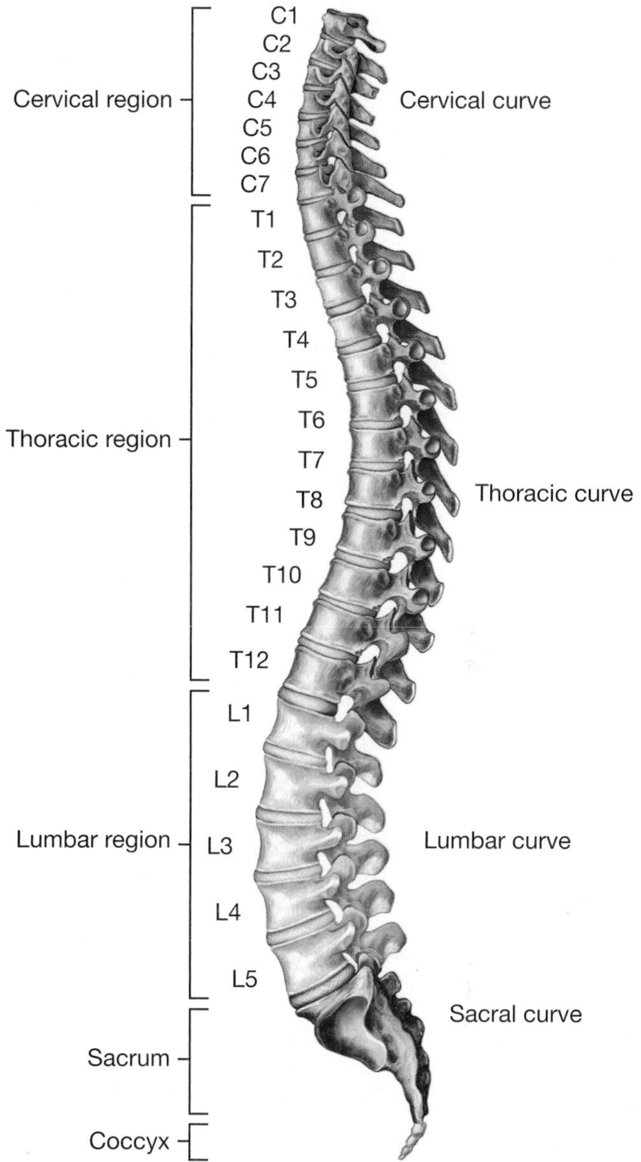

Figure 5.13 The vertebral column (spine).

Regions of the Spine

There are five named sections of the spine. These include the cervical, thoracic, and lumbar regions, as well as the sacrum, and coccyx.

The ***cervical region*** (neck) includes the upper seven vertebrae that enable the head to nod up and down and rotate to the right and left. The first cervical vertebra, the ***atlas***, is specialized to provide the connection between the occipital bone of the skull and the spinal column (**Figure 5.14**). (The atlas is so-called after the mythical Greek Titan named Atlas, who was condemned to hold up the weight of the world for an eternity.) The second cervical vertebra, the ***axis***, is also specialized, with an upward projection called the *odontoid process* or *dens*, on which the atlas rotates. The cervical vertebrae are the smallest of the vertebrae, and they are characterized by relatively short spinous processes. They include large vertebral foramina, as well as foramina that serve as passageways for the vertebral arteries connecting upward to the brain region.

The ***thoracic region*** encompasses the next 12 vertebrae, which extend through the chest region and articulate (connect) with the ribs. The thoracic vertebrae are larger than those in the cervical region. They have large, thick bodies and prominent spinous and transverse processes. Costal facets on these vertebrae articulate with the heads of the ribs.

The ***lumbar region*** includes the five vertebrae found in the lower back. These are the largest of the vertebrae with the thickest bodies. Lumbar vertebrae are well designed for supporting all the weight of the trunk, head, and arms.

The ***sacrum*** consists of five fused vertebrae that form the posterior portion of the pelvic girdle, articulating with the L5 vertebrae above and the coccyx below (**Figure 5.15**). Laterally, the alae of the sacrum articulate with the hip bones, forming the sacroiliac joints. The fused spinous processes form a prominent ridge, known as the ***median sacral crest***, down the midline of the posterior surface, with posterior sacral foramina on either side. The ***sacral canal*** ends with a large opening called the ***sacral hiatus***, which is the point of administration for certain anesthetics.

The ***coccyx***, or tailbone, is located at the bottom of the spine. It includes three to five irregularly shaped, fused vertebrae.

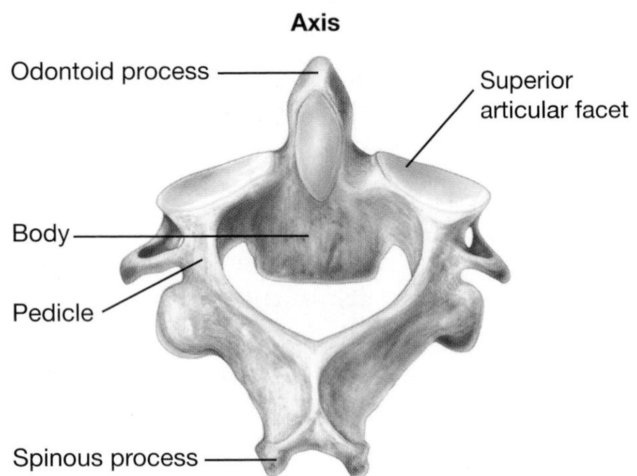

Figure 5.14 The first and second cervical vertebrae, the atlas and the axis.

Structures of the Vertebrae

Although no two vertebrae are exactly alike, most of the vertebrae have several structural features in common (**Figure 5.16**):

- The vertebral body is the thick, disc-shaped portion that bears weight and forms the anterior portion of the vertebra.
- The vertebral arch is the round projection of bone on the posterior aspect of the vertebra. It surrounds a hole known as the *vertebral foramen* (foh-RAY-mehn), through which the spinal cord passes.
- The transverse processes are bony projections on the lateral sides of the vertebral arch.
- The spinous process is a bony projection that extends posteriorly.
- The superior and inferior articular processes are indentations or facets where a vertebra articulates, or joins, with the vertebrae immediately above and below it. These articulations are called *facet joints*.

There is a progressive increase in vertebral size from the cervical region down through the lumbar region (**Figure 5.17**). This gradual size increase serves a functional purpose. When the body is in an upright

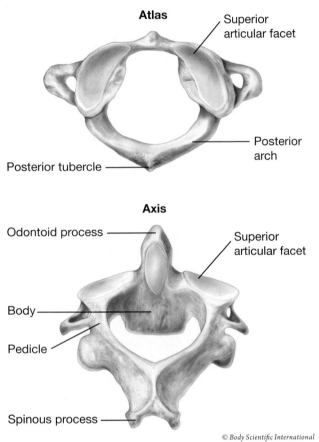

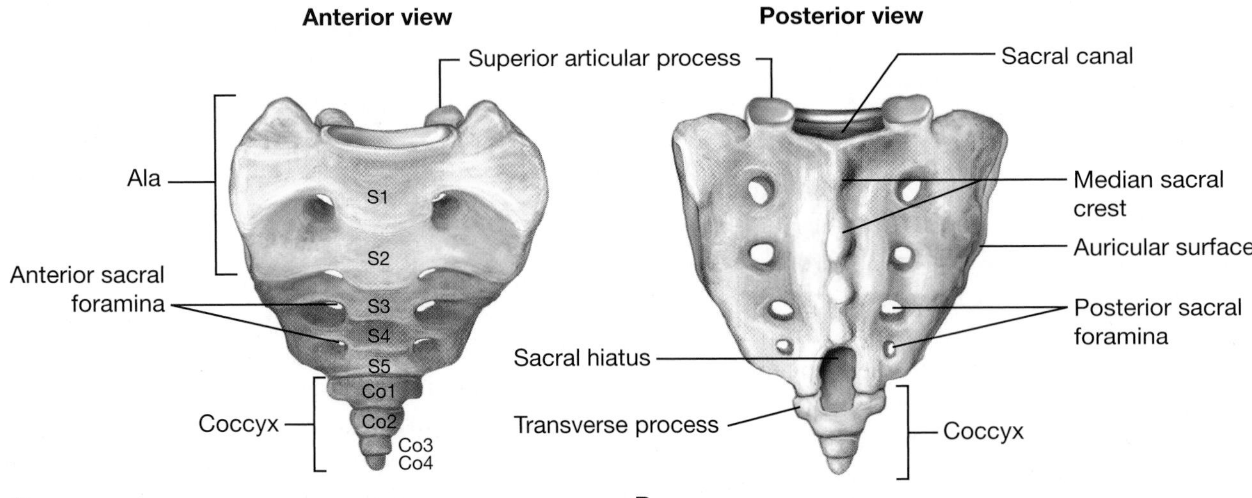

Figure 5.15 The sacrum and coccyx. A—Anterior view. B—Posterior view.

position, each vertebra must support the weight of all of the body parts positioned above it. Think about what this means. While a cervical vertebra supports only the weight of the head and neck, a lumbar vertebra supports the weight of the head, neck, arms, and the entire trunk positioned above that vertebra.

The size and angulation of the vertebral processes also vary throughout the spinal column. This changes the orientation of the facet joints, which interconnect the vertebrae and serve to limit range of motion in the different spinal regions.

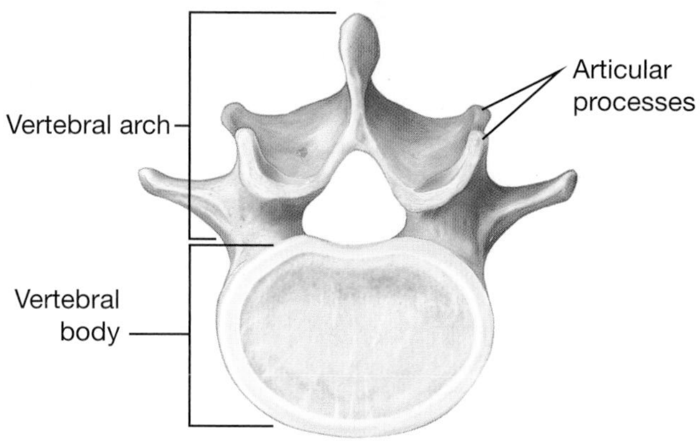

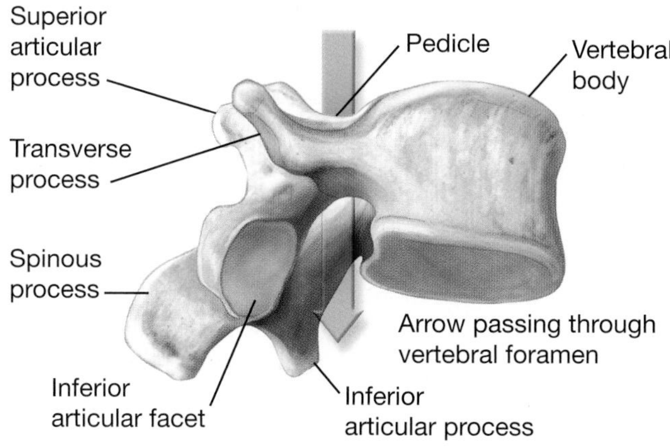

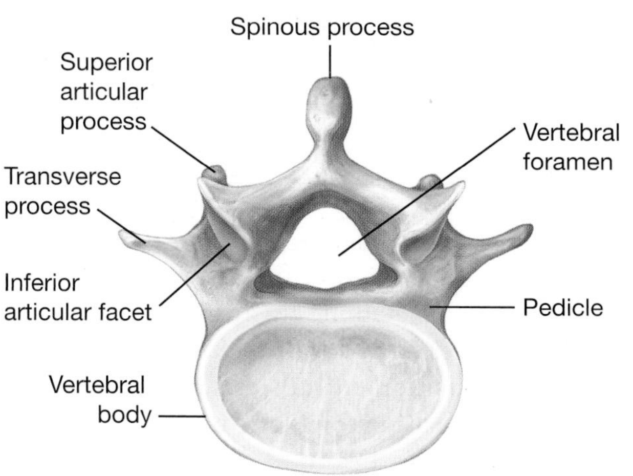

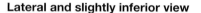

Figure 5.16 Three views of a typical vertebra.

The Spinal Curves

The characteristic shapes of the vertebrae in the different spinal regions also form the normal spinal curves. As **Figure 5.13** shows, the cervical and lumbar curves are posteriorly concave, while the thoracic, sacral, and coccyx curvatures are anteriorly concave. These alternating curves make the spine stronger and better able to resist potentially injurious forces than if it were straight.

The thoracic and sacral curves are known as *primary spinal curves* because they are present at birth. The lumbar and cervical curves are referred to as *secondary spinal curves*. They develop after the baby begins to raise the head, sit, and stand, as increased muscular strength enables the young child to shift body weight to the spine.

Abnormal spinal curvatures can develop due to genetic or congenital abnormalities, or as a result of the spine being habitually subjected to asymmetrical forces (**Figure 5.18**). Exaggeration of the lumbar curve is called *lordosis*, accentuation of the thoracic curve is called *kyphosis*, and any lateral deviation of the spine is known as *scoliosis*.

Intervertebral Discs

Intervertebral discs composed of fibrocartilage provide cushioning between all articulating vertebral bodies that are not fused. These discs serve as shock absorbers and allow the spine to bend. The differences in the anterior and posterior thicknesses of these discs produce the normal cervical, thoracic, and lumbar curves.

In a normal adult, the discs account for approximately one-quarter of the height of the spine. When a person is lying in bed during overnight sleep, the discs absorb water and expand slightly. During periods of upright standing and sitting, when the discs are bearing weight, they lose a small amount of fluid and compression occurs. For this reason, people may be as much as three-fourths of an inch taller when they first arise in the morning. Injury and progressive

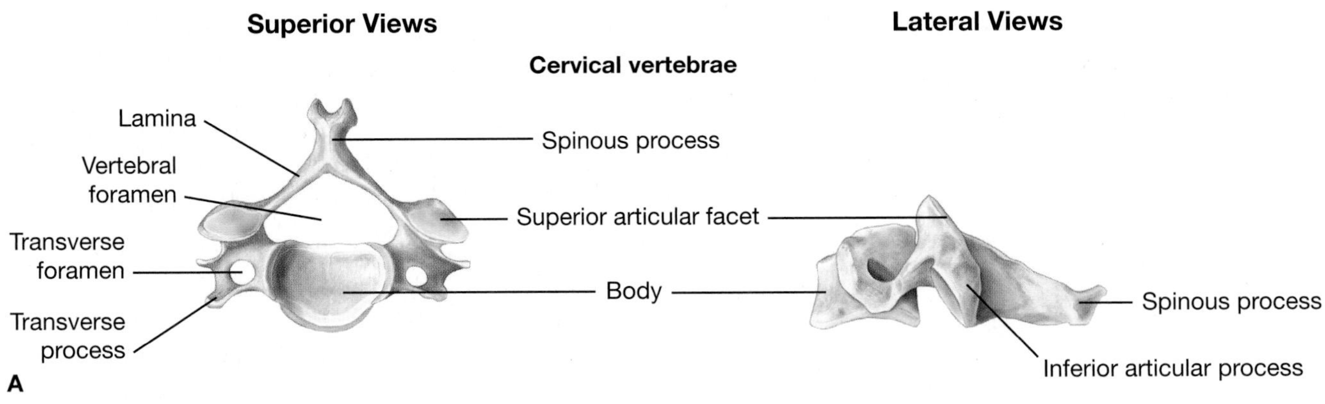

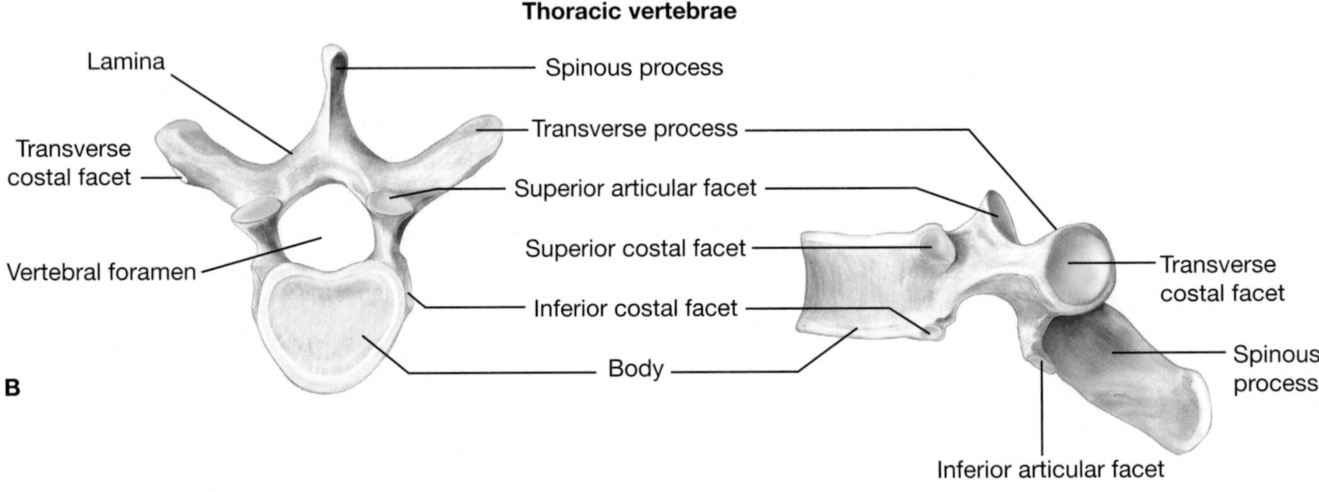

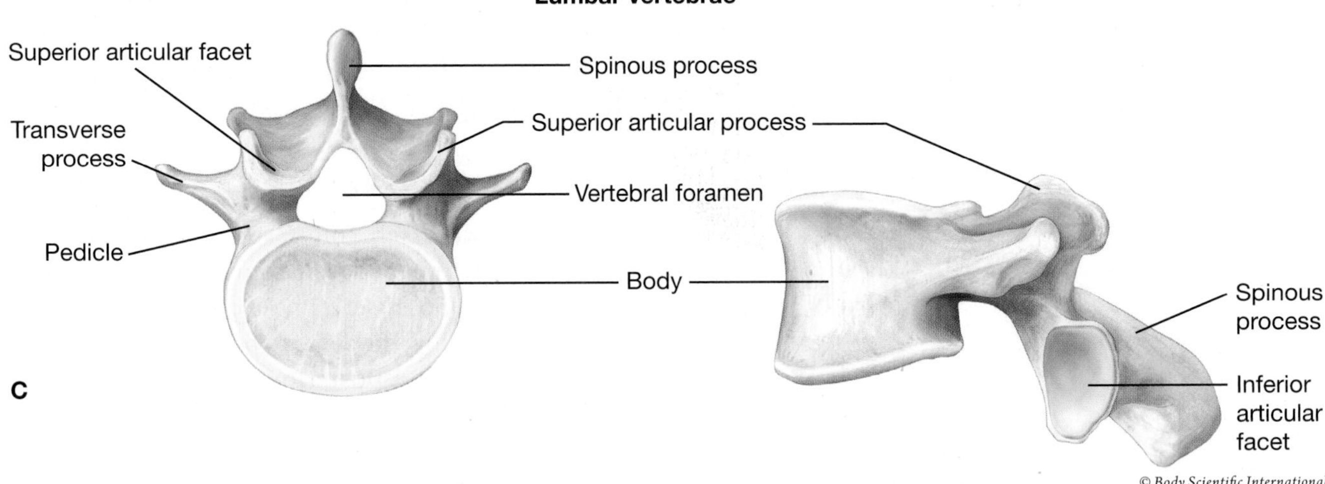

Figure 5.17 Superior and left lateral views of typical cervical (A), thoracic (B), and lumbar (C) vertebrae.

aging reduce the water retention capability of the discs, accounting for diminished standing height in elderly individuals.

Because the discs receive no blood supply, they must rely on changes in posture and body position to produce a pumping action that brings in nutrients and flushes out metabolic waste products with an influx and outflow of fluid. Because maintaining a fixed body position curtails this pumping action, sitting in one position for a long period of time can negatively affect disc health.

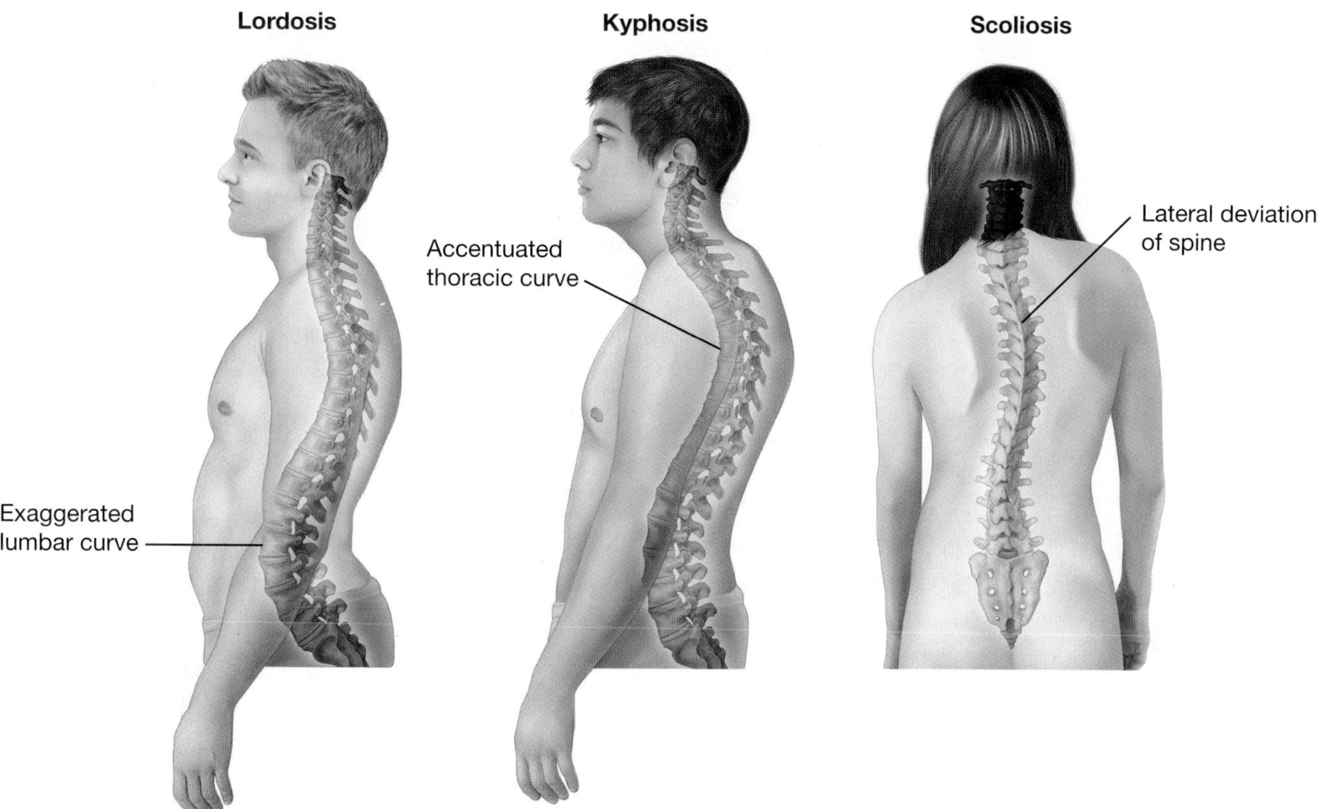

Figure 5.18 Three types of abnormal spinal curvature.

SELF CHECK

1. List the five regions of the vertebral column, from upper to lower.
2. What is the functional purpose for the increasing size of vertebrae from the cervical region down to the lumbar region?
3. What is the function of the intervertebral discs?

Thoracic Cage

The ribs, sternum, and thoracic vertebrae are collectively known as the ***thoracic cage***, or bony thorax, because together they form a protective, bony "cage" that surrounds the heart and lungs in the thoracic cavity, as shown in **Figure 5.19**. The breastbone, or ***sternum***, includes three regions:

- Manubrium—the upper portion of the sternum; it has articulations to the left and right bones of the clavicle, as well as to the first and second ribs
- Body—the remainder of the bony portion of the sternum
- Xiphoid process—projection at the lower end of the sternum

The sternum has three notable bony features. The jugular notch is a readily palpable indentation at the superior end of the sternum. The sternal angle is a slightly elevated transverse ridge occurring where the body of the sternum joins the manubrium at a small angle. The xiphisternal joint is, as the name suggests, the junction between the sternal body and xiphoid process at the level of the ninth thoracic vertebrae.

There are 12 pairs of ribs in the thoracic cage, as shown in **Figure 5.19**. The first seven pairs (1–7) attach directly to the sternum and are, therefore, called *true ribs*. The next three pairs of ribs (8–10) are called *false ribs* because they have cartilaginous attachments to the cartilage of the seventh rib, rather than attaching directly to the sternum. The lowest two pairs of ribs (11–12) are known as *floating ribs*, because they do not attach to bone or cartilage in front of the body.

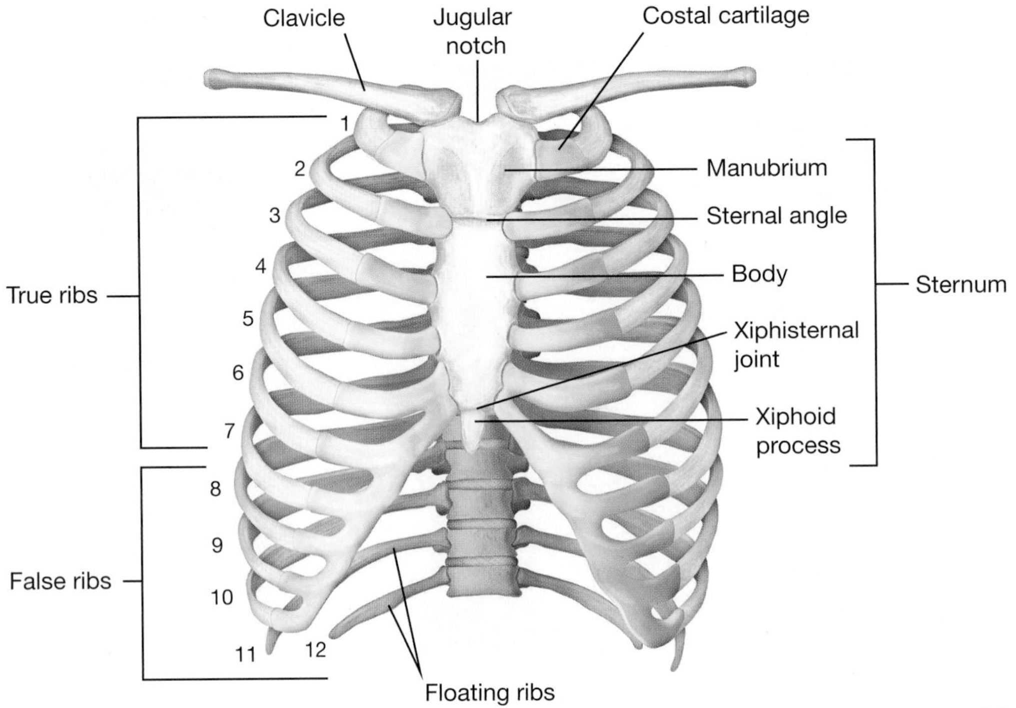

Figure 5.19 The thoracic cage.

SECTION 5.2

REVIEW

Mini-Glossary

atlas the first cervical vertebra; specialized to provide the connection between the occipital bone of the skull and the spinal column

axial skeleton the central portion of the skeletal system, consisting of the skull, spinal column, and thoracic cage

axis the second cervical vertebra; specialized with an upward projection called the *odontoid process*, on which the atlas rotates

cervical region the first seven vertebrae, comprising the neck

coccyx the four vertebrae at the base of the spine that are fused to form the tailbone

cranium collective term for the fused, flat bones surrounding the back of the head

facial bones bones of the face

fontanel an opening in the infant skull through which the baby's pulse can be felt; these openings enable compression of the skull during birth and brain growth during late pregnancy and early infancy

intervertebral discs fibrocartilaginous cushions between vertebral bodies that allow bending of the spine and help to create the normal spinal curves

lumbar region five vertebrae comprising the low back region of the spine

mandible jaw bone

maxillary bones two fused bones that form the upper jaw, house the upper teeth, and connect to all other bones of the face, with the exception of the mandible

median sacral crest prominent elevation formed by the fused spinous processes of the upper four sacral vertebrae

sacral canal continuation of the vertebral canal in the sacral region

sacral hiatus prominent opening at the inferior end of the sacral canal

sacrum collective term for five fused vertebrae that form the posterior of the pelvic girdle

skull the part of the skeleton composed of all of the bones of the head

sternum breastbone

sutures joints in which irregularly grooved, articulating bone sheets join closely and are tightly connected by fibrous tissues

thoracic cage the bony structure surrounding the heart and lungs in the thoracic cavity; composed of the ribs, sternum, and thoracic vertebrae

thoracic region the 12 vertebrae located in the middle of the back

vertebra one of the bones making up the spinal column

(continued)

Review Questions

1. Explain the function of the axial skeleton and list the bones included in it.
2. The bones of the skull are often divided into two groups. Name those two groups.
3. In what respect are sutures and fontanels similar?
4. List the five named sections of the spine and state how many vertebrae are included in each of these sections.
5. Name at least five structural features common to most vertebrae.
6. Which bone of the skull is freely movable?
7. Why is it important to protect and cradle a baby's head when you are holding the baby?
8. Compare and contrast lordosis, kyphosis, and scoliosis.
9. How does the composition of an intervertebral disc relate to its functions of acting as a shock absorber and allowing the spine to bend?
10. Explain the different ways in which ribs are attached to the sternum.
11. What are the primary and secondary spinal curves? Explain why and distinguish between them.

SECTION 5.3 The Appendicular Skeleton

Objectives

- Identify the bones and joints of the upper extremity and describe their motions.
- Identify the bones and joints of the lower extremity and describe their motions.

Key Terms

appendicular skeleton
calcaneus
carpal bones
clavicle
false pelvis
femur
fibula
humerus
lower extremity
metacarpal bones
metatarsal bones
patella
pectoral girdle
pelvis
phalanges
radius
scapula
shoulder complex
tarsal bones
tibia
true pelvis
ulna
upper extremity

The ***appendicular skeleton***, as the name suggests, includes the body's appendages. These include both the bones of the ***upper extremity*** (the shoulder complex, arms, wrists, and hands) and those of the ***lower extremity*** (the pelvic girdle, legs, ankles, and feet). Altogether, there are approximately 126 bones in the appendicular skeleton. The appendicular skeleton is built for motion.

Upper Extremity

The upper extremity is well designed for all of the tasks that people routinely ask it to perform. The muscles, bones, and joints of the upper extremity enable movements as diverse as carrying a load, throwing a ball, and threading a needle. The different movements of hammering a nail, texting on a cell phone, and performing a handspring are also made possible by this unique design.

Shoulder Complex

The bones surrounding the shoulder are referred to as the shoulder girdle, or ***pectoral girdle***. This structure includes the left and right ***clavicle***, or collarbone, and a left and right ***scapula***, or shoulder blade (**Figure 5.20**). These bones serve as sites of attachment for the numerous muscles that enable the arms to move in so many different directions at the shoulders.

As **Figure 5.21** shows, there are two bony projections on the scapula, known respectively as the *acromion* and the *coracoid process*. The prominent suprascapular notch, which cradles nerves, is found just medial to the coracoid process. The lateral end of the clavicle attaches to the acromion process to form the acromioclavicular joint (**Figure 5.20**). The medial end of the clavicle attaches to the sternum to form the sternoclavicular joint.

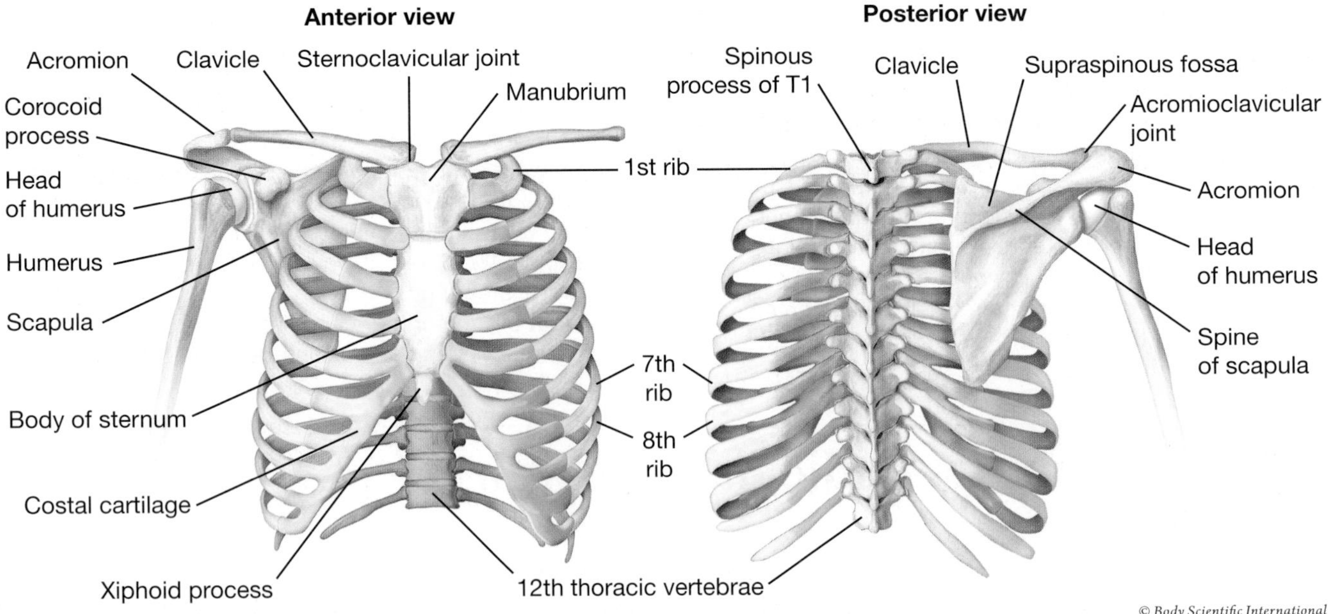

Figure 5.20 Anterior and posterior views of the shoulder girdle, ribs, and humerus.

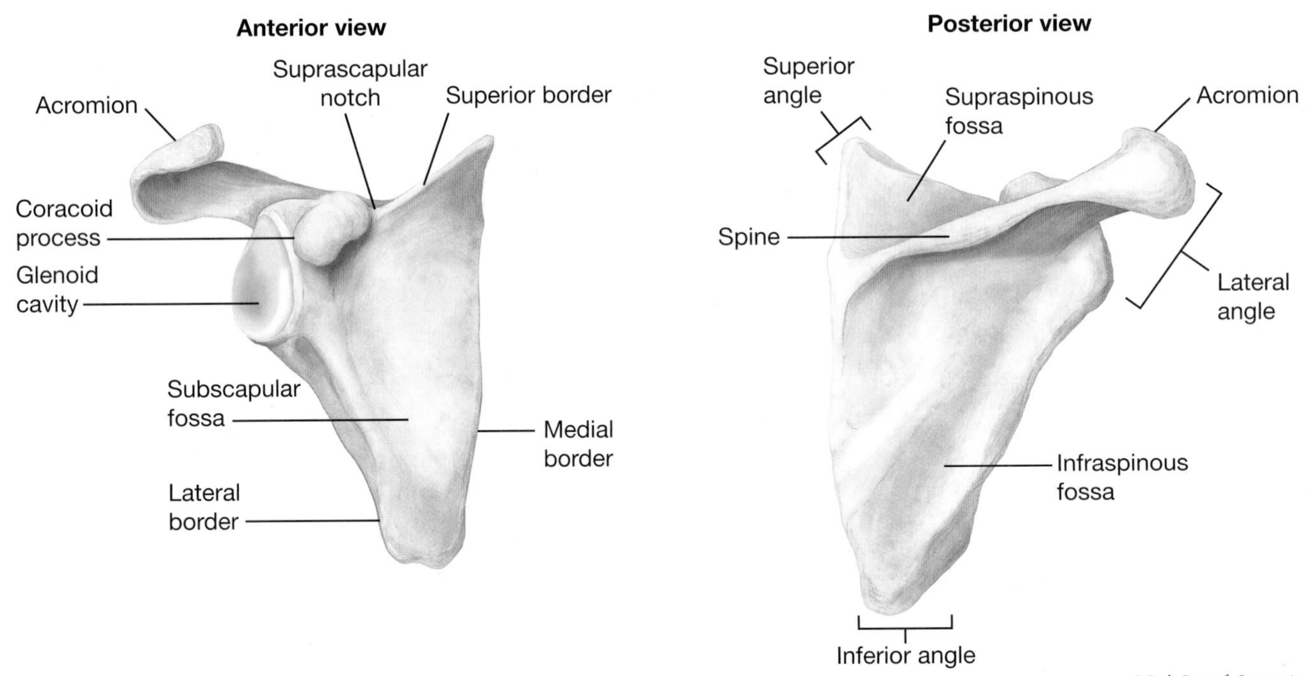

Figure 5.21 Anterior and posterior views of the scapula.

The acromioclavicular joint primarily allows you to raise your arm so that you can perform movements above your head. The sternoclavicular joint enables you to move your clavicle and scapula for motions such as shrugging your shoulders, raising your arms, and swimming.

The clavicle serves as a brace for positioning the shoulder laterally away from the trunk. Although there are no bony articulations between the scapulae and the posterior aspect of the trunk, the region between each scapula and the underlying tissues is sometimes referred to as the *scapulothoracic joint*.

The glenoid fossa (socket) of the scapula is a relatively shallow indentation that articulates, or joins, with the head of the ***humerus***, the bone in the upper arm, to form the glenohumeral joint, or shoulder joint. Because the glenoid fossa is less curved than the humeral head, the humerus is able to glide against the glenoid fossa, in addition to rotating. As a result, the glenohumeral joint allows motion in more directions than any other joint in the body.

The glenohumeral joint and the bones and joints of the shoulder girdle are collectively referred to as the ***shoulder complex***. Together these joints provide the significant range of motion present in a healthy shoulder. This large degree of mobility, however, comes at the cost of instability: the shoulder is one of the most frequently dislocated joints in the human body. **Figure 5.22** summarizes the joints of the shoulder complex.

Arm

The single bone of the upper arm is the humerus (**Figure 5.23**). The humerus is a large, strong bone, second in size only to the major bone of the upper leg. The upper end of the humerus forms a rounded head that articulates with the glenoid fossa of the scapula to form the glenohumeral joint. The humerus includes a number of bony landmarks:

- The anatomical neck is a slightly indented line that mostly circles the humeral head.
- The greater and lesser tubercles are bulbous projections that are lateral to the humeral head and are separated by a prominent indentation called the *intertubercular sulcus*.

Articulating Bones of the Shoulder Complex

Joint	Notched Bone	Joining Bone or Region
acromioclavicular joint	acromion of the scapula	clavicle
sternoclavicular joint	sternum	clavicle
scapulothoracic joint	scapula	thorax
glenohumeral (shoulder) joint	glenoid fossa of the scapula	humerus

Figure 5.22

Goodheart-Willcox Publisher

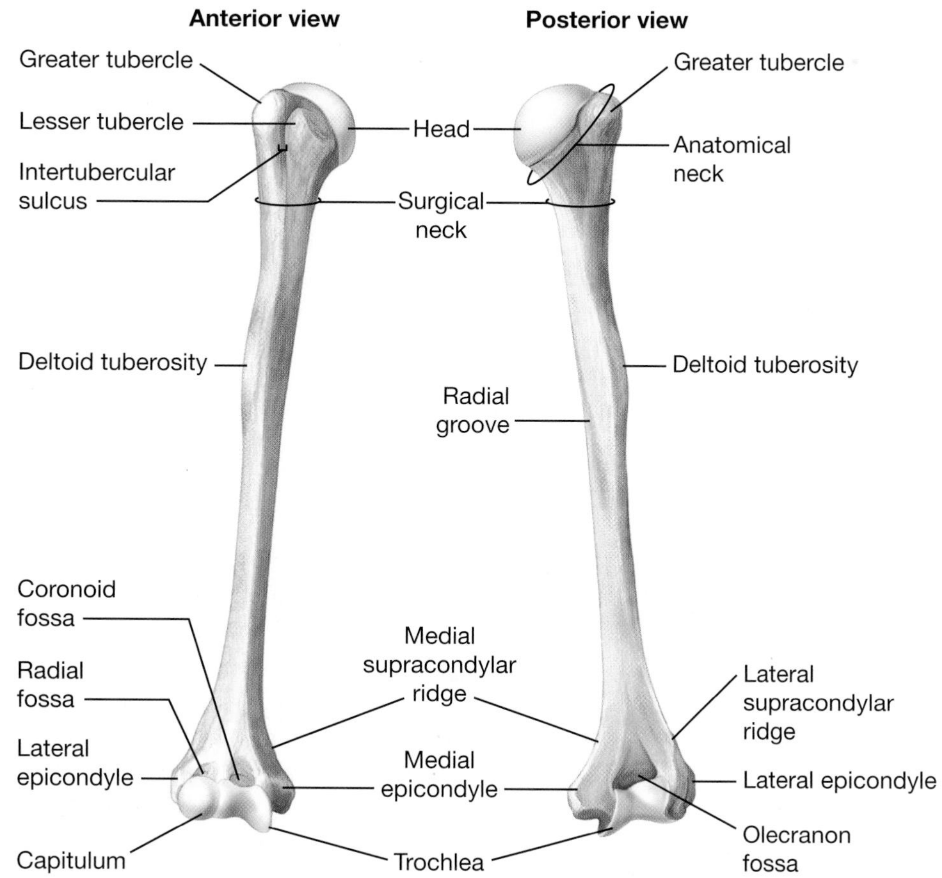

© Body Scientific International

Figure 5.23 Anterior and posterior views of the humerus.

- Just below (distal to) the tubercles is the surgical neck, so named because it is the most frequently fractured portion of the humerus.
- The mid-shaft of the humerus is marked by the radial groove, which underlies the radial nerve, and the deltoid tuberosity, to which the powerful deltoid muscle attaches.
- At the distal end of the humerus are the prominent and readily palpable medial and lateral condyles.
- Also at the distal end of the humerus and interior to the elbow joint are the trochlea on the medial side and the capitulum on the lateral side, both enabling free motion of the articulating ulna.
- Just superior to the trochlea are the posterior olecranon fossa and the anterior coronoid fossa, which serve as sites of muscle attachments.

As **Figure 5.24** shows, the framework for the forearm consists of two bones—the ***radius*** and ***ulna***. The radius is the bone that articulates with the wrist on the thumb side. The name *radius* comes from the ability of this bone to rotate "radially" around the ulna. This radial rotation is the familiar motion that enables the forearm and hand to rotate freely. Below the head and neck of the radius is the radial tuberosity, which is the attachment site for the biceps.

The ulna is larger and stronger than the radius, and it articulates with the humerus at the humeroulnar joint (elbow). The ulna attaches to the wrist on the "little finger" side. Two processes are located at the proximal end of the ulna. The olecranon (oh-LEHK-ra-nahn) on the posterior side is the elbow. On the anterior side is the coronoid process, which is separated from the olecranon process by the trochlear notch. The ulnar tuberosity serves as an attachment site for part of the brachialis.

The radius and ulna are connected along their entire lengths by an interosseus membrane. The two bones articulate at both ends, and these joints are known as the *proximal* and *distal radioulnar joints*.

At the distal (lower) ends of both the radius and ulna are styloid processes that are easy to see and feel with your fingers. The distal end of the radius unites with several of the carpal bones of the wrist to form the radiocarpal joint (**Figure 5.25**).

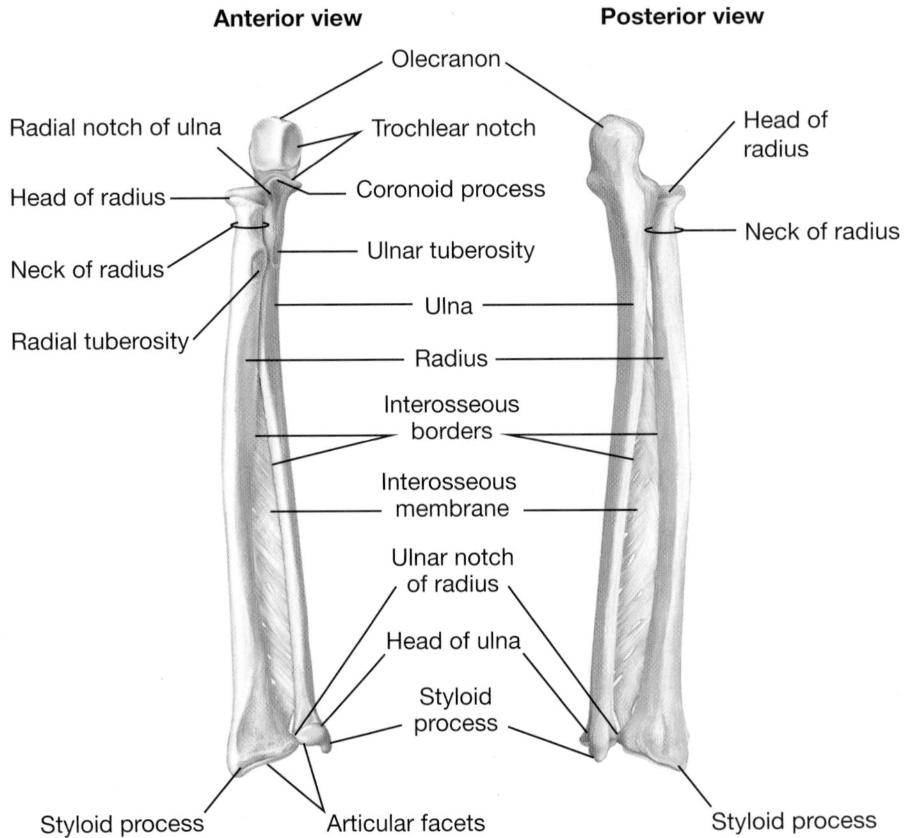

Figure 5.24 Anterior and posterior views of the radius and ulna.

Articulating Bones of the Arm and Wrist		
Joint	**Notched Bone**	**Joining Bone**
humeroulnar (elbow) joint	humerus	ulna
radioulnar joints (proximal and distal)	radius	ulna
radiocarpal (wrist) joint	radius	three carpal bones

Figure 5.25

Goodheart-Willcox Publisher

Wrist and Hand

Collectively, there are 54 bones in the wrists and hands—27 on the left hand and 27 on the right hand. This large number of bones enables a wide range of precise movements along with the important ability to grasp objects.

As **Figure 5.26** shows, the wrist includes eight ***carpal bones*** that are roughly arranged in two rows. The carpal bones are bound together by ligaments that allow a small amount of gliding motion at the intercarpal joints. However, the main function of the carpals is to provide a base for the bones of the hand.

Five ***metacarpal bones*** in each hand articulate with the carpal bones in the wrist. The ***phalanges***, or fingers, of each hand consist of 14 bones. Each of the four fingers has proximal, medial, and distal phalanges, but the thumb has only two.

Whereas the joints of the fingers permit motion in only one plane, the thumb has the ability to freely rotate and to stretch across the palm of the hand. This capability, known as an *opposable thumb*, is seen only in humans and other primates.

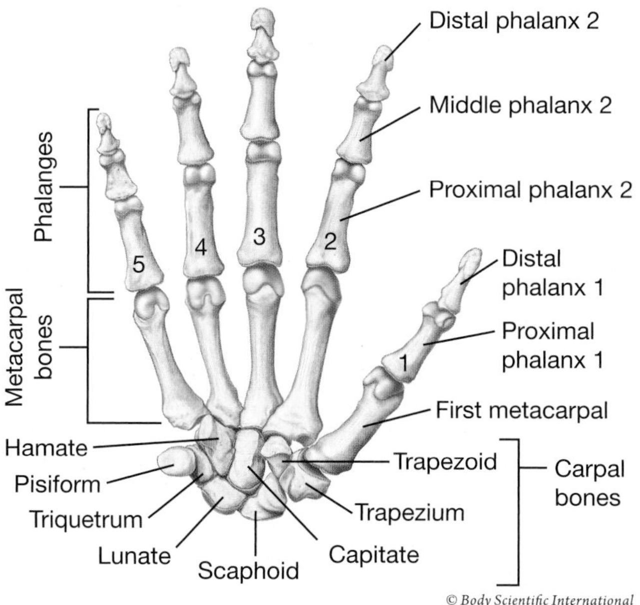

© Body Scientific International

Figure 5.26 Anterior view of the bones of the right hand.

SELF CHECK

1. Which bones make up the appendicular skeleton?
2. Which bones are included in the shoulder complex?
3. Which forearm bone enables rotation of the hand around the longitudinal axis of the arm?
4. How many bones are in each wrist and hand?

Lower Extremity

With large, strong bones, the lower extremity is well designed for its functions of weight bearing and gait, including walking and running. During sporting activities, the muscles, bones, and joints of the lower extremity also enable movements involved in jumping, skating, surfing, skiing, dancing, and many other activities.

Pelvic Girdle

As the name suggests, the pelvic girdle is a bony encasement of the pelvic region that shelters the reproductive organs, the bladder, and part of the large intestine. The pelvic girdle is formed by two large, strong coxal bones (hip bones) and the sacrum (**Figure 5.27**). These three bones, with the addition of the coccyx, comprise the ***pelvis***.

Each coxal bone in an adult is formed by the fusion of the ilium, ischium, and pubis. During childhood, these are three separate bones.

The ilium comprises most of each coxal bone, connecting posteriorly to the sacrum at the sacroiliac joint. The prominent upper edge of the ilium, which can usually be palpated (examined or felt by touch), is called the *iliac crest*. The opposite ends of the iliac crest are the anterior superior iliac spine (ASIS) and posterior superior iliac spine (PSIS).

The ischium (IS-kee-um), forming the inferior portion of each coxal bone, is the bone that supports

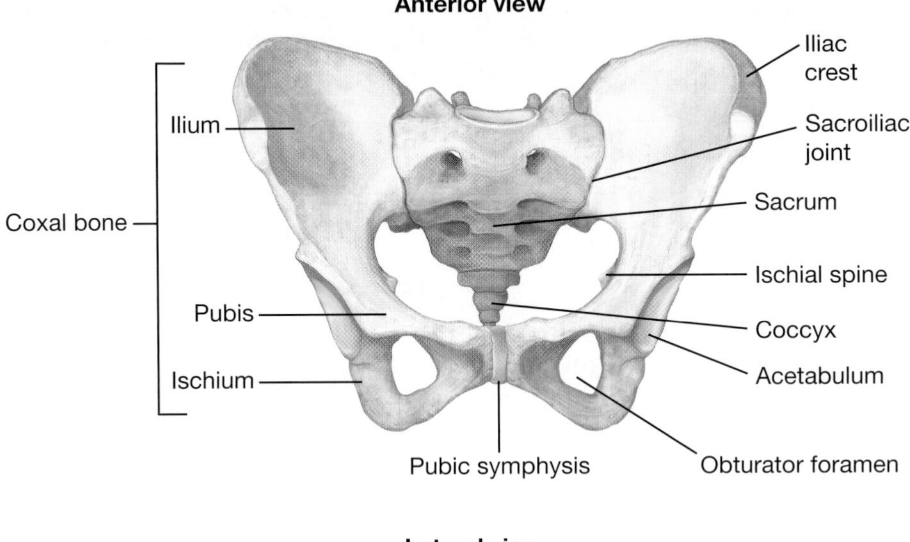

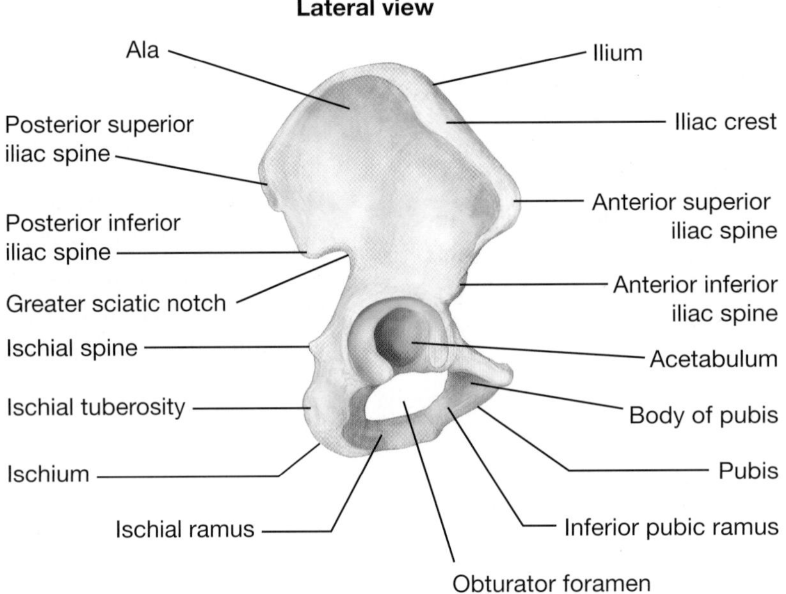

Figure 5.27 Bones of the pelvis.

the weight of the upper body during sitting. The ischium has several features:

- The greater sciatic notch is a prominent feature on the posterior hip at the junction of the ilium and ischium.
- The ischial spine is a projection inferior to the greater sciatic notch that narrows the passageway through which babies pass during birth.
- The ischial tuberosity is a raised area that directly supports upper body weight during sitting.
- The ischial ramus is the narrow bony connection between the ischium and the pubis.

The pubis is the anterior (front) portion of each coxal bone. The inferior pubic ramus is fused to the ischial ramus to enclose the obturator foramen, a large opening for blood vessels and nerves traversing to the anterior thigh. The two pubic bones fuse in the center front of the body at the pubic symphysis, where the bones are joined by a disc of hyaline cartilage.

The ilium, ischium, and pubis fuse to form the lateral and slightly anterior facing acetabulum (as-eh-TAB-yoo-lum). This is a deep, bony socket that receives the head of the thigh bone. The hip is an extremely stable joint thanks to the depth of the acetabulum and the strength of the large muscles surrounding the hip.

As shown in **Figure 5.28**, the part of the pelvic region above the pelvic inlet is called the ***false pelvis***. The ***true pelvis*** is the bony structure surrounding the pelvic inlet, the superior rim of the large central opening in the pelvis. The pelvic outlet is the inferior rim of this opening. The pelvic inlet and outlet are the boundaries of the passageway through which a baby's head must fit during normal childbirth.

You may have wondered what enables forensic experts to identify whether a skeleton is male or female. Certain differences in the pelvic region facilitate this identification. The female pelvis is characteristically distinguished from the male pelvis by the following features:

- a shallower, lighter structure
- a larger, more circular inlet
- a shorter sacrum
- more laterally spread ilia
- shorter ischial spines
- a larger angle of the pubic arch

There are, of course, individual variations and a whole range of bone configurations in all humans, but these differences are typical.

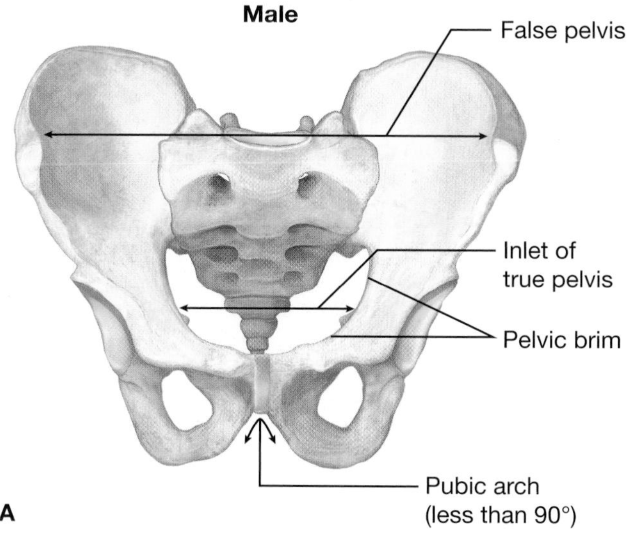

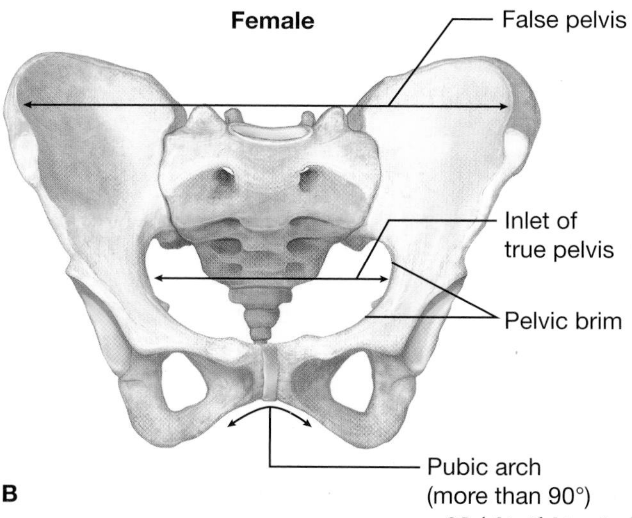

© Body Scientific International

Figure 5.28 Comparison of (A) male and (B) female pelvic characteristics.

Leg

The single bone of the upper leg, or thigh, is the ***femur***, which is the longest and strongest bone in the body. **Figure 5.29** shows the anatomical features of the femur. The head of the femur fits snugly into the acetabulum of the hip, making the joint extremely stable. The most vulnerable part of the femur is the neck, the site where hip fractures most often occur. The greater and lesser trochanters are separated by the intertrochanteric line on the anterior side and by the intertrochanteric crest on the posterior side. These trochanters, along with the gluteal tuberosity, are sites of muscle attachments.

The lower leg has two bones: the tibia and fibula (**Figure 5.30**). The thick, strong ***tibia***, or shinbone, bears most of the body's weight. The proximal head of the tibia includes medial and lateral condyles that articulate with the distal femur to form the knee joint. The intercondylar eminence separates the two condyles.

The ***patella***, or kneecap, is a small, flat, triangular-shaped bone (sesamoid bone) that protects the front of the knee. The patellar ligament attaches to the tibial tuberosity, a roughened prominence on the anterior aspect of the upper tibia. The anterior crest of the tibia, a sharp edge that is readily palpable, is the feature that gives the tibia its nickname—the "shinbone." Another easily felt portion of the tibia is the medial malleolus, which is the prominence on the inner side of the ankle.

Unlike the radius in the forearm, the ***fibula*** has no special motion capability and serves primarily as a site for muscle attachments. The fibula is not part of the

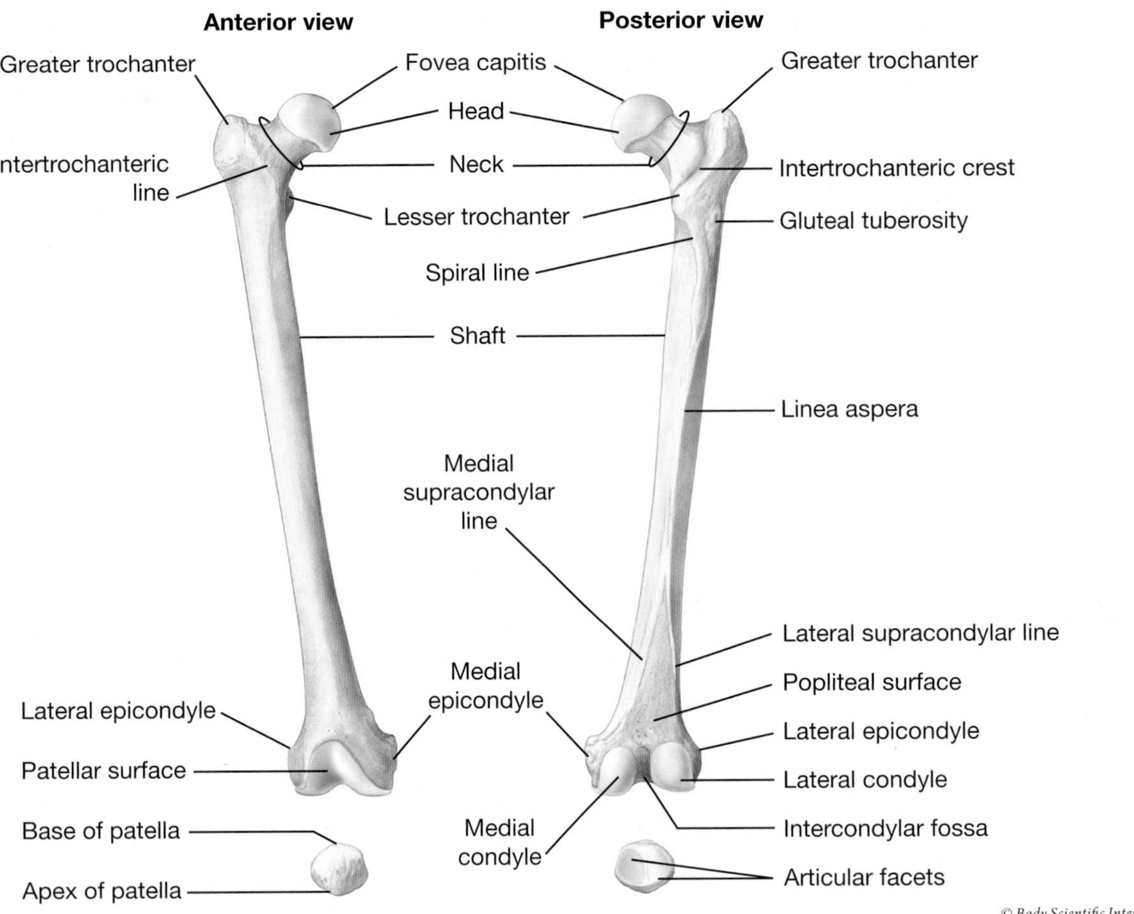

Figure 5.29 The right femur and patella.

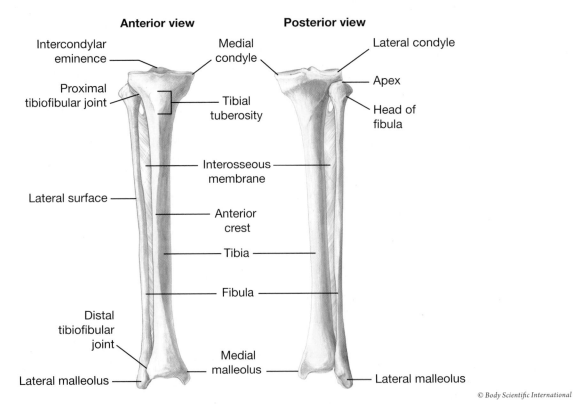

Figure 5.30 The right tibia and fibula, anterior and posterior views.

articulation with the femur at the knee joint, but the distal (lower) end of the fibula has a bony prominence called the *lateral malleolus*. You can readily touch and feel this prominence on the lateral (outer) side of the ankle. Like the radius and ulna in the forearm, the tibia and fibula are connected along their lengths by an interosseous membrane, and they articulate at both ends of the fibula (**Figure 5.31**).

Ankle and Foot

The ankle and foot serve the critically important functions of supporting body weight and enabling locomotion. The foot is so well designed that it assists with walking and running by acting like a spring that stores and releases energy.

As **Figure 5.32** shows, the hindfoot is constructed of ***tarsal bones***. The two largest, the talus (TAY-lus) and ***calcaneus*** (kal-KAY-nee-us), or heel bone, bear most of the weight of the body. The five ***metatarsal bones*** that support the midfoot region are similar to the metacarpals of the hand. Like the fingers, each toe has three phalanges, and like the thumb, the big toe has only two phalanges. The toes increase the area of the foot during weight-bearing activities, such as walking and running, thereby increasing body stability.

Articulating Bones of the Leg and Ankle

Joint	Notched Bone or Socket	Joining Bone or Region
iliofemoral (hip) joint	acetabulum	femur
tibiofemoral (knee) joint	tibia	femur
patellofemoral joint	patella	anterior knee
tibiofibular joints (proximal and distal)	tibia	fibula

Figure 5.31

Goodheart-Willcox Publisher

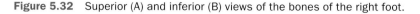

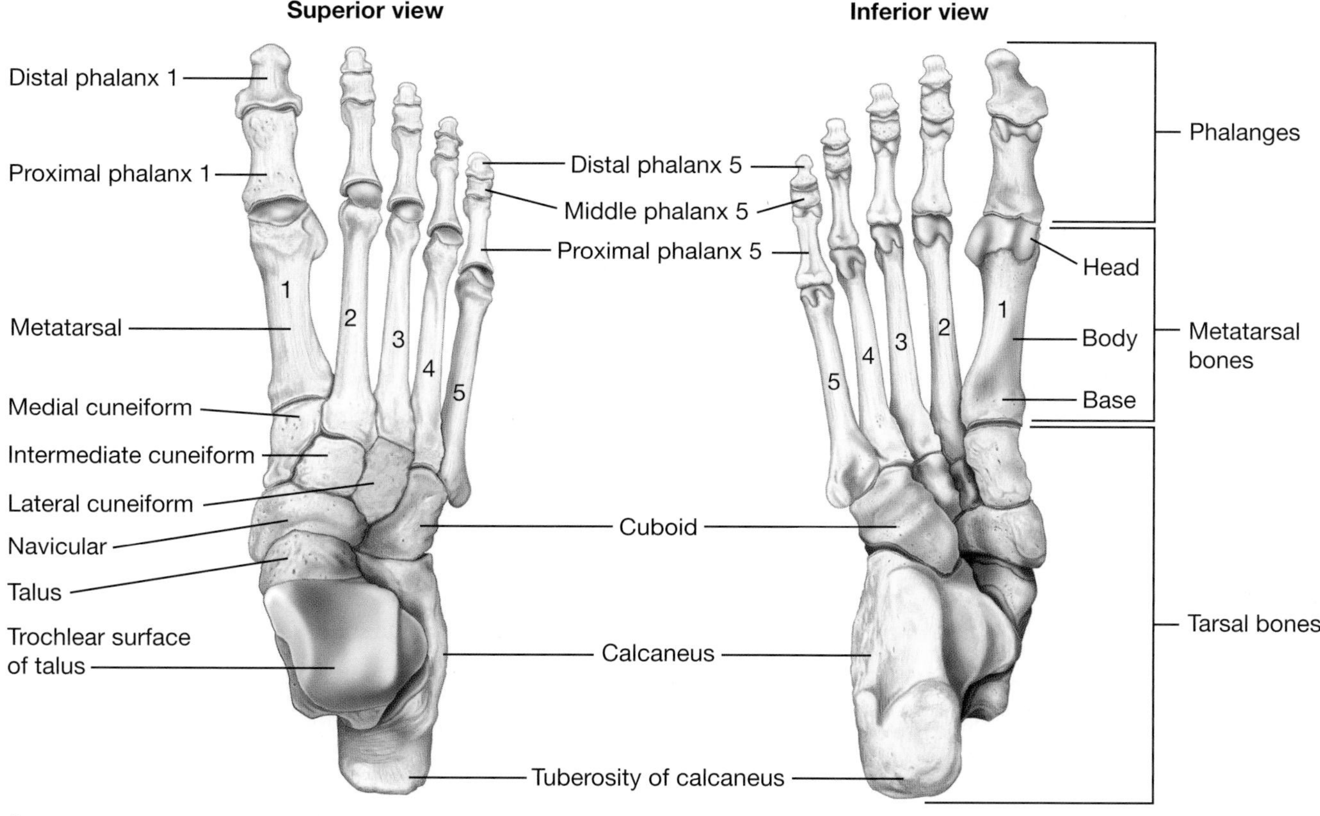

© Body Scientific International

Figure 5.32 Superior (A) and inferior (B) views of the bones of the right foot.

The configuration of the metatarsal bones forms two important arches (**Figure 5.33**). The longitudinal arch runs lengthwise from the calcaneus to the heads of the metatarsals. The transverse arch runs perpendicular to the longitudinal arch and typically causes the medial center of the bottom of the foot to be slightly elevated. It is these arches that compress somewhat during the weight-bearing phase of the human gait, but then act as springs when they rebound to their original shape during the propulsive (push-off) phase of the gait.

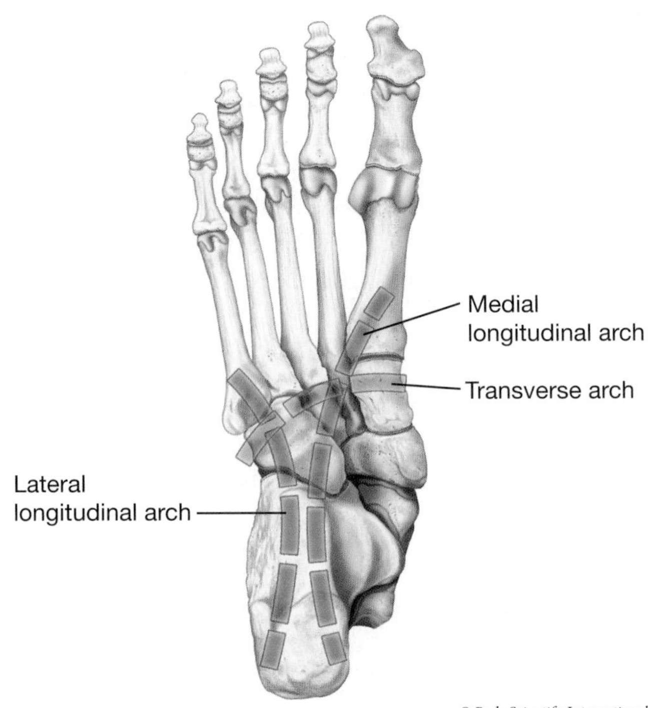

Figure 5.33 Arches of the foot, inferior view.

SECTION 5.3

REVIEW

Mini-Glossary

appendicular skeleton collective term for the bones of the body's appendages; the arms and legs
calcaneus the largest of the tarsal bones; referred to as the *heel bone*
carpal bones bones of the wrist
clavicle a doubly curved long bone that forms part of the shoulder girdle; also known as the *collarbone*
false pelvis the bony region of the pelvis that is located superior to the pelvic inlet
femur thigh bone
fibula bone of the lower leg that does not bear weight
humerus major bone of the upper arm
lower extremity the hips, legs, and feet
metacarpal bones the five interior bones of the hand that connect the carpals in the wrist to the phalanges in the fingers
metatarsal bones the small bones of the ankle
patella kneecap
pectoral girdle the bones surrounding the shoulder, including the clavicle and scapula
pelvis collective term for the bones of the pelvic girdle and the coccyx at the base of the spine
phalanges bones of the fingers
radius the smaller of the two bones in the forearm; rotates around the ulna
scapula shoulder blade
shoulder complex all of the joints surrounding the shoulder, including the acromioclavicular, sternoclavicular, and glenohumeral joints
tarsal bones bones of the ankle
tibia the major weight-bearing bone of the lower leg
true pelvis the region of the pelvis immediately surrounding the pelvic inlet
ulna larger bone of the lower arm
upper extremity the shoulders, arms, and hands

Review Questions

1. Explain how the bones of the pectoral girdle, along with various muscles and joints, allow movement in many different directions.
2. Which bone of the forearm is larger and stronger than the other?
3. Why is the pelvis of a female wider than the pelvis of a male?
4. Which bone of the lower leg is the stronger bone that bears most of the weight of the body above it?
5. Functionally, why does the pectoral girdle have much more range of motion than the pelvic girdle?
6. Why are there two bones in the forearm rather than just one?
7. Why would you not be able to walk properly if you had a fracture in one of the metatarsals or phalanges?

SECTION 5.4

Joints

Objectives

- Describe the general structures and functions of the three major categories of joints.
- Explain the purpose of the articular tissues, including tendons, ligaments, bursae, and articular cartilage.

Key Terms

amphiarthrosis
articular fibrocartilage
ball-and-socket joint
bursae
condylar joint
diarthrosis
gliding joint
hinge joint
ligament
pivot joint
saddle joint
symphysis
synarthrosis
synchondrosis
syndesmosis
synovial joint
tendon
tendon sheaths

The joints of the human body, also known as *articulations*, govern the extent and directions of movement of the bones that articulate (come together) at the joint. Although the range of motion at a given joint is affected by the tightness of the soft tissues crossing that joint, it is the structure of the bony articulation that determines the directions of motion permitted.

Anatomists classify joints in different ways based on joint complexity, the number of axes present, joint structure, and joint function. Joint function determines movement capability, and it is the most easily remembered classification, so it will be used in this section.

Types of Joints

There are three main categories of joints with regard to function: the immovable joints, the slightly movable joints, and the freely movable joints. Moving is the function of the arms, hands, legs, and feet, so most of the joints in the body appendages are freely movable. The axial skeleton's functions include stability and protection, so its joints are primarily immovable or slightly movable.

Synarthroses

The immovable joints are called ***synarthroses***. The prefix *syn-* means "together" and the root word *arthron* means "joint." Synarthroses are fibrous joints that can absorb shock but permit little or no movement of the articulating bones. There are two types of immovable joints: sutures and syndesmoses.

Sutures, which you read about earlier in this chapter, are joints in which irregularly grooved, articulating bone sheets join closely and are tightly connected by fibrous tissues. The fibers begin to ossify (turn to bone) in early adulthood and are eventually replaced completely by bone. The only sutures in the human body are the sutures of the skull.

Syndesmoses, meaning "held by bands," are joints in which dense, fibrous tissue binds the bones together, permitting extremely limited movement. Examples include the coracoacromial (kor-a-koh-a-KROH-mee-al) joint and the distal (lower) tibiofibular joints.

Amphiarthroses

The ***amphiarthroses*** are joints that permit only slight motion. These cartilaginous joints allow more motion of the articulating bones than the synarthrodial joints. This means they are somewhat better able to absorb shock. The two types of amphiarthroses are synchondroses and symphyses.

Synchondroses, meaning "held by cartilage," are joints in which the articulating bones are held together by a thin layer of hyaline cartilage. Examples include the sternocostal joints (between the sternum and the ribs) and the epiphyseal plates (growth plates).

Symphyses are joints in which thin plates of hyaline cartilage separate a disc of fibrocartilage from the bones. Examples include the vertebral joints and the pubic symphysis.

Diarthroses

Freely movable joints are called ***diarthroses***. They are also referred to as ***synovial joints*** because each joint is surrounded by an articular capsule with a synovial membrane lining that secretes a lubricant known as *synovial fluid* (**Figure 5.34**). There are six different types of diarthrosis; each is structured to permit different types of motion (**Figure 5.35**).

Figure 5.34 Anterior view of the knee, which is a synovial joint.

At ***gliding joints***, the articulating bone surfaces are nearly flat. The only movement these joints permit is gliding. Examples of gliding joints are the joints between some of the bones in the wrists and the ankles.

In ***hinge joints***, one articulating bone surface is convex (curved outward), and the other is concave (curved inward). Strong ligaments restrict movement to a planar, hinge-like motion, similar to the hinge on a door. The joint at the knee is an example of a hinge joint.

Pivot joints permit rotation around only one axis. Think of this movement as similar to moving around your stationary pivot foot in basketball. The joint between the first two vertebrae (the axis and atlas) is an example of a pivot joint.

At ***condylar joints***, one articulating bone surface is an oval, convex shape, and the other is a reciprocally shaped concave surface. Condylar joints allow flexion, extension, abduction, adduction, and circumduction.

Gliding joint (intercarpal)

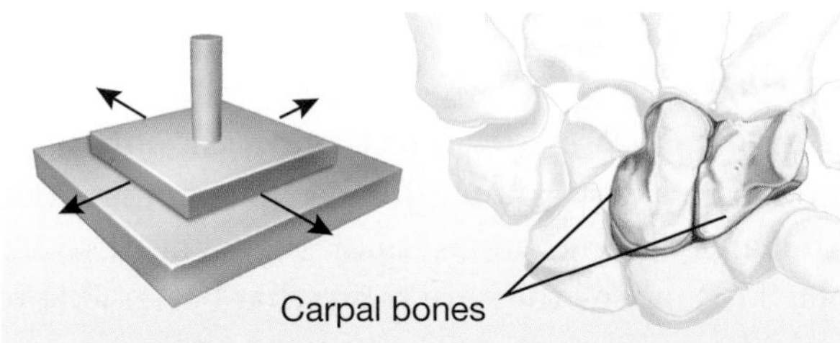

Hinge joint (humeroulnar)

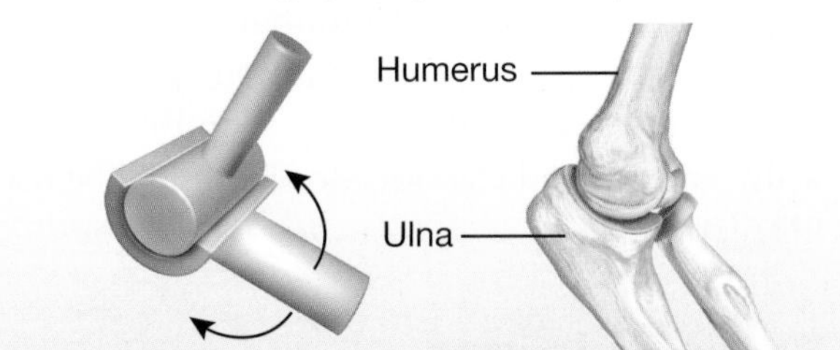

Pivot joint (radioulnar)

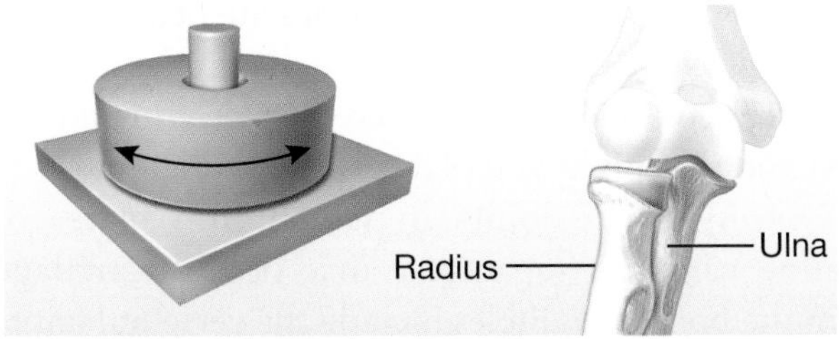

Condylar joint (metacarpophalangeal)

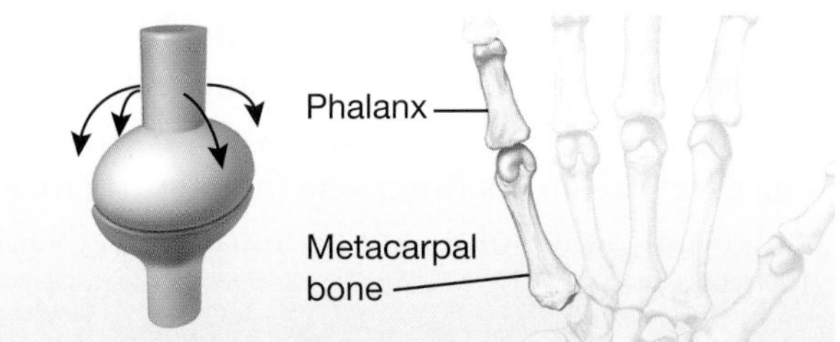

Saddle joint (trapeziometacarpal)

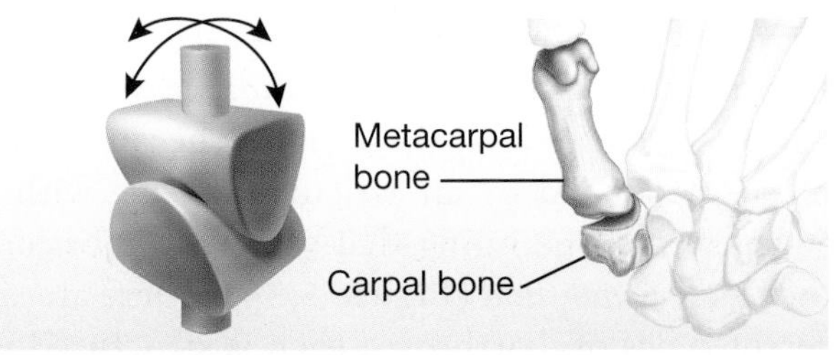

Ball-and-socket joint (humeroscapular)

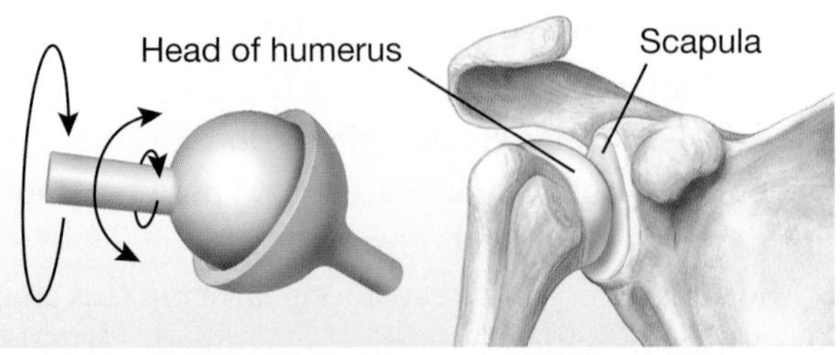

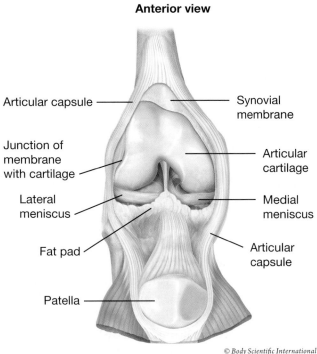

© Body Scientific International

Figure 5.35 Examples of the six different types of diarthroses.

One example of a condylar joint is the joint at the base of the index finger.

Saddle joints are so named because their articulating bone surfaces are both shaped like the seat of a riding saddle. Movement capability is the same as that of the condylar joint, but saddle joints have a greater range of movement. The joint at the base of the thumb is an example of a saddle joint.

Ball-and-socket joints are the most freely movable joints in the body. In these joints, the surfaces of the articulating bones are reciprocally convex and concave, with one bone end shaped like a "ball" and the other like a "socket." Rotation in all three planes of movement is permitted. In areas where the joint socket is relatively shallow, such as the shoulder, a large range of motion is permitted, but joint stability is sacrificed. Alternatively, the deep socket of the hip joint maximizes stability but allows much less range of motion than the shoulder.

Two structures often associated with diarthrodial joints are bursae and tendon sheaths. ***Bursae*** are small capsules lined with synovial membranes and filled with synovial fluid. Their purpose is to cushion the structures they separate. Most bursae separate tendons from bone, reducing the friction on the tendons during joint motion.

Tendon sheaths are double-layered synovial structures surrounding tendons that are subject to friction because of their proximity to bones. These sheaths secrete synovial fluid to promote free motion of the tendon during joint movement. Many long muscle tendons crossing the wrist and finger joints are protected by tendon sheaths.

SELF CHECK

1. What is the anatomical word for joints that permit only slight motion?
2. List two examples of ball-and-socket joints.
3. Explain the differences between a condylar joint and a saddle joint.
4. What is the purpose of a tendon sheath?

Articular Tissues

The joints of any mechanical device must be properly lubricated if the movable parts are to move freely and not wear against each other. In the human body, articular cartilage covers the ends of bones at diarthrodial joints and provides a protective lubrication. Articular cartilage cushions the joint and reduces friction and wear.

At some joints, ***articular fibrocartilage***, shaped like a disc or a partial disc called a *meniscus*, is also present between the articulating bones. The intervertebral discs and the menisci of the knee are examples. These discs and menisci help to distribute forces evenly over the joint surfaces and absorb shock at the joint.

Tendons, which connect muscles to bones, and ***ligaments***, which connect bones to other bones, are also present at the diarthrodial joints. Composed of collagen and elastic fibers, these tissues are slightly elastic and return to their original length after being stretched, unless overstretched to the point of injury. The tendons and ligaments crossing a joint play an important role in joint stability. The hip joints, in particular, are crossed by a number of large, strong tendons and ligaments.

SECTION 5.4 REVIEW

Mini-Glossary

amphiarthrosis a type of joint that permits only slight motion

articular fibrocartilage tissue shaped like a disc or a partial disc called a *meniscus* that provides cushioning at a joint

ball-and-socket joint a synovial joint formed between one bone end shaped roughly like a ball and a receiving bone reciprocally shaped like a socket

bursae small capsules lined with synovial membranes and filled with synovial fluid that cushion the structures they separate

condylar joint a type of diarthrosis in which one articulating bone surface is an oval, convex shape, and the other is a reciprocally shaped concave surface

diarthrosis a freely movable joint; also known as a *synovial joint*

gliding joint a type of diarthrosis that allows only sliding motion of the articulating bones

(continued)

hinge joint a type of diarthrosis that allows only hinge-like movements in forward and backward directions

ligament a band of collagen and elastic fibers that connects bones to other bones

pivot joint a type of diarthrosis that permits rotation around only one axis

saddle joint a type of diarthrosis in which the articulating bone surfaces are both shaped like the seat of a riding saddle

symphysis a type of amphiarthrosis in which a thin plate of hyaline cartilage separates a disc of fibrocartilage from the bones

synarthrosis a fibrous joint that can absorb shock, but which permits little or no movement of the articulating bones

synchondrosis a type of amphiarthrosis joint in which the articulating bones are held together by a thin layer of hyaline cartilage

syndesmosis a type of synarthrosis joint at which dense, fibrous tissue binds the bones together, permitting extremely limited movement

synovial joint a diarthrodial joint

tendon a band of collagen and elastic fibers that connects a muscle to a bone

tendon sheaths double-layered synovial structures surrounding tendons that are subject to friction because they are located so close to bones; secrete synovial fluid to promote free motion of the tendons during joint movement

Review Questions

1. What does it mean to say that bones articulate with each other?
2. Give two examples of immovable joints and state where they are found in the body.
3. Give two examples of slightly movable joints and state where they are found in the body.
4. Give six examples of freely movable joints and state where they are found in the body.
5. Why is it important to have a layer of cartilage between bones that articulate with each other?
6. Why does the human body need joints that permit little to no movement in the skeleton?
7. What happens when articular cartilage begins to erode from excessive wear and stress on a joint?

SECTION 5.5 Injuries and Disorders of the Skeletal System

Objectives

- Identify the different types of bone and epiphyseal injuries, and explain the forces that can cause each of these injuries.
- Discuss osteoporosis, including contributing factors, groups at risk, consequences, and prevention strategies.
- Describe the common types of joint injuries, including the structures affected, symptoms, and common treatments.
- Explain what is involved with arthritis and describe specific types of arthritis.

Key Terms

amenorrhea
anorexia nervosa
apophysis
arthritis
bulimia nervosa
bursitis
dislocation
female athlete triad
fracture
osteoarthritis
osteopenia
osteoporosis
rheumatoid arthritis
sprain

Considering all of the important functions performed by bone, bone health is a vital part of general health. Bone health can be diminished by injuries and pathologies.

Common Bone Injuries

Perhaps the most common, and often the most visible, types of bone injuries are fractures of various types. However, other types of injuries, such as epiphyseal injuries, are also possible.

Fractures

A ***fracture*** is a break or crack in a bone. The nature of a fracture depends on the size, direction, and duration of the injurious force, as well as the health and maturity of the bone.

Fractures are classified as simple when the bone ends remain within the surrounding soft tissues, and compound when one or both bone ends protrude from the skin. When the bone is splintered, the fracture is said to be *comminuted*. See **Figure 5.36**.

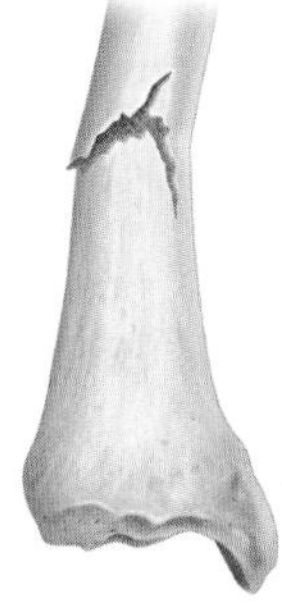

A *greenstick fracture* is incomplete. The break occurs on the convex surface of the bend in the bone.

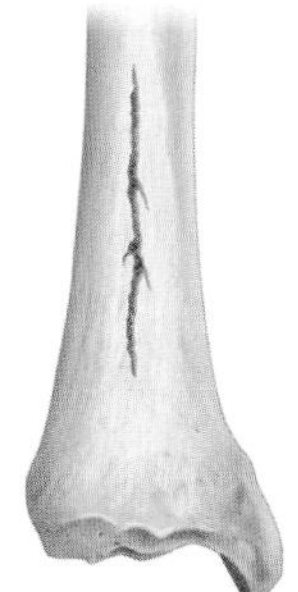

A *stress fracture* involves an incomplete break.

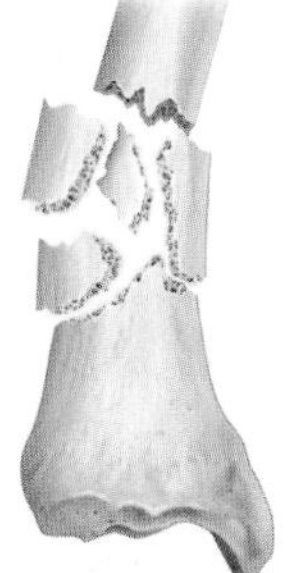

A *comminuted fracture* is complete and splinters the bone.

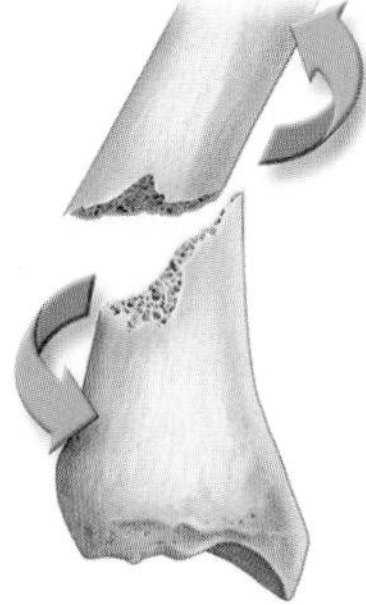

A *spiral fracture* is caused by twisting a bone excessively.

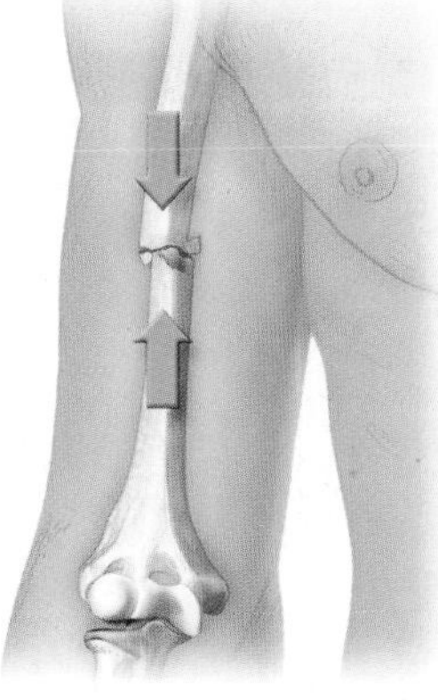

An *impacted fracture* involves compression of a long bone along the longitudinal axis, forcing the broken ends together.

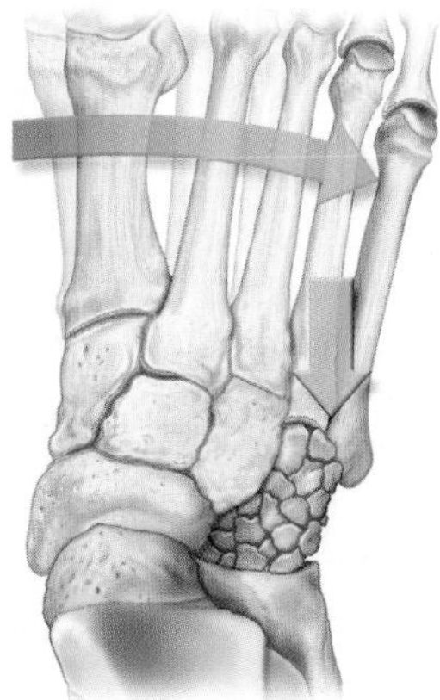

A *crush fracture* is one in which a bone fails under a compressive load.

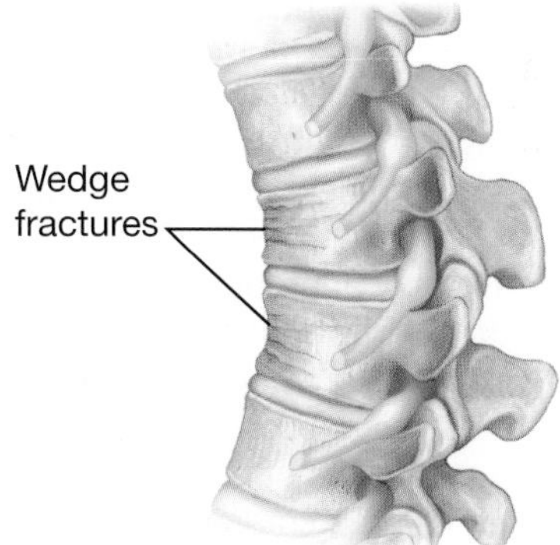

A *wedge fracture* occurs vertically in the spinal column, resulting in a wedge-shaped vertebra.

Figure 5.36 Types of fractures.

Compression fractures result when bone fails under a compressive force. There are several variations of compression fractures, based on the direction of the compressive force and the resulting injury to the bone. An impacted fracture is one in which the compressive force is directed along the longitudinal axis of a long bone, causing the broken ends of the bone to be forced together. Crush fractures occur most often in the weakened osteoporotic spine when the internal trabecular bone fails under a compressive load directed down the length of the spinal column, resulting in a loss of vertebral height. Vertebral crush fractures caused by postural loading are known as *wedge fractures*. These result from compression directed down the anterior side of the spine, often result in a wedge-shaped vertebral body with the narrow portion to the front.

Avulsions are fractures caused when a tendon or ligament pulls away from its attachment to a bone, taking a small chip of bone with it. Explosive throwing and jumping movements may cause avulsion fractures of the medial epicondyle of the humerus and the calcaneus.

Forceful bending and twisting movements can produce spiral fractures of the long bones. A common example occurs during downhill skiing. When a ski is planted in one direction, and the skier rotates while falling in a different direction, a spiral fracture of the tibia can result.

The bones of children contain relatively larger amounts of collagen than the bones of adults. For this reason, children's bones are more flexible and are generally less likely to fracture than adult bones.

Consequently, greenstick fractures, or incomplete fractures, are more common in children than in adults. A greenstick fracture is caused when a bone bends or twists but does not break all the way through.

Stress fractures are tiny, painful cracks in bone that result from overuse. Under normal circumstances, bone responds to stress-related injury by remodeling. Osteoclasts resorb the damaged tissue, and then osteoblasts deposit new bone at the site, resulting in repair of the injury. However, when overuse is repeated or continuous, the remodeling process cannot keep up with the damage being done. When this happens, the condition progresses to a stress fracture. Runners are prone to stress fractures, particularly in the tibia and the metatarsals.

Clinical Application Bone Tissue Engineering

Fractures and malformations of the skull and face can result from birth defects, infections, cancers, or traumatic injury. These can be dangerous for patients and often require costly healthcare procedures. Current approaches to repair and reconstruction include rigid fixation of an artificial plate, bone grafting, and transfer of new bone tissue to the region. However, these techniques often involve complications, such as poor fitting of the plate or graft failure.

Bone tissue engineering, one of the most challenging and exciting new fields for scientists and clinicians, offers some creative new approaches. Engineered therapies for enhanced healing and regeneration of craniofacial bone typically involve a combination of live stem cells and growth factors applied over artificial, biodegradable scaffolds. The success of bone tissue engineering relies on understanding the complex interactions among live stem cells, the regulatory signals, and the platforms used to deliver them. All of these components are collectively known as the *tissue engineering triad*.

The live cells employed are typically mesenchymal stem cells combined with bone marrow. A surgeon harvests a small amount of mesenchymal stem cells from the patient's iliac crest. These cells are then carefully cultured in a growth medium until they become larger cell colonies that can differentiate into cells that form bone.

More recently, scientists have discovered that stem cells can also be extracted from fat. These adipose stem cells can be collected in large quantities with little patient discomfort, in contrast to the invasive and painful extraction techniques used to obtain bone marrow mesenchymal cells. Although promising, more studies are needed to standardize and refine the techniques for harvesting and culturing adipose stem cells.

Whatever the source, the live bone cells are cultured and then implanted on a biomaterial scaffold. Many different growth factor delivery techniques and scaffold compositions have been explored, although none has yet emerged as universally recommended. Scientists have discovered that the size of the pores in the scaffolding material can greatly influence the ability of the cells to attach and colonize. Different scaffold materials also exert different biomechanical forces, which can profoundly affect bone cell development. Identifying biomaterials that are optimally capable of responding to physiological and mechanical changes inside the human body remains an important challenge in bone tissue engineering.

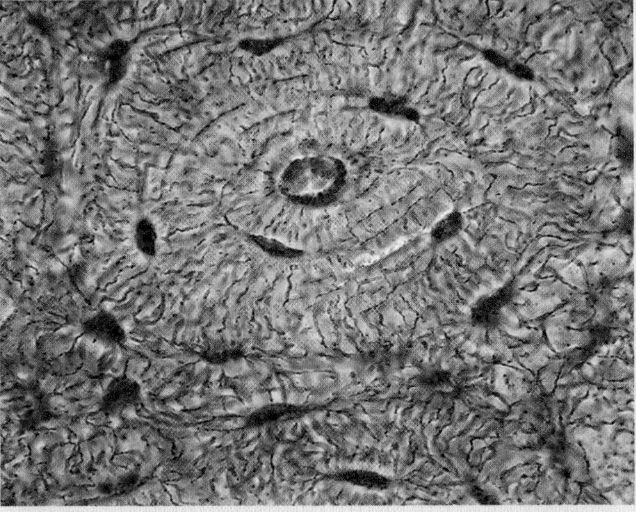

Jose Luis Calvo/Shutterstock.com

Growing new bone tissue is quite a complicated process, as evidenced by this microscopic view of bone structure showing osteons and Haversian canals.

Once the cells have been implanted on the scaffold, a surgeon inserts the bone cell colony and scaffold material into the site of bone damage. At this point, new challenges arise, including promoting the development of a blood supply to the implant and ensuring the survival of the live cells. Achieving long-term repair requires infusion of antibiotics and growth factors in appropriate amounts and with optimal timing during the healing and repair processes. Utilization of nanoparticles for delivery of drugs and growth factors to the region is one promising approach.

Another new approach begins with a CT scan of the bone defect and extraction of a small sample of fat from the patient. The CT scan is used to create a precise, three-dimensional model of the site that requires repair. The model is then placed in a growth chamber along with stem cells from the patient's fat sample. Ideally, in a few weeks, a perfectly fitting bony replacement part will grow from the patient's own cells. This promising approach is currently being developed in animals.

Epiphyseal Injuries

Epiphyseal injuries include injuries to the epiphyseal plate, articular cartilage, and the apophysis. An ***apophysis*** is a site at which a tendon attaches to a bone. Both acute and overuse-related injuries can damage the growth plate, potentially resulting in premature closure of the epiphyseal junction and termination of bone growth.

Osteochondrosis, also known as *Osgood-Schlatter disease*, is another form of bone injury. The powerful quadriceps muscle group on the front of the thigh attaches distally to the upper tibia. When the quadriceps is used a lot in sports activities during the adolescent growth spurt, the area of the tibia around the attachment site becomes irritated or swollen, causing pain. The condition is believed to be a result of overuse injuries that occur before the area has finished growing.

Osteochondrosis is common in adolescents who play soccer, basketball, and volleyball, and in those who participate in gymnastics. Males are more often affected than females. The primary symptom is a painful region of swelling at the muscle attachment site, which can occur on one or both legs. The pain worsens with physical activity.

SELF CHECK

1. List and describe the following types of fractures: simple, compound, comminuted, avulsion, spiral, greenstick, stress, impacted, crush, and wedge.
2. Explain osteochondrosis.
3. Why is it important for children to avoid activities that could cause damage to an epiphyseal plate?

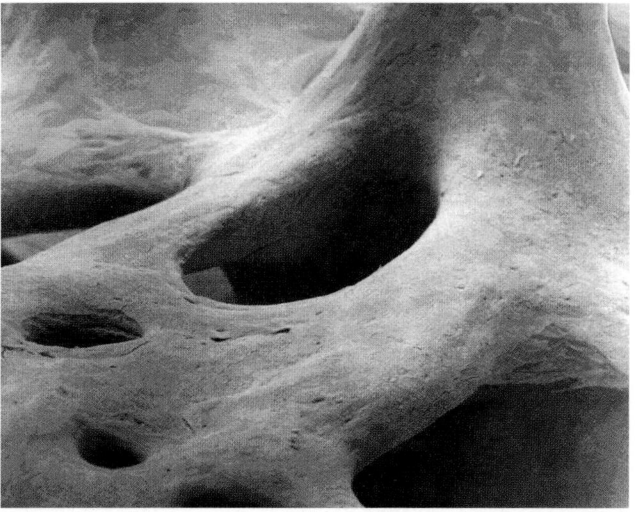

A

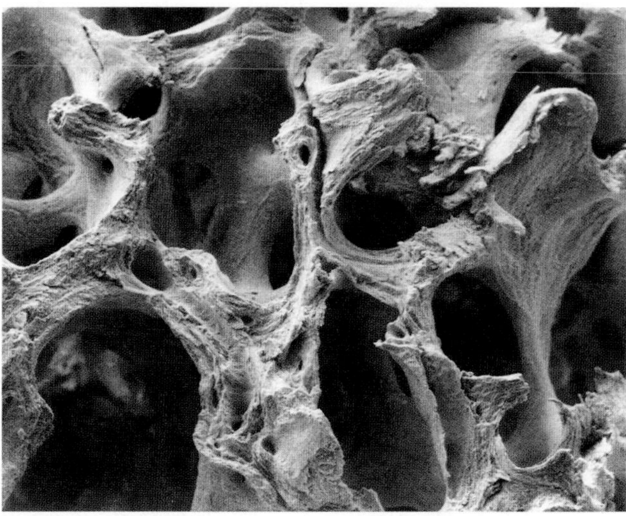

B

Dee Breger/Science Source [both images]

Figure 5.37 Compare the normal trabecular bone (A) with the brittle, degraded bone (B) characteristic of osteoporosis. As the bone becomes more brittle, it is more likely to fracture.

Osteoporosis

Osteoporosis is a condition in which bone mineralization and strength are so abnormally low that regular daily activities can result in painful fractures. With its honeycomb structure, trabecular bone is the most common site of osteoporotic fractures (**Figure 5.37**).

Age-Related Osteoporosis

Osteoporosis occurs in most elderly individuals, with earlier onset in women. The condition begins as ***osteopenia***, which is characterized by reduced bone mass without the presence of a fracture. The osteopenia often progresses to osteoporosis, with fractures present. Although once regarded as primarily a health issue for women, the increasing age of the general population means that osteoporosis is now also becoming a concern for older men as well.

In type I osteoporosis, also known as *postmenopausal osteoporosis*, fractures usually begin to occur about 15 years after menopause. The femoral neck, vertebrae, and wrist bones are the most common fracture sites. Type II osteoporosis, also called *age-associated osteoporosis*, affects most women, and also affects men over 70 years of age. After 60 years of age, the majority of fractures in both men and women are osteoporosis-related. In the elderly population fractures of the femoral neck, in particular, often trigger a downward health spiral that leads to death.

The most common symptom of osteoporosis, however, is back pain derived from crush-type fractures of the weakened trabecular bone of the vertebrae. These fractures can be caused by activities as simple as picking up a bag of groceries or a bag of trash. Vertebral crush fractures frequently cause reduction of body height and tend to accentuate the kyphotic curve in the thoracic region of the spine.

The Female Athlete Triad

Unfortunately, osteoporosis is not confined to the elderly population. It can also occur in female athletes at the high school and collegiate levels who strive to maintain an excessively low body weight.

Striving for an extremely low weight can cause a dangerous condition known as the ***female athlete triad***. This condition involves a combination of disordered eating, ***amenorrhea***—having no period or menses—and osteoporosis. Because the triad can cause negative health consequences ranging from irreversible bone loss to death, friends, parents, coaches, and physicians need to be alert to the signs of this condition.

Female athletes participating in endurance or appearance-related sports are most likely to be affected by the female athlete triad. Disordered eating can take the form of anorexia nervosa or bulimia nervosa.

Symptoms of ***anorexia nervosa*** in girls and women include a body weight that is 15% or more below the minimal normal weight range, extreme fear of gaining weight, an unrealistic body image, and amenorrhea. ***Bulimia nervosa*** involves a minimum of two eating binges per week for at least three months; an associated feeling of lack of control; use of self-induced vomiting, laxatives, diuretics, strict dieting, or exercise to prevent weight gain; and an obsession with body image.

Research Notes Preventing Osteoporosis

Osteoporosis is not inevitable with advancing age. It is typically the result of a lifetime of habits that are erosive to the skeletal system. Simply stated, it is easier to prevent osteoporosis than to treat it.

The single most important strategy for preventing or delaying the onset of osteoporosis is maximizing bone mass during childhood and adolescence. Weight-bearing exercise such as running, jumping, and even walking is particularly important prior to puberty because of the high level of growth hormone present during this period. Growth hormone makes exercise particularly effective in increasing bone density.

Diet also plays an important role in bone health. Physicians now recognize that a predisposition for osteoporosis can begin in childhood and adolescence when a poor diet interferes with bone mass development. Adequate dietary calcium is particularly important during the teenage years, but unfortunately the typical American girl falls below the recommended daily intake of 1,200 mg per day by 11 years of age. A modified diet or calcium supplement can be critical for the development of peak bone mass among adolescent females who have this dietary deficiency.

The role of vitamin D is also important, because vitamin D enables bone to absorb calcium. In North America, more than 50% of women being treated for low bone density also have a vitamin D deficiency.

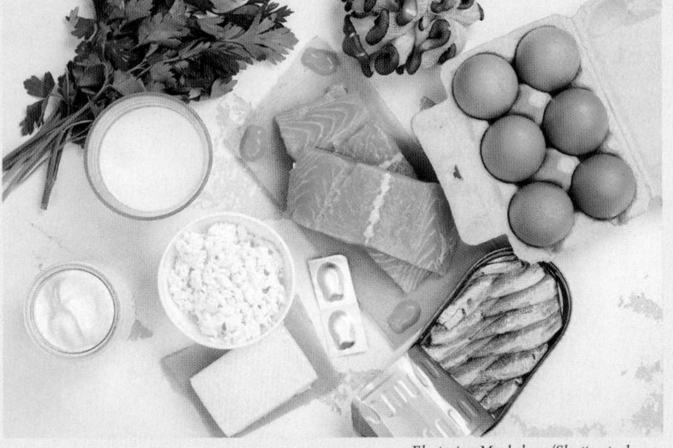

Ekaterina Markelova/Shutterstock.com

Common sources of calcium and vitamin D. Eating a balanced diet that includes a variety of foods like these helps young people achieve normal, healthy bone mass.

Other lifestyle factors also affect bone mineralization. Risk factors for developing osteoporosis include a sedentary lifestyle, weight loss or excessive thinness, and smoking tobacco.

To help prevent later development of osteoporosis, young women are encouraged to engage in regular physical activity and to avoid the lifestyle factors that negatively affect bone health.

Although the incidence of osteoporosis among female athletes is unknown, the consequences of the female athlete triad are potentially tragic. Amenorrheic, premenopausal female athletes are known to have an elevated rate of stress fractures. More important, the loss of bone that occurs may be irreversible, and osteoporotic wedge fractures of the vertebrae can ruin posture for life.

SELF CHECK

1. How does osteoporosis differ from osteopenia?
2. What is the female athlete triad?

Common Joint Injuries

The freely movable joints of the human body are subjected to significant wear over the course of a lifetime. Both acute and overuse injuries affect the joints.

Sprains

Sprains are injuries caused by abnormal motion of the articulating bones that results in overstretching or tearing of ligaments, tendons, or other connective tissues crossing a joint. The most common site of sprain is the ankle, and the most common mechanism is injury to the lateral ligaments.

Lateral ankle sprains occur frequently because the ankle is a major weight-bearing joint and because there is less ligamentous support on the lateral than on the medial side of the ankle. Pain and swelling are the symptoms of joint sprains. Immediate treatment should include intermittent icing and elevation.

Dislocations

When one of the articulating bones is displaced from the joint socket, the injury is called a ***dislocation*** of that joint. Dislocations usually result from falls or forceful collisions.

Common dislocation sites include the shoulders, fingers, knees, elbows, and jaw. Signs and symptoms include visible joint deformity, pain, swelling, and some loss of movement capability.

Bursitis

Bursitis is the inflammation of one or more bursae, the fluid-filled sacs that provide cushioning of the moving tissues around a joint. Bursitis is an overuse injury that results in irritation and inflammation of the bursae due to friction. For example, runners who overtrain may experience inflammation of the bursa between the Achilles tendon and the calcaneus. Symptoms of bursitis include pain and sometimes swelling.

SELF CHECK

1. Which structures are affected when a joint is sprained?
2. What types of actions may result in dislocations?
3. What are the causes and symptoms of bursitis?

Arthritis

Arthritis is a common pathology associated with aging. It is characterized by joint inflammation accompanied by pain, stiffness, and sometimes swelling. Arthritis is not a single condition but a large family of pathologies. Over one hundred different types of arthritis have been identified.

Rheumatoid Arthritis

Rheumatoid arthritis is an autoimmune disorder in which the body's own immune system attacks healthy joint tissues (**Figure 5.38**). It is the most debilitating

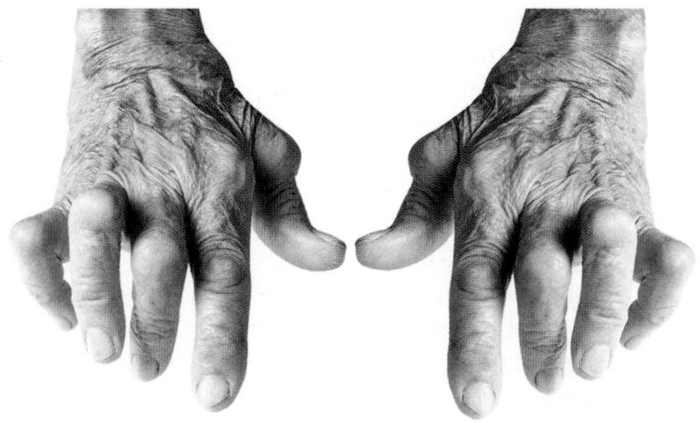

Chaowalit Seeneha/Shutterstock.com

Figure 5.38 This person's hands have been disfigured by rheumatoid arthritis. Most patients take medication for the intense pain.

and painful form of arthritis. Rheumatoid arthritis is more common in adults but occasionally occurs in children (juvenile rheumatoid arthritis).

Symptoms of rheumatoid arthritis include inflammation and thickening of the synovial membranes and breakdown of the articular cartilage. The results are extremely limited joint motion and, in extreme cases, complete fusing of the articulating bones. Associated symptoms can include anemia, fatigue, and muscular atrophy.

Osteoarthritis

Arthritis also takes a noninflammatory form as ***osteoarthritis***, a degenerative disease of articular cartilage. Onset of osteoarthritis is characterized by progressive roughening of the normally smooth joint cartilage, with the cartilage eventually completely wearing away. Pain, swelling, range-of-motion restriction, and stiffness are all symptoms, with the pain typically relieved by rest and the joint stiffness improved by activity.

SECTION 5.5 REVIEW

Mini-Glossary

amenorrhea absence of a menstrual period in women of reproductive age

anorexia nervosa condition characterized by body weight 15% or more below the minimal normal weight range, extreme fear of gaining weight, an unrealistic body image, and amenorrhea

apophysis site at which a tendon attaches to bone

arthritis a family of more than 100 common pathologies associated with aging; characterized by joint inflammation accompanied by pain, stiffness, and sometimes swelling

bulimia nervosa condition characterized by a minimum of two eating binges a week for at least three months; an associated feeling of lack of control; use of self-induced vomiting, laxatives, diuretics, strict dieting, or exercise to prevent weight gain; and an obsession with body image

bursitis inflammation of one or more bursae

dislocation injury that involves displacement of a bone from its joint socket

female athlete triad combination of disordered eating, amenorrhea, and osteoporosis

fracture any break or disruption of continuity in a bone

osteoarthritis degenerative disease of the articular cartilage; characterized by pain, swelling, range-of-motion restriction, and stiffness

osteopenia condition characterized by reduced bone mass without the presence of a fracture

osteoporosis condition in which bone mineralization and strength are so abnormally low that regular, daily activities can result in painful fractures

rheumatoid arthritis autoimmune disorder in which the body's own immune system attacks healthy joint tissues; the most debilitating and painful form of arthritis

sprain injury caused by abnormal motion of the articulating bones that result in overstretching or tearing of ligaments, tendons, or other connective tissues crossing a joint

Review Questions

1. What is an avulsion?
2. At what point in a person's life is osteochondrosis most likely to occur?
3. What is the most common symptom of osteoporosis?
4. Which joint in the skeleton is the most commonly sprained?
5. What happens to healthy joint tissue in a person with rheumatoid arthritis?
6. Explain how the remodeling of a bone and a stress fracture are related.
7. Why are females who participate in certain sports more vulnerable to the condition known as the *female athlete triad*?
8. A 17-year-old soccer player has sustained several fractures to different parts of her body. When her bone density was tested, she was found to be on the low end of the normal range. What would you suggest that she do to increase her bone strength?

Medical Terminology: The Skeletal System

By understanding the word parts that make up medical words, you can extend your medical vocabulary. This chapter includes many of the word parts listed below. Review these word parts to be sure you understand their meanings.

a-	no, not, loss of
arthr/o	joint
cortic/o	cortex, outer part
epi-	above, upon
hemato-	blood
hyper-	above, excessive
hypo-	below, insufficient
inter-	between
men/o	menses, menstruation
oste/o	bone
peri-	around
-physis	to grow
-poiesis	formation
-rrhea	flow, discharge
-trophy	condition

Now use these word parts to form valid medical words that fit the following definitions. Some of the words are included in this chapter. Others are not. When you finish, use a medical dictionary to check your work.

1. formation of blood
2. outer layer of bone
3. around the bone
4. to grow upon
5. condition of above-normal density or growth rate
6. between the vertebrae
7. condition of bone loss
8. lack of menstrual flow
9. inflammation of a joint
10. bone and joint inflammation

Chapter 5 Summary

- The five functions of the skeletal system are support, protection, movement, storage, and blood cell formation.
- The four categories (by shape) of bones are long bones, short bones, flat bones, and irregular bones.
- Throughout a person's life, osteoblasts build new bone tissue, and osteoclasts resorb damaged bone tissue.
- Remodeling of bones continues throughout life to keep bones strong.
- The skull contains eight cranial bones and fourteen facial bones.
- The five sections of the spine are the cervical region, thoracic region, lumbar region, sacrum, and coccyx.
- The thoracic cage surrounds and protects the heart and lungs.
- The upper extremity includes the shoulder complex, arms, wrists, and hands.
- The lower extremity includes the pelvic girdle, legs, ankles, and feet.
- The three main categories of joints, with regard to function, are the immovable joints, the slightly movable joints, and the freely movable joints.
- Articular tissues include articular fibrocartilage, tendons, ligaments, and bursae.
- The nature of a fracture depends on the size, direction, and duration of the injurious force, as well as the health and maturity of the bone.
- Osteoporosis is a condition in which bone mineralization and strength are critically low, often leading to fractures.
- Sprains, dislocations, and bursitis are common joint injuries.
- Arthritis is characterized by joint inflammation accompanied by pain, stiffness, and sometimes swelling.

Chapter 5 Review

Understanding Key Concepts

1. Name the five functions of the skeletal system.
2. The term for blood cell formation is:
   A. osteocyte
   B. hematopoiesis
   C. osteogenesis
   D. osteoblast
3. Strong, dense bone tissue is called ______.
   A. trabecular bone
   B. coxal bone
   C. cortical bone
   D. hard bone

4. What are the five shape categories of bones?
5. The shaft, or middle, of a bone is called the ______; the ends of a bone are called the ______.
6. Specialized bone cells that break down bone are called ______.
   A. osteocytes
   B. osteoclasts
   C. osteoblasts
   D. osteons
7. Specialized bone cells that build new bone are called ______.
   A. osteocytes
   B. osteoclasts
   C. osteoblasts
   D. osteons
8. Which spinal region includes the vertebrae of the neck?
   A. thoracic
   B. lumbar
   C. sacral
   D. cervical
9. Which spinal region connects to the ribs?
   A. thoracic
   B. lumbar
   C. sacral
   D. cervical
10. Which condition causes a lateral (sideways) curvature of the spine?
    A. lordosis
    B. kyphosis
    C. scoliosis
    D. neurosis
11. Which of the following is *not* part of the thoracic cage?
    A. the ribs
    B. the thoracic vertebrae
    C. the sternum
    D. the sacrum
12. Which of the following is *true* about the false ribs?
    A. They do not attach directly to the sternum.
    B. They do not attach directly to the vertebrae.
    C. They do not attach directly to anything.
    D. They do not exist.
13. Which structures make up the axial skeleton?
    A. the arms and legs
    B. the head and trunk
    C. the thoracic cage
    D. the spinal column
14. Which structures are part of the appendicular skeleton?
    A. the head and trunk
    B. the spinal column
    C. the arms and legs
    D. the thoracic cage
15. Which bone is always on the "little finger" side of the forearm?
    A. humerus
    B. radius
    C. ulna
    D. tibia
16. What is the term for the prominent upper edge of the hip bone?
    A. sacroiliac joint
    B. acetabulum
    C. ischium
    D. iliac crest
17. What is the longest, strongest bone in the body?
    A. sternum
    B. humerus
    C. femur
    D. tibia
18. Which of the following is the heel bone?
    A. talus
    B. femur
    C. patella
    D. calcaneus
19. The shoulder girdle consists of the right and left ______ and the right and left ______.
20. There are ______ bones in each wrist and hand.
21. What three bones fuse to form each coxal bone?
22. Which of the following are immovable joints?
    A. sutures of the skull
    B. gliding joints
    C. pivot joints
    D. hinge joints

23. Which of the following is *not* a function of articular cartilage?
    A. cushions the joint
    B. reduces wear to the joint
    C. reduces friction at the joint
    D. helps distribute forces evenly
24. Another term for freely movable joints is ______.
25. ______ are small sacs filled with synovial fluid that cushion the structures they separate.
26. ______ connect muscle to bone, while ______ connect bone to bone.
27. Which term describes a fracture in which the ends of a bone protrude from the skin?
    A. comminuted
    B. compound
    C. simple
    D. avulsion
28. Which type of fracture is more common in children than in adults?
    A. compound
    B. avulsion
    C. greenstick
    D. simple
29. Injuries to which of the following can stop the growth of a long bone?
    A. intervertebral disc
    B. meniscus
    C. epiphyseal plate
    D. sutures
30. ______ fractures are tiny, painful cracks in a bone that result from overuse.
31. The site where a tendon attaches to a bone is known as the ______.
32. ______ is an autoimmune disorder in which the body's own immune system attacks healthy joint tissues.

Thinking Critically

33. Given your knowledge of the intervertebral discs, what activities should a person avoid to promote disc health? Name at least two activities and explain why each should be avoided.
34. If a forensic scientist finds skeletal remains after a house fire, how might she determine whether the individual was a male or female?
35. Give reasons why you either would or would not want all of your joints to be ball-and-socket joints.
36. A 10-year-old boy and his 42-year-old father were building a tree house when the branch they were standing on broke away from the tree. The father sustained two broken ribs, but the boy had only a few bruises. What might explain the difference in the severity of their injuries?

Clinical Case Study

Read again the Clinical Case Study at the beginning of this chapter. Use the information provided in the chapter to answer the following questions.

37. Among the conditions described in this chapter, what do you think might be going on with Dana?
38. Which condition do you think is most likely? Why?

Analyzing & Evaluating Data

Astronauts who spend an extended amount of time in space may lose 1% to 2% of their bone mass each month if they do not perform regular resistance exercises.

39. If the astronaut spends three months in space and never exercises, what percentage of his bone mass might he lose?
40. You read in this chapter that bones account for about 15% of body weight. If this astronaut weighs 170 pounds, how much do his bones weigh?
41. If he fails to exercise for 6 months in space, how much weight might this astronaut lose in bone mass?

Investigating Further

42. Choose one of the following topics: anorexia nervosa, bursitis, dislocation, female athlete triad, fracture, osteoporosis, rheumatoid arthritis, sprain, or stress fracture. Using this textbook as a starting point, research your topic and prepare a report on causes and treatments.

6 The Muscular System

Clinical Case Study

Mike played varsity basketball in high school and now, in his second year of college, he still enjoys an occasional pick-up game with his friends. In a friendly game just yesterday he had an opening to break around two defenders and sprinted to make a layup shot. But he did not make it to the basket because in mid-stride he suddenly felt a sharp pain on the mid-posterior aspect of his right thigh.

Today Mike cannot walk without limping, although he does not have any swelling in his thigh. He decides to head over to the student health center to find out what to do. Based on the description of his situation and symptoms, what diagnoses are possible, and which seems most likely? Given the description, what grade is his injury?

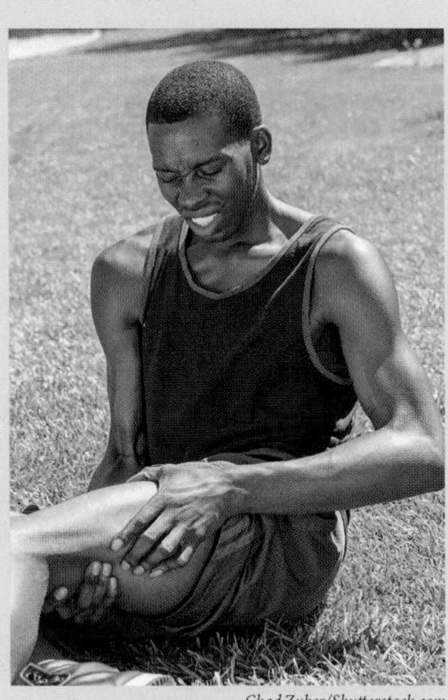

Chad Zuber/Shutterstock.com

Chapter 6 Outline

Muscle is the only human tissue capable of shortening, or contracting. This unique ability is what makes purposeful body movements possible. Without muscle, the powerful movements required in athletic performances would be impossible, as would the finely tuned, graceful movements needed to send a text message or play a musical instrument. Muscles also control the movements of the eyes, the movement of food through the digestive system, and the beating of the heart.

What enables muscle to be so versatile? This chapter describes the different types, properties, and structures of muscle and examines the effects of different kinds of physical training on skeletal muscle. It also discusses some of the common muscle injuries and disorders, how these problems tend to occur, and how their likelihood, in some cases, can be reduced.

SECTION 6.1

Types and Functions of Muscle Tissue

Objectives

- Describe the structural characteristics of the three categories of muscle.
- Explain the functions of each type of muscle tissue.

Key Terms

agonist
antagonist
aponeurosis
concentric contraction
contractility
eccentric contraction
elasticity
endomysium
epimysium
extensibility
fascicle
irritability
isometric contraction
muscle fiber
perimysium
sarcolemma

The human body has several different types of muscles, each with different structural characteristics. Each type of muscle is adapted to perform different physiological functions.

Muscle Categories

The three major categories of muscles are skeletal, smooth, and cardiac muscle. This section examines the important structural and functional differences among the three types of muscles.

Skeletal Muscle

The skeletal muscles attach to bones and are largely responsible for voluntary body movements. Skeletal muscle is also known as *striated muscle* due to the prominent cross-stripes, or striations, that can be seen when examining this tissue under a microscope (**Figure 6.1A**). A third name, *voluntary muscle,* is appropriate because this type of muscle is stimulated by consciously directed nerve activity.

An individual skeletal muscle cell is referred to as a ***muscle fiber*** because of its thread-like shape. Muscle fibers include many nuclei and vary considerably in length and diameter. Some fibers run the entire length of a muscle; others are much shorter.

The number of muscle fibers in a given person is genetically determined and does not change as a person ages, except for the occasional loss of fibers resulting from injury. Although the number of fibers does not change, skeletal muscle fibers grow in length and diameter from birth to adulthood. Adults can increase their fiber diameter, and their strength, through resistance training with a few repetitions of heavy loads on a regular basis over a period of time.

As **Figure 6.2** shows, skeletal muscle is highly organized. The cell membrane of the muscle fiber is called the ***sarcolemma***. The sarcolemma of each muscle fiber is covered by the ***endomysium***, a fine, protective sheath of connective tissue. Groups of muscle fibers are bundled together by a strong fibrous membrane called a ***perimysium*** into a unit known as a ***fascicle***.

All of the fascicles in a muscle are enclosed by the ***epimysium***, which is a thick, tough connective tissue. The epimysium connects at both ends of the muscle with either a cordlike tendon composed of extremely strong connective tissue or a flat, sheetlike ***aponeurosis***.

Tendons and aponeuroses directly connect each muscle to a bone, cartilage, or other connective tissue. Recall from Chapter 5 that tendons differ from ligaments in that ligaments connect bone to bone.

Smooth Muscle

In contrast to skeletal muscle fibers, smooth muscle cells are small, spindle-shaped, and nonstriated. These muscles are involuntary (not under conscious control), and they have a single nucleus (**Figure 6.1B**). Also known as *visceral muscle,* this type of muscle is found in the walls of many internal organs, such as the stomach, intestines, urinary bladder, arteries, and respiratory passages.

Smooth muscle cells are arranged in layers, with one layer running lengthwise and the other surrounding the organ in which the muscles are contained. The coordinated, alternate contracting and relaxing of these layers changes the size and shape of the organ and can aid in moving the contents of the organ. Moving food through the digestive system, emptying the bladder, and changing the diameter of the blood

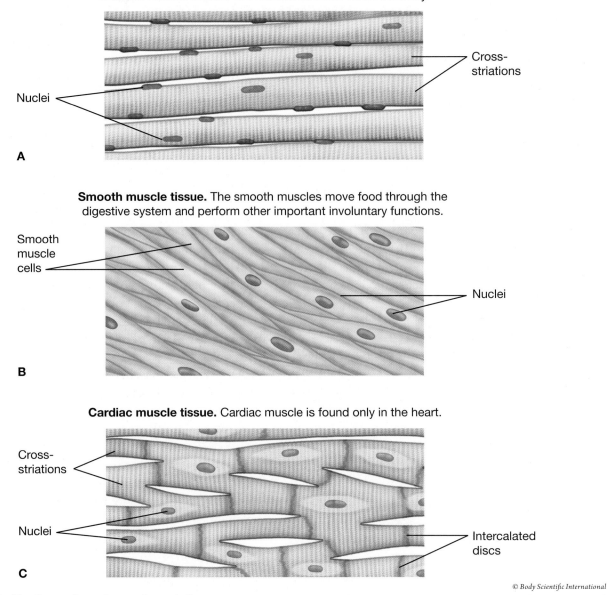

Skeletal muscle tissue. The skeletal muscles move the body.

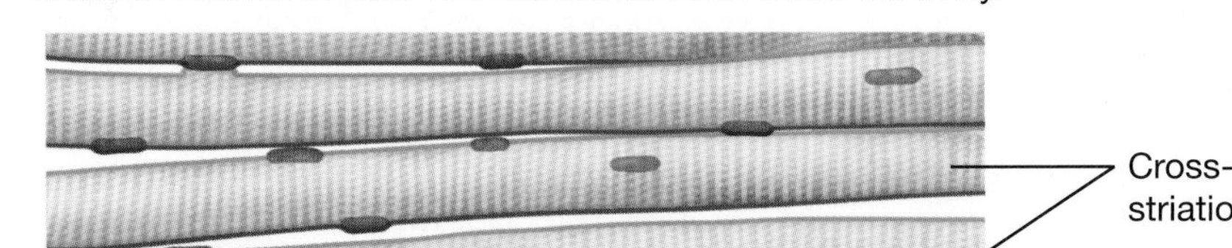

Smooth muscle tissue. The smooth muscles move food through the digestive system and perform other important involuntary functions.

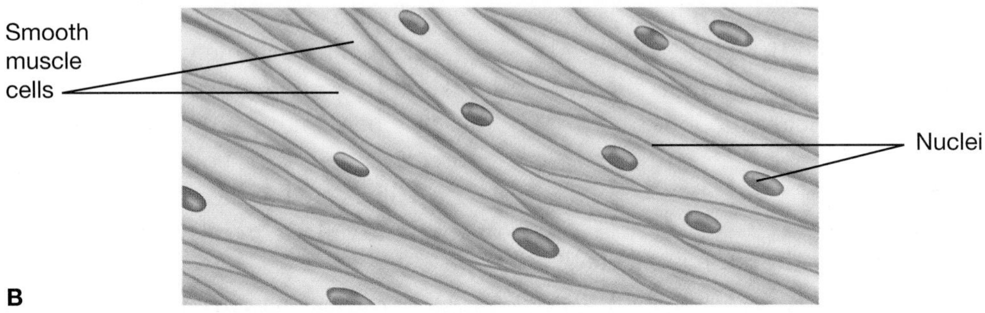

Cardiac muscle tissue. Cardiac muscle is found only in the heart.

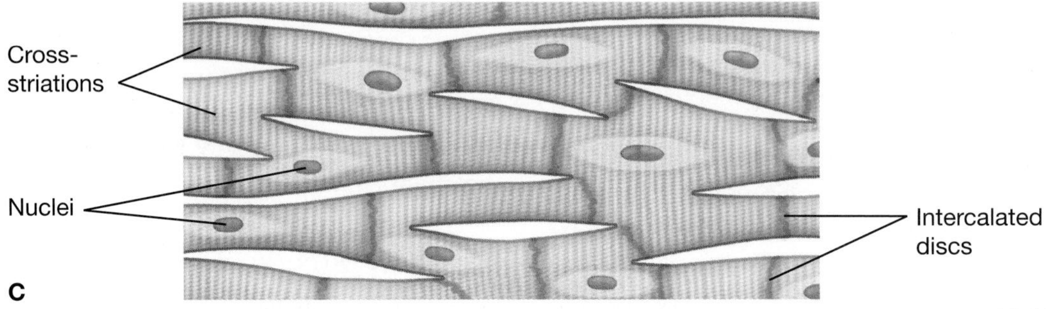

Figure 6.1 The three primary types of muscle tissue.

vessels are examples of the important functions of smooth muscles.

The autonomic nervous system controls smooth muscle activity. Unlike the skeletal muscles, smooth muscles can sustain contraction for long periods of time without becoming fatigued.

Cardiac Muscle

As the name suggests, cardiac muscle is located solely in the walls of the heart. Cardiac muscle cells are branched, striated, and involuntary, and are under the control of the autonomic nervous system (**Figure 6.1C**). Cardiac cells are arranged in an interconnected network of figure-eight- or spiral-shaped bundles that join together at structures called *intercalated* (in-TER-kah-lay-tehd) *discs*. This arrangement enables simultaneous contraction of neighboring cells to produce the heartbeat.

The table in **Figure 6.3** summarizes the major characteristics of each category of muscle tissue. Although all three types of muscle are important and, in fact, essential for human life, this chapter focuses primarily on the skeletal muscles. Cardiac muscle is described in more detail in Chapter 12, and smooth muscle is described in Chapter 14.

SELF CHECK

1. What is the difference between voluntary and involuntary muscles?
2. Categorize each muscle type as voluntary or involuntary.
3. What are the three layers of tissue that run the length of a skeletal muscle?

Functions of Muscles

Despite the different properties of the three types of muscle, certain behavioral characteristics are common to all muscle tissue. In addition, skeletal muscles contribute to various movements of the body.

Behavioral Properties

All muscle tissues have four behavioral characteristics in common: irritability, extensibility, elasticity, and

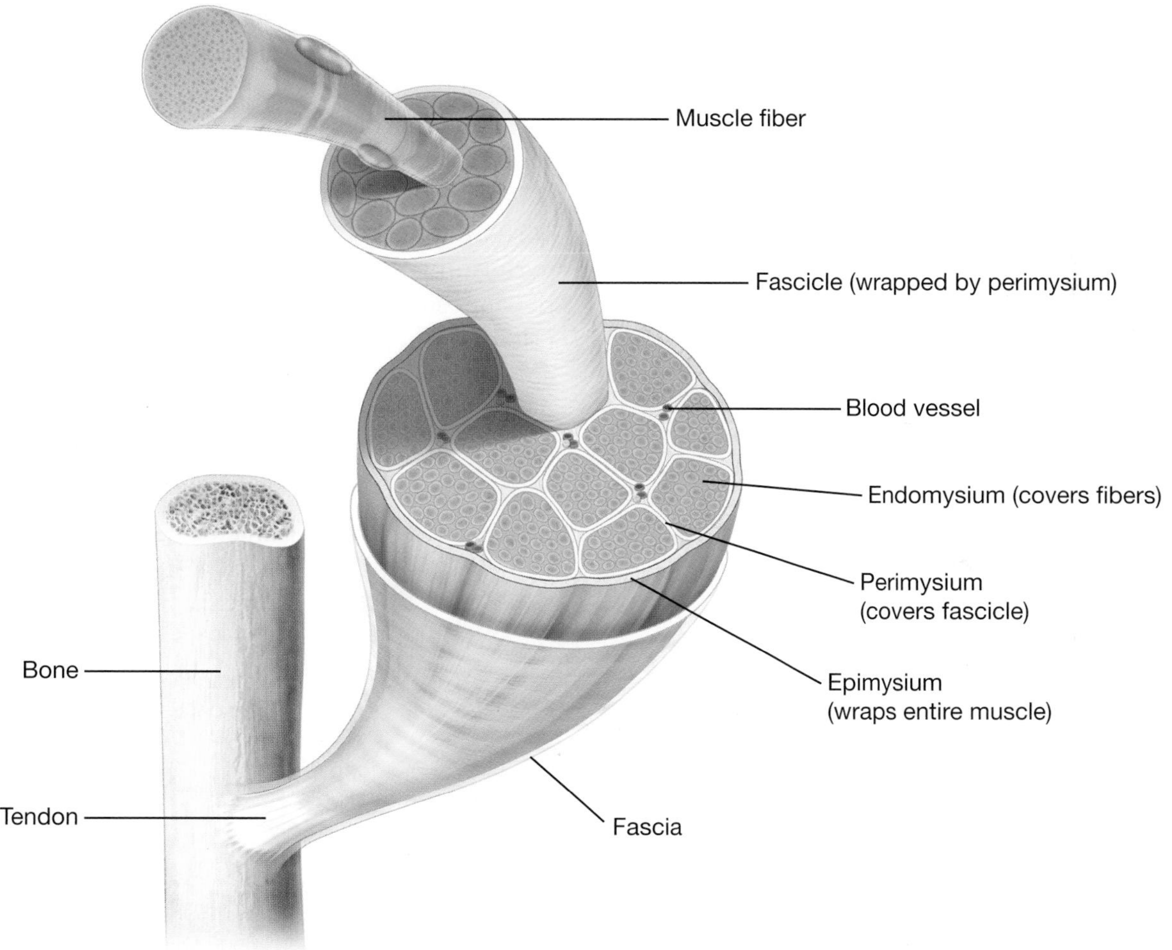

© Body Scientific International

Figure 6.2 The organization of skeletal muscle. The sarcolemma (membrane of muscle fiber) is not shown in this view.

Muscle Categories				
Type of Muscle	**Cell Structure**	**Nucleus**	**Control**	**Location**
Skeletal	varying lengths, thread-shaped, striated	multinucleate	voluntary	most attach to bones; some facial muscles attach to skin
Smooth	short, spindle-shaped, no striations	one nucleus	involuntary	walls of internal organs other than the heart
Cardiac	branching interconnected chains, striated	one nucleus	involuntary	walls of the heart

Figure 6.3

Goodheart-Willcox Publisher

contractility. Two of these—***extensibility***, the ability to be stretched, and ***elasticity***, the ability to return to normal length after being stretched—are common not just to muscle, but to many types of biological tissues. As an example, when a muscle group, such as the hamstrings (on the posterior side of the thigh), are stretched over a period of time, the muscles lengthen, and the range of motion at the hip increases, making it easier to touch the toes. The stretched muscles do not return to resting length immediately, but shorten over a period of time.

Another characteristic common to all muscle is ***irritability***, or the ability to respond to a stimulus. Muscles are routinely stimulated by signals from the nerves that supply them. Muscles can also be mechanically stimulated, such as by an external blow to a muscle. A muscle's response to all forms of stimulus is contraction.

Contractility, the ability to contract or shorten, is the one behavioral characteristic unique to muscle tissue. Most muscles have a tendon attaching to a bone at one end and another tendon attaching to a different bone at the other end. When a muscle contracts, it pulls on the bones to which it is attached. This pulling force is called a *tensile force*, or tension. The amount of tension developed is constant throughout the muscle, tendons, and attachment sites.

Skeletal Muscle Contraction

Although the term *contraction* (which implies shortening) is commonly used to mean that tension has developed in a muscle, muscles do not always shorten when they develop tension. When a skeletal muscle develops tension, one of three actions can occur: the muscle can shorten, remain the same length, or actually lengthen. The familiar large muscle groups—the biceps and triceps, on the anterior and posterior sides of your upper arm—provide examples of these three different types of tension.

When the biceps muscle develops tension and shortens, your hand moves up toward your shoulder (**Figure 6.4A**). This is called a ***concentric contraction***, or shortening, contraction of the biceps. The biceps is performing the role of ***agonist***, or prime mover, and the opposing muscle group, the triceps, is playing the role of ***antagonist***. The antagonist muscles may be completely relaxed or may develop a slight amount of tension, depending on the requirements of the movement.

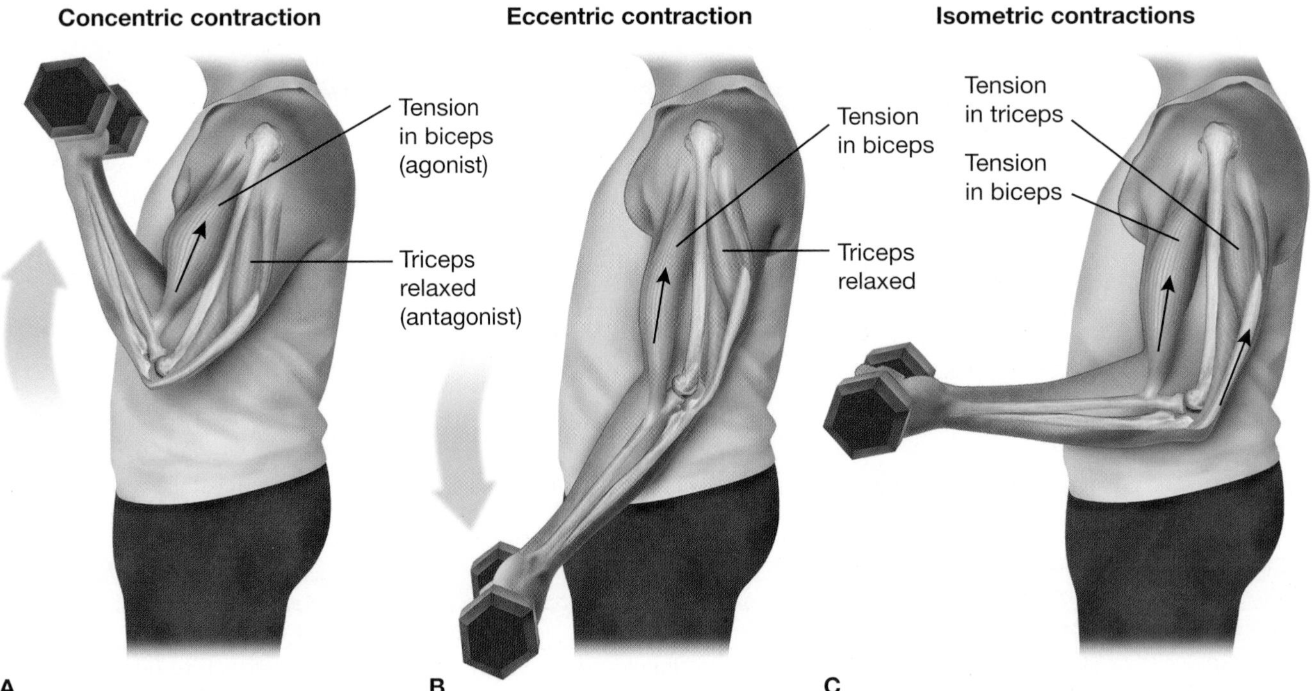

Figure 6.4 Muscle contraction. A—In concentric contraction, the agonist biceps contracts and the antagonist triceps relaxes. B—The biceps is eccentrically contracting (lengthening) while serving as a brake to control the downward motion of the weight. C—In isometric contractions, both the biceps and triceps develop tension, but neither muscle shortens, and there is no motion.

A muscle can also lengthen while developing tension. Suppose someone were to place in your hands a weight that was too heavy for you to hold in position. At first, your biceps would develop tension in an effort to hold the weight in place. But because the weight is too heavy to manage, you would lower the weight, and your biceps would lengthen. This type of action is known as an ***eccentric contraction***, or lengthening, contraction (**Figure 6.4B**). In this case, the force of gravity (not the triceps) acting on the weight causes the weight to lower.

In a third scenario (**Figure 6.4C**), you "flex" the muscles in your arm, developing tension in both the biceps and triceps, but there is no movement. This is called an ***isometric contraction*** of both the biceps and triceps. During an isometric contraction, no change in muscle length occurs.

The versatility of the arrangements of human muscles in agonist and antagonist pairs around joints enables the different movements of the human body. These versatile arrangements also help to stabilize joints and maintain body posture.

Heat Production

Everyone knows that vigorous exercise is typically accompanied by an increase in body temperature and sweating. This happens because the working muscles generate heat. Even when you are not exercising, the muscles, comprising approximately 40% of body mass, generate heat, and this heat helps maintain normal body temperature.

How does this happen? Muscles require energy in the form of adenosine triphosphate (ATP) to function. You may recall from your study of Chapter 2 that ATP is generated within muscle cells. The ATP is then released to provide energy when the muscle is stimulated, generating heat in the process.

SECTION 6.1 REVIEW

Mini-Glossary

agonist role played by a skeletal muscle in causing a movement

antagonist role played by a skeletal muscle acting to slow or stop a movement

aponeurosis a flat, sheetlike fibrous tissue that connects muscle or bone to other tissues

concentric contraction a type of contraction that results in shortening of a muscle

contractility the ability to contract or shorten

eccentric contraction a type of contraction that results in lengthening of a muscle

elasticity the ability to return to normal length after being stretched

endomysium a fine, protective sheath of connective tissue that surrounds a skeletal muscle fiber

epimysium the outermost sheath of connective tissue that surrounds a skeletal muscle

extensibility the ability to be stretched

fascicle a bundle of muscle fibers

irritability the ability to respond to a stimulus

isometric contraction a type of contraction that involves no change in muscle length

muscle fiber an individual skeletal muscle cell

perimysium a connective tissue sheath that envelops each primary bundle of muscle fibers

sarcolemma the delicate membrane that surrounds each striated muscle fiber

Review Questions

1. Starting with a muscle fiber and working from the inside out, name each part of the skeletal muscle structure.
2. Describe the role of each type of muscle tissue (cardiac, smooth, and skeletal).
3. Explain the difference between irritability and contractility.
4. What is the difference between extensibility and elasticity?
5. Give three examples of how you use isometric contractions during a typical day.
6. What do you think would happen if your antagonist muscles no longer functioned?

SECTION 6.2

Skeletal Muscle Physiology

Objectives

- Describe a motor unit and explain the functional differences between motor units that contain large and small numbers of muscle fibers.
- Describe the differences between slow-twitch and fast-twitch skeletal muscle fibers.
- Discuss the concepts of muscular strength, power, and endurance.
- Describe and give examples of the types of body motions that occur in the sagittal, frontal, and transverse planes.

Key Terms

abduction
acetylcholine
action potential
adduction
all-or-none law
axon
axon terminals
circumduction
cross bridges
dorsiflexion
eversion
extension
fast-twitch
flexion
hyperextension
insertion
inversion
lateral rotation
medial rotation
motor neuron
motor unit
neuromuscular junction
opposition
origin
parallel fiber architecture
pennate fiber architecture
plantar flexion
pronation
sarcomeres
slow-twitch
supination
synaptic cleft
tetanus

The development of tension in a skeletal muscle is influenced by a number of variables, including signals from the nervous system, the properties of the muscle fibers, and the arrangement of fibers within the muscle. This section describes how muscle actions contribute to muscular strength, power, and endurance.

Motor Units

Muscle tissue cannot develop tension unless it is stimulated by one or more nerves. Because of the dependent relationship between the muscular system and the nervous system, the two are often referred to collectively as the *neuromuscular system*.

A nerve that stimulates skeletal muscle, which is under voluntary control, is known as a ***motor neuron***. A single motor neuron and all of the muscle cells that it stimulates is known as a ***motor unit*** (**Figure 6.5**). The motor unit is the functional unit of the neuromuscular system.

One motor neuron supplying impulses to a muscle may connect to anywhere between 100 and nearly 2,000 skeletal muscle fibers, depending on the size and function of the muscle. The small muscles responsible for finely tuned movements, such as those in the eyes and fingers, have small motor units with few fibers per motor unit. Large, powerful muscles, such as those surrounding the hips, have large motor units with many fibers. Motor units are typically contained within a portion of a muscle, but may also be interspersed with the muscle cells of other motor units.

Action Potentials

How does a motor neuron communicate with the muscle cells to stimulate them? As **Figure 6.5** shows, a long, thin fiber called an ***axon*** connects the motor neuron cell body with the muscle fibers included in the motor unit. Close to the fibers, the axon branches into ***axon terminals***, which in turn branch into individual muscle fibers. Each link between an axon terminal and a muscle fiber is called a ***neuromuscular junction***. The axon terminal and fiber are separated by a tiny gap known as the ***synaptic cleft***, which is filled with interstitial fluid (**Figure 6.6**).

When a nerve impulse reaches the end of an axon terminal, a chemical called a *neurotransmitter* discharges and diffuses across the synaptic cleft to attach to receptors on the muscle fiber's sarcolemma. The neurotransmitter that stimulates muscle is ***acetylcholine***.

The effect of acetylcholine is to make the sarcolemma temporarily permeable. This opens channels that allow positive sodium ions (Na+) to rapidly invade the fiber at the same time that positive potassium ions (K+) rush out of the fiber. Because more Na+ enters than K+ exits, the net effect is the creation of a relatively positive charge inside the muscle fiber.

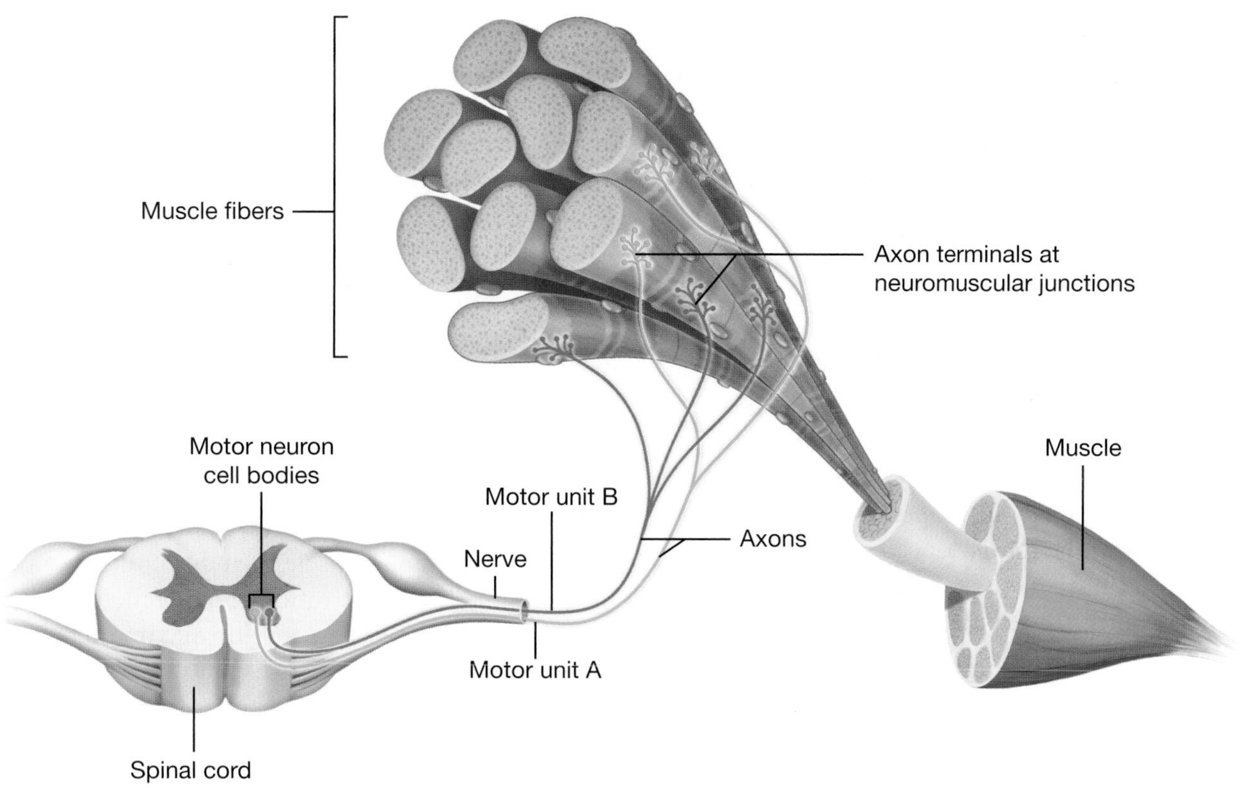

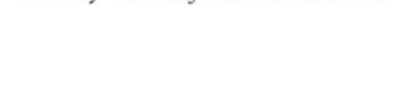

Figure 6.5 Each motor unit includes a motor neuron and all the muscle fibers it activates.

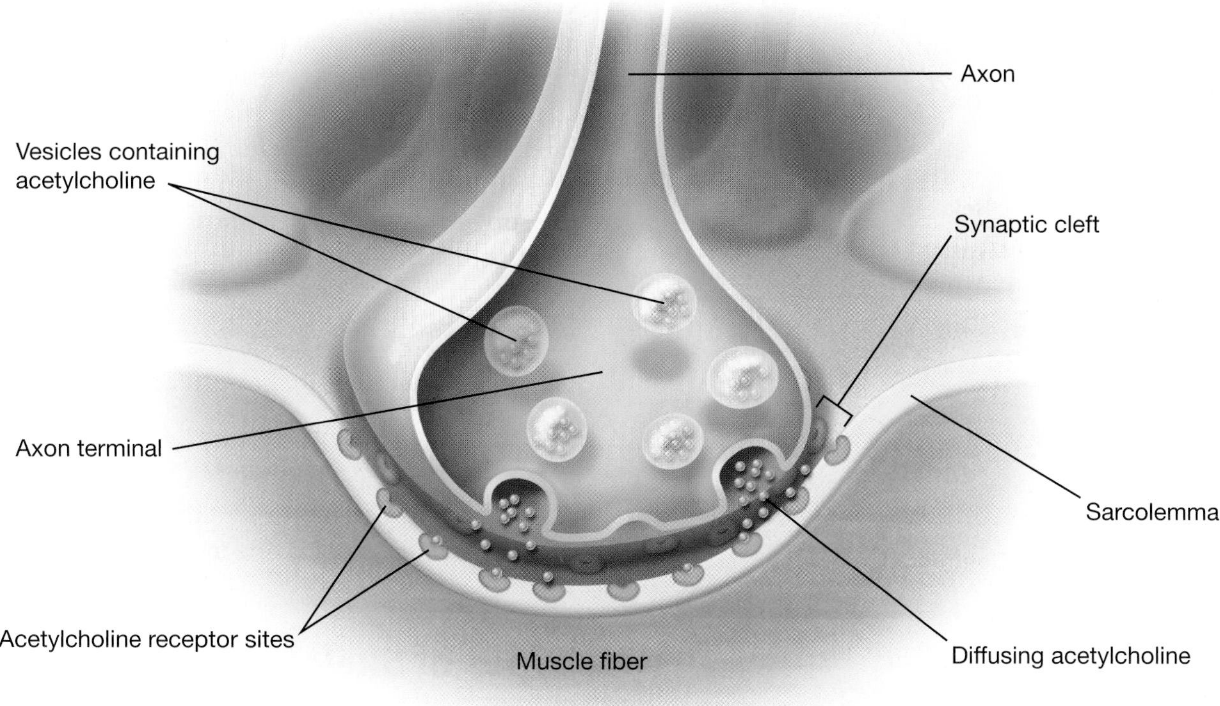

Figure 6.6 The neuromuscular junction is the site at which nerve impulses are transmitted to muscle.

This change in electrical charge is known as *depolarization*. Depolarization triggers the opening of additional channels in the fiber membrane that allow only entry of additional Na+. The flood of positive ions into the fiber generates an electrical charge called an ***action potential***.

Sarcomere Contraction

Glucose stored in the form of glycogen within the muscle cell provides the energy for creating an action potential. Phosphocreatine within the cell enables the transfer of energy to protein filaments known as *actin* and *myosin*. Actin and myosin are contractile proteins that reside in functional units called ***sarcomeres*** inside the muscle fiber. The release of calcium ions (Ca++) triggers the actin filaments to slide over the myosin filaments, resulting in a contraction of the sarcomere (**Figure 6.7**).

Notice in **Figure 6.7** that the myosin filaments are encircled by small protrusions called *heads*. When the sarcomere is activated by an action potential, these heads attach to receptor sites on the actin filaments, forming ***cross bridges***. The cross bridges contract, pulling the actin filaments toward the center of the sarcomere. During the process of sarcomere contraction, the cross bridges attach, pull, and release multiple times. The Ca++ ions released with the arrival of the action potential enable the myosin heads to attach to the actin filaments.

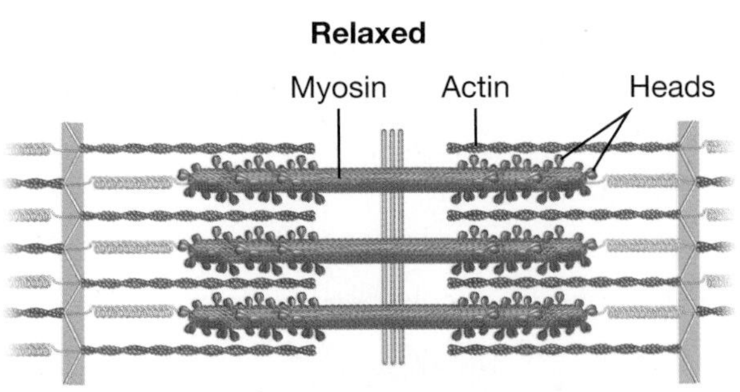

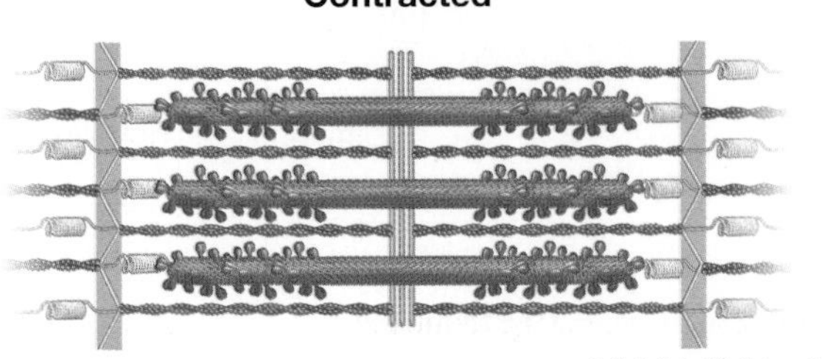

© Body Scientific International

Figure 6.7 The sarcomere is the contractile unit of muscle. When the muscle is stimulated, the actin filaments slide together, producing contraction of the sarcomere.

The neuromuscular system can produce slow, gentle movements as well as fast, forceful movements. This is accomplished by regulating the number of motor units activated, as well as the number and frequency of action potentials. Only a small number of action potentials are needed for slow, gentle movements, while fast or forceful movements require a large number of action potentials, released rapidly.

Maximum Tension and Return to Relaxation

When it receives an action potential, a motor unit always develops maximum tension. This physiological principle is known as the ***all-or-none law***. However, because each whole muscle includes multiple motor units, simultaneous activation of many motor units is required for the muscle to develop maximum tension. The diagram in **Figure 6.8** displays the relationship between the number and frequency of action potentials and the development of tension in the muscle. With high-frequency stimulation, the muscle develops a sustained, maximal level of tension called ***tetanus***.

Almost all skeletal motor units develop tension in a twitch-like fashion, generating maximum tension very briefly and then immediately relaxing. After the action potential has traveled the length of the muscle fiber, chemical processes return the fiber to its resting state. Sodium ions diffuse back out of the cell into the interstitial fluid, and calcium ions return to storage sites within the cell. The actin filaments slide back to their original positions as the cross bridges release them, and the muscle fiber returns to a state of relaxation.

SELF CHECK

1. What structures make up a motor unit?
2. Describe the neuromuscular junction.
3. What is an action potential?
4. Why is a small motor unit more suitable than a large one for fine motor skills?

Types of Skeletal Fibers

Have you ever noticed that some athletes are especially good at events or tasks that require endurance, whereas others excel at activities that require explosive strength or speed? The reason may have something to do with the ways in which these individuals train, but that is only a small part of the explanation. In fact, a big part

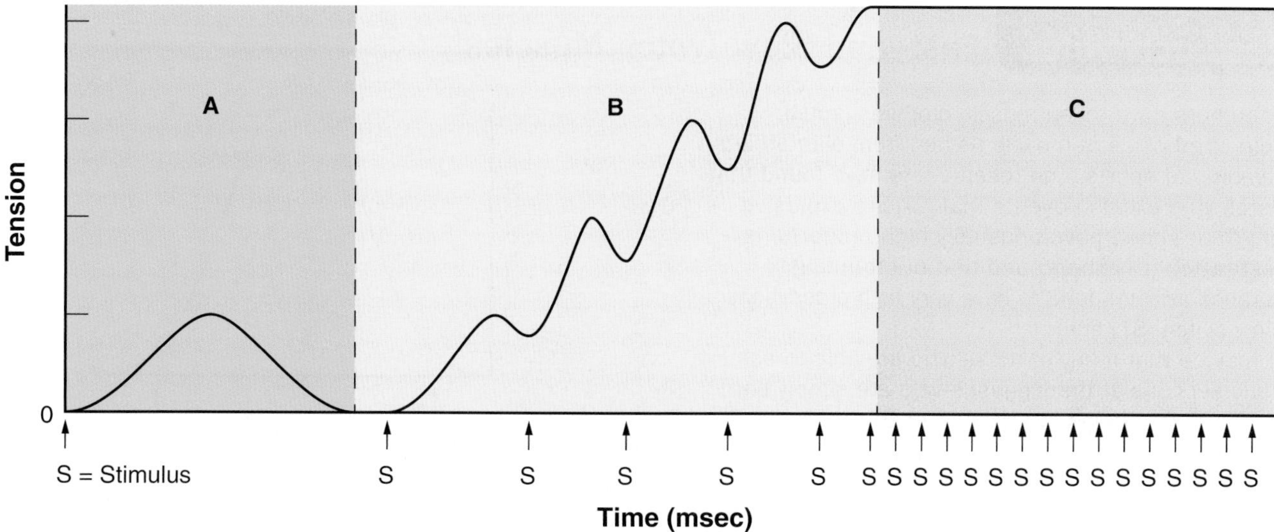

Goodheart-Willcox Publisher

Figure 6.8 Tension developed in a muscle in response to a single stimulus (A), in response to repetitive stimulation (B), and in response to high-frequency stimulation, or tetanus (C).

of why some people are better at particular activities and sports may be due to the characteristics of their skeletal muscle fibers.

Slow-Twitch and Fast-Twitch Fibers

Skeletal muscle fibers can be divided into two umbrella categories: ***slow-twitch*** (Type I) and ***fast-twitch*** (Type II). As the names suggest, the fast-twitch fibers contract much faster than slow-twitch fibers.

Because sufficient variation exists among the fast-twitch fibers, they too have been divided into two categories: Type IIa and Type IIb. The contraction speed of Type IIa fibers falls somewhere between the slow-twitch fibers and Type IIb fibers, which are the classic fast-twitch fibers. Type IIb fibers contract very rapidly, in about one-seventh the time required for slow-twitch fibers to contract. As a result, Type IIb fibers also fatigue rapidly. Although all of the muscle fibers in a motor unit are of the same type, most skeletal muscles include motor units of both fast-twitch and slow-twitch fibers. The fast-twitch/slow-twitch ratio varies from muscle to muscle and from person to person.

Fiber Architecture

Another factor that affects functions of skeletal muscles is fiber architecture. *Fiber architecture* refers to the ways in which fibers are arranged within the muscle. The two major categories of muscle fiber arrangement are parallel and pennate.

Parallel Fiber Architecture

In ***parallel fiber architecture***, the fibers run largely parallel to each other along the length of the muscle. As **Figure 6.9A** shows, this arrangement may result

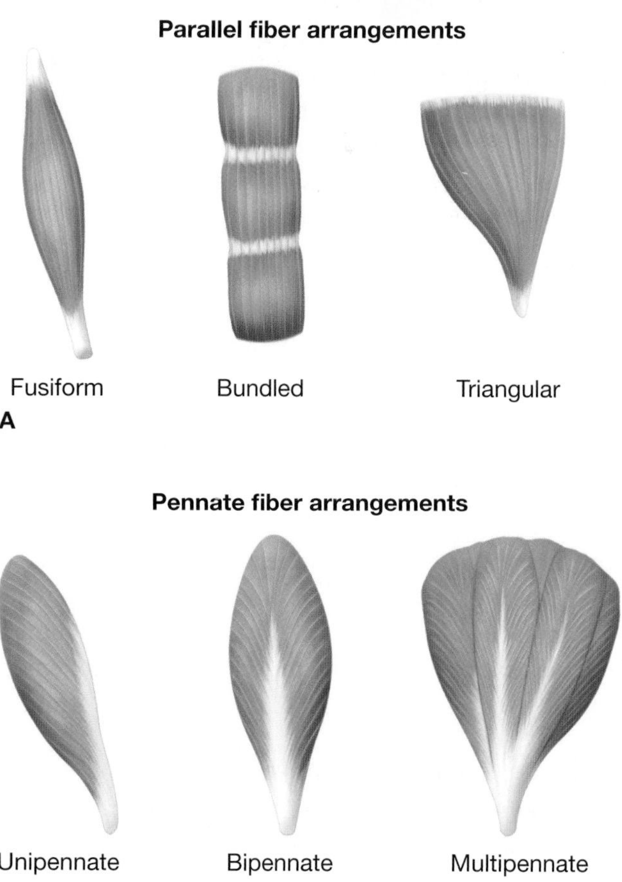

© Body Scientific International

Figure 6.9 Fibers within a muscle may be arranged so that they are largely parallel (A) or pennate (B).

Research Notes Fast- and Slow-Twitch Muscles

Researchers have taken muscle biopsies (small, needle-sized plugs of muscle tissue) from elite athletes in a variety of sports. The researchers have found that athletes who excel in events that require explosive strength or speed have unusually high proportions of fast-twitch (FT) fibers, and that outstanding endurance athletes tend to have very high proportions of slow-twitch (ST) fibers.

It may be that many of those who are able to achieve athletic success at the highest levels are simply born with high percentages of either FT or ST fibers. Once these individuals have experienced success in a particular sport or event, it is likely that they gravitate toward that sport or event.

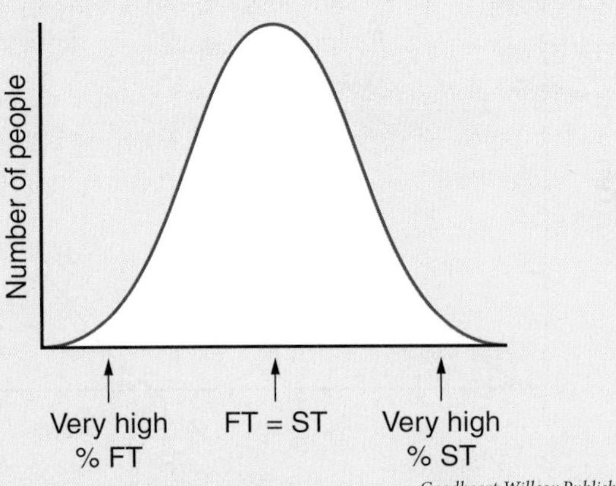

Goodheart-Willcox Publisher

The percentages of fast-twitch (FT) and slow-twitch (ST) fibers in the general population are normally distributed.

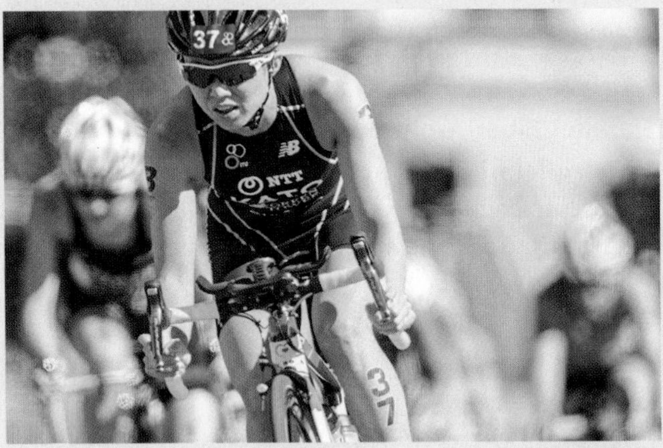

Stefan Holm/Shutterstock.com

Elite sprint cyclists tend to have high percentages of fast-twitch muscle fibers.

Of course, certain individuals within the general population of untrained people also have high percentages of FT or ST muscles. The distribution of FT/ST ratios among the general population is represented by the normal, bell-shaped curve.

Research also indicates that FT-fiber types can change over time. FT fibers can be converted to ST fibers with years of endurance training. No evidence exists, however, that any form of training can convert ST fibers to FT fibers. It has been documented, however, that a progressive loss of FT motor units and fibers occurs as people age, although this loss can be minimized by regular, high-intensity exercise throughout life.

in muscle shapes that are fusiform (wide in the middle and tapering on both ends), bundled, or triangular. Examples of muscles with this type of architecture are the *biceps brachii* (fusiform), *rectus abdominis* (bundled), and *pectoralis major* (triangular).

The individual fibers in the parallel architecture typically do not run the entire length of the muscle. Instead, the individual parallel fibers are connected to neighboring fibers, which promotes contraction when the muscle is stimulated. This fiber arrangement enables shortening of the muscle and the movement of body segments through large ranges of motion.

Pennate Fiber Architecture

In a ***pennate*** (featherlike) ***fiber architecture***, each fiber attaches obliquely to a central tendon, and in some cases, to more than one tendon. As **Figure 6.9b** shows:

- Fibers that are aligned in one direction to a central tendon are unipennate.
- Fibers that attach to a central tendon are bipennate.
- Fibers that attach to a central tendon in more than two directions are multipennate.

Certain muscles of the hand are unipennate, the *rectus femoris* (a member of the quadriceps group in the thigh) is bipennate, and the *deltoid* is multipennate.

A muscle with a pennate fiber arrangement does not shorten as much upon contraction as a muscle with a parallel fiber arrangement. However, the pennate arrangement makes it possible to pack more fibers into the muscle. This means that the muscle can generate more force.

SELF CHECK

1. What is the difference between fast-twitch and slow-twitch fibers?
2. Which fiber type helps a sprinter get out of the blocks quickly?
3. Why can pennate-arranged fibers generate more force than parallel-arranged fibers?

Strength, Power, and Endurance

In everyday conversation, people sometimes use the words *strength* and *power* interchangeably. However, muscular strength and muscular power are quite different concepts. This section examines that difference, as well as muscle fatigue and the related concept of muscular endurance, which is a little more complicated.

Muscular Strength

It may be tempting to think that muscular strength is the amount of force a given muscle can produce. It is impossible, however, to measure muscle force directly without penetrating the body. So to avoid invasive procedures, researchers use external measures, such as the amount of resistance a person can move, to establish an indirect measure of muscle strength.

Remember that most joints in the human body are crossed by more than just one muscle. Additionally, many exercises involve more than one joint. This

Clinical Application Supplements You Do Not Want to Take

Some athletes and bodybuilders have succumbed to the temptation to take drugs to increase their muscle size, strength, and power production. The results have included devastating physiological and psychological side effects, as well as ruined professional careers and public disgrace. Famous athletes such as Lance Armstrong, Mark McGwire, Alex Rodriguez, José Canseco, Ben Johnson, and Marion Jones have been exposed for using banned drugs.

The World Anti-Doping Code prohibits supplementing with all forms of anabolic agents at all times for athletes. *Anabolic* means "building up," and refers to increasing bone and muscle mass. Different types of anabolic drugs have been developed for medical treatment of certain conditions. They are *not* intended for use by athletes and bodybuilders to build muscle.

For example, anabolic androgenic steroids are synthetic versions of the male hormone testosterone. These drugs are designed for medical treatment of delayed puberty, some forms of impotence, and diseases that cause wasting of muscle tissue. When used inappropriately, however, these drugs can cause severe, long-lasting, and sometimes irreversible negative effects on health, including:

- liver damage, including blood-filled cysts and tumors
- kidney failure
- elevated blood pressure and other cardiovascular effects contributing to early heart attack and stroke
- stunted growth due to premature closure of epiphyses in long bones
- abnormally increased aggressiveness
- depression and suicide

In children, these steroids can disrupt puberty. In adolescents, stunted growth and accelerated puberty changes can result from steroid use. Males may experience breast development, shrinking of the testicles, impotence, reduced sperm production, and an increased risk of prostate cancer. Females may experience irreversible deepening of the voice, cessation of breast development, male pattern hair growth, enlarged clitoris, and abnormal menstrual cycles.

Another banned anabolic agent is human growth hormone (HGH). Synthetic human growth hormone is approved by the FDA for specific uses in children and adults. In children, HGH injections are approved for treating medical conditions that impair normal growth. In adults, HGH is used to treat conditions that prevent normal absorption of nutrients in the intestines or cause muscle wasting. Negative side effects of HGH include severe headaches, vision loss, acromegaly, high blood pressure, heart failure, diabetes, tumors, and crippling arthritis.

Diuretics are also banned for use as anabolic agents. However, they are medically used for treatment of hypertension, kidney disease, and congestive heart failure. These drugs are sometimes taken by athletes trying to reduce body weight, notably in sports that classify competition by weight. The side effects of diuretics are dehydration, muscle cramps, dizziness or fainting, low blood pressure, and a loss of coordination and balance.

Use of all of these drugs for purposes other than medical treatment is not only inadvisable, but also dangerous. Many of the identified side effects can also result in death. The intelligent, safe way to increase muscle size and strength is through a program of progressive resistance training.

means that an index-of-strength measure such as maximum bench press actually assesses the collective work of several muscles that cross the shoulder and elbow (**Figure 6.10**). The main muscles that work during execution of a bench press include the pectoralis major, pectoralis minor, anterior deltoid, and triceps brachii.

A more precise assessment of the strength of a muscle group at a given joint is the amount of *torque,* or rotary force, that the muscles can generate. Torque is the product of the size of a force and the perpendicular distance of that force from an axis of rotation. For the joint shown in **Figure 6.11**, the torque produced by a muscle is the product of muscle force and the perpendicular distance from the muscle attachment to the center of rotation at the joint.

The more torque a muscle generates at a joint, the greater the tendency for movement of the bones at the joint. Machines called *dynamometers* measure joint torque. Joint torque, which is a measure of strength, is based solely on the resistance moved or matched. The speed with which a resistance is moved is not relevant to the strength measurement.

Muscular Power

The definition of *mechanical power* is force multiplied by velocity (force × velocity). Muscular power, then, is muscle force multiplied by muscle-shortening velocity during contraction. Notice, however, that neither muscle force nor shortening velocity can be measured from outside the body. Research dynamometers generate estimates of muscular power based on the resistance moved and the speed of the movement.

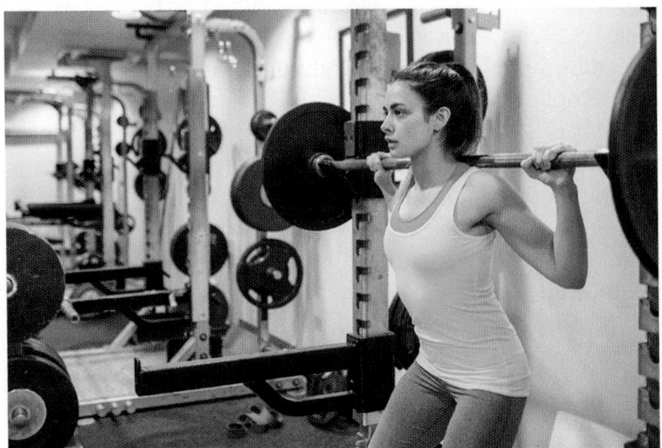

wavebreakmedia/Shutterstock.com

Figure 6.10 The amount of weight being lifted is an indirect measure of this woman's muscular strength.

Like muscular strength, muscular power is typically generated by several different muscles working collectively. Sprinting, along with the jumping and throwing events in track and field, are good examples of activities that require muscular power. Because force production and movement speed contribute equally to muscular power, the sprinter with the greatest leg strength may not necessarily be the fastest.

Muscular Endurance

Muscular endurance is the ability of a muscle to produce tension over a period of time. The tension may be constant (for example, when a gymnast holds a motionless handstand), or it may vary cyclically (for example, during running, cycling, or rowing). Generally, the longer the physical activity is maintained, the greater the required muscular endurance. Because the force and speed requirements of different movements can vary significantly, the definition of muscular endurance is specific to each physical activity.

In general, muscle fatigue can be thought of as the opposite of muscular endurance. The faster a muscle fatigues, the less endurance it has. A variety of factors affect the rate at which a muscle fatigues, including the nature of the work or exercise being done, how often the muscle is used, the muscle fiber composition of the muscle, and the temperature and humidity of the environment.

In general, muscle fatigue can be thought of as the opposite of muscular endurance. The faster a muscle fatigues, the less endurance it has. A variety of factors affect the rate at which a muscle fatigues, including the nature of the work or exercise being done, how often the muscle is used, the muscle fiber composition of the muscle, and the temperature and humidity of the environment.

SELF CHECK

1. What is measured to determine muscular strength?
2. What is measured to determine muscular power?
3. What is muscular endurance?
4. What influences muscular endurance?

Directional Motions

Skeletal muscles have attachments at both ends; the most common attachments are tendon connections to bone. The end of a muscle that attaches to a relatively fixed structure is called the ***origin***. The end of a muscle that attaches to a bone, which typically moves when the muscle contracts, is called the ***insertion***.

For an example of origin and insertion, consider the brachialis muscle, which crosses the anterior side of the elbow. Its origin is on the humerus, and its insertion is on the ulna in the forearm. When the brachialis contracts, the forearm (ulna) is pulled toward the upper arm while the upper arm (humerus) remains stationary.

Calculating Muscle Force

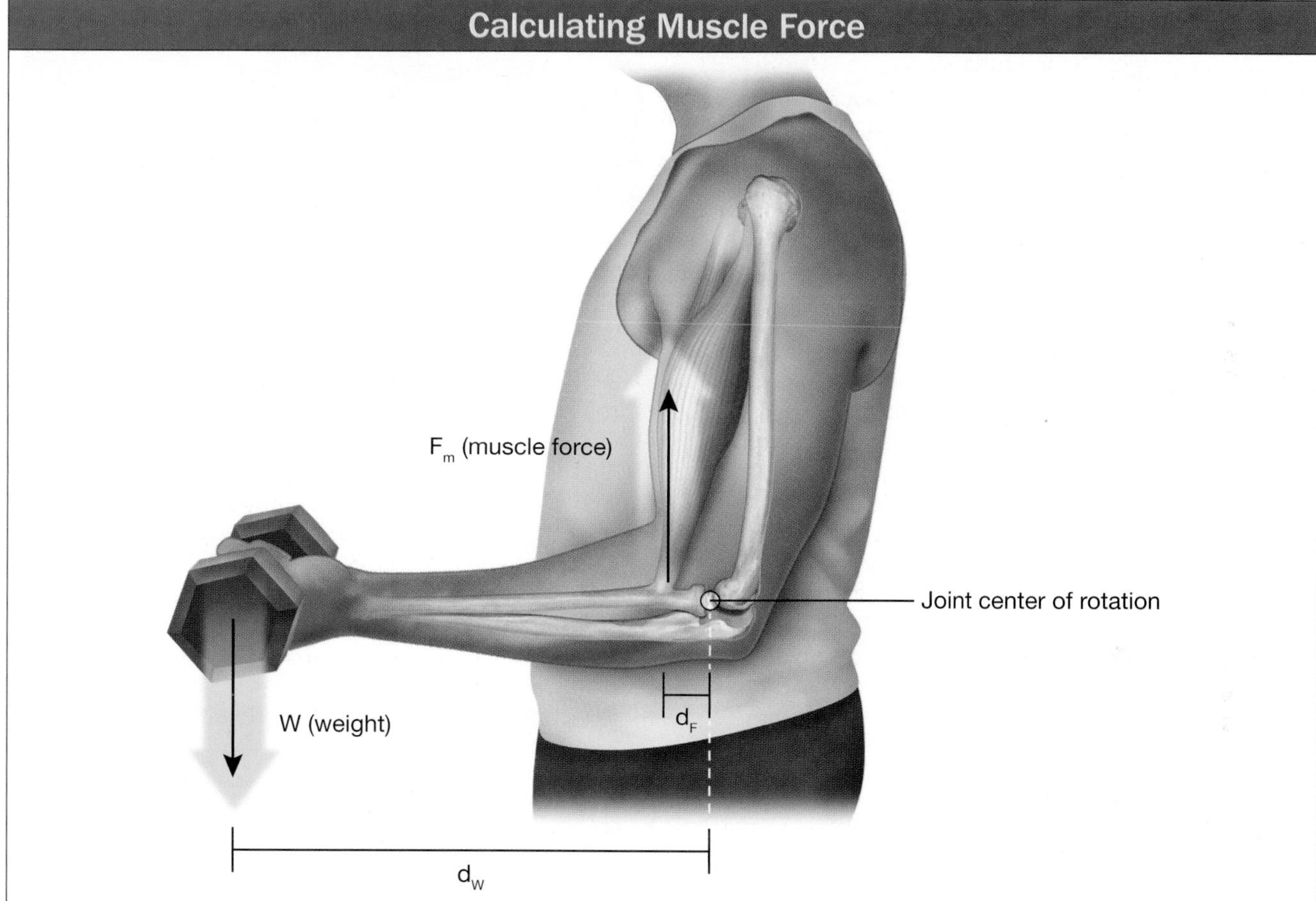

Do you know how much force your muscle must generate to hold a 5-pound weight in the position shown in the illustration? To hold the weight in this position, the torque at the elbow joint generated by the muscle (muscle torque) must balance the torque produced by the weight (weight torque) at the elbow.

Muscle torque is the product of muscle force and the perpendicular distance of that force from the center of rotation at the joint. The formula is:

$$T_m = F_m \times d_F$$

where T_m = muscle torque, F_m = muscle force, and d_F = the perpendicular distance.

Weight torque is the product of the weight and the perpendicular distance of that weight from the center of rotation at the joint. This formula is:

$$T_W = W \times d_W$$

where T_W = weight torque, W = weight, and d_W = the perpendicular distance.

Suppose that the weight in the illustration is 5 pounds, and that it is being held at a distance (d_W) of 12 inches from the center of the joint. The distance of the muscle attachment from the joint center (d_F) is 1 inch. How much force must the muscle produce to support the weight?

$$T_m = T_W$$
$$F_m \times d_F = W \times d_W$$
$$F_m \times 1'' = 5 \text{ lb} \times 12''$$
$$F_m = 60 \text{ lb}$$

Are you surprised? To support just 5 pounds in the hand, the muscle must generate 60 pounds of force. Because muscles attach so closely to joints, the human musculoskeletal system is designed more for movement speed than for strength.

Now you try: Suppose that the weight (W) in this picture is 10 pounds, the d_W is 15 inches, and the d_F is 1 inch. What is the F_m?

Figure 6.11

Research Notes Sarcopenia

You may have observed that older individuals typically do not have as much muscular strength as younger individuals. This age-related loss of skeletal muscle mass, strength, and function is called *sarcopenia*.

Sarcopenia is one of the factors responsible for a progressive decline in elderly individuals' functional capacity and their ability to live independently. This condition is associated with slowed walking speed, greater risk of falling, increased incidence of hospitalization, and a high mortality rate.

Sarcopenia is characterized by a decline in muscle mass resulting from reductions in both the number of muscle fibers and muscle fiber size. The reduction in fiber size occurs almost exclusively in Type II fibers through a remodeling process that results in denervation of Type II fibers. There is also a decline in muscle quality; one researcher reports a 34% reduction in the force-generating capability of the muscle fibers.

Many of the age-related changes contributing to this loss of mass and force-generating capacity in skeletal muscle occur at the cellular and molecular levels. These include reductions in muscle fiber activation, excitation-contraction coupling, actin-myosin cross-bridge interaction, energy production, and capacity for repair and regeneration. Changes in central nervous system drive, dysfunction of the peripheral nerve, and alterations in neuromuscular junction structure and function also contribute.

Although all of these age-related changes in muscle have been scientifically documented, the cause of sarcopenia is currently not well understood. Recent research suggests a number of potential contributors, including a sedentary lifestyle, low protein intake, hormone imbalance, chronic inflammation, reduced neural stimulation, and decreased capillary blood flow. There is promising evidence that exercise combined with dietary strategies, including adequate intake of protein and vitamin D, can slow the onset of sarcopenia. Resistance exercise, in particular, can maintain or increase muscle strength for individuals of all ages.

As the population of the world's developed countries continues to age, the growing incidence of sarcopenia is of increasing concern. Notably, by 2050, the percentage of population over 60 years of age is projected to double from approximately 11% to 22%, resulting in 2 billion people 60 years of age or older living on Earth. While this increase occurs, the need for healthcare workers is likely to increase as well.

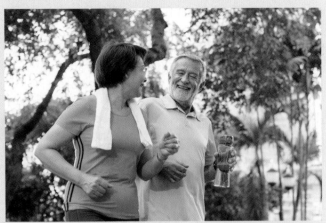

Rawpixel.com/Shutterstock.com

One way to help reduce the effects of sarcopenia or delay its onset is to engage in regular weight-bearing exercise.

Remember—when stimulated to develop tension, muscles can only pull. They are incapable of pushing. In addition, remember from Chapter 1 that three major planes through the center of the body are used to describe the human body and its movements:

- Forward and backward motions take place in the sagittal plane.
- Sideways motions occur in the frontal plane.
- Rotational movements occur in the transverse plane.

The frame of reference for all movement is the anatomical position. In this position, the human body is erect with the hands at the sides and the palms facing forward. As you read this section, refer to the illustrations in **Figure 6.12**.

Movements in the Sagittal Plane

The primary movements within the sagittal plane are flexion, extension, and hyperextension. ***Flexion*** describes forward-bending motion of the head, trunk, upper arm, forearm, hand, and hip. Flexion also includes backward motion of the lower leg at the knee. In flexion movements, body surfaces are coming together. ***Extension*** returns body segments from a position of flexion to the anatomical position. ***Hyperextension*** continues the extension motion past the anatomical position.

Two movements of the foot also occur primarily in the sagittal plane. Bringing the top of the foot toward the lower leg is called ***dorsiflexion***, and moving the foot in the opposite direction, away from the lower leg, is called ***plantar flexion***.

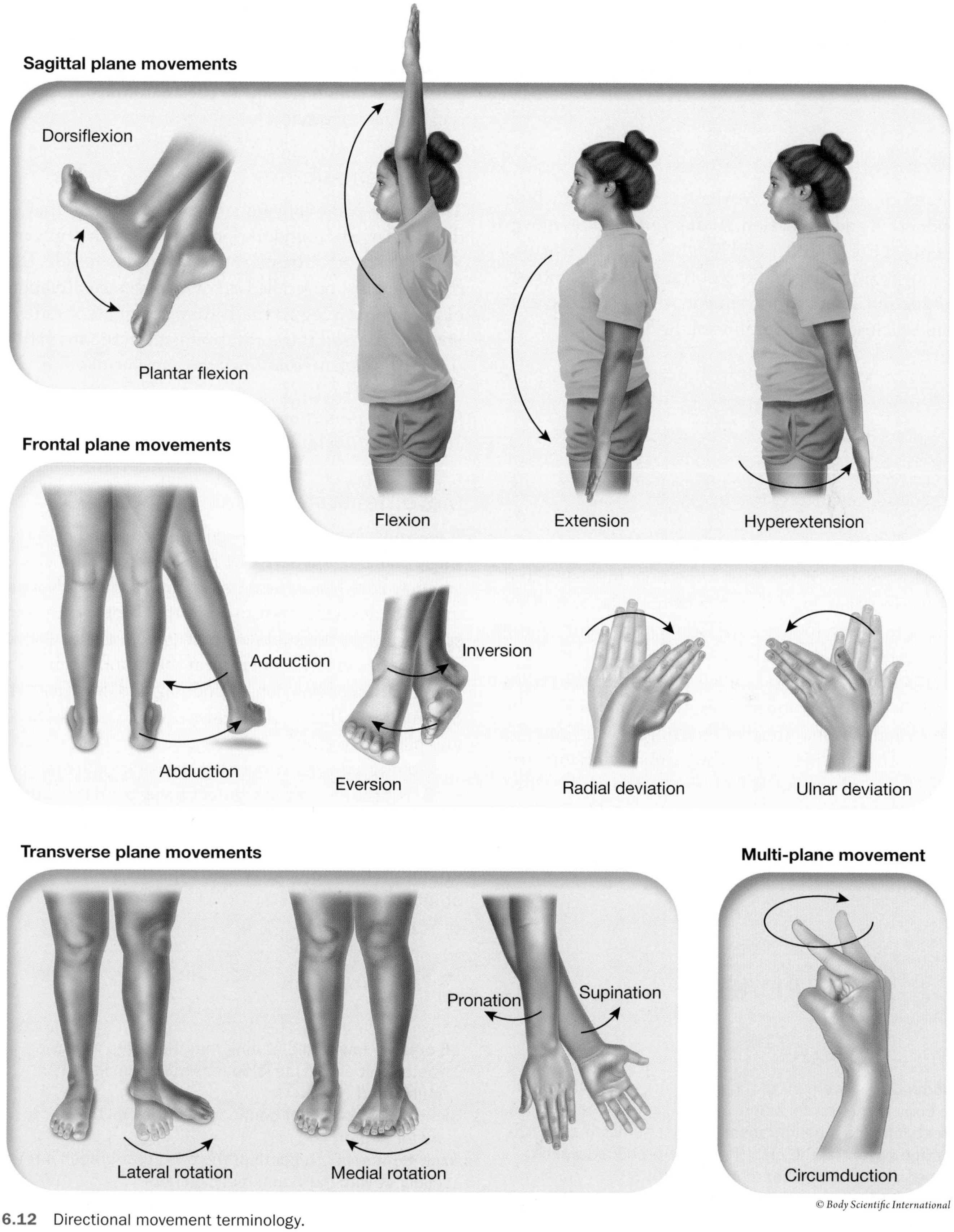

Sagittal plane movements
Dorsiflexion
Plantar flexion
Flexion
Extension
Hyperextension
Frontal plane movements
Adduction
Abduction
Inversion
Eversion
Radial deviation
Ulnar deviation
Transverse plane movements
Lateral rotation
Medial rotation
Pronation
Supination
Multi-plane movement
Circumduction
© Body Scientific International

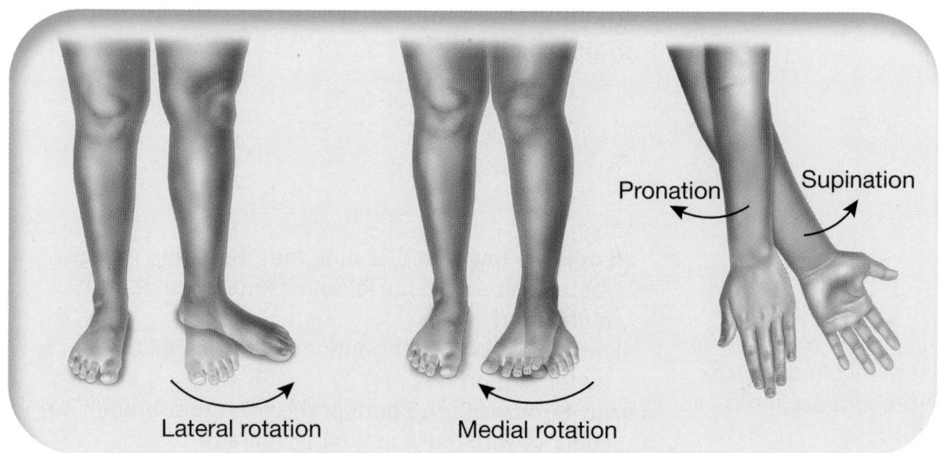

6.12 Directional movement terminology.

Understanding Medical Terminology

Planting the ball of the foot is the motion involved in *plantar* flexion.

Movements in the Frontal Plane

Common movements in the frontal plane include abduction and adduction. ***Abduction*** includes movements at the shoulder and hip that take the arm and leg away from the midline of the body. In contrast, ***adduction*** refers to movements that bring the arm and leg closer to the midline of the body.

Understanding Medical Terminology

Just as *abduct* means "to take away," abduction takes a body segment away from the body. Just as *add* means "to bring back," adduction returns a body segment closer to the body.

Movements of the foot known as inversion and eversion occur mainly in the frontal plane. Rolling the sole of the foot inward is ***inversion***, and rolling the sole of the foot outward is ***eversion***.

Recall that the forearm has two bones: the radius and the ulna. The radius is on the thumb side of the hand, and the ulna is on the "little finger" side. From the anatomical position, with the palms facing forward, abduction of the hand toward the thumb is called *radial deviation*, and adduction of the hand toward the little finger is called *ulnar deviation*.

Trunk and neck motions directed away from anatomical position in the frontal plane are called *lateral flexion* and *side bending*. Movement that returns from a position of lateral flexion to the anatomical position is called *lateral extension*.

Movements in the Transverse Plane

Transverse plane movements involve rotation that is directed largely around the long axis of a body segment. When the head or trunk rotates from side to side, the movement is simply called *left* or *right rotation*. Rotation of an arm or a leg in the transverse plane is called ***medial rotation*** if the rotation is directed medially (inward), or ***lateral rotation*** if the movement is directed laterally (outward). The terms used for rotation of the forearm are ***pronation*** for medial (palm down) rotation and ***supination*** for lateral (palm up) rotation.

Movements in Multiple Planes

A few movements of body segments do not fall within a single plane. If you have ever purchased running shoes, you may have heard the terms *pronation* and *supination* used to describe motions of the foot occurring specifically at the subtalar joint (where the heel and ankle bones meet). Pronation at the subtalar joint is a combination of eversion, abduction, and dorsiflexion. Supination at this joint includes inversion, adduction, and plantar flexion.

Moving a finger, arm, or leg in a rotational manner such that the end of the segment traces a circle is called ***circumduction***. Finally, touching any of your four fingers to the thumb is known as ***opposition***. Having an opposable thumb gives humans the all-important ability to grasp objects.

SECTION 6.2 REVIEW

Mini-Glossary

abduction movement of a body segment away from the body in the frontal plane

acetylcholine a neurotransmitter that stimulates muscle

action potential the electric charge produced when a nerve or muscle fiber is stimulated

adduction movement of a body segment closer to the body in the frontal plane

all-or-none law a rule stating that the fibers in a given motor unit always develop maximum tension when stimulated

axon a long, thin fiber connected to the cell body of a motor neuron

axon terminals offshoots of the axon that branch out to connect with individual muscle fibers

circumduction rotational movement of a body segment such that the end of the segment traces a circle

(continued)

cross bridges connections between the heads of myosin filaments and receptor sites on the actin filaments
dorsiflexion movement of the top of the foot toward the lower leg
eversion movement in which the sole of the foot is rolled outward
extension movement that returns a body segment to anatomical position in the sagittal plane
fast-twitch a type of muscle that contracts quickly
flexion forward movement of a body segment away from anatomical position in the sagittal plane
hyperextension backward movement of a body segment past anatomical position in the sagittal plane
insertion the site of a muscle's attachment to a bone that tends to move when the muscle contracts
inversion movement in which the sole of the foot is rolled inward
lateral rotation outward (lateral) movement of a body segment in the transverse plane
medial rotation inward (medial) movement of a body segment in the transverse plane
motor neuron a nerve that stimulates skeletal muscle tissue
motor unit a single motor neuron and all of the muscle fibers that it stimulates
neuromuscular junction the link between an axon terminal and a muscle fiber
opposition the act of touching any of your four fingers to your thumb; this movement enables grasping of objects
origin the site of a muscle's attachment to a relatively fixed structure
parallel fiber architecture a muscle fiber arrangement in which fibers run mostly parallel to each other along the length of the muscle
pennate fiber architecture a muscle fiber arrangement in which each fiber attaches obliquely to a central tendon
plantar flexion downward movement of the foot away from the lower leg
pronation medial rotation of the forearm (palm down)
sarcomeres units composed of actin and myosin that contract inside the muscle fiber
slow-twitch type of muscle that contracts slowly and is resistant to fatigue
supination lateral rotation of the forearm (palm up)
synaptic cleft the tiny gap that separates the axon terminal from the muscle fiber
tetanus a sustained, maximal level of muscle tension that occurs with high-frequency stimulation

Review Questions

1. Explain the role of acetylcholine in muscle contractions.
2. What is measured to determine muscular power?
3. Discuss the differences between a large and small motor unit and their functions.
4. Describe parallel and pennate fiber patterns.
5. What is the difference between pronation and supination of the hand and the foot?
6. What are the directions of movement for the sagittal, frontal, and transverse planes?
7. Describe the difference between abduction and adduction.
8. Which fiber types do you think contribute to each of the following: muscular strength, power, and endurance? Explain your reasoning.
9. Is the strongest athlete the fastest? Why or why not?
10. Why do temperature and humidity increase the rate of muscle fatigue?
11. Do you think a soccer player has more fast-twitch or slow-twitch muscle fibers? Why?
12. Which joints in the upper and lower limbs can perform flexion and extension?

SECTION 6.3 Major Skeletal Muscles

Objectives

- Identify the locations and functions of the muscles of the head and neck.
- Identify the locations and functions of the trunk muscles.
- Identify the locations and functions of the muscles of the upper limb.
- Identify the locations and functions of the muscles of the lower limb.

Key Terms

agonist-antagonist pairs
diaphragm
linea alba
rectus sheath
rotator cuff

There are more than 650 skeletal muscles in the human body. This section presents only the most important muscles from the standpoint of functional movement. Almost all of these muscles are arranged in ***agonist-antagonist pairs***, causing opposing actions at one or more joints.

Muscles of the Head and Neck

The muscles of the head and neck can be divided into three groups: facial muscles, chewing muscles, and neck muscles. The difference between facial muscles and most other muscles is that the insertions of facial muscles connect them to other muscles or skin rather than a bone. When these muscles contract, pulling on the skin, they produce an array of facial expressions.

With the exception of the *orbicularis oris*, which encircles the mouth, and the sheetlike *platysma* on the front and sides of the neck, all of the head and neck muscles are paired—one on the right and one on the left. The head and neck muscles are displayed in **Figure 6-13**, and their locations and functions are summarized in **Figure 6-14**.

Facial Muscles

The *frontalis* muscle is so named because it covers the frontal bone of the skull. It attaches the epicranial aponeurosis to the skin above the eyebrows, enabling elevation of the eyebrows and wrinkling of the forehead. On the posterior side, the epicranial aponeurosis is attached to the temporal bone by the *occipitalis* muscle. Contraction of the occipitalis pulls the scalp posteriorly.

The *orbicularis oculi* and *orbicularis oris* respectively surround the eyes and mouth. The *orbicularis oculi* enables closing and squinting of the eyes. *Orbicularis oris* contracts to close the mouth and extend the lips as in kissing.

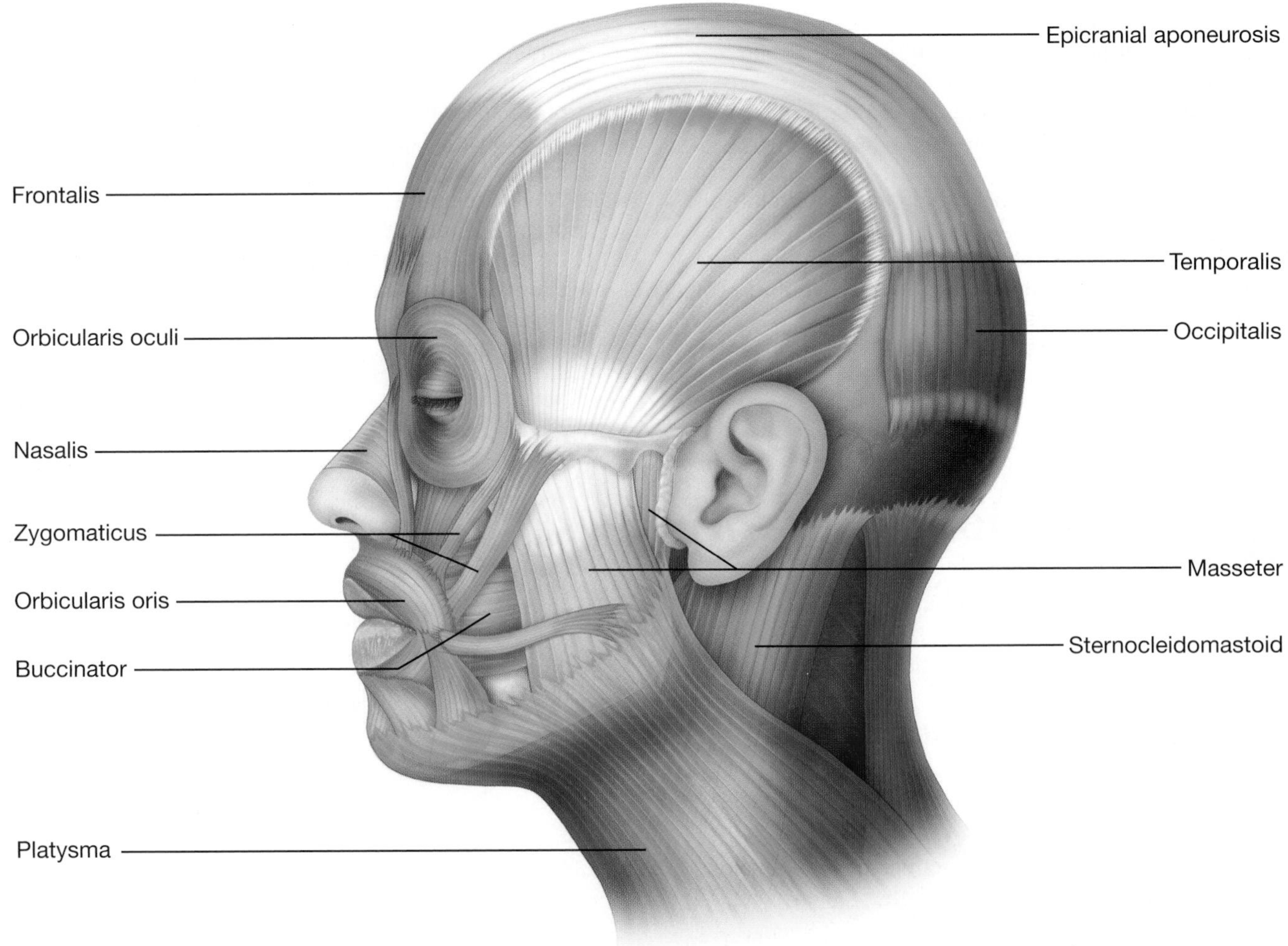

Figure 6.13 Major muscles of the head and neck.

Muscles of the Head and Neck			
Facial Muscles			
Muscle	**Origin**	**Insertion**	**Primary Functions**
Frontalis	epicranial aponeurosis	skin above eyebrows	raises eyebrows, wrinkles forehead
Occipitalis	temporal bone	epicranial aponeurosis	pulls scalp posteriorly
Orbicularis oculi	frontal bone and maxilla	tissue encircling eyes	closes eyes, enables squinting
Nasalis	maxilla lateral to nose	bridge and cartilage of nose	modifies size of nostrils
Orbicularis oris	mandible and maxilla	skin and muscle around mouth	closes lips, produces kissing motion
Buccinator	maxilla and mandible	orbicularis orbis	compresses cheek
Zygomaticus	zygomatic bone	skin and muscle at corners of mouth	the "smiling" muscle
Platysma	connective tissue over chest muscles	tissue around mouth	pulls corners of mouth down, opens mouth wide
Chewing Muscles			
Muscle	**Origin**	**Insertion**	**Primary Functions**
Masseter	zygomatic arch of temporal bone	mandible	closes the jaw
Temporalis	temporal bone	mandible	assists masseter with closing jaw
Neck Muscles			
Muscle	**Origin**	**Insertion**	**Primary Functions**
Sternocleidomastoid	two heads arise from the sternum and clavicle	mastoid process of temporal bone	flexion of head, rotation of head toward opposite side of contraction

Figure 6.14

Goodheart-Willcox Publisher

The *buccinator* and *zygomaticus* muscles form part of the sides of the face. The buccinator extends from the maxilla and mandible to the *orbicularis oris*. When it contracts, this muscle compresses the cheek. *Zygomaticus* is named after its origin on the zygomatic bone. It attaches to the skin and muscle around the corners of the mouth; contraction of the *zygomaticus* produces smiling.

Chewing Muscles

The major muscle used for chewing is the *masseter,* which connects the zygomatic process of the temporal bone to the mandible, or jaw bone. Contraction of the masseter elevates the mandible, bringing the teeth together. An assistive muscle for chewing is the *temporalis,* which covers a large portion of the temporal bone and connects the temporal bone to the mandible. The *buccinators* also assist with chewing when they contract to hold the cheeks firm.

Neck Muscles

The paired *sternocleidomastoid* muscles are primary supporters and movers of the head. Each muscle has two heads—one that originates on the sternum, and one that originates on the clavicle. The heads fuse into a single large muscle that inserts on the mastoid process of the temporal bone. Contracting together, the *sternocleidomastoid* muscles produce flexion of the head and neck. When one muscle contracts alone, the result is rotation of the head toward the opposite side.

The *platysma* is a single, thin, flat, superficial muscle that blankets the entire anterior and lateral portions of the neck. It originates in the connective tissue covering the chest muscles and inserts in the tissues around the mouth. Contraction of the *platysma* pulls the corners of the mouth downward. It is also activated when opening the mouth wide.

SELF CHECK

1. In what way are facial muscles different from most other muscles?
2. Which muscles assist with chewing?
3. What movements result from contraction of the *sternocleidomastoid* muscles?

Muscles of the Trunk

The trunk muscles provide stability for the vertebral column. They are also responsible for maintaining upright posture. American football players train to strengthen their neck and trunk muscles in an effort to maximize spinal stability and minimize risk of injury to the delicate spinal cord and internal organs (**Figure 6.15**). Conversely, gymnasts train to enhance the flexibility of the spine and are capable of extraordinary spinal hyperextension, especially during balance-beam and floor-exercise routines.

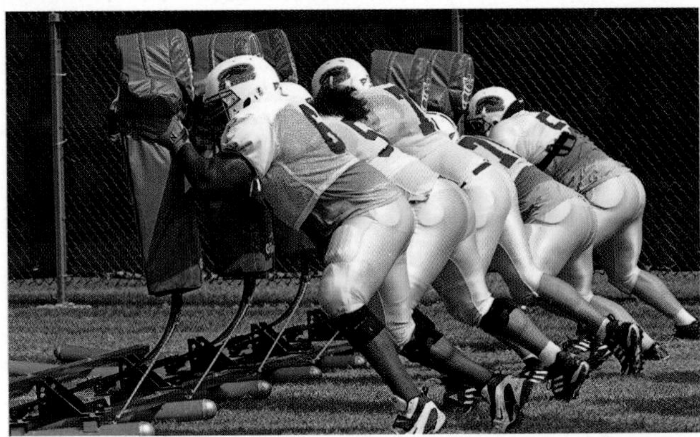

Tomasz Symanski/Shutterstock.com

Figure 6.15 Football players work to condition their trunk muscles to help prevent injury.

Collectively, the trunk muscles enable flexion, extension, hyperextension, lateral flexion, and rotation of the head and trunk. From a functional perspective, the anterior abdominal muscles also assist with urination, defecation, forced expiration during breathing, and childbirth. The all-important diaphragm muscle regulates breathing. The trunk muscles also serve as a protective sheath for the organs of the thoracic and abdominal cavities. The locations and primary functions of the major muscles of the anterior and posterior trunk are summarized in the table in **Figure 6.16** and are shown in **Figure 6.17**.

Anterior Trunk Muscles

Running the entire length of the anterior abdomen, the superficial, paired *rectus abdominis* muscles are flat and encased in a connective tissue called the ***rectus sheath***. The muscles are separated by a longitudinal band of connective tissue called the ***linea alba***. This, in combination with several lateral bands of connective tissue, divides the muscle into eight muscle bellies,

Muscles of the Trunk			
Anterior Muscles			
Muscle	**Origin**	**Insertion**	**Primary Functions**
Rectus abdominis	pubic crest	sternum and ribs 5–7	flexion and lateral flexion of trunk
External oblique	ribs 5–12	anterior iliac crest and pubis	flexion, lateral flexion, and rotation to opposite side of trunk
Internal oblique	anterior iliac crest	ribs 10–12	flexion, lateral flexion, and rotation to same side of trunk
Posterior Muscles			
Muscle	**Origin**	**Insertion**	**Primary Functions**
Trapezius	occipital bone, nuchal ligament, and vertebrae C7–T3	clavicle and scapular spine	extension and hyperextension of head; elevation, depression, and adduction of scapula
Erector spinae: iliocostalis	ilium and ribs	ribs and transverse processes of vertebrae	extension, lateral flexion, and rotation to opposite side
Erector spinae: longissimus	inferior aspect of transverse processes of vertebrae	superior aspect of transverse processes of vertebrae	extension, lateral flexion, and rotation to opposite side
Erector spinae: spinalis	inferior aspect of spinous processes	superior aspect of spinous processes	extension, lateral flexion, and rotation to opposite side
Quadratus lumborum	iliac crests	upper lumbar vertebrae	individually assist lateral flexion; together assist trunk extension
Muscles for Breathing			
Muscle	**Origin**	**Insertion**	**Primary Functions**
Diaphragm	(separates thoracic and abdominal cavities)		enlarges thoracic cavity for inhalation
Internal intercostals	(between ribs)		decrease thoracic cavity volume during forced expiration
External intercostals	(between ribs)		help enlarge thoracic cavity volume during inhalation

Goodheart-Willcox Publisher

Figure 6.16

Anterior view

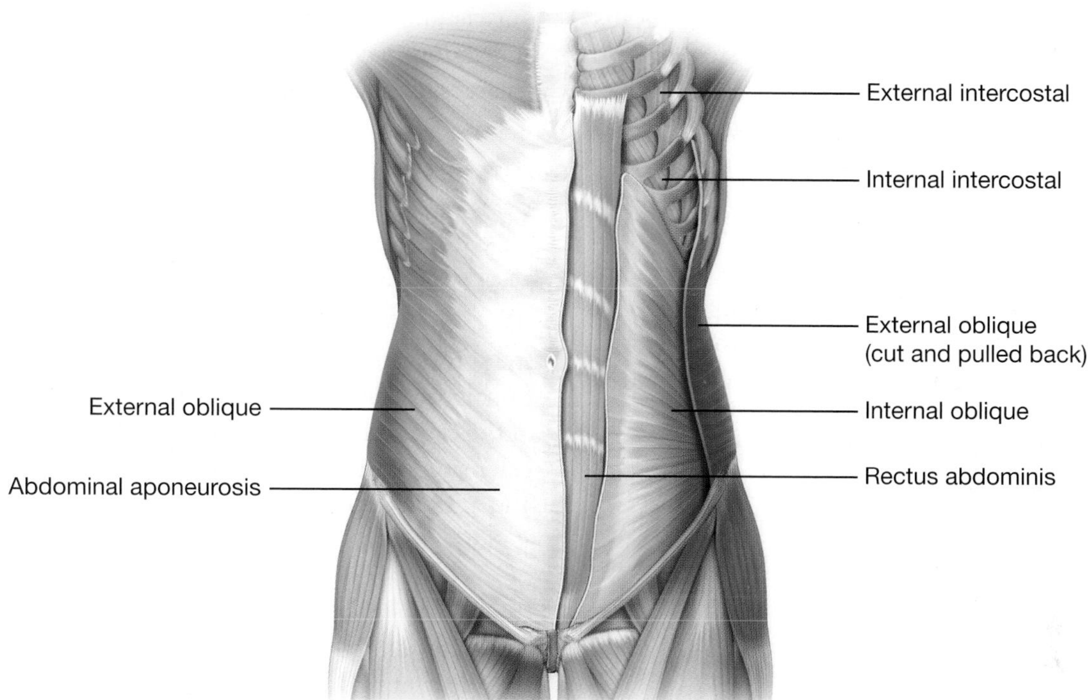

Posterior view of superficial muscles

Trapezius

Erector spinae muscle group

Posterior view of deep muscles

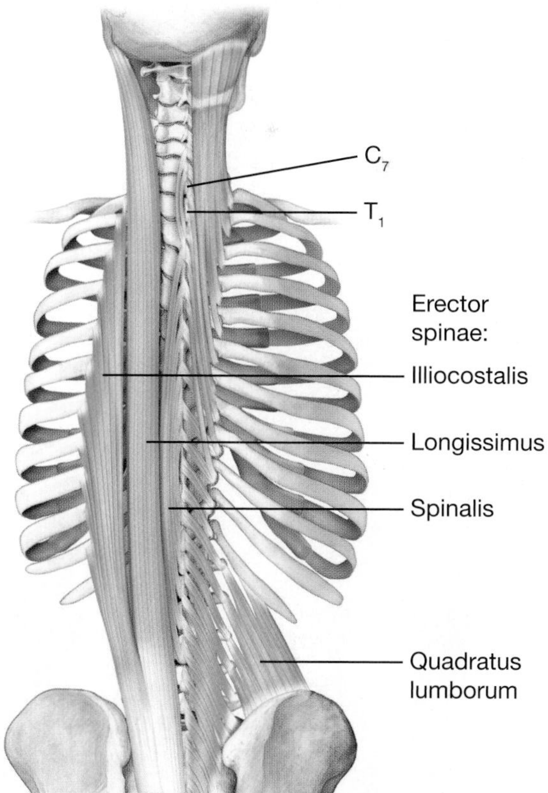

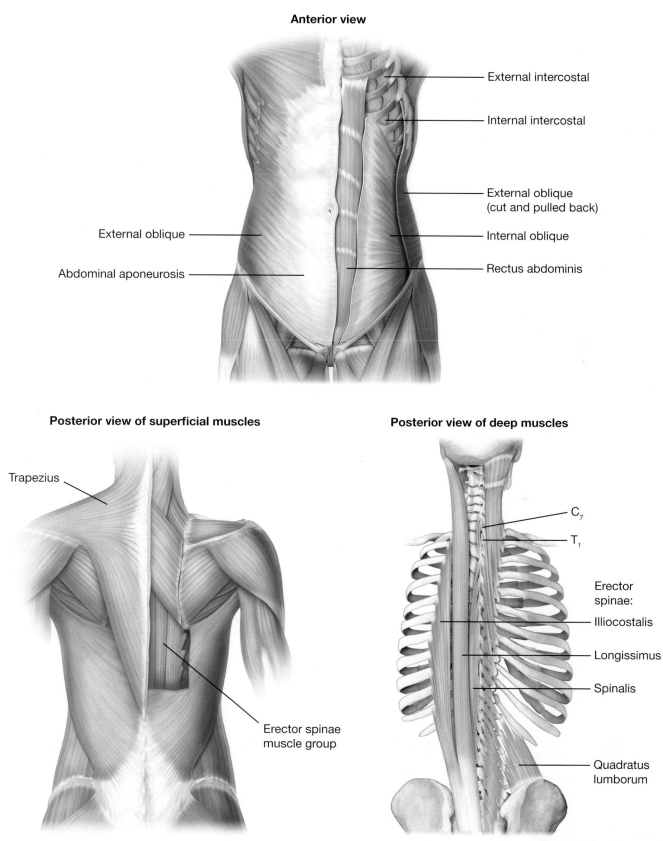

Figure 6.17 Major muscles of the trunk.

which are visible in individuals with well-developed abdominal muscles (**Figure 6.18**). The rectus abdominis connects the pubic crest to the sternum and ribs 5 through 7. Contraction of both muscles produces flexion of the trunk, and unilateral contraction assists with lateral flexion of the trunk.

The paired *external oblique* muscles are also superficial in the abdominal region. Running from rib 512 to the anterior iliac crest and pubis, these muscles form the lateral walls of the abdomen. Working together, the *external obliques* contribute to trunk flexion. Individually, they produce lateral flexion of the trunk and rotation to the opposite side.

Lying deep to the *external obliques* are the *internal obliques*. Connecting the iliac crest to ribs 10–12, these muscles are positioned at right angles to the external obliques. Functionally, these muscles produce the same movement as the external obliques.

The external and internal *intercostal* muscles are located between the ribs. Contraction of the external intercostals pulls the ribs outward, enlarging the thoracic cavity for inhalation. Contraction of the internal intercostals pulls the ribs inward, compressing the lungs for forced exhalation.

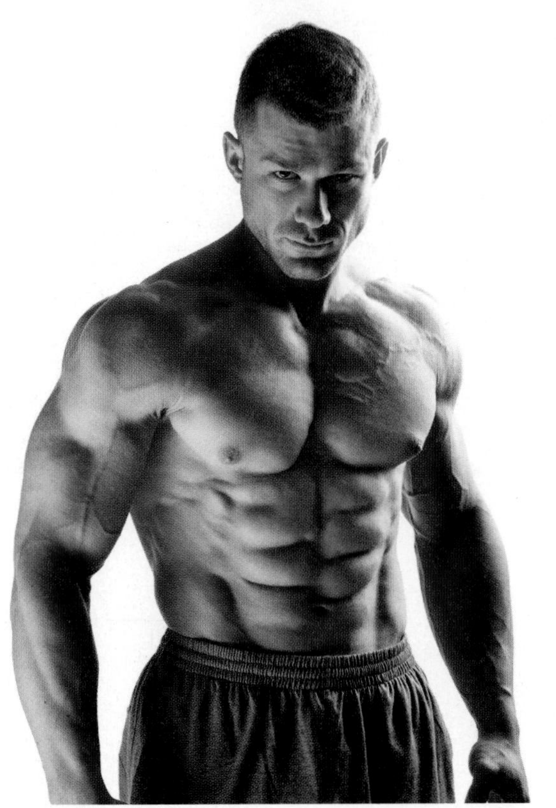

Aleksandr Petrunovskyi/Shutterstock.com

Figure 6.18 The paired *rectus abdominis* muscles are divided into eight muscle bellies by the linea alba, running longitudinally, and bands of connective tissue running laterally.

The ***diaphragm*** is a dome-shaped sheet of muscle and fibrous tissue that separates the thoracic and abdominal cavities. Contraction of the diaphragm enlarges the thoracic cavity, drawing air into the lungs.

Posterior Trunk Muscles

The superficial, paired *trapezius* muscles cover a large, kite-shaped expanse of the upper back and neck. The origin of each muscle runs from the occipital bone of the skull, down the nuchal ligament, and attaches to the spinous processes of vertebrae C7–T3. The insertion is on the clavicle and scapular spine. Actions of the trapezius muscles include extension and hyperextension of the head, as well as elevation, depression, and adduction of the scapula.

The *erector spinae* group includes three columns of muscle running most of the length of the spine: the *iliocostalis, longissimus,* and *spinalis*. The *iliocostalis* originates on the ilium and the ribs, and it connects to the adjacent ribs and transverse processes. *Longissimus* connects the transverse processes of adjacent vertebrae. As the name suggests, *spinalis* connects the adjacent spinous processes of the vertebrae. Functionally, these muscles serve as the primary extensors of the trunk. They also produce lateral flexion to the same side when contracting unilaterally.

The *quadratus lumborum* also acts as an extensor of the trunk. This muscle originates on the iliac crest and inserts on the upper lumbar vertebrae. These bilateral muscles function like the *erector spinae* group.

SELF CHECK

1. Why does training for gymnasts differ from training for football and other contact sports?
2. What is the purpose of the rectus sheath?
3. Explain the function of the intercostal muscles.

Muscles of the Upper Limb

The joints of the upper limb include those of the shoulder, elbow, wrist, and fingers. This section includes information about the major muscles that cross the shoulder and elbow joints. **Figure 6.19** shows the major muscles of the upper limb, and the table in **Figure 6.20** summarizes their locations and functions.

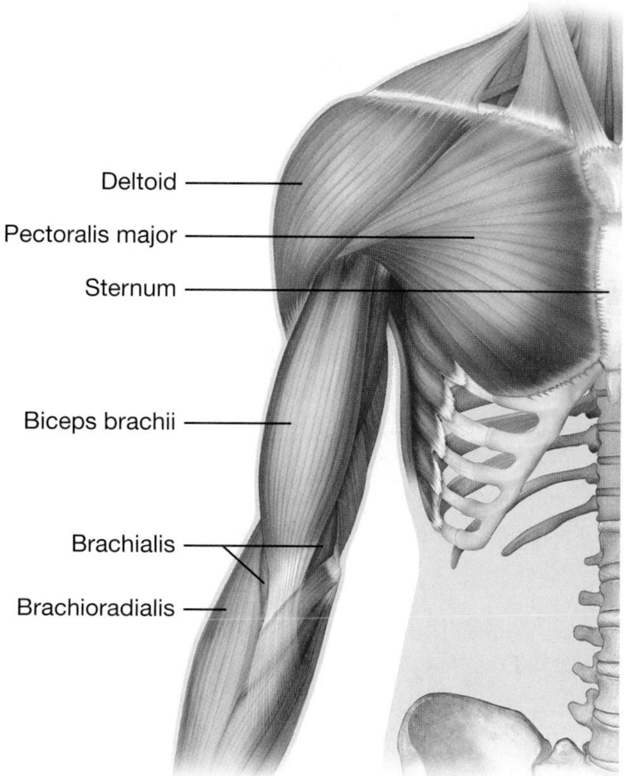

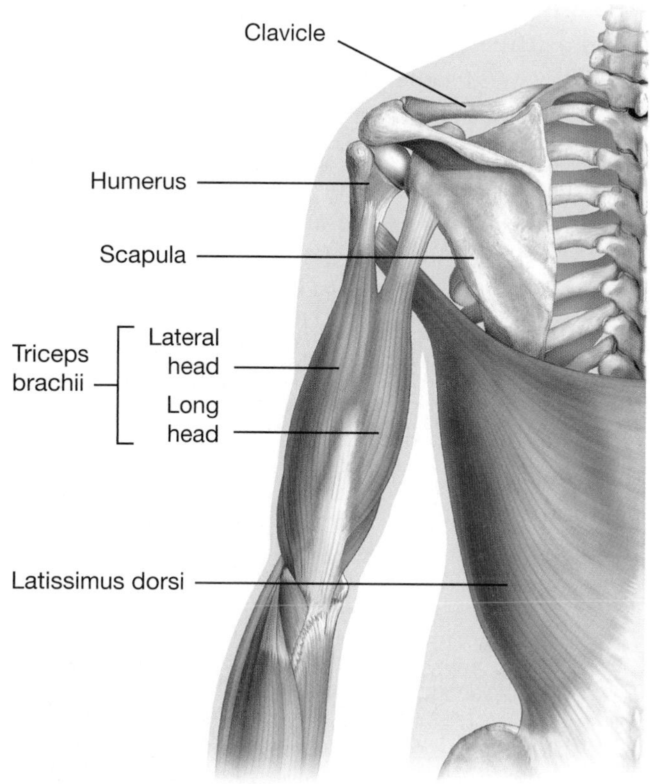

© Body Scientific International

Figure 6.19 Muscles of the upper limb. The medial head of the *triceps* shares the proximal tendon of the lateral head, so the muscle is concealed behind the lateral and long heads in this illustration.

Muscles of the Upper Limb			
Shoulder Muscles			
Muscle	**Origin**	**Insertion**	**Primary Functions**
Pectoralis major	sternum, clavicle, and ribs 1–7	proximal humerus	adduction and flexion of arm
Deltoid	scapular spine, acromion, and clavicle	deltoid tuberosity of humerus	prime mover for abduction; assists with flexion, extension, and rotation of arm
Latissimus dorsi	lower 6 thoracic and all lumbar vertebrae, ribs 10–12, sacrum, and iliac crest	anterior humerus	extension, adduction, and medial rotation of arm
Elbow Muscles			
Muscle	**Origin**	**Insertion**	**Primary Functions**
Biceps brachii	superior glenoid fossa and coracoid process	radial tuberosity	assists with flexion and supination of forearm
Brachialis	humerus	ulna	flexion of forearm
Brachioradialis	distal styloid process of the radius	lateral supracondylar ridge of the humerus	flexion of forearm
Triceps brachii	inferior glenoid fossa and entire humeral shaft	olecranon process of ulna	extension of forearm

Figure 6.20

Goodheart-Willcox Publisher

Muscles Acting at the Shoulder

Because the shoulder is a ball-and-socket joint and the most freely movable joint in the human body, the movement capabilities of the upper limb are impressive. This large range of motion is achieved because the bone structure of the glenohumeral joint provides little to no stability. Although this gives the shoulder a large range of motion, it also makes the shoulder susceptible to dislocation. Therefore, it is up to the large, powerful muscles surrounding the shoulder to maintain the stability and integrity of the joint.

Sizable muscles inserting on the humerus include the *pectoralis major* on the anterior side of the joint, the *latissimus dorsi* on the posterior side of the joint, and the *deltoid* covering the lateral aspect of the joint. The pectoralis originates on the sternum, clavicle, and ribs 1–7, positioning it to contribute to adduction and flexion of the arm. The *latissimus* originates on the lower 6 thoracic vertebrae, all of the lumbar vertebrae, ribs 10–12, the sacrum, and the iliac crest, enabling extension, adduction, and medial rotation of the arm. The deltoid originates on the scapular spine, acromion, and clavicle, making it a prime mover for arm abduction.

Four muscles attaching the humerus to the scapula also contribute to glenohumeral joint stability and produce rotational movements of the humerus. Because these muscles and their tendons form a cuff where they insert around the head of the humerus, they are collectively known as the ***rotator cuff***. **Figure 6.21** shows these muscles, and **Figure 6.22** describes their locations and functions.

The muscles of the rotator cuff are nicknamed the "SITS muscles," after the first letter of each of their

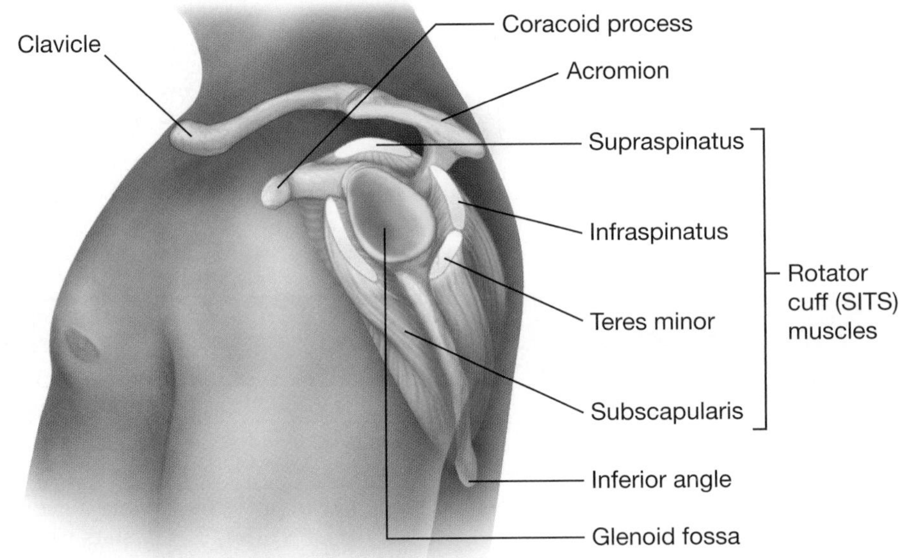

Figure 6.21 Lateral view of the rotator cuff muscles.

Rotator Cuff Muscles			
Muscle	**Origin**	**Insertion**	**Primary Functions**
Supraspinatus	supraspinous fossa of scapula	greater tubercle of humerus	assists arm abduction, stabilizes humeral head against downward slippage
Infraspinatus	infraspinous fossa of scapula	greater tubercle of humerus	lateral rotation of humerus, stabilizes humeral head against upward slippage
Teres minor	lateral border and posterior scapula	greater tubercle of humerus	lateral rotation of humerus, stabilizes humeral head against upward slippage
Subscapularis	subscapular fossa of scapula	lesser tubercle of humerus	medial rotation of humerus, stabilizes humeral head against upward slippage

Figure 6.22

names: *supraspinatus, infraspinatus, teres minor,* and *subscapularis. Supraspinatus,* named after its origin in the supraspinous fossa of the scapula, assists with arm abduction. *Infraspinatus,* named after its origin in the infraspinous fossa of the scapula, contributes to lateral rotation of the humerus. *Teres minor,* originating on the lateral posterior scapula, also laterally rotates the humerus. Emanating from the subscapular fossa or the scapula, *subscapularis* medially rotates the humerus.

Muscles Acting at the Elbow and Wrist

The arm muscles enable strong, controlled movements in sports such as gymnastics, rowing, and archery, as well as fast, powerful movements in weightlifting, boxing, and throwing. The *biceps brachii* and *triceps brachii* are superficial muscles on the anterior and posterior aspects of the arm, respectively, that are typically well developed in bodybuilders. One head of the biceps originates on the superior side of the glenoid fossa, and the other originates on the coracoid process. Both heads insert on the radial tuberosity, enabling the biceps to assist with supination and flexion of the forearm. The three heads of the *triceps brachii* cover the posterior aspect of the arm, with origins on the inferior glenoid fossa and entire humeral shaft. The insertion is on the olecranon. The triceps contracts to extend the arm at the elbow.

Other anterior arm muscles include the *brachialis* and *brachioradialis,* which also contribute to flexion of the forearm. The brachialis connects the humerus and ulna, and the *brachioradialis* connects the radius and humerus.

There are nine muscles that cross the wrist, and ten muscles contained entirely within the hand, many of which branch to several of the fingers. The names of many of these muscles describe their functions as well as their locations. For example, the *flexor carpi ulnaris* causes flexion at the wrist and crosses the wrist on the ulnar (little finger) side. The *extensor digitorum superficialis* and *extensor digitorum profundus* cause extension of the digits, or fingers.

SELF CHECK

1. What is sacrificed at the shoulder to allow greater range of motion?
2. Which four muscles make up the rotator cuff?

Muscles of the Lower Limb

While the structure of the upper limb lends itself well to activities that involve large ranges of motion, the lower limb is well designed for its primary jobs of standing and walking. Running, jumping, kicking, climbing, skipping, hopping, and dancing are just a few of the additional capabilities of the lower limb.

The lower limb includes the joints of the hip, knee, and ankle, along with numerous joints in the foot. This section includes the major muscles of the hip, knee, and ankle, but omits a number of small muscles that play assistive roles. The table in **Figure 6.23** outlines the locations and primary functions of the major muscles of the lower limb. **Figure 6.24** shows these muscles.

Muscles Acting at the Hip

The hip is surrounded by large, powerful muscles that make it an extremely stable joint but also tend to limit its range of motion. The large, superficial *gluteus maximus,* extending from the sacrum and iliac to the gluteal tuberosity of the femur, is the primary extensor muscle of the hip. This muscle also contributes to lateral rotation of the leg. It is usually activated only when the hip is in flexion, stretching the muscle slightly, as during cycling or climbing stairs.

Just deep to *gluteus maximus* is the *gluteus medius.* Connecting the posterior ilium to the greater trochanter of the femur, this muscle is responsible for abduction and medial rotation of the leg. It also serves the important function of stabilizing the pelvis during the support phase of walking and running or when standing on one leg.

The primary flexor of the hip is the *iliopsoas complex,* consisting of the *iliacus* (originating from the iliac fossa and sacrum) and the *psoas* (originating from the 12th thoracic and all of the lumbar vertebrae). These muscles join to insert on the lesser trochanter of the femur.

Adduction at the hip is the function of the *adductor* muscles, which extend from the pubis to the linea aspera of the femur. The *adductors* are active during the swing phase of gait to bring the foot under the body's center of gravity.

The longest muscle in the human body is the *sartorius,* a thin strap muscle that originates on the anterior superior iliac spine and inserts on the proximal tibia. *Sartorius* assists with flexion and lateral rotation of the thigh at the hip.

Muscles Acting at the Knee

Notice the muscle groups on the anterior side and posterior side of the thigh, described in **Figure 6.23** and shown in **Figure 6.24**. The anterior group, the *quadriceps,* includes the *rectus femoris, vastus lateralis, vastus medialis,* and *vastus intermedius,* which lies under the *rectus femoris.* These four muscles are often referred to as a group because they all attach to the tibia via the patellar tendon. Collectively, they are the prime extensors of the leg at the knee.

Muscles of the Lower Limb			
Hip Muscles			
Muscle	**Origin**	**Insertion**	**Primary Functions**
Gluteus maximus	sacrum and iliac	gluteal tuberosity of femur	extension and lateral rotation of leg
Gluteus medius	posterior ilium	greater trochanter of femur	abduction and medial rotation of leg
Iliopsoas **(fusion of *iliacus* and *psoas* muscles)**	iliac fossa and sacrum, 12th thoracic and all lumbar vertebrae	lesser trochanter of femur	flexion of leg at hip
Adductor muscles ***magnus*** ***longus*** ***brevis***	pubis	linea aspera of femur	adduction and medial rotation of leg
Sartorius	anterior superior iliac spine	proximal tibia	assists with flexion and lateral rotation of leg
Knee Muscles			
Muscle	**Origin**	**Insertion**	**Primary Functions**
Quadriceps: rectus femoris	anterior inferior iliac spine	tibia via patellar tendon	extension of leg at knee
Quadriceps: vastus lateralis	greater trochanter and linea aspera	tibia via patellar tendon	extension of leg at knee
Quadriceps: vastus intermedius	anterior femur	tibia via patellar tendon	extension of leg at knee
Quadriceps: vastus medialis	linea aspera	tibia via patellar tendon	extension of leg at knee
Hamstrings: semitendinosus	ischial tuberosity	proximal medial tibia	flexion of leg at knee; medial rotation
Hamstrings: semimembranosus	ischial tuberosity	proximal medial tibia	flexion of leg at knee; medial rotation
Hamstrings: biceps femoris	long head originates on ischial tuberosity; short head originates on linea aspera	lateral condyle of tibia and head of fibula	flexion of leg at knee; lateral rotation
Ankle/Foot Muscles			
Muscle	**Origin**	**Insertion**	**Primary Functions**
Gastrocnemius	posterior medial and lateral femoral condyles	calcaneus (heel bone) via Achilles tendon	plantar flexion of foot, flexion of leg at knee
Soleus	fibula and tibia	calcaneus via Achilles tendon	plantar flexion of foot
Tibialis anterior	tibia	first cuneiform and first metatarsal in foot	dorsiflexion and inversion of foot
Extensor digitorum longus	lateral condyle of tibia and proximal ¾ of fibula	phalanges of toes 2–5	dorsiflexion, eversion, toe extension
Fibularis longus brevis tertius	fibula	metatarsals	plantar flexion, eversion

Figure 6.23

Goodheart-Willcox Publisher

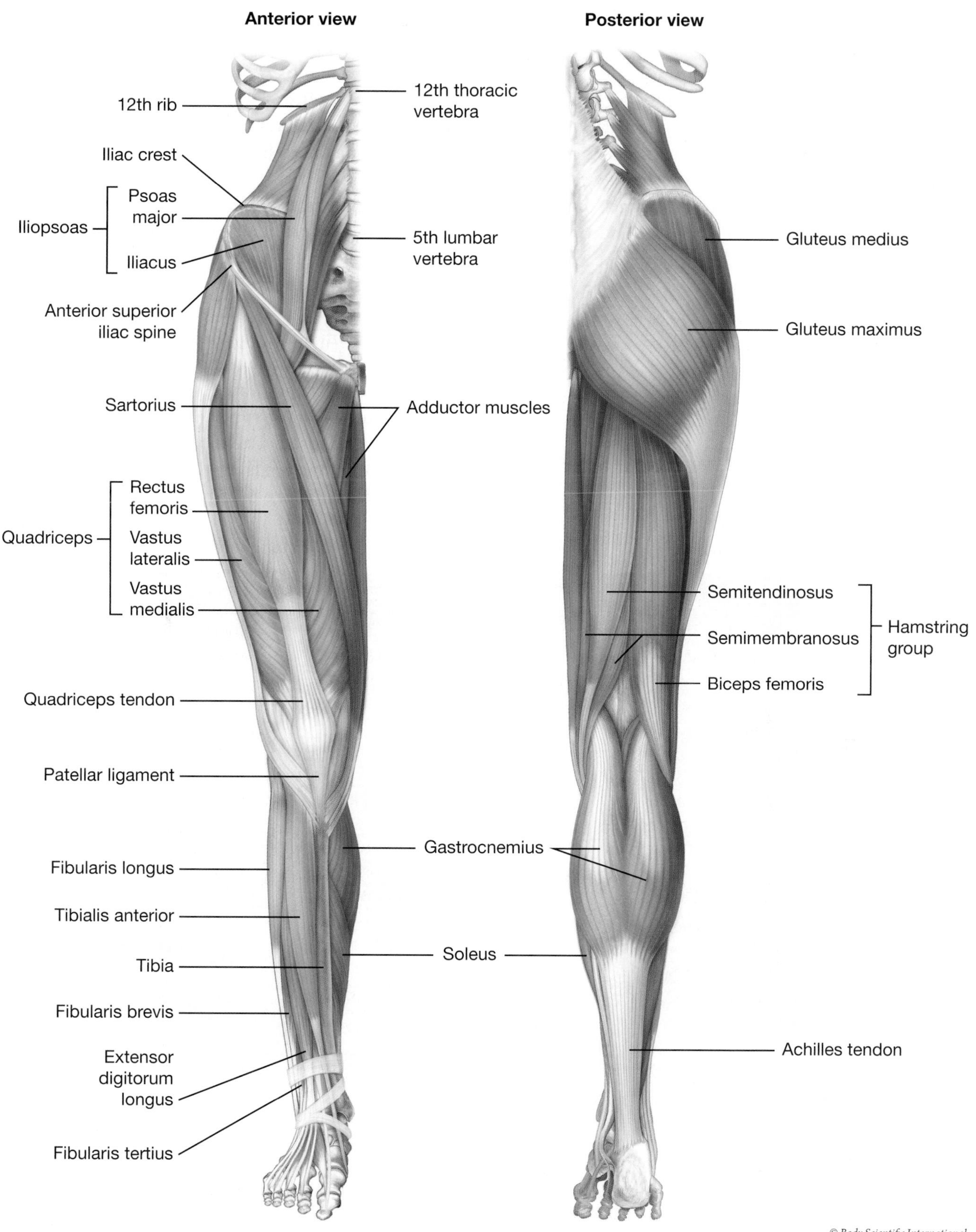

Figure 6.24 Major muscles of the lower limb.

The posterior group, the *hamstrings,* includes the *biceps femoris, semimembranosus,* and *semitendinosus.* What these muscles have in common, besides their general location and common origin on the ischial tuberosity, is strong, stringlike tendons that can be felt on either side of the back of the knee. Collectively, they are the prime flexors of the leg at the knee. The term *hamstrings* comes from the fact that hams consist of thigh and hip muscles, and butchers use the tendons of these muscles to hang the hams for smoking.

Muscles Acting at the Ankle

The primary movements occurring at the ankle are the sagittal plane motions of plantar flexion and dorsiflexion. The plantar flexors are the *gastrocnemius* and *soleus* muscles on the posterior aspect of the lower leg. The superficial *gastrocnemius* extends from the posterior medial and lateral femoral condyles. The underlying *soleus* extends from the fibula and tibia. Both muscles insert on the calcaneus via the Achilles tendon. The three branches of the *fibularis* muscle are the *longus, brevis,* and *tertius.* These muscles connect the fibula to the metatarsals and assist with plantar flexion and eversion.

Dorsiflexion is produced by the *tibialis anterior* and *extensor digitorum longus* on the anterior aspect of the lower leg. The *tibialis anterior,* connecting the tibia to the first cuneiform and first metatarsal, also acts to invert the foot. The *extensor digitorum longus,* extending from the lateral tibia and fibula to the metatarsals, also contributes to eversion.

As discussed throughout the sections on the upper and lower limbs, many superficial muscles are readily palpable when tensed. The superficial muscles of both the upper and lower extremities are displayed by the bodybuilder in **Figure 6.25**.

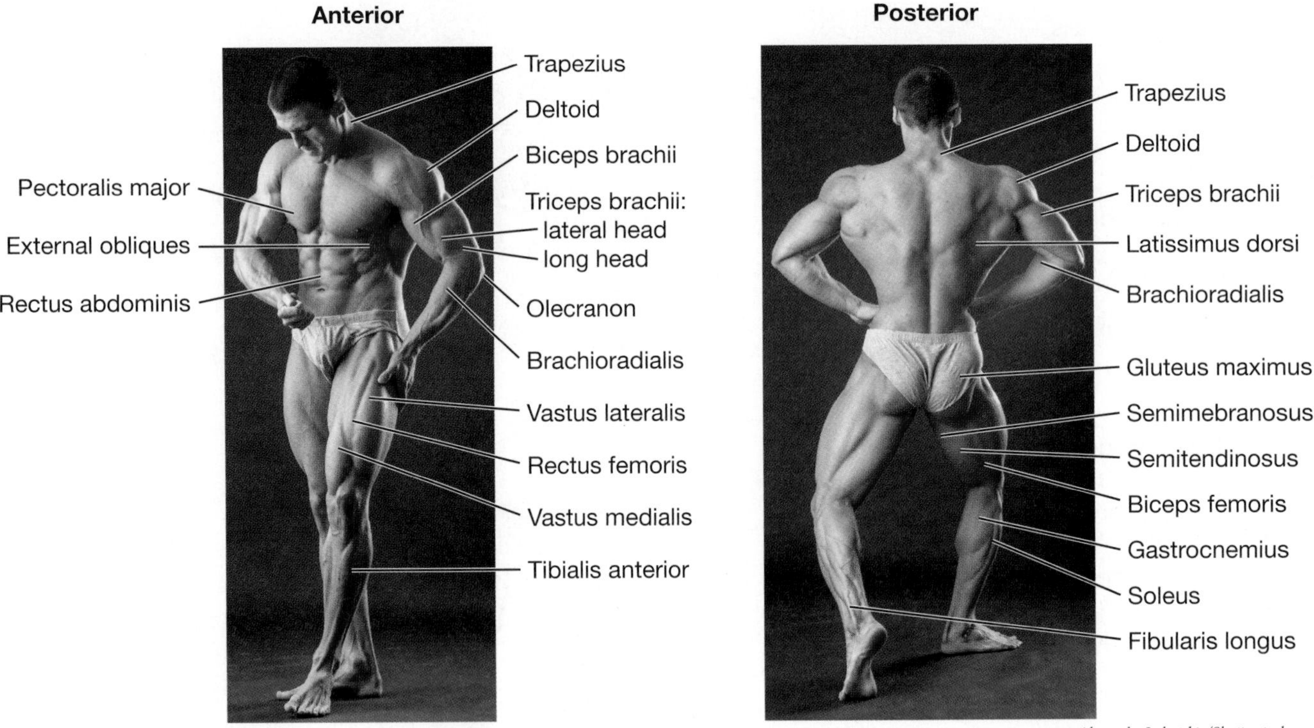

Figure 6.25 Anterior and posterior views of the major superficial muscles.

SECTION 6.3

REVIEW

Mini-Glossary

agonist-antagonist pairs pairs of muscles that cause opposing actions at a joint

diaphragm a dome-shaped sheet of muscle and fibrous tissue that separates the thoracic and abdominal cavities

linea alba a longitudinal band of connective tissue that separates the *rectus abdominis* muscles

rectus sheath connective tissue that encases the *rectus abdominis* muscles

rotator cuff the four muscles that attach the humerus to the scapula and their tendons

Review Questions

1. List the major muscles of the face.
2. What are the major functions of the trunk muscles?
3. Explain the purpose of the diaphragm.
4. Using the drawings and tables in this lesson, identify the agonist/antagonist pairs for abduction/adduction of the hip and plantar flexion/dorsiflexion of the ankle.
5. What type of motor units do you think the forearm and hands have? Why?
6. Compare and contrast inversion and eversion of the foot and supination and pronation of the hand.
7. Try writing the answers to one of the questions at the left without using your thumb. Why is opposition important?
8. What position are you in if all of your joints that can perform flexion do so at the same time?
9. In a push-up, what movements are happening at the shoulder and elbow when you are moving up? Which muscles are performing these movements? What movements occur when you move down? Which muscles cause these movements?

SECTION 6.4

Common Muscle Injuries and Disorders

Objectives

- Explain the causes of common muscular injuries.
- Describe the causes and symptoms of major muscle disorders.

Key Terms

contusion
delayed-onset muscle soreness (DOMS)
hernia
muscle cramps
muscle strain
muscular dystrophy (MD)
myositis ossificans
shin splint
tendinitis
tendinosis

Although common, most muscle injuries are relatively minor. Fortunately, the healthy human body has considerable ability to self-repair a variety of injuries, such as those inflicted on muscles. This section describes some of the common muscle injuries and disorders.

Muscle Injuries

Many people think about muscle injuries as being associated with sport participation. Although injuries do occur during sport competitions, the fact is, muscle injuries also occur as people go about their daily activities. The injuries described in this section are typical.

Strains

A ***muscle strain*** occurs when a muscle is stretched beyond its usual limits. Someone who has a large degree of flexibility at a particular joint has a much lower risk of straining those muscles than someone with extremely "tight" muscles crossing that same joint.

Another factor affecting muscle strains is the speed with which the muscles are stretched. Many strains to the hamstrings, for example, result from participating in activities that involve running, accelerating, and changing direction all at the same time. Strains of the hamstrings are a frequent problem for athletes because these injuries are slow to heal and tend to recur. One-third of all hamstring strains recur within the first year of returning to a sport or an activity.

Strains are classified as Grade I, II, or III:

- Grade I (mild) strains result in muscle tightness the day after the injury, but nothing more.
- Grade II (moderate) strains produce pain caused by a partial tear in the muscle. Associated weakness and temporary loss of function may also occur.
- Grade III (severe) strains result in damage and symptoms that are significantly greater than those accompanying Grades I and II. Grade III strains involve a tearing of the muscle, loss of function, internal bleeding, and swelling.

Understanding Medical Terminology

The terms *strain* (to muscles or tendons) and *sprain* (to a ligament at a joint) are very similar. Remember that *T*ight muscles and *T*endons get s*T*rains.

Contusions

A ***contusion*** is a bruise or bleeding within a muscle, resulting from an impact. When an already injured muscle is repeatedly struck, a more serious condition called ***myositis ossificans*** can develop.

Myositis ossificans involves the formation of a calcium mass within the muscle over a period of three to four weeks. After six or seven weeks, the mass usually begins to dissolve and is resorbed by the body. In some cases, a bony lesion may remain in the muscle.

Cramps

Muscle cramps involve moderate to severe muscle spasms that cause pain. The cause of cramps is unknown; in fact, there may be numerous causes. Some of the possible causes include an electrolyte imbalance; deficiency in calcium, magnesium, or potassium; and dehydration.

Research Notes Low Back Pain

Low back pain (LBP) is a major health problem. Approximately 80%–85% of people experience it at some time during their lives. Back injuries are also the most common and most expensive of all worker's compensation claims. Second only to the common cold in causing absences from work, the incidence of LBP has steadily increased in the United States for the past 15 years. This is likely due, in part, to the increasing proportion of overweight and obese individuals. LBP is significantly associated with excess weight in men and women of all ages.

Nearly 30% of children in the United States experience LBP. The likelihood that children will experience LBP increases with age. By age 16, the percentage of children with LBP has reached the adult incidence of 80%–85%. Children who are more physically active tend to incur LBP more often than sedentary children.

Athletes of all ages have a much higher incidence of LBP than nonathletes. In fact, more than 9% of college athletes receive treatment for LBP. Gymnasts (particularly those who are female) have an even higher incidence of LBP. Studies show that as many as 85% of competitive gymnasts experience this health problem.

What causes LBP? Although injuries and certain disorders may cause LBP, 60% of LBP cases are of unknown origin. In some cases, the low back pain is caused by muscle strain or other injury. In many cases, however, the pain may be due to a *sympathetic contraction* of the low back muscles. This means that the muscles involuntarily contract as the body attempts to stabilize an underlying injury of the spinal column.

Fortunately, most LBP is self-limiting—75% of patients are back to normal within three weeks.

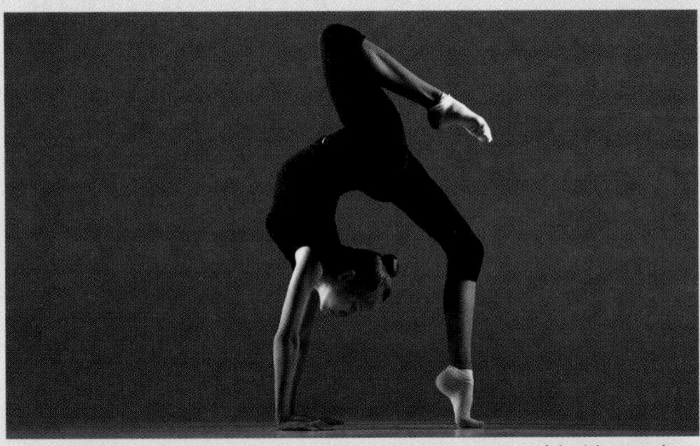

fizkes/Shutterstock.com

Repeated, extreme lumbar hyperextension increases the likelihood that female gymnasts will develop low back pain.

Approximately 90% of patients recover within two months, with or without medical treatment.

What can you do to avoid developing LBP? Known risk factors for LBP include the following:

- sitting for prolonged periods
- standing for long periods in an unchanging position
- working in an unnatural posture
- working with one hand
- encountering sudden or unexpected motions
- performing heavy manual labor

Taller and heavier individuals are at increased risk for developing LBP. Cigarette smoking is also associated with increased risk of LBP, most likely because habitual smoking can contribute to degeneration of the intervertebral discs.

Delayed-Onset Muscle Soreness

Muscle soreness is common and typically arises shortly after unaccustomed activity. ***Delayed-onset muscle soreness (DOMS)*** follows participation in a particularly long or strenuous activity, with the soreness beginning 24 to 72 hours after the activity. DOMS involves multiple, microscopic tears in the muscle tissue and causes inflammation, pain, swelling, and stiffness.

Tendinitis and Tendinosis

Tendons are the bands of tough, fibrous connective tissue that connect muscles to bones. ***Tendinitis*** is inflammation of a tendon, usually accompanied by pain and swelling.

Both acute and overuse injuries can cause tendinitis. The condition can also occur with age, as tendons wear and elasticity decreases. Diseases such as diabetes and rheumatoid arthritis can also promote the development of tendinitis. Tendinitis can occur in any part of the body, but common sites include the shoulder, elbow, and wrist, and the Achilles tendon of the heel. These areas are often subject to injury that causes tendinitis.

Treatments for tendinitis include rest and application of heat or cold. Pain relievers such as aspirin and ibuprofen can reduce pain and inflammation. In severe cases, steroid injections into the tendon can help control pain. Once the pain is reduced, physical therapy to stretch and strengthen both the muscle and the tendon promotes healing and can help prevent reinjury.

If untreated, chronic tendinitis can progress to ***tendinosis***. It is believed that tendinosis, or degeneration of a tendon, is caused by microtears in the tendon's connective tissue, which decrease the tendon's strength. This weakened condition increases the likelihood that the tendon will rupture.

Although tendinosis is painful, no inflammation is present. Once tendinosis has developed, recovery takes months to years, during which only minimal use is permitted. In many cases, physical therapy can help.

Rotational Injuries of the Shoulder

Repetition of forceful overhead motions at the shoulder (as in throwing in baseball, spiking in volleyball, and serving in tennis) can lead to inflammation of or tears in the muscles and muscle tendons surrounding the shoulder (**Figure 6.26**). A similar condition experienced among competitive swimmers is known as *swimmer's shoulder.*

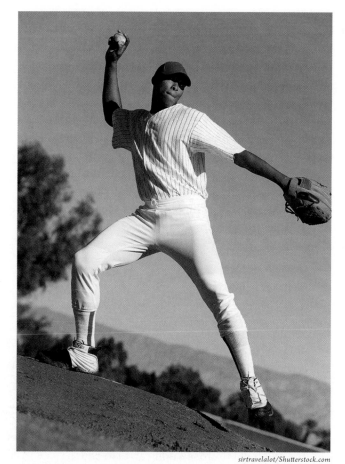

sirtravelalot/Shutterstock.com

Figure 6.26 Sports such as baseball can sometimes lead to overuse injuries of the shoulder muscles.

Improper motion mechanics increase the likelihood of these types of shoulder injuries. The symptoms include pain and stiffness that accompany overhead or rapid movements of the shoulder. If not treated, the pain can become constant. Treatment includes application of ice, rest, and, when necessary, surgical repair.

Overuse Injuries of the Elbow

Epicondylitis involves inflammation and sometimes microtearing of the muscle tendons that cross the lateral and medial sides of the elbow. If untreated, the condition can worsen, leading to swelling and then scarring of the tendons near the elbow. Lateral epicondylitis, which is reported in 30%–40% of tennis players, is known as *tennis elbow,* although it also can result from activities such as swimming, fencing, and repetitious hammering. Medial epicondylitis, known as *Little Leaguer's elbow,* can result from repeated throwing, especially with improper pitching mechanics. Both lateral and medial epicondylitis commonly occur among amateur golfers.

Understanding Medical Terminology

The suffix *-itis* means "inflammation." Numerous medical conditions involve inflammation of a part of the body. The names for all of those conditions contain the *-itis* suffix.

Shin Splints

The term ***shin splint*** is often used to describe pain localized to the medial lower leg. The condition is an overuse injury that typically arises from running or dancing—particularly running on a hard surface or uphill. The cause of the pain is believed to be micro-damage to the muscle tendons that attach to the tibia or inflammation of the periosteum of the tibia. The muscles potentially involved include the *soleus, tibialis anterior,* and *extensor digitorum.*

Whiplash Injuries

Whiplash injuries to the neck are fairly common, often resulting from automobile accidents in which the victim's car is rear-ended. Such injuries result

Focus On Tennis Elbow

Cause

Tennis elbow is the common name for lateral epicondylitis, or inflammation of the tendons on the lateral side of the elbow. A common cause of this condition is repeated twisting motions of the arm, as when hitting a backhand with poor technique in racquet sports. Other repetitive motions in activities such as painting, carpentry, plumbing, and yard work can also lead to lateral epicondylitis. A direct blow to the lateral elbow or a fall on an outstretched arm can also cause the condition.

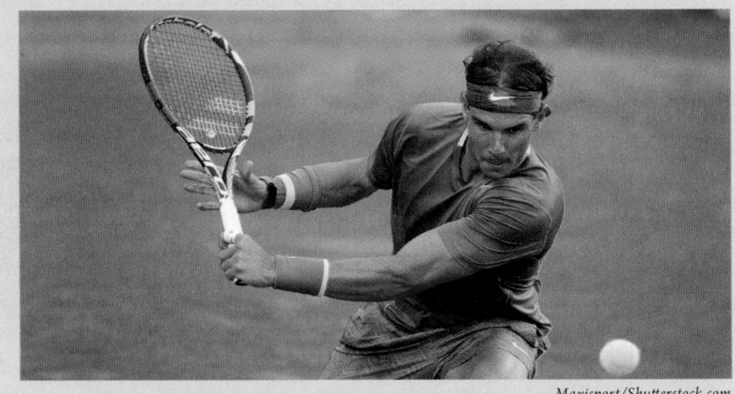

Maxisport/Shutterstock.com

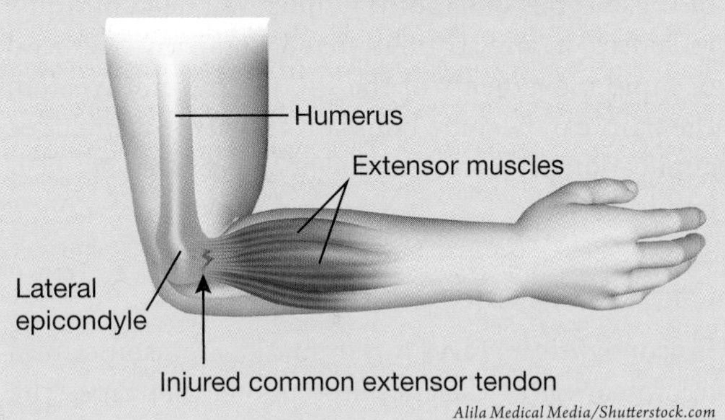

Alila Medical Media/Shutterstock.com

Symptoms

The onset of symptoms is usually gradual, with soreness or a dull ache around the lateral elbow that disappears within 24 hours following activity. With repeated occurrences, the pain may persist longer as the tendons are further damaged. In serious cases, any use of the arm during daily activities can cause pain. The pain may also spread to the hand, wrist, and other parts of the arm, shoulder, or neck. Sometimes the pain increases later in the day, making sleep difficult.

Treatment

The key to successful treatment is cessation of the activity that caused the irritation. Rest! Depending on the severity of the microtears in the tendons, weeks or months of rest may be needed. Applying ice packs for 10–15 minutes at a time several times a day can help relieve pain. Over-the-counter pain medications can also be used judiciously. Severe cases may require surgery. Elbow splints and sleeves have not been shown to help.

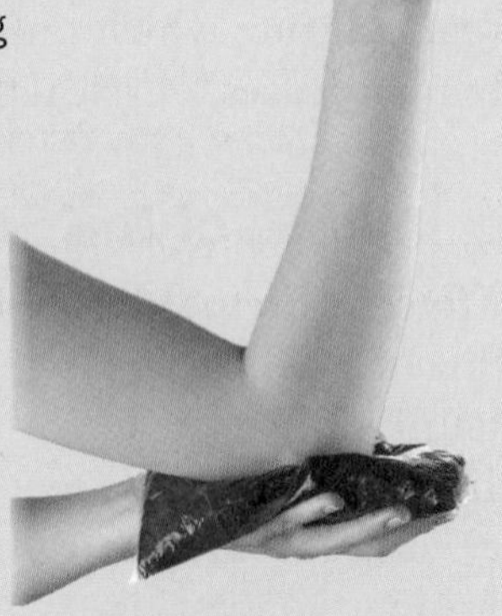

Melodia plus photos/Shutterstock.com

from abnormal motion of the cervical vertebrae, accompanied by rapid, forceful contractions of the neck muscles as the neuromuscular system attempts to stabilize and protect the spine. Symptoms may include neck muscle pain; pain or numbness extending down to the shoulders, arms, and even the hands; and headache.

SELF CHECK

1. Describe the differences among the three classifications of muscle strains.
2. Why are athletes more likely than others to have problems with strains?
3. What causes swimmer's shoulder?
4. What is the difference between tennis elbow and Little Leaguer's elbow?
5. What is the role of the neuromuscular system in whiplash injuries?

Muscle Disorders

In addition to injuries, the muscular system is subject to a variety of disorders and conditions. Two of the more common disorders are discussed in this section.

Muscular Dystrophy

Muscular dystrophy (MD) is a group of similar, inherited disorders characterized by progressively worsening muscle weakness and loss of muscle tissue. Depending on the specific type, the onset of MD may occur during either childhood or adulthood, and the symptoms vary.

Some forms of MD affect only certain muscle groups, whereas other forms affect all of the muscles. The more severe types of MD begin in childhood; symptoms may include intellectual disability, delayed development of motor skills, frequent falling, drooling, and drooping of the eyelids. Some forms of MD also affect the heart muscle, resulting in an irregular heartbeat.

There are no known cures for the various muscular dystrophies; the goal of treatment is to control symptoms. Some types of muscular dystrophy lead to a shortened life; others cause little disability, allowing for a normal life span.

Hernia

A ***hernia*** is a balloon-like section of tissue that protrudes through a hole or weakened section of a muscle, most commonly in the abdomen. A hernia can be caused by heavy lifting, or by any activity or medical problem that increases pressure on the tissue. In most cases, however, no specific cause is evident. Some hernias are present at birth, and some occur in infants and children. A hernia that is present at birth may not become noticeable until later in life.

Most hernias produce no symptoms, although some are accompanied by discomfort or pain that intensifies with heavy lifting or other activities that produce strain. A large hernia may strangulate, or cut off, the blood supply to the tissue inside the hernia. A strangulated hernia requires immediate surgery.

Small hernias that cause no symptoms do not necessarily require treatment. Larger hernias and those that cause discomfort can be permanently remedied with surgery.

SECTION 6.4 REVIEW

Mini-Glossary

contusion bruising or bleeding within a muscle as a result of an impact

delayed-onset muscle soreness (DOMS) muscle pain that follows participation in a particularly long or strenuous activity; begins 24–73 hours after activity and involves multiple, microscopic tears in the muscle tissue that cause inflammation, pain, swelling, and stiffness

hernia a balloon-like section of tissue that protrudes through a hole or weakened section of a muscle

muscle cramps moderate to severe muscle spasms that cause pain

muscle strain an injury that occurs when a muscle is stretched beyond the limits to which it is accustomed

muscular dystrophy (MD) a group of similar, inherited disorders characterized by progressively worsening muscle weakness and loss of muscle tissue

myositis ossificans a condition in which a calcium mass forms within a muscle three to four weeks after a muscle injury

shin splint pain that is localized to the anterior lower leg

(continued)

tendinitis inflammation of a tendon; usually accompanied by pain and swelling

tendinosis degeneration of a tendon believed to be caused by microtears in the tendon's connective tissue

Review Questions

1. What causes a muscle strain?
2. What can you do to increase your chances of avoiding muscle strains?
3. What is myositis ossificans? What problems can it cause?
4. What do shoulder, elbow, and shin injuries have in common?
5. What is the main cause of DOMS?
6. Why is it important to treat chronic tendinitis?
7. What is believed to be the main cause of shin splints?
8. Name an activity often associated with hernias.
9. If obesity is a major cause of LBP, why do gymnasts experience this health problem?
10. How do poor body mechanics contribute to overuse injuries such as swimmer's shoulder and tennis elbow? Describe and analyze the effect of torque in these injuries.

Medical Terminology: The Muscular System

By understanding the word parts that make up medical words, you can extend your medical vocabulary. This chapter includes many of the word parts listed below. Review these word parts to be sure you understand their meanings.

-al	pertaining to
-bradia	slowness
-clonus	twitching
dorsi-	back
dys-	bad, difficult, abnormal
flex/o	bend or flex
-genesis	birth, formation of
-ion	process
leio-	smooth
muscul/o	muscle
my/o	muscle
myom/o	muscle tumor
mysi/o	muscle fiber
neur/o	nerve
peri-	surrounding
-trophy	condition of

Now use these word parts to form valid medical words that fit the following definitions. Some of the words are included in this chapter. Others are not. When you finish, use a medical dictionary to check your work.

1. surrounding a muscle (fiber)
2. process of bending backward
3. condition of abnormal muscles
4. pertaining to both a muscle and a nerve
5. formation of a muscle
6. pertaining to both the muscles and the skeleton
7. tumor in smooth muscle
8. process of bending
9. muscle twitching
10. muscle slowness

Chapter 6 Summary

- The three major categories of muscle fibers are smooth, cardiac, and skeletal (striated).
- Muscles are either voluntary or involuntary and have four common behavioral characteristics: extensibility, elasticity, irritability, and contractility.
- Skeletal muscles work in an agonist/antagonist relationship and can experience concentric, eccentric, or isometric contractions.
- The motor unit is the functional unit of the neuromuscular system and is made up of the neuron and the muscle fibers that the neuron stimulates.
- Skeletal muscle fibers are classified as fast-twitch fibers, which are powerful and fatigue quickly, and slow-twitch fibers, which are fatigue-resistant.
- Sagittal plane movements are forward and backward actions; frontal plane movements take the body part toward or away from the midline of the body; and transverse plane movements are actions that move side to side or rotate around a longitudinal axis.
- The muscles of the head and neck can be divided into three groups: facial muscles, chewing muscles, and neck muscles.

- The trunk muscles provide stability for the vertebral column and help maintain posture.
- The upper limb sacrifices stability for increased range of motion when compared with the lower limb.
- The lower limb is designed for its primary jobs of standing and walking.
- Causes of muscular injuries include not only sports mishaps, but also accidents and overuse of muscles during everyday activities.
- Common muscle disorders include muscular dystrophy and hernias.

Chapter 6 Review

Understanding Key Concepts

1. The individual skeletal muscle cell is referred to as a(n) ______.
2. The three layers of muscle tissue, from the inside out, are ______, ______, and ______.
3. Skeletal muscle is connected to bone by either ______ or aponeuroses.
4. ______ muscle is found in organs and blood vessels.
5. The heart is made up of ______ muscle cells.
6. The ability of a muscle and other tissue to be stretched is the behavioral characteristic known as ______.
   A. extensibility
   B. elasticity
   C. irritability
   D. contractility
7. The ability of a muscle to respond to stimuli is the behavioral characteristic known as ______.
   A. extensibility
   B. elasticity
   C. irritability
   D. contractility
8. A nerve that stimulates skeletal muscle is called a(n) ______.
9. The functional unit of the neuromuscular system is the ______.
10. A(n) ______ is an electrical charge that creates tension within a muscle fiber.
11. ______-twitch muscle fibers contract powerfully but fatigue quickly.

Instructions: *Write the **letter** of the name of the **muscle** next to the corresponding number.*

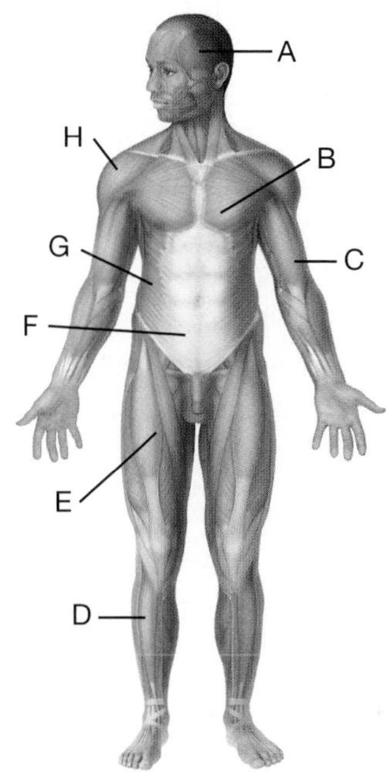

12. Deltoid
13. Abdominal aponeurosis
14. Biceps brachii
15. Rectus femoris
16. Temporalis
17. Pectoralis major
18. Tibialis anterior
19. External oblique
20. A muscle strain is classified as ______, ______, or ______.
21. A(n) ______ is a bruise or bleeding within a muscle.
22. A complication that can arise from a contusion is ______.
    A. sarcolemma
    B. myositis ossificans
    C. neuroma
    D. spondylosis
23. Which of the following is *not* a typical cause of cramps?
    A. electrolyte imbalance
    B. dehydration
    C. deficiency in minerals such as calcium or potassium
    D. lack of aerobic exercise

Thinking Critically

24. Discuss in depth the differences between concentric, isometric, and eccentric contractions and provide examples of how each one is used in daily life.
25. What do you think would be the pros and cons of body organs being made up exclusively of voluntary muscle (no involuntary muscle)? Provide specific examples and some pros and some cons for each.
26. Describe the structure of skeletal muscle.
27. Discuss muscle fiber arrangements that contribute to the force a muscle can generate.
28. How do you think slow-twitch muscle fibers are usually arranged? Give reasons for your answer.
29. Who generates more power: An Olympic weightlifter who must lift 400 pounds from the ground to a position over his head very rapidly, or a power lifter who must squat down and stand up with 800 pounds on his back? Defend your answer.
30. Discuss how torque is used to measure the strength of a muscle group at a specific joint.
31. Compare and contrast the sagittal and frontal planes. Be sure to discuss the movements that occur in each plane.
32. In circumduction, through which planes does the limb move, and what actions do you think are being utilized to make the conical/circular motion?
33. Do agonists and antagonists have to perform their actions in the same plane? Why?
34. If being active is considered healthy, why do you think active people and athletes have a significantly higher incidence of LBP than inactive, sedentary people?

Clinical Case Study

Read again the Clinical Case Study at the beginning of this chapter. Use the information provided in the chapter to answer the following questions.

35. What diagnoses are possible?
36. Which diagnosis is most likely given the description?
37. Given the description, what grade is this injury?

Analyzing and Evaluating Data

Use the bar graph to answer the following questions.

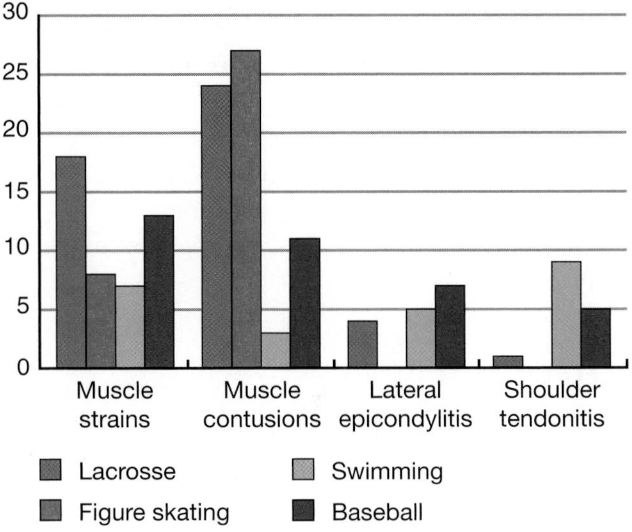

38. Which sport involves the most muscle strains?
39. Which sport involves the most muscle contusions?
40. What percentage of swimming injuries is attributed to muscle strains?
41. What is the approximate ratio of muscle contusions in figure skating to muscle contusions in baseball?
42. Compare the total number of swimming injuries with the total number of figure skating injuries.

Investigating Further

43. Consider the physiology involved in doing a push-up. Which muscles experience concentric contractions? Which muscles experience eccentric contractions? Which muscles experience isometric contractions? Through which plane(s) does the shoulder move? What actions occur at the shoulder, elbow, and wrist?
44. Try to switch the common ("normal") origin and insertion points of as many muscles as you can. Focus on the most frequent, everyday movements. Make a list and describe what you did to switch them. Hint: Compare origin and insertion points when doing straight-leg sit-ups and straight-leg leg lifts.

7 The Nervous System

Clinical Case Study

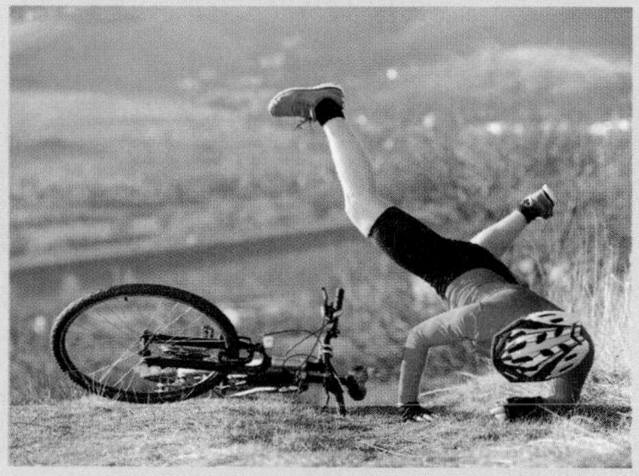
Halfpoint/Shutterstock.com

Julie and Miles are students at their local community college who were drawn together by their mutual love of cycling. As often as their schedules and the weather permit, they enjoy going for long rides on weekends.

Yesterday they were enjoying a nice ride on a back road when a pickup truck came barreling around a curve, causing them to have to swerve sharply and veer off the road to avoid being hit. Although Julie managed to stay upright on her bike, Miles hit a large rock and crashed, hitting his head. Fortunately, Miles was wearing a cycling helmet. But when he tried to stand up, he found that he was dizzy and within a short time he developed a bad headache.

Today Miles feels much better, but Julie insists that he visit the student health center to be checked out. Among the conditions listed in the chapter, which might Miles have sustained and which is most likely? Given the description, what grade was Miles' injury?

Chapter 7 Outline

To understand the nervous system, start by thinking of your body as a biological machine that runs on electricity. In fact, this is true! Your brain is the control center that sends and receives electrical impulses, or signals, throughout your body. The sophisticated communication system that delivers these electrical signals to and from the brain is your nervous system.

With all of this electrical activity going on, why doesn't the body light up? The answer is that the electrical charges within the body are very tiny. In the eighteenth century, Italian scientist Luigi Galvani discovered that muscle produces a detectable electric current, or voltage, when developing tension. But it was not until the twentieth century that technology became sophisticated enough to detect and record the extremely small electrical charges that move through the nervous system.

The activities performed by the nervous system are crucial. This chapter describes the anatomical structures that enable the nervous system to perform these functions so efficiently. The chapter also discusses some of the common injuries and disorders of the nervous system, along with their symptoms and treatments.

SECTION 7.1 Anatomy of the Nervous System

Objectives

- Explain the general organization of the human nervous system.
- Describe the types of tissue present in the nervous system and identify the general role of each.

Key Terms

afferent nerves
autonomic nervous system
axon
cell body
central nervous system (CNS)
dendrites
efferent nerves
myelin sheath
neurilemma
neuroglia
neuron
nodes of Ranvier
peripheral nervous system (PNS)
somatic nervous system
synapse
synaptic cleft

The human nervous system has an amazing ability to direct a whole host of different functions simultaneously. The nervous system not only controls voluntary movement by activating skeletal muscle, but it also directs the involuntary functions of smooth muscle in internal organs and cardiac muscle in the heart.

By automatically controlling the functions of smooth muscle and cardiac muscle, the nervous system ensures that these life functions can occur without conscious thought. At the same time that your heart is beating and your latest meal is making its way through your digestive tract, you may be talking to a friend, walking to a class, or even reading this book.

In addition to its interaction with the muscular system, the nervous system also plays a role in the sensory system. The senses—the ability to see, hear, smell, taste, feel pressure, and feel pain—all depend on sensory electrical input from specialized receptors.

For the purpose of discussion, the nervous system is organized into structural and functional subdivisions. This organization makes it easier to learn about the activities directed by the various parts of the nervous system, and how these parts interact.

Nervous System Organization

Because the nervous system is complex, it helps to discuss its components from both a structural perspective and a functional perspective. This section describes these two different approaches to the organization of the nervous system. The structure and function of the parts of the system are examined in greater detail later in the chapter. **Figure 7.1** presents a schematic overview of the structural and functional aspects of the nervous system.

Structural Divisions

The human nervous system has two major structural divisions: the central nervous system and the peripheral nervous system. The ***central nervous system (CNS)*** includes the brain and spinal cord. The CNS directs the activity of the entire nervous system. Injuries to either the brain or the spinal cord have serious consequences and can be life threatening. Fortunately, these delicate structures are well protected inside the skull and vertebral column.

The parts of the nervous system other than the brain and spinal cord make up the ***peripheral nervous system (PNS)***. The PNS includes spinal nerves that transmit information to and from the spinal cord and cranial nerves that transmit information to and from the brain. The PNS also includes specialized nerve endings called *sensory receptors*, which respond to stimuli such as pressure, pain, and temperature.

Functional Divisions

The nervous system also has two functional classifications. Nerves that transmit impulses from the sensory receptors in the skin, muscles, and joints to the CNS are known as ***afferent*** (sensory) ***nerves***. Those that carry impulses from the CNS out to the muscles and glands are ***efferent*** (motor) ***nerves***.

Understanding Medical Terminology

Afferent nerves tell the body how it is being *affected* by stimuli such as light, heat, and pressure. *Efferent* nerves stimulate muscles to produce *effort*.

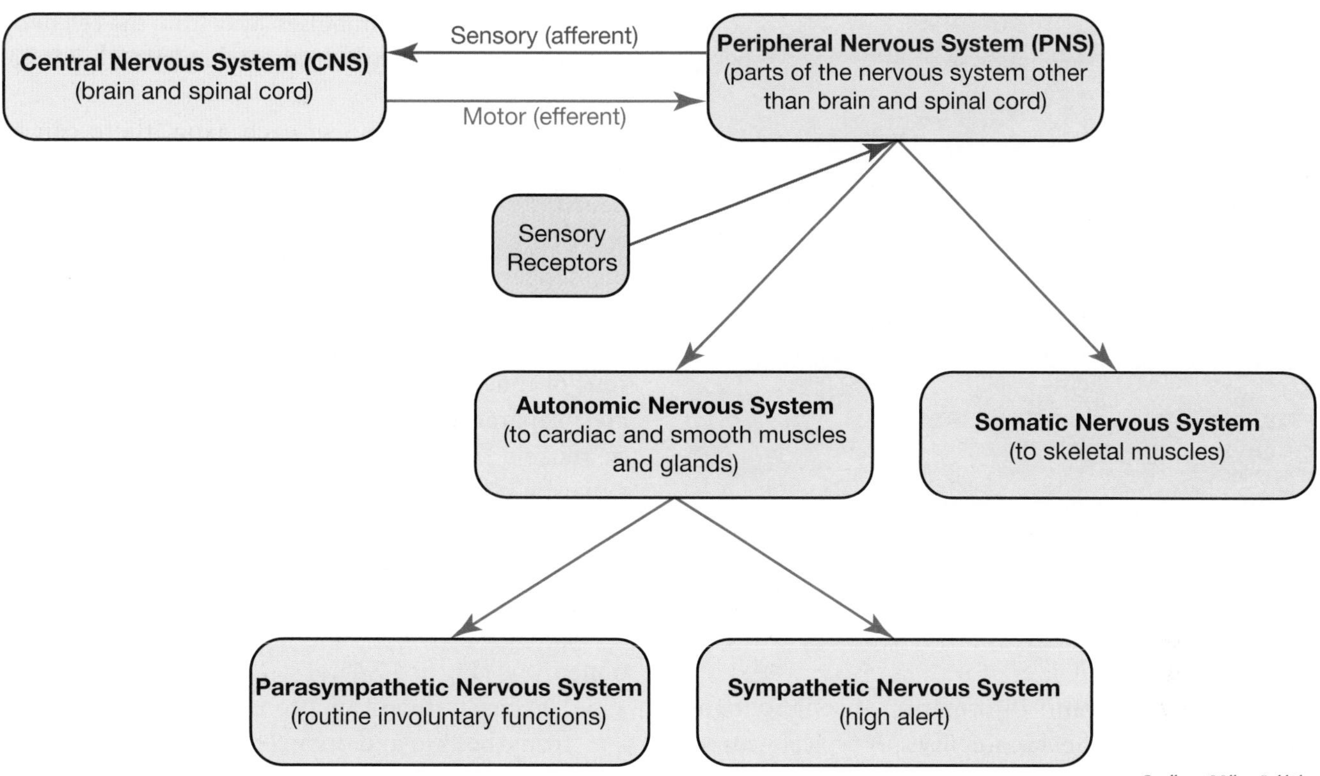

Figure 7.1 This diagram represents the organization of the nervous system and summarizes the relationships among the subdivisions.

The Afferent Nerves

Afferent, or sensory, nerves deliver information in the form of electrical impulses from sensory receptors located all over the body to the central nervous system. Nerve fibers transmitting impulses from receptors in the skin, muscles, and joints are known as *somatic sensory fibers*. Impulses originating in the visceral organs are transmitted by *visceral sensory fibers*.

The Efferent Nerves

The efferent, or motor, nerves have two functional subdivisions. The ***somatic*** (voluntary) ***nervous system*** stimulates the skeletal muscles, causing them to develop tension. The ***autonomic*** (involuntary) ***nervous system*** controls the cardiac muscle of the heart and the smooth muscles of the internal organs. The autonomic nervous system prompts the heart to beat faster during exercise and causes the smooth muscle activities that move food through the digestive system. Thanks to the autonomic nervous system, people do not have to think about everyday body functions that sustain life.

Under certain circumstances, such as when you inadvertently touch a hot surface, the efferent neurons can trigger involuntary action of the skeletal muscles through a reflex arc. The sympathetic and parasympathetic branches of the autonomic nervous system are discussed later in the chapter.

Becoming aware of these various subdivisions will help you learn and understand the nervous system's various functional capabilities. Keep in mind, however, that the nervous system functions as a single, remarkably coordinated unit.

SELF CHECK

1. Which structures make up the central nervous system (CNS)?
2. Which structures make up the peripheral nervous system (PNS)?
3. For which function is the somatic nervous system responsible?
4. For which functions is the autonomic nervous system responsible?

Cells of the Nervous System

Two specialized types of cells exist within the nervous system. These cell types are neurons and supporting cells called *neuroglia* (**Figure 7.2**).

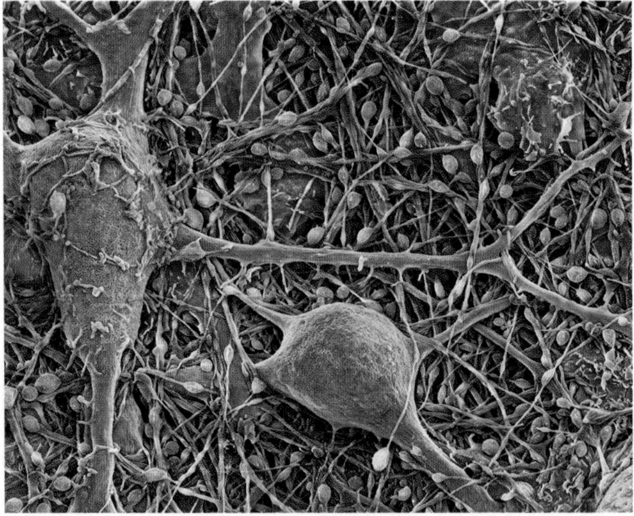

Figure 7.2 A scanning electromicrograph of neurons and neuroglia.

Neurons

The ***neurons*** transmit information throughout the body in the form of nerve impulses. A typical neuron, or nerve cell, consists of a cell body surrounded by branching dendrites and a long, tail-like projection called an *axon* (**Figure 7.3**).

Like all cell bodies, the ***cell body*** of a neuron includes a nucleus, mitochondria, and other organelles. Centrioles, however, are not present in neurons because most neurons are not capable of replication. The ***dendrites*** collect stimuli and transport them to the cell body. ***Axons*** transmit impulses away from the cell body. A neuron may have hundreds of dendrites, but it has only one axon.

At the terminal end of each axon, there can be thousands of axon terminals that connect with other neurons or muscles. These axon terminals are filled with tiny sacs, or vesicles, that contain chemical messengers called *neurotransmitters*. The function of neurotransmitters is described later in this chapter.

Axon terminals do not actually touch adjacent neurons or muscles. A microscopic gap called a ***synaptic cleft*** separates axon terminals from other neurons or muscle fibers. This intersection, including the synaptic cleft, is known as a ***synapse***. As you may recall from Chapter 6, the synapse between an axon terminal and a muscle fiber is called the *neuromuscular junction*.

When classified by function, there are three types of neurons (**Figure 7.4**):

- Sensory (afferent) neurons carry impulses from the skin and organs to the spinal cord and brain, providing information about the external and internal environments.
- Motor (efferent) neurons transmit impulses from the brain and spinal cord to the muscles and glands, directing body actions.
- Interneurons, association neurons, form bridges to transmit impulses to other neurons.

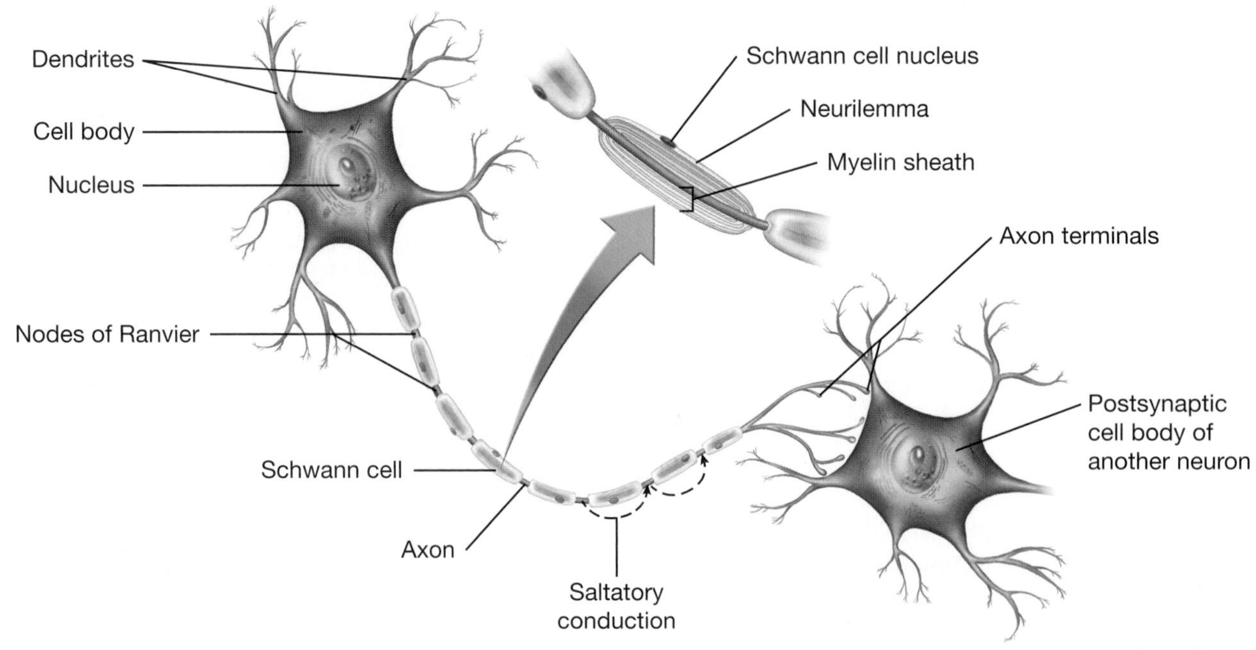

Figure 7.3 A typical neuron.

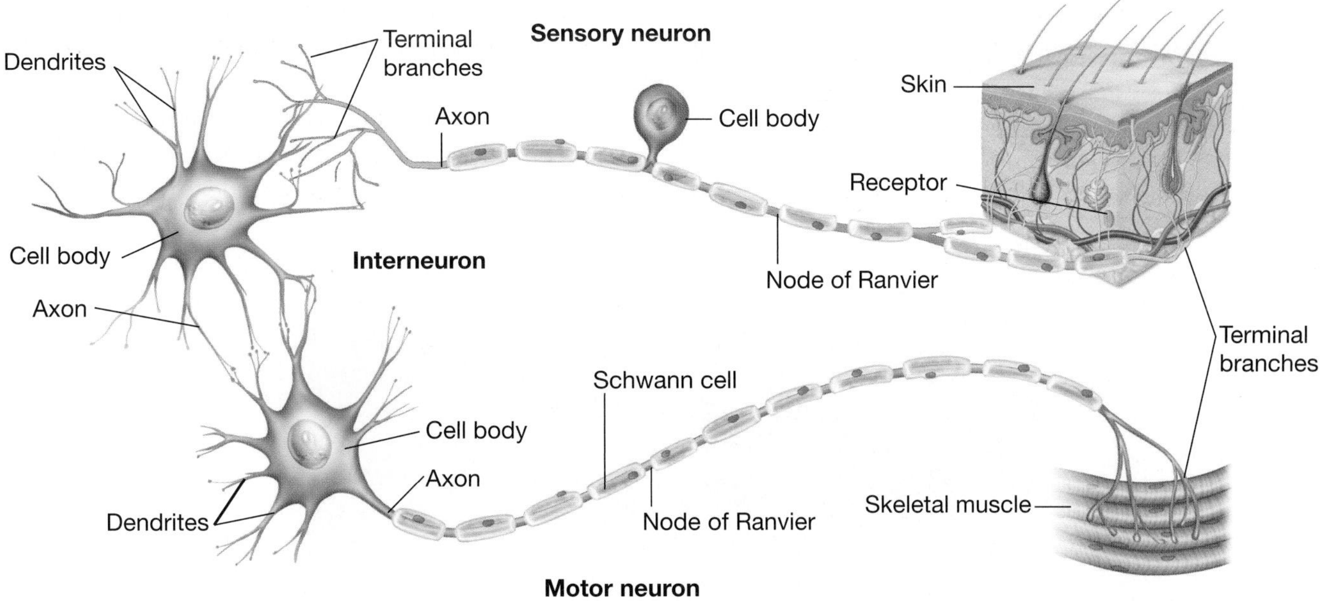

© Body Scientific International

Figure 7.4 The three types of neurons are sensory neurons, interneurons, and motor neurons.

As shown in **Figure 7.5**, there are also three different neuron structures:

- *Bipolar neurons* have one axon and one dendrite. These are sensory processing cells such as those found in the eyes and nose.
- *Unipolar neurons* have a single axon with processes that extend in opposite directions. They have dendrites on the peripheral end and axon terminals on the central end. The peripheral process carries impulses to the cell body, while the central process carries impulses to the central nervous system. Some of the sensory neurons in the PNS are unipolar.
- *Multipolar neurons* have one axon and multiple dendrites. All motor neurons and interneurons are multipolar.

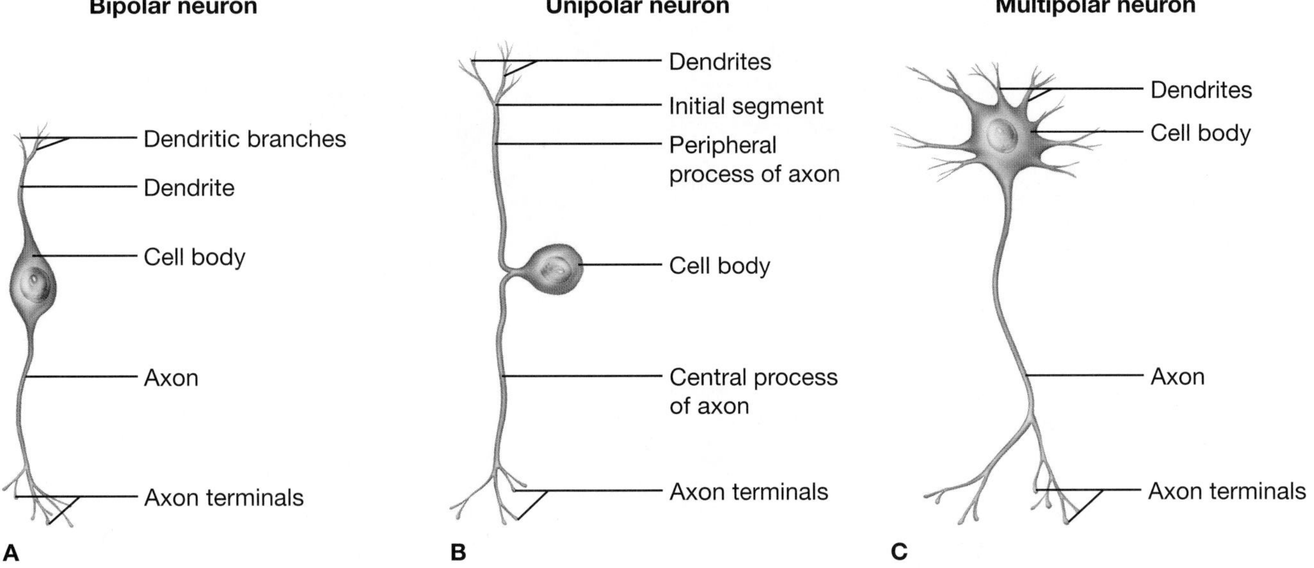

© Body Scientific International

Figure 7.5 Different neuron structures. A—Bipolar neurons have an axon with two processes: a central process that carries impulses to the CNS, and a peripheral process that carries impulses to the cell body. B—Unipolar neurons have a single axon process, with the cell body in the middle and to the side. C—Multipolar neurons have a single axon and multiple dendrites.

Neuroglia

The ***neuroglia*** (ner-ROHG-lee-a), also known as *glial* (GLIGH-al) *cells,* are specialized cells that perform support functions (**Figure 7.6**). Four types of glial cells occur only in the CNS:

- Astrocytes are positioned between neurons and capillaries; they link the nutrient-supplying capillaries to neurons and control the chemical environment to protect the neurons from any harmful substances in the blood. Astrocytes account for nearly half of all neural tissue.

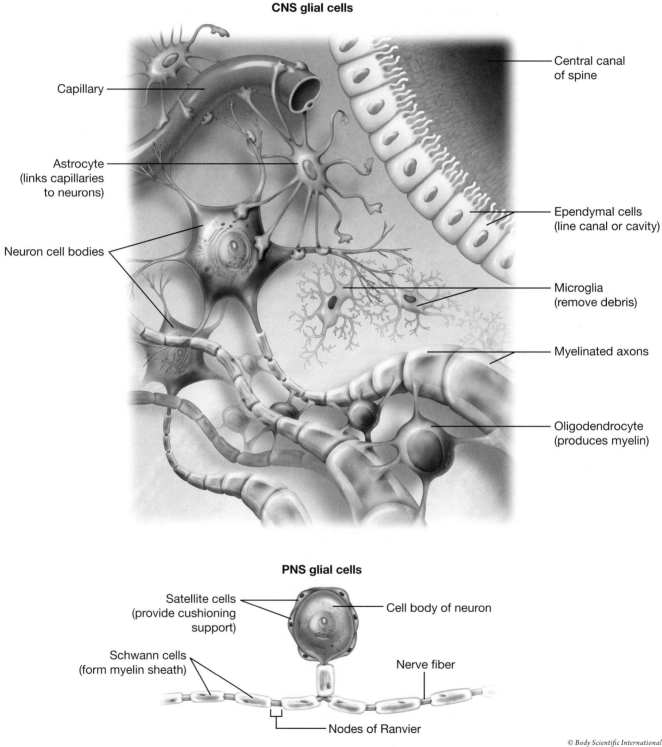

CNS glial cells

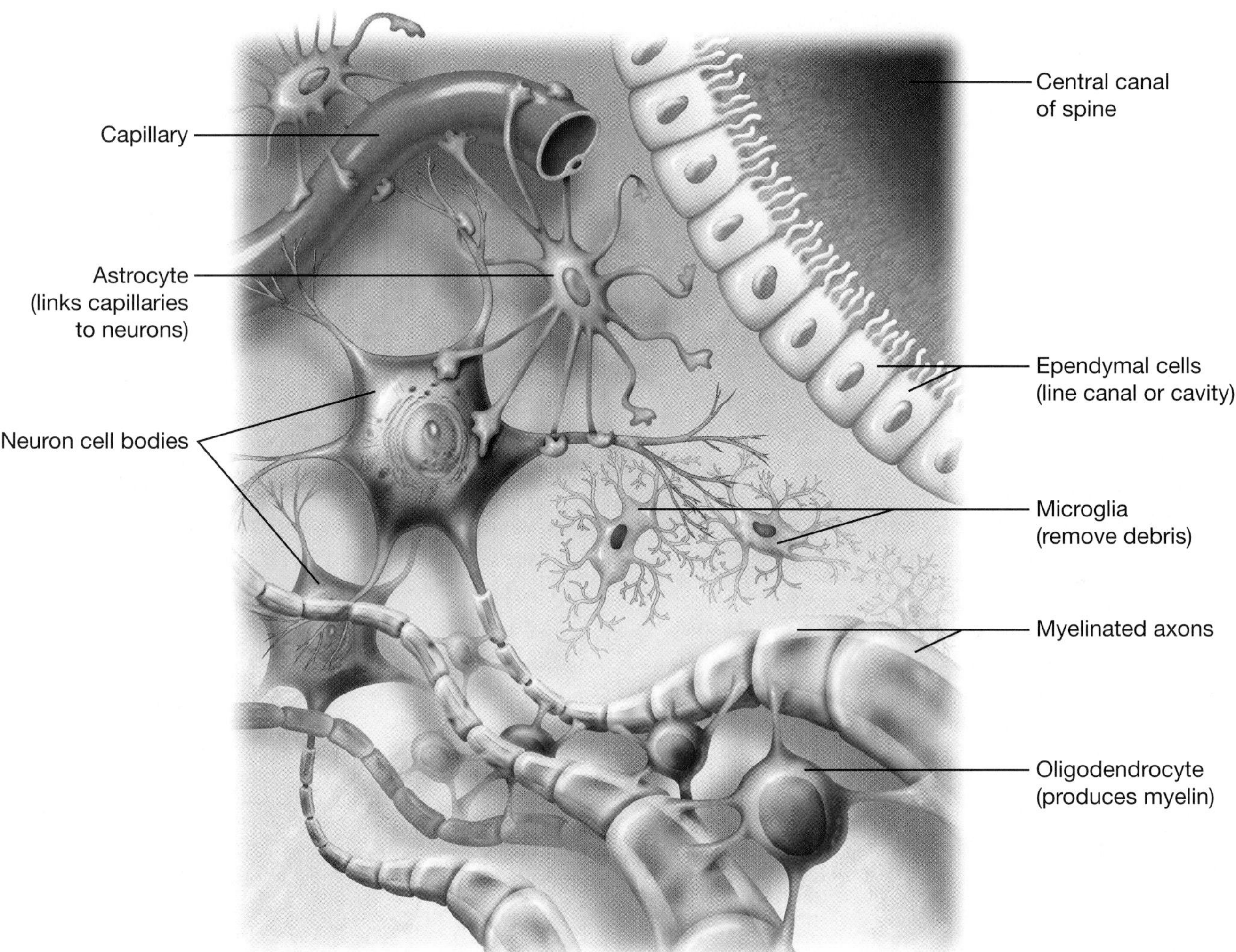

PNS glial cells

Figure 7.6 The glial cells of the central nervous system and peripheral nervous system.

- Microglia absorb and dispose of dead cells and bacteria.
- Ependymal cells form a protective covering around the spinal cord and central cavities within the brain.
- Oligodendrocytes wrap around nerve fibers and produce a fatty insulating material called *myelin.*

Two types of glial cells occur only in the PNS:

- Satellite cells serve as cushioning supports for neurons.
- Schwann cells form the fatty myelin sheaths around nerve fibers in the PNS.

Schwann cells wrap around the axon of a neuron, covering most of it with a fatty ***myelin sheath***. The myelin sheaths serve an important purpose: to insulate the axon fibers, which increases the rate of neural impulse transmission.

The external covering of a Schwann cell, outside the myelin sheath, is called the ***neurilemma***. The uninsulated gaps, where the axon is exposed between the Schwann cells, are known as the ***nodes of Ranvier*** (rahn-vee-AY). The myelin sheaths are white, giving rise to the term *white matter* to describe tracts of myelinated fibers within the CNS. *Gray matter* is the term for unmyelinated nerve fibers. Bundles of nerve fibers (axons) are called *tracts* when they are located within the CNS. In the PNS, bundles of nerve fibers are simply called *nerves.*

SECTION 7.1 REVIEW

Mini-Glossary

afferent nerves sensory transmitters that send impulses from receptors in the skin, muscles, and joints to the central nervous system

autonomic nervous system the branch of the nervous system that controls involuntary body functions

axon a long, tail-like projection found on a typical nerve that transmits impulses away from the cell body

cell body the part of an axon that contains a nucleus and other common organelles

central nervous system (CNS) division of the nervous system that includes the brain and spinal cord

dendrites branches of a neuron that collect stimuli and transport them to the cell body of a neuron

efferent nerves motor transmitters that carry impulses from the central nervous system to the muscles and glands

myelin sheath the fatty band of insulation surrounding an axon fiber

neurilemma the thin, membranous sheath enveloping a nerve fiber

neuroglia cells that form the interstitial or supporting elements of the CNS; also known as *glial cells*

neuron specialized nerve cell that transmits information throughout the body in the form of electrical impulses

nodes of Ranvier the uninsulated gaps in the myelin sheath of a nerve fiber, where the axon is exposed

peripheral nervous system (PNS) the division of the nervous system that contains all parts of the nervous system external to the brain and spinal cord

somatic nervous system the branch of the nervous system that stimulates the skeletal muscles

synapse the intersection between two neurons, or between a neuron and a muscle, gland, or sensory receptor

synaptic cleft a microscopic gap that separates neurons

Review Questions

1. Explain how the nervous system is organized, including subdivisions of each component.
2. What is a sensory receptor?
3. Which nerves—the afferent or efferent—are also referred to as *motor nerves*? Why?
4. List the three parts of a typical neuron and state the function of each part.
5. What do the tiny sacs inside axon terminals contain?
6. Identify two ways of classifying neurons.
7. Explain the difference among bipolar, unipolar, and multipolar neurons.
8. Describe a synapse using the terminology presented in this chapter.
9. Explain the negative effects on a neuron when the myelin sheath is damaged or destroyed by a demyelinating disorder.

SECTION 7.2

Impulse Transmission

Objectives

- Explain what action potentials are and how they are generated.
- Explain the factors that influence the speed of neural impulse transmission.
- Describe the role of neurotransmitters in transmitting impulses across synapses.
- Describe the three types of reflexes and explain how they work.

Key Terms

action potential
autonomic reflexes
conductivity
depolarized
neurotransmitter
polarized
reflexes
refractory period
repolarization
saltatory conduction
somatic reflexes

Neurons have one behavioral property in common with muscles: irritability, or the ability to respond to a stimulus. However, neurons have an aspect of irritability that muscles do not have: the ability to convert a stimulus into a nerve impulse. ***Conductivity***, the other behavioral property of neurons, is the ability to transmit nerve impulses. A nerve impulse is a tiny electrical charge that transmits information between neurons. This section explores the processes by which nerve impulses are created and spread throughout the nervous system.

Action Potentials

When a neuron is inactive or at rest, there are potassium (K^+) ions inside the cell and sodium (Na^+) ions outside the cell membrane. The overall distribution of ions is such that the inside of the membrane is more negatively charged than the outside. Because of this difference in electrical charge, the cell membrane is said to be ***polarized***. When the membrane is polarized and more negative inside than outside, the neuron is inactive.

Many different stimuli can activate a neuron. A bright light in the eyes, a bitter taste on the tongue, or the reception of neurotransmitter chemicals from another neuron are all possible stimuli. In all cases, if a stimulus exceeds a critical voltage, hundreds of gated sodium channels in the cell membrane briefly open. This allows the sodium ions outside the cell to rapidly diffuse into the neuron. As a result, the area inside the membrane becomes more positively charged and the cell membrane is ***depolarized***.

Depolarization of the cell membrane opens more gated ion channels in the membrane, generating a wave of depolarization along the neuron. This wave of electrical charge is known as a *nerve impulse*, or ***action potential***, which executes in an all-or-none fashion. This means that the electrical charge of the action potential is always the same size, and once initiated, it always travels the full length of the axon.

Following the discharge of the action potential, the membrane becomes permeable to (accepting of) potassium ions, which rapidly diffuse out of the cell. This begins the process of restoring the membrane to its original, polarized resting state, a process called ***repolarization***. Until the cell membrane is repolarized, it cannot respond to another stimulus. The time between the completion of the action potential and repolarization is called the ***refractory period***. During the refractory period, the neuron is temporarily "fatigued," and is unresponsive to further excitation.

SELF CHECK

1. What electrical conditions exist when a cell membrane is polarized?
2. What is a refractory period?

Transmission Speed

Two factors have a major impact on the speed at which a nerve impulse travels: the presence or absence of a myelin sheath and the diameter of the axon. Because the fatty myelin sheath is an electrical insulator, action potentials in a myelinated axon "jump over" the myelinated regions of the axon. Depolarization occurs only at the nodes of Ranvier, where the axon is exposed. This process, which is known as ***saltatory conduction***, results in significantly faster impulse transmission than is possible in nonmyelinated axons.

Impulse transmission is also much faster in nonmyelinated axons with larger diameters than in those with smaller diameters. The larger the axon, the greater the number of ions there are to conduct a current. This is somewhat like the advantage of a large-diameter pipe versus a small-diameter pipe when transferring water from one place to another.

A third factor that influences transmission speed is body temperature. Warmer temperatures increase ion diffusion rates, whereas local cooling, which occurs when holding an ice cube, for example, decreases ion diffusion rates.

The type and size of the nerve axon have much to do with the speed of nerve impulses. Impulses that signal limb position to the brain travel extremely fast—up to 119 meters per second (m/s). Information or impulses from the objects people touch travel more slowly, at around 76 m/s. The sensation of pain moves even more slowly, at less than 1 m/s. Thought signals, which are happening right now as you are reading, transmit at 20–30 m/s. For a nerve to transmit impulses at speeds greater than 1 m/s, it must have a myelinated axon.

SELF CHECK

1. What conditions cause a cell membrane to be polarized?
2. Do action potentials occur when neuron cell membranes are polarized or depolarized?
3. What factors influence the speed at which a nerve impulse travels?

Neurotransmitters

Communication between most neurons occurs at synapses, with a chemical neurotransmitter relaying the impulse from one neuron to the next. Because the action potential is electrical, and the process at the synapse is chemical, transmission of nerve impulses across synapses is said to be an electrochemical event.

When an action potential reaches an axon terminal, the terminal depolarizes, the calcium gates open, and calcium (Ca^{++}) ions flow into the terminal. The axon terminal is filled with tiny vesicles containing ***neurotransmitter*** chemicals (**Figure 7.7**). The influx of calcium causes these vesicles to join to the cell membrane adjacent to the synaptic cleft. Pores then form in the membrane, allowing the neurotransmitter to diffuse across the synapse to receptors on the membrane of the adjoining neuron or muscle fiber.

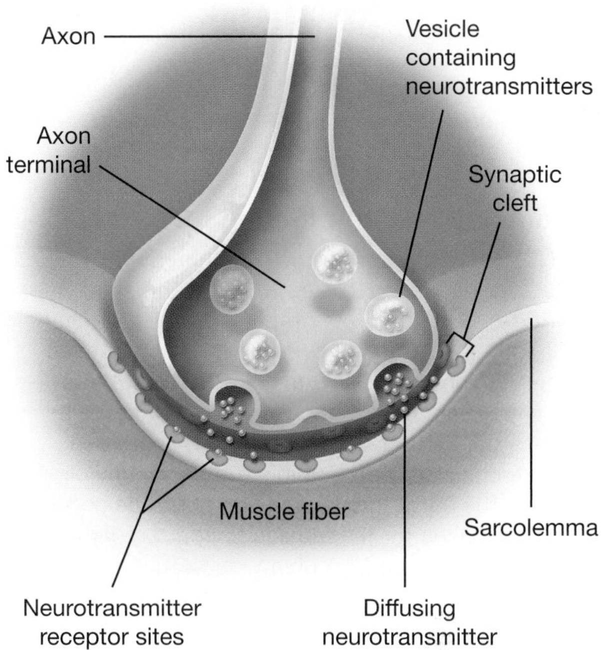

© Body Scientific International

Figure 7.7 The synapse is the site at which the neurotransmitter is released from the nerve axon terminal. The neurotransmitter then diffuses across the synaptic cleft to receptor sites on the next nerve cell body, or to a muscle fiber.

The nervous system uses several different neurotransmitters, and each has a different effect. For example, neurotransmitters can have an excitatory effect or an inhibitory effect on the receiving cell. An example of an excitatory neurotransmitter is acetylcholine, the chemical that activates muscle fibers. By contrast, endorphins are neurotransmitters released to inhibit nerve cells from discharging more pain signals.

The final step in communication between nerves at a synapse is the removal of the neurotransmitter, usually by an enzyme, to prevent ongoing stimulation of the receptor cell. Acetylcholine, for example, is deactivated by the enzyme acetylcholinesterase.

In some specialized nerve cells, communication occurs in the absence of a neurotransmitter through direct transfer of electrical charges at electrical synapses. Located within sites called *gap junctions,* these synapses are much narrower than chemical synapses. The intercalated discs between cardiac muscle fibers, for example, serve as gap junctions.

Research Notes: Measuring Nerve Impulses

How do scientists and clinicians measure the speed and function of nerve impulses? One common method is to use a nerve conduction velocity (NCV) test.

Conducting and Interpreting NCV Tests

The NCV test begins with the attachment of three small, flat, disc-shaped electrodes to the skin. One electrode is attached over the nerve being studied, and another is attached over the muscle supplied by the nerve. The third electrode is attached over a bony site, such as the elbow or ankle, to serve as an electrical ground.

The technician then administers short, tiny electrical pulses to the nerve through the first electrode and records the time it takes for the muscle to contract, as sensed by the second electrode. Computer software calculates the NCV as the distance between the stimulating and sensing electrodes divided by the elapsed time between stimulation and contraction.

Adjustments may be made to this general procedure to gather different information. Placing stimulating electrodes at two or more different locations along the same nerve makes it possible to determine the NCV across different segments of the nerve. To test for sensory neuron function, the stimulating electrode is placed over a region of sensory receptors, such as a fingertip. The recording electrode is then placed at a distance up the limb.

How are the results of a clinical NCV test interpreted? An NCV that is significantly slower than normal suggests damage to the myelin sheath. Alternatively, if the NCV is slow but close to the normal range, damage to the axons of the involved neurons may be suspected. Evaluation of the overall pattern of responses can serve as a diagnostic tool that helps a clinician determine the pathology involved in an abnormal NCV.

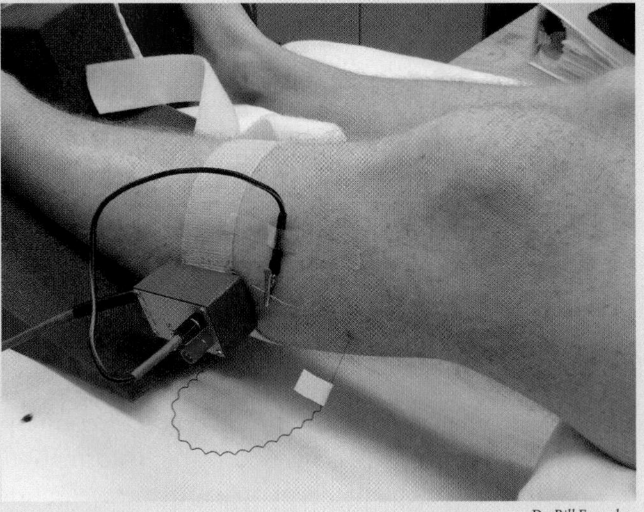

Dr. Bill Farquhar

Microneurography is a technique involving insertion of fine wire electrodes into a nerve for direct recording of electrical impulse activity.

Microneurography

Scientists have used a similar but more sophisticated procedure called *microneurography* to record electrical activity from single sensory fibers. This technique involves the direct insertion of fine-tipped wire electrodes into the nerve being studied.

The use of microneurography has enabled scientists to develop their current understanding of the sympathetic nervous system. Topics studied include various reflexes, interactions within the sympathetic nervous system, metabolism, hormones, and the effects of drugs or anesthesia during operative procedures. Sympathetic recordings have also been used to study the effects of performance at high altitudes, as well as in space.

SELF CHECK

1. Which neurotransmitter activates muscle fibers?
2. In what ways are electrical synapses different from chemical synapses?

Reflexes

Reflexes are simple, rapid, involuntary, programmed responses to stimuli. The transmission of impulses follows a reflex arc that includes both PNS and CNS structures (**Figure 7.8**). There are two types of reflexes.

Somatic reflexes are those that involve stimulation of skeletal muscles. For example, have you ever quickly withdrawn your hand from something hot, even before you realized that it was hot? If so, you were experiencing a somatic reflex. In such a situation, the motion of your hand occurs so quickly because a motor nerve has been directly stimulated by a sensory neuron, by way of an interneuron in the spinal cord. The signal between neurons is so fast because it does not have to travel to the brain and back.

Autonomic reflexes are those that regulate the cardiac muscle of the heart and the smooth muscle of internal organs. These activities include digestion, elimination, sweating, and blood pressure.

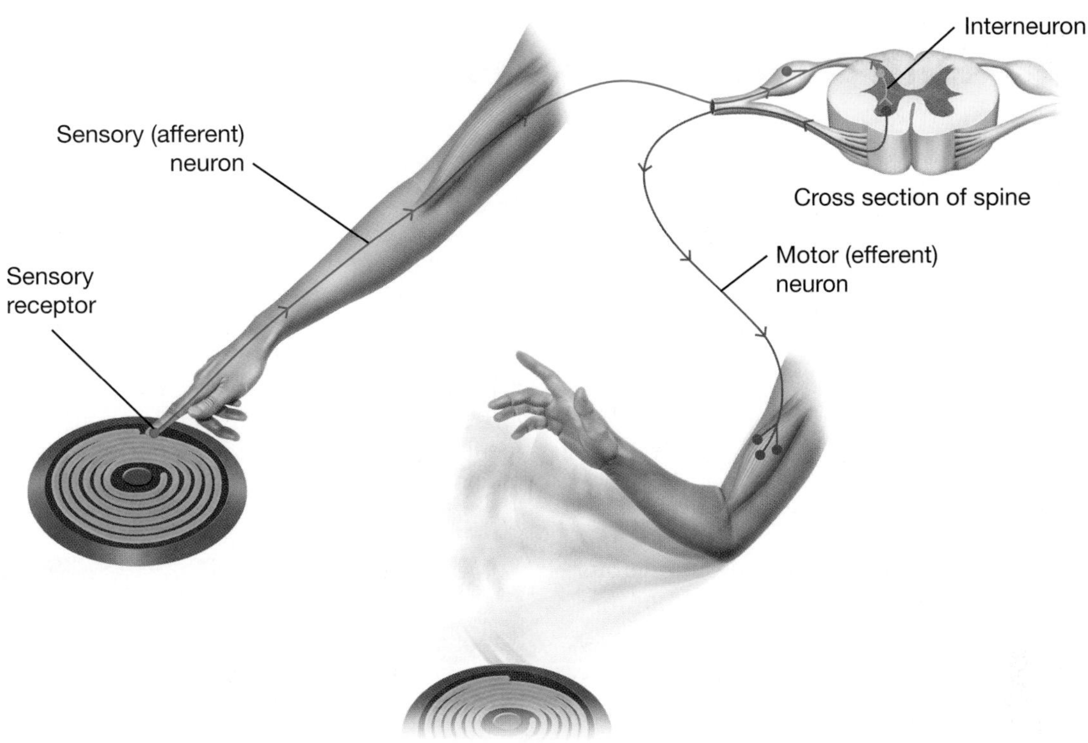

© Body Scientific International

Figure 7.8 A sensory receptor is stimulated by a hot surface, sending an afferent signal to the spinal cord. The signal is then transferred by an interneuron directly to a motor neuron, stimulating quick removal of the hand from the hot surface.

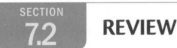

SECTION 7.2 REVIEW

Mini-Glossary

action potential an electrical charge that travels along a nerve fiber when stimulated

autonomic reflexes involuntary stimuli transmitted to cardiac and smooth muscle

conductivity the ability of a neuron to transmit a nerve impulse

depolarized a condition in which the inside of a cell membrane is more positively charged than the outside

neurotransmitter chemical used to pass along a message by carrying a signal from an axon to a receptor cell

polarized a condition in which the inside of a cell membrane is more negatively charged than the outside

reflexes simple, rapid, involuntary, programmed responses to stimuli

refractory period the time between the completion of the action potential and repolarization

repolarization the reestablishment of a polarized state in a cell after depolarization

saltatory conduction the process in which an action potential rapidly skips from node to node on myelinated neurons

somatic reflexes involuntary stimuli transmitted to skeletal muscles from neural arcs in the spinal cord

Review Questions

1. Name two behavioral properties of a nerve impulse.
2. Describe a neuron at rest compared to a neuron activated by a stimulus.
3. What has to happen before a cell membrane can respond to a second stimulus?
4. What effect does a myelin sheath have on nerve impulses?
5. How does body temperature affect the conduction speed of an electrical impulse?
6. What are the two categories of reflexes?
7. How would submerging a person in a tub of cold water affect the conduction speeds of the person's nerve impulses?
8. Is conduction of nerve impulses always faster in axons with a larger diameter compared to axons with a smaller diameter? Explain.
9. Aside from touching a hot surface, in what other circumstances might a sensory receptor bypass the brain and stimulate an interneuron to instigate quick action?

SECTION 7.3

Central Nervous System

Objectives

- Identify and describe the major parts of the brain, including the cerebrum, diencephalon, brain stem, cerebellum, meninges, and blood-brain barrier.
- Explain the structure and functions of the spinal cord.

Key Terms

cerebellum
cerebrum
diencephalon
epithalamus
fissures
frontal lobes
hypothalamus
lobes
medulla oblongata
meninges
midbrain
occipital lobes
parietal lobes
pons
primary motor cortex
primary somatic sensory cortex
spinal cord
temporal lobes
thalamus

The central nervous system includes numerous anatomical structures with specialized functions. Using sophisticated imaging techniques, scientists have been able to identify which structures control or contribute to various physiological processes and actions.

Brain

As you might expect, given its all-important role in directing the activity of the entire nervous system, the brain is structurally and functionally complex. The adult human brain weighs between 2.25 and 3.25 pounds and contains approximately 100 billion neurons and even more glial cells. Recent research indicates that the size of a person's brain does have some relationship to intelligence; about 6.7% of individual variation in intelligence is attributed to brain size. The four major anatomic regions of the brain are the cerebrum, diencephalon, brain stem, and cerebellum. The primary functions of these structures are summarized in **Figure 7.9.**

Functions of the Brain	
Cerebral Lobes	
Part of Brain	**Primary Functions**
frontal lobe	memory, intelligence, behavior, emotions, motor function, smell
parietal lobe	somatic sensations (pain, touch, hot/cold), speech
occipital lobe	vision, speech
temporal lobe	hearing, smell, memory, speech
Diencephalon	
Part of Brain	**Primary Functions**
thalamus	relays sensory impulses up to the sensory cortex
hypothalamus	autonomic center regulating metabolism, heart rate, blood pressure, thirst, hunger, energy level, and body temperature
epithalamus	regulates hormones secreted by pineal gland
Brain Stem	
Part of Brain	**Primary Functions**
midbrain	relays sensory and motor impulses
pons	assists with regulation of breathing
medulla oblongata	regulates heart rate, blood pressure, and breathing, and controls the reflexes of coughing, sneezing, and vomiting
reticular formation	regulates waking from slumber and heightened states of awareness
Cerebellum	
Part of Brain	**Primary Functions**
cerebellum	coordinates body movements and balance

Figure 7.9 *Goodheart-Willcox Publisher*

Cerebrum

The left and right cerebral hemispheres are collectively referred to as the ***cerebrum***, which makes up the largest portion of the brain. The outer surface of the cerebrum, known as the *cerebral cortex*, is composed of nonmyelinated gray matter. The internal tissue is myelinated white matter, with small, interspersed regions of gray matter called *basal nuclei*.

As you can see in **Figure 7.10**, the surface of the brain is not smooth; instead, it is convoluted. Each of the curved, raised areas is called a *gyrus* (JIGH-rus), and each of the grooves between the gyri is called

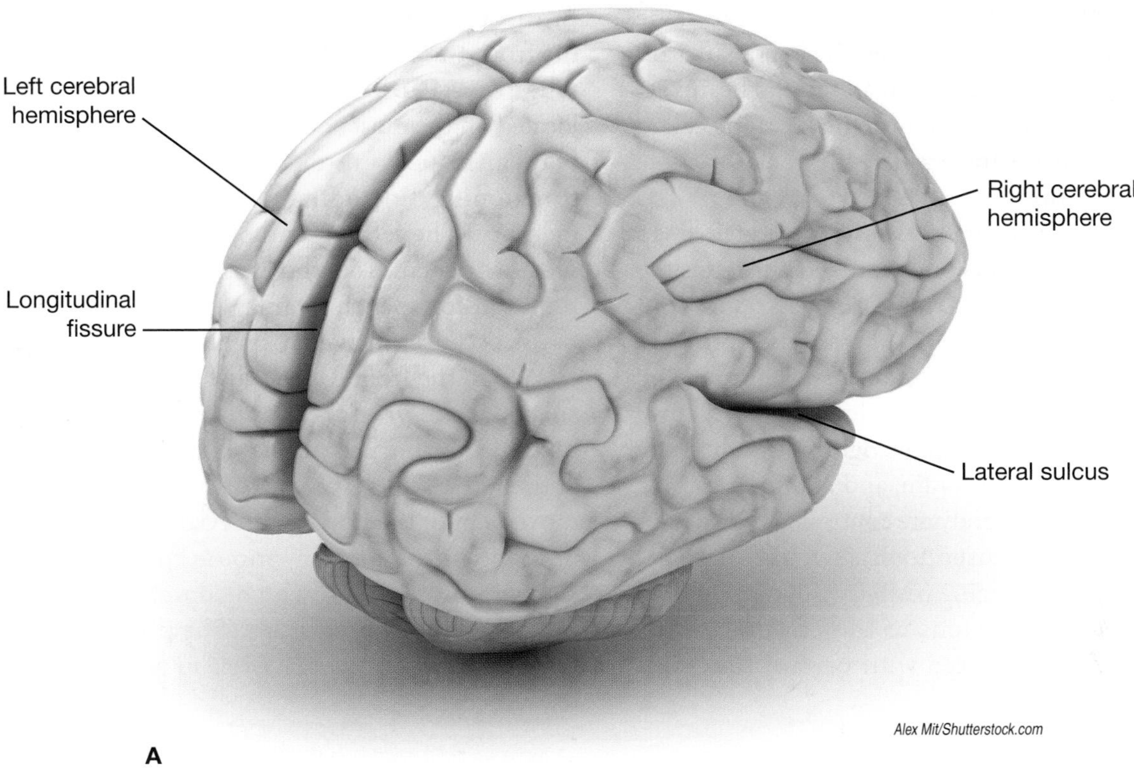

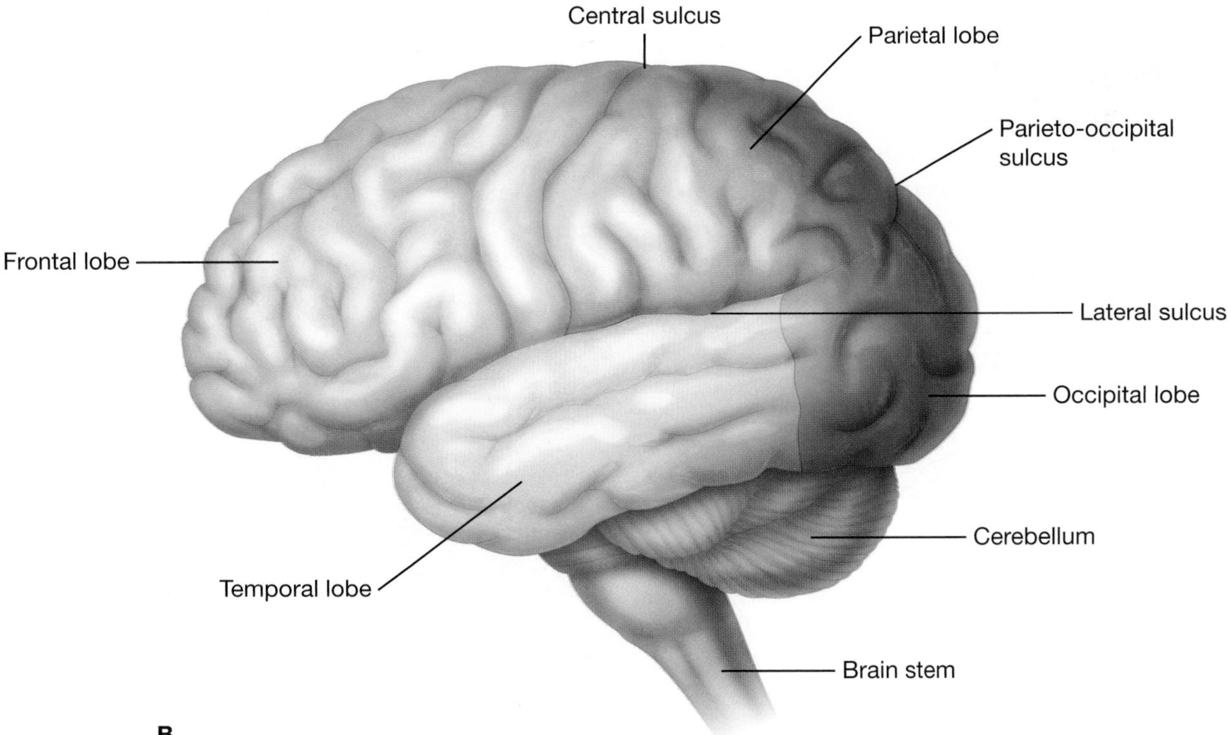

© Body Scientific International

Figure 7.10 A—The hemispheres of the cerebrum. B—The four lobes of the cerebrum are separated by sulci.

a *sulcus*. Together, these structures are referred to as *convolutions*. No two brains have exactly the same pattern of convolutions. However, the major sulci are arranged in the same pattern on all human brains.

The sulci divide the brain into four regions called ***lobes***. The four lobes of the brain are the frontal, parietal, occipital, and temporal.

Like sulci, ***fissures*** are uniformly positioned, deep grooves in the brain. The longitudinal fissure runs the length of the brain and divides it into left and right hemispheres. The left and right hemispheres are connected by the corpus callosum, a large, myelinated tract containing over 200 million axons. Neural communications to and from the right side of the body are controlled by the left brain, and communications with the left side of the body are controlled by the right brain. Scientists have used tools such as functional magnetic resonance imaging (fMRI) to observe injured brains and identify regions of the cerebral cortex that seem to be associated with certain functions (**Figure 7.11**).

The ***frontal lobes***, located behind the forehead in the anterior portion of the brain, are sectioned off from the rest of the brain by the central sulcus (**Figure 7.10B**). The anterior association cortex, located on the most anterior portion of the frontal lobe, plays an important role in higher order intellectual functioning, including planning, reasoning, and memory. The left frontal lobe also includes Broca's area, which controls the tongue and lip movements required for speech. Damage to this area in stroke patients causes difficulty speaking.

Within the frontal lobes, just anterior to the central sulcus, is the ***primary motor cortex***. This structure sends neural impulses to the skeletal muscles to initiate and control the development of muscle tension and movement of the body parts. Axons descending from neurons in the primary motor cortex join to form the pyramidal tracts, which communicate with the brain stem and spinal cord. The premotor cortex is believed to play an assistive role in planning voluntary movements.

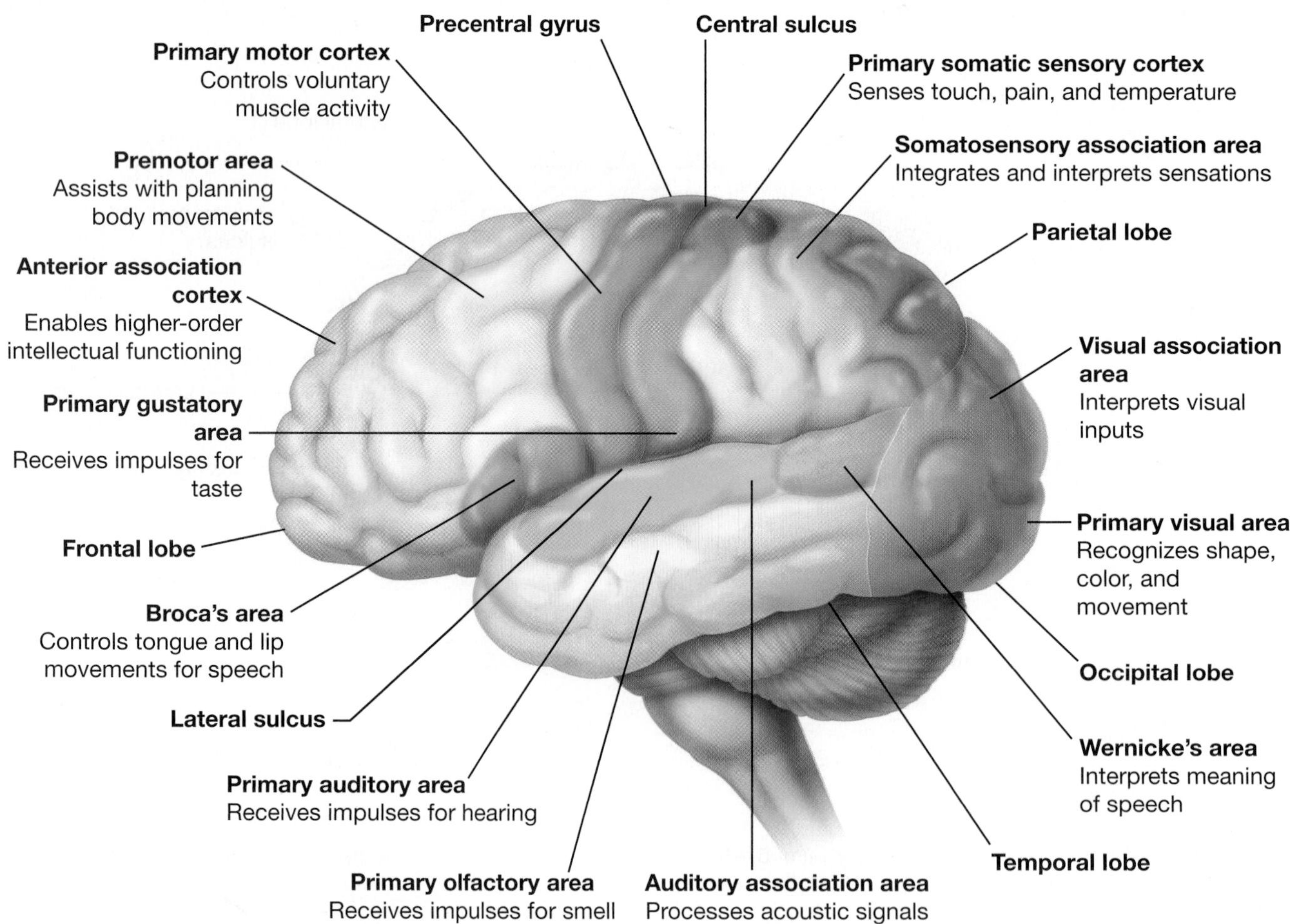

Figure 7-11 Functional regions of the brain.

As **Figure 7.12** shows, scientists have mapped the primary motor cortex to establish which body parts are controlled in each region of the cortex. Notice that relatively small regions of the cortex control major body segments, such as the trunk, pelvis, thigh, and arm. Much larger regions of the cortex are allocated for control of smaller body segments, such as the hands, lips, and tongue. The body parts associated with larger areas of the motor cortex are the ones capable of the more fine-tuned movements. Such movements require the activation of more nerves.

Focus On Memory

Have you ever challenged yourself to remember a phone number or other information without writing it down? Have you always been successful? If this is something you are good at, you might enjoy memory sport.

Memory sport is a competition in which participants memorize amazingly large amounts of information and then present it back to judges, in accordance with the rules of the competition. The World Memory Sports Council has organized the World Memory Championships since 1991. Several countries, including the United States, Germany, India, and the United Kingdom, have held national competitions.

Nelson Dellis is a four-time USA Memory Champion and is the holder of multiple US memory records. Dellis holds the US national record for memorizing the order of a deck of shuffled cards in 63 seconds, as well as the US national record for memorizing the largest number of ordered digits (303) in five minutes. However, Dellis's worldwide ranking for these accomplishments is not as impressive as you might think—in 2015, he ranked 15th in the world for card memorization and 24th in the world as an overall memory athlete.

How do Dellis and other memory athletes accomplish such feats? Most of these individuals, known as *mnemonists*, use some version of a technique that involves building a "memory palace." The technique relies on placing new items of information to be remembered into discrete locations within a mental framework, or memory palace. Subsequently, the mnemonist moves sequentially through the palace locations to retrieve the information. For example, competitor Ben Pridmore was able to memorize 28 decks of cards in order over the course of one hour by utilizing 28 memory palaces.

All mnemonists use some variation of an encoding technique that helps make each item to be remembered more personally memorable. Another way to think about this is to associate mundane, unmemorable things with something that is striking and memorable to you. Cueing the brain to recall the memorable item calls forth the unmemorable. For example, to remember the name of someone you just met who is named Jack, and who is wearing an orange shirt, you might think of a jack-o-lantern, a quaint name for a carved pumpkin.

Memory is the ability to store and recall information received from the senses. Recalling memories involves activation of some of the same neural pathways originally used in sensing the experience and, in particularly strong recollections, may almost recreate the event. However, multiple areas of the brain are involved in extracting the essence of sensed experiences and forming personally meaningful concepts. To further complicate things, a given memory is not simply formed and stored for future recollection. Studies confirm that memories can change over time in terms of both strength and nature as they are influenced by new experiences.

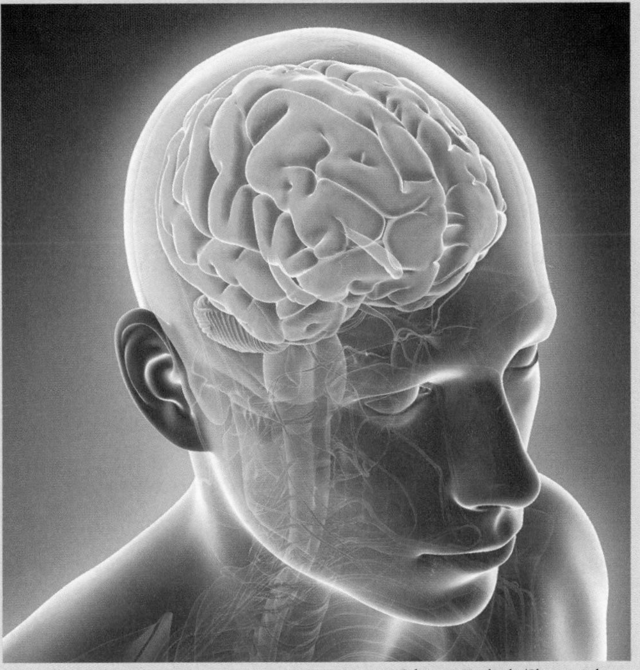

Sebastian Kaulitzki/Shutterstock.com

The two hippocampi, highlighted here, are the brain structures that scientists have documented as being critical for memory formation.

Through studies of brain scans, scientists have been able to determine which structures in the brain are involved in creating memories. Short-term memories, lasting only up to a minute or so, are processed in the highly developed prefrontal lobe. The process of translating short-term memory into long-term memory is a more complicated, involved process. The structure in the brain that is clearly instrumental in this process is the hippocampus. The hippocampus, Latin for "seahorse," is named after its shape. There is a hippocampus located deep and medially within each of the temporal lobes.

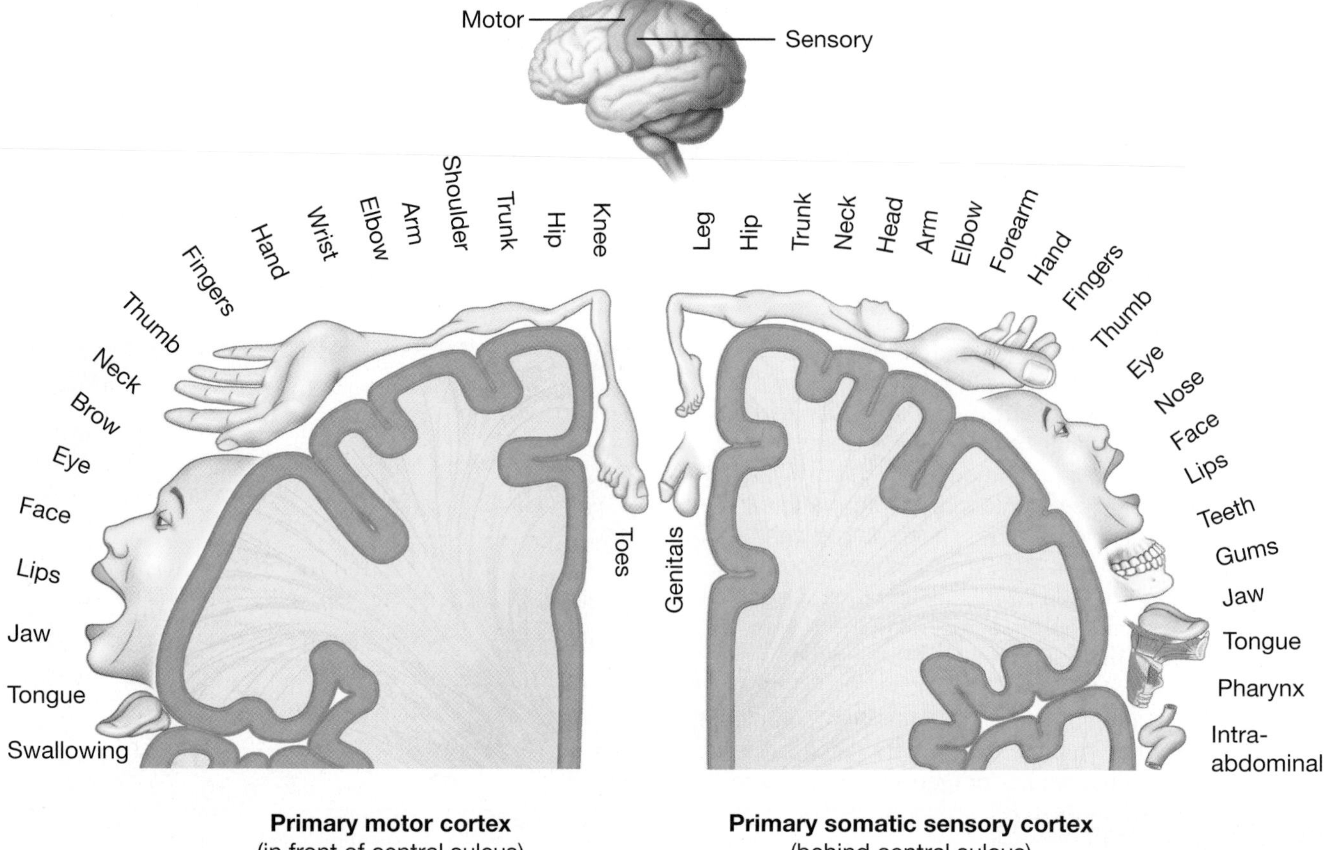

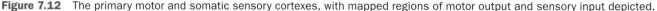

Figure 7.12 The primary motor and somatic sensory cortexes, with mapped regions of motor output and sensory input depicted.

The ***parietal lobes*** are immediately posterior to the frontal lobes. The parietal lobes include the ***primary somatic sensory cortex***, which interprets sensory impulses received from the skin, internal organs, muscles, and joints. The somatic sensory cortex illustration in **Figure 7.12** represents the density, or amount, of sensory neural input received from different parts of the body. Notice that the fingertips and lips, in particular, occupy large portions of the sensory cortex. This is because these parts have many sensory receptors. The parietal lobes also include the somatosensory association area, which plays a role in integrating and interpreting sensations.

The ***occipital lobes***, posterior to the parietal lobes, are responsible for vision. They include the primary visual area, where visual sensory inputs are received, and the visual association area, where these visual inputs are interpreted.

The lateral sulci divide the ***temporal lobes***, the most inferior lobes, from the frontal and parietal lobes above them. The temporal lobes include the primary olfactory area, which receives impulses for smell; the primary auditory area, which receives impulses for hearing; the auditory association area, where acoustic signals are processed; and Wernicke's area, which interprets speech.

Diencephalon

The ***diencephalon***, also known as the *interbrain*, is located deep inside the brain, enclosed by the cerebral hemispheres (**Figure 7.13**). It includes several important structures: the thalamus, hypothalamus, and epithalamus.

- The ***thalamus*** serves as a relay station for communicating both sensory and motor information between the body and the cerebral cortex. It also plays a major role in regulating the body's states of arousal, including sleep, wakefulness, and high-alert consciousness.
- Only the ***hypothalamus***, which is only about the size of a pearl, is a key part of the autonomic nervous system, regulating functions such as metabolism, heart rate, blood pressure, thirst, hunger, energy level, and body temperature. The centers for sex, pain, and pleasure also lie within the hypothalamus.

Anterior view

Diencephalon (thalamus in view)

Midbrain

Pons

Brain stem

Medulla oblongata

Spinal cord

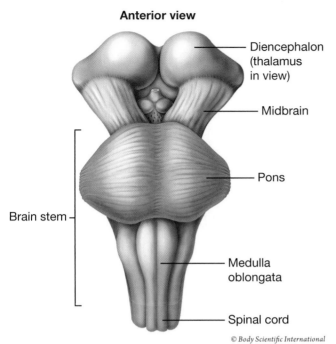

© Body Scientific International

Figure 7.13 The diencephalon includes the thalamus (exterior), and the hypothalamus and epithalamus (both interior). The brain stem includes the midbrain, pons, and medulla oblongata.

- The ***epithalamus*** includes the pineal gland, which secretes hormones that regulate the sleep cycle.

Brain Stem

Approximately the size of a thumb, the brain stem is shaped somewhat like a stem, and it includes three structures: the midbrain, pons, and medulla oblongata.

- The ***midbrain***, located on the superior end of the brain stem, serves as a relay station for sensory and motor impulses. Specifically, it relays information concerning vision, hearing, motor activity, sleep and wake cycles, arousal (alertness), and temperature regulation.
- The ***pons***, located immediately below the midbrain, plays a role in regulating breathing.
- The ***medulla oblongata*** is inferior to the pons. It regulates heart rate, blood pressure, and breathing, and controls the reflexes for coughing, sneezing, and vomiting.

Research Notes Studying the Brain

An increasing variety of approaches is available for studying the functional roles of different parts of the central nervous system. As technology advances, more sophisticated techniques emerge.

fMRI Scans

One procedure extremely useful for both scientific and clinical evaluation of the brain is called *functional magnetic resonance imaging (fMRI)*. This technology creates images of changes in blood flow to activated brain structures. This is made possible by the slightly different magnetic properties of oxygenated and deoxygenated blood. The individual undergoing the brain scan is presented with certain tasks that can cause activation (increased blood flow) in the regions of the brain responsible for perception, thought, and a stimulated motor action, such as raising an arm or smiling. The fMRI images show which brain structures are activated during each task, as well as the amount of time the structures are activated.

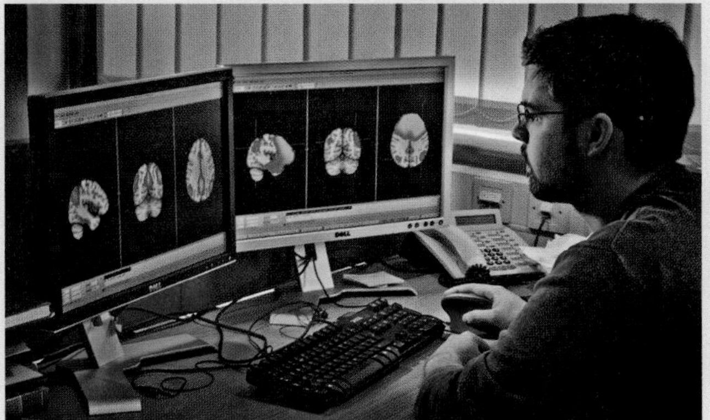

James King-Holmes/Science Source

Functional magnetic resonance imaging (fMRI) scans of the brain show different areas of activation.

Increasingly, physicians are using fMRI to diagnose disorders and diseases of the brain. With a fine sensitivity to changes in blood flow, fMRI is particularly useful for evaluating patients who may have suffered a stroke. Early diagnosis of stroke is important because treatment can be significantly more effective the earlier it is given.

PET Scans

Another approach to studying brain function involves positron emission tomography (PET). This procedure tracks the locations of radioactively labeled chemicals in the bloodstream. PET scans can show blood flow, oxygen absorption, and glucose absorption in the brain, indicating which areas of the brain are active and inactive. Although fMRI has largely replaced PET for the study of brain activation patterns, PET scans still provide the advantage of showing where particular neurotransmitters are concentrated in the brain. PET scans are also still widely used in diagnosing various forms of brain disease because they can be analyzed and interpreted more quickly than fMRI scans.

The reticular formation is a collection of interconnected gray matter that extends the length of the brain stem. A group of neurons within the reticular formation, known as the *reticular activating system (RAS)*, is involved in regulating states of waking, slumber, and heightened awareness. Damage to the RAS can result in coma. Individuals with severe brain injuries can continue to live as long as the brain stem remains functional and they receive sufficient hydration and nutrition.

Cerebellum

The ***cerebellum***, found below the occipital lobes, looks similar to the cerebrum with its outer gray cortex, convolutions, and dual hemispheres. The cerebellum serves the important role of coordinating body movements, including balance.

To coordinate body movements and balance, the cerebellum receives input from the eyes, inner ears, and sensory receptors throughout the body. It also continuously monitors body segment positions and motions, and sends out signals to make adjustments when necessary. For example, if you were to lose your balance on a slippery surface, the cerebellum would send nerve impulses to your legs to move in a way to prevent a fall.

As you might guess, research has shown that the cerebellums of accomplished athletes are better developed in terms of size and amount of neural connections than those of nonathletes.

Meninges

Three protective membranes, known as the ***meninges***, surround the brain and spinal cord (**Figure 7.14**). The outer membrane is called the *dura mater*, meaning "hard mother." This membrane is a tough, double-layered membrane that lies beneath the skull and surrounds the brain. The inner layer of the dura mater extends down to enclose the spinal cord.

The middle membrane, called the *arachnoid mater*, is composed of web-like tissue. Beneath this membrane is the subarachnoid space, which is filled with cerebrospinal fluid (CSF). This fluid cushions the brain and spinal cord. The composition of CSF is similar to the plasma in the blood, but it has a different electrolyte balance and contains more vitamin C and less protein.

The innermost layer of the meninges attaches directly to the surface of the brain and spinal cord. This delicate layer is called the *pia mater*, meaning "gentle mother."

Blood-Brain Barrier

A rich network of blood vessels supplies the brain. Like all tissues of the body, the brain depends on a circulating blood supply to provide nutrients and carry away the waste products of cell metabolism. At any given time, roughly 20%–25% of the blood in your body is circulating in the region of the brain.

The capillaries that supply the brain, however, are different from other capillaries in the body. They are impermeable to many substances that freely diffuse

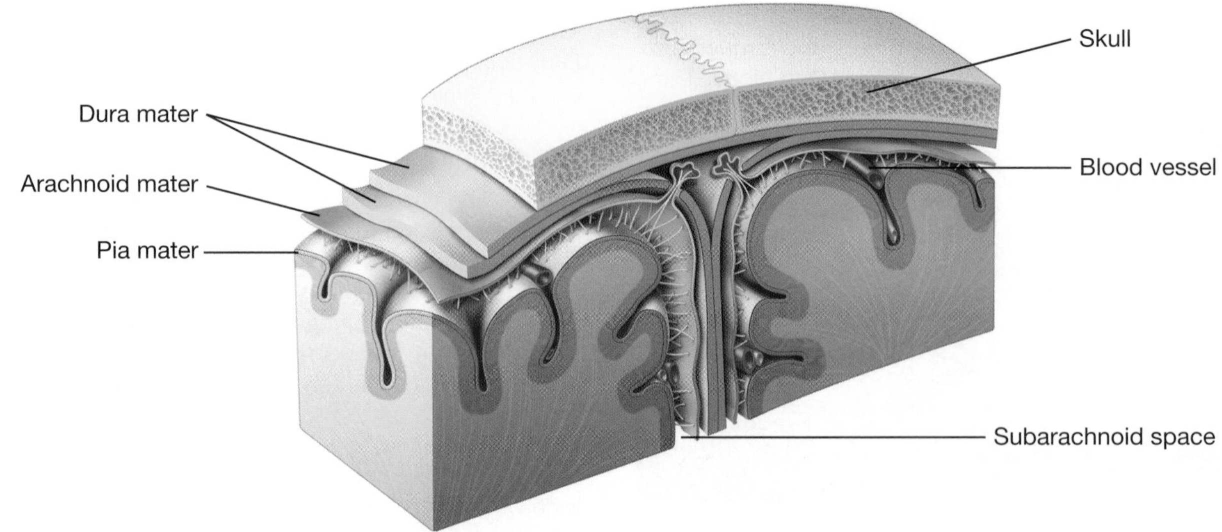

Figure 7.14 The three meninges (the protective linings of the brain and spinal cord) include the double-layered dura mater, the arachnoid mater, and the pia mater.

through the walls of capillaries in other body regions. This property of impermeability has given rise to the term *blood-brain barrier.*

The blood-brain barrier protects the brain against surges in concentrations of hormones, ions, and some nutrients. Water, glucose, and essential amino acids are allowed to pass through the capillaries. Other substances that can penetrate the blood-brain barrier include blood-borne alcohol, nicotine, fats, respiratory gases, and anesthetics.

SELF CHECK

1. List the four major anatomic regions of the brain.
2. List the four lobes of the brain and state the function(s) of each lobe.
3. Name the three structures that make up the diencephalon and state their functions.
4. Name the three structures that make up the brain stem and state their functions.
5. Where is the cerebellum located, and what is its function?

Spinal Cord

The ***spinal cord*** extends from the brain stem down to the beginning of the lumbar region of the spine. It serves as a major pathway for relaying sensory impulses to the brain and carrying motor impulses from the brain. The spinal cord also provides the neural connections involved in reflex arcs. Like the brain, the spine is surrounded and protected by the three meninges and cerebrospinal fluid.

When viewed in cross section, the exterior of the spinal cord is made up of myelinated white matter, with butterfly-shaped gray matter, composed of neuron cell bodies and interneurons in the center (**Figure 7.15**). The regions of white and gray matter in the spinal cord are named after their locations—ventral (anterior), lateral, and dorsal (posterior). The dorsal columns of white matter carry sensory impulses to the brain, while the lateral and ventral columns transmit both sensory and motor impulses. The dorsal, lateral, and ventral projections of gray matter are called *horns*. The central canal that contains cerebrospinal fluid runs through the middle of the gray matter. **Figure 7.15** also shows the formations of the spinal nerves. These will be discussed in the next section.

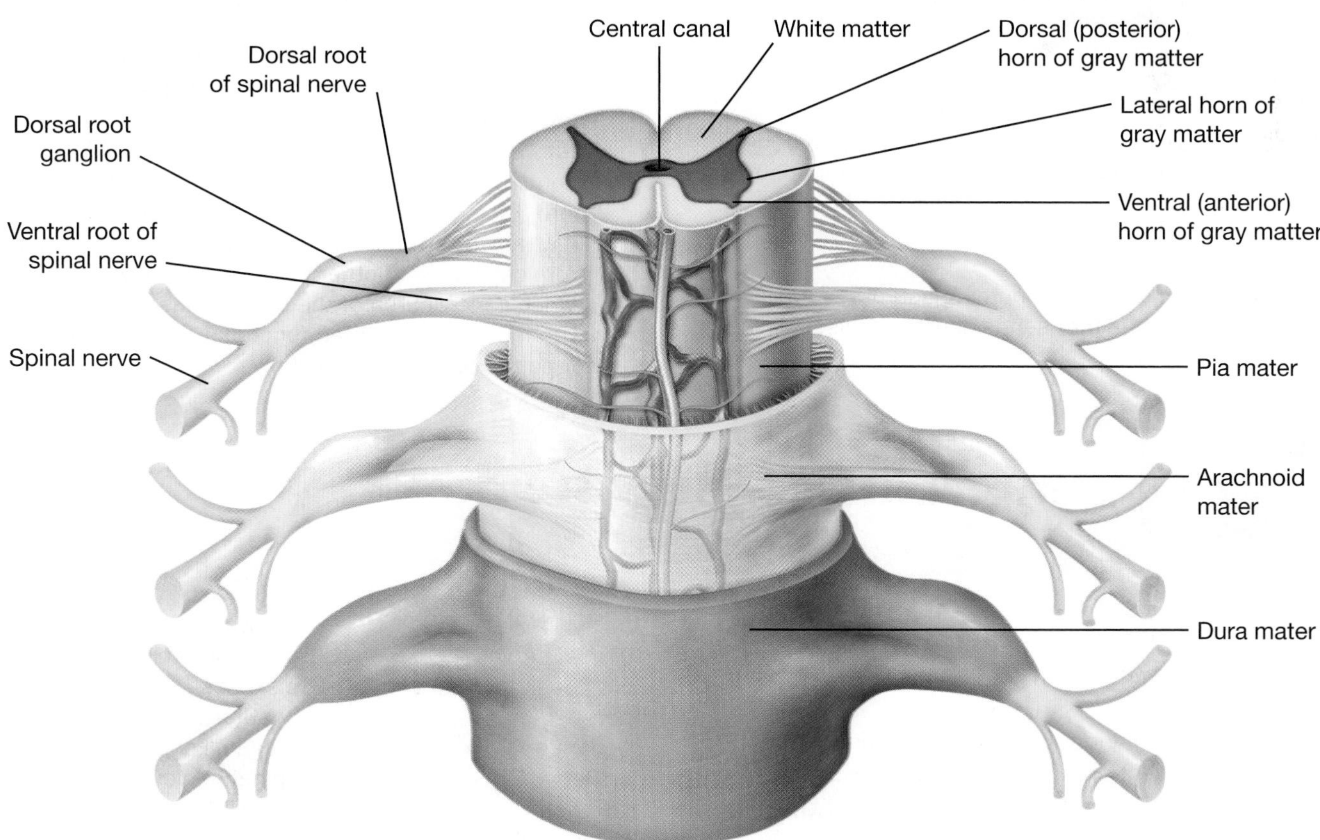

Figure 7.15 Layers and regions of the spinal cord.

SECTION 7.3 REVIEW

Mini-Glossary

cerebellum the section of the brain that coordinates body movements, including balance

cerebrum the largest part of the brain, consisting of the left and right hemispheres

diencephalon the area of the brain that includes the epithalamus, thalamus, and hypothalamus; also known as the *interbrain*

epithalamus the uppermost portion of the diencephalon, which includes the pineal gland and regulates sleep-cycle hormones

fissures the uniformly positioned, deep grooves in the brain

frontal lobes the regions of the brain located behind the forehead; include areas that control higher order intellectual functioning and speech

hypothalamus the portion of the diencephalon that regulates functions such as metabolism, heart rate, and blood pressure

lobes the regions of the brain; include the frontal, parietal, occipital, and temporal lobes

medulla oblongata the lower portion of the brain stem, which regulates heart rate, blood pressure, and breathing, and controls several reflexes

meninges the three protective membranes that surround the brain and spinal cord

midbrain the relay station for sensory and motor impulses; located on the superior end of the brain stem

occipital lobes the regions of the brain located behind the parietal lobes; responsible for vision

parietal lobes the regions of the brain located behind the frontal lobes; integrate sensory information from the skin, internal organs, muscles, and joints

pons the section of the brain stem that plays a role in regulating breathing

primary motor cortex the outer region of the brain in the frontal lobes that sends neural impulses to the skeletal muscles

primary somatic sensory cortex the outer region of the brain in the parietal lobes that interprets sensory impulses received from the skin, internal organs, muscles, and joints

spinal cord a column of nerve tissue that extends from the brain stem to the beginning of the lumbar region of the spine

temporal lobes the most inferior portions of the brain; responsible for speech, hearing, vision, memory, and emotion

thalamus the largest portion of the diencephalon; communicates sensory and motor information between the body and the cerebral cortex

Review Questions

1. Into how many lobes and hemispheres is the brain divided?
2. What is the difference between gray matter and white matter in the brain? Where is each found?
3. Explain why someone might say that the brain is convoluted.
4. Are major body segments, such as the trunk and pelvis, controlled by large or small regions of the brain's primary motor cortex?
5. Which area of the brain has probably been damaged if a stroke patient has difficulty speaking?
6. Like the brain, the spinal cord contains gray and white matter. Identify the responsibilities of both the gray matter and the white matter in the spinal cord.
7. Compare and contrast the three protective membranes surrounding the brain and spinal cord. Discuss their structures and functions.
8. In what way are the capillaries in the brain different from capillaries in other parts of the body?
9. Which general area of the brain is associated with more sophisticated functions—the anterior or posterior region? Explain.

SECTION 7.4 Peripheral Nervous System

Objectives

- Describe the basic structure of a nerve.
- Identify the twelve cranial nerves and the purpose of each.
- Explain the organization of the spinal nerves, the dorsal and ventral rami, and the plexuses.
- Differentiate between the functions of the sympathetic and parasympathetic nerves within the autonomic nervous system.

Key Terms

acetylcholine
cranial nerves
craniosacral division
dorsal ramus
endoneurium
epineurium
ganglion
norepinephrine
paravertebral ganglia
perineurium
plexuses
postganglionic neuron
preganglionic neuron
spinal nerves
thoracolumbar division
ventral ramus

The peripheral nervous system (PNS) transmits information to the CNS and carries instructions from the CNS. It achieves these functions through a network of nerves outside of the CNS.

Nerve Structure

Each nerve consists of a collection of axons (nerve fibers) and nutrient-supplying blood vessels, all bundled in a series of protective sheaths of connective tissue. As shown in **Figure 7.16**, each axon is covered by a fine ***endoneurium***. In myelinated axons, the endoneurium surrounds the myelin sheath as well as the nodes of Ranvier.

Groups of these sheathed fibers are bundled into fascicles surrounded by a protective ***perineurium***. Finally, groups of fascicles and blood vessels are encased in a tough ***epineurium***. This structural arrangement provides a cordlike strength that helps nerves resist injury.

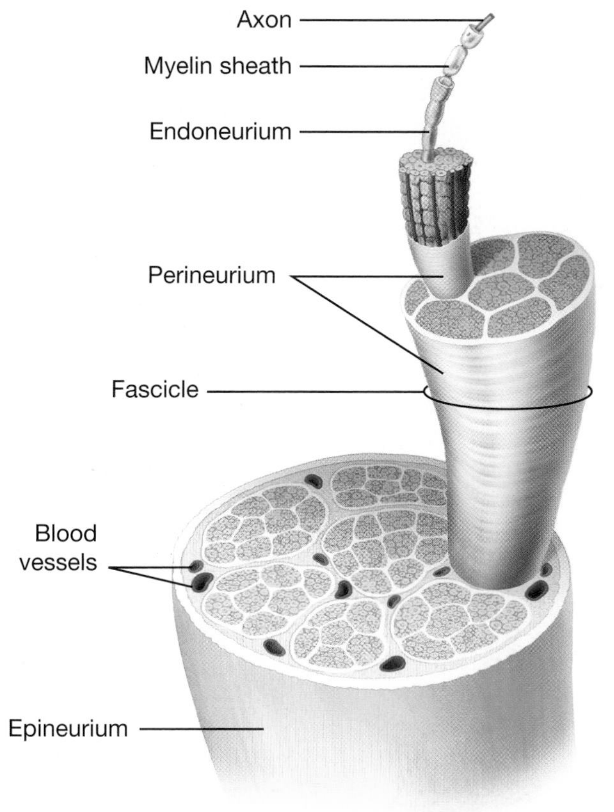

Figure 7.16 Structure of a nerve showing the protective, fibrous tissue sheaths.

SELF CHECK

1. Describe the basic structure of a nerve.
2. What is the purpose of the perineurium?

Cranial Nerves

Twelve pairs of ***cranial nerves*** relay impulses to and from the left and right sides of the brain. These pairs are referred to by both a name and a number (**Figure 7.17**). The names of these nerves indicate their functions. The functions of the cranial nerves are summarized in **Figure 7.18**.

Some of these nerves contain only afferent (sensory) fibers, some contain only efferent (motor) fibers, and others—the mixed nerves—contain both kinds of fibers. Mixed nerves also transmit both sensory and motor impulses.

SELF CHECK

1. How many pairs of cranial nerves does the body have?
2. What kind of impulses do mixed nerves carry?

Spinal Nerves and Nerve Plexuses

Thirty-one pairs of ***spinal nerves*** branch out from the left and right sides of the spinal cord. Each pair is named for the vertebral level from which it originates. As explained in Chapter 5, the vertebral levels include the cervical, thoracic, and lumbar regions, as well as the sacrum. All of the spinal nerves are mixed nerves, so they all carry both afferent and efferent information.

The spinal nerve cell bodies are located within the gray matter of the spinal cord. The axons of spinal nerve cells extend out of the spinal cord and eventually connect with muscles. Because the spinal cord does not extend the entire length of the vertebral column, the spinal nerves at the inferior end of the cord extend part of the way down the vertebral canal before exiting. This collection of nerve fibers in the inferior vertebral tunnel is called the *cauda equina*, literally translated as "horse's tail," after its appearance. As shown earlier in **Figure 7.15**, dorsal (posterior) and ventral (anterior) spinal nerve roots unite to form the left and right spinal nerves that exit at each spinal level.

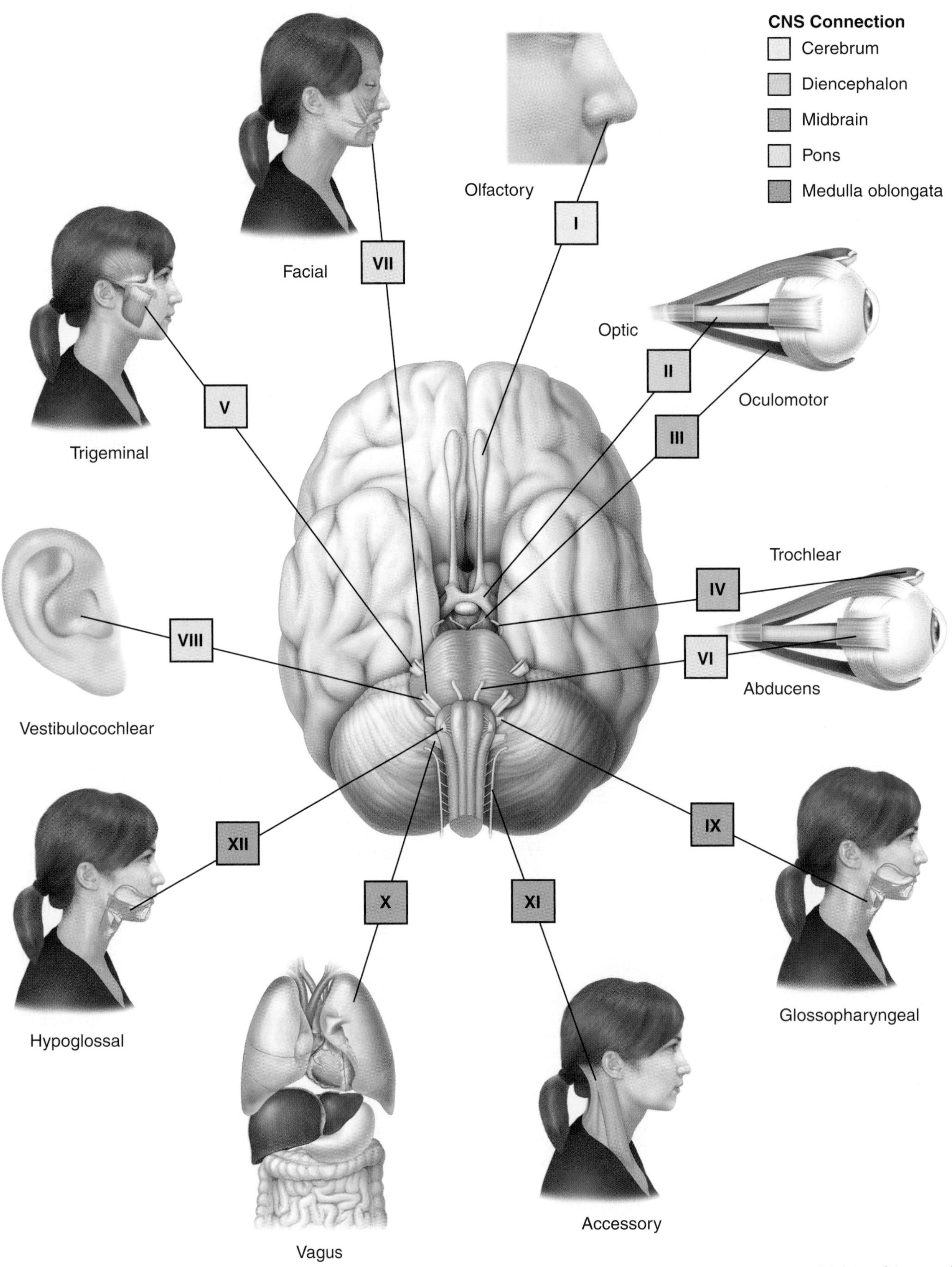

Figure 7.17 The cranial nerves.

Functions of the Cranial Nerves			
Nerve	**Number**	**System**	**Function**
olfactory	I	sensory	smell
optic	II	sensory	sight
oculomotor	III	both	eye movements
trochlear	IV	both	eye movements
trigeminal	V	both	facial sensation, jaw motion
abducens	VI	both	eye movements
facial	VII	both	facial movements, taste
vestibulocochlear	VIII	sensory	hearing, balance
glossopharyngeal	IX	both	throat muscle movements, taste
vagus	X	both	autonomic control of heart, lungs, digestion, taste, communication between brain and organs
accessory	XI	mostly motor	trapezius movements, sternocleidomastoid movements
hypoglossal	XII	both	tongue muscle movements, tongue sensation

Figure 7.18

Goodheart-Willcox Publisher

The spinal nerve fibers exiting the vertebral column are only about one-half inch long, and they immediately divide into a ***dorsal ramus*** (plural *rami*) and ***ventral ramus*** (**Figure 7.19**). The dorsal and ventral rami carry nerve impulses to the muscle and skin of the trunk.

All of the rami are mixed nerves, carrying both afferent and efferent signals:

- The small dorsal rami, running the length of the spine, transmit motor impulses to the posterior trunk muscles and relay sensory impulses from the skin of the back.

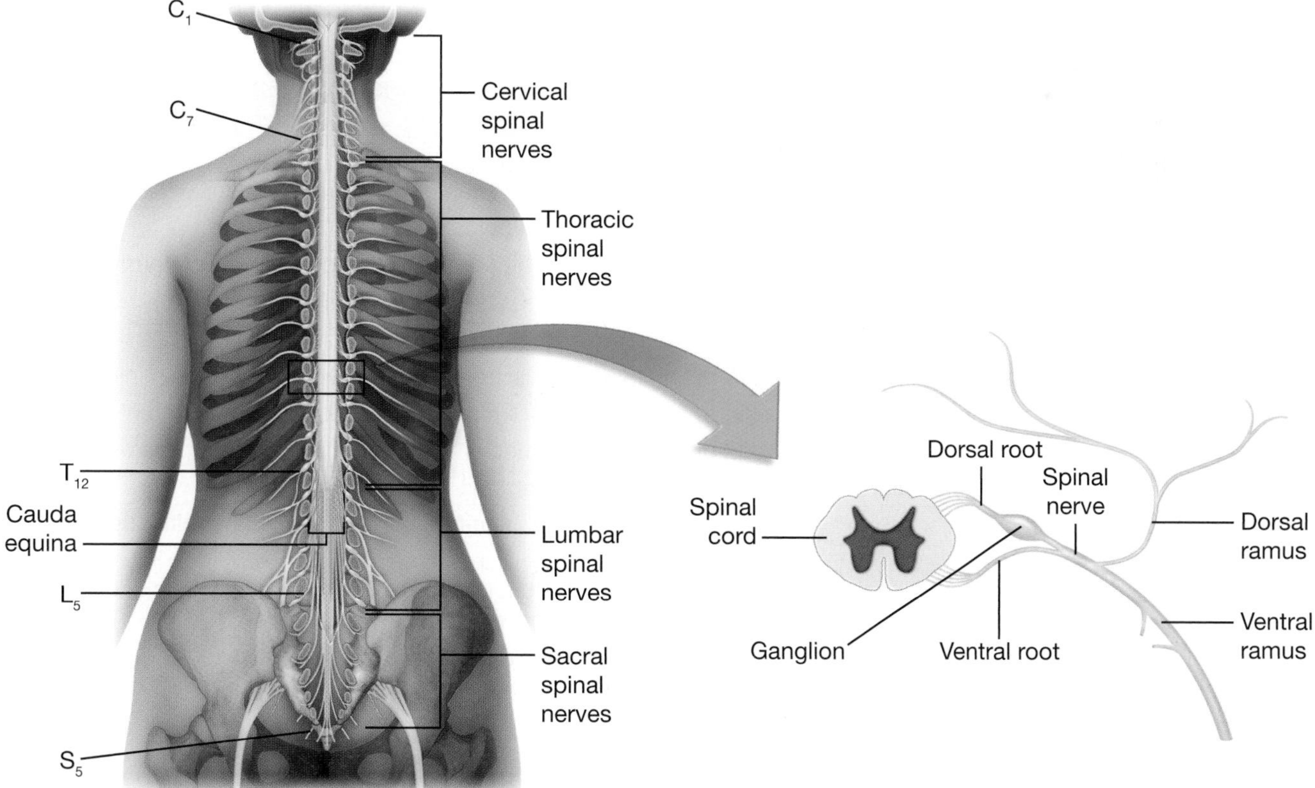

© Body Scientific International

Figure 7.19 The spinal nerves, formed from dorsal and ventral roots, immediately branch into dorsal and ventral rami.

- The ventral rami in the thoracic region of the spine (T1–T12) become the intercostal nerves (running between the ribs). They communicate with the muscles and skin of the anterior and lateral trunk.
- The ventral rami in the cervical and lumbar regions of the spine branch out to form complex interconnections of nerves called ***plexuses***. Most of the major efferent nerves in the neck, arms, and legs originate in the plexuses.

The four plexuses in the body are summarized in **Figure 7.20**. To see how the major nerves branch out from the lower three plexuses, refer to **Figure 7.21**.

SELF CHECK

1. How many pairs of spinal nerves does the human body have?
2. What part of the spinal nerves is located in the gray matter of the spinal cord?
3. Name the four plexuses in the body.

Autonomic Nervous System

As described earlier in the chapter, the efferent nerves have two divisions: the somatic nervous system and the autonomic, or involuntary, nervous system. The somatic nervous system sends impulses to activate the skeletal muscles. The autonomic nervous system is programmed by the CNS to control the heart, smooth muscles, and glands.

Within the autonomic system, two neurons connect the CNS to each of the organs it activates. The cell body of the first neuron originates in the gray matter of the brain or spinal cord. Autonomic cell bodies that originate in the spinal cord reside in the lateral horn of the gray matter. The myelinated axons of the first neuron terminate at a synapse with a second neuron in an enlarged junction called a ***ganglion***. The second, unmyelinated neuron then courses from the ganglion to supply the cardiac muscle, smooth muscle, or gland.

As you might suspect, the first neuron in the sequence just described is called the ***preganglionic neuron***. The second is called the ***postganglionic neuron*** (**Figure 7.22**).

The two divisions of the autonomic nervous system are the sympathetic and parasympathetic divisions. These divisions are described in the following sections.

Spinal Nerve Plexuses			
Plexus	**Spinal Nerves**	**Exiting Nerves**	**Region Supplied**
cervical	c1–c5	phrenic	diaphragm, skin and muscles of neck and shoulder
brachial	c5–c8 and t1	axillary	skin and muscles of shoulder
		radial	skin and muscles of lateral and posterior arm and forearm
		median	skin and flexor muscles of forearm, some hand muscles
		musculocutaneous	skin of lateral forearm, elbow flexor muscles
		ulnar	skin of hand, flexor muscles of forearm, wrist and some hand muscles
lumbar	l1–l4	femoral	skin of medial and anterior thigh, anterior thigh muscles
		obturator	skin and muscles of medial thigh and hip
		saphenous	skin of the medial thigh and medial lower leg
sacral	l4–l5 and s1–s4	sciatic	two of the hamstrings (semimembranosus, semitendinosus), adductor magnus
		tibial	muscles of knee flexion, plantar flexion, and toe flexion; skin of the posterior lower leg and sole of the foot
		common fibular	biceps femoris, tibialis anterior, muscles of toe extension, skin of the anterior lower leg, superior surface of foot, and lateral side of foot
		superior and inferior gluteal	gluteal muscles
		posterior femoral cutaneous	skin of posterior thigh and posterior lower leg

Figure 7.20 Goodheart-Willcox Publisher

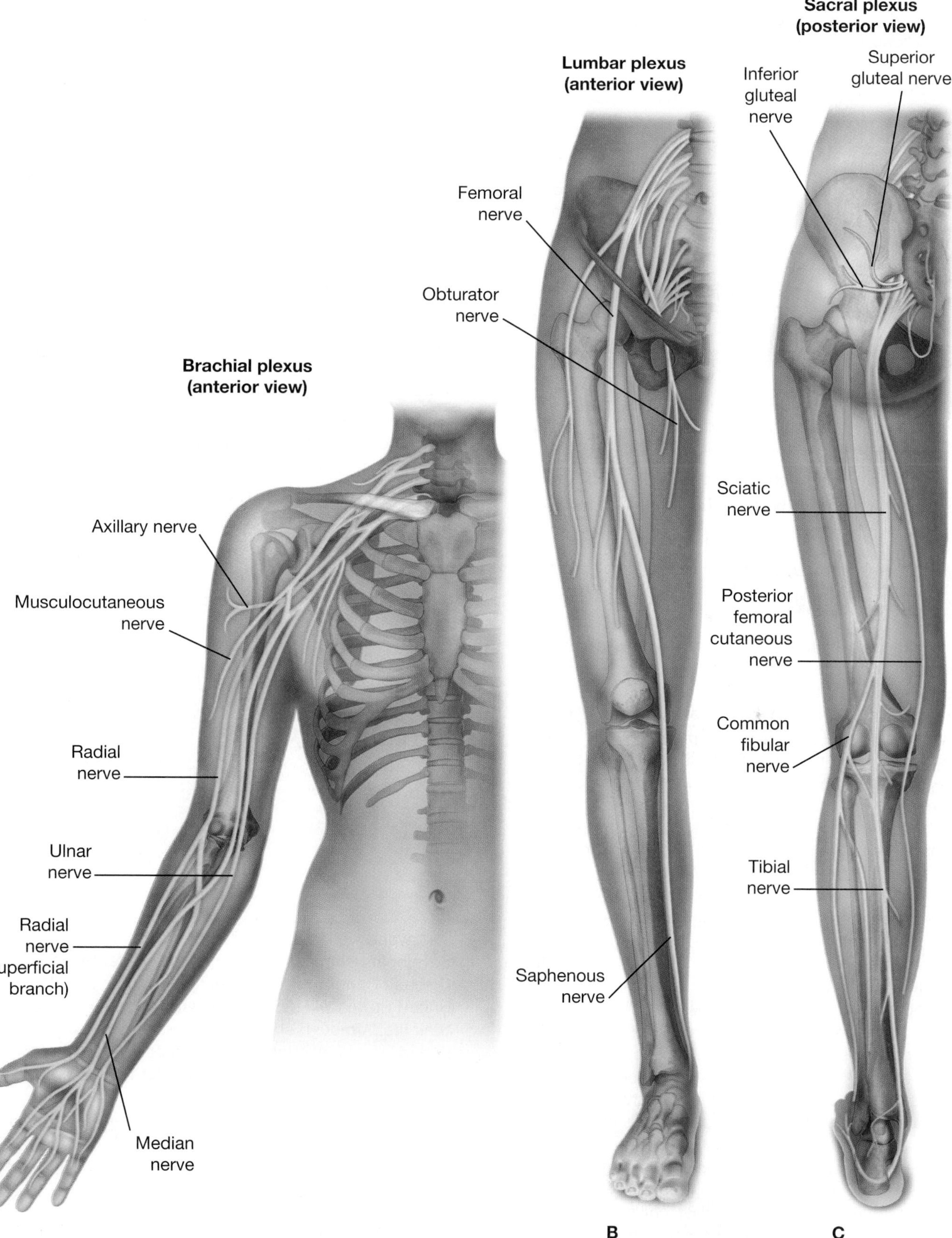

Figure 7.21 Major nerves emanate from the brachial, lumbar, and sacral plexuses. The word *plexus* is derived from the Latin *plectere*, meaning "to braid."

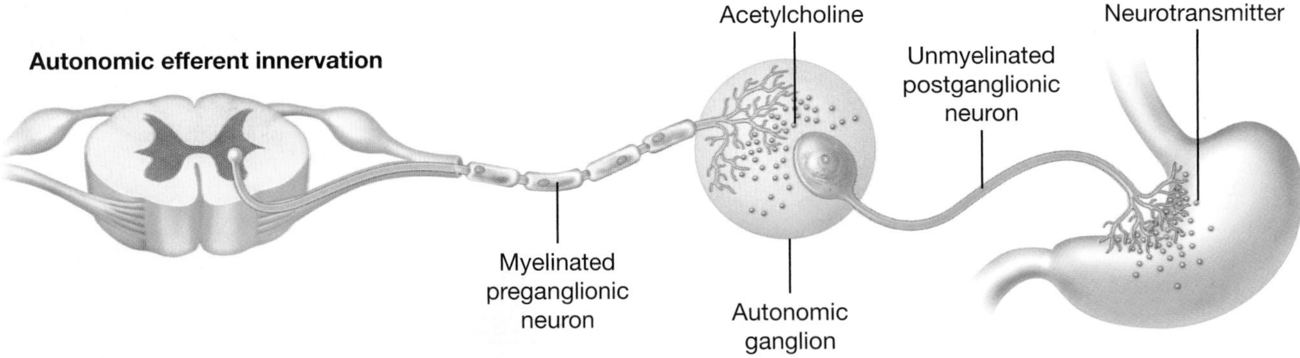

© Body Scientific International

Figure 7.22 Pre- and postganglionic neurons stimulating the smooth muscle of the stomach (an effector organ). The postganglionic neurotransmitter is norepinephrine in sympathetic fibers and acetylcholine in parasympathetic fibers.

Sympathetic Nerves

The sympathetic nerves activate the fight-or-flight response by stimulating the adrenal gland to release epinephrine, a hormone that is also known as *adrenaline.* In primitive times, when a person was confronted by a predator, the fight-or-flight response—characterized by increased heart and breathing rates and sweating—supposedly prepared the individual to either fight or run. In modern times, this sympathetic response is physiologically the same, but it can be triggered by any type of situation that is perceived as stressful. You will learn more about the fight-or-flight response in Chapter 9.

Clinical Application Shingles

Chickenpox, which is caused by the *varicella zoster* virus, was once a common childhood disease. It is highly contagious and can be spread through airborne mechanisms such as sneezing or coughing, or by direct contact with the skin rash. The primary symptom of chickenpox is an itchy rash that persists for about 5–10 days. Other symptoms include fever, headache, sore throat, cough, and decreased appetite. In individuals with weakened immune systems, symptoms can be more severe. Today, chickenpox infections are much less prevalent due to the *varicella* vaccine. Childhood immunization is routine in many countries.

A much more serious and painful expression of the *varicella zoster* virus is the condition known as *shingles*. When a person recovers from chickenpox, although the chickenpox symptoms disappear, the virus remains in the body for life, harboring in the posterior root ganglia. In healthy individuals, the immune system keeps the virus in check. Any immune insufficiency can cause the virus to break out and travel along the sensory nerve fibers, leaving a rash of extremely painful, fluid-filled vesicles in a swath along the path of the nerve.

Outbreaks of shingles usually occur around the waist or chest area on one side of the body, and sometimes on the face. Infection of an eye can result in loss of vision. Other symptoms may include fever, chills, headache, and upset stomach. A more serious complication can be severe pain that persists in the areas of the shingles outbreak for weeks or months, and as long as years in some people.

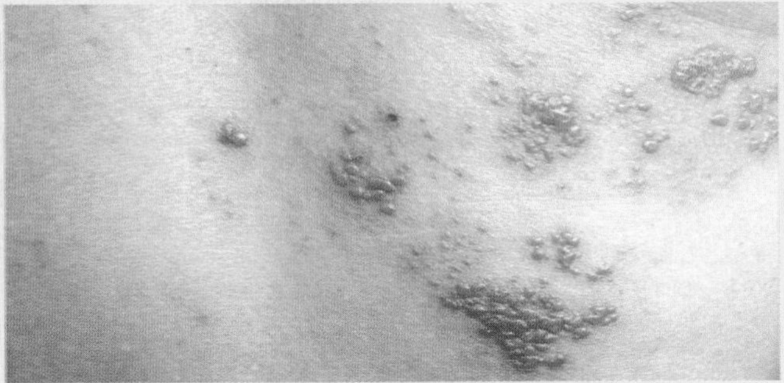

komkrit Preechachanawate/Shutterstock.com

Shingles rash.

Anyone who has had chickenpox is at risk for developing shingles. According to the Centers for Disease Control (CDC), nearly one in three people in the United States will develop shingles at some time during their life. Although shingles outbreaks can occur at any age, the incidence increases with age. Approximately half of all cases occur in adults older than 60 years of age. Although most people experience only one outbreak of shingles, second or even third outbreaks are possible. The shingles vaccine, which is effective for approximately five years, is recommended for people 60 years of age and older.

Shingles cannot be passed from one person to another. However, if someone who is susceptible to chickenpox comes in direct contact with weeping shingles blisters, that person can contract chickenpox. Until the shingles rash is crusted over, it should be covered.

The preganglionic neurons in the sympathetic system arise from the spinal segments extending from T1–L2. For this reason, the sympathetic system is also called the ***thoracolumbar division***.

Neurons in this system secrete acetylcholine to stimulate the postganglionic neurons in the ***paravertebral ganglia***. The paravertebral ganglia are named after their location; they lie parallel to the spinal cord. The postganglionic neurons release the neurotransmitter ***norepinephrine***, which plays a role in triggering the fight-or-flight response.

Parasympathetic Nerves

In contrast to the sympathetic nervous system, the parasympathetic nervous system controls all of the automatic, everyday functions of the circulatory, respiratory, and digestive systems. Because of this, the system is sometimes called the *resting and digesting system*. In addition, after a fight-or-flight situation, the parasympathetic nervous system produces a calming effect that returns the body to a normal state.

Preganglionic parasympathetic neurons originate in one of two separate regions—the brain stem or the sacral (lowermost) region of the spinal cord. For this reason, the parasympathetic system is also known as the ***craniosacral division***.

Activation of both preganglionic and postganglionic neurons in this system triggers the release of the neurotransmitter ***acetylcholine***. Although acetylcholine stimulates skeletal muscle, it also inhibits activity in cardiac and smooth muscle. This helps the body calm down after a fight-or-flight response.

SECTION 7.4 REVIEW

Mini-Glossary

acetylcholine a neurotransmitter that stimulates skeletal muscle and inhibits activity in cardiac and smooth muscle

cranial nerves twelve pairs of nerves that originate in the brain and relay impulses to and from the PNS

craniosacral division the parasympathetic nervous system; includes nerves that originate in the brain stem or sacral region of the spinal cord

dorsal ramus the division of posterior spinal nerves that transmit motor impulses to the posterior trunk muscles and relay sensory impulses from the skin of the back

endoneurium a delicate, connective tissue that surrounds each axon, or nerve fiber, in a nerve

epineurium the tough outer covering of a nerve

ganglion a mass of nervous tissue that is composed mostly of nerve cell bodies and acts as an enlarged junction between neurons

norepinephrine a neurotransmitter that is released by postganglionic neurons in the sympathetic nervous system and plays a role in triggering the fight-or-flight response

paravertebral ganglia mass of nerve cell bodies that lie parallel to the spinal cord

perineurium a protective sheath that surrounds a bundle of nerve fibers, or fascicle

plexuses complex interconnections of nerves

postganglionic neuron the second neuron in a series that transmits impulses from the CNS

preganglionic neuron the first neuron in a series that transmits impulses from the CNS

spinal nerves thirty-one pairs of nerves that branch from the left and right sides of the spinal cord

thoracolumbar division the sympathetic system; includes nerves that originate from the thoracic and lumbar regions of the spine

ventral ramus the anterior division of spinal nerves that communicate with the muscle and skin of the anterior and lateral trunk

Review Questions

1. Explain the function of the peripheral nervous system.
2. What is the major purpose shared by the endoneurium, perineurium, and epineurium?
3. How would you describe cranial nerves in terms of sensory and motor fibers?
4. Where do the majority of cranial nerves originate?
5. Are spinal nerves efferent, afferent, or mixed?
6. Which division of efferent nerves sends impulses to the heart?
7. Why is the parasympathetic nervous system also known as the *craniosacral division*?
8. Explain the difference between a preganglionic neuron and a postganglionic neuron.
9. Explain how the structure of a nerve decreases the chances of nerve damage.
10. When is the fight-or-flight response activated by sympathetic nerves?
11. Neurons meet at junctions called *ganglions*. Explain the purpose of a ganglion and describe how these structures help transmit nerve impulses throughout the body.
12. What determines whether a cranial nerve is a sensory fiber, a motor fiber, or both?

SECTION 7.5

Nervous System Injuries and Disorders

Objectives

- Describe the symptoms and recovery strategies for someone who has suffered a traumatic brain or spinal cord injury.
- Describe common diseases and disorders of the nervous system.

Key Terms

Alzheimer's disease (AD)
cerebral palsy (CP)
dementia
epilepsy
Huntington's disease (HD)
meningitis
multiple sclerosis (MS)
paraplegia
Parkinson's disease (PD)
quadriplegia
traumatic brain injury (TBI)

Given the critical roles played by the central nervous system, injuries and disorders of the CNS can have potentially serious consequences. This section describes some of the more common injuries and disorders of the CNS.

Injuries to the Brain and Spinal Cord

The brain and spinal cord are well protected. They are encased, respectively, in the skull and vertebral column, and both are surrounded by the three meninges and cerebrospinal fluid. Unfortunately, violent injuries can still cause mild to severe damage to these structures.

Traumatic Brain Injury

Traumatic brain injury (TBI) can occur as a result of violent blows to the head, particularly when the skull is pierced or fractured and bone fragments penetrate the brain. These injuries are classified as mild, moderate, or severe, with increasing levels of damage to the nervous system, particularly the cells and tissues of the brain.

In the case of a mild TBI, a person may remain conscious or lose consciousness for a short time. Symptoms may include any of the following: headache, confusion, dizziness, disturbed vision, ringing in the ears, bad taste in the mouth, fatigue, abnormal sleep patterns, behavioral changes, and trouble with intellectual functions.

Symptoms of moderate to severe TBI include all of those listed above, as well as more serious symptoms such as prolonged headache, repeated nausea or vomiting, convulsions or seizures, inability to awaken from sleep, dilation of one or both pupils of the eyes, slurred speech, weakness or numbness in the extremities, loss of coordination, confusion, and agitation.

Cases of moderate and severe TBI require immediate medical care in order to prevent further brain injury. X-rays and imaging tests may be performed to help assess the nature and extent of the damage. Maintaining proper blood pressure and flow of oxygenated blood to the brain and throughout the body are priorities. About 50% of severe TBI cases require surgical repair.

Case Study: Phineas Gage

A miraculous story of survival from a significant TBI is the case of Phineas Gage, a railroad construction foreman who was injured in 1848 when he was 25 years old. Gage and his crew were blasting rock to make way for railroad construction outside the town of Cavendish, Vermont, when a 3½-foot iron rod was accidentally blasted through Gage's skull. The iron entered below the left cheekbone and exited through the top of the skull. The blast was of such force that the rod landed approximately 80 feet away.

Amazingly, within a few minutes Gage was able to speak, walk, and ride upright in a cart back to his home, where he received medical attention. Gage's recovery was slow, with advances and declines, including time spent in a coma due to brain swelling. Nevertheless, his physical recovery was complete.

Accounts of Gage's mental recovery vary, but they suggest that his personality was negatively altered. Gage survived for 12 years after the accident. He began to suffer a series of increasingly severe seizures that eventually resulted in his death. The case of Phineas Gage is still discussed in medical and neurology classes.

Current Treatment and Prevention

Today, follow-up care for TBI involves individualized rehabilitation programs that may include physical, occupational, and speech-language therapies; psychiatric evaluation; and social support. The prognosis for those who have suffered from a traumatic brain injury varies greatly, with a potential for lingering problems with intellectual functioning, sensation, and behavior. Serious head injuries can also result in an unresponsive state or a coma.

Research is being conducted in scientific and clinical settings to achieve a clearer understanding of the biological effects of TBI. One goal of this research is to develop strategies and interventions that limit the brain damage that occurs during the first few days after a head injury. Another goal is to develop more effective therapies for facilitating the recovery of brain function.

Research Notes Concussions

The most common form of traumatic brain injury is a concussion. Symptoms may include headache as well as problems with concentration, memory, judgment, balance, and coordination. Fortunately, these effects are usually temporary. Although a concussion can cause a loss of consciousness, most concussions do not. Thus, many people experience mild concussions without realizing it.

The most common cause of concussion is a blow to the head. However, concussions can also occur when the head and upper body are violently shaken. In fact, the word *concussion* comes from the Latin term *concutere*, which means "to shake violently."

Concussions in Sports

Injuries that produce concussions are of particular concern for participants in American football, boxing, and soccer, although they also occur in other sports. According to the Centers for Disease Control (CDC), as many as 3.8 million sports- and recreation-related concussions occur in the United States each year. Concussions also result from car, bicycle, and diving accidents, work injuries, and falls.

Because all concussions injure the brain to some extent, it is crucial that these injuries be allowed sufficient time to heal. Healing time is particularly important for athletes in contact sports, which involve higher risks of reinjury to the brain. For this reason, researchers are focusing their attention on the consequences of repeated concussions.

Recent Research

A recent study showed that retired professional football players appear to be at a higher risk of death from diseases of the brain, compared to the general US population. In the study, which was sponsored by the National Institute for Occupational Safety and Health (NIOSH), researchers examined the medical records of 3,439 former National Football League (NFL) players with an average age of 57. At the time of the analysis, only 10% of the players had died, which is about half the death rate of men that age in the general population. This indicated that the study participants were in better-than-average general health.

The medical records also showed, however, that an NFL player's risk of death from Alzheimer's disease or amyotrophic lateral sclerosis (ALS), also known as *Lou Gehrig's disease*, was almost four times higher than in the general population. Furthermore, players in "speed" positions—such as wide receiver, running back, and quarterback—accounted for most of these deaths. The researchers emphasized that the data in this type of study do not establish a cause-effect relationship. They hypothesized, however, that the players in "speed" positions had likely experienced more high-speed collisions, and possibly repeated concussions, than the "non-speed" players.

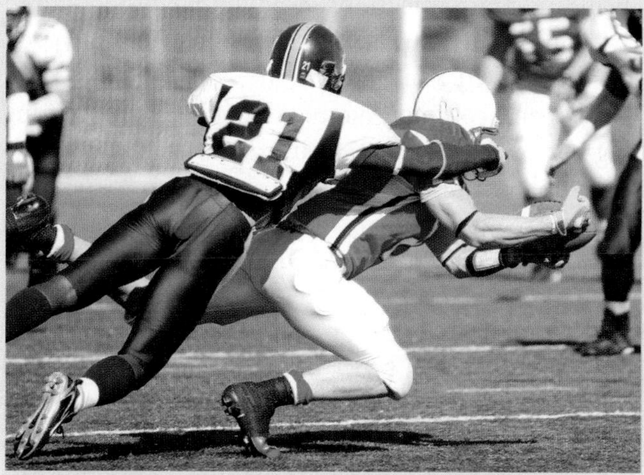

Daniel Padavona/Shutterstock.com

Research funded by the NFL may help find ways to prevent or reduce the effects of common sports injuries.

NFL Takes Action

The NFL has donated $30 million to help establish the Sports and Health Research Program within the National Institutes of Health (NIH). This initiative provides funding for research on concussions and other common injuries in athletes across all sports, as well as members of the military.

The NFL also has taken steps to help prevent concussions, such as fining players for dangerous hits, notably helmet-to-helmet tackles. Rule changes at both the professional and collegiate levels now prevent players diagnosed with concussions from returning to play until they have been declared free of symptoms by a medical doctor.

Cerebral Palsy

Cerebral palsy (CP) is a group of nervous system disorders caused by damage to the brain before or during birth, known as a *congenital defect,* or in early infancy. Congenital defects that can cause CP include an abnormal brain shape or structure, or damaged nerve cells and brain tissues. Infections such as rubella in a woman during pregnancy can produce CP in her baby. During the first two years, while the infant's brain is still developing, several conditions—including brain infections, head injury, and impaired liver function—can cause CP. Sometimes, however, the cause of CP is unknown.

The most common symptoms of CP involve varying degrees of motor function impairment, but can also include hearing, vision, and cognitive impairment. The degree of impairment may be barely noticeable or very severe (**Figure 7.23**). One or both sides of the body may be affected, and the arms, legs, or both may be involved.

Several different types of cerebral palsy exist, and some individuals may have mixed symptoms. The most common form is spastic CP, with symptoms that include very tight muscles and joints, muscle weakness, and a gait (manner of walking) in which the arms are held close to the body with the elbows in flexion, the knees touch or cross, and the individual walks on tiptoes.

In other types of cerebral palsy, motor function degradation may include twisting or jerking movements; tremors; unsteady gait; impaired coordination; and excessive, floppy movements. Sensory and cognitive symptoms may include learning disabilities or diminished intelligence, problems with speech, problems with hearing or vision, seizures, pain, and problems with swallowing and digestion. Other symptoms may include slowed growth, drooling, breathing irregularities, and incontinence.

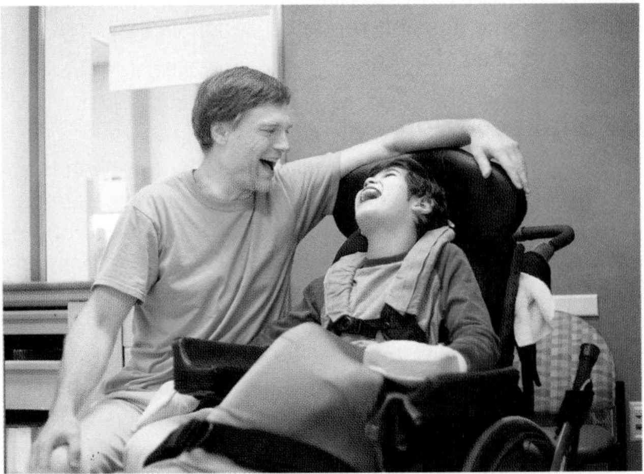

Jaren Jai Wicklund/Shutterstock.com

Figure 7.23 The severity of CP symptoms varies from mild to severe.

There is no cure for cerebral palsy, so the goal of treatment in moderate to severe cases is to promote quality of life and, when possible, independent living. In some cases, surgical intervention can improve gait, alleviate spasticity or pain, or restore joint range of motion.

Spinal Cord Injury

Fractures or displacements of the vertebrae can result in injury to the spinal cord. Such injuries most commonly occur during automobile accidents or participation in high-speed or contact sports. Although injuries to the spinal cord can occur at any level, they most commonly develop in the cervical region because of the flexibility of the neck compared to that of the trunk.

A complete severing of the spinal cord produces permanent paralysis, with a total lack of sensory and motor function below the point of injury. The level of the spine at which the cord is severed determines the extent of the injury:

- C1–C3—usually fatal
- C1–C4—***quadriplegia***, characterized by loss of function below the neck
- C5–C7—complete paralysis of the lower extremities, and partial loss of function in the trunk and upper extremities
- T1–L5—***paraplegia***, characterized by loss of function in the trunk and legs

Fortunately, most spinal cord injuries do not completely sever the spinal cord. In an incomplete injury, the ability of the spinal cord to transmit sensory and motor impulses is not completely lost. This allows some degree of sensory and/or motor function to remain below the point of injury. The prognosis in such cases is typically uncertain; some patients achieve nearly complete recovery, whereas others suffer complete paralysis.

Spinal cord injuries are medical emergencies. Immediate, aggressive treatment and follow-up rehabilitation can help minimize damage and preserve function. Because movement of a fractured or displaced vertebra can cause more damage to the spinal cord after the injury, it is critical that the head, neck,

Clinical Application Neuroprosthetics

Many individuals with missing or paralyzed limbs find it difficult to carry out activities of daily living. Quadriplegics, who constitute the most extreme example of impaired neurological function, must rely completely on others to feed, groom, and otherwise care for them. Scientists and clinicians have been working on different approaches to enable these individuals to harness their thoughts to move external objects, such as a computer cursor or a robotic arm. The ability to move these devices can translate into at least a small degree of increased functionality. For quadriplegics and others with lesser neurological loss, even small improvements in functional capability can make significant differences in quality of life and emotional outlook.

Neuroprosthetics are tiny transducers implanted within the brain to convert neural transmissions into the motion of an artificial limb or other device controlled by the patient. With neuroprosthetics positioned in the motor cortex, patients have successfully produced movement of a robotic limb. In the case of amputees, the robotic limb is connected to the patient's body. In the case of a paraplegic or quadriplegic individual, the artificial limb is separate from the body. Although this approach has been successful, the movements of robotic limbs arising from impulses in the motor cortex have been somewhat awkward and jerky, lacking the fluidity of most natural human movements.

In thinking about ways to improve this approach and enable individuals to generate more normal movement patterns with prosthetics, scientists have considered what is known about the functional regions of the brain. Whereas the motor cortex enables execution of commands such as "lift the arm," "extend the arm," and "grasp the pencil," a normal individual does not typically think about each of these components of the movement. Instead, an individual thinks, "I want to pick up the pencil."

In terms of brain function, picking up a pencil begins with a visual signal ("I see a pencil on the desk") that is processed in the primary visual area and interpreted in the visual association area of the occipital lobe. The signal then moves up to the somatosensory association area in the posterior parietal cortex, where the *intention* to pick up the pencil is formulated. This intention is transmitted to the motor cortex through the spinal cord, and then to the muscles where contractions are required to execute the movements.

This understanding has led scientists to select the posterior parietal cortex as the site of implantation for a new generation of neuroprosthetics. This newer, more advanced technique utilizes two small silicon chips, each containing a matrix of 96 microscopic electrodes. Researchers estimate that each chip can simultaneously read the activity being generated in approximately 100 neurons. The chips are connected by wires to computers that process the signals, decode the intention for movement, and translate that intention into the motions of output devices such as a computer cursor or robotic arm.

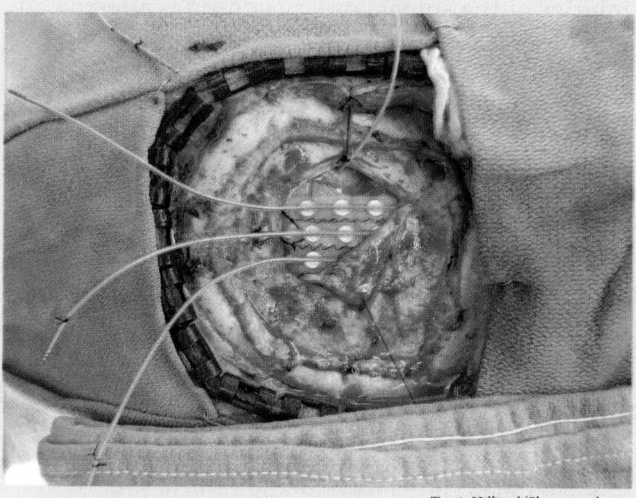

Travis Hilliard/Shutterstock.com

Neuroprosthetics implanted in the brain are revolutionizing the capabilities of robotic limb prosthetics.

To test the safety and effectiveness of this new system, surgeons implanted the silicon chips in two areas of the posterior parietal cortex of a quadriplegic patient who had been paralyzed for over 10 years. The patient was successfully trained to control a computer cursor and a robotic arm with his thoughts. Continued training has enabled the patient to further refine his control of the arm and the cursor, while at the same time giving the researchers more insight into the workings of the posterior parietal cortex.

The general goal of this work is to develop means by which individuals with missing or paralyzed limbs can lead lives that are more typical and functional. Enabling control of a computer cursor provides the ability to interact with a computer. Control of a robotic arm provides the potential for performing daily activities such as combing hair, drinking from a glass, and eating unassisted.

Although the silicon chips described above are now commercially available and approved by the US Food and Drug Administration, much remains to be done before this approach can be broadly utilized in practical therapeutic interventions. Some of the current challenges include improving the durability of the implants, refining the ability to isolate single nerve cells, and optimizing computational algorithms for interpreting signals and converting them into actions. The silicon chips also need to be refined so that they can communicate wirelessly with a computer, as the hard-wire connections present an avenue for infection. Despite these challenges, the use of neuroprosthetics is clearly promising for the future.

and trunk be immobilized before a victim is moved (**Figure 7.24**). In about one-third of severe neck injuries of the spinal cord, breathing is affected and respiratory support is necessary. Surgery is often warranted to remove bone fragments or realign vertebrae to alleviate pressure on the spinal cord.

Ongoing research aims to develop techniques for repairing injured spinal cords. Researchers are also working to advance the understanding of which rehabilitation approaches will be optimally successful at restoring lost function. Promising new rehabilitation techniques are helping patients with spinal cord injuries become more mobile.

SELF CHECK

1. Evaluate the causes of traumatic brain injury (TBI).
2. List the conditions that can cause cerebral palsy (CP).
3. Describe the usual result of a spinal cord injury that occurs at each of the following levels: C1–C3, C1–C4, C5–C7, and T1–L5.

Diseases and Disorders of the Central Nervous System

This section explores some of the common diseases and disorders that affect the central nervous system (CNS). These include meningitis, multiple sclerosis, epilepsy, Parkinson's disease, Huntington's disease, and dementia and Alzheimer's disease.

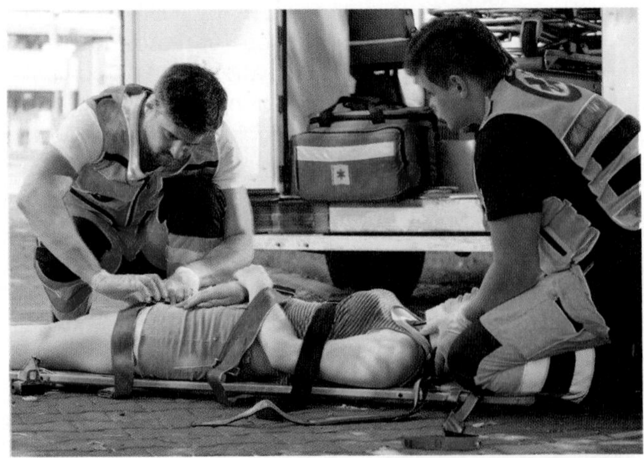

Photographee.eu/Shutterstock.com

Figure 7.24 It is critically important that the head, neck, and trunk be immobilized before transporting a patient with a potential spinal cord injury.

Meningitis

Meningitis is an inflammation of the meninges surrounding the brain and spinal cord. Swelling of these tissues, which is caused by an infection, often produces the signature symptoms of headache, fever, and a stiff neck.

Most infections that cause meningitis are viral, but meningitis can also be caused by bacterial and fungal infections. Viral meningitis, the milder form, can resolve on its own. Bacterial meningitis is much more serious and potentially life-threatening. Fortunately, bacterial meningitis can be treated with antibiotics. In either case, a person should seek immediate medical attention if meningitis is suspected.

Multiple Sclerosis

Multiple sclerosis (MS) is an autoimmune disease in which the body's own immune system causes inflammation that destroys the myelin sheath of nerve cell axons. This damage to the myelin sheath, which may occur in any part of the brain or spinal cord, impairs the ability of the affected nerves to transmit impulses. MS can occur at any age, but it is most commonly diagnosed between 20 and 40 years of age. MS occurs with greater frequency in women than in men. The cause of MS is unknown.

The symptoms of MS vary widely, depending on the location of damaged nerves within the CNS and the severity of each episode. Symptoms may include the following:

- impairments in motor function—difficulties with balance, coordination, and movement of the arms and legs; tremors; weakness; muscle spasms; and difficulty speaking or swallowing
- sensory impairments—numbness, tingling, pain, double vision, uncontrollable eye movements, and loss of vision or hearing
- impairments in autonomic function—difficulties with urination, defecation, and sexual function
- associated cognitive issues— decreased attention span, difficulty with reasoning, loss of memory, and depression

An active attack of MS can last for days, weeks, or months. Periods during which the symptoms vanish or diminish are called *remissions*. Exposure to heat and stress can trigger or worsen attacks.

There is no known cure for multiple sclerosis, so treatments are designed to help control symptoms and maintain quality of life. Exercise is often beneficial during the early stages. General recommendations for MS patients include sufficient rest, sound nutrition, avoidance of hot temperatures, and minimization of stress. Although MS is a chronic condition, life expectancy can be normal. Many individuals with MS continue functioning well in their jobs until retirement.

Epilepsy

Epilepsy is a group of brain disorders characterized by repeated seizures over time. A seizure is triggered by abnormal electrical activity in the brain that causes widely varying symptoms. Symptoms range from changes in attention span or behavior to uncontrolled convulsions, depending on the type of epilepsy and area of the brain affected.

Epilepsy may be caused by a disease or injury that affects the brain, although in many cases the cause is unknown, and genetics may play a role. Onset of epilepsy can happen at any age but occurs most frequently in infants and the elderly.

The nature of epileptic seizures is relatively consistent in a given individual. Before a seizure, some people experience an unusual sensation such as tingling, a strange smell, or an emotional change. This signal is referred to as an *aura*.

Epilepsy can be controlled with medication in most, but not all, people. Some types of epilepsy completely disappear after childhood. However, medication fails to control seizure incidence in more than 30% of people with epilepsy. If epileptic seizures are caused by an observable problem, such as a tumor, abnormal blood vessels, or bleeding in the brain, surgery to address these issues may eliminate further seizures.

Parkinson's Disease

Parkinson's disease (PD) is one of the most common nervous system disorders among the elderly. It is characterized by tremors, difficulty with initiating movements—especially walking—and deficits in coordination. PD typically develops after the age of 50, although a genetic form of the disease may occur in younger adults. Men and women are equally affected by this disease.

The characteristic symptoms of PD are caused by slow but progressive destruction of the brain cells responsible for production of the neurotransmitter dopamine, which plays a role in motor function. Without dopamine, the cells in the affected part of the brain cannot initiate nerve impulses, leading to progressive loss of muscle function. The cause of Parkinson's disease is unknown.

The symptoms of PD tend to begin with a mild tremor, or a slight stiffness or weakness in one or both of the legs or feet. As brain cell destruction progresses, symptoms of motor dysfunction affecting one or both sides of the body may include:

- difficulty initiating and continuing movements
- problems with balance and gait
- stiff, painful muscles and tremors
- slowed movement, including blinking
- loss of fine motor control in hand movements
- slowed speech, drooling, and difficulty swallowing
- loss of facial expression
- stooped posture

Autonomic and cognitive functions can also be impaired, as characterized by:

- sweating and fluctuations in body temperature
- fainting and inability to control blood pressure
- constipation
- confusion or dementia
- anxiety or depression

There is currently no cure for Parkinson's disease. The goal of treatment is control of symptoms. If untreated, the disorder will progress, resulting in deterioration of all brain functions and early death. The medications prescribed for Parkinson's patients are designed to increase the levels of dopamine in the brain.

Huntington's Disease

Huntington's disease (HD) is caused by a genetic mutation that is passed down through families. Each child of a parent with HD has a 50% chance of receiving the defective gene. Children who do not inherit the HD gene will not develop the condition and cannot pass it on to their children. Those who do receive the gene, however, will develop HD and their children have a 50% chance of receiving the defective gene.

The HD gene causes degeneration of neurons in the brain, resulting in an inability to control movements, loss of intellectual capacity, and emotional disturbance. Early symptoms of HD include mood swings, depression, irritability, and difficulty with tasks such as driving, learning new things, remembering facts, or making decisions. As the disease progresses, daily activities become difficult, and patients may have difficulty feeding themselves and swallowing.

The age of onset and rate of progression of Huntington's disease vary from person to person. When onset occurs before the age of 20, the disease is called *juvenile Huntington's disease*, and the progression of symptoms is more rapid.

The neuromuscular disorders that characterize Huntington's disease include involuntary movements and the inability to control voluntary movements. Examples include:

- involuntary jerking or writhing movements (known as *chorea*)
- muscle rigidity or muscle contracture (known as *dystonia*)
- slow or abnormal eye movements
- impaired gait, posture, and balance
- difficulty controlling tongue movements for speech or swallowing

Intellectual impairments often associated with Huntington's disease include the following:

- difficulty organizing, prioritizing, or focusing on tasks
- the tendency to become overly focused on a thought, behavior, or action
- lack of impulse control that can result in outbursts
- lack of awareness of one's own behaviors
- slowed processing of thoughts
- difficulty learning new information

The most common psychiatric disorder associated with Huntington's disease is depression, which results from degenerative changes in the brain. Specific symptoms may include feelings of irritability, sadness, or apathy; social withdrawal; insomnia; fatigue and loss of energy; and thoughts of death, dying, and suicide.

Several medications can help control the emotional issues and movement problems associated with HD. In 2008, the US Food and Drug Administration approved tetrabenazine to treat the disease's involuntary writhing movements (Huntington's chorea), making it the first drug approved for use in the United States specifically to treat HD. Genetic engineering holds the promise of future repair or replacement of the genetic mutation that causes HD.

Dementia and Alzheimer's Disease

Dementia is a condition involving loss of function in two or more areas of cognition including memory, thinking, judgment, behavior, perception, and language. Dementia usually occurs after the age of 60, and risk of developing the condition increases with age. Although forgetfulness is often the first sign of dementia, occasional forgetfulness alone does not qualify as dementia.

Dementia can be caused by disruption in the blood supply to the brain, as in stroke or related disorders. However, the single most common cause of dementia is Alzheimer's disease.

Alzheimer's disease (AD), or senile dementia, is a progressive loss of brain function with major consequences for memory, thinking, and behavior. In one form of the disease, called *early onset AD*, symptoms appear before age 60. This type of AD tends to worsen quickly and is believed to involve genetic predisposition. The more common form, known as *late onset AD*, occurs after age 60. The cause of AD is currently unknown.

Early symptoms of AD may include difficulty with tasks that were previously routine; difficulty learning new ideas, concepts, or tasks; becoming lost in familiar territory; difficulty recalling the names of familiar objects; misplacing objects; a flat mood and loss of interest in activities; personality changes; and loss of social skills.

Worsening symptoms can include difficulty performing activities of daily living, progressive loss of short- and long-term memories, depression and agitation, delusions and aggressive behavior, inability to speak coherently, loss of judgment, and change in sleep patterns. Advanced symptoms include the inability to understand language and recognize family members. Although no cure currently exists for Alzheimer's disease, medications can help slow the worsening of symptoms.

SECTION 7.5

REVIEW

Mini-Glossary

Alzheimer's disease (AD) a condition involving a progressive loss of brain function with major consequences for memory, thinking, and behavior

cerebral palsy (CP) a group of nervous system disorders resulting from brain damage before or during birth, or in early infancy

dementia an organic brain disease involving loss of function in two or more areas of cognition

epilepsy a group of brain disorders characterized by repeated seizures over time

Huntington's disease (HD) a genetic disease that causes degeneration of neurons in the brain, resulting in an inability to control movements, a loss of intellectual capacity, and emotional disturbance

meningitis an infection-induced inflammation of the meninges surrounding the brain and spinal cord

multiple sclerosis (MS) a chronic, slowly progressive disease of the central nervous system that destroys the myelin sheath of nerve cell axons

paraplegia a disorder characterized by loss of function in the lower trunk and legs

Parkinson's disease (PD) a chronic nervous system disease characterized by a slowly spreading tremor, muscular weakness, and rigidity

quadriplegia a disorder characterized by loss of function below the neck

traumatic brain injury (TBI) mild or severe trauma that can result from a violent impact to the head

Review Questions

1. Describe the body functions that may be affected by cerebral palsy (CP).
2. What is meant by the term *incomplete injury* as it relates to a spinal cord injury?
3. What are the two types of meningitis and which is easier to treat?
4. What happens to the body of a person with multiple sclerosis (MS)?
5. Describe Parkinson's disease.
6. What autoimmune disease did you learn about in Chapter 5? How are that disease and multiple sclerosis similar?
7. Explain what happens in the brain when a person has a seizure.

Medical Terminology: The Nervous System

By understanding the word parts that make up medical words, you can extend your medical vocabulary. This chapter includes many of the word parts listed below. Review these word parts to be sure you understand their meanings.

-al	pertaining to
-ar	pertaining to
arachn/o	spider-like
astro-	star-shaped
crani/o	brain, brain stem
-cyte	cell
-graphy	process of recording
hypo-	below, underneath
-ic	pertaining to
-lemma	sheath, covering
micro-	small
myel/o	spinal cord, bone marrow
neur/o	nerve
-oid	resembling
-otomy	incision
-phthisis	wasting away, atrophy
-poiesis	formation of
post-	after
sacr/o	sacrum
somat/o	body

Now use these word parts to form valid medical words that fit the following definitions. Some of the words are included in this chapter. Others are not. When you finish, use a medical dictionary to check your work.

1. pertaining to the body
2. pertaining to both the nerves and the muscles
3. pertaining to a synapse
4. star-shaped cell
5. external covering of a nerve (Schwann cell)
6. spinal cord incision
7. chemical that transmits nerve impulses
8. atrophy of the spinal cord

9. process of recording small nerves
10. below the thalamus
11. tissue that resembles a spider's web
12. pertaining to both the brain stem and the sacrum
13. pertaining to after a ganglion
14. formation of bone marrow

Chapter 7 Summary

- The structures within the nervous system are divided into two major divisions: the central nervous system and the peripheral nervous system.
- The nervous system contains two types of tissue: neuroglia and neurons.
- Stimuli bring about depolarization, which creates a nerve impulse, or action potential.
- Factors that influence the speed at which a nerve impulse travels include the presence of a myelin sheath, the diameter of the axon, the purpose of the nerve impulse, and body temperature.
- Chemical neurotransmitters conduct impulses across synapses.
- Reflexes are simple, rapid, involuntary, programmed responses to stimuli.
- The brain consists of four major anatomical regions: the cerebrum, diencephalon, brain stem, and cerebellum.
- The spinal cord serves as a major pathway for relaying sensory and motor impulses.
- The peripheral nervous system includes cranial nerves, spinal nerves, and nerve plexuses.
- Within the autonomic nervous system, the sympathetic nerves activate the fight-or-flight response; the parasympathetic nerves control day-to-day functions.
- The brain and spinal cord are well-protected, but injuries do occur, and they can have serious consequences.
- Some common disorders and diseases of the CNS include meningitis, multiple sclerosis (MS), epilepsy, Parkinson's disease (PD), cerebral palsy (CP), dementia, Huntington's disease, and Alzheimer's disease.

Chapter 7 Review

Understanding Key Concepts

1. The central nervous system (CNS) includes the _____ and the _____.
2. The peripheral nervous system (PNS) is made up of _____ nerves and _____ nerves.
3. Nerves that transmit impulses from sensory receptors to the CNS are known as _____.
4. Nerves that transmit impulses from the CNS to the muscles and glands are known as _____.
5. The two subdivisions of the efferent nerves are the _____ nervous system and the _____ nervous system.
6. What are the four types of glial cells in the CNS?
7. The main function of an axon's myelin sheath is to _____.
8. The two behavioral properties of a neuron are _____ and _____.
9. Because of the difference in electrical charge between the inside and outside of a resting cell, the cell membrane is said to be _____.
10. Which of the following factors does *not* influence the speed of a nerve impulse?
    A. body temperature
    B. diameter of the axon
    C. presence of a myelin sheath
    D. body weight
11. Communication between cells occurs through direct transfer of electrical signals. The point at which this transfer occurs is called the _____.
12. A rapid, involuntary, programmed response to a stimulus is known as a(n) _____.
13. _____ reflexes send involuntary stimuli to the cardiac muscle of the heart and the smooth muscle of internal organs.
14. The adult human brain weighs approximately _____ pounds, and it contains about _____ neurons.
15. *True or False?* Recent evidence suggests that the size of a person's brain is related to intelligence.

16. Each curved, raised area of the brain is called a ______.
    A. sulcus
    B. gyrus
    C. neuron
    D. lobe
17. Each of the grooves between the gyri in the brain is called a ______.
    A. sulcus
    B. gyrus
    C. neuron
    D. lobe
18. The four lobes of the brain are the frontal, occipital, temporal, and ______.
    A. cervical
    B. ependymal
    C. parietal
    D. ventral
19. The diencephalon is also called the ______.
    A. interbrain
    B. midbrain
    C. left brain
    D. outer brain
20. The three protective membranes that surround the brain are the ______.
    A. fascicles
    B. synapses
    C. perineuria
    D. meninges
21. In a nerve, each axon fiber is covered by a fine sheath called the ______.
    A. endoneurium
    B. peritoneum
    C. epineurium
    D. perineurium
22. Groups of sheathed nerve fibers are bundled into fascicles surrounded by the ______.
    A. endoneurium
    B. peritoneum
    C. epineurium
    D. perineurium
23. Groups of fascicles and blood vessels are surrounded by the ______.
24. Mixed nerves carry both ______ impulses and ______ impulses.
25. How many pairs of cranial nerves does a person have?
26. How many pairs of spinal nerves does a person have?
27. Each spinal nerve is divided into a ______ ramus and a ventral ramus.
    A. cranial
    B. superior
    C. dorsal
    D. posterior
28. The ______ nervous system controls all of the automatic functions of the cardiovascular, respiratory, and digestive systems.
    A. sympathetic
    B. parasympathetic
    C. central
    D. parietal
29. Name at least five symptoms of mild traumatic brain injury.
30. *True or False?* Cerebral palsy can be caused by several disorders or conditions.
31. Meningitis is inflammation of the ______ that surround the brain and spinal cord.
32. *True or False?* Multiple sclerosis (MS) is considered an autoimmune disease.
33. Alzheimer's disease is a progressive loss of brain function with consequences for ______, thinking, and ______.

Thinking Critically

34. Create a flowchart that shows the main components or structures of the nervous system and each of its subdivisions. List the functions and processes that each component controls.
35. Recalling what you have learned about nerve impulses, how do you think each of the following substances affects conduction speeds: caffeine, sedatives, and energy drinks?

36. If a person has extremely low blood calcium levels, will that affect the transmission of electrical signals from one cell to another? Explain your answer.
37. If one component or structure in the brain becomes damaged, do you think the other structures can compensate enough for the person to function fairly normally? Explain your answer.
38. Examine the importance of the blood-brain barrier. Explain what you think would happen if this protective measure were no longer in place.
39. Explain what happens physiologically when the fight-or-flight response is activated in the body.
40. Evaluate the causes and effects of cerebral palsy on the structure and function of cells, tissues, organs, and systems.
41. Explain the range of problems that can result from injuries to different parts of the spinal column.
42. Evaluate the causes and effects of TBI on the structure and function of cells, tissues, organs, and systems.

Clinical Case Study

Read again the Clinical Case Study at the beginning of this chapter. Use the information provided in the chapter to answer the following questions.

43. What diagnoses are possible and which is most likely?
44. Given the description, what grade is this injury?

Analyzing and Evaluating Data

The bar graph to the right shows approximate transmission speeds for several different types of nerve impulses. Use the graph to answer the following questions.

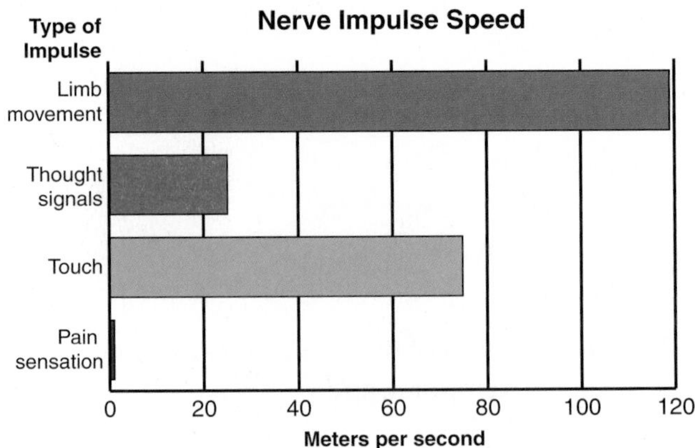

45. About how much faster do you *think* than *feel* pain?
46. Do nerve impulses signaling the sense of touch travel at approximately two, three, or four times the speed of thought impulses?
47. Assume that rising temperatures increase all the nerve impulse speeds by 5%. If the limb movement speed shown is 119 meters per second (m/s), what will it be at the higher temperature?
48. Give approximate feet-per-second (fps) speeds for each type of nerve transmission shown in the graph. (Use the conversion chart in the appendices if necessary.)

Investigating Further

49. Choose one of the diseases or disorders described in this chapter and find out more about current research regarding its diagnosis and/or treatment.
50. Conduct further research into neurotransmitters in the human body. Create a table that lists each neurotransmitter and its function.

8 The Sensory Systems

Clinical Case Study

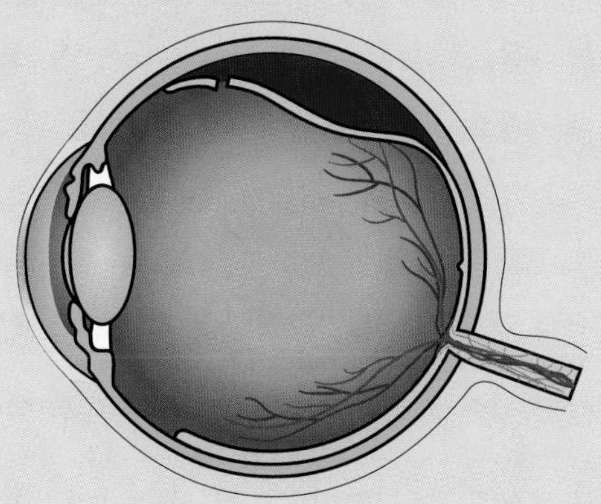
By Mrs_Bazilio/Shutterstock.com

Jenny is living in a dormitory at her college, but she often drives home on weekends to visit her parents and younger brother. It also happens to be convenient to do her laundry at her parents' house.

This past weekend Jenny's mother, Sally, was helping her fold her clean clothes when Sally mentioned that she kept seeing a tiny flash of light on the extreme right side of her vision. Once the clothes were folded, the light flash did not reoccur and so both Jenny and Sally stopped thinking about it.

Later, however, Jenny started thinking again about the light flashes and she worried that they might be indicative of a medical issue. Thinking further, she realized that this condition was mentioned in a chapter in her anatomy and physiology textbook. Jenny strongly encouraged her mother to see her ophthalmologist right away. Among the diseases and disorders of the eye discussed in this chapter, which conditions are possible, and which is most likely?

Chapter 8 Outline

To capture a picture or video, you might use a camera or smartphone. If you want to listen to music on a phone or portable music player, you might use earphones. As useful as these items are, the human eyes, ears, nose, and mouth far exceed the ability of modern technology to capture and transmit special sensory information to the brain.

The special senses, including vision, hearing, smell, and taste, involve extraordinarily well-designed sensory pathways in the nervous system. For each of the senses, highly specialized receptor cells communicate with neurons to begin the virtually instantaneous process of sending sensory messages to the brain. Once in the brain, messages from the sensory systems are rapidly integrated and interpreted.

This chapter examines the anatomical structures and physiological capabilities of the components of the sensory systems. In addition, it describes some of the common injuries and disorders of these systems, including their symptoms and current treatments.

SECTION 8.1

The Eye

Objectives

- Describe the external and internal anatomical structures of the human eye and how they work together to produce vision.
- List and describe eye injuries, vision disorders, and diseases of the eye.

Key Terms

aqueous humor
choroid
ciliary body
ciliary glands
cones
conjunctiva
cornea
extrinsic muscles
fovea centralis
iris
lacrimal glands
lens
optic chiasma
optic nerve
optic tracts
pupil
retina
rods
sclera
suspensory ligaments
tarsal glands
vitreous humor

According to an old English proverb, "The eyes are the windows to the soul." Whether or not this is true, some people do have expressive eyes that help convey their emotional states. Eyes "twinkling with amusement" or "flashing with anger" are familiar descriptive phrases. A person can also be described as *bright-eyed, dark-eyed, shifty-eyed,* or *eagle-eyed,* all of which suggest distinctive images or characteristics.

The eyes are important parts of human anatomy, because vision is an extremely useful sense. This section describes the anatomical components of the eye and explains how they function together to produce the remarkable ability to see.

Anatomy and Physiology of the Eye

The adult eye is about 1 inch (2.5 cm) in diameter, and it has a slightly oblong spherical shape. A variety of external structures protect the eye, and internal structures send sensory signals to the brain, enabling vision.

External Structures

The eye is a delicate structure that, fortunately, is well protected. The eye is encased in the bony orbital socket of the skull and is covered by an eyelid. The eyebrows also function as protection; they help shield the eyes from dripping sweat on hot days, for example. The eyelashes and eyelids provide considerable protection from circulating dust particles. The visible region of the eye, between the eyelids, is called the *palpebral fissure.*

Several structures work together to lubricate the eyes (**Figure 8.1**). ***Tarsal glands*** in the eyelids produce an oily secretion. Modified sweat glands called ***ciliary glands***, which are located between the eyelashes, produce sweat for lubrication. The ***conjunctiva***, a delicate external membrane that covers the exposed eyeball and lines the eyelid, also secretes lubricating mucus.

The lacrimal apparatus includes the structures that bathe the eyes in tears. The ***lacrimal glands*** are located above the lateral commissure, or the outer end of each eye. Excretory ducts in these glands continually release the familiar, salty solution known as *tears.* Because tears contain antibodies and an enzyme called *lysozyme* that attacks bacteria, they not only lubricate the surface of the eye but also keep it clean.

Tears are flushed into tiny canals called *lacrimal canaliculi* in the medial commissure, or inside corner of each eye. These canaliculi then drain into the nasolacrimal duct, which empties into the nasal cavity.

Irritation to the eye produces extra tearing, which helps wash away foreign substances. Under stressful conditions, tears may be produced at such a high rate that they cannot be drained away fast enough and spill over onto the cheeks.

Six ***extrinsic muscles*** attach to the outer surface of the eye and are responsible for moving the eye within the orbital socket (**Figure 8.2**). The specific functions of these muscles are listed in the table in **Figure 8.3**.

© Body Scientific International

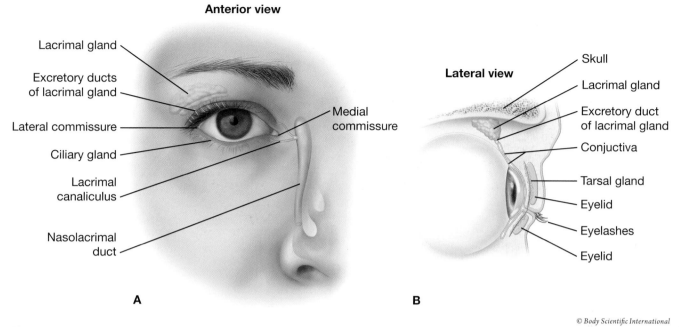

Figure 8.1 Lubricating structures of the eye. A—Anterior view. B—Lateral view.

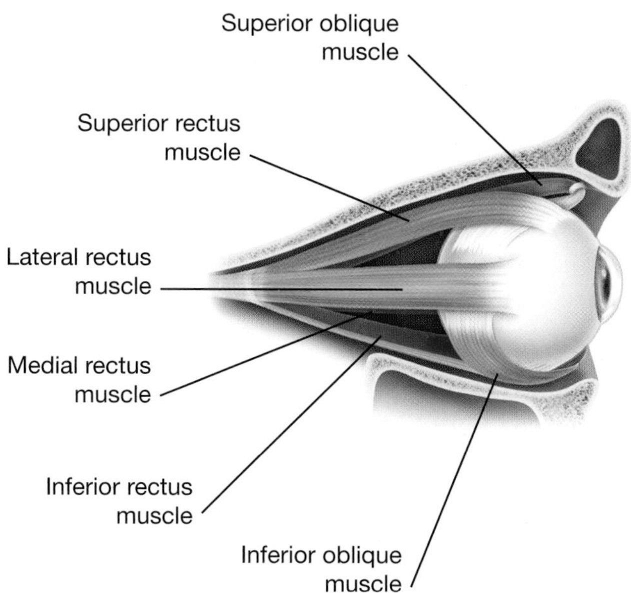

© Body Scientific International

Figure 8.2 Lateral view of the extrinsic muscles of the eye.

Internal Structures

The eye is a hollow chamber, somewhat oblong in shape, filled with fluids called *aqueous* and *vitreous humors*. These fluids help the eyeball maintain its shape (**Figure 8.4**).

Three layers of tissue form the walls of the eyeball. The tough, fibrous ***sclera*** makes up the outer layer of the eye. The sclera includes the "white of the eye" as well as the transparent ***cornea*** located over the anterior center of the eye. The cornea is called the *window of the eye* because light passes through it. The cornea has no blood supply and, therefore, is the only body tissue that can be transplanted from one person to another without concern about rejection.

The middle layer of the eye, called the ***choroid***, contains a rich supply of blood vessels that provide nourishment to the eye. These blood vessels contribute to a crimson-purple pigmentation that darkens the interior of the eye, preventing light reflections. On its anterior side, the choroid also includes the ***iris***, which gives the eye its color. The iris can widen or narrow to control the size of the ***pupil***, the opening through which light passes into the interior of the eye.

Two sets of muscles within the iris work to control the amount of light admitted to the eye. The sphincter pupillae contracts in the presence of bright light, as well as when the eye focuses on an object within close range. This contraction causes the pupil to grow smaller and allow less light into the eye. In the presence of dim

The Extrinsic Eye Muscles

Muscle	Action
superior rectus	upward eye motion
inferior rectus	downward eye motion
lateral rectus	lateral eye motion
medial rectus	medial eye motion
superior oblique	downward and lateral eye motion
inferior oblique	upward and lateral eye motion

Figure 8.3 Goodheart-Willcox Publisher

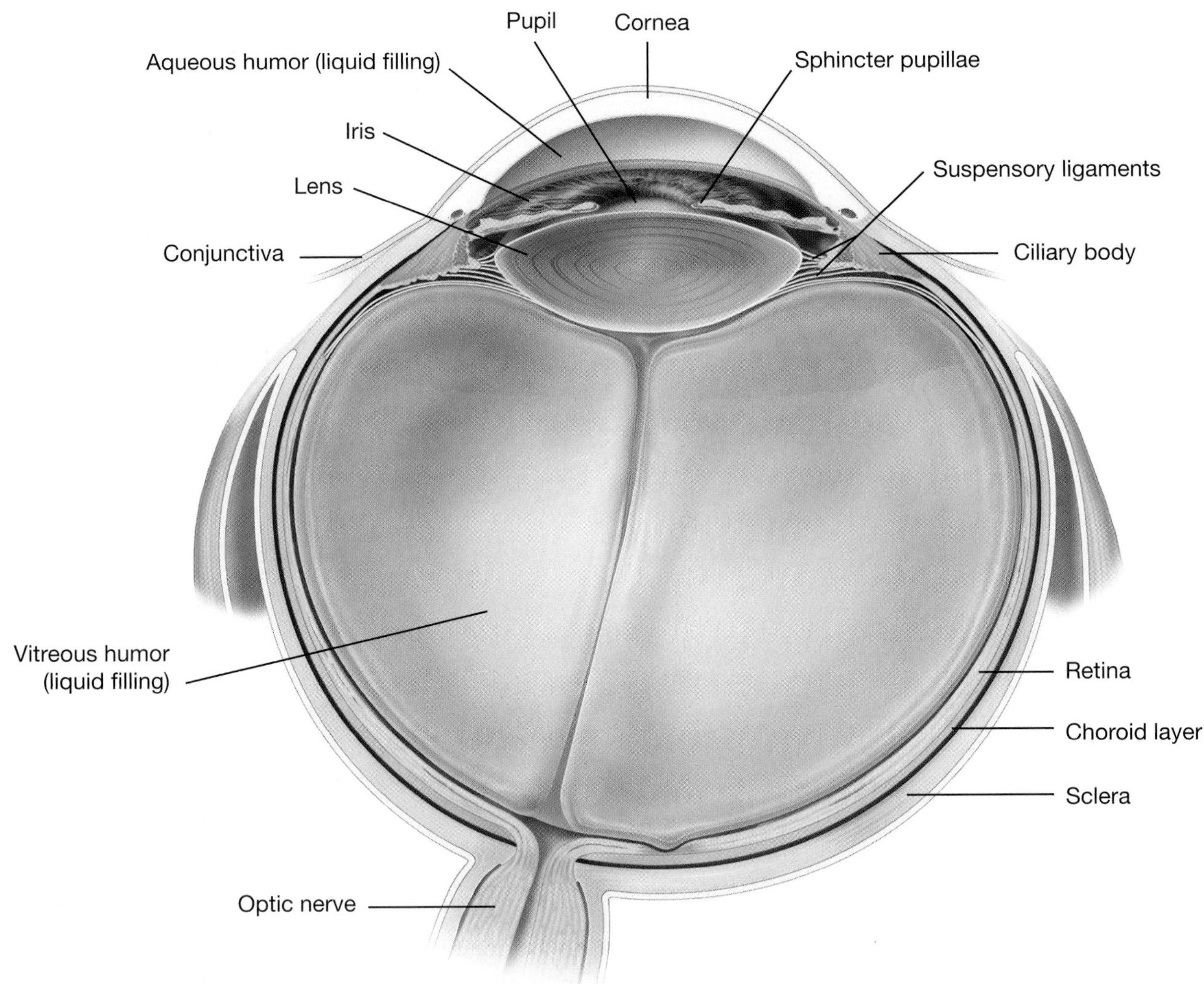

Figure 8.4 Internal structures of the eye.

light, and when the eye focuses on a distant object, the dilator pupillae muscle contracts, causing dilation of the pupil and allowing more light to enter the eye.

The innermost layer of the eye, known as the ***retina***, is located only around the posterior portion of the eye, anterior to the choroid. The retina is composed of two layers. The outer layer, or pigmented layer, includes pigmented cells that absorb light, store vitamin A, and serve as phagocytes to remove damaged receptor cells on the inner layer. The inner layer, or neural layer, of the retina is dense in specialized, light-sensitive nerve endings. These nerve endings send impulses through the optic nerve to the occipital lobe of the brain, where images are interpreted.

The sensory receptor cells in the neural layer of the retina are called *rods* and *cones* (**Figure 8.5**). The ***rods*** are activated in dim light; the ***cones*** are sensitive to bright light and also provide color vision. The rods are most densely distributed around the periphery of the retina. They provide peripheral vision and enable perception of shades of gray in dim light. The cones are most densely distributed in the center of the retina, with decreasing distribution toward the periphery.

The ***fovea centralis*** is a tiny spot near the center of each retina that contains only cones. This is the point of greatest visual acuity, or clarity, so it is the spot where the eye tends to focus when trying to view something clearly. As displayed in **Figure 8.6**, there are three types of cones, with each type responding to a different spectrum of light—blue, green, or green and red. Since the green-and-red-sensitive cones are the only ones responding to red light, they are simply called *red cones*. Nerve ganglions and bipolar neurons provide connections between the retina and the rods and cones.

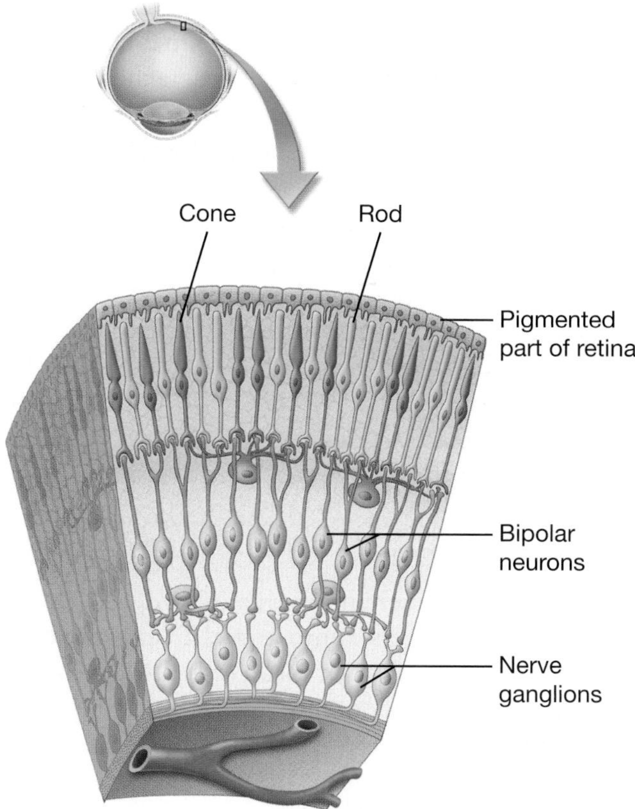

Figure 8.5 Rods and cones in the retina.

People sometimes reference a "blind spot" in their vision. A physiological blind spot called the *optic disc* appears on each retina. The optic disc is the junction between the optic nerve and the eye. Because there are no rods and cones in the optic disc, this tiny area is unable to transmit visual information—hence the term *blind spot.*

Under normal circumstances, people do not perceive the blind spot because the brain fills in the visual information from the other eye. Given the separation between the two eyes, the blind spots are missing different pieces of the combined visual field.

The ***lens*** of the eye is located behind the iris. It is a transparent, flexible, crystal-like structure that curves outward on both sides. The lens is held in place by the tiny ***suspensory ligaments*** that surround it. These ligaments attach to the ***ciliary body,*** which merges with the choroid layer.

The lens separates the anterior and posterior chambers of the eye. The anterior chamber is filled with the clear, watery ***aqueous humor.*** Continually secreted by the choroid, the aqueous humor provides nutrients to the avascular (without blood vessels) lens and cornea and helps maintain normal pressure inside the eye (intraocular pressure). The posterior chamber of the eye is filled with the gel-like ***vitreous humor,*** which also contributes to intraocular pressure.

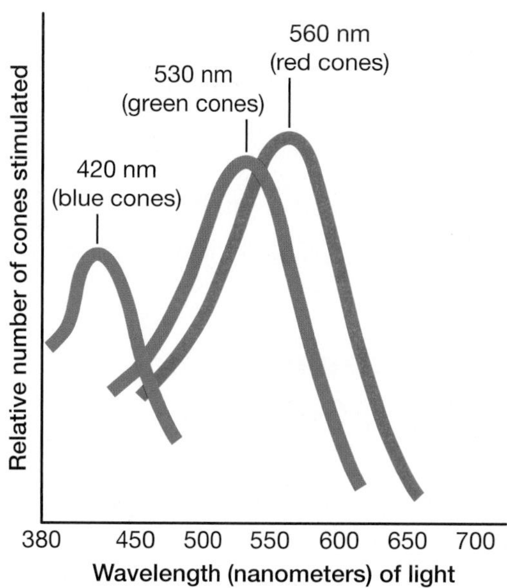

Figure 8.6 The three types of cones are stimulated by different regions of the spectrum of visible light.

When at rest, the eye is focused for distance vision. For the eye to clearly view objects closer than about 20 feet, the muscles of the ciliary body contract to change the shape of the lens. This process of contraction, known as *accommodation,* makes the lens thicker, enabling it to focus incoming light rays on the surface of the retina.

After about 40 years of age, the ability of the ciliary body muscles to appropriately contract diminishes. In the absence of other visual corrections, this causes people who are older than 40 years of age to need reading glasses for up-close vision.

Vision

The eye perceives an object when the light reflected from that object passes through the cornea, pupil, and lens to the retina. The rods and cones in the retina are stimulated and send impulses to the ***optic nerve,*** which transmits sensory signals to the brain.

The two optic nerves (one from each eye) cross at the ***optic chiasma.*** The nerve fibers exiting the optic chiasma are called ***optic tracts.*** The optic tracts carry visual stimuli to the occipital lobe of the brain.

SELF CHECK

1. What do the tarsal glands produce?
2. Describe two different ways in which tears clean the eyes.
3. Name the three layers of the eye.
4. What is the function of the optic nerve?

Injuries, Diseases, and Disorders of the Eye

The eyes are vulnerable to various injuries, diseases, and disorders. This section examines some common examples.

Eye Injuries

The structure of the face and eyes helps protect the eyes from injury. The bony socket in which the eyeball is encased, the eyelid, the eyebrows, and the eyelashes all provide a barrier to foreign objects. In fact, these features are so effective in protecting the eye that many eye injuries affect the surrounding tissues and structures rather than the eyeball itself. Still, certain injuries can damage the eyeball, causing impairment or loss of vision.

Usually, minor irritants are flushed from the eye through tear production. Irritating chemicals, however, should be flushed with large quantities of water. Fragments of glass or other solid particles that become lodged in the eye should be removed only by a medical professional.

The cornea is well supplied with pain and touch receptors. Consequently, corneal injuries (abrasions or tears) are extremely painful. Fortunately, the cornea has an astonishing self-repairing ability; most injuries to the cornea resolve themselves within 24 hours.

Trauma to the eye can cause a detached retina, in which the retina separates from the underlying support tissue. The detachment may be partial in the beginning, but it can rapidly progress to complete detachment if not treated. The associated vision loss can progress from minor to severe and even to blindness within a few hours or days.

Surgical techniques such as lasers, air bubbles, or a freezing probe can be used to reattach the retina. In most cases, surgery can restore good vision. If left unrepaired, a detached retina can cause loss of peripheral vision and subsequently loss of central vision.

Vision Disorders

A variety of relatively minor, common eye defects can impair vision, as summarized in the table in **Figure 8.7**. Three common vision disorders are shown in **Figure 8.8**. Many of these disorders can be completely corrected with prescription lenses (**Figure 8.9**).

Myopia

Commonly known as *nearsightedness*, myopia results from an elongated eyeball shape, which causes the lens to focus objects in front of the retina rather than directly upon it (**Figure 8.8B**). Nearby objects can be seen clearly, but distant objects appear blurry.

A Snellen chart or other chart similar to it is used to diagnose myopia. This familiar chart includes rows of letters, with each successive row printed smaller than the one above. These charts are used only as a first step in diagnosing myopia. Medical eye specialists perform a number of tests before they prescribe corrective lenses for visual defects. Laser surgery techniques also can be performed to correct myopia.

Characteristics of Common Vision Disorders		
Condition	**Description**	**Cause**
myopia	nearsightedness	elongated eyeball
hyperopia	farsightedness	shortened eyeball
presbyopia	age-related farsightedness	stiffness of the lens
astigmatism	blurred vision	irregular curvature of cornea or lens
amblyopia	lazy eye	abnormal dominance of one eye
diplopia	double vision	abnormal alignment of the eyes
strabismus	crossed eyes	muscles in one eye do not coordinate with those in the other eye
color blindness	inability to distinguish colors	disorder of the cone cells in the retina
night blindness	difficulty seeing at night	disorder of the rod cells in the retina

Figure 8.7

Goodheart-Willcox Publisher

Hyperopia

By contrast, in hyperopia, also known as *farsightedness*, the distance from the lens to the retina is shortened because the eyeball has a more flattened shape (**Figure 8.8C**). This means that light rays focus behind the retina instead of directly upon it. As a result, objects at a distance can be seen clearly, but objects nearby appear blurry. Prescription lenses can correct this condition.

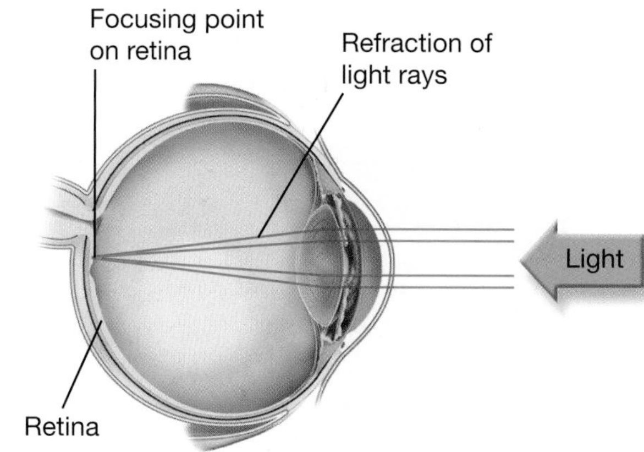

A Normal vision: light rays focus on the retina

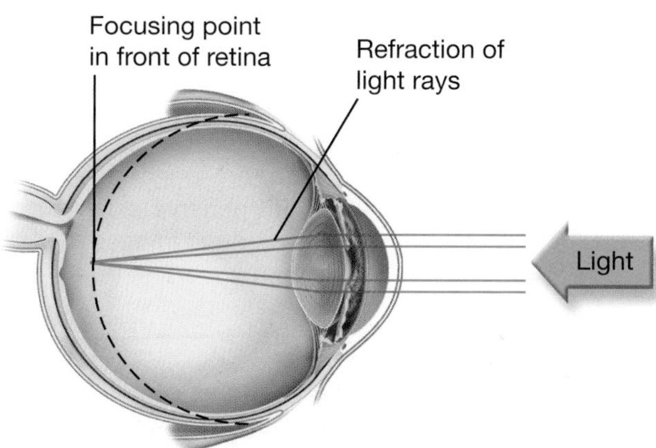

B Myopia (nearsightedness): light rays focus in front of the retina

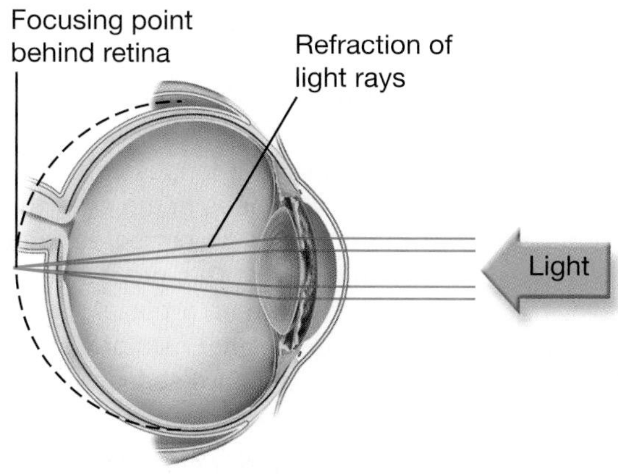

C Hyperopia (farsightedness): light rays focus beyond the retina

© Body Scientific International

Figure 8.8 Common vision disorders.

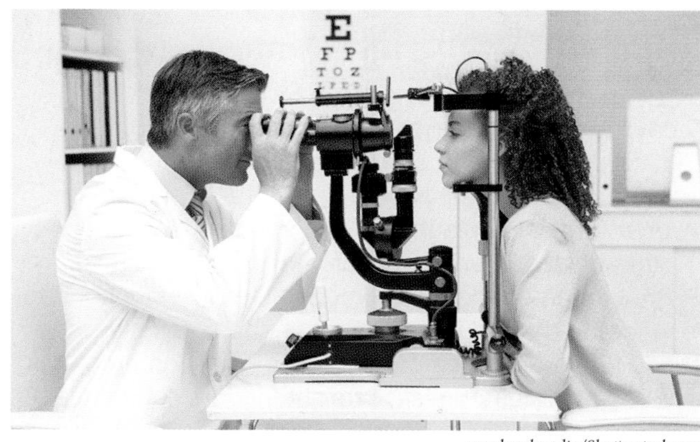

wavebreakmedia/Shutterstock.com

Figure 8.9 Have your eyes examined on a regular basis and as soon as possible if you experience any of the problems discussed in this chapter. Many problems can be remedied if treated early but can be very damaging if left untreated.

Presbyopia

Presbyopia is an age-related version of farsightedness. Onset of presbyopia commonly occurs between 40 and 45 years of age because of age-related changes in the body that stiffen and discolor the lens of the eye. Presbyopia causes blurring of up-close vision that impedes the ability to read printed material or text on a computer screen.

Astigmatism

Irregular curvature of the cornea or lens causes astigmatism, another common eye disorder. The result is blurred vision. Depending on the nature and extent of the curvature, vision may be proportionally affected. Corrective lenses can partially or completely correct astigmatism.

Understanding Medical Terminology

You may have heard middle-aged individuals joke that they are "getting old" because they need reading glasses. The word *presbyopia* comes from *presby-*, a combining form meaning "old," and *-opia*, a root word that means "visual defect or condition." The term was adopted in the late eighteenth century, when people in their forties were considered old!

The root *-opia* is also used in conjunction with other combining forms to describe various eye disorders (*myopia*, *hyperopia*, and *amblyopia*, for example).

Clinical Application Vision Correction Surgeries

Today, certain surgical procedures can reduce or eliminate the need for corrective lenses. Some of these techniques entail reshaping the eye itself, and others involve surgical implantation of corrective lenses.

Refractive surgery procedures reshape the curvature of the cornea so that light entering the eye is optimally focused on the retina and vision is sharp and clear. These procedures can correct common vision problems such as nearsightedness, farsightedness, astigmatism, and presbyopia.

LASIK

The refractive surgery procedure used most widely today is called *Laser-Assisted In Situ Keratomileusis (LASIK)*. This procedure permanently changes the shape of the cornea, correcting vision in people with myopia, hyperopia, and astigmatism.

The LASIK procedure begins with the surgeon using a mechanical microkeratome (a device that includes a tiny, extremely sharp blade) or a laser keratome (a laser-based device) to cut an ultrathin, hinged flap in the outer layer of the cornea. This flap is then folded back, and a laser is used to reshape the underlying corneal tissue to properly focus light on the retina. Some procedures utilize an excimer laser, which uses ultraviolet light to vaporize and remove tissue from the surface of the eye. A procedure involving the precise measurement of distortions in light passing through the cornea, called *wavefront analysis*, can assist with precise topographical mapping of the cornea.

Finally, the corneal flap is returned to its original position, and the surgery is complete. LASIK is typically performed while the patient is under local anesthesia administered in eye drops. The procedure takes approximately 10 minutes per eye to complete.

Patients have reported advantages and disadvantages of LASIK surgery. On the plus side, according to the American Society of Cataract and Refractive Surgery, 96% of patients achieve corrected vision within 24 hours of the nearly painless surgery with no stitches or bandages required. However, creation of the corneal flap occasionally causes complications that can permanently affect vision.

Photorefractive Keratectomy

A procedure known as *photorefractive keratectomy (PRK)* is one alternative to LASIK surgery. In PRK, the surgeon uses a laser to reshape the eye by focusing a cool pulsing beam of ultraviolet light directly onto the surface of the cornea. In contrast to LASIK, PRK does not involve cutting a flap in the surface of the cornea.

As with LASIK, PRK has advantages and disadvantages. PRK seems to enable faster nerve regeneration in the surface of the eye, which could help reduce dry eye and other complications that may occur during the healing process. The PRK procedure occurs purely on the eye's surface, so there is no surgical flap or its related complications. PRK also appears to be a safer procedure in instances when the cornea may be too thin for LASIK surgery to be successful. However, recovery time and the time it takes for vision to clear are longer after PRK than LASIK. In addition, some PRK patients experience sensitivity to light and mild halos around images, which are effects that can be permanent.

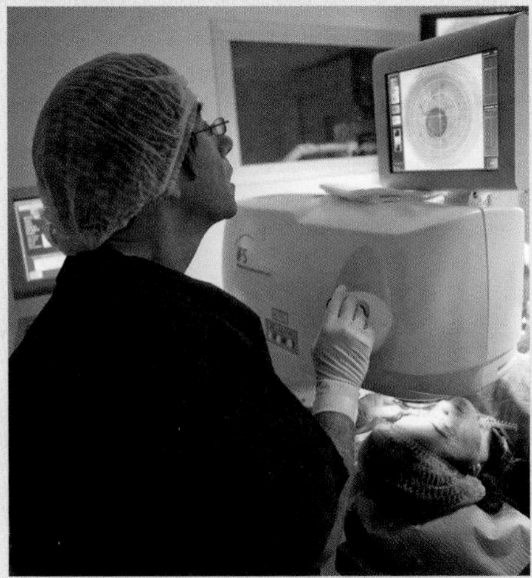

Amélie Benoist/Science Source

A surgeon using computer-assisted imagery to guide reshaping of the cornea in a LASIK operation.

Conductive Keratoplasty

A refractive surgery procedure known as *conductive keratoplasty (CK)* can be used to address hyperopia and presbyopia. In this procedure, the surgeon applies dots of low-heat radio waves around the periphery of the cornea to enhance curvature. CK was approved for use in the United States in 2002.

Implants

Multiple vision problems may also be corrected by implanting artificial lenses within the eye. For individuals with extreme myopia, corrective lenses can be surgically implanted over the natural lenses in the eyes to correct vision. Extreme hyperopia may be corrected through refractive lens exchange (RLE). This procedure involves replacing the natural lens with an artificial lens that is differently shaped. Due to a higher risk for complications, RLE is reserved for people who have serious vision deficits.

Vision correction for cataracts can be accomplished with lens implants called *multifocal intraocular lenses*, or *multifocal IOLs*. These advanced lens implants not only restore vision, but also correct presbyopia, myopia, and hyperopia.

Amblyopia

Amblyopia, or lazy eye, usually appears during childhood when one eye is extremely dominant, and the other eye—the lazy eye—develops poor vision. If this condition is not corrected, the lazy eye can become blind. Treatment generally consists of covering the "good" eye, which forces the extrinsic muscles of the lazy eye to function and strengthen.

Diplopia

Diplopia, or double vision, occurs when one eye is misaligned, causing two images of an object to be perceived simultaneously. Treatment may involve wearing a temporary patch over the affected eye, using corrective lenses, or undergoing surgery.

Strabismus

Strabismus is the medical term for crossed eyes. A person with strabismus has an eye that drifts in different directions due to malfunctioning extrinsic muscles in that eye. This condition is treated with eye exercises, corrective lenses, or surgery.

Color Blindness

Color blindness affects the cone cells on the retina, impairing an individual's ability to distinguish colors. Red-green color blindness, the inability to distinguish red from green, is a common form of this disorder.

Color blindness is an inherited condition. For a man to be color blind, he needs to inherit the gene for color blindness only from his mother. By contrast, for a woman to be color blind, she must inherit the gene from both parents. This explains why men have a higher incidence of color blindness compared to women.

Night Blindness

In a person with night blindness, the rods in the retina do not function optimally, making it difficult for the person to see well at night. Night blindness is associated with aging.

Eye Diseases and Disorders

Many diseases and disorders can affect the eye. This section briefly examines some of the more common eye conditions that require professional care.

Conjunctivitis

Commonly known as "pinkeye," conjunctivitis is a painful inflammation of the conjunctiva. Symptoms include redness, pain, swelling, and mucus discharge. Some forms of conjunctivitis are caused by harsh chemicals or allergens, but others, caused by viruses, bacteria, or fungi, can be highly contagious. Conjunctivitis that is caused by a bacterial infection can be treated with antibiotics.

Cataracts

A cataract is a progressive clouding of the transparent lens of the eye, causing obstruction of light. The result is blurred vision, poor night vision, yellowing of colors, and "halos" around lights. Cataracts are associated with aging and frequently occur in people older than 70 years of age. Exposure to bright sunlight can speed the development of cataracts. Cataracts are treated with laser surgery.

Glaucoma

Glaucoma is a condition of increased pressure within the eyeball caused by overproduction of aqueous humor or blockage of normal aqueous humor drainage. The onset of symptoms is gradual and includes aching eyes, poor vision in dim light progressing to blurred vision, and the appearance of halos around lights.

As the condition progresses, tunnel vision (loss of peripheral vision) occurs, and blindness eventually follows. Untreated glaucoma is a common cause of blindness. Glaucoma occurs in about 20% of adults older than 40 years of age. Early detection is a must! Glaucoma can be readily treated with medication or surgery.

Macular Degeneration

A progressive loss of central vision, the hallmark symptom of macular degeneration, occurs in about 10% of elderly people. Peripheral vision, however, remains unaffected. There are two types of macular degeneration: dry and wet.

Dry macular degeneration is caused by progressive thinning of the retina. Although there is currently no treatment, most individuals with this condition do not completely lose their eyesight and are able to function with vision aids. Wet macular degeneration involves leakage of small blood vessels within the eye. Some individuals with this condition respond favorably to medication or laser surgery (**Figure 8.10**).

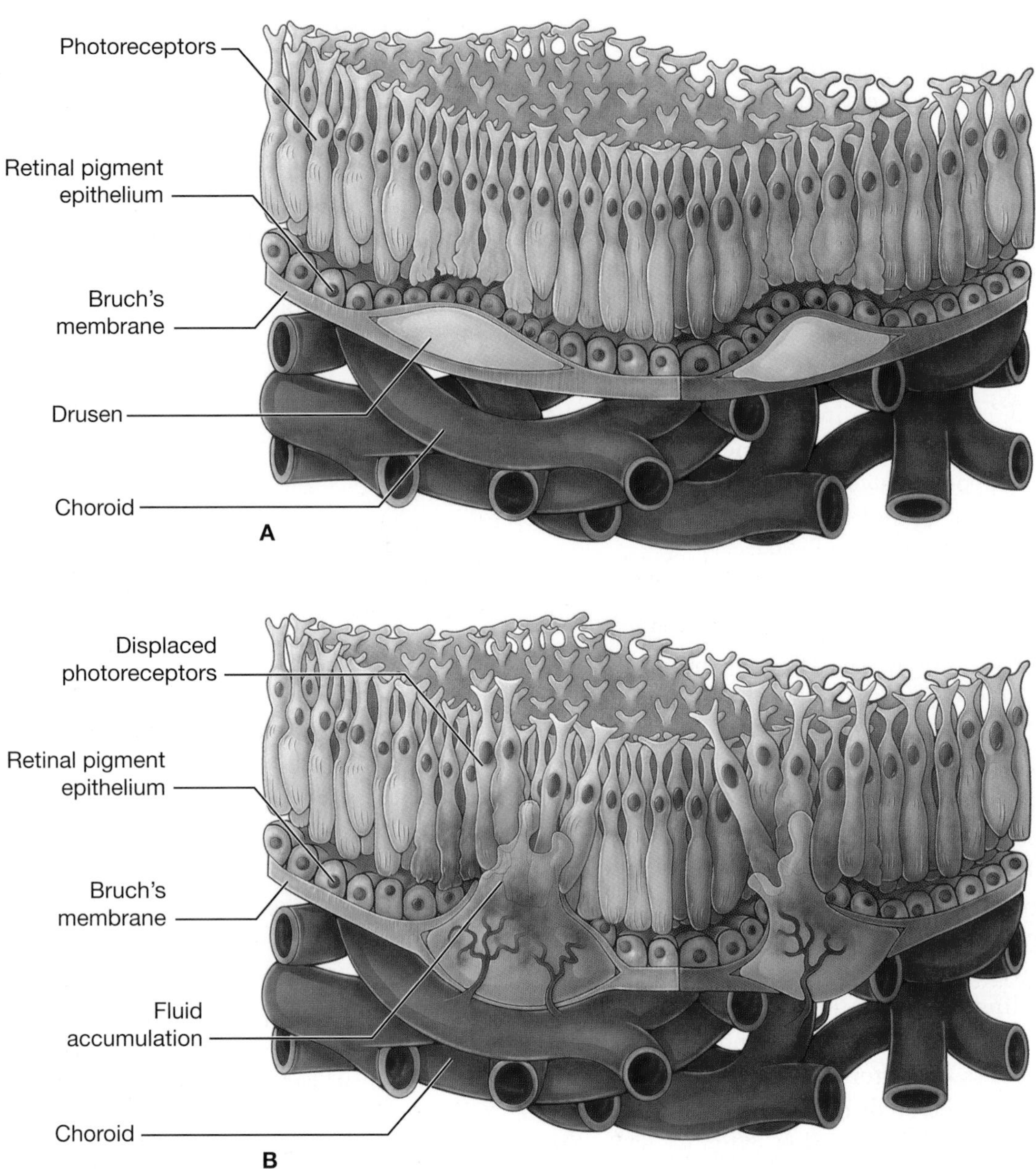

Evan Oto/Science Source

Figure 8.10 Macular degeneration takes two forms: A—dry, and B—wet.

Diabetic Retinopathy

Damage to the retina caused by long-term diabetes is called *diabetic retinopathy*. This condition is becoming increasingly prevalent and is currently the leading cause of blindness in American adults. Diabetic retinopathy involves swelling and leaking of the vessels that supply blood to the retina.

When diabetic retinopathy is sufficiently advanced, bleeding occurs in the eye, causing the affected individual to see red spots. Laser surgery is typically effective in treating diabetic retinopathy when it is caught early enough.

Vitreous Floaters

Vitreous floaters are small, irregularly shaped specks that drift around within the field of vision. Floaters form when tiny chunks of the gel-like vitreous humor break off and float in the aqueous humor in the center of the eyeball.

Although sometimes distracting, ordinary eye floaters are common and normally not a cause for alarm. However, the sudden appearance of multiple floaters accompanied by what appear to be flashes of light on the lateral periphery of the eye can be symptoms of a retinal tear or retinal detachment. In such cases, immediate medical attention is required.

SECTION 8.1 REVIEW

Mini-Glossary

aqueous humor a clear, watery substance in the anterior chamber of the eye that provides nutrients to the lens and cornea and helps maintain normal intraocular pressure

choroid the middle layer of the wall of the eye

ciliary body the structure between the choroid and the iris that anchors the lens in place

ciliary glands modified sweat glands located between the eyelashes

cones sensory cells in the retina that are sensitive to bright light and provide color vision

conjunctiva a delicate external membrane that covers the exposed eyeball and lines the eyelid

cornea a transparent tissue located over the anterior center of the eye

extrinsic muscles the muscles that are attached to the outer surface of the eye and are responsible for changing the eye's direction of viewing

fovea centralis a tiny spot near the center of each retina that contains only cones and is the point of greatest visual acuity

iris the anterior portion of the choroid, which gives the eye its color

lacrimal glands the glands that are located above the lateral end of each eye and secrete tears

lens a transparent, flexible structure that curves outward on both sides

optic chiasma the point at which the optic nerves cross

optic nerve the transmitter of visual sensory signals to the occipital lobe of the brain

optic tracts the portion of the optic nerve fibers that extend beyond the optic chiasma

pupil the opening through which light rays enter the eye

retina the innermost layer of the eye, which contains light-sensitive nerve endings that send impulses through the optic nerves to the brain

rods sensory cells in the retina that are activated in dim light

sclera the tough, fibrous outer layer of the eye

suspensory ligaments tiny structures that attach the lens of the eye to the ciliary body

tarsal glands the glands that are located in the eyelids and secrete an oily substance

vitreous humor a gel-like substance in the posterior chamber of the eye that helps maintain intraocular pressure

Review Questions

1. What part of the eye is called the *window of the eye*?
2. Which layer of the eye contains rods and cones?
3. Describe the pathway of vision.
4. Where are the extrinsic muscles located, and what is their purpose?
5. List the anatomical features that protect the eye from injury.
6. Which glands produce the salty solution known as *tears*?
7. Which part of the eye has many pain receptors and is able to repair itself quickly?
8. Compare and contrast myopia, hyperopia, and presbyopia.
9. Derrick has had to do a lot of reading in college. He never had a problem with his vision in the past, but lately he has had trouble reading the print in his textbook. When he noticed that he was holding his book farther and farther away from his eyes to see better, he decided to see an ophthalmologist. What do you think the doctor told Derrick? Which injury, disorder, or disease that you read about in this chapter is the most likely diagnosis? What treatment do you think the doctor prescribed?

SECTION 8.2 The Ear

Objectives

- Describe the major anatomical structures of the outer ear, the middle ear, and the inner ear.
- Explain the functions of the ear, including the hearing process and the process of maintaining equilibrium.
- Describe common disorders and infections of the ear.

Key Terms

auditory canal
auricle
bony labyrinth
ceruminous glands
cochlea
cochlear duct
endolymph
Eustachian tube
incus
malleus
membranous labyrinth
organ of Corti
ossicles
oval window
perilymph
semicircular canals
stapes
tympanic membrane
vestibule
vestibulocochlear nerve

The human ear is remarkable in its ability to capture, amplify, and transmit sounds of varying loudness and pitch (high versus low tones) to the brain. In addition to these functions, the ears play a central role in maintaining physical balance and even in recognizing which direction is up. This section examines the anatomy of the ear and explains how the functions of hearing and balance are carried out.

Anatomy of the Ear

The ear includes three anatomical regions—the external (outer) ear, the tympanic cavity (middle ear), and the internal (inner) ear. The external ear and tympanic cavity contribute to the ability to hear. The internal ear plays roles in both hearing and equilibrium (balance).

External Ear

The irregularly shaped outer portion of the ear is called the ***auricle***, or *pinna*. In many animal species, the outer ear serves to channel sound waves into the ear, but this function is minimal in the human species. As **Figure 8.11** shows, the auricle connects with the ***auditory canal***, also known as the *external acoustic meatus*.

The auditory canal is a short, tubelike structure that is about 1 inch long and 1/4 inch in diameter. The walls of this canal are lined with skin that contains ***ceruminous glands***. The ceruminous glands secrete cerumen, also known as *earwax*. Earwax helps to clean, lubricate, and protect the ear.

The ***tympanic membrane***, commonly known as the *eardrum*, is located at the end of the auditory canal. Sound waves entering the ear cause the tympanic

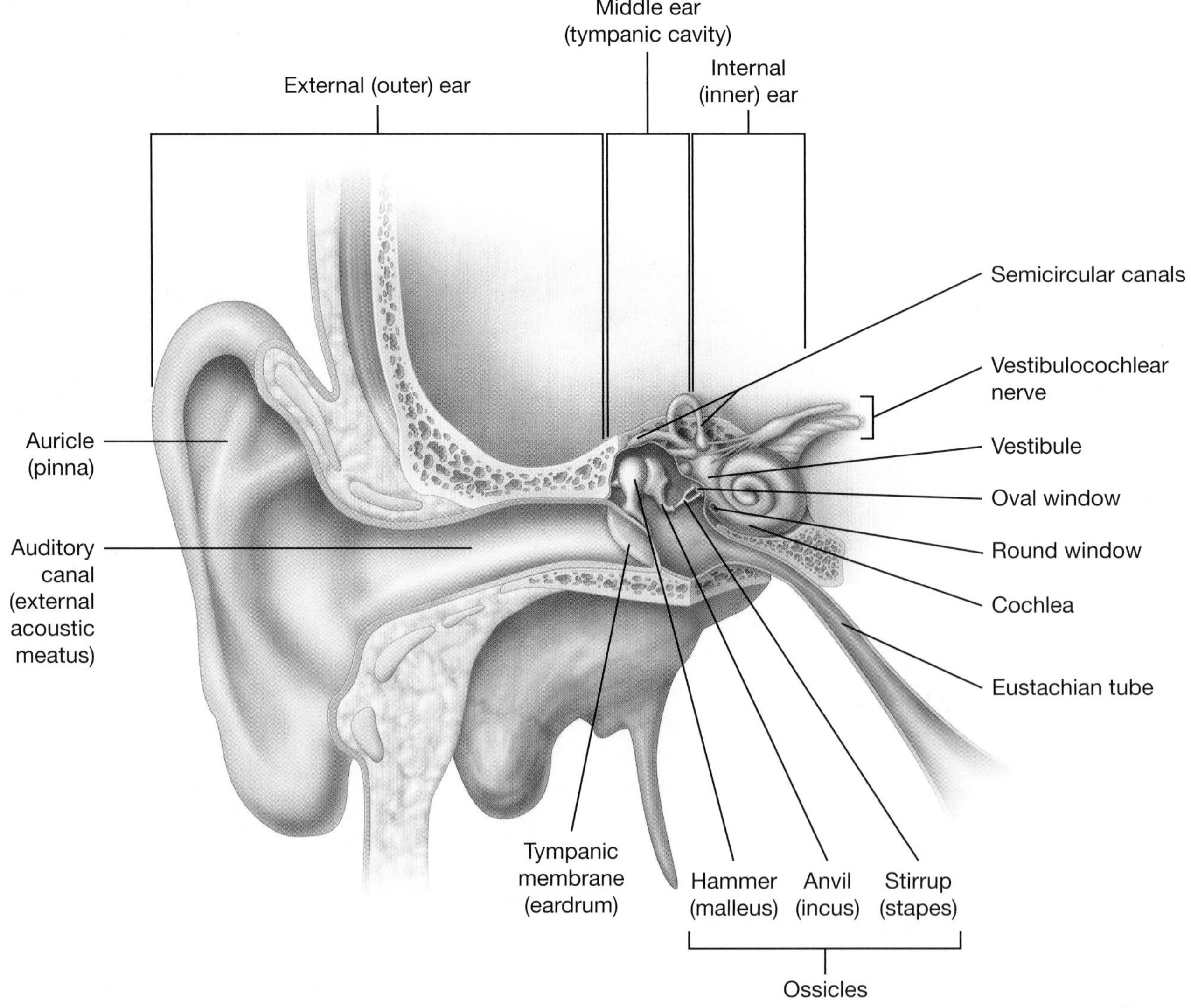

Figure 8.11 Anatomy of the ear.

membrane to vibrate, which initiates the process of hearing. The eardrum also separates the outer ear from the tympanic cavity.

Tympanic Cavity

The middle ear, or tympanic cavity, is a small, open chamber in the temporal lobe of the skull. The tympanic membrane is located on the lateral side of the cavity. The medial side is mostly bone, with a membrane-covered opening known as the ***oval window***. Beneath the oval window is a round window, which allows fluid in the inner ear to move.

The tympanic cavity houses the three smallest bones in the body—the ***ossicles***. The ossicles include the ***malleus***, or hammer; the ***incus***, or anvil; and the ***stapes***, or stirrup. Together, these bones connect the tympanic membrane to the membrane of the oval window. The hammer attaches to the tympanic membrane, the anvil attaches to the hammer, and the stirrup attaches to the anvil on one side and to the oval window on the other. Because of their mechanical arrangement, the ossicles not only transmit sound waves, but also amplify them.

The ***Eustachian tube*** connects the tympanic cavity to the pharynx. The pharynx is the part of the throat that connects the mouth and nasal cavity to the esophagus. The Eustachian tube serves to equalize pressure on either side of the tympanic membrane. Yawning widely is a way of bringing pressure in the pharynx, Eustachian tube, and tympanic cavity to the same level of pressure found outside the ear. This is a good strategy to use when air (barometric) pressure changes rapidly, such as during an airplane's descent or while driving down a mountain road.

Internal Ear

The oval window connects the tympanic cavity with the inner ear. The inner ear structures reside in a hollow tunnel that winds and twists like a bowl of interconnected spaghetti noodles. **Figure 8.12** shows a representation of this winding tunnel, known as the ***bony labyrinth***. As this figure indicates, the three components of the inner ear are the ***cochlea***, the ***vestibule***, and the ***semicircular canals***.

The cochlear nerve and the vestibular nerve transmit sensory information from the cochlea and vestibule, respectively. The cochlear nerve carries information about hearing, and the vestibular nerve carries information about balance. These two nerves join to form a single cranial nerve, the ***vestibulocochlear nerve***.

Filled with a clear fluid called ***perilymph***, the bony labyrinth contains membrane-covered tubes called the ***membranous labyrinth***, which follow the course of the bony labyrinth. The membranous labyrinth is filled with a thicker fluid called ***endolymph***.

SELF CHECK

1. What are the two functions of the ear?
2. What is the function of cerumen?
3. List the ossicles and explain why they are important.
4. What is the significance of the Eustachian tube?

Physiology of the Ear

The function of the ears is to detect sounds in the environment. Many people are surprised to learn that the ears also help the body maintain its balance, or equilibrium. This section discusses these two important functions of the ear.

Hearing

The ability to hear resides deep within the snail-shaped cochlea of the inner ear. The portion of the membranous labyrinth inside the cochlea is called the ***cochlear duct***. Within the cochlear duct is the spiral-shaped ***organ of Corti***, which contains hearing receptors called *hair cells* (**Figure 8.13**). Some hair cells are short and others are long. The short, stiff

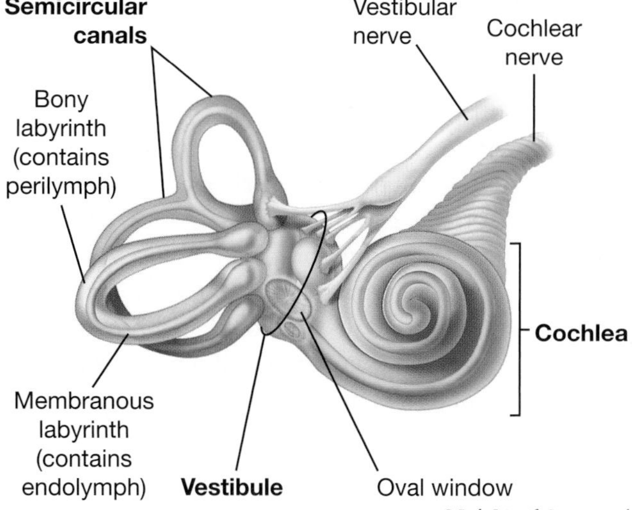

Figure 8.12 Structures of the inner ear.

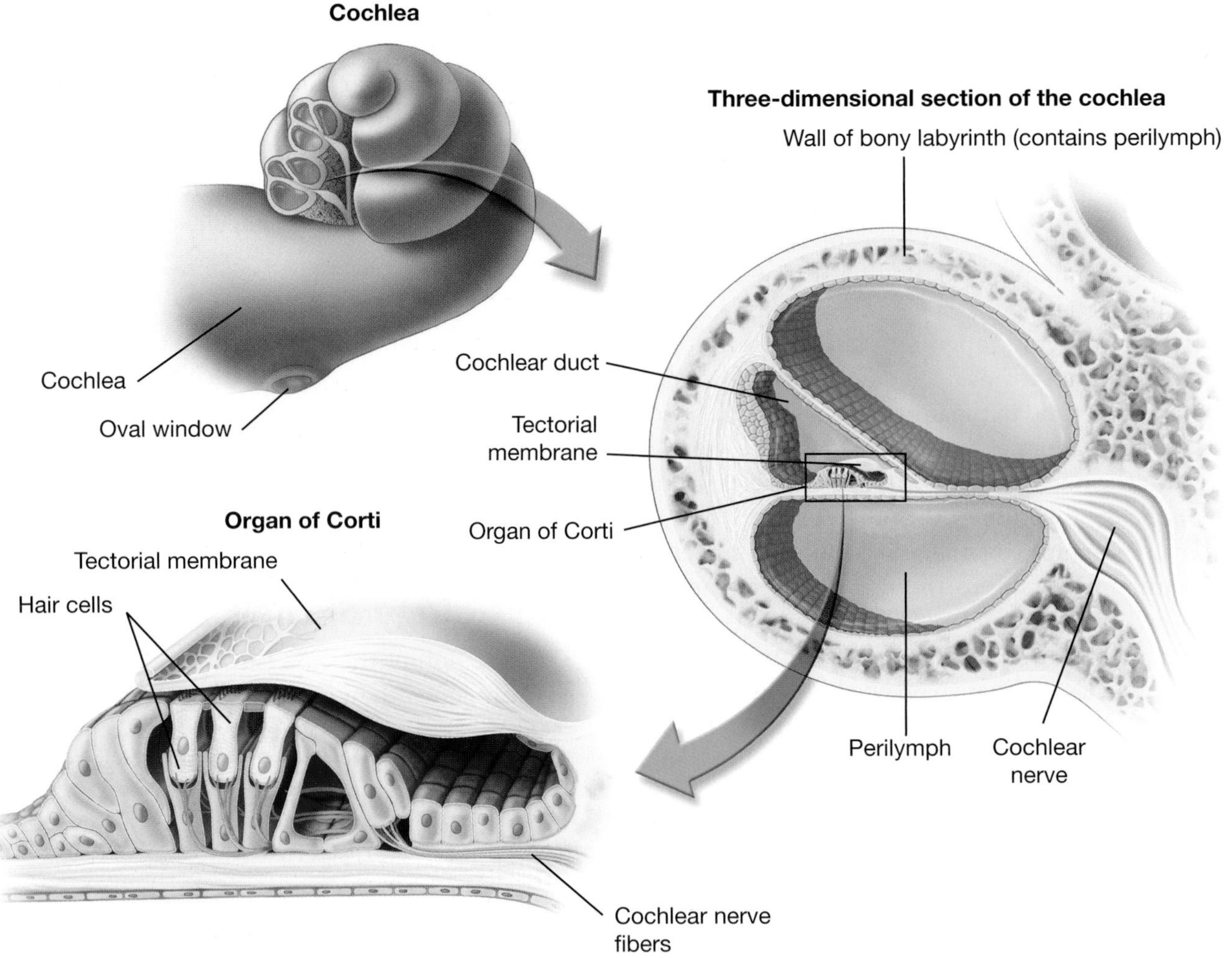

Figure 8.13 Anatomy of the cochlea.

hair cells are stimulated by high-pitched sounds; the longer, more flexible hair cells are stimulated by low-pitched sounds.

When sound waves enter the ear, they are transmitted through the auditory canal, causing the tympanic membrane to vibrate. This motion stimulates the malleus, incus, and stapes to amplify and transmit these vibrations to the membrane of the oval window. This process of amplification and transmission sets in motion the fluids of the inner ear.

Motion of the endolymph in the cochlear duct causes the tectorial membrane to move. Movement of the tectorial membrane stimulates the hair cells, which in turn stimulate the cochlear branch of the vestibulocochlear nerve. The vestibulocochlear nerve then transmits electrical impulses to the auditory region of the brain in the temporal lobe.

Have you ever noticed that a loud and noisy environment seems less loud after some time? This is because the auditory neurons accommodate loud noise levels by discharging smaller amounts of neurotransmitter. Upon returning to a quieter environment, the auditory nerves resume discharging normal amounts of neurotransmitter when stimulated. This homeostatic mechanism helps prevent depletion of neurotransmitter, which could result in temporary deafness.

Equilibrium

People tend to take equilibrium, or the ability to balance, for granted. Only when they are dizzy or disoriented do they truly appreciate balance. The ability to balance comes from specialized structures in the inner ear.

The vestibule of the inner ear contains three semicircular canals. The hair cells in the semicircular canals are stimulated by movement of the endolymph in the canals, much like the hair cells in the organ of Corti are stimulated by motion of the endolymph in the cochlear duct. The hair cells in the semicircular canals, however, stimulate the vestibular branch of the vestibulocochlear nerve, which communicates with the cerebellum to provide information about the orientation and motion of the head. The cerebellum receives input from the eyes, inner ears, and sensory receptors throughout the body to monitor body position and respond with impulses that help maintain balance. The semicircular canals play an important role in balance whether a person is stationary or moving.

SELF CHECK

1. What is the function of the organ of Corti?
2. Which structure in the inner ear controls equilibrium?

Ear Disorders and Infections

A variety of conditions can affect hearing or balance. This section addresses some of the most common disorders and infections of the ear.

Deafness

Deafness is the term applied to any loss of hearing, ranging from a slight to a complete inability to hear. Injuries that affect the structures of the middle or inner ear can cause deafness. Regular exposure to extremely loud sounds, such as construction noise or loud music, can damage the hair cells in the organ of Corti, leading to hearing loss. Other causes of deafness include excessive earwax, scarring of the tympanic membrane following inflammation, and damage to the auditory nerve or auditory region of the brain.

Presbycusis is the term for age-related hearing loss. Presbycusis can usually be improved through the use of hearing aids.

Hearing aids amplify and change sounds so that the wearer can better hear them. Some hearing aids amplify all sounds, while others specifically boost low- or high-frequency sounds. For elderly individuals with hearing deficits, use of a hearing aid not only improves hearing, but also improves the ability to balance. Scientists are studying this recently discovered phenomenon to try to understand how it works.

Hearing aids are available in a variety of styles and sizes (**Figure 8.14**), and price ranges vary considerably. This is why you should carefully analyze all

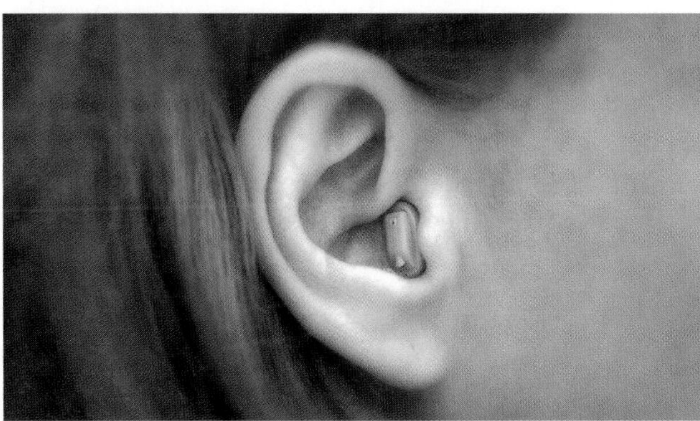

A

Andrey_Popov/Shutterstock.com

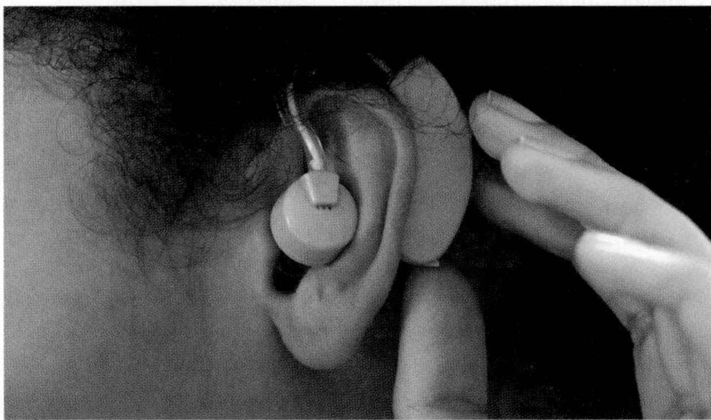

B

Pavel_D/Shutterstock.com

Figure 8.14 Typical hearing aids. A—"In-the-canal" model. B—"Behind-the-ear" model.

Research Notes Tone Deafness

You may have noticed that some people have difficulty singing in key with music. It is typically said that these people cannot "carry a tune."

A person who sings off-key has amusia. Amusia is characterized by the inability to determine differences in pitch (that is, how high or low a tone is), as well as the inability to remember melodies. Amusia is present in about 3% of people from birth, but it can also result from a brain injury.

Researchers studying this condition have tried to train amusic children to develop the ability to hear and reproduce musical tones. One method entails having the children repeatedly listen to popular music for one month. This training, however, has had no apparent effect. Studies of brain activity in amusic individuals indicate that their difficulty in processing musical tones is caused by poor neural connections between the auditory center in the brain and other related areas of the brain.

information received from healthcare workers and promotional materials before making inferences about the best products and services for you or the person you are helping with the purchase.

"In-the-canal" hearing aids are custom-molded to fit inside an individual's auditory canal. This type of hearing aid is recommended for mild to moderate hearing loss.

"Half-shell" hearing aids are custom-fit to sit inside the small, inner, bowl-shaped area of an individual's outer ear. These hearing aids are recommended for mild to moderately severe hearing loss.

Somewhat larger "in-the-ear" hearing aids are custom-designed to fill most of the bowl of an individual's outer ear. This type of hearing aid is recommended for mild to severe hearing loss.

Finally, "behind-the-ear" hearing aids, designed to be worn behind the ear, are capable of greater amplification than the other types of hearing aids. This model, which transmits amplified sound to a molded piece inside the auditory canal, is recommended for most types of hearing loss.

Tinnitus

Tinnitus is a condition that causes a sound like ringing to be heard in the ear. Tinnitus occurs when the hair cells in the organ of Corti, which stimulate the auditory nerve, are damaged. Normal movement of these hair cells is triggered by sound waves. When the hair cells have been damaged, however, they sometimes move randomly, generating the ringing sound.

What damages these hair cells? Certain diseases, disorders, and injuries, as well as prolonged use of certain medications can cause tinnitus. However, the most common culprit is repeated exposure to loud

Clinical Application: Cochlear Implants

A cochlear implant is a surgically implanted electronic device for individuals who are deaf or severely hearing-impaired. A cochlear implant consists of several components:

- a microphone to detect sounds
- a speech processor, which refines sounds picked up by the microphone
- a transmitter and receiver/stimulator, which convert signals from the speech processor into electric impulses
- an array of electrodes that send impulses from the transmitter to different regions of the cochlear (auditory) nerve

Unlike a hearing aid, which amplifies sounds for damaged structures in the ear to process, cochlear implants bypass those damaged structures to directly stimulate the cochlear nerve. Although the brain is able to recognize the signals that are generated as sound, stimulation by the implant device is different from stimulation of the nerve during the normal hearing process. Consequently, hearing through a cochlear implant is different from normal hearing, and it requires time to learn. People who use cochlear implants usually perceive words by their syllables and rhythms.

Although an implant does not provide normal hearing, it can give a deaf person the ability to detect sounds and the opportunity to learn to understand speech. Speech-language pathologists and audiologists can assist with this learning process.

Cochlear implants are approved for deaf children beginning at 12 months of age. Researchers have found that children who receive implants and intensive therapy before 18 months of age can better hear and understand sounds, and also learn to speak better, than children who receive implants when they are older. Research has also shown that children who receive a cochlear implant at a young age are able to develop language skills at a rate comparable to children with normal hearing, and many succeed in mainstream classrooms.

Researchers are working to improve cochlear implants by fine-tuning their signal processing and developing processing algorithms that are more sophisticated. One goal is to enable people with a hearing impairment to better hear music. Specifically, researchers hope to improve the ability to detect pitch (melody and intonation) and timbre (quality of sound in different instruments).

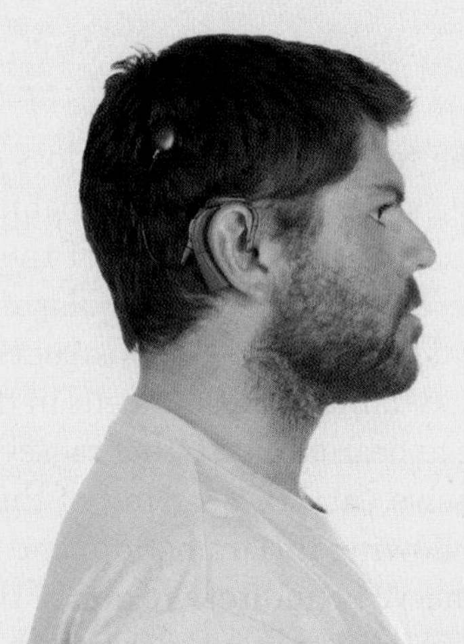

Elsa Hoffmann/Shutterstock.com

The external components of a cochlear implant.

noise, such as loud music. Tinnitus is a common and growing problem. According to the American Tinnitus Association, some 50 million people in the United States suffer from the disorder.

Otitis Externa

Have you ever gone swimming in a lake and later developed an earache? You might have had swimmer's ear, formally known as *external otitis*. This bacterial or fungal infection of the auditory canal is caused by immersion in contaminated water. Symptoms may include pain, fever, and, in extreme cases, temporary hearing loss.

External otitis can be prevented by thoroughly cleaning and drying the ear canal with an alcohol-based solution after swimming, or by avoiding immersion of the ears.

Otitis Media

Otitis media is an infection of the middle ear caused by bacteria or a virus. It is usually associated with an upper respiratory tract infection. Otitis media is relatively common in infants and toddlers because their Eustachian tubes are not yet fully developed. Symptoms of a middle ear infection may include swelling and production of pus, which may cause a painful elevation of pressure in the middle ear.

A mild to moderate middle ear infection caused by bacteria is treated with antibiotics. Serious bacterial infections do not respond well to antibiotics, and they are frequently treated by a surgical procedure. During the surgery, tiny tubes are inserted into the tympanic membrane. These small tubes alleviate the elevated pressure in the inner ear.

Viral infections do not respond to antibiotics at all. However, they often improve with time.

Otitis Interna

Otitis interna, also known as labyrinthitis, is an infection of the inner ear that produces inflammation. This condition affects the semicircular canals in particular and can disrupt their normal function, causing vertigo (severe dizziness), nausea, and vomiting. Individuals with vertigo are unable to stand because their sense of orientation is severely compromised.

Chronic inflammation of the semicircular canals of the inner ear is called *Ménière's disease*. This disease causes periodic but severe vertigo as well as progressive hearing loss.

An ear infection that causes vertigo is treated with antibiotics, if the infection is bacterial. If the ear infection is viral, certain medications may be prescribed to ease the discomfort caused by vertigo.

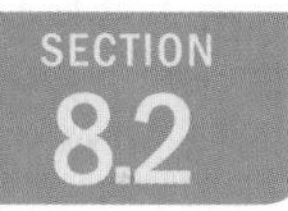

REVIEW

Mini-Glossary

auditory canal a short, tubelike structure that connects the outer ear to the eardrum

auricle the irregularly shaped outer portion of the ear; also known as the *pinna*

bony labyrinth term that describes the winding tunnel located in the inner ear

ceruminous glands the glands that secrete cerumen (earwax) and are located in the auditory canal

cochlea a snail-shaped structure in the inner ear that enables hearing

cochlear duct the portion of the membranous labyrinth located inside the cochlea

endolymph a thick fluid that fills the membranous labyrinth

Eustachian tube a channel that connects the middle ear to the pharynx and serves to equalize pressure on either side of the tympanic membrane

incus a tiny bone within the middle ear that transmits sound from the malleus to the stapes; sometimes called the *anvil* because of its shape

malleus a tiny bone in the middle ear that transmits sound from the tympanic membrane (eardrum) to the anvil; sometimes called the *hammer* because of its shape

membranous labyrinth term that describes the membrane-covered tubes located inside the bony labyrinth

organ of Corti a spiral-shaped ridge of epithelium in the cochlear duct, which is lined with hair cells that serve as hearing receptors

ossicles the body's three smallest bones—the hammer, anvil, and stirrup; found in the middle ear

oval window a membrane-covered opening that connects the middle ear to the inner ear

perilymph a clear fluid that fills the bony labyrinth

(continued)

semicircular canals channels located in the inner ear, which contain hair cells that play an important role in balance

stapes a tiny bone in the middle ear that attaches to the anvil on one side and the oval window on the other; sometimes called the *stirrup* because of its shape

tympanic membrane a sheet of tissue found at the end of the auditory canal; also known as the *eardrum*

vestibule a chamber in the inner ear that contains the three semicircular canals

vestibulocochlear nerve a cranial nerve comprising the cochlear nerve and the vestibular nerve

Review Questions

1. What are the three anatomical regions of the ear?
2. Name the two terms used to describe the outer portion of the ear.
3. Where are the ceruminous glands located?
4. The Eustachian tube connects the ____ to the ____.
5. Define *equilibrium*.
6. Which part of the brain controls equilibrium?
7. Compare and contrast the function of the short, stiff hairs and the long, flexible hairs in the organ of Corti.
8. Describe the pathway of hearing.
9. What is the main function of the semicircular canals?
10. Describe the differences among otitis externa, otitis media, and otitis interna.

SECTION 8.3 Smell and Taste

Objectives

- Describe the anatomy of the olfactory region and explain how it functions.
- Discuss common injuries and disorders related to the nose.
- Describe the major anatomical structures of the gustatory sense and explain their functions.
- Discuss common disorders related to the tongue.

Key Terms

antihistamines
gustatory cells
gustatory hairs
histamines
limbic system
olfactory bulb
olfactory hairs
olfactory nerve
olfactory receptor cells
olfactory region
papillae
septum
tastants
taste buds
taste pores

Why does the smell of your favorite food cooking cause your mouth to water? The sense of smell can stimulate the mouth to secrete saliva. Smell and taste are closely connected. Just imagine a perfectly cooked, scrumptious meal without the ability to smell or taste it.

The senses of smell and taste enable you to enjoy what you eat and drink. These senses can also alert you when food or drink has gone bad, as in the case of sour milk. In addition, the sense of smell can alert you to environmental dangers. For example, you would immediately leave an area if you smelled toxic fumes or another undesirable or potentially harmful scent.

How is the human body able to interpret odors and tastes so rapidly? This section explores the anatomy and physiology of the sensory pathways of smell and taste.

Olfactory Sense

You may have noticed that when you have a cold, your ability to smell is considerably lessened. The sensors responsible for smell are located in two dime-sized areas called the ***olfactory regions***, one on top of each nasal cavity (**Figure 8.15**). These sensors are called ***olfactory receptor cells***. When the nasal cavity becomes congested with mucus from a cold, the olfactory receptors are covered and partially blocked. As a result, odor molecules from foods that would normally trigger the sense of smell cannot reach the olfactory receptor cells.

The olfactory receptor cells are neurons. (For a definition of *neuron*, see Chapter 7.) Tiny ***olfactory hairs*** extend from these neurons into the nasal cavity, where they are covered by a thin, protective layer of mucus. Whenever you inhale an odor, the chemicals that caused the odor dissolve in the mucous layer surrounding the olfactory hairs. This dissolving action stimulates the olfactory receptor cells, which send impulses through the olfactory filaments that make up the ***olfactory nerve***. The olfactory filaments feed impulses to the ***olfactory bulb***, which is the thickened end of the olfactory nerve. The olfactory nerve sends impulses to the olfactory cortex of the brain.

The nerve pathway between the nose and the brain travels through the ***limbic system***, the part of the brain responsible for emotions. As a result, a smell may

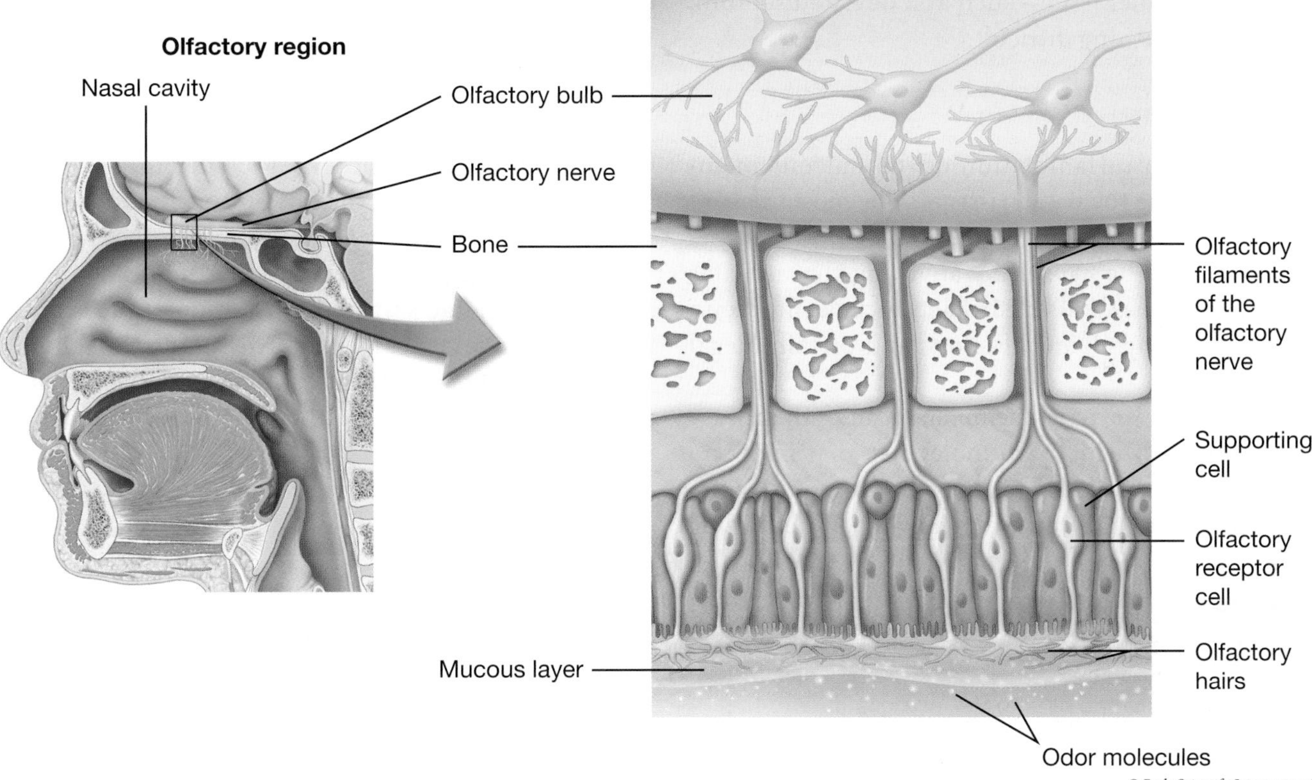

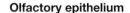

Figure 8.15 The olfactory region.

trigger a positive or negative emotion because you have associated a particular experience with that scent. For instance, the scent of cookies baking in an oven may remind you of family, bringing about a positive emotion. By contrast, the smell of antiseptic ointment may remind you of an injury that you experienced, which could trigger a negative emotion.

Although most animals have a much stronger sense of smell than humans do, human olfactory receptors are actually quite sensitive. It takes only a few molecules of an inhaled odor to stimulate the olfactory receptors, which then fire a nerve impulse. Thus, the olfactory receptors can easily become used to an odor to which they are repeatedly exposed. This explains why people who habitually wear a certain perfume or cologne, for example, tend not to smell it on themselves.

Why might different people prefer or dislike different perfumes and other scented products? On a biological level, the answer has to do with individual differences in olfactory receptors. A given smell activates different olfactory receptors in different people.

When scientists compared olfactory receptors across a group of people, they found that any two individuals are likely to be approximately 30% different. This may seem surprising, but given that there are about 400 genes, with 900,000 variations, coding the olfactory receptors, a certain level of interindividual differences should be expected.

How many different basic odors do you suppose there are? Although many smells are derived from a combination of basic odors, scientists have isolated 10 basic odor qualities from analysis of olfactory perception data. These basic odors are sweet, fragrant, woody/resinous, fruity (non-citrus), chemical, minty/peppermint, popcorn, lemon, decaying, and pungent.

SELF CHECK

1. Where are the sensors for smell located?
2. Explain the connection between smell and emotions.

Injuries and Disorders of the Nose

The nose is important to overall health. It acts as a filter to remove dust, irritants, and germs from the air that people breathe. When a pathogen or irritant gets through this filter, an illness such as the common cold can result. Other issues, such as a deviated septum, can make breathing difficult.

Rhinitis

Rhinitis is an inflammation of the mucous membranes that line the nasal passages. The most frequent cause of rhinitis is the common cold. However, the condition can be caused by anything that irritates these membranes. Possible irritants include infections, allergies, strong chemical odors, and certain illegal drugs.

Irritation of the nasal membranes causes the release of ***histamines***, which are molecules that trigger a reaction that produces nasal congestion and drainage. Treatment of rhinitis requires removing or minimizing the original irritant and taking medications that contain ***antihistamines*** to curb the activity of histamines.

Septum Problems

The ***septum*** of the nose is the structure made of cartilage that divides the nose into left and right air passages. It is normal for the septum to be not perfectly centered; a slight deviation to one side is common. However, a large shift in the position of the septum away from the center is called a *deviated septum*. Injury is usually, but not always, the cause of a deviated septum. When warranted, a deviated septum can be surgically repaired.

The septum may also develop one or more holes due to injury, an ulcer, long-term exposure to toxic

Research Notes Sense of Smell in Animals

How does the human olfactory sense compare to that of animals and fish? The human sense of smell is sufficiently powerful that it can detect the presence of a skunk with only 0.000,000,000,000,071 of an ounce of scent present. However, because the sense of smell among many species of animals and fish is related to survival, a larger portion of their brains is devoted to receiving and interpreting scents.

Dogs, for example, have about 125 to 220 million olfactory receptor cells. This is roughly 20 times the number of receptors that humans have. Dogs bred for hunting have even more olfactory receptors; the bloodhound, for instance, has nearly 300 million. In fact, the percentage of a dog's brain that is responsible for smell is 40 times greater than the corresponding percentage of the human brain.

The dog's wet nose assists with scent detection by capturing odor particles. With all of these advantages, a dog's sense of smell is estimated to be 100 thousand to 1 million times more sensitive than that of a human, and a bloodhound's olfactory sense may be up to 100 million times more sensitive. This is why the bloodhound, referred to as "a nose with a dog attached," is often used in law enforcement to track down missing persons and criminals.

A horse's olfactory sense is not as sharp as a dog's, but it is still stronger than a human's sense of smell. Horses use their olfactory sense to identify other horses, people, predators, pastures, feeds, and water sources. A mare's sense of smell is so discriminating that it enables her to pick out her own foal in a group of foals.

Fish such as salmon also have an extremely well-developed sense of smell. Salmon are born in small, freshwater streams. They then swim to the ocean, where they spend one to three years. After this period, they generally return to the same stream where they were born to lay eggs.

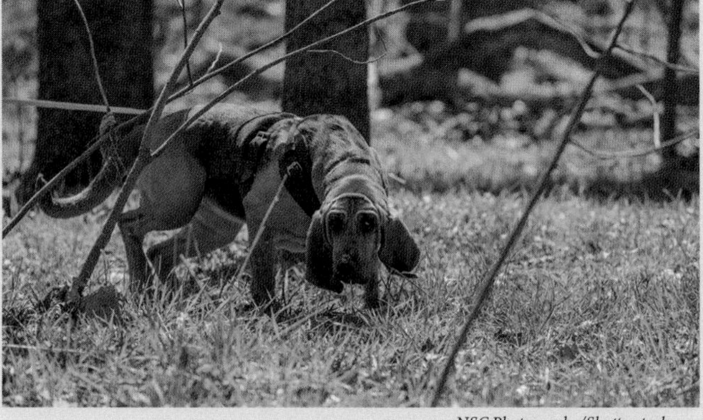

NSC Photography/Shutterstock.com

The bloodhound has an extraordinarily well-developed sense of smell, making it ideal for law enforcement applications such as tracking missing persons and criminals.

How does each salmon locate the exact same stream in which it was born? One hypothesis is that the newborn salmon brain is imprinted with the distinctive odor of the water from the stream of its birth. Researchers tested this hypothesis by tagging a large number of young salmon and recording the location of their births. They then plugged the nostrils of 50% of these salmon to block their ability to smell. When the salmon returned to fresh water to lay their eggs, the researchers discovered that the salmon with plugged nostrils did not return to the same stream where they were born. By contrast, most of the salmon with unplugged nostrils returned to the site of their births. Although other factors may influence the salmon's remarkable ability to return to its birth stream, its sense of smell clearly plays a key role.

fumes, or illegal drug abuse. This condition is known as a *perforated septum*. A perforated septum can be surgically treated to close the open areas.

SELF CHECK

1. What is the most common cause of rhinitis?
2. What are the two basic treatments for rhinitis?
3. What might cause a perforated septum?

Gustatory Sense

The human mouth contains approximately 10,000 sensory receptors for taste. These ***taste buds*** are scattered throughout the interior of the mouth, including on the lips and the sides, top, and back of the mouth. The majority of taste buds, however, reside on the familiar tiny bumps on the tongue known as ***papillae***. Within each taste bud, ***gustatory cells*** send tiny ***gustatory hairs*** up through very small openings in the tops of the taste buds known as ***taste pores*** (**Figure 8.16**).

When you eat food, the food is mixed in your mouth with saliva produced by the salivary glands. Chemical molecules from food dissolve in the saliva to produce compounds called ***tastants***. The tastants stimulate the gustatory hairs to send nerve impulses to the brain. Three of the cranial nerves—the facial nerve, the glossopharyngeal nerve, and the vagus nerve—are responsible for transmitting taste sensations to the brain.

Although people enjoy many foods and beverages because of the complex taste sensations they generate, the gustatory sense comprises only five basic tastes. These are sweet, salty, sour, bitter, and umami. Umami is the taste of beef as well as the taste of monosodium glutamate (MSG), a seasoning commonly added to processed foods to enhance their taste. Some have also proposed fat, termed *oleogustus*, as a sixth basic taste. Although a single gustatory cell responds to only one of the five or six taste sensations, individual taste buds contain 50 to 100 gustatory cells, which typically include all five or six taste sensations.

The flavors that people detect in foods and beverages are influenced by sensations from the taste buds, but they are also strongly influenced by the sense of smell. An estimated 75% to 90% of what people attribute to taste is actually due to what they smell. In the absence of smell, a person would be able to distinguish only the five basic tastes—sweet, salty, sour, bitter, and umami. With the assistance of smell, the average person is able to distinguish approximately 10,000 different flavors (**Figure 8-17**).

The human mouth contains no taste receptors for the distinctly recognizable tastes of peach, tomato, lime, or chocolate, for example. Each of these flavors is produced by a combination of taste and smell. The brain receives sensory information from the receptors for both taste and smell, and then translates this information into the flavors that people recognize.

Flavor is actually a combination of taste, smell, texture or consistency, and temperature. Many people have aversions to foods and beverages because they simply do not find their consistency appealing. A hot food or drink gives off odors that strongly activate

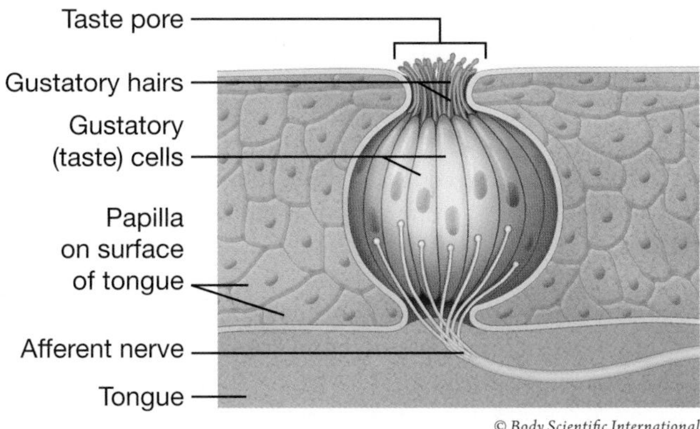

© Body Scientific International

Figure 8.16 Anatomy of a taste bud.

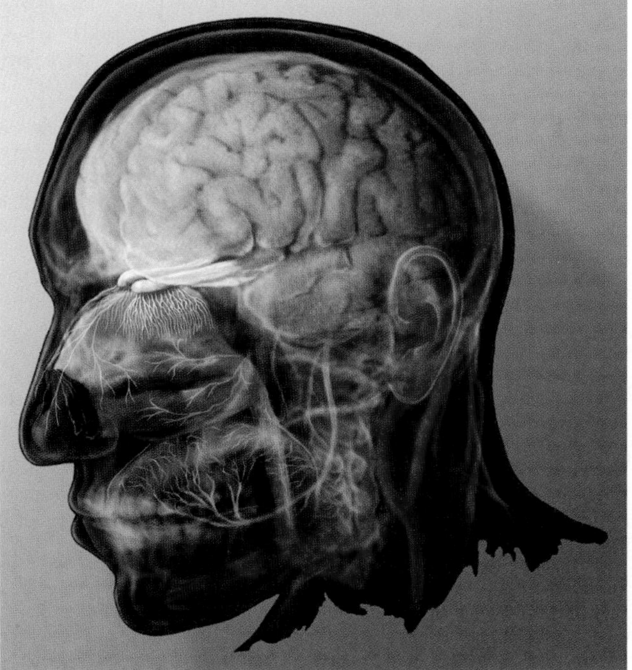

Anatomical Travelogue/Science Source

Figure 8.17 The senses of smell and taste work closely together to inform the brain of various flavors.

the neural pathways for smell, whereas the same cold food or beverage gives off a much weaker odor, making it less appealing. Spicy foods stimulate not only gustatory cells but also pain receptors in the mouth. Because everyone perceives pain differently, some people enjoy the sensation of spicy foods and others do not.

SELF CHECK

1. What are papillae?
2. List the three nerves responsible for sending taste sensory signals to the brain.
3. Explain the relationship between the senses of smell and taste in detecting flavors.

Tongue Disorders

The powerful muscles of the tongue enable people to speak and to chew and swallow food. As discussed earlier, taste buds on the surface of the tongue allow people to experience different taste sensations. A variety of disorders, including infections, injuries, and abnormal tissue growth, can affect the appearance and function of the tongue. Some tongue disorders are short-lived and can be remedied with antibiotics. Other disorders require ongoing treatment for an underlying physical condition.

Infection of the tongue may follow severe biting of the tongue, or it may be associated with piercing of the tongue. Antibiotics are used to treat a tongue infection. Fortunately, the human tongue tends to heal quickly. In fact, it heals more quickly than any other part of the body.

Certain conditions can promote unnatural growth of the gustatory hairs of the tongue, resulting in the look and feel of a "hairy tongue." The most common cause is inadequate oral hygiene, but other causes include use of certain medications, excessive drinking of coffee or tea, frequent tobacco use, and radiation treatments to the head or neck region. Good oral

Focus On Taste Testing

Businesses that are growing, developing, or marketing food or beverages regularly use taste testing to help guide their decisions about which products to market. Consider the soda industry, in which big players Coca-Cola and PepsiCo have produced dueling product lines based on consumer taste tests since 1898. That year, Pepsi first entered the market to challenge Coca-Cola, which was then selling 1 million gallons per year. The variety of soft drinks offered by both companies over the years have been rigorously researched through taste testing and other market analysis techniques to strategically select and position products in the market.

In a taste test, people serving as "tasters" sample and provide feedback on the food or beverage they are given. The purpose of the taste test may be to compare similar products or to ensure consistency in a given product. In food or beverage competitions, taste testing is done to rate the product and select winners.

Taste testing of foods is typically performed blind, so that tasters do not know what they are tasting before they answer questions about the product. In some cases, the tasters may actually be blindfolded, but they are more typically offered different samples that have been staged to be as identical as possible. In a double-blind test, the samples have been coded so that neither the samplers nor the researchers are aware of which product is which until the sampler feedback has been recorded. This procedure helps to ensure the objectivity of the test results.

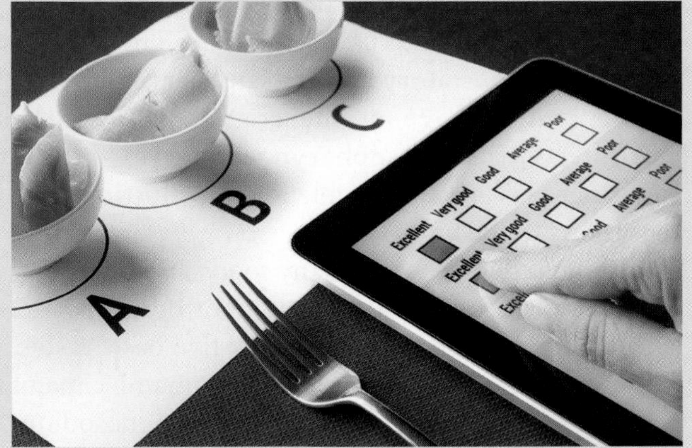

Beeldbewerking/iStock.com

Tasters follow a methodical procedure to evaluate all aspects of the food or beverage being tested.

Although the term *taste testing* suggests that it is all about taste, all of the senses may actually be involved in evaluating the desirability of a food or beverage. As discussed in this chapter, the senses of taste and smell are intimately related. The neutrally transmitted messages about taste and smell converge to produce what people perceive as a flavor. Vision and touch enable people to evaluate the desirability of a food or beverage's appearance and consistency. Even hearing can be involved in the case of foods that "crunch."

hygiene, including brushing the tongue as well as the teeth, is both a prevention and cure for hairy tongue.

Burning mouth syndrome, as the name suggests, involves a sensation of moderate to severe burning in the mouth that may continue for months or even years. When the pain persists, anxiety and depression may develop. Related symptoms may include tingling, numbness, or dryness of the mouth and a bitter or metallic taste. The condition can arise from a variety of causes, including damage to the taste and pain receptors in the mouth, chronically dry mouth, nutritional deficiencies, hormonal changes, acid reflux, and infection in the mouth.

Treatment of burning mouth syndrome is based on the cause, so it may involve addressing an underlying disorder with nutritional supplements, hormone therapy, antibiotics, or other remedies. When no underlying disorder is apparent, treatment is designed with the goal of reducing the pain associated with burning mouth syndrome.

SECTION 8.3 REVIEW

Mini-Glossary

antihistamines medications that help curb the activity of histamines

gustatory cells sensory receptors located within taste buds

gustatory hairs tiny threads in taste buds that send nerve impulses to the brain

histamines molecules that trigger a reaction to irritation of the nasal membranes, producing nasal congestion and drainage

limbic system the part of the brain responsible for emotions

olfactory bulb the thickened end of the olfactory nerve, which sends sensory impulses to the olfactory region of the brain

olfactory hairs tiny threads that extend from the olfactory receptor cells into the nasal cavity

olfactory nerve a cranial nerve that sends impulses to the olfactory cortex of the brain

olfactory receptor cells the sensors responsible for smell

olfactory region a dime-sized area found on top of each nasal cavity that houses the olfactory receptor cells

papillae tiny bumps on the tongue that house taste buds

septum the structure made of cartilage that divides the nose into left and right air passages

tastants compounds that stimulate the gustatory hairs to send nerve impulses to the brain

taste buds the sensory receptors for taste

taste pores very small openings in the top of the taste buds through which gustatory hairs project

Review Questions

1. Define *histamines* and explain the importance of antihistamines.
2. Which part of the brain is responsible for emotions related to scent?
3. What causes the blockage of the olfactory receptor cells when you have a cold?
4. What is the name of the structure that separates the right and left air passages of the nose?
5. The sense of taste is affected by the sense of _____.
6. Which disorder causes a bitter or metallic taste in the mouth?
7. Describe in detail how you are able to taste food.
8. List the five basic recognized tastes and give examples of each taste.
9. Natural gas has no smell. Explain why utility companies add an unpleasant smell to natural gas.
10. What is the difference between taste and flavor?

Medical Terminology: The Sensory Systems

By understanding the word parts that make up medical words, you can extend your medical vocabulary. This chapter includes many of the word parts listed below. Review these word parts to be sure you understand their meanings.

a-	without
-acusis	hearing
-al	pertaining to
ambly/o	dull, dim
aque/o	water
-ar	pertaining to
aur/o	ear
hyper-	above, excessive
-ic	pertaining to
intra-	within
lacrim/o	tear, tear duct
ocul/o	eye
ophthalm/o	eye
-opia	vision defect
-ous	pertaining to
presby/o	old age
vascul/o	blood vessels

Now use these word parts to form valid medical words that fit the following definitions. Some of the words are included in this chapter. Others are not. When you finish, use a medical dictionary to check your work.

1. without blood vessels (avascular)
2. inside the eye (intraocular)
3. pertaining to water (aqueous)
4. pertaining to tears (lacrimal)
5. condition of having dim vision (amblyopia)
6. hearing loss pertaining to the aging process (presbycusis)
7. pertaining to the eye (ophthalmic)
8. within the ear (intra-aural)
9. abnormally good hearing (hyperacusis)
10. pertaining to the ear (aural)

Chapter 8 Summary

- A variety of external structures protect the eye, and internal structures send sensory signals to the brain, enabling vision.
- Common eye problems include eye injuries, various vision disorders, and eye diseases and disorders including conjunctivitis, cataracts, glaucoma, macular degeneration, diabetic retinopathy, and vitreous floaters, which may indicate a retinal tear or detachment.
- The ear is divided into three parts—the external ear, middle ear, and internal ear.
- The inner ear is responsible for hearing and equilibrium.
- Common ear problems include deafness, tinnitus, otitis externa, otitis media, and otitis interna.
- The olfactory receptor cells send impulses to the olfactory nerve, which then sends the stimuli to the olfactory cortex of the brain.
- Injuries and disorders of the nose include the common cold, rhinitis, and septum problems.
- The senses of smell and taste involve highly specialized, sensitive receptors that provide information to the facial nerve, glossopharyngeal nerve, and vagus nerve which, in turn, transmit sensory impulses from the taste receptors to the brain.
- Tongue disorders include infections, "hairy tongue," and burning mouth syndrome.

Chapter 8 Review

Understanding Key Concepts

1. The white of the eye is called the ______.
2. Which of the following four words does *not* belong? Why?
   A. retina
   B. rods
   C. cones
   D. choroid
3. Which of the following four words does *not* belong? Why?
   A. cornea
   B. sclera
   C. retina
   D. extrinsic muscles
4. The conjunctiva is a membrane that lines the ______.
   A. eyelid
   B. innermost part of the eye
   C. iris
   D. rods and cones

5. The eyeball has three layers: the sclera, the choroid, and the ______.
   A. iris
   B. lens
   C. orbit
   D. retina
6. Maria wears contact lenses to see the whiteboard at school. She probably has an eye disorder called ______.
   A. strabismus
   B. hyperopia
   C. myopia
   D. presbyopia
7. Which part of the eye is removed during cataract surgery?
   A. iris
   B. lens
   C. sclera
   D. cornea
8. Which of the following describes the correct pathway of vision?
   A. cornea, retina, optic nerve, pupil, lens
   B. pupil, lens, retina, cornea, optic nerve
   C. cornea, pupil, lens, retina, optic nerve
   D. cornea, pupil, retina, lens, optic nerve
9. Another name for the eardrum is the ______.
10. The outer part of the ear is known as the ______, or pinna.
11. In which structure of the ear is the organ of Corti located?
12. Where would you find cerumen?
    A. pinna
    B. Eustachian tube
    C. auditory canal
    D. middle ear
13. Which part of the ear carries sound impulses to the brain?
    A. pinna
    B. tympanic membrane
    C. cochlear nerve
    D. auditory nerve
14. In the pathway of hearing, sound waves travel from the tympanic membrane to the ______.
    A. ossicles
    B. cochlea
    C. Eustachian tube
    D. auditory nerve
15. What is the purpose of the Eustachian tube?
    A. to carry sound waves to the middle ear
    B. to carry sound waves to the inner ear
    C. to equalize pressure in the middle ear
    D. to protect the inner ear from microorganisms
16. An audiologist would examine someone with ______.
    A. hearing loss
    B. a sore throat
    C. blurred vision
    D. chest pain

Instructions: *Write the **letter** of the name of the **part of the ear** on your answer sheet next to the corresponding number.*

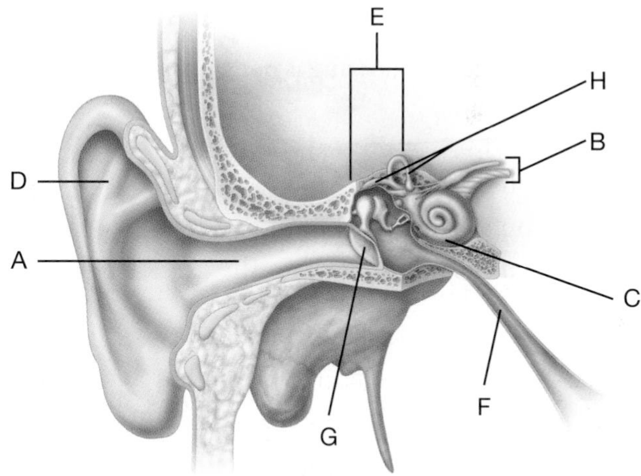

17. auditory canal
18. middle ear
19. semicircular canals
20. auricle
21. vestibulocochlear nerve
22. tympanic membrane
23. cochlea
24. Eustachian tube

25. What percentage of a person's perception of flavor is supplied by smell?
26. Describe at least three functions of your nose and sense of smell.
27. The gustatory sense comprises only five basic tastes. What are they?
28. A person has burned his tongue and has trouble tasting food. Which structures of his mouth were damaged?
    A. stapes
    B. pinna
    C. papillae
    D. palate
29. How can people prevent hairy tongue disorder?
30. What is the most common cause of rhinitis?
31. Which of the following would *not* cause a perforated septum?
    A. illegal drug use
    B. injury
    C. histamines
    D. an ulcer
32. Give two examples of foods that have the taste of umami.
33. Which of the following is *not* a possible location for taste buds?
    A. in the nose
    B. on the tongue
    C. on the lips
    D. on the roof of the mouth

Thinking Critically

34. Compare the anatomy and functions of the iris and the pupil.
35. What would happen if a person had no lacrimal glands, or if the person's lacrimal glands were clogged?
36. What would be the result of the vitreous humor leaking out of the eyeball?
37. Explain why a particular smell might trigger a memory. Use the anatomy and physiology described in this chapter to support your hypothesis.

Clinical Case Study

Read again the Clinical Case Study at the beginning of this chapter. Use the information provided in the chapter to answer the questions at the end of the scenario.

38. What diagnoses are possible?
39. Which diagnosis is most likely?

Analyzing and Evaluating Data

The chart to the right shows the average percentage of hearing loss in males and females in various age ranges. Use the chart to answer the following questions:

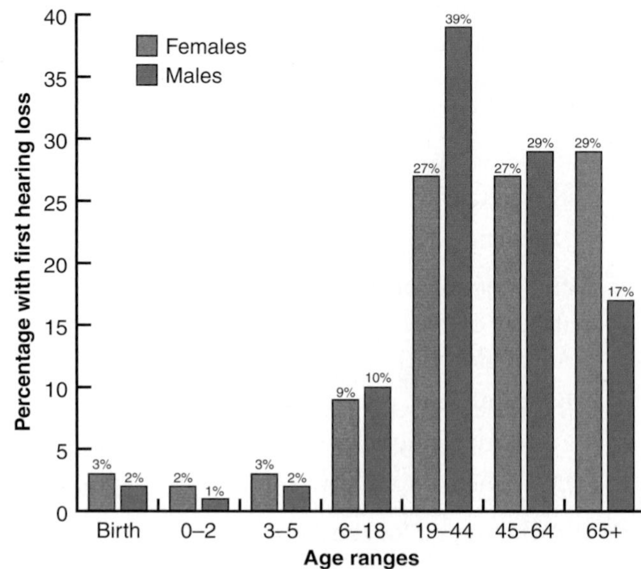

40. Which age range has the highest percentage of people (male and female combined) experiencing their first hearing loss?
41. Which group—men or women—tends to lose their ability to hear at an earlier age?

Investigating Further

42. With a group of friends, taste various foods. Discuss and compare your sensitivity to the five basic tastes with your friends' sensitivity to these tastes. How would you describe your sense of taste compared with theirs?
43. Conduct research to find out more about otitis media in infants and toddlers. What can caregivers do to help minimize the risk of infection in this susceptible population?

9 The Endocrine System

Clinical Case Study

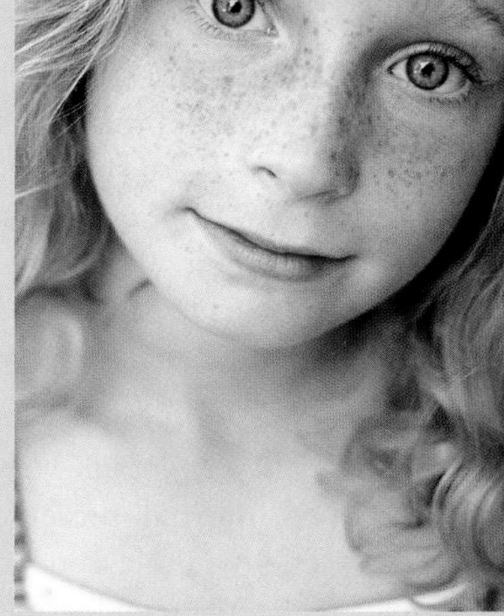
sianc/Shutterstock.com

Caitlyn, age 10, had always been a healthy, physically active, energetic youngster. Fair-haired and freckle-faced, she started playing soccer when she was five and has exceled in it since then. Caitlyn's family is currently staying with their grandmother, Beth, who works as a school health nurse. Grandma Beth's home is busting at the seams with three grandchildren, their parents, and their dog underfoot.

Since the move to Gran's, Caitlyn has increasingly been complaining of feeling tired, and she seemed lethargic to her family. She always seemed to be hungry and thirsty, and she appeared thinner. Just to be sure that Caitlyn wasn't getting a cold or the flu, Gran Beth checked her vital signs, but her heart rate, blood pressure, and body temperature were all normal.

Due to the cramped conditions at the house, Caitlyn has been sleeping on an air mattress in her grandmother's room. Beth noticed that Caitlyn gets up several times a night to use the bathroom. After a week, Beth decided that Caitlyn needed to be seen by their family physician. Among the medical conditions and disorders discussed in this chapter, what are the possible causes of Caitlyn's ailment, and which one would be the most likely diagnosis? What types of tests would help evaluate Caitlyn's condition?

Chapter 9 Outline

In 2010, the *Guinness Book of World Records* named Sultan Kosen, a 29-year-old man from Turkey, the world's tallest man, measuring 8 feet, 3 inches. Kosen also achieved the records for the largest hands (11.22 inches, or 28.5 centimeters) and largest feet (14.4 inches, or 36.5 centimeters). A basketball player may read about this and think, *"Awesome!"*

Kosen's size is not normal, however. A tumor caused Kosen's pituitary gland to secrete excessive amounts of growth hormone, resulting in gigantism, a condition in which a person grows to an exceptionally large size. The only way to treat this condition is to stop the secretion of growth hormone.

In 2010, doctors at the University of Virginia's Medical Center put Kosen on medication to balance his hormone levels. Then they used a gamma knife, which emits focused beams of radiation, to target the tumor on his pituitary gland. Because the tumor was too deep for conventional surgery, the gamma knife was their best option. The surgery was a success, and Sultan stopped growing.

Sultan's story highlights the overwhelming effects that the small but powerful endocrine glands and organs can have on the body. This chapter describes these glands and organs, as well as some diseases and disorders that can occur in the endocrine system.

SECTION 9.1

Anatomy and Physiology of the Endocrine System

Objectives

- Describe the basic anatomy of the endocrine system.
- Describe the functions of hormones, and explain how hormones move through the body.
- Explain the three types of hormonal control that help maintain homeostasis.

Key Terms

amino acid-derived hormones
cyclic adenosine monophosphate (cAMP)
downregulated
epinephrine
glucagon
hormonal control
hormones
humoral control
hypothalamic non-releasing hormones
hypothalamic releasing hormones
insulin
neural control
steroid hormones
upregulated

Like the nervous system, the endocrine system controls and monitors organs, glands, and processes in the body. The nervous and endocrine systems work together to regulate bodily functions, but they act in very different ways. The nervous system works quickly through electrical impulses, and the effects of those impulses are short lived. The endocrine system secretes hormones that are slower to react, but their effects are longer lasting.

Everyone experiences the "fight-or-flight" response at some point in their lives. This response occurs when a person encounters a potentially dangerous situation, such as almost being hit by a car or being startled by something unexpected. The body jumps into action to move the person out of the way of a speeding vehicle or other impending danger—that's the nervous system at work. After the danger has passed, a racing heartbeat, an increased respiratory rate, and a thin layer of sweat on the skin may persist for a time. This slower, longer-lasting response is the work of the endocrine system.

Endocrine System Anatomy

The endocrine system is a collection of organs and small glands that directly or indirectly influence all functions of the body. Some of the endocrine glands are also part of the nervous system. These include the hypothalamus, pituitary, adrenal, and pineal glands. This overlap allows the two systems to integrate their responses.

For example, when body temperature drops below the normal level, the sympathetic nervous system (SNS) springs into action. The SNS wants the thyroid gland to release heat-producing hormones to raise the body temperature, but the SNS cannot directly act on the thyroid. Instead, the hypothalamus receives sensory input from the SNS, which triggers the secretion of hypothalamic releasing hormones. These hormones cause the pituitary gland to secrete other hormones that ultimately cause the thyroid to release the heat-producing hormones desired by the SNS.

Endocrine Glands

The endocrine system is made up of ductless glands called *endocrine glands*. Endocrine glands are glands of internal secretion. They secrete ***hormones***, or chemical messengers, directly into the bloodstream. The major endocrine glands include the hypothalamus, pancreas, pituitary gland, adrenal glands, thyroid gland, parathyroid glands, pineal gland, testes (male), and ovaries (female).

The organs and glands of the endocrine system are spread throughout the body, and they regulate many functions. **Figure 9.1** illustrates the location of the major endocrine glands.

Exocrine Glands

Exocrine glands are glands of external secretion. Unlike endocrine glands, exocrine glands each have a duct through which secretions are carried to the body's surface or to other organs. Examples of exocrine glands and their secretions include:

- sweat glands (sweat)
- salivary glands (saliva)
- mammary glands (breast milk)
- lacrimal glands (tears)
- pancreas gland (digestive enzymes)

The pancreas is unique because it functions as both an exocrine gland and an endocrine gland. The pancreas releases hormones that regulate blood glucose levels in the body. It also secretes digestive enzymes through a duct into the small intestine.

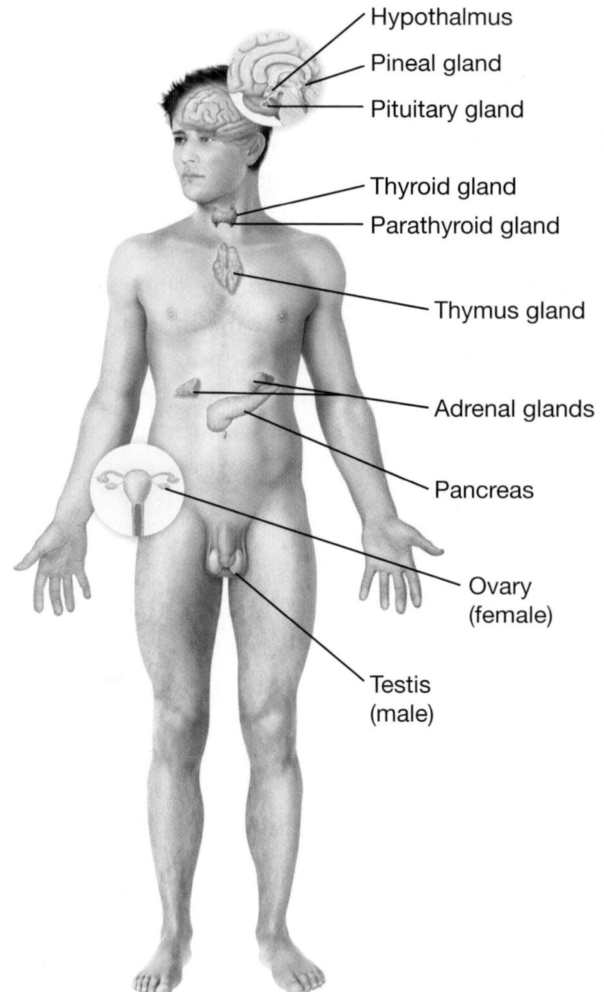

Figure 9.1 The glands and organs of the endocrine system are located throughout the body.

SELF CHECK

1. Which endocrine glands are also part of the nervous system?
2. What is the difference between endocrine and exocrine glands?

Hormones

Have you ever wondered why you get hungry and thirsty? When the hypothalamus gland is stimulated by hormones secreted by the adipose tissue and gastrointestinal tract, you feel hungry or thirsty. Do you feel energized, refreshed, and happier after getting a good night's sleep? You can thank the pineal gland for secreting melatonin, a hormone that induces sleep. You may be filled with energy some days, and feel sluggish and tired on others. The thyroid gland secretes several hormones that affect your energy level.

Generally, hormones regulate carbohydrate, fat, and protein metabolism; water and electrolyte balance; reproductive activity; growth and development; and energy balance. Hormones also aid in the body's response to infection and stress. These are just a few of the ways in which the endocrine system affects everyday functions, emotions, and behaviors.

Understanding Medical Terminology

The term *hormone* is derived from the Greek word *hormôn*, which means "to excite" or "to activate."

Target Cells

Hormones are transported throughout the body by the blood, which comes into contact with all of the body's tissues and organs. Although hormones pass by many sites in the body, each hormone affects only the cells of tissues and organs that have matching protein receptors. Cells that have the specific protein receptors that match a hormone are referred to as the hormone's *target cells*. Receptors are located on the cell membrane's surface or inside the cell (intracellular receptor). Target cells can be located close to or far away from the gland secreting the hormone (**Figure 9.2**).

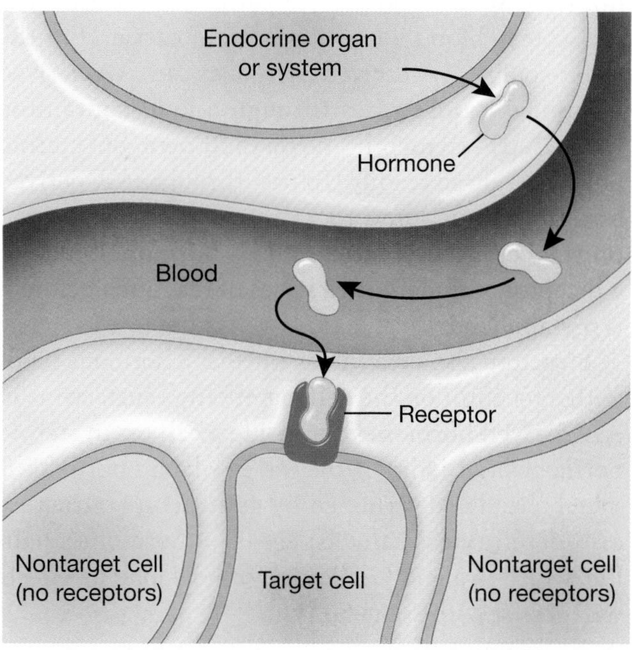

Figure 9.2 Hormones travel through the bloodstream to reach their target cells.

When a hormone binds with its protein receptor, the connection is similar to a lock and key. Once this hormone-receptor complex is complete, it influences the activity of the target cell by changing the cell membrane's permeability, increasing or decreasing enzyme activity, increasing protein synthesis or glycogen breakdown, or stimulating mitosis and secretory activity.

Some hormones, such as ***epinephrine***, have receptors at many different sites, making their effects widespread. Other hormones have fewer target sites, limiting their effects.

Types of Hormones

Hormones are usually classified according to their chemical structure. Fat-soluble lipid hormones are called ***steroid hormones***. Water-soluble hormones that are composed of protein or protein-related substances such as peptides are called ***amino acid-derived hormones***. Most hormones are amino acid-derived hormones (AA-derived hormones), except those secreted by the adrenal cortex and the reproductive glands.

A hormone's structure determines how it travels through the bloodstream. AA-derived hormones travel alone, but steroid hormones require a helper known as a *protein carrier*. To understand how fat- and water-soluble hormones function, consider the analogy of oil and water. The substances just don't mix! Fat-soluble hormones cannot move through the watery blood without a protein carrier, but the water-soluble AA-derived hormones can. AA-derived hormones cannot pass through a lipid-containing (fat-based) cell membrane on their own, but steroid hormones do so readily. To pass through, AA-derived hormones must bind to a protein receptor located on the cell's membrane. After a hormone binds to a receptor, it undergoes a series of reactions before it is metabolized.

Structure also determines whether a hormone binds with a receptor on the cell membrane's surface (as in AA-derived hormones) or inside a cell (as in steroid hormones). In addition, the way in which a hormone is metabolized is determined by its structure. Structure also determines many aspects of a hormone's half-life, which is a good indication of how long its effects will persist within the body.

Functions of Steroid Hormones

Steroid hormones and AA-derived hormones function differently based on where they bind to protein receptors. Steroid hormones, which are lipid soluble, can diffuse through the target cell's membrane and bind to the receptor located in the cytoplasm or nucleus of the cell. AA-derived hormones are not lipid soluble, so they cannot diffuse through the target cell's membrane. Instead, they must bind to a receptor located on the cell membrane.

Steroid hormones are secreted by the reproductive glands and the adrenal cortex, and they are transported in the blood by protein carriers. Once a steroid hormone reaches a target cell, it binds to the protein receptor inside the cell and forms a hormone-receptor complex that enters the nucleus of the cell. The hormone-receptor complex binds with DNA in the nucleus and "turns on" certain genes in a process known as *direct gene activation*. In this process, messenger RNA (mRNA) is produced. The mRNA travels into the cytoplasm and stimulates protein synthesis. **Figure 9.3** illustrates the actions of steroid hormones and their intracellular receptors.

Functions of Amino Acid-Derived Hormones

By contrast, the receptors for AA-derived hormones are found on the cell membrane on the surface of a cell. AA-derived hormones cannot enter the cell, so a second messenger inside the cell is needed. This process can be likened to a "tag team" in which the AA-derived hormone is the first messenger. **Figure 9.4** illustrates this process. The process begins when a hormone binds with the surface receptor to form a hormone–receptor complex and creates a series of reactions, which ultimately activates an enzyme. The activated enzyme generally creates a second messenger, which works inside the cell to produce a variety of responses.

In **Figure 9.4**, an AA-derived hormone binds with a surface receptor, causing reactions that activate the enzyme adenylate cyclase. Adenylate cyclase stimulates the formation of ***cyclic adenosine monophosphate (cAMP)***, an important second messenger in this process. cAMP activates the protein kinases with energy supplied by ATP, producing a

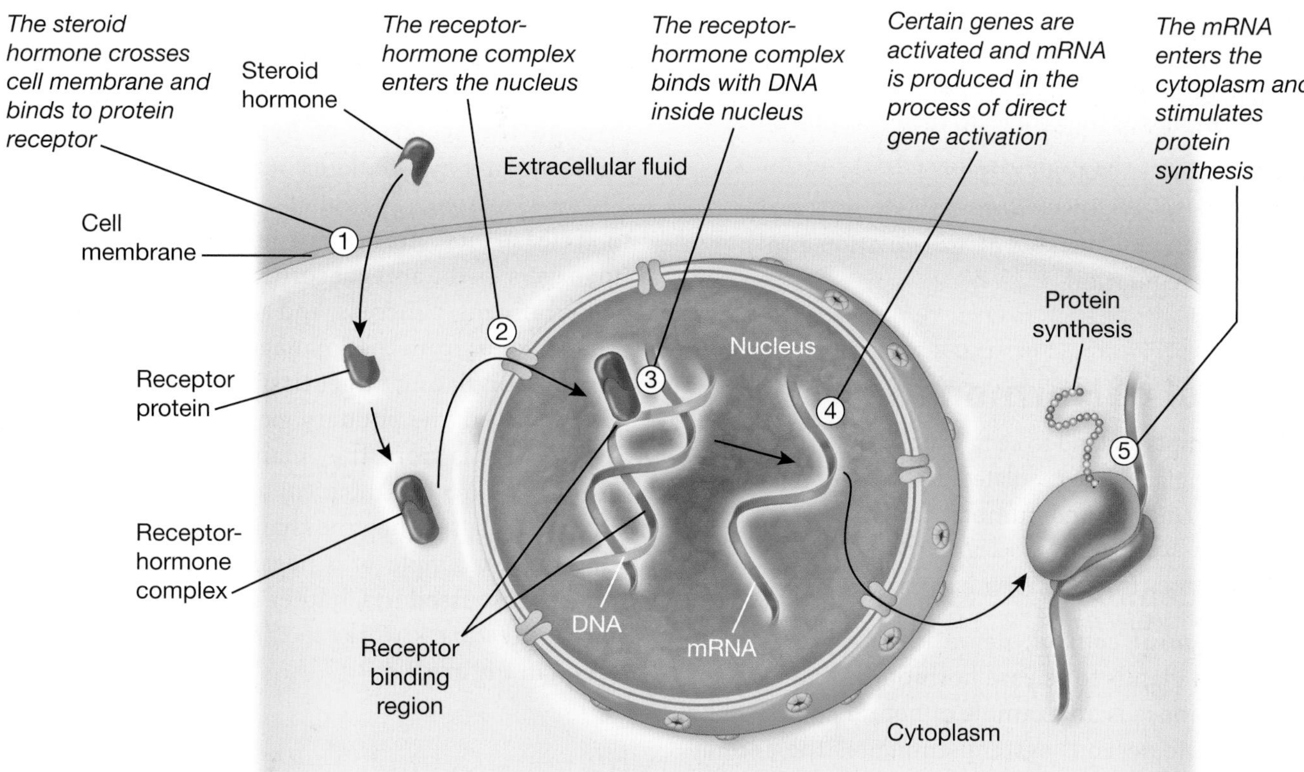
The steroid hormone crosses cell membrane and binds to protein receptor
Steroid hormone
The receptor-hormone complex enters the nucleus
The receptor-hormone complex binds with DNA inside nucleus
Certain genes are activated and mRNA is produced in the process of direct gene activation
The mRNA enters the cytoplasm and stimulates protein synthesis
Extracellular fluid
Cell membrane
1
2
3
4
5
Nucleus
Protein synthesis
Receptor protein
Receptor-hormone complex
DNA
mRNA
Receptor binding region
Cytoplasm

© Body Scientific International

Figure 9.3 Mechanism of action of steroid hormones.

cascade of responses that can range from activating cellular enzymes, to causing protein synthesis and glycogen breakdown. Examples of hormones that use cAMP as a second messenger are epinephrine and glucagon, which stimulate glycogen breakdown in the muscle and liver, respectively. There are many other secondary messengers, including cyclic guanine monophosphate (cGMP), inositol triphosphate (IP3), and calcium (Ca^{++}).

Upregulation and Downregulation

The activity of hormone receptors can be ***upregulated*** (increased) or ***downregulated*** (decreased), making them more or less sensitive to hormones. Exercise upregulates insulin receptors, making them more sensitive to ***insulin*** (a hormone that promotes the uptake of glucose in body tissues). Due to this process, less insulin is needed to promote glucose uptake in people who are physically active. However, obesity downregulates insulin receptors, so more insulin must be present to promote glucose uptake by cells in those who are obese. These two glucose-uptake scenarios have important implications for diabetics, particularly those who are overweight.

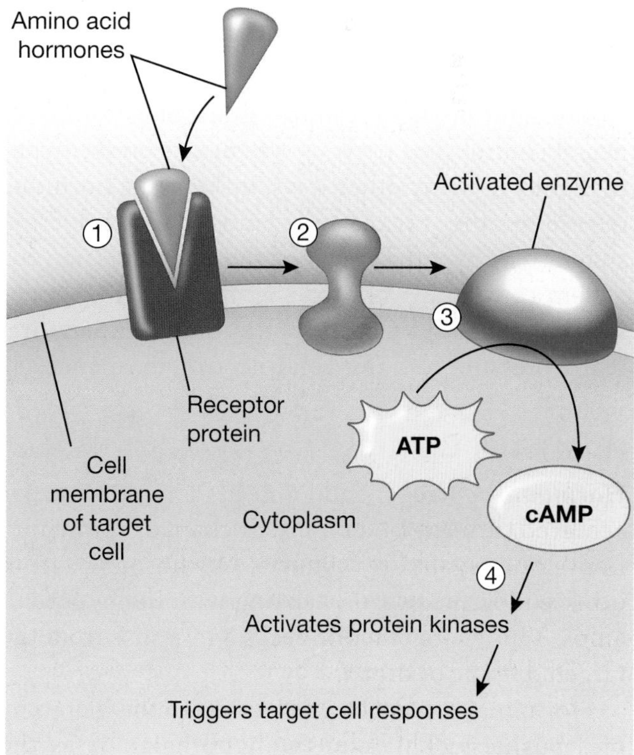
Amino acid hormones
Activated enzyme
1
2
3
Receptor protein
Cell membrane of target cell
ATP
Cytoplasm
cAMP
4
Activates protein kinases
Triggers target cell responses

© Body Scientific International

Figure 9.4 Mechanism of action of amino acid-derived hormones.

SELF CHECK

1. What serves as the transport system for hormones as they travel to their receptor sites?
2. Where are the receptors for steroid and amino acid-derived hormones located?
3. Explain the concepts of upregulation and downregulation.

Control of Hormone Secretion

What prompts a gland to secrete or inhibit a hormone? Endocrine glands are regulated in three different ways: neural, hormonal, and humoral control.

Neural Control

During ***neural control***, nerve fibers stimulate the endocrine glands to release hormones. The fight-or-flight response is an example of neural control. The sympathetic nervous system stimulates the adrenal medulla to release epinephrine and norepinephrine. These hormones prime the body to fight or flee from a stressful situation by increasing heart rate, blood pressure, respiration, and blood flow to muscles, while also decreasing blood flow to organs that are not essential in a fight-or-flight situation, such as the digestive organs.

The fight-or-flight response is just one example of neural control. The nervous system acts on the hypothalamus in many other ways, influencing hormone release in other organs and glands of the endocrine system. The hypothalamus and the autonomic nervous system constantly work together to maintain homeostasis of numerous factors such as body temperature, blood pressure, and fluid and electrolyte balance.

Hormonal Control

Hormonal control of endocrine glands and organs is achieved through a hierarchy, or chain of command. Endocrine organs are stimulated by hormones from other endocrine organs, starting with the hypothalamus. This chain reaction seeks a response from the targeted tissue or organ.

Hormonal control can be likened to the hierarchy of a business. Think of the hypothalamus as the president of the company, the pituitary gland as the vice president, and the other endocrine glands and organs as managers (**Figure 9.5**).

As "president" of the endocrine system, the hypothalamus directs the activities of the pituitary gland (the "vice president"). The hypothalamus does this through the secretion of ***hypothalamic releasing hormones*** and ***hypothalamic non-releasing hormones***. These hormones stimulate the pituitary gland to release its many hormones to direct the "managers"—the adrenal cortex, thyroid gland, reproductive organs, pancreas, and adrenal medulla.

Hormones from the "managers" have an end goal, such as stimulating target tissues. Once the goal has been achieved, the pituitary gland and hypothalamus receive signals from the "manager" hormones that inhibit, or turn off, the pituitary and hypothalamic hormones, thus ending the chain of hormonal control. This is an example of a negative feedback loop, a concept discussed in Chapter 1. A summary of how negative feedback works in the endocrine system is shown in **Figure 9.6**.

Humoral Control

The endocrine system achieves ***humoral control*** by monitoring the levels of various substances in body fluids, such as the blood. If it detects a homeostatic imbalance, it initiates corrective actions to help the body regain homeostasis.

For example, when blood glucose levels rise, the pancreas secretes insulin, stimulating the absorption of glucose in body tissues. Greater absorption of glucose in body tissues lowers blood glucose levels. By contrast, when blood glucose levels drop, the pancreas secretes the hormone ***glucagon***. Glucagon causes the breakdown of glycogen stored in the liver. The glycogen then enters the bloodstream, which increases blood glucose levels.

Hormones and Homeostasis

The body is constantly monitoring all of its systems to ensure that everything is working normally. This functional balance is called *homeostasis*. If the function of any organ system deviates from the normal range (homeostatic imbalance), the body takes corrective measures to restore homeostasis.

Neural, hormonal, and humoral controls trigger the release of hormones during homeostatic imbalance. Increased hormone levels affect the sites where imbalance occurs, initiating actions that restore homeostasis. Homeostatic balance and rising hormone

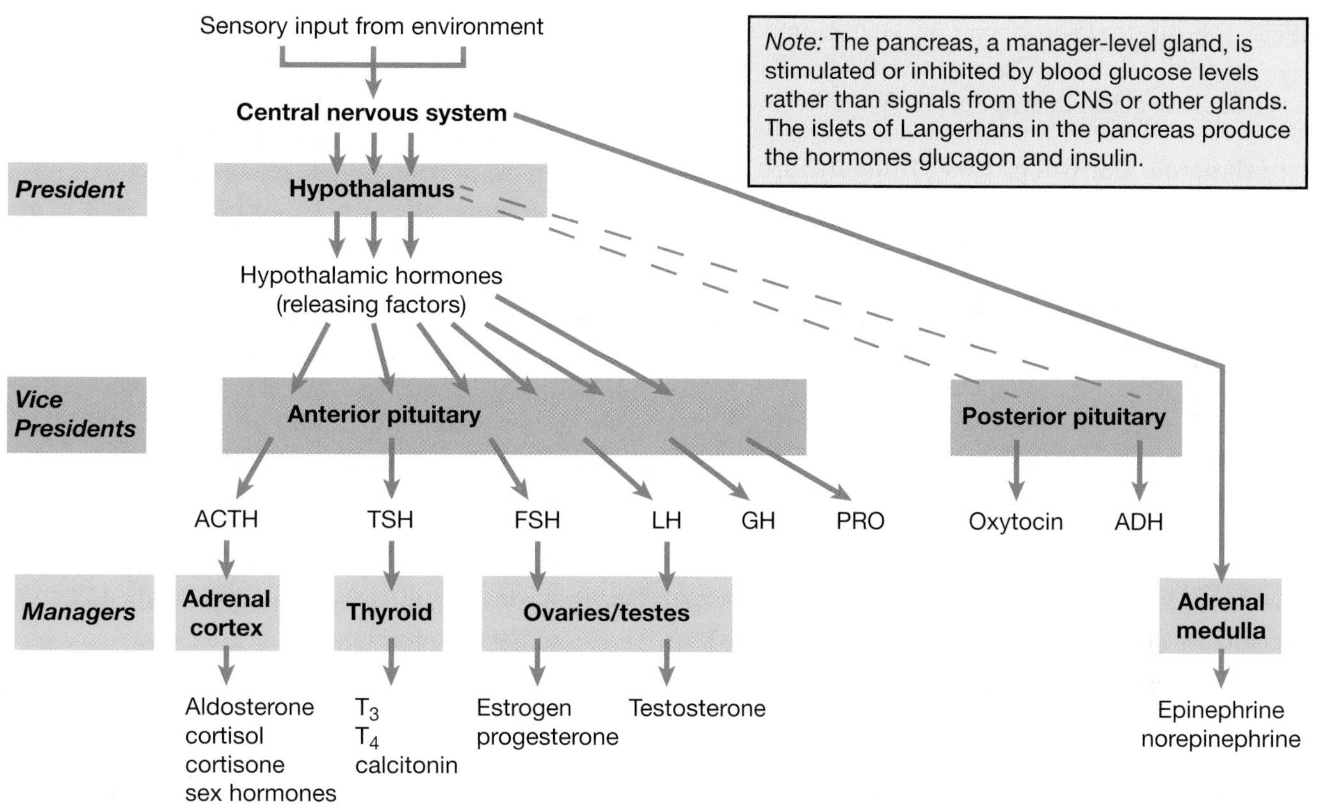

© Body Scientific International

Figure 9.5 Hierarchy of hormonal control in the endocrine system. Each gland in the hierarchy controls the activities of the gland or glands below it, and each gland is controlled by the gland or glands above it.

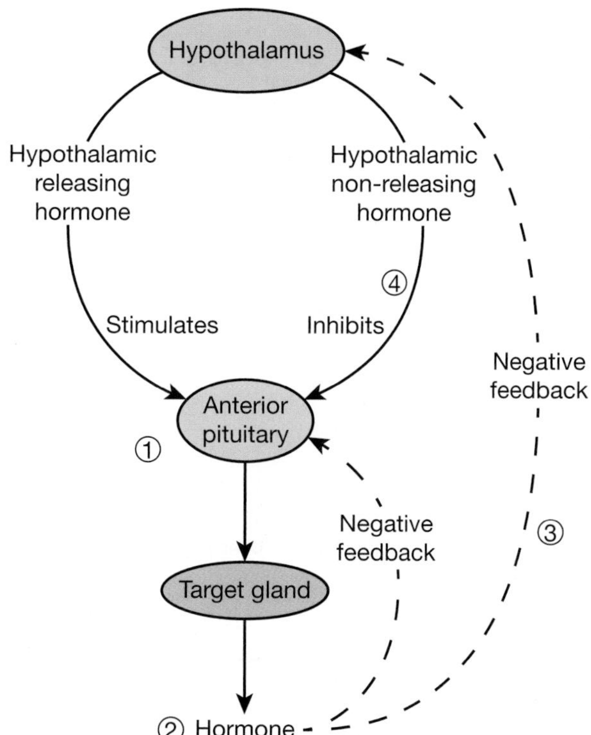

© Body Scientific International

Figure 9.6 Negative feedback in the endocrine system. 1—The hypothalamus and the pituitary gland direct the target gland to release hormones. 2—The target gland releases hormones to achieve a goal, such as the stimulation of target tissues. 3—After the goal is achieved, the target gland sends signals to the hypothalamus and the pituitary gland. 4—The hypothalamus inhibits the production of additional hypothalamic and anterior pituitary hormones.

levels inhibit further hormone secretions via a negative feedback loop. The negative feedback causes the endocrine gland to stop secreting the hormone.

Hypothalamic Control of Body Temperature

The thermostat in a home functions much like the negative feedback loop in the human body. When the temperature falls below the point set on the thermostat, the furnace turns on. When the home reaches the desired temperature, the furnace turns off. As **Figure 9.7** shows, the hypothalamus functions as a thermostat for the body, working to maintain the body's temperature at the set point of 98.6°F (37°C). If body temperature drops below 98.6°F (37°C), the hypothalamus sets in motion a series of responses by releasing hormones that act on the thyroid gland. The thyroid gland produces thyroxine, a hormone that increases metabolic rate and heat production. The hypothalamus also stimulates the SNS, which initiates shivering and decreased blood flow to the skin. Shivering increases heat production and helps the body maintain core temperature.

When body temperature has been restored to its hypothalamic set point (homeostasis), the hypothalamus signals the thyroid gland to stop releasing thyroxine. The hypothalamus also signals the SNS to send messages to the body that stop shivering and restore blood flow to the skin.

When the body's thermal receptors sense an increase in body temperature above 98.6°F (37°C), the hypothalamus stimulates the SNS to increase sweat production by stimulating the sweat glands and widening the blood vessels of the skin, increasing blood flow to the area. In addition, the thyroid gland decreases thyroxine secretion to slow down metabolic rate and heat production.

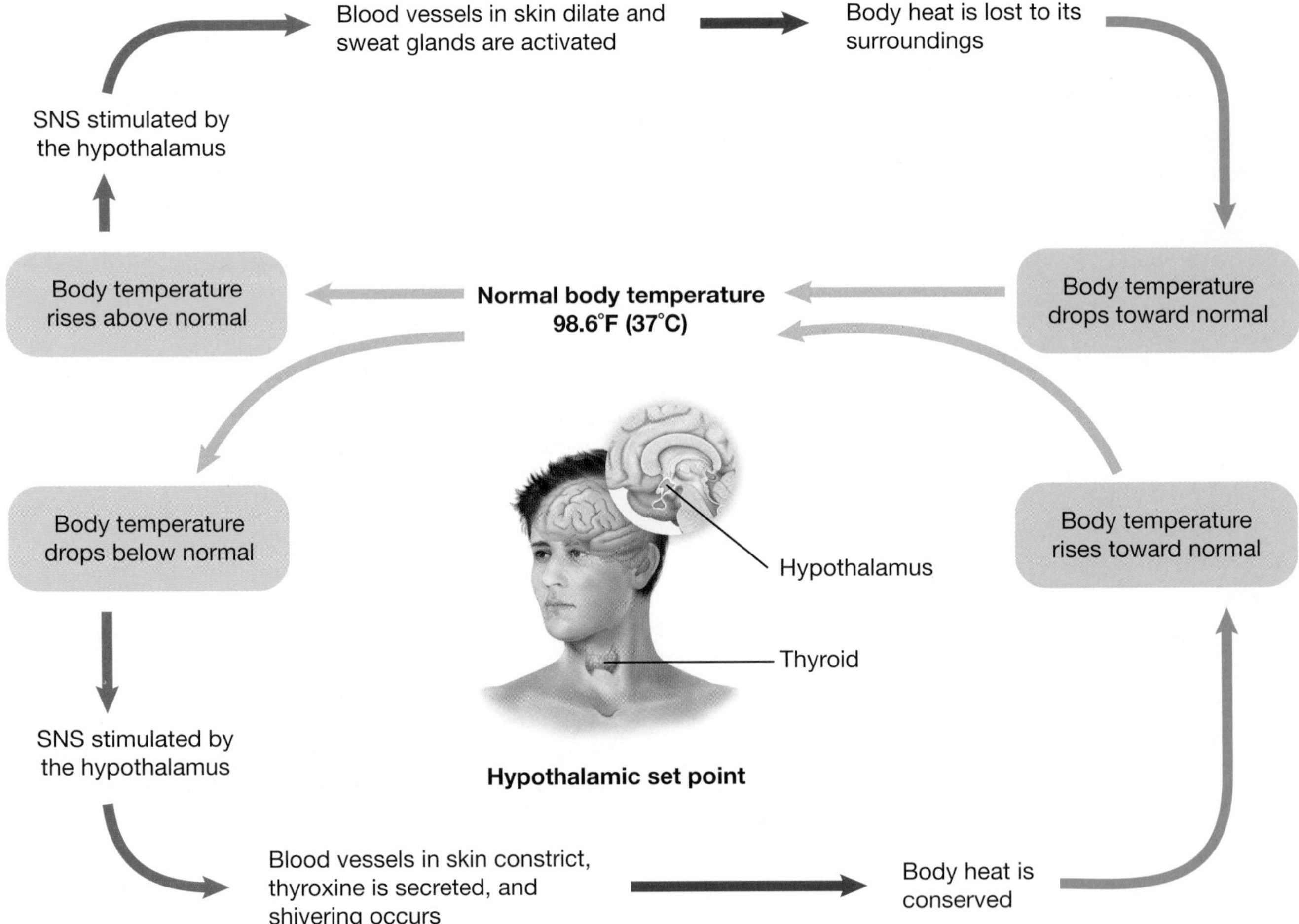

Figure 9.7 The hypothalamus performs temperature regulation, which is one example of how the body maintains functional balance.

Case Study: Jordan Romero

When Jordan Romero decided that he wanted to become the youngest person to climb Mount Everest at 13 years of age, he and his dad embarked on a training program to get Romero's body into shape. The 29,029-foot (8,848-meter) climb would challenge Romero's body, particularly because lower oxygen concentration in the air at high altitudes diminishes blood oxygen levels.

While at sea level, Romero spent many hours in an altitude tent, where he was exposed to a hypoxic environment (one with low oxygen content). The hypoxic environment of the altitude tent simulated the environment near the peak of Mount Everest. The low oxygen content of the air that Romero was breathing stimulated his kidneys to secrete the hormone erythropoietin. Erythropoietin stimulates stem cells in the bone marrow to produce red blood cells (RBCs).

As a result of this process, the effects of the hypoxic environment near the peak of Mount Everest were not as fatiguing or harmful to Romero. Thanks to this hormone response, Romero achieved his goal of becoming the youngest person to climb Mount Everest.

SECTION 9.1 REVIEW

Mini-Glossary

amino acid-derived hormones water-soluble hormones composed of proteins or protein-related substances

cyclic adenosine monophosphate (cAMP) a chemical derived from ATP that serves as a messenger to activate protein kinases, which in turn trigger a variety of responses in the cell, such as protein synthesis and glycogen breakdown.

downregulated decreased

epinephrine the chief neurohormone of the adrenal medulla; used as a heart stimulant, vasoconstrictor (narrows the blood vessels), and bronchodilator (relaxes the bronchial tubes in the lungs)

glucagon a hormone secreted by the pancreas that causes the breakdown of glycogen stored in the liver

hormonal control the type of endocrine control in which endocrine organs are stimulated by hormones from other endocrine organs, starting with the hypothalamus

hormones chemical messengers secreted by the endocrine glands

humoral control the type of endocrine control in which levels of various substances in body fluids are monitored for homeostatic imbalance

hypothalamic non-releasing hormones the hormones that are produced in the hypothalamus and carried by the blood to the anterior pituitary, where they stop certain hormones from being released; also known as *hypothalamic inhibiting hormones*

hypothalamic releasing hormones the hormones that are produced in the hypothalamus and carried by the blood to the anterior pituitary, where they stimulate the release of anterior pituitary hormones

insulin a hormone that promotes glucose uptake in body tissues

neural control the type of endocrine control in which nerve fibers stimulate endocrine organs to release hormones

steroid hormones lipid (fat-based) hormones

upregulated increased

Review Questions

1. What is the endocrine system?
2. Which gland has both endocrine and exocrine functions?
3. Which gland is "president" of the endocrine system? Which is "vice president"?
4. What are the three ways in which hormone secretions are controlled?
5. Identify similarities and differences between the nervous and endocrine systems.
6. Describe how the activity of a hormone receptor can be upregulated or downregulated.
7. Explain the role of neural control in a fight-or-flight response.
8. Following a December snowstorm in Wisconsin, Mark's parents ask him to help shovel the sidewalk in front of their home. After spending some time outside in the cold, Mark begins to shiver. In what other ways is Mark's body responding as his endocrine system works to raise his body temperature?

SECTION 9.2

Endocrine Organs

Objectives

- Identify the functions of the hypothalamus.
- Identify the hormones secreted by the anterior and posterior pituitary gland.
- Describe the location and function of the thyroid gland.
- Explain the function of the parathyroid glands.
- Describe the location and function of the adrenal glands.
- Explain the endocrine and exocrine functions of the pancreas.
- List other hormone-producing organs and tissues.

Key Terms

adrenal cortex
adrenal glands
adrenal medulla
anterior pituitary
ovaries
pancreas
parathyroid glands
pineal gland
pituitary gland
posterior pituitary
scrotum
testes
thymus
thyroid gland
tropic hormones

As you may recall from the previous section, the endocrine system is run by the hypothalamus. The hormones of this tiny gland stimulate the pituitary gland, starting a chain reaction that affects organs and hormones throughout the endocrine system. Each organ and gland plays an important role in ensuring that the endocrine system runs smoothly.

Hypothalamus

The hypothalamus is a very small gland (about 4 grams) buried deep in the brain, below the thalamus. The job of the hypothalamus is to collect information from each body system and integrate the responses of the nervous and endocrine systems to maintain homeostatic balance. Recall from Chapter 7 that the hypothalamus is a part of the nervous system that plays an important role in regulating everyday functions such as metabolism, heart rate, energy level, body temperature, thirst, hunger, nutrient intake, blood pressure, and blood composition. It even plays a role in emotions and, to some degree, regulates sleep.

Although the hypothalamus is part of the nervous system, it is also a key part of the endocrine system because it produces hypothalamic releasing hormones and hypothalamic non-releasing hormones. These hormones either stimulate or inhibit the release of hormones from the anterior pituitary gland, thereby directing its actions.

For example, the hypothalamus secretes thyrotropin-releasing hormone (TRH), which flows through a network of capillaries connecting the hypothalamus to the anterior pituitary, called the *hypothalamic-hypophyseal portal system*. Once TRH reaches the anterior pituitary, it stimulates the gland to release thyroid-stimulating hormone (TSH). TRH is a hypothalamic releasing hormone.

Conversely, growth hormone-inhibiting hormone (also called *somatostatin*) from the hypothalamus inhibits the release of growth hormone from the anterior pituitary. This is an example of a hypothalamic non-releasing hormone. The hypothalamus also produces antidiuretic hormone (ADH) and oxytocin, which are stored in the posterior pituitary and will be discussed later.

SELF CHECK

1. Through what two mechanisms, or classes of hormones, does the hypothalamus direct the endocrine system?
2. Which hormone inhibits the release of growth hormone from the pituitary?

Pituitary Gland

The ***pituitary gland*** is about the size of a pea and includes two lobes—the ***anterior pituitary*** and the ***posterior pituitary***. This gland is located in the depression of the sphenoid bone, and it is suspended from the underside of the hypothalamus by a short stalk called the *infundibulum*.

Besides producing hormones, the anterior pituitary also stores and releases hormones from the hypothalamus. These hormones are kept in the anterior pituitary until the hypothalamus stimulates their release. **Figure 9.8** summarizes the hormones of the hypothalamus and the pituitary gland, as well as their primary functions.

Hormones of the Anterior Pituitary

Hormones secreted by the anterior pituitary gland function in two ways. They can act directly on target tissue to cause a specific metabolic response, or they can stimulate other endocrine glands (the manager-level glands discussed earlier in the chapter) to release their own hormones (**Figure 9.9**). Pituitary hormones that stimulate other endocrine glands are called ***tropic hormones***, or *tropins*.

The anterior pituitary gland secretes six hormones:

- growth hormone (GH)
- prolactin (PRO)

Hormones of the Hypothalamus and Pituitary Gland		
Gland	**Hormones**	**Functions**
Hypothalamus 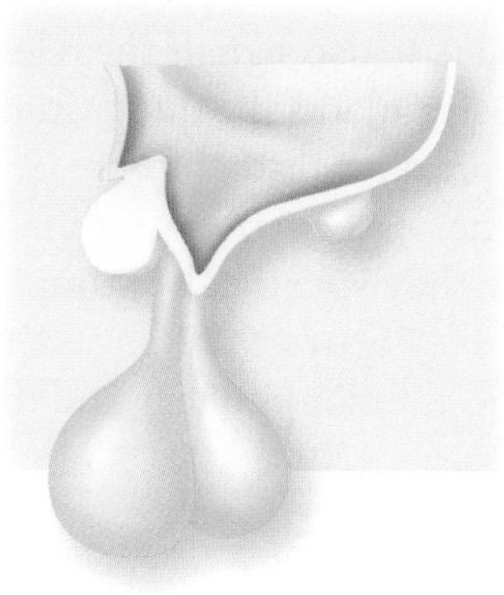	hypothalamic releasing hormones	stimulate secretion of hormones by the pituitary gland
	hypothalamic non-releasing hormone	inhibit secretion of hormones by the pituitary gland
Pituitary gland: anterior lobe 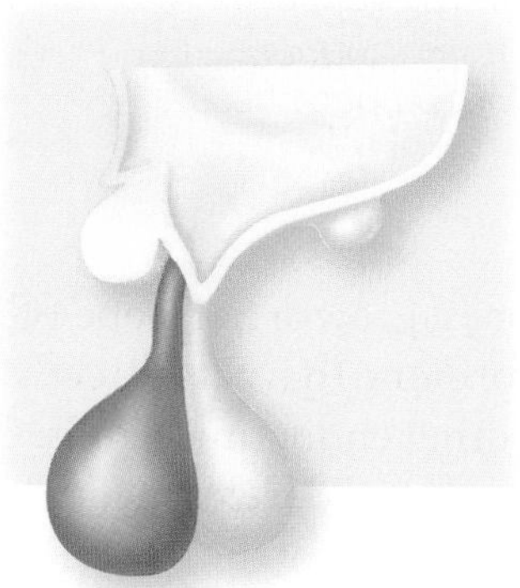	growth hormone (GH)	stimulates the growth and development of muscles, cartilage, and long bones
	prolactin (PRO)	stimulates the growth of mammary glands and the production of milk
	follicle-stimulating hormone (FSH)	females: stimulates the production of estrogen and ova males: stimulates the production of sperm
	luteinizing hormone (LH)	stimulates the reproductive organs to produce sex hormones
	thyroid-stimulating hormone (TSH)	stimulates the thyroid to secrete the thyroid hormones T_3 and T_4
	adrenocorticotropic hormone (ACTH)	stimulates the adrenal cortex to secrete steroid hormones
Pituitary gland: posterior lobe (hormones produced by the hypothalamus) 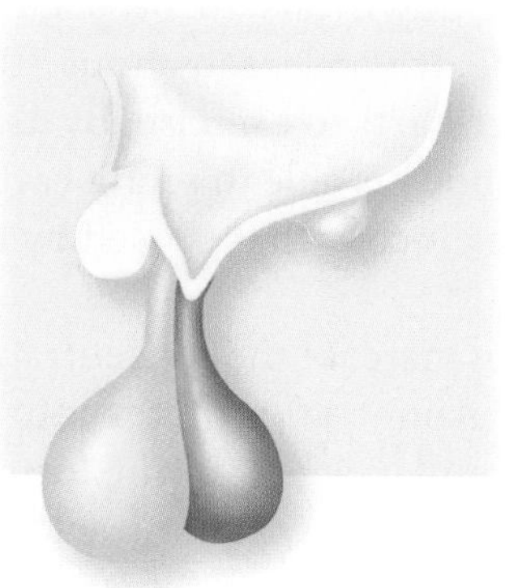	oxytocin	stimulates uterine contractions and breast milk secretion
	antidiuretic hormone (ADH)	stimulates the kidneys to increase water reabsorption and return the fluid to the blood

Figure 9.8

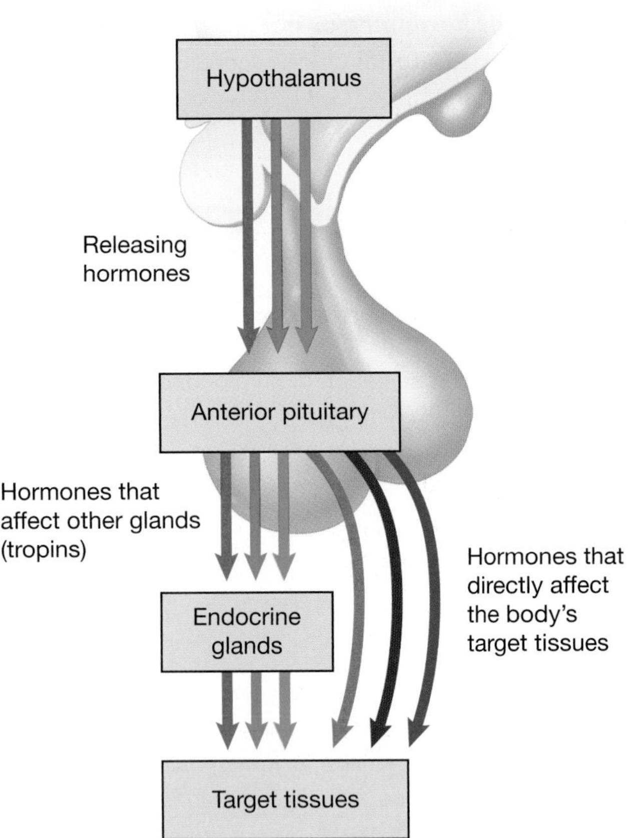

Figure 9.9 Some anterior pituitary hormones act on other glands, while others act directly on the body's tissues.

- adrenocorticotropic hormone (ACTH)
- thyroid-stimulating hormone (TSH; also called *thyrotropin*)
- follicle-stimulating hormone (FSH)
- luteinizing hormone (LH)

Understanding Medical Terminology

To remember the six hormones secreted by the anterior pituitary gland, try remembering the saying, "Pro Amateur Golfers Take Long Flops," with each word representing one of the six anterior pituitary hormones:

PRO = prolactin
Amateur = adrenocorticotropic hormone
Golfers = growth hormone
Take = thyroid-stimulating hormone
Long = luteinizing hormone
Flops = follicle-stimulating hormone

Tropic Hormones

Of the six hormones secreted by the anterior pituitary, four of these are tropic hormones:

- ACTH acts on the adrenal cortex to stimulate release of steroid hormones.
- TSH acts on the thyroid gland to stimulate release of two thyroid hormones—thyroxine (T_4) and triiodothyronine (T_3).
- FSH stimulates the ovaries to produce estrogen and eggs in women and stimulates the testes to develop sperm in men.
- LH acts on the ovaries to produce progesterone and estrogen in women. It also signals the release of eggs. In men, LH stimulates the interstitial cells of the testes to produce testosterone.

FSH and LH are further categorized as gonadotropic hormones because they specifically stimulate the gonads, or sex glands. **Figure 9.10** shows the hormones produced by the anterior pituitary and their target glands or tissues.

Understanding Medical Terminology

ACTH, TSH, FSH, and LH are called *tropic hormones* because they are produced by gonadotropes, cells in the anterior pituitary. Tropic hormones act on other endocrine glands, *not* on body tissue.

Growth Hormone

Unlike the tropic hormones, growth hormone (GH) is an anterior pituitary hormone that acts directly on body tissues rather than other endocrine glands. GH is responsible for the growth and development of the muscles, cartilage, and long bones of the body. Recall the discussion of Sultan Kosen, the world's tallest man in the chapter introduction. Kosen's record-breaking height, hand size, and feet size are the result of excessive amounts of GH.

GH also helps break down fats to be used by the body as a fuel source. It is released about 30 to 45 minutes after a person starts to exercise. By using fats as a fuel source, the body is able to retain carbohydrates, which provide glucose that is used by the brain for energy.

Additionally, GH helps increase the concentration of glucose in the body. About 80 minutes into an exercise session, GH stimulates fats (in the form of glycerol) and proteins (in the form of amino acids) to be converted into glucose by the liver. This process is called *gluconeogenesis*.

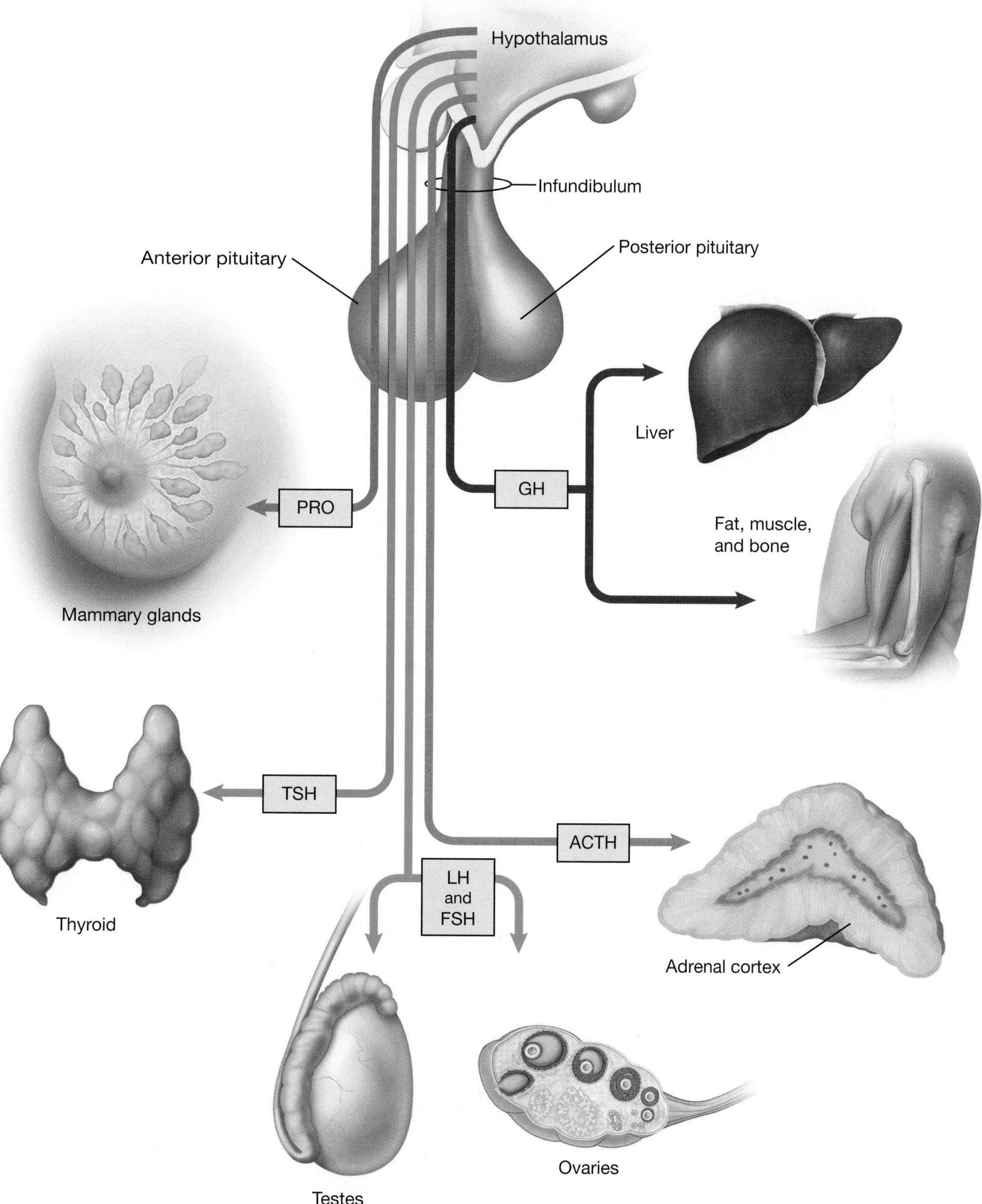

Figure 9.10 Hormones secreted by the anterior pituitary affect many parts of the body.

By stimulating the use of fats and proteins as a fuel source, growth hormone plays an important role in the ability to maintain prolonged physical activity, such as running a marathon.

Prolactin

Prolactin stimulates the growth of mammary glands and the production of milk in a nursing mother. This hormone is named for its function: the prefix *pro-* means "for," and the combining form *lact/o* means "milk." Prolactin is also present in males, but its role is unclear.

> **Understanding Medical Terminology**
>
> Gluconeogenesis, the process by which the liver converts fat and protein into glucose, can be easily remembered by examining its word parts. *Gluc/o* refers to glucose, *neo-* means "new," and *-genesis* means "creation." Put the parts together, and you have the definition of *gluconeogenesis*!

Hormones of the Posterior Pituitary

The posterior pituitary is actually an extension of the hypothalamus. Instead of producing its own hormones, the posterior pituitary *stores* two hormones produced by the hypothalamus—antidiuretic hormone (ADH) and oxytocin. These hormones are transported along the neurosecretory network of cells that connects the hypothalamus to the posterior pituitary gland.

Because it does not produce its own hormones, the posterior pituitary is not a true endocrine gland. Secretion of hormones from the posterior pituitary is the result of hypothalamic neuroendocrine input, or nervous system stimulation of the hypothalamus (**Figure 9.11**).

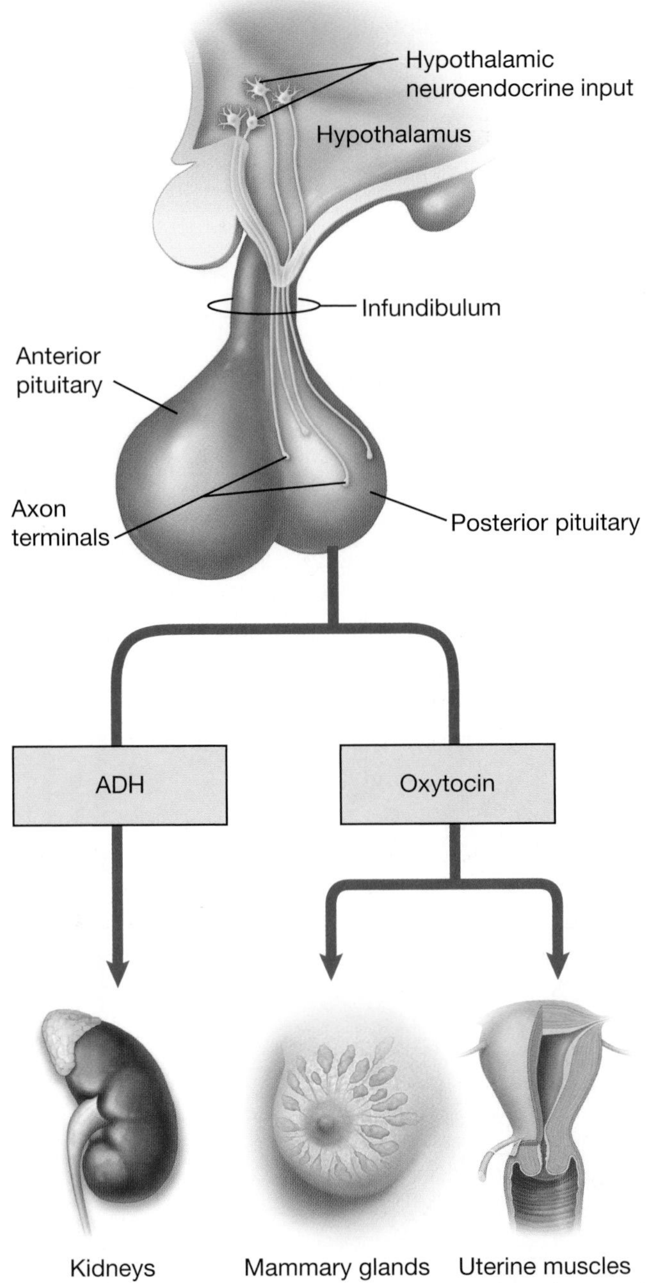

Figure 9.11 The posterior pituitary stores ADH and oxytocin secreted by the hypothalamus. These hormones help maintain the body's fluid balance. In addition, they stimulate uterine contractions in pregnant women and milk production in nursing women.

Antidiuretic Hormone

Diuretics are substances that stimulate urine production to decrease fluid retention in the body. Antidiuretic hormone (ADH) does the opposite—it decreases urine output, which increases body fluid volume.

ADH travels in the blood to reach its target organs, including the kidneys and the sweat or eccrine glands. ADH stimulates the kidneys to increase water reabsorption and return the fluid to the blood. ADH also decreases sweating, which causes retention of water. People who engage in regular physical activity have an increased sensitivity to ADH. As a result, they have a higher volume of blood plasma (the liquid portion of blood).

ADH is subject to humoral control. It is secreted when plasma volume decreases due to dehydration or profuse sweating during exercise. ADH is also secreted when the solid particles in the blood (blood cells and platelets) become too concentrated.

ADH also plays an important role in blood pressure regulation. Arterial blood pressure is the tension or force of the blood on the walls of arteries. ADH can raise blood pressure by causing vasoconstriction, or narrowing of the arteries, which increases their resistance to blood flow. Due to this effect, ADH is also called *vasopressin*. At the same time, blood volume increases because ADH causes greater reabsorption of fluid and sodium by the kidneys. The combination of increased blood volume and narrowed arteries leads to higher blood pressure because more blood is flowing through the smaller vessels.

Alcohol inhibits ADH, which leads to increased urination, dehydration, and a dry mouth the morning after a person drinks alcoholic beverages. Caffeine and foods such as asparagus also inhibit ADH, and they act as diuretics.

Oxytocin

Pregnant women produce oxytocin during labor, and the hormone stays in their bodies until they are finished nursing the child. Oxytocin facilitates childbirth by stimulating the muscles of the uterus to contract. Oxytocin release is also stimulated by the sucking mechanism of a nursing infant, causing the mammary glands to secrete breast milk from the mammary ducts. Perhaps you have heard of a pitocin drip. This is a synthetic, intravenous form of oxytocin that is administered to induce, or speed up, delivery of a baby.

SELF CHECK

1. Describe the role of the hypothalamus in the endocrine system.
2. What does *FSH* stand for, and what is its purpose?
3. Which parts of the body does growth hormone help to grow and develop? Name an additional function of GH.
4. Which two hormones are stored in the posterior pituitary?

Thyroid Gland

The ***thyroid gland*** is located inferior to the larynx at the base of the throat. This butterfly-shaped gland is two inches long and lies at the front and sides of the trachea (**Figure 9.12A**). The two lobes of the thyroid gland are divided by a band of tissue called the *isthmus*.

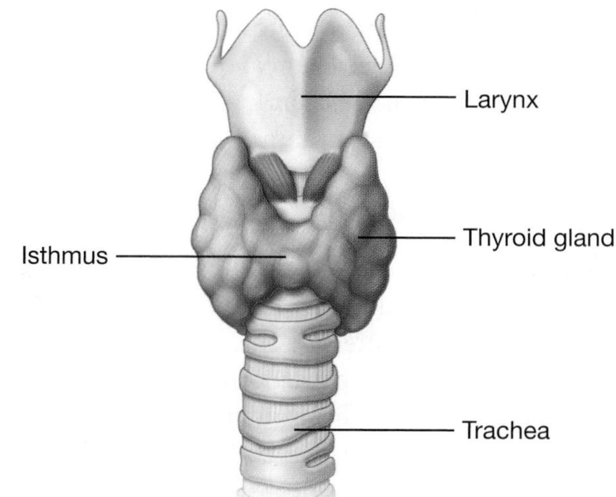

A Location of the thyroid gland

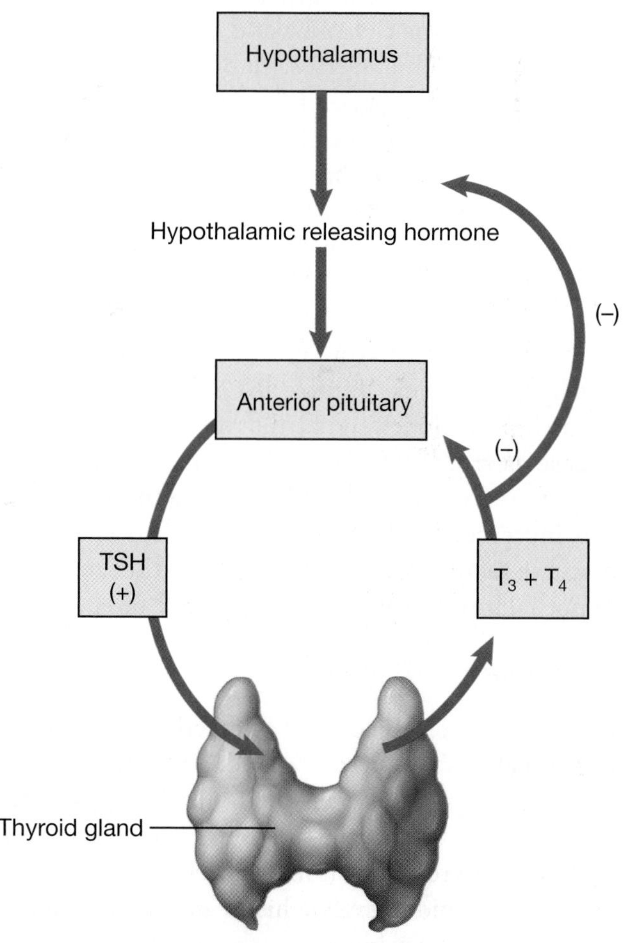

B Regulation of thyroid hormone release

Figure 9.12 The thyroid gland. A—The thyroid gland is located below the larynx and above the trachea. B—The thyroid gland produces thyroid hormone when signaled by the hypothalamus and anterior pituitary.

The thyroid gland secretes three hormones: two closely related hormones often collectively called *thyroid hormone* and *calcitonin*. These hormones drive metabolism.

Thyroxine and Triiodothyronine

"Thyroid hormone" includes the hormones thyroxine (T_4) and triiodothyronine (T_3). These hormones are secreted by the follicular cells of the thyroid and are responsible for controlling the body's rate of energy metabolism and heat production. Every cell in the body is affected by the thyroid hormones because every living cell needs energy to survive. These hormones also play a vital role in growth, development, and maturation. People often blame an underactive thyroid gland for their overweight condition, but the thyroid gland is rarely the reason that people become overweight or obese.

T_4 and T_3 are formed from two linked tyrosine amino acids with iodine atoms attached. T_4 has four iodine atoms, and T_3 has three iodine atoms. T_3 is the more powerful of the two hormones. The iodine required to make T_4 and T_3 comes from dietary intake, which is why salt is fortified with iodine in many countries.

Release of the thyroid hormones is controlled by the hypothalamus (**Figure 9.12B**). Hypothalamic releasing hormones signal the anterior pituitary to release thyroid-stimulating hormone (TSH). TSH triggers secretion of T_3 and T_4 by the thyroid gland. The increased levels of circulating T_3 and T_4 trigger a negative feedback loop, inhibiting further release of hypothalamic releasing hormones and TSH.

Calcitonin

Calcitonin is produced and released by the parafollicular cells of the thyroid gland. The parafollicular cells are located between the follicular cells in the connective tissue of the thyroid. Calcitonin, along with parathyroid hormone (PTH) (produced by the parathyroid glands), helps maintain calcium homeostasis in the body.

When blood calcium levels rise, the thyroid gland releases calcitonin. Calcitonin causes calcium in the blood to be deposited and absorbed into the bone. As a result, blood calcium levels decrease. Calcitonin also reduces the absorption of calcium by the intestines and kidneys. Once a person reaches adulthood and has fully developed bones, little (if any) calcitonin is released by the thyroid gland.

SELF CHECK

1. Which three hormones are secreted by the thyroid gland?
2. Which chemical element found in certain foods is necessary for thyroid hormone production?

Parathyroid Glands

The ***parathyroid glands*** are two pairs of glands located on the posterior aspect of the thyroid gland. These four tiny glands, each of which is the size of a grain of rice, secrete parathyroid hormone (PTH) in response to low blood calcium levels. Parathyroid hormone increases blood calcium levels in three ways:

- by stimulating breakdown of bone tissues by osteoclasts, thus moving calcium from the bone into the blood
- by increasing calcium absorption in the intestines during digestion with the aid of vitamin D
- by stimulating the kidneys to reabsorb calcium from urine and excrete phosphorus

Figure 9.13 illustrates the regulation of blood calcium levels by both PTH and calcitonin. **Figure 9.14** summarizes the hormones of the thyroid and parathyroid glands.

SELF CHECK

1. How many parathyroid glands do humans have, and where are they located?
2. How does parathyroid hormone (PTH) increase blood calcium levels?

Adrenal Glands

As **Figure 9.15** shows, the ***adrenal glands*** are a pair of glands, with one sitting on top of each kidney. Each of the adrenal glands is actually two organs: the ***adrenal cortex*** functions as a gland, whereas the ***adrenal medulla*** is part of the nervous system.

The adrenal cortex makes up the outer layer of each adrenal gland. The adrenal cortex itself comprises three sublayers, each of which secretes a

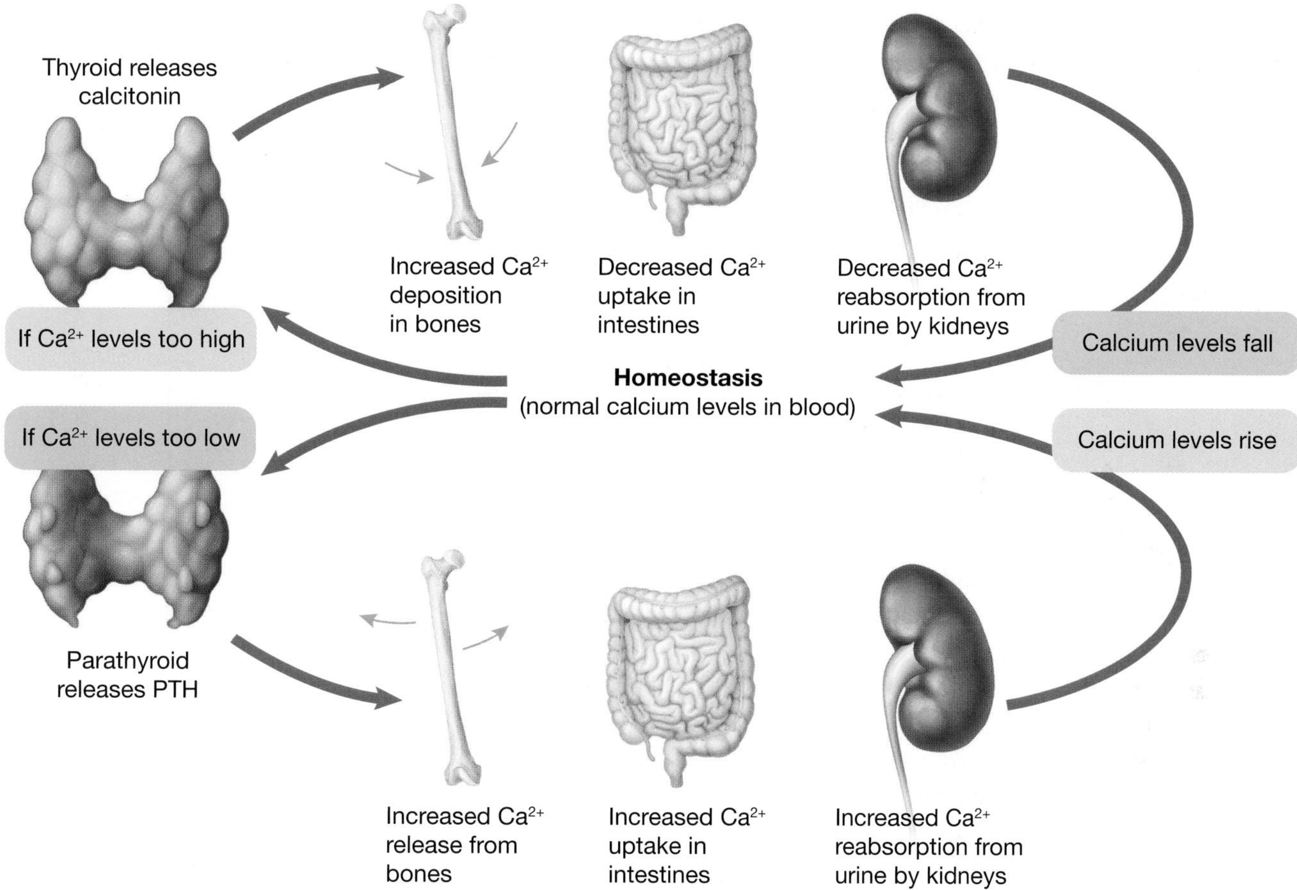

© Body Scientific International

Figure 9.13 The thyroid and parathyroid glands act together to maintain healthy blood calcium levels.

Hormones of the Thyroid and Parathyroid Glands

Gland	Hormones	Functions
Thyroid gland	thyroxine (T_4) triiodothyronine (T_3)	control the body's rate of energy metabolism and heat production
	calcitonin	helps maintain calcium homeostasis
Parathyroid glands	parathyroid hormone (PTH)	increases blood calcium level

Figure 9.14

© Body Scientific International

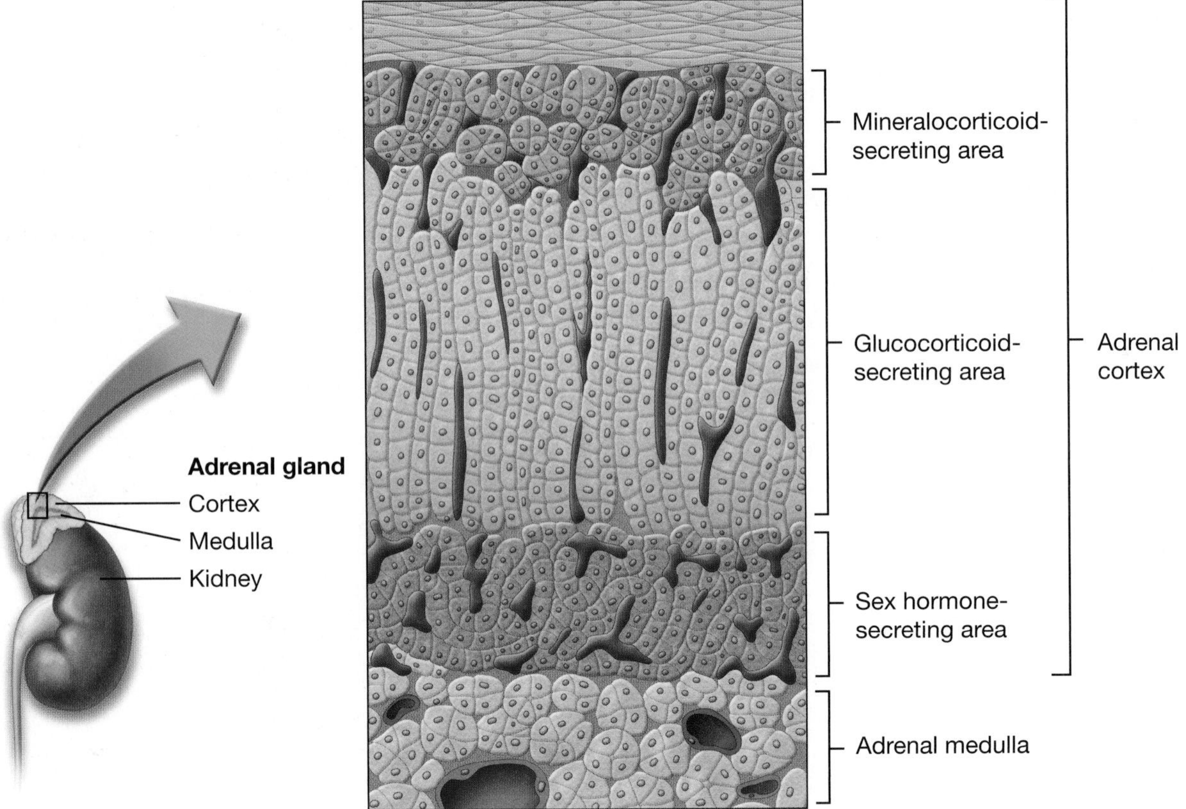

Figure 9.15 The adrenal glands are located on top of each kidney. The adrenal cortex (outer layer) is divided into three layers. The inner layer is the adrenal medulla. Hormones released by the adrenal medulla are integral in initiating an "adrenaline rush."

steroid hormone. The adrenal medulla makes up the inner layer, and it is stimulated by the sympathetic branch of the autonomic nervous system (ANS). **Figure 9.16** summarizes the hormones released by the adrenal glands.

Hormones of the Adrenal Cortex

The adrenal cortex includes three sections, each of which produces a different type of steroid hormones:

- mineralocorticoids, which regulate sodium concentrations
- glucocorticoids, which regulate glucose (blood sugar)
- sex hormones, which regulate sex hormone levels

The anterior pituitary controls the release of these corticoid hormones, or hormones of the adrenal cortex. Like all steroid hormones, they are made from cholesterol and are lipid soluble (that is, they can dissolve in fats). Many of the corticoid hormones are vital to survival, so a decrease in their production can be life threatening.

Understanding Medical Terminology

The three substances regulated by the hormones of the adrenal cortex all start with an *S*: **S**odium, **S**ugar, and **S**ex hormones.

Mineralocorticoids

The principal mineralocorticoid hormone is aldosterone. Aldosterone stimulates the kidneys to reabsorb sodium and water from urine, and to eliminate potassium from the body. Through this process, aldosterone plays a major role in regulating blood pressure and plasma volume levels. When sodium and water are reabsorbed by the kidneys, the plasma volume increases, raising blood pressure. Aldosterone also regulates the concentration of blood electrolytes, such as sodium and potassium.

The secretion of aldosterone is regulated by several factors (**Figure 9.17**). Decreased blood volume and/or blood pressure stimulates the kidneys to secrete renin, which causes a cascade of events that convert angiotensin I to angiotensin II. Angiotensin II is a potent stimulant for aldosterone secretion by the adrenal cortex. The other primary regulatory factor

Hormones of the Adrenal Glands		
Gland	**Hormones**	**Functions**
Adrenal cortex 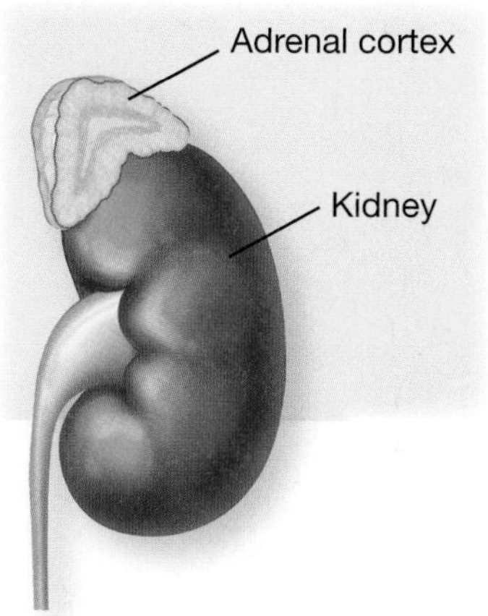 (Adrenal cortex; Kidney)	mineralocorticoids (aldosterone)	stimulate the kidneys to reabsorb sodium and water from urine, and to eliminate potassium from the body
	glucocorticoids (cortisone, cortisol)	help maintain blood glucose levels
	sex hormones (testosterone, estrogen)	essential for the development and maintenance of male and female reproductive organs
Adrenal medulla 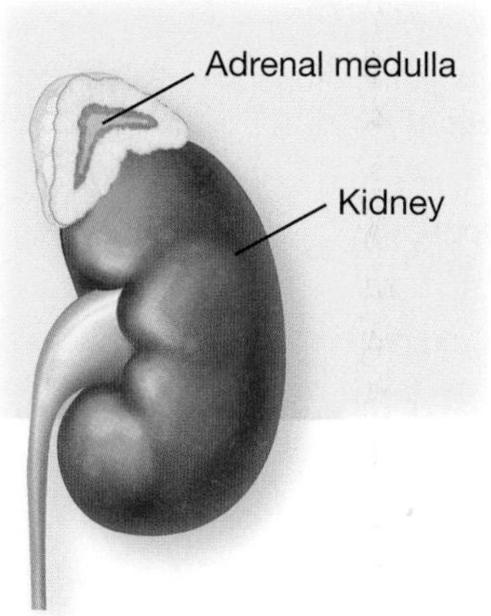 (Adrenal medulla; Kidney)	epinephrine norepinephrine	increase metabolic rate, glucose production, heart rate, breathing rate, and blood pressure

Figure 9.16

that increases aldosterone secretion is an elevated level of potassium or lowered level of sodium in the blood.

To a lesser degree, stress can alter aldosterone secretion by the adrenal cortex. Stress stimulates the hypothalamus to release corticotropin-releasing hormone (CRH), which directs the anterior pituitary to release adrenocorticotropic hormone (ACTH). ACTH promotes aldosterone secretion from the adrenal cortex (**Figure 9.18**).

Increased blood pressure and blood volume also alter aldosterone secretion. Increases in blood pressure and/or blood volume cause the atria fibers of the heart to stretch, which stimulates the release of atrial natriuretic peptide hormone (ANP). ANP inhibits the release of aldosterone, which causes less sodium reabsorption and therefore less water retention in the blood. This in turn causes a reduction in blood volume and decreases the elevated blood pressure and/or blood volume levels.

Glucocorticoids

The main glucocorticoid hormones, cortisone and cortisol, maintain blood glucose levels by converting fats and amino acids into glucose via gluconeogenesis. This ensures that the brain and nervous system have a constant supply of glucose, which is their only fuel source.

Glucocorticoid hormones also have anti-inflammatory properties that diminish the swelling, redness, and pain associated with inflammation. This is why prednisone and other corticosteroids are used to treat inflammatory conditions such as arthritis, cancer, lupus, and multiple sclerosis. Glucocorticoid

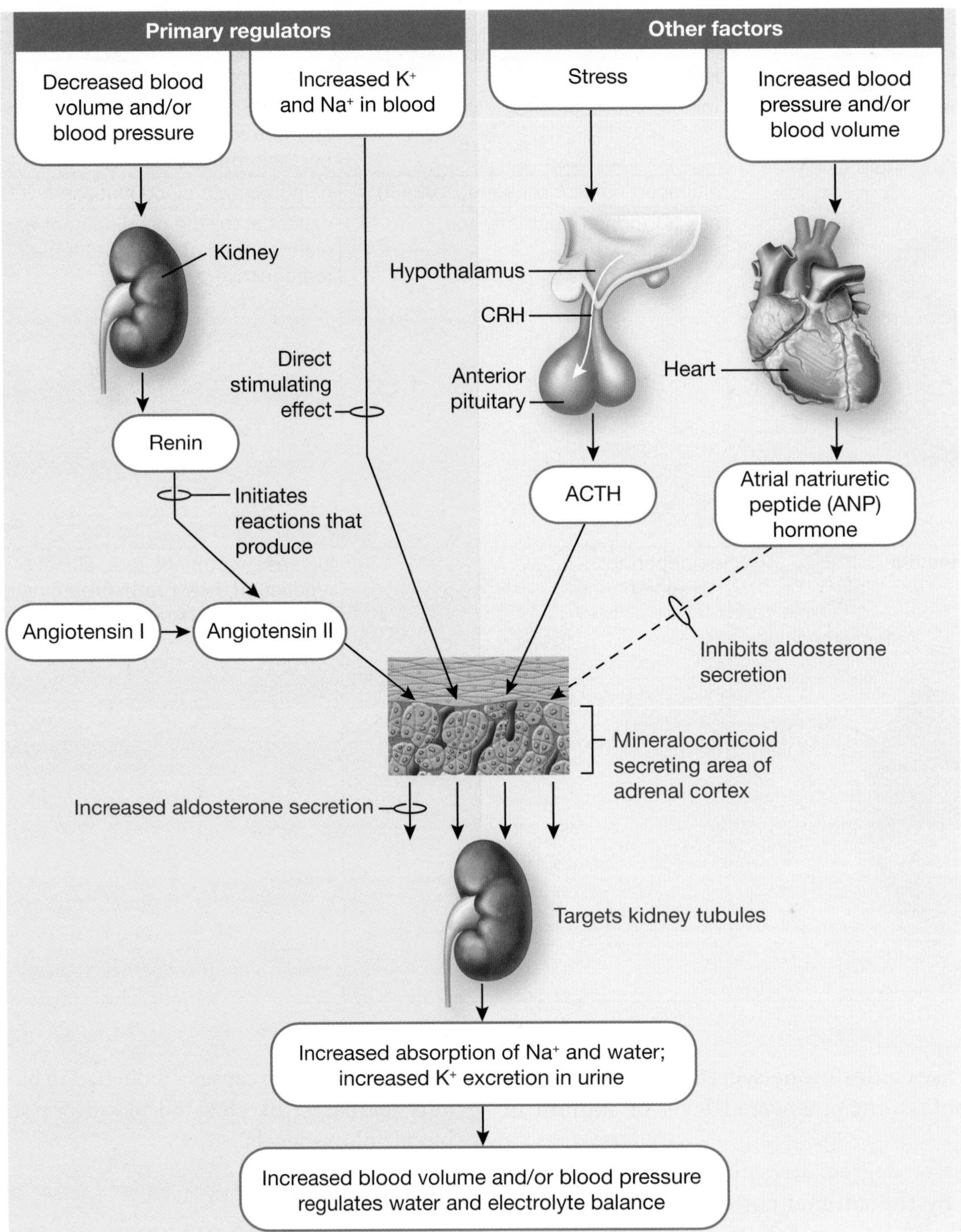

Figure 9.17 Regulation of aldosterone secretion.

hormones also decrease the immune response, so they are often administered to transplant patients to decrease the risk of organ rejection.

Cortisol is considered the universal stress hormone because it becomes elevated when individuals are subjected to psychological or physical stressors. This hormone springs into action (along with epinephrine) during the fight-or-flight response by increasing blood glucose to boost the energy available for the impending "fight" or "flight." Cortisol also diminishes activities of the immune system. This is helpful when a person experiences acute danger such as an organ transplant, but when exposed to stressors for prolonged periods of time, the body can sustain damage in innumerable ways.

Chronic stress exposure can come from many sources. These include ongoing work or school pressures; long-term relationship problems; caring for

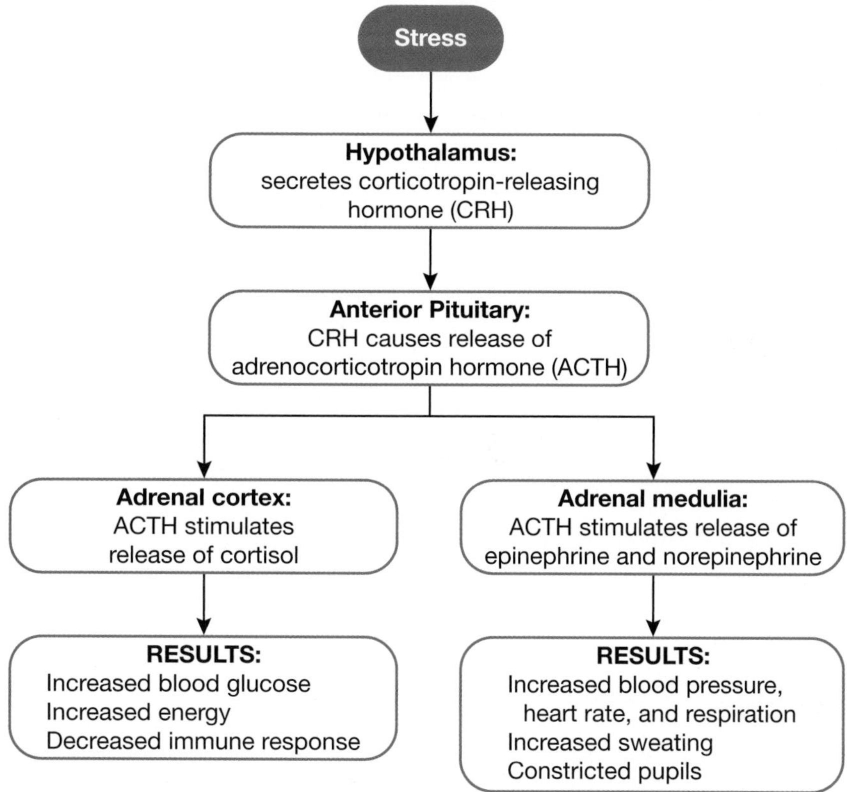

Figure 9.18 When the body is stressed, the hypothalamus releases corticotropin-releasing hormone, which triggers a cascade of hormonal responses.

children, the sick, or ailing older adults; loneliness; and financial troubles. Chronic stress can cause increased incidence of heart disease, stroke, gastrointestinal disorders, diabetes, reproductive disorders, and anxiety, as well as a lower cancer survival rate.

Sex Hormones

The adrenal cortex produces small amounts of estrogens (female sex hormones). However, most of the sex hormones secreted by the adrenal cortex are androgens (male sex hormones), primarily testosterone.

The reproductive organs also produce sex hormones. The effects of sex hormones produced by the reproductive organs (discussed in Chapter 16) usually mask the effects of sex hormones produced by the adrenal cortex in younger people because the reproductive organs secrete higher volumes of hormones earlier in life. As people age, their reproductive organs secrete smaller quantities of sex hormones. The adrenal cortex, however, continues to produce the same amount of sex hormones. This means the effects of these hormones may become more noticeable with age. For example, because the adrenal cortex secretes high quantities of androgen, some females develop facial hair and other masculine traits as they age.

Hormones of the Adrenal Medulla

The fight-or-flight response occurs when the adrenal medulla secretes two hormones: epinephrine (commonly referred to as *adrenaline*) and norepinephrine (also known as *noradrenalin*). Epinephrine and norepinephrine are both catecholamines, which are hormones that are released into the blood during times of physical or emotional stress.

The release of these hormones begins when stress stimulates the hypothalamus to release corticotropin-releasing hormone (CRH). CRH triggers the anterior pituitary to release adrenocorticotropin hormone (ACTH). This stimulates the adrenal medulla to release epinephrine and norepinephrine, and the adrenal cortex to release cortisol.

The body's response to increased catecholamine levels is called an *adrenaline rush*. The telltale signs of an adrenaline rush include increased heart rate, blood pressure, and breathing. Other changes also occur. For example, blood flow is shunted to the heart, and the muscles prepare to fight or take flight. Increased metabolic rate and glucose production in the liver make more energy available for the potential brush with danger.

Understanding Medical Terminology

To remember the hormones of the adrenal medulla, just remember the acronym *AMEN*: **A**drenal **M**edulla secretes **E**pinephrine and **N**orepinephrine.

SELF CHECK

1. Which component of the adrenal gland is actually part of the nervous system?
2. What three substances are regulated by the hormones of the adrenal cortex?
3. Which mineralocorticoid is responsible for regulating blood pressure and plasma volume?

Pancreas

The ***pancreas*** is a long, thin organ located posterior to the stomach in the upper part of the abdominal cavity. It functions as an endocrine gland by secreting hormones that control blood glucose levels. The pancreas also functions as an exocrine gland by secreting digestive enzymes. Chapter 14 describes the exocrine function of the pancreas in more detail.

The hormone-secreting cells of the pancreas are called the *islets of Langerhans*. The islets of Langerhans include alpha cells and beta cells. The alpha cells secrete glucagon, which increases blood glucose levels, and the beta cells secrete insulin, which lowers blood glucose levels. The alpha and beta cells work together to maintain blood glucose levels within the normal range of 70 and 105 mg/dL.

Clinical Application "Bionic" Pancreas Receives FDA Approval

In the past, type I diabetics managed their diabetes by carefully planning and timing periodic insulin injections. This process could be inconvenient, and it disrupted the activities of daily living for millions of diabetic patients. Recently, the FDA approved a hybrid closed-loop insulin delivery system, which combines a continuously monitoring glucose device with an insulin pump. This device is being heralded as a milestone in diabetes management and as a significant improvement in the quality of life for diabetic individuals. Type I diabetics will be able to live more freely, without having to monitor their glucose levels and administer insulin injections manually.

This "bionic pancreas" uses an advanced algorithm that is capable of delivering variable dosages of insulin 24 hours a day to better maintain normal blood glucose levels. The device is designed to detect how much insulin is needed based on blood glucose levels measured by an advanced glucose sensor. The sensor transmits the information to the insulin pump, which discharges the appropriate insulin dose.

The glucose sensor allows for seven-day continuous monitoring of glucose levels and also monitors its own functionality. If the glucose sensor malfunctions, the individual is notified. People wearing the closed-loop insulin delivery system must manually enter their carbohydrate intake at mealtime, accept bolus correction recommendations, and calibrate the sensor, but the system is otherwise fully automated.

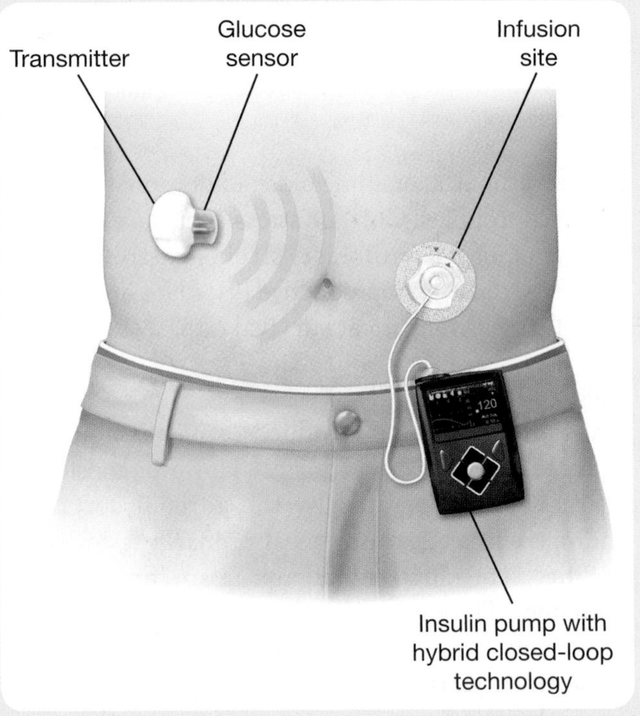

© Body Scientific International

Hybrid closed-loop insulin delivery system.

The FDA approved the closed-loop insulin delivery system after a 3-month multicenter study in which 124 patients between the ages of 14 and 75 used the system and had no episodes of severe hypoglycemia or ketoacidosis. Glycemic control among the participants went from "good" at the start of the study (hemoglobin A1c levels of 7.4%) to "excellent" at the end of the study (hemoglobin A1c levels of 6.9%).

Regulation of blood glucose levels by the pancreas is shown in **Figure 9.19**. When the body's blood glucose level is high (after a meal, for example), the pancreas secretes insulin to lower blood glucose levels. Insulin targets almost every cell in the body to promote glucose uptake and lower blood glucose levels. Once inside a cell, glucose is used for cellular energy. Insulin is essential for providing life-sustaining energy and health because it is the only hormone capable of getting glucose into body cells. Insulin also stimulates the liver to convert excess glucose into glycogen.

Glucagon has the opposite effect of insulin. When blood glucose level is low, the pancreas secretes glucagon, which increases the level of blood glucose. Glucagon secretion is achieved primarily through gluconeogenesis, or glycogen breakdown in the liver. Other hormones can increase the level of blood glucose, but glucagon is the most effective.

Understanding Medical Terminology

To remember the hormones secreted by the pancreas, just remember the acronym *PIG*: **P**ancreas secretes **I**nsulin and **G**lucagon.

SELF CHECK

1. What two types of cells in the pancreas secrete hormones?
2. What is the purpose of the hormones secreted by the pancreas?

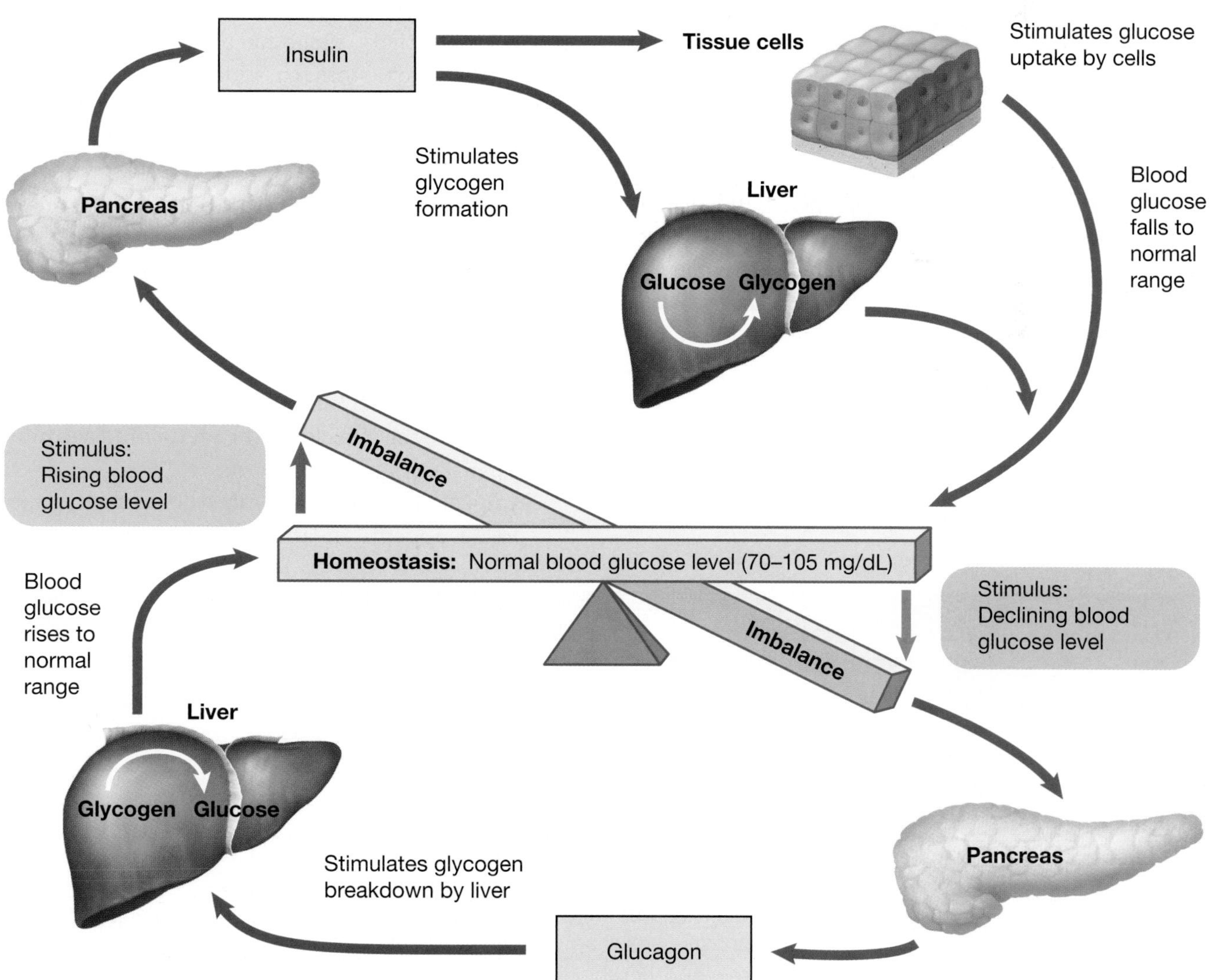

Figure 9.19 The pancreas secretes insulin and glucagon to regulate blood glucose levels.

Other Hormone-Producing Organs and Tissues

Several other organs and tissues also produce hormones to help regulate body systems. These include the thymus, pineal gland, sex glands, and some types of adipose tissue. **Figure 9.20** summarizes the hormones produced by the pancreas, thymus, pineal gland, and gonads.

Thymus

The ***thymus*** is both an endocrine gland and a lymphatic organ. It lies under the sternum, anterior to the heart. During childhood, the thymus gland is quite large, but it becomes smaller as people age. At the onset of puberty, the thymus begins to shrink, and it is barely visible by adulthood.

The thymus secretes thymosin, a hormone that is essential for the development of white blood cells known as *T lymphocytes*, or *T cells*. T cells play a key role in the body's immune system.

Pineal Gland

The ***pineal gland*** is a pinecone-shaped gland located in the brain. Its exact function remains unclear. However, researchers have discovered that when the body is exposed to darkness, the pineal gland releases the hormone melatonin, causing sleepiness. Melatonin levels are highest at night.

Gonads

Gonads are sex glands. In men, gonads are called ***testes***; in women, they are called ***ovaries***.

The paired, oval testes are encased by the ***scrotum***, a sac located outside the body. The testes produce sperm and androgens such as testosterone. Testosterone is responsible for sperm production, development of the male reproductive system, and the emergence of male secondary sex characteristics during puberty. The testes release testosterone when they are stimulated by luteinizing hormone (LH) from the anterior pituitary gland.

The ovaries, which are located inside the female pelvic cavity, produce eggs and the hormones estrogen and progesterone. Estrogen plays a key role in the development of the female reproductive glands and secondary sex characteristics. Along with progesterone, estrogen regulates the menstrual cycle and promotes breast development.

Hormones Produced in Other Locations

Hormones are produced by other tissues in the body, such as adipose (fatty) tissue and tissues that line organs such as the heart, stomach, kidneys and intestines. Hormone secretion is not the primary role of these organs and tissues; nonetheless, they do secrete hormones. For example:

- The kidneys secrete erythropoietin, a hormone that stimulates red blood cell production.
- Fatty tissue throughout the body secretes prostaglandins, which act at or near their site of production. Prostaglandins perform many roles: they regulate the smooth muscle cells that line the blood vessels and respiratory passages, stimulate the muscles of the uterus, and activate the inflammatory response.
- Adipose cells produce leptin, a hormone that suppresses appetite and increases energy production.

Pancreatic and Other Hormones

Gland	Hormones	Functions
Pancreas	insulin	decreases blood glucose level
	glucagon	increases blood glucose level
Thymus	thymosin	essential for the development of T cells
Pineal gland	melatonin	controls circadian rhythms (sleep cycle)
Gonads		
Testes	testosterone	responsible for sperm production, development and maintenance of the male reproductive system, and emergence of secondary sex characteristics
Ovaries	estrogen	responsible for the development of the female reproductive glands and secondary sex characteristics; regulates menstrual cycle
	progesterone	responsible for the development of the uterus and mammary glands; regulates menstrual cycle

Figure 19.20

Goodheart-Willcox Publisher

SECTION 9.2 REVIEW

Mini-Glossary

adrenal cortex the outer layer of the adrenal glands, which has three sublayers that secrete steroid hormones

adrenal glands a pair of glands that sit on top of the kidneys; consist of the adrenal cortex and adrenal medulla

adrenal medulla the inner layer of the adrenal glands, which functions as a part of the nervous system; secretes epinephrine and norepinephrine during the fight-or-flight response

anterior pituitary the anterior lobe of the pituitary gland, which secretes six different hormones: growth hormone, prolactin, adrenocorticotropin hormone, thyroid-stimulating hormone, follicle-stimulating hormone, and luteinizing hormone

ovaries the female sex glands

pancreas a long, thin organ located posterior to the stomach; secretes insulin and glucagon as an endocrine gland; secretes digestive enzymes as an exocrine gland

parathyroid glands four tiny glands that are located on the posterior aspect of the thyroid gland and secrete parathyroid hormone in response to low blood calcium levels

pineal gland a pinecone-shaped gland that is located in the brain and releases the sleep-inducing hormone melatonin

pituitary gland a pea-sized gland that activates a metabolic response in target tissues and stimulates other endocrine glands to release hormones

posterior pituitary the posterior lobe of the pituitary gland, which stores two hormones produced by the hypothalamus: antidiuretic hormone and oxytocin

scrotum a sac that encases the testes

testes the male sex glands

thymus an organ that secretes thymosin; functions as both an endocrine gland and a lymphatic organ

thyroid gland a gland that is located below the larynx and secretes thyroid hormones (T_3 and T_4) and calcitonin

tropic hormones pituitary hormones that act on other endocrine glands; also known as *tropins*

Review Questions

1. Which tropic hormones are secreted by the anterior pituitary gland?
2. Which hormones are secreted when TSH acts on the thyroid gland?
3. What is the purpose of gluconeogenesis?
4. What two roles does prolactin play in a nursing mother?
5. Which two hormones regulate the menstrual cycle?
6. Compare and contrast the adrenal cortex and the adrenal medulla.
7. Explain why the thyroid hormones affect all cells in the body.
8. Describe the regulation of calcium in the body.
9. Lena, a 70-year-old woman, visits her doctor because she is concerned about the slight appearance of hair on her face. Explain why it is not unusual for older women to develop masculine traits such as facial hair.

SECTION 9.3 Disorders and Diseases of the Endocrine System

Objectives

- List and describe disorders of the pituitary gland.
- Discuss the difference between hypothyroidism and hyperthyroidism and name the disorders associated with each.
- Identify disorders and diseases of the parathyroid glands.
- Describe disorders caused by malfunction of the adrenal glands.
- Explain the difference between type I and type II diabetes mellitus.

Key Terms

acromegaly
Addison's disease
Cushing's syndrome
diabetes insipidus
diabetes mellitus (DM)
dwarfism
goiter
Graves' disease
hypercalcemia
hyperglycemia
hyperthyroidism
hypothyroidism
insulin resistance
myxedema
neonatal hypothyroidism
peripheral neuropathy
tetanus
thyroiditis
type I diabetes mellitus
type II diabetes mellitus

Because the endocrine system is hierarchical in nature, many of its glands depend on one another, but they also act independently. Therefore, when an endocrine gland is not functioning properly, the effects of its malfunction may be felt either throughout the body or at a specific site. This section describes some common disorders and diseases of the endocrine system.

Pituitary Disorders

The pituitary gland releases many important hormones. Thus, an underactive or overactive pituitary gland can have widespread effects.

Hyperfunction of the Pituitary Gland

When the pituitary gland secretes excessive amounts of a specific hormone, it is said to be hyperfunctioning. One of the most common disorders caused by hyperfunction of the pituitary is ***acromegaly***, or gigantism, which is a rare condition that causes an increase in overall body size, especially in the extremities.

Acromegaly is usually caused by a noncancerous tumor pressing on the pituitary gland. Pressure from the tumor can also cause headaches, vision disturbances, loss of vision, seizures, and fatigue. This disorder most often affects middle-aged adults, but it may also affect children. In children, acromegaly causes unusually tall height, large hands, and large feet. In adults, acromegaly causes thickened bones and enlarged facial features, hands, and feet. Diagnosis of acromegaly in adults may take years because its effects appear gradually.

Treatment of acromegaly includes medications to shrink the tumor and to decrease GH levels. Surgery may be performed to remove the tumor if it is operable. Surgeons may operate on a patient using a gamma knife if the tumor is located in a hard-to-reach place. Although medications and surgery will stop excessive growth, the effects of acromegaly cannot be reversed. Unfortunately, acromegaly places a great strain on the body, which often leads to a shortened life span.

Hypofunction of the Pituitary Gland

Hypofunction of the pituitary is the secretion of inadequate amounts of hormones. Hypofunction can cause several disorders, including dwarfism and diabetes insipidus.

Dwarfism

Hyposecretion of GH by the pituitary gland can cause ***dwarfism***, a condition in which adult height reaches less than four feet (**Figure 9.21**). Dwarfism affects only a person's physical size; intellectual ability is normal.

Dwarfism may be congenital, or acquired during development in the uterus. It can also be caused by a brain injury or a medical condition such as growth hormone deficiency. When diagnosed at an early age, dwarfism is usually treated with supplemental growth hormones.

Diabetes Insipidus

Hyposecretion of ADH from the posterior pituitary causes ***diabetes insipidus***. ADH normally targets the kidneys, causing them to reabsorb water from urine. ADH deficiency can cause a large loss of water and electrolytes. People with diabetes insipidus experience excessive thirst, or polydipsia.

Diabetes insipidus is different from diabetes mellitus, which is the pancreatic disorder commonly referred to simply as *diabetes*. Diabetes mellitus is described later in this section.

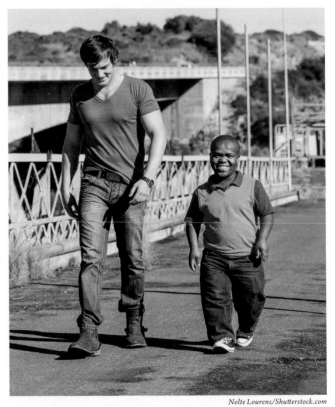

Nolte Lourens/Shutterstock.com

Figure 9.21 Dwarfism is caused by inadequate secretion of growth hormone by the pituitary.

SELF CHECK

1. Which condition results from hypofunction of the pituitary gland?
2. Which endocrine disorder is caused by an ADH deficiency?

Thyroid Disorders

The hormones T_4 and T_3 control the metabolism of every living cell in the body. When the thyroid secretes inadequate or excessive levels of these hormones, the result is a thyroid disorder.

Hyperthyroidism

Hyperthyroidism, or overactive thyroid, is characterized by a visibly enlarged thyroid gland in the neck (**Figure 9.22**). An enlarged thyroid is called a ***goiter***. A goiter may be caused by insufficient amounts of iodine, a chemical element necessary for the production of thyroid hormones. A goiter may also be caused by noncancerous growths or inflammation.

Iodine is not produced by the body, so it is important to eat foods containing iodine. This is one of the reasons that most countries, including the United States, add iodine to salt. An overactive thyroid works hard to secrete the hormones T_3 and T_4, but without adequate iodine from the diet, production of thyroid hormones is impaired.

Low levels of T_3 and T_4 cannot complete the negative feedback loop to stop secretions by the hypothalamus and the pituitary glands. As a result, the hypothalamus and pituitary gland continue to produce thyroid-releasing hormone and thyroid-stimulating hormone (TSH).

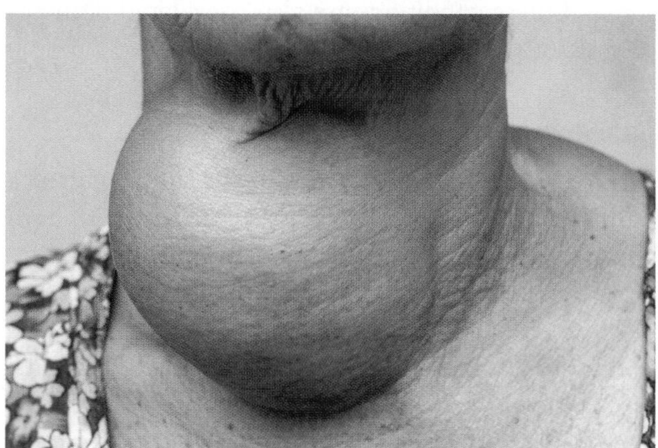

chatuphot/Shutterstock.com

Figure 9.22 This woman has a goiter large enough to cause difficulty breathing and swallowing.

An excess of TSH causes the thyroid gland to enlarge, resulting in the characteristic goiter. Increased heart rate, elevated body temperature, hyperactivity, weight loss, diarrhea, and difficulty concentrating are other side effects of hyperthyroidism.

Treatments for hyperthyroidism include surgery to remove part, or all, of the thyroid gland or the tumor affecting the gland. Radioactive iodine may also be used to destroy thyroid cells, or thyroid drugs may be administered to reduce thyroid hormones.

The most common cause of hyperthyroidism is ***Graves' disease***, an autoimmune disorder. This condition develops when a tumor grows on the thyroid gland, causing oversecretion of the thyroid hormones.

Graves' disease also causes the eyes to bulge outward, a condition called *exophthalmos*. This may make it difficult or impossible to close the eyelid, which can lead to drying and scarring of the cornea. Loss of vision may result from this condition.

Hypothyroidism

Hypothyroidism (underactive thyroid) is usually caused by ***thyroiditis***, or inflammation of the thyroid cells. Thyroiditis can be caused by the common cold, other respiratory infections, certain prescription drugs, or a condition in which the immune system attacks the thyroid. In addition, a specific type of thyroiditis, known as *postpartum thyroiditis*, can occur after pregnancy.

Hypothyroidism is most common in women and in people of both genders older than 50 years of age. Symptoms of hypothyroidism include fatigue, pale and dry skin, thin hair, brittle fingernails, increased sensitivity to cold temperatures, constipation, and weight gain. Treatment involves replacing the T_3 and T_4 hormones through supplemental hormone therapy. Most people with hypothyroidism require lifelong supplemental hormone therapy to manage the disease.

Myxedema

Adults with undiagnosed or untreated hypothyroidism will develop ***myxedema***. Myxedema is a severe form of hypothyroidism that causes weight gain; a swollen, puffy face; low body temperature; dry skin; and decreased mental acuity. This condition can be treated with an oral form of thyroxine.

Neonatal Hypothyroidism

Sometimes newborn children may develop ***neonatal hypothyroidism***. This thyroid deficiency may develop congenitally (before birth) or soon after birth. Often, children with neonatal hypothyroidism have a poorly developed thyroid gland or ineffective thyroid hormones.

Untreated neonatal hypothyroidism can lead to mental and physical disability. Dull, dry skin and dry, brittle hair are also common. Early diagnosis is essential because the effects of this disorder can be reversed. Like myxedema, neonatal hypothyroidism is treated with oral thyroxine.

SELF CHECK

1. What is an enlarged thyroid gland called?
2. Which thyroid disorder causes exophthalmos?
3. How is myxedema treated?

Parathyroid Disorders

Recall that the parathyroid glands secrete parathyroid hormone (PTH) and the thyroid gland secretes calcitonin. These hormones work together to regulate blood calcium levels. Malfunction of the parathyroid glands can result in conditions characterized by an imbalance of blood calcium levels.

Hypercalcemia

Hypersecretion of PTH causes high blood calcium, a condition known as ***hypercalcemia***. Hypercalcemia leads to increased calcium absorption by the kidneys and changes in the bones, which develop holes and become brittle. Excess calcium in the kidneys causes kidney stones to form. Hypercalcemia can also affect the nervous and cardiovascular systems, causing depression, decreased heart rate, and fatigue.

Hypocalcemia

Hyposecretion of PTH causes hypocalcemia, or low blood calcium, which leads to unstable nerve and muscle membranes that continuously fire electrical signals. The result is a condition known as ***tetanus***, which results in a sustained muscular contraction known as *tetany* (**Figure 9.23**). If left untreated, tetanus can affect the respiratory muscles, leading to asphyxiation and death. Treatment for hypocalcemia includes PTH replacement therapy, as well as administration of vitamin D and calcium. Blood tests to monitor calcium levels are also helpful in managing this disease.

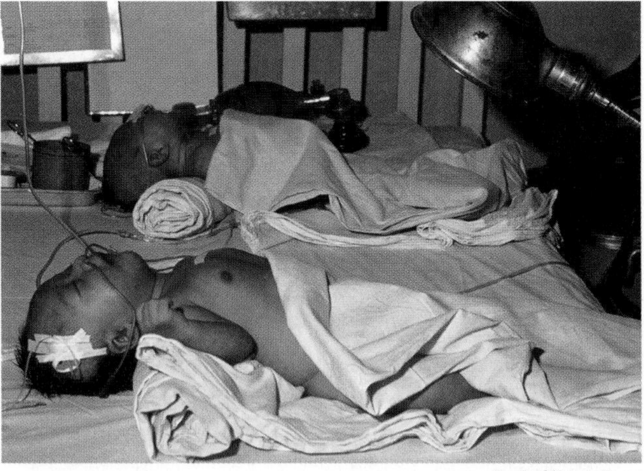

Sue Ford/Science Source

Figure 9.23 Tetanus results in tetany—a sustained muscular contraction that, in extreme or untreated cases, can result in a typical "bowed" appearance, extreme pain, and death.

SELF CHECK

1. Which glands secrete hormones that regulate blood calcium levels?
2. What happens when too much PTH is secreted?

Adrenal Disorders

Disorders related to the adrenal glands vary depending on whether they originate in the adrenal medulla or the adrenal cortex. In addition, because the adrenal glands receive orders from the pituitary hormones, some of these conditions are also considered pituitary disorders.

Disorders of the Adrenal Medulla

In rare cases, individuals develop a tumor called a *pheochromocytoma* on the adrenal medulla. A pheochromocytoma causes the adrenal medulla to hypersecrete the hormones epinephrine and norepinephrine.

High amounts of epinephrine and norepinephrine in the bloodstream can produce life-threatening results: high blood pressure, rapid heart rate, weight loss, nervousness, and sleep disturbances. These symptoms are experienced intermittently and usually resolve within 15 to 20 minutes.

Pheochromocytoma is diagnosed through an abdominal CT or MRI scan, catecholamine tests of the blood or urine, or an adrenal biopsy. Treatment involves immediate lowering of blood pressure through prescription or IV medications, and the removal of the tumor.

Disorders of the Adrenal Cortex

As with other disorders of the endocrine system, disorders of the adrenal cortex can result from several factors. These factors include tumors or growths on the adrenal gland, irregular secretion of hormones from glands (such as the pituitary gland) that act on the adrenal cortex, and hyposecretion or hypersecretion of adrenal cortex hormones.

Cushing's Syndrome

Cushing's syndrome is a disorder of the adrenal cortex caused by hypersecretion of cortisol. This syndrome can be caused by:

- oversecretion of ACTH by the pituitary gland, which stimulates hypersecretion of cortisol by the adrenal cortex.
- a tumor on the adrenal gland that stimulates hypersecretion of cortisol.
- prolonged use of steroid drugs, such as those prescribed to treat arthritis and other autoimmune disorders. Steroid drugs suppress the release of ACTH, thus preventing the production of cortisol.

Overproduction of cortisol causes many symptoms, including a rounded, moon-shaped face; weight gain (especially in the upper body); high blood glucose levels; hypertension; osteoporosis; reddish-purple abdominal stretch marks; difficulty concentrating; and facial hair in women (**Figure 9.24**).

Cushing's syndrome is diagnosed by measuring cortisol levels in the saliva each morning or by obtaining a 24-hour urine collection sample. Treatment of Cushing's syndrome caused by a tumor includes surgical removal of the tumor.

It is important to exercise caution when taking steroid drugs. Prolonged use of a steroid drug, whether for illness or to enhance athletic performance, can inhibit the release of ACTH by the anterior pituitary, leading to a lack of cortisol. This puts a patient at risk for developing Cushing's syndrome. Therefore, it is very important that patients be slowly weaned from steroid drugs, giving the anterior pituitary time to begin producing ACTH again.

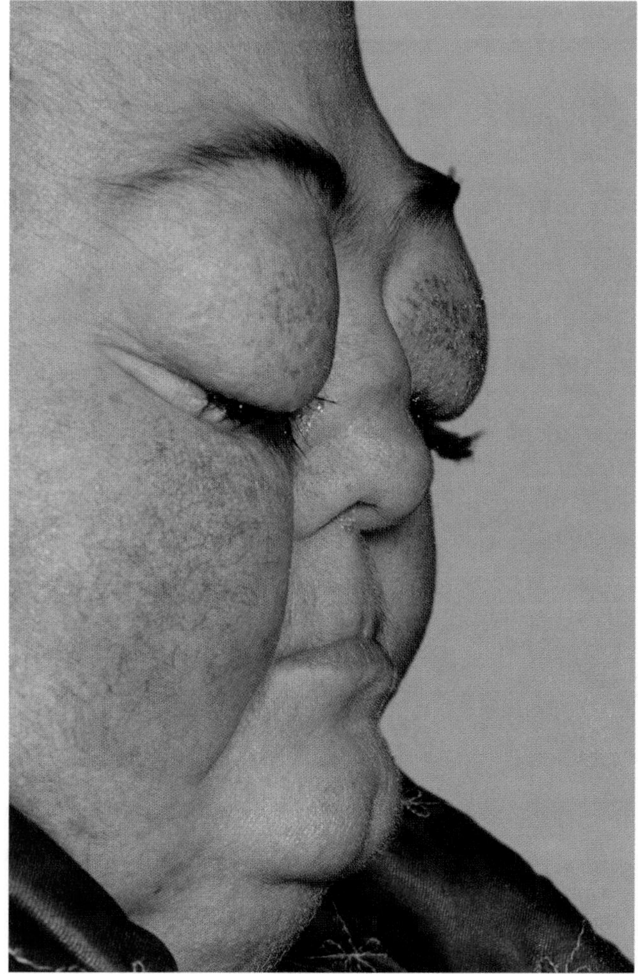

Biophoto Associates/Science Source

Figure 9.24 Cushing's syndrome is characterized by a rounded face, often with exophthalmos, and weight gain.

Athletes who use anabolic steroids often suffer numerous and long-lasting effects, including decreased heart function, elevated blood pressure, liver damage, premature bone plate closures, aggression, depression, impotence or decreased sperm count in males, and menstrual cycle abnormalities in females.

Addison's Disease

Damage to the adrenal cortex results in hyposecretion of adrenal corticoid hormones. This can cause ***Addison's disease***, which results in muscle atrophy, a bronze skin tone, low blood pressure, and kidney damage. Other symptoms include excessive levels of potassium in the blood (hypoglycemia), severe loss of fluids and electrolytes (especially sodium), and a general feeling of weakness. Addison's disease is life-threatening because it can lead to low blood volume, electrolyte disturbances, or shock. The usual treatment for Addison's disease is hormone replacement therapy.

SELF CHECK

1. What causes the formation of kidney stones in people with hypercalcemia?
2. What is the cause of Cushing's syndrome?
3. What life-threatening results may occur due to Addison's disease?

Diabetes Mellitus

Recall that the pancreas secretes two hormones that regulate blood glucose levels: insulin and glucagon. ***Diabetes mellitus (DM)*** is characterized by the body's inability to produce sufficient amounts of insulin to regulate blood glucose levels.

There are two types of diabetes—***type I diabetes mellitus*** and ***type II diabetes mellitus***. In the United States, 90% to 95% of diabetes cases are type II; the remaining 5% to 10% are type I. This disease is so common that almost everyone knows someone with diabetes. In 2010, the National Institutes of Health (NIH) reported that approximately 27% of adults 65 years of age and older were diabetic, and the numbers were rising. Diabetes is the seventh leading cause of death in the United States. It is also the leading cause of kidney failure, nontraumatic lower limb amputation, and new cases of blindness. Diabetes is also a major contributor to heart disease and stroke.

Symptoms and Diagnosis

Diabetes mellitus is diagnosed using the following blood tests:

- Blood glucose test—a blood glucose level of 126 mg/dL or higher after an eight-hour fast is considered positive for diabetes.
- Glucose tolerance test—in this oral glucose tolerance test, a person's blood glucose level is measured two hours after drinking a liquid that contains 75 grams of glucose. A blood glucose level of 200 mg/dL or greater is in the diabetic range.
- HbA1c test—also known as a glycosylated hemoglobin test, this test measures average blood glucose levels over a three-month period. A glucose level of 5.6% or less is normal, 5.7%–6.4% is prediabetic, and 6.5% or greater indicates diabetes.

Generally, a family history of diabetes mellitus or symptom onset prompts people to be tested for this disorder. The primary symptoms of diabetes include:

- polyuria—excessive urination to eliminate glucose
- polydipsia—excessive thirst to replenish water lost through polyuria
- polyphagia—increased hunger to replace fats and proteins used by the body as fuel sources.

Other symptoms of diabetes may include unexplained weight loss or gain, blurred vision, nausea, and slow-healing wounds.

Type I Diabetes Mellitus

Type I diabetes mellitus is an autoimmune disorder in which the immune system attacks and kills the insulin-secreting beta cells of the pancreas. Destruction of these cells causes insulin production to decrease or stop altogether. As a result, blood glucose levels rise from their normal circulating levels of 70–105 mg/dL to dangerously high levels exceeding 500 mg/dL.

Type I diabetics may need to receive insulin through several injections over the course of a day. Insulin dosage levels are based on self-administered blood glucose checks. If blood glucose levels are high, a higher insulin dose is administered; if blood glucose levels are low, less insulin is taken (**Figure 9.25**). Type I diabetics may also regulate their blood glucose levels through an externally worn insulin pump that continuously monitors glucose and delivers appropriate dosages of insulin.

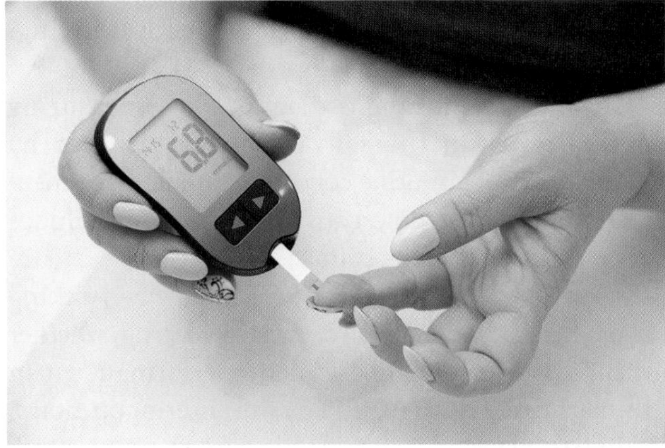

Parilov/Shutterstock.com

Figure 9.25 Diabetics use a device called a *glucometer* to monitor fluctuations in their blood glucose levels.

It's unclear what causes the immune system to attack the insulin-secreting beta cells of the pancreas. However, it is clear that type I diabetes mellitus is a hereditary condition. People with this disorder are usually diagnosed at a young age.

Type II Diabetes Mellitus

In people with type II diabetes, the pancreas secretes insulin, but the body's insulin receptors are downregulated—a condition called ***insulin resistance***. Insulin-resistant receptors do not take up glucose even when insulin is present, so blood glucose levels become elevated, a condition known as ***hyperglycemia***. When glucose builds up in the blood, it is absorbed by the kidneys and excreted in urine.

It is unclear what causes the body's cells to become insulin resistant but insulin resistance is associated with obesity, physical inactivity, family history of diabetes, and old age. In fact, the NIH estimates that 80% of type II diabetics are overweight or obese.

Although large amounts of glucose are available in the body for energy production, diabetics are unable to use this glucose either because insulin is unavailable or because the body's cells are insulin resistant.

When the body's cells are unable to use glucose as a fuel source, they use fats and proteins instead. Using fats for fuel produces ketone bodies that decrease the pH of the blood, making it dangerously acidic. This condition is called *ketoacidosis*. If left untreated, ketoacidosis can lead to diabetic coma and death. People with ketosis—high levels of ketones in the body—also have fruity-smelling breath because of the presence of acetone. If adopting a healthful diet and getting adequate exercise are not sufficient for managing type II diabetes mellitus, oral hypoglycemic agents or injectable insulin are available.

Living with Diabetes Mellitus

Patient education is very important for diabetic care. People with diabetes who develop ***peripheral neuropathy***, which causes loss of feeling in the extremities, must take particularly good care of their feet. As a result of peripheral neuropathy, diabetics may be unaware when they get a cut or wound on their foot. Unnoticed cuts or wounds can become infected. Severely infected wounds may result in amputation of the affected limb.

There is no known cure for diabetes mellitus. Since there is no cure, the goal for patients is learning how to successfully manage this disorder. The cornerstones of managing diabetes mellitus are a healthful diet, physical activity to increase insulin sensitivity of the body's cells, weight loss, and taking medications as prescribed.

Research Notes: Managing Diabetes with Diet and Exercise

Type II diabetes mellitus has reached epidemic proportions in the United States, largely because of the increased rate of obesity and lack of physical activity. The Centers for Disease Control estimates there are about 86 million prediabetic cases among adults in the United States.

Recently, a study of 3,000 diabetic and prediabetic people investigated the effect of diet and exercise on type II diabetes. Specifically, participants in the study ate a low-fat diet and engaged in 30 minutes of moderately intense exercise five days a week.

Most of the study participants chose walking as their exercise activity, and the results were dramatic. On average, participants lost 5% to 7% of their body weight. In addition, the simple but effective lifestyle changes reduced the incidence of type II diabetes in the sample group by nearly 60%.

Another study examined the association between strength training and the incidence of type II diabetes over a ten-year period. This study found that women who reported engaging in strength training experienced a 30% reduction in the incidence of type II diabetes. Thus, participation in both aerobic exercise and strength training are beneficial for managing diabetes mellitus.

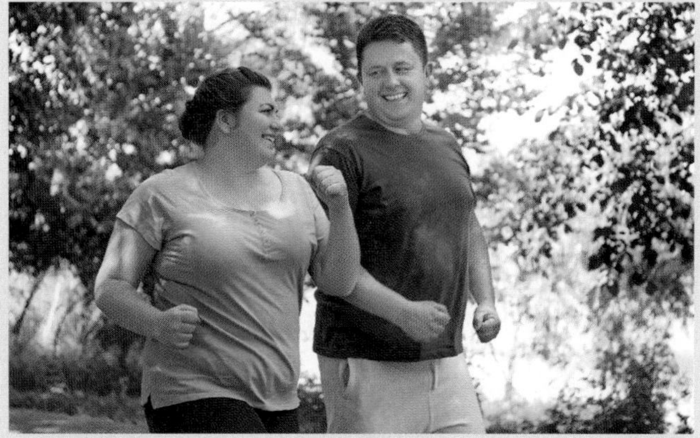

Africa Studio/Shutterstock.com

Regular exercise can decrease a person's risk of developing diabetes mellitus, particularly if the person is overweight.

SECTION 9.3

REVIEW

Mini-Glossary

acromegaly a condition in which the anterior pituitary hypersecretes growth hormone (GH), causing an increase in overall body size; also known as *gigantism*

Addison's disease a condition caused by hyposecretion of adrenal corticoid hormones

Cushing's syndrome a disorder of the adrenal cortex caused by hypersecretion of cortisol

diabetes insipidus a disorder caused by hyposecretion of antidiuretic hormone (ADH) by the posterior pituitary

diabetes mellitus a disease that results from the body's inability to regulate blood glucose levels; see *type I diabetes mellitus* and *type II diabetes mellitus*

dwarfism a condition in which the pituitary gland hyposecretes growth hormone (GH), resulting in an adult height of less than four feet

goiter an enlarged thyroid gland

Graves' disease an autoimmune disorder that causes an overactive thyroid gland and outward bulging of the eyes

hypercalcemia a condition characterized by increased blood calcium levels and increased calcium absorption by the kidneys; caused by the hypersecretion of parathyroid hormone (PTH)

hyperglycemia a condition in which blood glucose levels are elevated

hyperthyroidism the condition caused by an overactive thyroid gland; characterized by a visibly enlarged thyroid gland in the neck

hypothyroidism the condition of an underactive thyroid gland

insulin resistance a condition present in type II diabetes in which the pancreas secretes insulin, but the body's insulin receptors are downregulated, causing elevated blood glucose levels

myxedema a severe form of hypothyroidism that occurs when hypothyroidism goes undiagnosed or untreated

neonatal hypothyroidism a form of hypothyroidism that occurs in infants and children; may develop congenitally or soon after birth

peripheral neuropathy a disease or degenerative state of the peripheral nerves often associated with diabetes mellitus; marked by muscle weakness and atrophy, pain, and numbness

tetanus a condition in which muscles are in a state of tetany, or sustained muscular contraction

thyroiditis inflammation of the thyroid gland

type I diabetes mellitus an autoimmune disorder in which the immune system attacks the insulin-secreting beta cells of the pancreas, causing insulin production to decrease or stop completely

type II diabetes mellitus a condition in which the body's insulin receptors are downregulated

Review Questions

1. What causes diabetes insipidus?
2. Why are goiters uncommon in the United States today?
3. What are the symptoms of hypothyroidism?
4. Which disease is caused by the hyposecretion of adrenal corticoid hormones?
5. Which tests are used to diagnose diabetes mellitus?
6. Compare and contrast type I and type II diabetes mellitus.
7. Why does hypercalcemia cause brittle bones?

Medical Terminology

The Endocrine System

By understanding the word parts that make up medical words, you can extend your medical vocabulary. This chapter includes many of the word parts listed below. Review these word parts to be sure you understand their meanings.

-al	pertaining or relating to
cortic/o	cortex (cerebral or adrenal)
-crine	to secrete, secretion
-emia	blood condition
endo-	in, within, internal
exo-	out, away from
gonad/o	sex gland
home/o	unchanging, constant
hyper-	above normal
hypo-	below normal, under
-ic	pertaining to
-ism	condition, process
-stasis	to stop or control
thalam/o	thalamus
-therm	temperature, warmth
-tropin	stimulate, act on

Now use these word parts to form valid medical words that fit the following definitions. Some of the words are included in this chapter. Others are not. When you finish, use a medical dictionary to check your work.

1. pertaining to the thalamus
2. internal secretion
3. pertaining to below the thalamus
4. to control at a constant value
5. a hormone that acts on the sex glands
6. condition of being very large
7. related to both the thalamus and the cerebral cortex
8. pertaining to a constant temperature
9. above-normal concentration of lipoprotein in the blood
10. a hormone that acts on the adrenal cortex

Chapter 9 Summary

- The endocrine system is a collection of organs and glands that produce hormones that directly or indirectly influence all functions of the body.
- Hormones are chemical messengers that bind with receptors in or on a cell; the hormone can influence the activity of the cell in various ways.
- Endocrine glands are stimulated or inhibited in three different ways: neural control, hormonal control, and humoral control.
- The hypothalamus collects information from each body system and integrates the responses of the nervous and endocrine systems to maintain homeostatic balance.
- The anterior pituitary secretes six different types of hormones. The posterior pituitary gland stores antidiuretic hormone and oxytocin.
- The thyroid gland secretes three hormones: thyroxine and triiodothyronine, which drive the body's metabolism, and calcitonin, which helps maintain calcium homeostasis.
- The parathyroid glands produce parathyroid hormone, which works with calcitonin to maintain calcium levels in the blood.
- The adrenal cortex secretes three steroid hormones, which regulate sodium, sugar, and sex hormone levels.
- The pancreas secretes hormones that regulate blood glucose levels.
- Other hormone-producing organs and tissues include the thymus, pineal gland, sex glands, and some types of adipose tissue.
- Major disorders of the pituitary gland include acromegaly, dwarfism, and diabetes insipidus.
- Major disorders of the thyroid gland include hyperthyroidism (including goiter and Graves' disease) and hypothyroidism.
- Disorders of the parathyroid glands affect calcium levels in the blood.
- A tumor on the adrenal medulla can cause life-threatening hypersecretion of epinephrine and norepinephrine; disorders related to the adrenal cortex include Cushing's syndrome and Addison's disease.
- Diabetes mellitus results from the body's inability to regulate blood glucose levels.

Chapter 9 Review

Understanding Key Concepts

1. The chemical messengers secreted by the endocrine glands are known as ______.
   A. electrolytes
   B. enzymes
   C. hormones
   D. lacrimals
2. Which of the following is *not* an example of an exocrine gland?
   A. salivary gland
   B. sweat gland
   C. mammary gland
   D. adrenal gland
3. Which term describes lipid-based hormones?
   A. steroid hormones
   B. hypothalamic hormones
   C. amino acid-derived hormones
   D. mineralocorticoid hormones
4. Receptors for ______ hormones are found on the surfaces of cells.
5. Which endocrine gland maintains the homeostatic set point for body temperature at 98.6°F (37°C)?
   A. hypothalamus
   B. pituitary gland
   C. adrenal glands
   D. pancreas

6. Another name for the hormone epinephrine is ______.
7. ______ glands have ducts and are the counterparts to endocrine glands.
8. TSH is secreted by the pituitary gland and acts on the ______.
   A. pancreas
   B. testes
   C. thymus gland
   D. thyroid gland
9. The hormone prolactin, which stimulates milk production in a nursing mother, is produced by the ______.
   A. adrenal glands
   B. ovaries
   C. pituitary gland
   D. thyroid gland
10. Parathyroid hormone increases the concentration of ______ in the blood.
   A. calcium
   B. endorphins
   C. iron
   D. iodine
11. *True or False?* Antidiuretic hormone increases urine output and decreases body fluid volume.
12. The adrenal cortex produces three groups of steroid hormones: sex hormones, mineralocorticoids, and ______.
13. ______ is the hormone responsible for sperm production and the development of the male reproductive system.
   A. Progesterone
   B. Testosterone
   C. Estrogen
   D. Glycogen
14. Which endocrine gland is located in front of the trachea?
   A. adrenal gland
   B. thymus gland
   C. pituitary gland
   D. thyroid gland
15. Which two hormones are stored in the posterior pituitary?
   A. ADH and oxytocin
   B. ADH and LH
   C. TSH and oxytocin
   D. LH and oxytocin
16. The hormone-secreting cells of the pancreas are called the ______.
17. Where is the hypothalamus located?
   A. just below and to the right of the liver
   B. behind the sternum, above the diaphragm
   C. deep inside the brain
   D. inside the thyroid gland
18. *True or False?* The hormones secreted by the pituitary gland act directly on target tissues and also stimulate other endocrine glands.
19. Of the six hormones secreted by the anterior pituitary gland, which two are *not* considered tropic?
20. Which of the following glands does *not* secrete any hormones?
   A. parathyroid
   B. hypothalamus
   C. thyroid
   D. posterior pituitary
21. *True or False?* The adrenal cortex is part of the nervous system.
22. Which of the following glands secretes the hormone commonly referred to as *adrenaline*?
   A. pineal gland
   B. adrenal cortex
   C. pancreas
   D. adrenal medulla
23. Which of the following organs plays a key role in maintaining proper blood glucose levels?
   A. kidneys
   B. thymus
   C. pancreas
   D. gonads

24. Unusually tall height, along with enlargement of the hands, feet, and facial features, are common symptoms of ______.
    A. acromegaly
    B. Graves' disease
    C. hypothyroidism
    D. goiter
25. Which of the following disorders is *not* associated with growth hormone imbalance?
    A. acromegaly
    B. diabetes
    C. dwarfism
    D. gigantism
26. When diagnosed at a young age, dwarfism is treated by ______.
    A. removing the thyroid gland
    B. administering radiation therapy
    C. administering supplemental growth hormones
    D. administering iodine supplements
27. *True or False?* The pituitary gland controls the metabolism of every living cell in the human body.
28. A goiter is caused by a lack of ______ in the diet.
    A. sodium
    B. iodine
    C. calcium
    D. potassium
29. *True or False?* A person suffering from hypothyroidism would most likely have a goiter.
30. Hypocalcemia can cause ______.
    A. diabetes
    B. leukemia
    C. elevated blood sugar levels
    D. tetanus
31. Which of the following is *not* a common symptom of Cushing's syndrome?
    A. weight gain
    B. moon-shaped face
    C. enlarged thyroid
    D. hypertension
32. Normal blood glucose levels fall between 70 and ______ mg/dL.
    A. 500
    B. 105
    C. 80
    D. 135

Thinking Critically

33. The body's fight-or-flight response can be triggered in situations that pose no real physical threat or danger. For example, think about the last time you were very anxious in a social situation. What physical sensations did you feel? Relate your sensations to this chapter's description of the fight-or-flight response.
34. Compare and contrast the three control systems of the endocrine system.
35. Both antidiuretic hormone and aldosterone play major roles in blood pressure regulation. Explain the role of each hormone.
36. Explain the relationship between insulin and glucagon with regard to blood glucose levels.
37. A young woman is brought into a medical clinic by her husband. She complains of hyperactivity and weight loss. She also appears to be mentally sluggish and has difficulty concentrating when questioned by a nurse. There is a slight swelling in the anterior region of her neck. Which condition might you suspect? What are some possible causes and treatment options?

Clinical Case Study

38. Among the topics discussed in the chapter, what may be happening to Caitlyn? Which diagnosis is most likely?
39. What types of tests would help evaluate Caitlyn's condition?

Analyzing and Evaluating Data

Use the bar graph from the Centers for Disease Control shown here to answer the following questions.

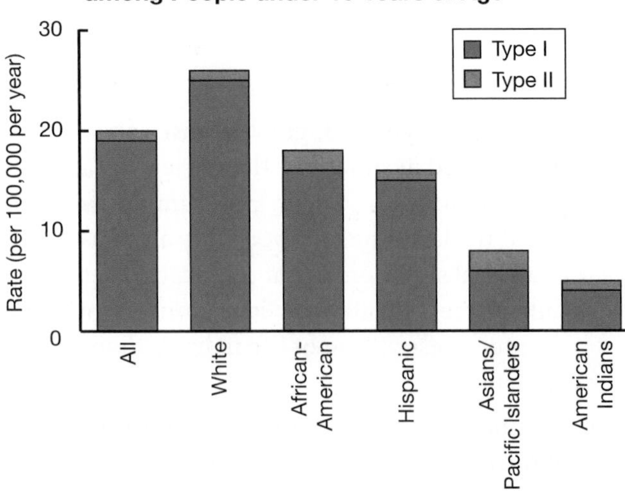

40. How many new cases of type I diabetes mellitus occurred per 100,000 children younger than 10 years of age? How many cases of type II diabetes occurred in this age group? What conclusion can you make from this data?
41. Which ethnic group experienced the most new cases of type I diabetes? Which group experienced the fewest new cases?
42. The number of new cases of type II diabetes increases dramatically in the 10 to 19 age group, as compared to the younger than 10 age group. Based on your reading of this chapter and any research you might need to do, develop reasons why new cases of type II diabetes mellitus are more prevalent in the older age group.

Investigating Further

43. In the competitive world of professional sports, athletes are sometimes tempted to take performance-enhancing drugs. One such drug is human growth hormone, a manufactured version of growth hormone. Research the use of human growth hormone by professional athletes. Identify an athlete who recently tested positive for human growth hormone. How did this revelation affect his or her career? Excessive amounts of growth hormone can lead to acromegaly. What other negative side effects does this drug have on the body?
44. Research current trends in obesity and diabetes in the United States, including any possible connection between these two issues and potential remedies.
45. Choose one of the following triggers: hunger, thirst, cold temperature, hot temperature, exhaustion, fear. Research how the endocrine system responds to the trigger you chose.

10 The Respiratory System

Clinical Case Study

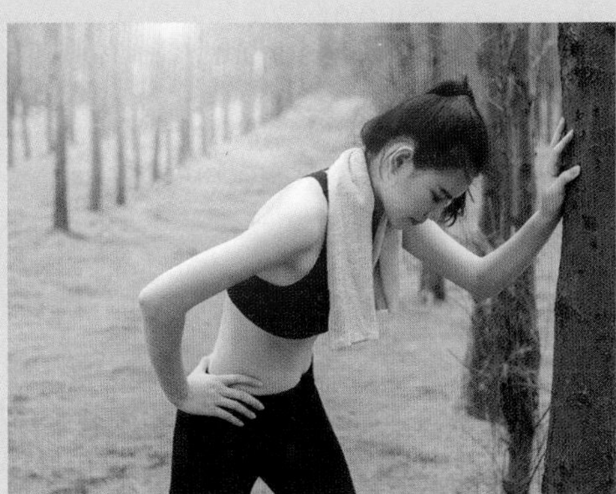
Zodiacphoto/Shutterstock.com

Jenna is an 18-year-old runner who is starting her freshman year of college with a track scholarship. She is looking forward to living in a cold-weather climate after growing up in Florida. As a child, Jen was relatively healthy and only had seasonal allergies that were relieved by over-the-counter medication.

In the fall, she started school and had a lot of success with her running. She consistently placed in the top three in her event. In late October, she was doing her normal cross-country workout and felt invigorated by the colder weather. Halfway through her workout, though, she felt her chest tighten up, so she decreased her pace and was able to complete the long run. Over the next month, Jen began to experience chest tightness during almost every practice, and she also began coughing after her workouts. Her running performance began to deteriorate and her symptoms became worse as the winter approached. Running was always her passion but now she was anxious and nervous about what might happen to her when she ran. The sports medicine physician referred her to a pulmonologist for further evaluation. Among the medical conditions and disorders discussed in this chapter, what are the possible causes of Jenna's ailment, and which one would be the most likely diagnosis? What types of tests would help evaluate Jenna's condition?

Chapter 10 Outline

Every breath that you take puts your respiratory system in direct contact with the environment. Have you ever stopped to think about what your lungs are exposed to on a daily basis? Commuting to school on a busy street causes you to breathe in exhaust fumes from other cars. Friends, family, or even strangers in public places expose your lungs to secondhand smoke. Through its anatomical structures and respiratory reflexes, such as sneezing and coughing, the respiratory system filters everything that you breathe in from the environment.

The respiratory system has a big job to do; appropriately, it is one of the largest organ systems in the body. The system includes about 1,500 miles of airways and almost 1,000 miles of capillaries in the lungs. If you were to spread out the 300 million air sacs found in the lungs, they would cover nearly the entire surface of a tennis court. In fact, the surface area of the lungs is about 80 times greater than the surface area of the skin.

Because the body cannot go without oxygen for long, the respiratory system is vital to survival. Working with the cardiovascular system, the respiratory system ensures that a supply of fresh oxygen is always available, while removing harmful waste gases, such as carbon dioxide, from the body.

SECTION 10.1

Anatomy of the Respiratory System

Objectives

- Identify the main structures of the upper respiratory tract.
- Describe the anatomy of the lower respiratory tract.

Key Terms

alveoli
bronchioles
cardiopulmonary system
ciliated epithelium
epiglottis
larynx
mediastinum
nares
nasal conchae
olfactory receptors
palate
pharynx
pleural sac
pores of Kohn
primary bronchi
sinuses
surfactant
thyroid cartilage
tonsils
trachea

Humans can survive for weeks without food and days without water, but only minutes without oxygen. In most cases, the brain will cease to function, and death will occur, after the brain has been deprived of oxygen for five to six minutes. However, there have been incidents in which individuals have survived for longer durations with effective cardiopulmonary resuscitation (CPR) and emergency medical treatment.

The main purpose of the respiratory system is to provide a constant supply of oxygen while eliminating carbon dioxide, a waste product, from the body. This process is called *gas exchange*. Most people understand why humans need sufficient amounts of oxygen, but they don't realize that removal of carbon dioxide from the body is equally important. Excessive levels of carbon dioxide can be toxic to the body, causing damage to cells and organs, and even resulting in death.

The respiratory system (sometimes called the *pulmonary system*) works cooperatively with the cardiovascular system to conduct gas exchange. These two systems are often collectively referred to as the ***cardiopulmonary system***. The blood is pumped through the body by the cardiovascular system, acting as a transport vehicle for oxygen and carbon dioxide. Through the blood, fresh oxygen from the lungs is delivered to all cells of the body. The body's cells discharge carbon dioxide into the bloodstream, which then carries the carbon dioxide back to the lungs for elimination.

The major organs of the respiratory system include the nasal cavity, pharynx, larynx, trachea, bronchi, bronchioles, and lungs (**Figure 10.1**). The respiratory system is divided into two parts: the upper respiratory tract and the lower respiratory tract.

Upper Respiratory Tract

The upper respiratory tract includes the nose, mouth, nasal cavity, pharynx, and larynx (**Figure 10.2**). The lower respiratory tract consists of the trachea, bronchi, bronchioles, and lungs. The lungs contain *alveoli* (al-VEE-oh-ligh), which are the air sacs in which the important gas exchange function occurs.

The structures of the upper respiratory tract not only serve as a passageway for air moving into and out of the lungs (breathing), but also perform other vital functions:

- filtering and removing foreign particles from inspired (inhaled) air
- humidifying and controlling the temperature of inspired air
- producing sound (voice)

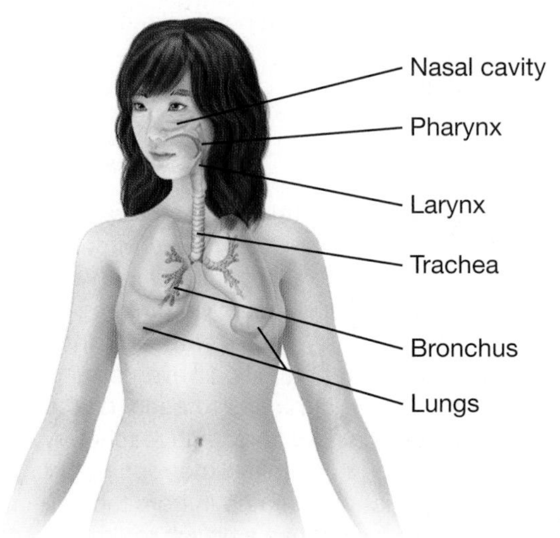

Figure 10.1 Simplified overview of the major respiratory structures.

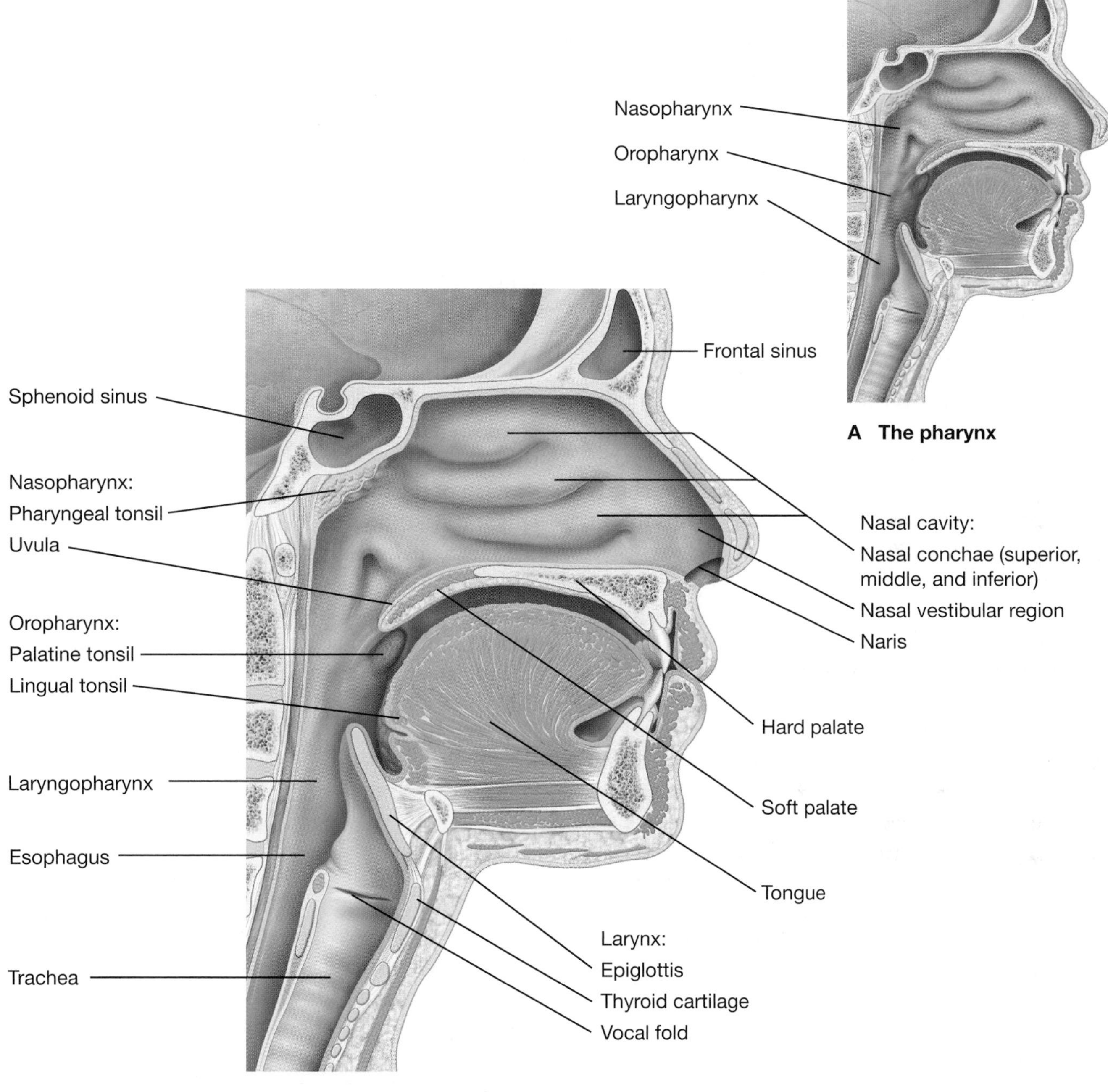

Figure 10.2 A—Regions of the pharynx. B—Structures of the upper respiratory tract.

- providing a sense of smell
- aiding in immune defense

As a result of these functions, the air that reaches the structures of the lower respiratory tract is warm, moist, and filtered—important qualities for lung health.

Nose and Nasal Cavity

The nose is the only part of the respiratory system that is external to the body. During inspiration (inhalation), air enters the nose through two openings called ***nares***, or nostrils.

The nose comes in many shapes and sizes. Some noses have bumps and others are small and turned up at the end. The nose's prominent location makes rhinoplasty (surgical modification of the nose) one of the most commonly performed plastic surgeries.

The nasal cavity occupies the space behind the nose. It is divided into right and left chambers by the nasal septum.

The nasal cavity is lined with mucous membranes that filter and purify inspired air. At the front of the nasal cavity, just inside each naris (the singular form of *nares*), is the vestibular region. This region contains oily, coated nasal hairs called *cilia*, which trap and prevent particles from entering the nose.

Along the mucous membrane that lines the roof of the nasal cavity is an area called the *olfactory region*. ***Olfactory receptors*** located in this region provide the sense of smell, which is closely tied to the sense of taste. When you have a stuffy nose and your sense of taste seems "off," an accumulation of mucus on your olfactory receptors may be the culprit.

The rest of the nasal cavity is called the *respiratory cavity*, despite the fact that no respiration occurs there. The respiratory cavity is lined with a mucosal membrane occupied by a dense network of thinly walled veins. This mucosal membrane warms the air that you breathe, but the thin walls of these veins, as well as their location, can cause nosebleeds.

Conchae

Three uneven, scroll-like ***nasal conchae*** (KAHN-kee) bones extend down through the nasal cavity. The conchae are named according to their location in the nasal cavity: superior, middle, and inferior conchae. These bones create three passageways that greatly increase the surface area available for filtering inspired air.

The conchae also increase the turbulence of the airflow in the nasal passage. This movement of air allows more particles to be trapped in the mucous membranes that line the nasal cavity and the conchae. When an airplane is subjected to turbulent airflow, the ride is bumpy. The erratic movement of a plane in turbulence is similar to the movement of inspired air when it enters the conchae.

Palate

The ***palate*** (PAL-at) is the roof of the mouth, which separates the nasal cavity from the oral cavity, or mouth. The anterior part of the palate is supported by bone, so it is called the *hard palate*. The posterior part of the palate is called the *soft palate* because it is composed of soft muscle and tissue and is unsupported by bone.

At the end of the soft palate is the uvula, a small, conical mass of connective tissue and muscle fibers. The uvula is believed to play a small role in speech, but it also helps prevent food from entering the nasal cavity.

When the two parts of the palate do not completely fuse together during fetal development, the result is a cleft (separated) palate. The upper lip can also be cleft. A cleft palate or lip leaves an opening in the roof of the mouth or a gap between the lip and nose. This condition occurs in about 1 out of every 700 babies. Surgery to close and repair the cleft palate or lip typically fixes this problem.

Sinuses

The ***sinuses*** are air-filled cavities that surround the nose. They are lined with mucous membranes and are connected to the nasal cavity by ducts that drain into the nose.

Each of the four sinuses is named for the bone on which it lies: the frontal sinus, the ethmoidal sinus, the sphenoidal sinus, and the maxillary sinus. Refer to Chapter 5, "The Skeletal System," for more information about the paranasal sinuses.

The sinuses reduce the weight of the head; warm and moisten inspired air; and amplify, or strengthen, the tone of the voice. Have you ever noticed how "nasal" a person's voice becomes during a sinus infection? This is because an infection causes the sinuses to become swollen and filled with fluid and germs, preventing the voice from projecting in its normal tone.

Pharynx

The ***pharynx*** is a muscular passage that transports air, food, and liquids from the nasal and oral cavities to the trachea and esophagus. Thus, the pharynx is part of both the respiratory system and the digestive system. The pharynx, commonly called the *throat*, is approximately 5 inches (12.7 centimeters) long.

Parts of the Pharynx

As shown in **Figure 10.2A**, the pharynx is composed of an upper section called the *nasopharynx*, a middle section called the *oropharynx*, and a lower region called the *laryngopharynx*. The nasopharynx is located behind the nasal cavity, superior and posterior to the soft palate. The Eustachian tubes of the middle ear drain into the nasopharynx. Because of this connection, an inner ear infection can cause an upper respiratory infection, or vice versa.

Whereas air is the only thing that passes through the nasopharynx, the oropharynx and laryngopharynx serve as passageways for air, food, and liquid. The oropharynx is posterior to the oral cavity, at the level of the hyoid bone. The laryngopharynx starts at the level of the hyoid bone, with its inferior end opening to the esophagus and the larynx. The sections of the pharynx are shown in relation to other upper respiratory structures in **Figure 10.2B**.

Tonsils

The ***tonsils*** are clusters of lymphatic tissue located in the pharynx. The pharyngeal tonsil is located in the upper part of the nasopharynx. The palatine and lingual tonsils lie in the upper portion of the oropharynx.

The tonsils are the respiratory system's first line of defense against infection. When bacteria and other pathogens enter the throat, they become trapped in the tonsils. This is why the tonsils themselves can become infected and inflamed, causing a condition called *tonsillitis*.

Larynx

The ***larynx***, or voice box, directs air and food to the proper passageways and houses the structures that produce speech. It is a triangular space located inferior to the pharynx. The larynx is composed of eight cartilaginous plates. The largest plate, the ***thyroid cartilage***, is commonly called the *Adam's apple*.

A flap of cartilaginous tissue called the ***epiglottis*** lies between the root of the tongue and the larynx. The epiglottis acts as a "gatekeeper" by controlling the destination of ingested food and liquid and inspired air. As food or liquid is swallowed, the epiglottis covers the opening of the larynx, preventing the substance from entering the trachea. If food or liquid does enter the trachea, a cough is triggered to expel the substance so that it does not enter the lungs. When you are not swallowing food or liquid, the epiglottis allows air to flow freely into the trachea and the lower respiratory tract.

The structures that produce each person's distinctive voice are located in the larynx. The larynx is lined with a mucous membrane that forms a pair of folds called the *vocal cords*. One of these folds is shown in **Figure 10.2**. Between the vocal cords is a space called the *glottis*, which gives the vocal cords room to vibrate. When air enters the vocal cords, they vibrate, producing sound.

SELF CHECK

1. List the structures that make up the respiratory system.
2. Besides serving as a passageway for air, what functions do the structures of the upper respiratory tract perform?
3. What is the only external part of the respiratory system?
4. Which two structures does the palate separate?
5. Where is the uvula located?
6. Which two body systems include the pharynx?

Lower Respiratory Tract

The lower part of the respiratory system consists of the trachea, the bronchi and bronchioles, and the lungs. This is the "working" part of the respiratory system, which accomplishes the gas exchange.

Trachea

The ***trachea***, also called the *windpipe*, is about 4 inches (10 centimeters) long and extends from the end of the larynx to about the fifth thoracic vertebra (mid-chest). The walls of the trachea are lined with a mucous membrane that contains ***ciliated epithelium***, a cellular covering that is embedded with tiny, hair-like structures known as *cilia* (**Figure 10.3**). The cilia continuously sweep foreign matter, such as dust, up toward the larynx and pharynx, where it can be swallowed or coughed up.

The walls of the trachea are reinforced by a series of cartilaginous, C-shaped rings (**Figure 10.4**). The C-shaped rings on the anterior side of the trachea contain rigid cartilage that provides support and prevents the airway from collapsing. The two sides of each C-shaped ring are connected on the posterior side of the trachea by the trachealis muscle (**Figure 10.5**). This muscle allows the trachea to be flexible and expand when large food particles pass through the esophagus.

Bronchi

At its bottom end, the trachea divides into right and left ***primary bronchi***. The primary bronchi are branches that conduct air to the right and left lungs, respectively. The bronchus (singular form of *bronchi*) on the right is wider, shorter, and lies more vertically than the left bronchus. Because of these structural differences, inhaled substances are more likely to become lodged in the right bronchus. Knowledge of the structure and layout of the bronchi has helped physicians quickly locate and remove inhaled objects, preventing many choking deaths.

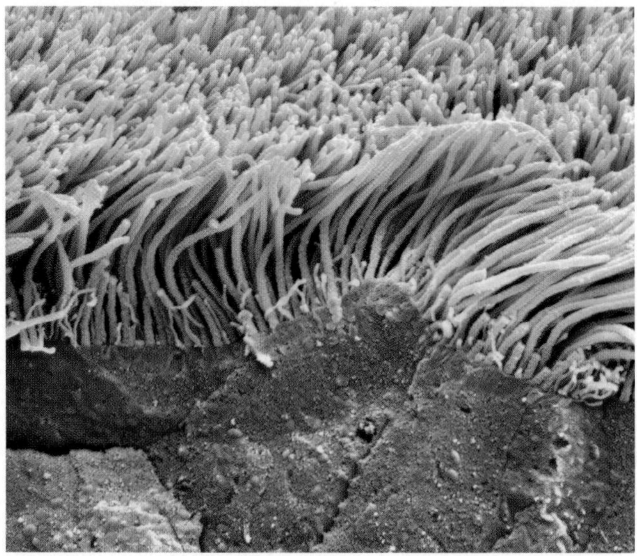

© Body Scientific International

Figure 10.3 This section through the tracheal wall, taken through a scanning electron microscope, clearly shows the ciliated epithelial cells that help move foreign particles upward and out of the trachea.

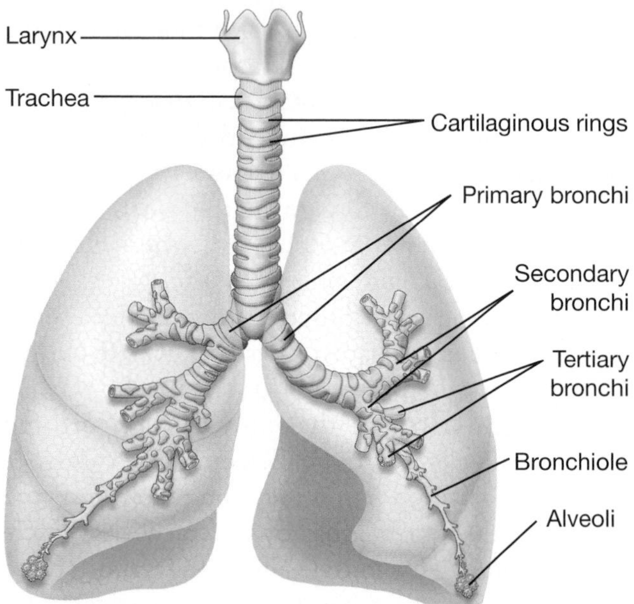

© Body Scientific International

Figure 10.4 The cartilaginous rings of the trachea continue throughout the primary, secondary, and tertiary bronchi, but are not present in the bronchioles.

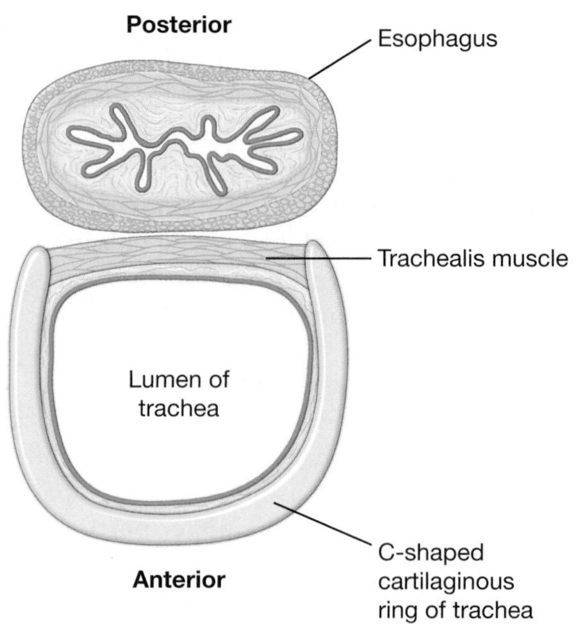

© Body Scientific International

Figure 10.5 The trachea lies anterior to the esophagus. Its front and sides are protected by the C-shaped cartilage, while the back is flexible to allow the esophagus to expand to accommodate swallowing food particles.

Bronchioles

The primary bronchi subdivide into smaller, Y-shaped branches called the *secondary* and *tertiary bronchi*, until they end in the smallest conducting passageways—the ***bronchioles***. The walls of the bronchial branches—but not the walls of the bronchioles—are reinforced by cartilaginous rings. The increasingly smaller branches of the bronchi are often compared to the branches of a tree. This is why the lungs and associated structures are sometimes referred to as the *respiratory tree* or *bronchial tree*.

Alveoli

The bronchi and bronchioles are collectively known as the *conducting zone* because they conduct air to and from the lungs. The terminal bronchioles lead into the *respiratory zone*, which contains the respiratory bronchioles, the alveolar ducts, and grape-like clusters of ***alveoli***. A limited amount of gas exchange occurs in the bronchioles, which are connected to the clusters of alveoli by the alveolar ducts.

The alveoli are air-filled sacs that serve as the main sites of gas exchange in the lungs. Millions of clusters of alveoli make up the bulk of the lung tissue. The alveolar walls are composed of very thin, squamous (flattened) epithelial cells. The interior of the alveoli is coated with ***surfactant***, a phospholipid. Surfactant reduces surface tension in the alveoli and prevents them from collapsing.

The internal environment of the alveoli is kept clean and healthy by bacteria-ingesting cells called *macrophages*. Gases and macrophages travel between alveoli via the ***pores of Kohn***, which are small openings in the alveolar wall.

The Lungs

The lungs are large organs that occupy almost the entire thoracic (chest) cavity (**Figure 10.6**). The ***mediastinum*** (mee-dee-as-TIGH-num) is the central area of the thoracic cavity, which lies between the lungs. This area houses the heart, great blood vessels, trachea, esophagus, thoracic duct, thymus gland, and other structures. The mediastinum creates a deep, concave indentation along the border of the left lung.

Lobes of the Lungs

The upper part of each lung, called the *apex*, is located just below the clavicles, or collarbone. The broad base of each lung rests on the diaphragm. The lungs are divided into lobes by fissures. The right lung has three divisions: the superior, middle, and inferior lobes. The left lung has only two divisions: the superior left lobe and inferior left lobe.

Most of the tissue in the lungs is filled with air. In fact, the average human lung weighs only 2.5 pounds, and it would float if placed in water.

The Pleural Sac

The lungs are surrounded by a thin, double-walled ***pleural sac*** composed of two slippery, serous membranes. One membrane, called the *parietal pleura*, lines the thoracic wall and the diaphragm. The other membrane, called the *visceral pleura*, covers the lungs and dips into their fissures. Both pleural membranes secrete a serous (watery) fluid that allows them to slide smoothly against each other as the lungs expand and contract during respiration. The serous fluid also acts as glue, keeping the two linings from pulling apart (**Figure 10.7**).

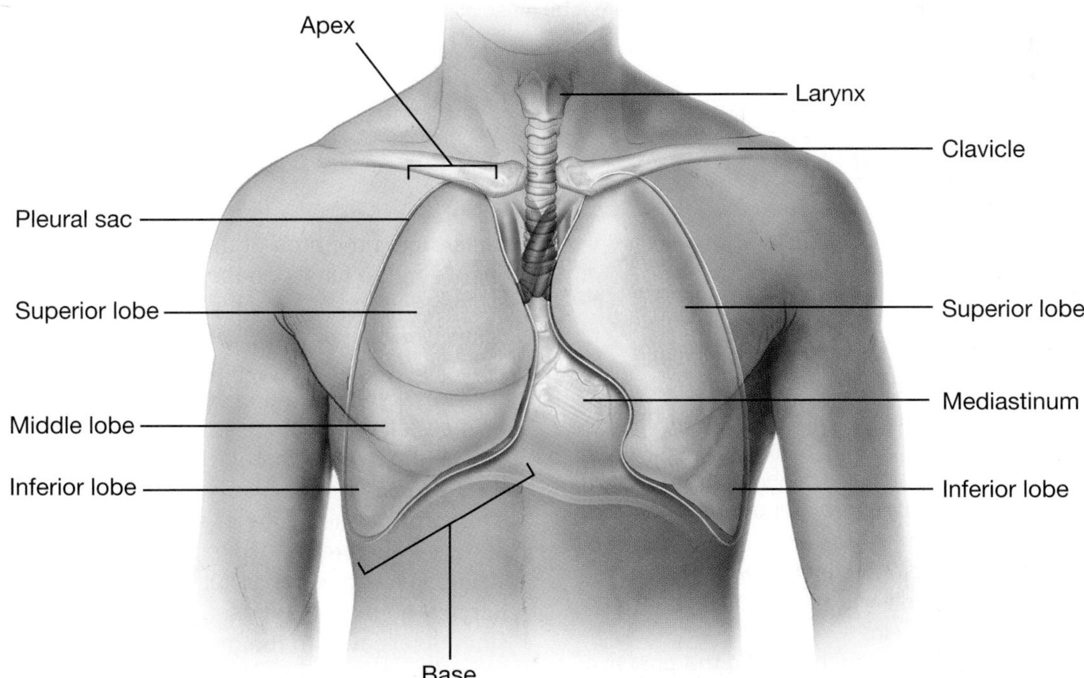

Figure 10.6 The right lung has three lobes, but the left lung has only two lobes.

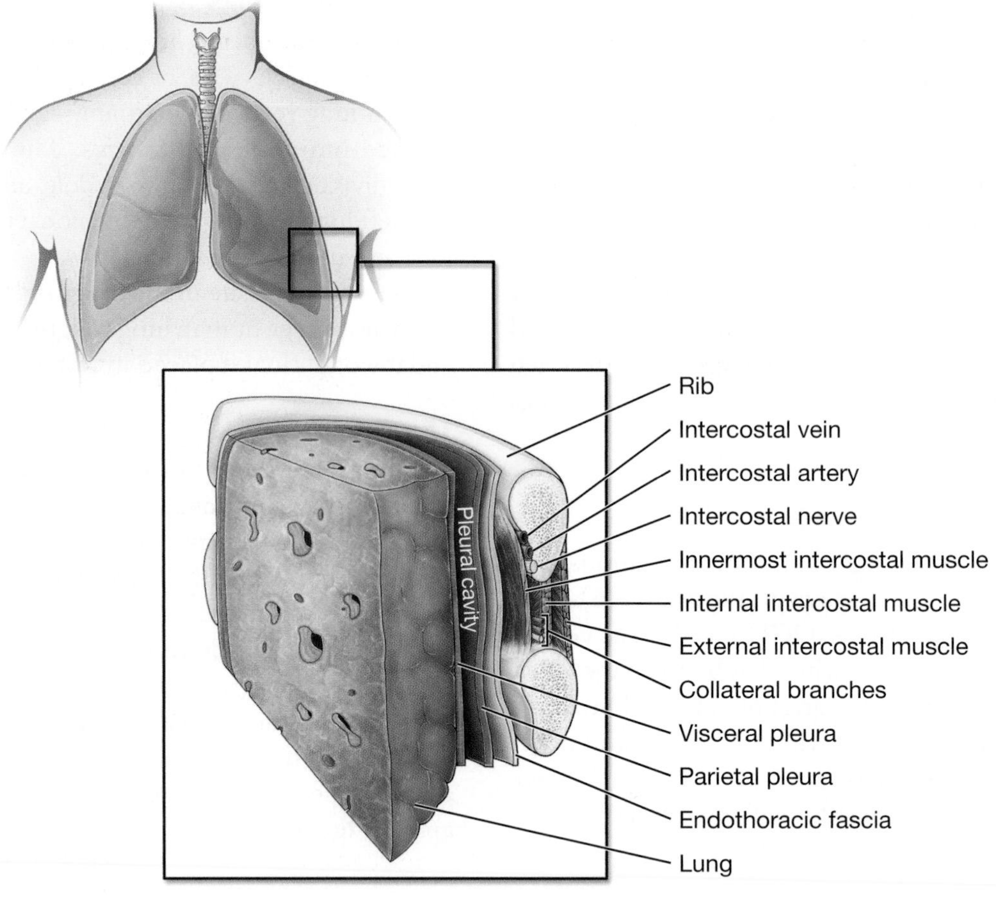

Evan Otto/Science Source

Figure 10.7 Each lung is separated from the ribs and intercostal muscles by the double-walled pleura, which reduces friction and allows the lungs to move freely within the chest.

SECTION 10.1 REVIEW

Mini-Glossary

alveoli air sacs that serve as the main sites of gas exchange in the lungs

bronchioles the thin-walled, smallest air-conducting passageways of the bronchi

cardiopulmonary system the collective name for the respiratory and cardiovascular systems

ciliated epithelium a cellular covering embedded with tiny, hair-like cilia that brush foreign particles upward and out of the trachea

epiglottis a flap of cartilaginous tissue that covers the opening to the trachea; diverts food and liquids to the esophagus during swallowing

larynx a triangular-shaped space inferior to the pharynx that is responsible for routing air and food into the proper passageways and producing speech; also known as the *voice box*

mediastinum the area of the thoracic cavity located between the lungs; houses the heart, great blood vessels, trachea, esophagus, thoracic duct, thymus gland, and other structures

nares the two openings in the nose through which air enters; also known as *nostrils*

nasal conchae three uneven, scroll-like nasal bones that extend down through the nasal cavity

olfactory receptors sensory cells in the olfactory region that provide the sense of smell

palate a structure that consists of hard and soft components and separates the oral and nasal cavities

pharynx the muscular passageway that extends from the nasal cavity to the mouth and connects to the esophagus

pleural sac the thin, double-walled serous membrane that surrounds the lungs

pores of Kohn small openings in the alveolar walls that allow gases and macrophages to travel between the alveoli

(continued)

primary bronchi the two passageways that branch off the trachea and lead to the right and left lungs
sinuses the air-filled cavities that surround the nose
surfactant a phospholipid that reduces surface tension in the alveoli and prevents them from collapsing
thyroid cartilage the largest cartilaginous plate in the larynx; commonly known as the *Adam's apple*
tonsils clusters of lymphatic tissue located in the pharynx that function as the respiratory system's first line of defense against infection
trachea the air tube that extends from the larynx into the thorax, where it splits into the right and left bronchi; commonly known as the *windpipe*

Review Questions

1. What is the main purpose of the respiratory system?
2. Why are the bronchi and bronchioles collectively called the *conducting zone*?
3. How many lobes does each lung have?
4. What is the function of the ciliated epithelium in the nasal cavity?
5. Which structures are housed in the larynx?
6. Which structures provide rigid support for the trachea and prevent it from collapsing?
7. Explain why a person's sense of taste is diminished when he or she has a stuffy nose.
8. Imagine that you are a physician and one of your patients recently gave birth to an infant with a cleft palate. How would you explain this condition and the treatment required?
9. Why is the epiglottis considered a "gatekeeper"?
10. Explain the three reasons that the process of gas exchange occurs so rapidly.

SECTION 10.2 Physiology of the Respiratory System

Objectives

- Understand the mechanics of respiration.
- Describe nonrespiratory causes of air movement in the body.
- Explain how breathing is affected by neural, chemical, and emotional factors, as well as by conscious control.
- Identify different methods of measuring lung volume, and explain how each method works.

Key Terms

alveolar capillary membrane
chemoreceptors
expiration
expiratory reserve volume (ERV)
external respiration
forced expiratory volume in one second (FEV_1)
forced expiratory volume in one second/forced vital capacity (FEV_1/FVC)
functional residual capacity (FRC)
Hering-Breuer reflex
inspiration
inspiratory reserve volume (IRV)
internal respiration
mechanoreceptors
partial pressure
pulmonary ventilation
residual volume (RV)
respiration
respiratory gas transport
tidal volume (TV)
total lung capacity (TLC)
vital capacity (VC)

Every minute of every day, the respiratory system works hard to deliver oxygen to the body's cells and to dispose of carbon dioxide. Breathing may seem like a subconscious action—something you aren't even aware that you are doing—but there are actually many factors that control respiratory activity. This section explores the mechanics of breathing and the mechanisms by which it is controlled.

Respiration

The main function of the respiratory system is gas exchange, which is achieved through a process called ***respiration***, or breathing. The cardiovascular system and the respiratory system work together to accomplish respiration. Four key tasks are involved in this process:

- ***pulmonary ventilation***: air is continuously moved into (inspiration) and out of (expiration) the lungs

- ***external respiration***: fresh oxygen from outside the body fills the lungs and alveoli, allowing gas exchange between the alveoli and pulmonary blood
- ***respiratory gas transport***: the oxygen and carbon dioxide gases in the blood are transported between the lungs and different body tissues; oxygen is brought from the lungs to the body tissues, and carbon dioxide waste from the tissues is brought to the lungs to be released to the outside world
- ***internal respiration***: gas exchange occurs *inside* the body between the tissues and capillaries

Boyle's Law

The mechanics of breathing can be explained by Boyle's law, which states that the volume of a gas is inversely proportional to its pressure. In simpler terms, as the volume of a gas increases, the pressure of the gas decreases.

Boyle's law affects breathing because of differences between atmospheric (outside) air pressure and intrapulmonary (inside the lung) air pressure. At rest, both atmospheric and intrapulmonary air pressures are 760 millimeters of mercury (mmHg). When these pressures are the same, lung volume, or the amount of air in the lungs, does not change. At this point, there is no airflow (**Figure 10.8**).

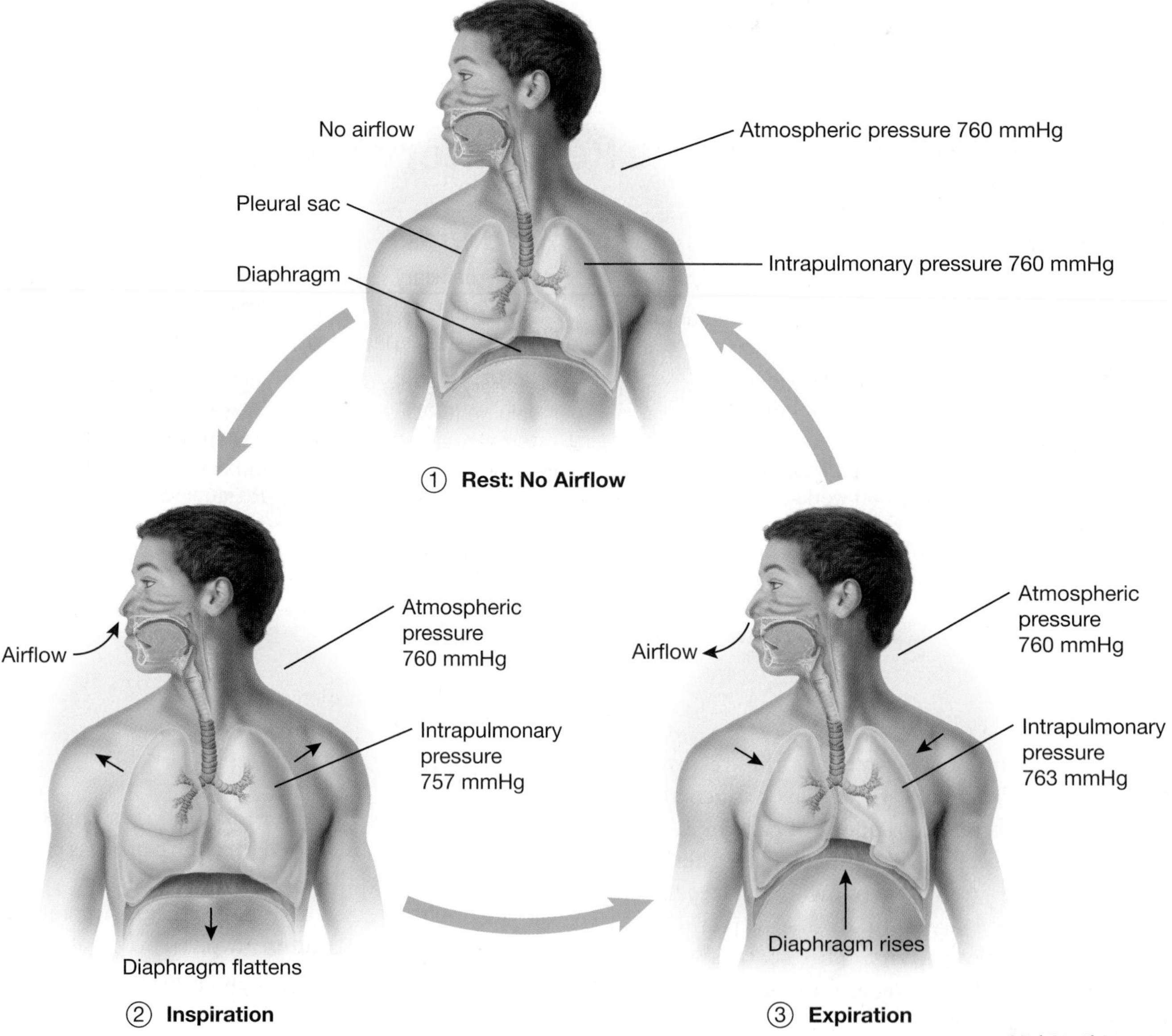

Figure 10.8 Changes in intrapulmonary and atmospheric pressure allow air to flow into and out of the lungs.

For the lungs to be able to take in air, the intrapulmonary pressure must be *less than* the atmospheric pressure. When the direction of airflow is reversed to expel air from the lungs, the intrapulmonary pressure must be *greater than* the atmospheric pressure.

Pulmonary Ventilation

During pulmonary ventilation, air is continuously being moved into and out of the lungs. This involves the processes of inspiration and expiration. ***Inspiration***, also called *inhalation*, is the process by which air flows into the lungs. Inspiration begins when the external intercostal muscles contract, lifting the ribs upward and outward. At the same time, the dome-like diaphragm muscle contracts downward and flattens. Both of these maneuvers expand the thoracic cavity, decreasing its internal pressure. As the thoracic cavity expands, it pulls the lungs with it, and the lungs also expand.

As the lungs expand, the intrapulmonary pressure falls below the atmospheric pressure. When the intrapulmonary pressure is lower than the atmospheric pressure, a vacuum is created. This vacuum sucks air into the lungs until the intrapulmonary pressure is equal to the atmospheric pressure.

The process by which air is expelled from the lungs is called ***expiration***, or *exhalation*. Expiration begins when the external intercostal muscles and the diaphragm relax, decreasing the space in the thoracic cavity. Intrapulmonary pressure rises to 763 mmHg.

Clinical Application **Easier Breathing**

After exercise, athletes and people with COPD often bend forward and assume a T-shaped position. This position facilitates breathing and helps promote blood flow back to the heart. This, in turn, increases ventilation and cardiac output.

When the intrapulmonary pressure exceeds the atmospheric pressure, air is forced out of the lungs.

It is important to note that expiration does not require muscular contraction. This is because normal expiration is a passive process. When asthma or mucus accumulation narrows the respiratory passageways, or when the respiration rate increases during exercise, expiration becomes an active process. Active expiration requires the internal intercostal muscles to forcibly depress the rib cage and contract the abdominal muscles toward the diaphragm, thereby expelling air from the lungs.

External Respiration

During external respiration, fresh oxygen from outside the body fills the lungs and alveoli, and carbon dioxide is transported from the lungs to the outside of the body. For oxygen to reach the body's tissues and carbon dioxide to leave the body, gas exchange must occur in the ***alveolar capillary membrane***, which consists of the alveoli and the capillaries that surround them (**Figure 10.9**).

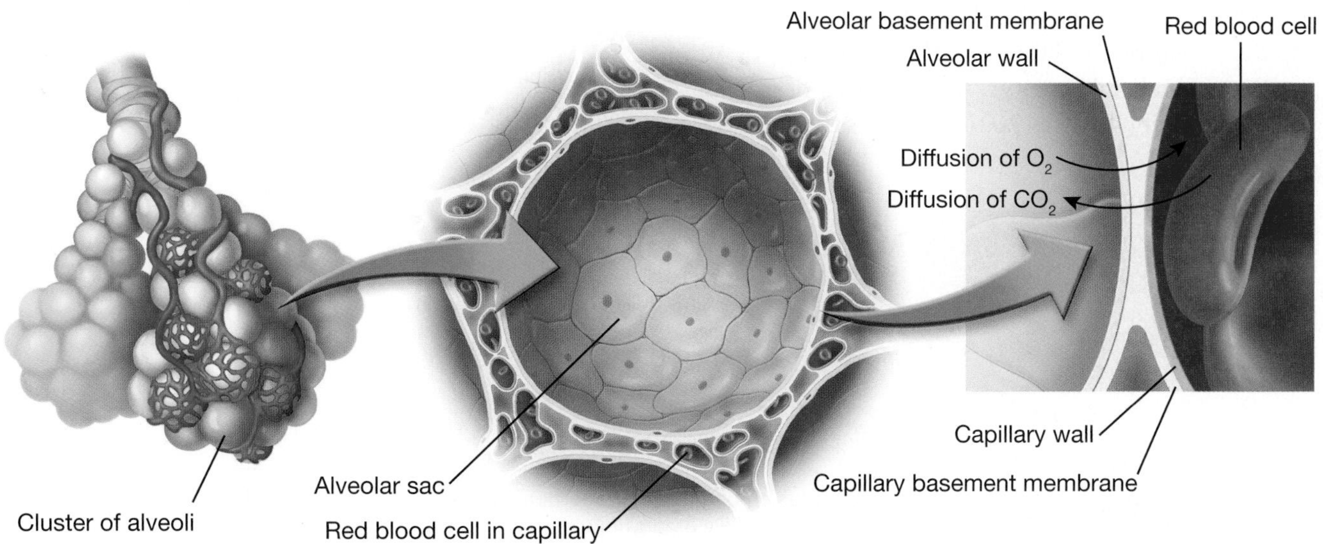

Figure 10.9 Lung tissue is made up of millions of alveoli clusters. Pulmonary gas exchange occurs rapidly because the capillary walls of the alveolar sacs are much thinner than even a sheet of tissue paper.

Under normal circumstances (in the absence of disease), blood becomes 98% oxygenated in 0.75 second—in about the blink of an eye. The factors that allow gas exchange to occur so quickly include surface area, the diffusion constant and partial pressures of oxygen and carbon dioxide, and the thickness of the tissue. The relationships among these factors are explained by Fick's Law of Diffusion.

Fick's Law of Diffusion states that the diffusion of oxygen (O_2) and carbon dioxide (CO_2) between the capillaries and the alveolar sacs is proportional to the surface area (S.A.) of the lungs, the diffusion constant (*D*) of each gas, and the difference in partial pressure between the capillary and the alveolar sac (P_1–P_2). According to this law, the diffusion of gases is also inversely related to the thickness of the tissues (T) involved. In simpler terms, thin-walled tissues allow for easier gas exchange (**Figure 10.10**).

Surface Area

The surface area of the lungs is immense. If you were to lay the alveolar sacs of the lungs side by side on the ground, they would almost cover an entire tennis court. These millions of alveolar sacs provide a huge number of sites for gas exchange between the blood and alveolar sacs. This vast number of available sites allows gas exchange to occur rapidly.

Diffusion Constant of Gases

The diffusion constant of a gas is proportional to its solubility but inversely related to the square root of its molecular weight (MW) (**Figure 10.10**). Oxygen has a lower molecular weight than carbon dioxide, so it should diffuse more quickly across the alveolar capillary membrane. However, the solubility of CO_2 is approximately 24 times greater than that of oxygen, so CO_2 actually diffuses 20 times faster than O_2.

Partial Pressure

The pressure that one gas in a mixture would exert if it occupied the same volume on its own is referred to as ***partial pressure***. Gases always flow from areas of high concentration to areas of low concentration. The difference between the partial pressure (P_1–P_2) of gas in the tissues and gas in the blood is called a *pressure gradient* (*PG*). The pressure gradient between the venous capillary blood and the alveolar sacs is 65 mmHg for O_2 and 6 mmHg for CO_2 during external respiration. Similarly, pressure gradients promote gas exchange between the arterial and venous blood and the body's tissues during internal respiration.

Tissue Thickness

The thickness of tissue affects how easily gases can diffuse from one area to another. The O_2 and CO_2 molecules involved in gas exchange travel from the red blood cells, through the capillary wall and its membrane, and then through the alveolar wall and its membrane during external respiration. These membranes are razor thin—even thinner than a sheet of tissue paper. This razor-thin quality makes it easy for oxygen and carbon dioxide to move freely between the alveoli and the bloodstream.

Respiratory Gas Transport

Respiratory gas transport involves transporting oxygen and carbon dioxide in the blood between the lungs and peripheral body tissues. In the lungs, oxygen is collected to take to peripheral tissues, and carbon dioxide is delivered from the peripheral tissues. In the peripheral tissues, carbon dioxide is collected to take to the lungs, and oxygen is delivered from the lungs. **Figure 11.11** illustrates both parts of this gas exchange.

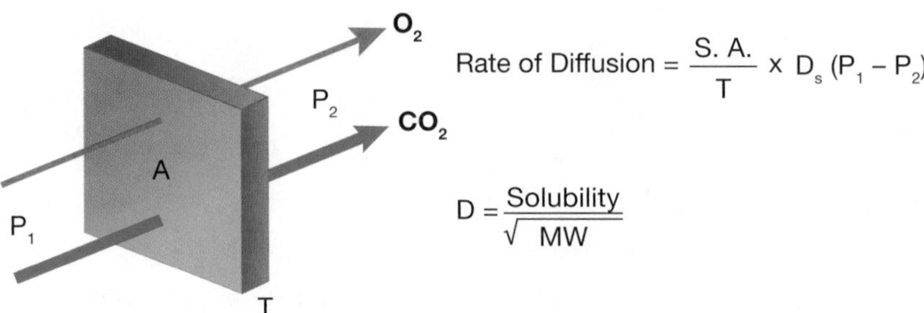

Figure 10.10 Fick's Law of Diffusion says that diffusion of a gas is proportional to the surface area (*A*), diffusion constant (*D*), and the difference in partial pressure (P_1–P_2), and is inversely proportional to the thickness of the tissue (*T*). *D* depends on the solubility and molecular weight (*MW*) of the individual gas.

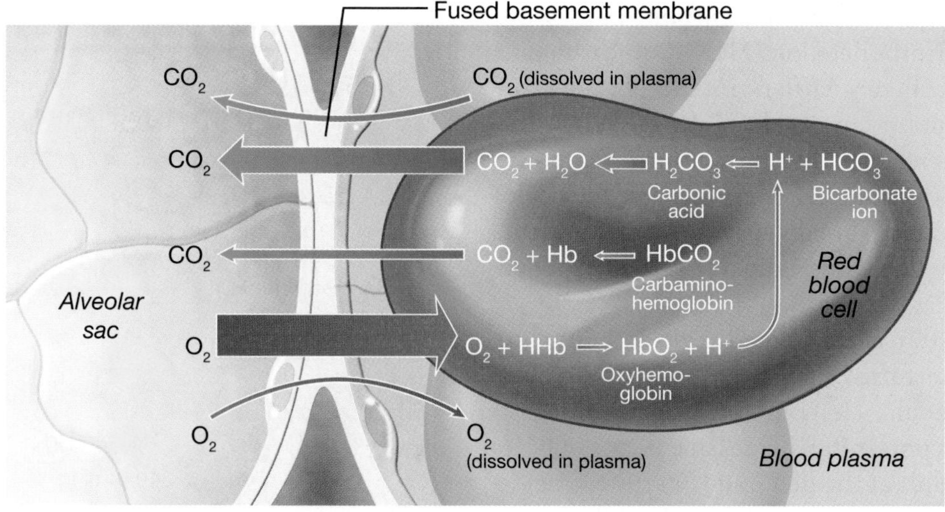

Figure 10.11 Respiratory gas transport. A—Gas exchange in the lungs. B—Gas exchange in the peripheral tissues.

Each gas is transported by binding to specific molecules. Oxygen is primarily transported by hemoglobin. Carbon dioxide is primarily transported by the bicarbonate ion, although hemoglobin also transports some carbon dioxide. Both gases are also transported by diffusion into the blood.

Oxygen Transport

Oxygen is transported in the bloodstream in two ways. More than 98% of oxygen is transported by hemoglobin, a protein found in the body's 20–30 million red blood cells. In the lungs, oxygen is picked up by hemoglobin for transport to the peripheral tissues.

Oxygen is "picked up" by binding to hemoglobin (Hb), forming an oxyhemoglobin (HbO_2) molecule. As the oxyhemoglobin molecule is transported throughout the body in the plasma, oxygen is dispensed to cells in the peripheral tissues that need oxygen to survive.

Exercise, which causes an increase in the body's pH and temperature, results in a greater unloading of oxygen. These factors help to meet the increased oxygen demands that occur during exercise.

Oxygen is also transported to peripheral tissues by dissolving in the plasma of the blood. However, this accounts for less than 2% of oxygen transport.

Carbon Dioxide Transport

Carbon dioxide is transported in one of three ways. In the peripheral tissues, carbon dioxide binds to bicarbonate ions, binds to hemoglobin, or dissolves into the plasma. Through these methods, carbon dioxide is carried to the lungs for expulsion.

Approximately 60–70% of carbon dioxide is bound to the bicarbonate ion (HCO_3^-). Bicarbonate is one of the primary buffers in the plasma, and it helps to maintain a normal pH range. When the bicarbonate ion reaches the lungs, it forms carbonic acid (H_2CO_3), which is a relatively unstable molecule. Carbonic acid rapidly breaks apart to form water and carbon dioxide. The carbon dioxide is then expelled during expiration.

About 20–30% of carbon dioxide is bound to hemoglobin to form the carbaminohemoglobin ($HbCO_2$) molecule. Hemoglobin has two binding sites: an iron-containing heme site and a globin site. Oxygen binds at the heme site. Carbon dioxide binds to amino acids on the globin site. Therefore, oxygen and carbon dioxide do not have to compete for a binding site. Both are easily transported by hemoglobin. Carbon dioxide binds to hemoglobin at the peripheral tissue and is transported to the lungs, where it dissociates from the hemoglobin and leaves the body.

The remaining 7–10% of carbon dioxide is dissolved in the blood plasma. The plasma carries it to the lungs, where it is expelled from the body.

Internal Respiration

Internal respiration is the process of gas exchange that occurs between blood in the tissue capillaries and the body's tissues (**Figure 10.12**). In internal respiration, carbon dioxide in the body tissues diffuses into the blood. Simultaneously, oxygen in the blood is released from the hemoglobin to which it was bound and diffuses into the tissues, which need oxygen to function. The venous blood returns to the heart and is pumped to the lungs, where the process of external respiration occurs. The deoxygenated blood becomes oxygenated, and carbon dioxide diffuses into the alveoli.

SELF CHECK

1. What is the main function of the respiratory system?
2. For inspiration to occur, what relationship must exist between intrapulmonary pressure and atmospheric pressure?
3. In what two ways is oxygen transported in the bloodstream?

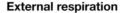

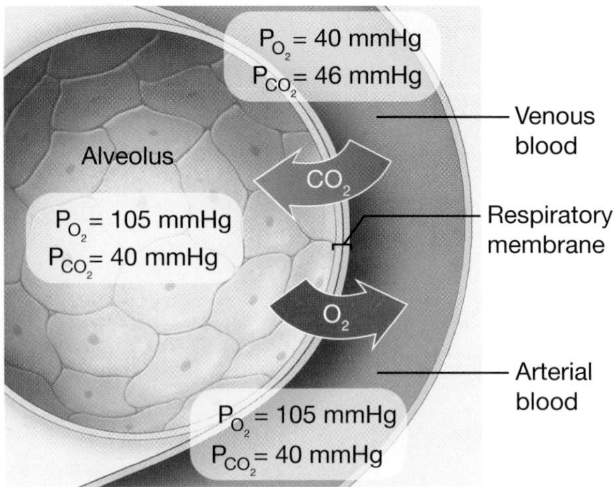

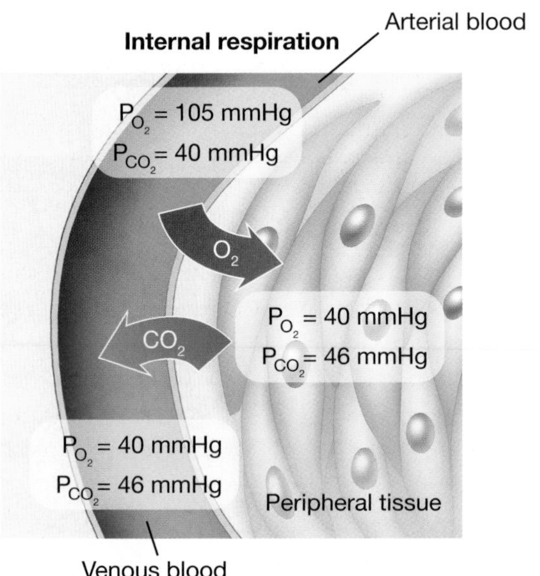

Figure 10.12 External vs. internal respiration. A—In external respiration, oxygen moves from the alveoli into the blood capillaries and carbon dioxide moves from the capillaries into the alveoli. B—In internal respiration, oxygen moves from the blood capillaries to the body cells and carbon dioxide moves from the body cells into the capillaries.

Other Causes of Air Movement

Besides breathing, there are other ways in which air moves into and out of the lungs. These are known as *nonrespiratory air maneuvers*. Everyone is familiar with coughing, sneezing, hiccupping, and yawning, but why do they happen?

These nonrespiratory maneuvers often occur as a reaction, or reflexive response, to a stimulus (such as dust or debris) entering the respiratory passages. **Figure 10.13** explains in more detail how and why these nonrespiratory air maneuvers occur.

SELF CHECK

1. What causes hiccups?
2. Compare and contrast the causes of coughing and sneezing. How are they alike? How are they different?

Controlling Respiration

Breathing is controlled mainly by neural, chemical, and to a certain extent, mechanical factors, although emotions and conscious control also play a small role. The average, at-rest respiratory rate for adults is 12 to 20 breaths per minute. Average respiratory rate can vary based on biological and physical factors.

One biological factor that affects the way people breathe is gender. In general, women have higher respiratory rates because they have a smaller lung capacity than men. Age is another important biological factor. Infants take between 40 and 60 breaths each minute because they have a very small lung capacity.

Respiratory rate may also be influenced by physical factors such as postural position (whether a person is sitting or standing). When a person moves from a reclining position to a standing position, breathing rate almost doubles. During maximal exercise, respiratory rate can increase dramatically—up to about 50 breaths per minute in the average person and higher in athletes. However, respiration does not usually limit the exercise ability of people with healthy lungs.

Neural Factors

Rate and depth of breathing are controlled by inspiratory and expiratory breathing centers in the brain (**Figure 10.14**). These centers are located in the medulla oblongata and the pons, which are parts of the brain stem.

The medulla oblongata and pons work as a team to make breathing a smooth, rhythmic process. The medulla is like the quarterback of the team, setting the normal breathing pace. By contrast, the pons is more of a utility player, fine-tuning respiratory rate and depth while also coordinating the transition between inspiration and expiration.

The medullary inspiratory center stimulates the diaphragm and the external intercostal muscles. This stimulation is achieved by afferent nerve impulses sent through the phrenic and intercostal nerves. Once stimulated, the external intercostal muscles and diaphragm contract, thus beginning inspiration.

As the lungs fill with air, stretch receptors in the bronchioles and alveoli trigger the ***Hering-Breuer reflex*** to prevent overinflation of the alveolar sacs. Once activated, the stretch receptors send nerve impulses to the medulla via the vagus nerve. These impulses alert the medulla to stop inspiration and start exhalation, which means the internal intercostals and diaphragm relax. The pons works to achieve smooth transitions between inspiration and expiration.

Chemical Factors

Most people don't think of oxygen and carbon dioxide as chemicals, but that is how they are classified when it comes to respiration. Oxygen (O_2) and carbon dioxide (CO_2) are chemicals that influence the inspiratory and expiratory centers of the brain. As **Figure 10.14** shows, oxygen and carbon dioxide influence the operation of chemoreceptors to affect respiration. ***Chemoreceptors*** are sensory cells that respond to chemical stimuli. Mechanoreceptors, which respond to mechanical stimuli, are indirectly affected by carbon dioxide.

Nonrespiratory Air Maneuvers		
Air Maneuver	**Cause**	**Result**
cough	a need to clear dust or other debris from the lower respiratory tract	a deep breath closes the epiglottis, and then a forceful exhalation is performed
sneeze	a need to clear the upper respiratory passageways of dust or other debris	stimulation of nerve endings in the nasal passages trigger a reflex in the brain, causing the forceful expulsion of air through the nose and mouth
hiccup	an irritation of the phrenic nerves that causes the diaphragm muscle to spasm	sudden inspirations against the vocal cords of a closed glottis cause the hiccupping sound
yawn	thought to be caused by a need for increased oxygen in the lungs	prolonged, deep inspirations (taken with the jaws widely open) saturate the alveoli with fresh air

Figure 10.13

Goodheart-Willcox Publisher

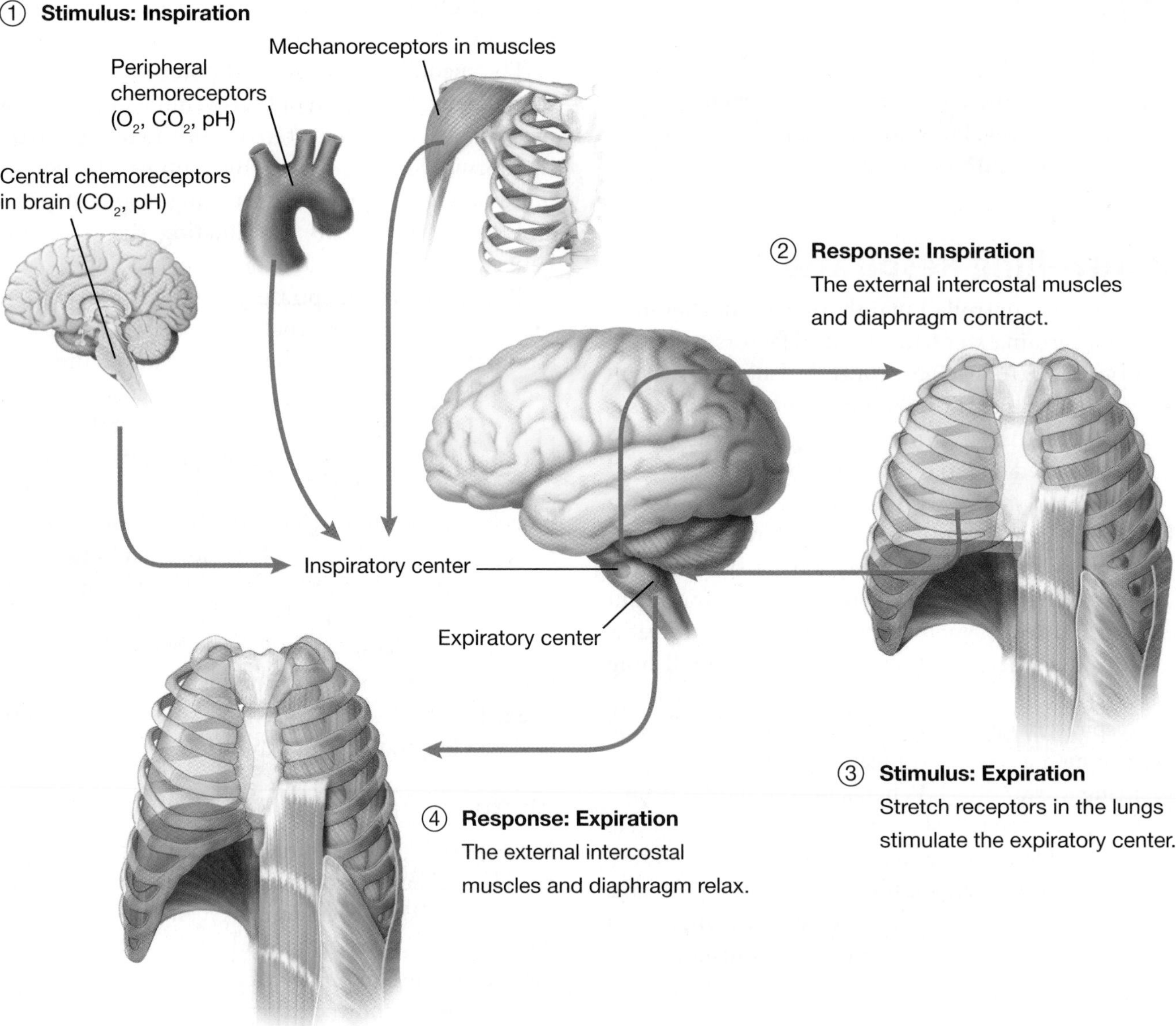
1 Stimulus: Inspiration
Mechanoreceptors in muscles
Peripheral chemoreceptors (O_2, CO_2, pH)
Central chemoreceptors in brain (CO_2, pH)
2 Response: Inspiration
The external intercostal muscles and diaphragm contract.
Inspiratory center
Expiratory center
3 Stimulus: Expiration
Stretch receptors in the lungs stimulate the expiratory center.
4 Response: Expiration
The external intercostal muscles and diaphragm relax.
© Body Scientific International

Figure 10.14 Regulation of breathing. The inspiratory and expiratory breathing centers, located in the medulla oblongata and pons, control the rate and depth of breathing. These centers are stimulated by sensory triggers (central chemoreceptors, peripheral chemoreceptors, and mechanoreceptors) and neural triggers (stretch receptors).

Central Chemoreceptors

Central chemoreceptors are located within the respiratory centers of the brain, in the medulla oblongata. These chemoreceptors constantly monitor changes in the partial pressure of carbon dioxide (P_{CO_2}) and the pH (acidity or alkalinity) of cerebrospinal fluid. A decrease in cerebrospinal fluid pH indicates high amounts of carbon dioxide in the body. High levels of carbon dioxide increase the number of hydrogen ions in the body. These hydrogen ions cause the pH of the cerebrospinal fluid to decrease. As the pH decreases, the body becomes more acidic.

When the central chemoreceptors sense a decrease in cerebrospinal fluid pH, they stimulate the brain's inspiratory center by sending impulses to the inspiratory center via the vagus and glossopharyngeal nerves. In response, the inspiratory center stimulates an increase in the rate and depth of breathing. The result is a fresh supply of oxygen and lower carbon dioxide levels, which helps raise and stabilize the body's pH. In this sense, carbon dioxide is the driving chemical force behind respiration.

Peripheral Chemoreceptors

Located in the aortic arch and carotid arteries, peripheral chemoreceptors are sensitive to changes in the partial pressure of oxygen (P_{O_2}), partial pressure of carbon dioxide (P_{CO_2}), and hydrogen ion (H^+) concentration in the blood. However, they are most sensitive to P_{O_2}. When the P_{O_2} decreases, or the P_{CO_2} and H^+ concentration increase, peripheral chemoreceptors stimulate respiration. Like the central chemoreceptors, peripheral chemoreceptors stimulate respiration by sending sensory information to the inspiratory center via the vagus and glossopharyngeal nerves.

Understanding Medical Terminology

Here is a simple way to remember which chemoreceptors are most sensitive to which chemicals. **C**entral chemoreceptors are sensitive to **c**arbon dioxide. Both of these terms start with *C*. **P**eripheral chemoreceptors are most sensitive to **o**xygen. *P* and *O* are close together in the alphabet.

Mechanical Factors

Mechanoreceptors are another type of sensory cell that plays a role in regulating respiration. Located in muscles and joints, mechanoreceptors detect muscle contraction and force generation during exercise. Mechanoreceptors are responsible for the quick increase in ventilation that occurs when you first begin to exercise. As exercise continues and carbon dioxide builds up, the chemoreceptors handle respiration regulation to move the excess carbon dioxide quickly out of the body.

SELF CHECK

1. What three types of factors control breathing?
2. What is the average breathing rate for adults?
3. How many breaths per minute does an infant take?
4. Where are the inspiratory and expiratory control centers located?
5. What processes do the inspiratory and expiratory centers control?

Lung Volume

Lung volume measurements are used to assess whether a person's lung capacity is normal. The total capacity for a pair of healthy adult lungs is about six liters of air. Abnormal lung capacities can indicate disease or disorder.

Lung volume varies according to age, height, weight, gender, and race. Therefore, it is important to use an appropriate set of normative values as a reference when measuring lung volume. There are two types of lung volume: static and dynamic. Static lung volume is a measure of volume at one instant only; dynamic lung volume is a measure of volume over time. For example, a dynamic lung volume measurement might assess the volume of air the lungs can forcibly expire in one second.

Static Lung Volume

Measuring static lung volume is important because it can be used to determine whether a person has a lung deficiency or disorder. Static lung volume is measured using a spirometer. The person performs a series of breathing maneuvers. First, the person is instructed to breathe normally into a spirometer for at least six breaths so that a measurement of ***tidal volume (TV)*** can be obtained. Tidal volume is the amount of air inhaled during a normal breath. Then, the person inspires maximally (breathes in as deeply as possible), followed by a maximal expiration into a spirometer. This helps identify the person's ***vital capacity (VC)***, which is the total amount of air that can be forcibly expired after a maximal inspiration.

The volume of air that never leaves the lungs, even after the most forceful expiration, is called the ***residual volume (RV)***. Residual volume is important because it allows gas exchange to occur continuously between inspiration and expiration. Residual volume cannot be measured by a spirometer; it requires advanced measurement techniques and calculations.

Other static lung volumes include the following:

- ***inspiratory reserve volume (IRV)***: the amount of air that can be inhaled immediately after a normal inspiration
- ***expiratory reserve volume (ERV)***: the amount of air that can be exhaled immediately after a normal expiration
- ***functional residual capacity (FRC)***: the amount of air that remains in the lungs after a normal expiration; ERV + RV
- ***total lung capacity (TLC)***: the total amount of air that the lungs can accommodate; a combination of the vital capacity and the residual volume; VC + RV (which usually measures about 6 liters of air)

All of these measurements can be obtained with a spirometer except for the FRC, which requires more sophisticated equipment. See **Figure 10.15** for an example of results from a static lung volume spirometer test. Test results are usually compared to normal values matched to the patient's age, height, weight, gender, and ethnicity.

Generally, lung volume does not predict the average athlete's performance. During maximal exercise, only about 65% of the lungs' vital capacity is used. Because high-intensity exercise does not require 100% of the lungs' vital capacity, lung volume is not a limiting factor for healthy individuals.

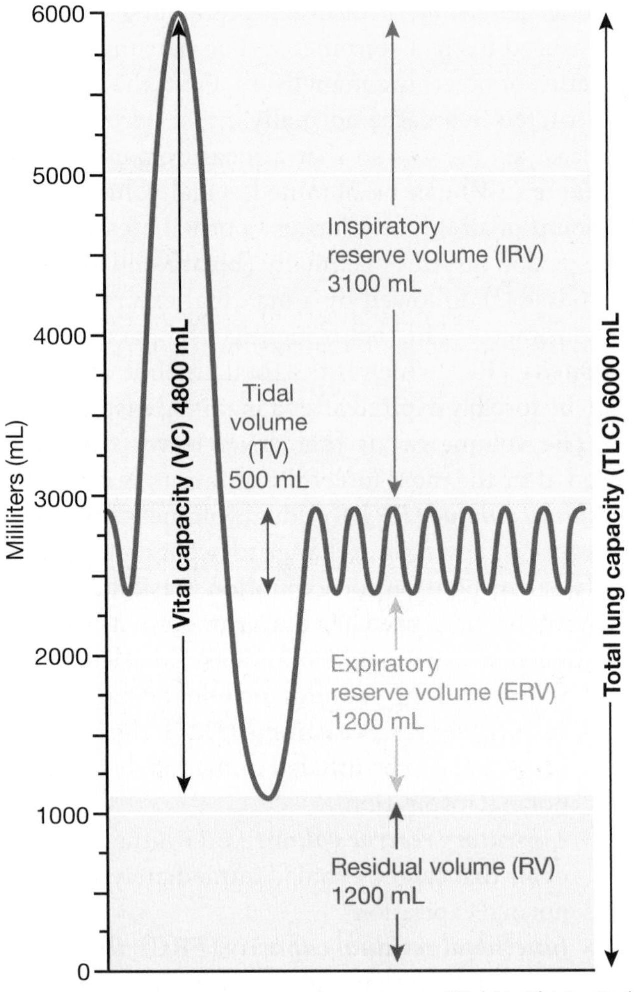

Figure 10.15 Lung volume chart. This lung volume tracing was obtained by a test using a spirometer.

Dynamic Lung Volume

Dynamic lung volume is a measurement of flow rate during a forced vital capacity maneuver. Pulmonary function testing is performed using a computerized flow-volume meter or a peak flow meter to measure dynamic lung volume. The pulmonary function test is very important because it can determine whether a person has asthma, obstructive lung disease, or restrictive lung disease.

During a test of dynamic lung volume, a person is instructed to breathe normally into a mouthpiece connected to a flow-volume meter. After several tidal (normal) respirations, the person is instructed to inspire maximally, and then to expire as long, hard, and fast as possible. The goal is for the person to breathe out for at least six seconds. This may not sound very hard, but most people cannot expire for six seconds on their first attempt. The most important measurements obtained from this test include the following:

- ***forced expiratory volume in one second*** **(*FEV_1*)**: the maximum amount of air that a person can expire in one second; measures the ability of the lungs to expel air
- ***forced expiratory volume in one second/forced vital capacity*** **(*FEV_1/FVC*)**: the proportion of vital capacity that an individual can exhale in the first second of forced exhalation; measures the overall expiratory power of the lungs

People with a chronic obstructive pulmonary disease (COPD), such as emphysema, asthma, or chronic bronchitis, often have increased airway resistance because of an obstruction. As a result, their FEV_1 and FEV_1/FVC values are less than 80% of those of healthy individuals.

People with restrictive lung disease, such as cystic fibrosis or pneumonia, have an increased stiffness in the lungs, which prevents the lungs from expanding normally. Lung stiffness causes static and dynamic lung volume values to be much lower than normal. Lung volumes indicative of some pulmonary disorders are discussed in greater detail later in this chapter.

SECTION 10.2

REVIEW

Mini-Glossary

alveolar capillary membrane a structure that contains the alveoli and the capillaries surrounding the alveoli; the site where gas exchange occurs

chemoreceptors sensory cells that respond to chemical stimuli

expiration the process by which air is expelled from the lungs; also known as *exhalation*

expiratory reserve volume (ERV) the additional amount of air that can be exhaled immediately after a normal exhalation

external respiration the process by which gas exchange occurs between the alveoli in the lungs and the pulmonary blood capillaries

forced expiratory volume in one second (FEV_1) the amount of air a person can expire in one second

forced expiratory volume in one second/forced vital capacity (FEV_1/FVC) ratio that indicates the overall expiratory power of the lungs

functional residual capacity (FRC) the amount of air that remains in the lungs after a normal expiration; ERV + RV

Hering-Breuer reflex an involuntary impulse that halts inspiration and initiates exhalation; triggered by stretch receptors in the bronchioles and alveoli

inspiration the process by which air flows into the lungs; also known as *inhalation*

inspiratory reserve volume (IRV) the amount of air that can be inhaled immediately after a normal inhalation

internal respiration the process by which gas exchange occurs between the tissues and the arterial blood

mechanoreceptors chemical receptor cells that detect muscle contraction and force generation during exercise; they quickly increase respiration rates when exercise begins

partial pressure the individual pressure of a gas in a mixture of gases

pulmonary ventilation the process by which air is continuously moved in and out of the lungs

residual volume (RV) the volume of air that never leaves the lungs, even after the most forceful expiration

respiration breathing; the process by which the lungs provide oxygen to body tissues and dispose of carbon dioxide

respiratory gas transport the process by which oxygen and carbon dioxide are transported to and from the lungs and tissues

tidal volume (TV) the amount of air inhaled in a normal breath

total lung capacity (TLC) a combination of the vital capacity and the residual volume; VC + RV

vital capacity (VC) the total amount of air that can be forcibly expired from the lungs after a maximum inspiration

Review Questions

1. What four key tasks does the cardiopulmonary system work to accomplish?
2. Describe the mechanics of a cough.
3. Why do women take more frequent breaths than men do?
4. How does posture affect your breathing rate?
5. Where are the neural centers for breathing located?
6. What does vital capacity measure?
7. What are stretch receptors, and what role do they play in the Hering-Breuer reflex?
8. Explain Boyle's law, and describe how it relates to breathing.
9. Imagine that you are a pediatrician. A frantic mother visits you in your office with her newborn son. The mother expresses concern that her baby's breathing rate is too high. She tells you that the baby takes many more breaths each minute than his older brother. After testing the baby's respiratory rate, you discover that it falls in the normal range for newborns. How do you explain this to the mother?

SECTION 10.3

Respiratory Disorders and Diseases

Objectives

- Identify common illnesses of the upper respiratory tract.
- Describe common illnesses of the lower respiratory tract.
- Identify the forms of chronic obstructive pulmonary disease and describe strategies for management of their symptoms.
- Explain the physiology of asthma and describe common treatments.
- Understand the causes and symptoms of lung cancer, as well as available treatment options.

(continued)

Key Terms

acute bronchitis
asthma
bronchospasms
chronic bronchitis
chronic obstructive pulmonary disease (COPD)
emphysema
hyperventilation
influenza
laryngitis
nasopharyngitis
pharyngitis
pneumonia
sinusitis
tonsillitis
tuberculosis (TB)

Just about everyone has had the common cold at some point—after all, it is called the *common* cold for a reason! Most people also have had the flu, have a friend with asthma, or know someone whose tonsils have been removed. But how do you prevent a cold or the flu? What causes your friend's asthma attacks?

This section describes the causes and symptoms of several respiratory disorders, as well as treatment options. Some of these disorders cannot be cured, but others can be prevented by behavior as simple as hand washing.

Illnesses of the Upper Respiratory Tract

Upper respiratory tract illnesses, or URIs, are the most common acute respiratory illnesses. Recall that the upper respiratory tract includes the nose, nasal cavity, sinuses, pharynx, and larynx. Infection and inflammation of the upper respiratory tract can lead to a variety of illnesses. The symptoms often overlap, and it is not uncommon for patients to have more than one simultaneously. **Figure 10.16** lists the causes and symptoms of common upper respiratory tract illnesses.

Pharyngitis and Nasopharyngitis

An inflammation of the pharynx, or throat, is known as ***pharyngitis***. When the nasal passages are also involved, the medical term is ***nasopharyngitis***. The common cold is one form of nasopharyngitis. However, the inflammation may be due to infection by any of several viruses or bacteria. When the infection is caused by group A streptococcus, it is called strep throat.

Symptoms of pharyngitis and nasopharyngitis commonly include a sore, scratchy throat; fever; headache; and swollen lymph nodes. Treatment depends on the source of the infection. If it is a viral infection, treatment is generally aimed at reducing the symptoms. Patients are encouraged to gargle with

Common Upper Respiratory Tract Illnesses

Upper Respiratory Tract Illness	Cause	Symptoms	Treatment
pharyngitis	infection from the common cold or flu virus; bacterium such as group A *streptococcus* (strep throat)	sore, scratchy throat; fever; headache; swollen lymph nodes	gargle with saline solution; drink warm fluids; suck on freezer pops or throat lozenges; take over-the-counter pain relievers; take antibiotics if strep is diagnosed
sinusitis	bacteria, viruses, fungi	sinus pain, nasal stuffiness and discharge, headache, fever, sore throat, postnasal drip, fatigue	drink fluids; apply warm, moist cloth to face; use humidifier and nasal saline spray; see a doctor about severe symptoms
laryngitis	infections such as the common cold or flu virus, bacterial infections, allergies, inhaled irritants	sore throat, hoarseness, loss of voice, fever	rest your voice; use humidifier, decongestants, or pain relievers
tonsillitis	viral or bacterial infection; group A *streptococcus* is the most common bacterial infection	red, swollen tonsils; white/yellow patches on tonsils; difficult, painful swallowing; bad breath; swollen neck glands	gargle with saline solution; drink warm fluids such as tea with honey; take over-the-counter pain medications (no aspirin for those younger than 21 years of age); take antibiotics if strep is diagnosed; surgery

Figure 10.16 Goodheart-Willcox Publisher

saline solution, drink warm fluids, or suck on freezer pops or throat lozenges to relieve a sore throat. They may also take over-the-counter pain relievers and fever reducers. (*Note:* Patients under the age of 21 should not take aspirin due to the possibility of Reyes syndrome.) If the source is a bacterial infection, such as strep throat, antibiotics are prescribed as well.

Sinusitis

Sinusitis is an inflammation of the sinuses that can be caused by bacteria, viruses, or fungi. Symptoms frequently include sinus pain, nasal stuffiness and discharge, headache, fever, sore throat, postnasal drip, and fatigue.

Treatment for sinusitis caused by nonbacterial microbes includes drinking fluids, using a humidifier or nasal saline spray, and applying a warm, moist cloth to the face. If symptoms are severe, a physician should be consulted; the infection may be bacterial and require an antibiotic.

Laryngitis

Inflammation of the larynx, or voice box, is called ***laryngitis***. Like pharyngitis and sinusitis, common causes include viral and bacterial infections. Laryngitis can also be caused by allergies or inhaled irritants, such as harsh chemicals or dust particles.

Symptoms include a sore throat, hoarseness or loss of voice, and fever. Treatment generally includes resting the voice, using a humidifier, and taking over-the-counter decongestants and pain relievers.

Tonsillitis

When inflammation occurs in the tonsils, ***tonsillitis*** is diagnosed. This, too, can be caused by viral or bacterial infection, including group A streptococcus. Symptoms include red, swollen tonsils; white or yellow patches on the tonsils; difficult, painful swallowing; bad breath; and swollen neck glands.

Treatment for tonsillitis is similar to that for other types of throat inflammation. Patients are encouraged to gargle with saline solution and drink warm fluids such as tea with honey. Over-the-counter pain relievers are often prescribed, as well as a prescription antibiotic if streptococcus or another type of bacteria is responsible for the infection. Surgery to remove the tonsils may also be recommended in severe cases.

Influenza

Influenza, or the flu, is a viral infection that affects the respiratory system. Unlike a cold, the symptoms of which come on slowly, the flu strikes quickly. Symptoms include a fever of 100°F (38°C) or higher, headache, nasal congestion, alternating chills and sweats, a dry cough, fatigue, and aching muscles, especially in the back, arms, and legs.

From November through March each year, the flu strikes the Northern Hemisphere in epidemic proportions. According to the Centers for Disease Control (CDC), 5% to 20% of the US population is infected with the flu each year, and more than 200,000 people are hospitalized because of flu-related complications. The CDC also reports that, on average, there are about 25,000 influenza-related deaths each year in the United States, although this number can vary greatly from year to year. The CDC estimates that school-aged children (5 to 17 years of age) in the United States miss 38 million days of school each year because of the flu.

The single best way to protect against seasonal flu is to get the seasonal influenza vaccine each year. It is necessary to be vaccinated on a yearly basis because there is not one, but hundreds or perhaps even thousands of flu viruses. The prevalent strains differ from year to year. Researchers attempt to predict which strains are most likely to affect people in a given year and prepare the vaccine to address those strains.

Avoiding URIs

Most people get between two and four colds per year. According to the Cleveland Clinic, there are 12 million medical visits for pharyngitis and 20 billion cases of bacterial sinusitis each year.

Transmission of upper respiratory illnesses such as nasopharyngitis occurs through direct hand-to-hand contact, by handling a contaminated object, and via airborne droplets produced by unprotected sneezing or coughing. Proper respiratory etiquette and hand hygiene are the most effective techniques for preventing URIs (**Figure 10.17** and **Figure 10.18**):

- Cover your nose and mouth with a tissue when you cough or sneeze and dispose of the tissue in the nearest waste container. If a tissue is unavailable, sneeze or cough into your hands and then immediately wash your hands thoroughly.

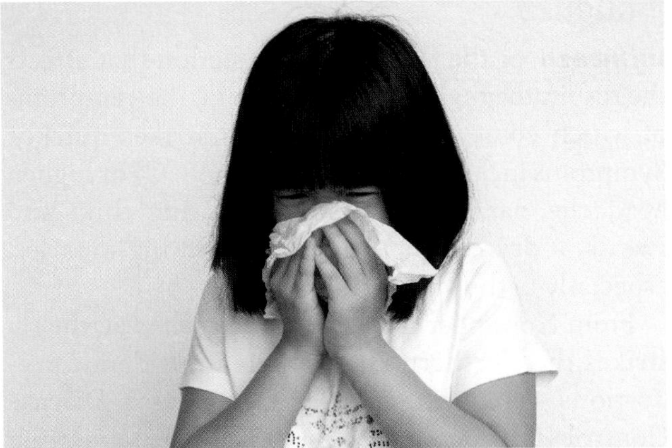

BlurryMe/Shutterstock.com

Figure 10.17 Cover your nose and mouth with a tissue when coughing or sneezing, and dispose of the tissue in the nearest waste container.

- Wash your hands often with soap and hot water. Use an alcohol-based hand sanitizer if soap and water are not available.
- Decrease the spread of germs by avoiding touching your eyes, nose, or mouth with your hands.
- If you suspect that you have a URI, avoid touching or shaking hands with other people.

SELF CHECK

1. How are treatment options different for infections caused by viruses and those caused by bacteria?
2. How many colds does the average person contract each year?
3. Which URI is characterized by red, swollen tonsils and swollen neck glands?

Illnesses of the Lower Respiratory Tract

Recall that the lower respiratory tract includes the trachea, bronchi, bronchioles, alveoli, and lungs. The most common diseases associated with the lower respiratory tract are bronchitis, pneumonia, and tuberculosis.

Acute Bronchitis

Generally, bronchitis is classified as either *acute* or *chronic*. ***Acute bronchitis*** is an inflammation of the mucous membranes that line the trachea and bronchial passageways. You will learn about chronic bronchitis later in this section.

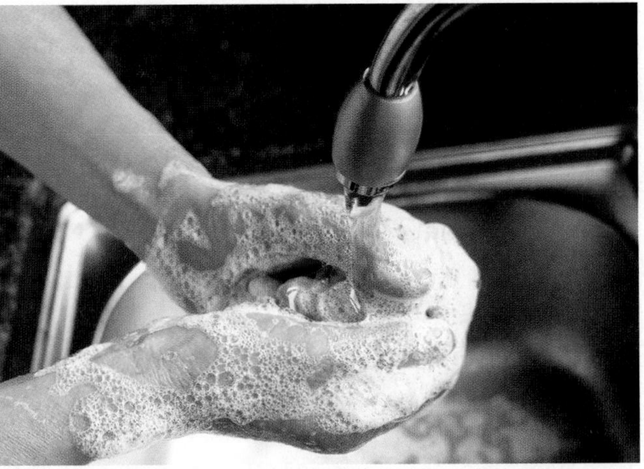

Liu Jixing/Shutterstock.com

Figure 10.18 Wash your hands with hot, soapy water for 20 seconds.

Acute bronchitis is characterized by a cough that may or may not produce mucus. This illness usually develops as a result of an ongoing viral infection, such as influenza or a cold, although it may also be caused by bacterial infection in some cases. Treatment for acute bronchitis varies based on the patient's symptoms. However, it often includes the use of nonsteroidal anti-inflammatory drugs (NSAIDs), decongestants, and expectorants (medications that expel mucus). Bacterial bronchitis also requires an antibiotic, but antibiotics are not prescribed for viral bronchitis because antibiotics are not effective against viruses.

Pneumonia

Pneumonia is an infection of the lungs. It is usually caused by a virus or bacterium, but some pneumonia infections are caused by a fungus or parasite.

The immune response to the invading virus or bacterium damages and sometimes kills the cells of the lungs. Fluid also builds up in the lungs, making gas exchange difficult. Symptoms of pneumonia include cough, fever, chills, fatigue, shortness of breath, nausea, vomiting, and diarrhea. Pneumonia is diagnosed through examination of chest X-rays and cell cultures. Treatment of pneumonia includes antibiotics, if the infection is caused by a bacterium, and supplemental oxygen, as necessary.

Tuberculosis

Tuberculosis (TB) is a highly contagious infection caused by *Mycobacterium tuberculosis*. This bacterium most commonly attacks the lungs, but it can spread to other organs, such as those in the digestive, nervous,

Clinical Application Assessing Someone for Breathing Disorders without Equipment

Being aware of certain clues or symptoms can help you determine whether a person has a breathing disorder. Ask yourself these questions when assessing people for breathing disorders:

- Is their breathing regular, labored, or are they using purse-lipped breathing?
- Are their lips or fingernails bluish?
- Are they leaning forward and resting their hands on their thighs?
- Are they able to speak, or is their breathing making it difficult to speak?
- Can you hear wheezing or gurgling during their breathing?

or lymphatic systems. TB is contracted by breathing in air droplets from the cough or sneeze of an infected person.

Symptoms of TB include fever, fatigue, unintentional weight loss, and excessive sweating, especially at night. People with TB also develop a cough that may produce mucus or blood.

Most forms of TB can be treated with antibiotics, but some new forms of the disease are drug resistant. Individuals with TB must be quarantined at home or in the hospital for 2 to 4 weeks to avoid spreading this contagious disease to others.

SELF CHECK

1. Name three common diseases associated with the lower respiratory tract.
2. What causes tuberculosis, and how can people catch this disease?

Chronic Obstructive Pulmonary Disease

The term ***chronic obstructive pulmonary disease (COPD)*** describes any lung disorder characterized by a long-term airway obstruction that makes it difficult to breathe. The CDC reports that COPD is the third leading cause of death in the United States and a major cause of long-term disability. According to the World Health Organization, COPD accounts for 5% of all deaths worldwide.

People with COPD are more likely to have frequent respiratory infections such as cold and flu viruses, pneumonia, or a cough that produces mucus. They also experience dyspnea (difficulty breathing), which progressively worsens as they live with COPD. Breathing—something that many people take for granted—is an exhausting experience for COPD patients. Difficulty breathing leaves many COPD patients unable to participate in everyday activities. The challenges associated with managing COPD can also cause patients to develop depression.

Two of the most common forms of COPD are emphysema and chronic bronchitis. Although they are both classified as obstructive lung disease, these diseases are quite different.

Emphysema

Emphysema is a form of COPD that leads to chronic inflammation in the lungs. Smoking is the most common cause. Other causes include exposure to air pollution and occupational exposure to dust and other irritants. The inflammation damages the air passages distal to the terminal bronchioles, particularly the alveolar ducts and alveolar sacs (**Figure 10.19**). The alveolar capillary membrane is also damaged. This damage decreases the surface area of the lungs, limiting the number of sites available for gas exchange. As emphysema progresses, the alveolar sacs rupture, leading to even less opportunity for gas exchange and a buildup of carbon dioxide in the lungs.

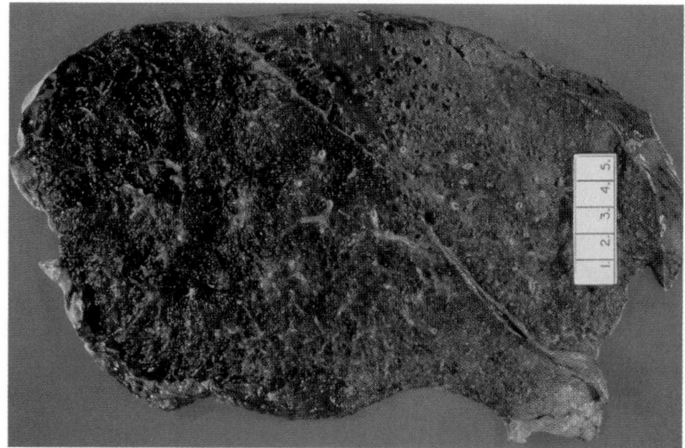

Dr. E. Walker/Science Source

Figure 10.19 A lung damaged by emphysema. Compare the damaged (black) area on the left with the normal lung tissue on the right.

To compensate for poor gas exchange, the body triggers ***hyperventilation***, which increases the respiratory rate. Hyperventilation is an attempt to bring in more oxygen while allowing the lungs to dispose of accumulated carbon dioxide.

People with emphysema work so hard to breathe normally that they often lose weight. Their exertion also causes their faces to develop a pink hue or color. The characteristic pink cheeks and labored breathing of COPD patients have resulted in the descriptive term "pink puffers" among those in clinical circles.

Chronic Bronchitis

Bronchitis is classified as *chronic* when a person has a cough that has lasted from three months to two years. People with ***chronic bronchitis*** have an obstructed airway due to inflammation of the bronchi and excessive mucus production. The excessive mucus limits respiration and gas exchange. It also increases the risk of infection because bacteria can become trapped in the warm, moist environment of the lungs and breed there. The body responds to the mucus accumulation by decreasing the respiratory rate and increasing cardiac output. Unlike emphysema, chronic bronchitis does not cause damage to the alveolar capillary membrane.

The face and lips of a person with chronic bronchitis develop a blue color due to *hypoxemia*, which is a condition characterized by lowered arterial blood oxygen content. Residual volume in the lungs also increases, causing a bloated appearance. These two side effects have led to the description of chronic bronchitis patients as "blue bloaters."

Causes of COPD

The most common cause of COPD is cigarette, cigar, or pipe smoking. The longer a person smokes, the more susceptible he or she becomes to COPD. However, not all people who have COPD are smokers. The risk of developing COPD is also increased by long-term, regular exposure to secondhand smoke or long-term exposure to chemical fumes, dust, or pollution.

Treatment for COPD

There is currently no cure for COPD. The main goals of treatment are to help patients manage their symptoms, improve their quality of life, slow the progression of their disease, and treat any related infections they contract. For many people, the key factor in achieving these goals is smoking cessation. Individuals with COPD who smoke *must* stop

Focus On Electronic Cigarettes and Hookahs

For years, the health issues caused by cigarettes and nicotine consumption have been widely known. Despite this knowledge, some people have continued to smoke. Recently, electronic cigarettes (ECs) have emerged as a possible "safe" alternative to regular cigarettes.

In particular, young people have been drawn to electronic cigarettes and other alternative forms of nicotine delivery. From 2013 to 2014, the use of ECs by youth tripled. In 2014, the use of ECs by youth surpassed the use of all other tobacco products, including cigarettes. How safe are electronic cigarettes?

While there have been no clinical trials on the safety of ECs, studies have shown that they deliver varying levels of nicotine. Just as with regular cigarettes, this can have a negative impact on fetal and adolescent brain development. In addition, cancer-causing carcinogens like formaldehyde, benzene, and nitrosamines have been found in the vapors breathed in via ECs. In some cases, these carcinogens also appear in the secondhand smoke of ECs. In addition, ECs with a higher voltage deliver higher levels of formaldehyde.

Hookahs, also called *nargiles* or *gozas*, are water pipes used to smoke specially formulated tobacco that comes in a variety of flavors. Hookahs are most often used by groups of people sharing a mouthpiece to smoke, and their use among young people doubled between 2013 and 2014. Hookah cafés and bars are gaining in popularity worldwide. About 15–20% of youths and 22–40% of college-aged individuals use hookahs.

While smoking one tobacco cigarette, an individual typically inhales 500–600 mL of smoke. During a 60-minute hookah group smoking session, individuals inhale approximately 90,000 mL of smoke, far more than by smoking one cigarette. In addition to nicotine delivery, the charcoal used to heat hookahs contains toxic agents (carbon monoxide, metals, and cancer-causing substances) that are linked to an increased risk of oral, lung, and bladder cancers, as well as other lung disorders and cardiovascular disease.

Researchers still have not determined the long-term health effects associated with ECs and hookahs. Therefore, doctors, researchers, and healthcare providers do not recommend their usage.

smoking. Anyone who has COPD should also avoid exposure to substances that may irritate their lungs.

COPD symptoms can be alleviated through a variety of methods. One technique, known as *purse-lipped breathing*, helps maximize breathing and ease shortness of breath. Patients using this technique are advised to inhale through their nose and then slowly release the air through pursed, or puckered, lips. Respiratory muscle training, pulmonary rehabilitation, and supplemental oxygen can also help reduce some COPD symptoms.

Pharmacological therapies such as bronchodilators, anti-inflammatory medications, and inhaled steroids can help expand airways, so these therapies are often prescribed for COPD patients. However, for smokers, none of these methods slows the progression of COPD more effectively than smoking cessation.

Pulmonary function tests, X-rays, bronchoscopies, and monitoring gas levels in arterial blood are used in the diagnosis and management of COPD. **Figure 10.20** illustrates typical results of a pulmonary function test for normal individuals and for people who have emphysema, chronic bronchitis, or other restrictive lung disease (any chest disease that reduces lung volumes). Note the concave expiration pattern for people who have emphysema and chronic bronchitis. This is due to air trapped in the lungs. Additionally, note that inspiration and expiration are limited in people with restrictive lung disease compared to normal individuals. This is because the lungs are stiff and unable to expand.

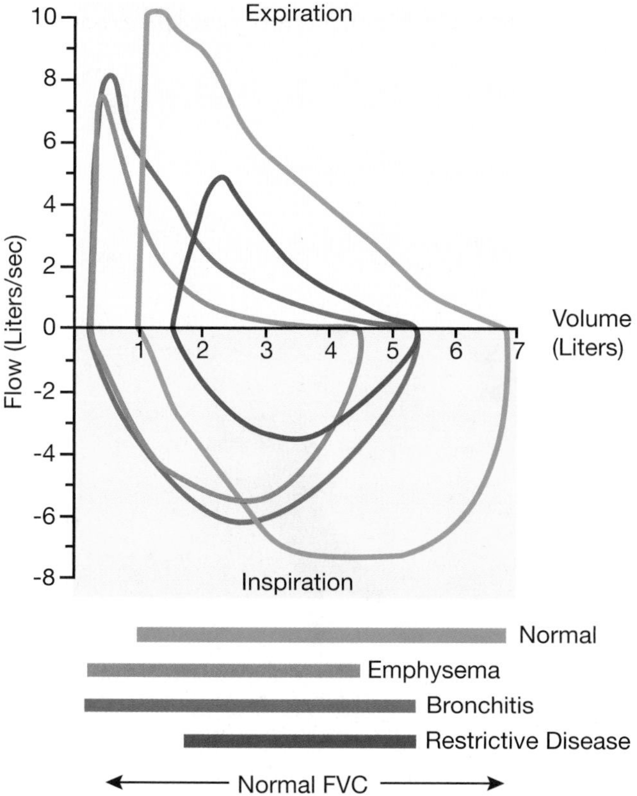

© Body Scientific International

Figure 10.20 Results of a pulmonary function test for healthy individuals, and for people diagnosed with emphysema, chronic bronchitis, and restrictive disease.

Clinical Application Effects of Smoking

Smoking causes 1 in 5 deaths annually, or 440,000 deaths each year. The CDC estimates that 25 million people alive today will die prematurely from the harmful effects of smoking. This includes 5 million people younger than 18 years of age. The nicotine in tobacco is more addictive than cocaine, so a person may experience several failed attempts at quitting smoking before success is achieved. The use of nicotine gum or patches increases the likelihood of smoking cessation, but they, too, can be addictive.

SELF CHECK

1. What is the difference between acute and chronic bronchitis?
2. How is tuberculosis contracted?
3. What is the most common cause of COPD?
4. Which respiratory disease is associated with the term "pink puffer"?

Asthma

Asthma is a respiratory disease in which the airways become narrow and inflamed during episodes called *asthma attacks*. During an asthma attack, the airways are temporarily constricted by ***bronchospasms***, or contractions of the smooth bronchial muscles. In addition, the lining of the inflamed airways produces mucus that causes further narrowing. Bronchospasms, inflammation, and excess mucus result in symptoms such as wheezing, breathlessness, coughing, and a feeling of tightness in the chest.

People with a family history of allergies are at an increased risk of developing asthma because many of the stimuli that trigger allergies also cause asthma attacks. A variety of substances and activities can trigger an asthma attack. Asthma triggers include cigarette smoke, mold, air pollution, pet hair and dander, cold air, exercise, dust, pollen, and emotional stress.

Early symptoms of asthma may include losing breath easily, feeling very tired or weak when exercising, wheezing and coughing after exercise, or experiencing a frequent cough (especially at night). A nurse or other healthcare professional can diagnose asthma using a peak flowmeter to measure the airflow from the lungs).

A physician may use a more detailed pulmonary function test to diagnose asthma. Proper diagnosis is important because it leads to treatment options that limit the frequency and severity of asthma attacks, enabling an asthmatic person to lead a healthy, productive life and participate in physical activities.

Treatments for asthma include limiting exposure to irritants that can trigger an asthma attack and using prescription medications such as bronchodilators, anti-inflammatory drugs, and inhaled steroids (**Figure 10.21**). These medications work by relaxing the muscles of the bronchi and expanding the airways.

The prevalence of asthma in the United States has increased dramatically in recent years, with 50% more cases in African-American children. In the general population, about 8% of adults and 9% of children have asthma. This respiratory disease can be fatal; it kills more than 3,500 people each year. In the United States, the costs associated with asthma treatments and lost productivity in the workplace amount to roughly $56 billion each year.

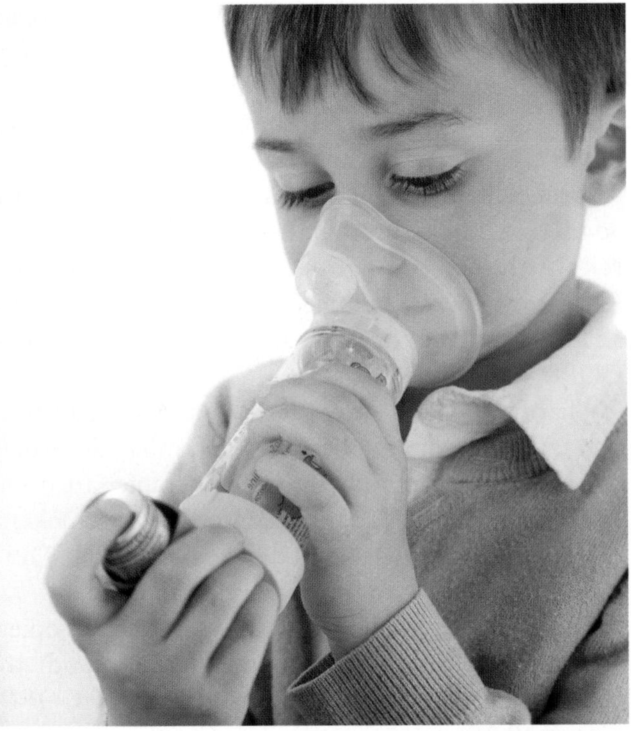

Gustoimages/Science Source

Figure 10.21 The spacer attached to this inhaler allows more of the medicine to get into the child's lungs.

SELF CHECK

1. What percentage of adults in the United States has asthma?
2. What are some treatments for asthma?

Research Notes Exercise-Induced Asthma

Asthma attacks triggered by exercise are called *exercise-induced bronchospasms (EIBs)*, or *exercise-induced asthma*. Exercise-induced asthma is not uncommon. Many people who exercise regularly have asthma, even professional athletes. For example, hundreds of athletes successfully compete at the Olympic Games despite having asthma.

Researchers investigated the incidence of EIBs among members of the US Olympic Winter Sports teams. The athletes tested for EIBs included members of seven different teams: biathlon, cross-country skiing, figure skating, ice hockey, Nordic combined events, long-track speed skating, and short-track speed skating.

All of the athletes in the study were tested for EIBs during actual or simulated competition. The overall incidence of EIBs was 23%. This percentage included nearly half of the cross-country skiing team, as well as winners of gold, silver, and bronze medals. This study demonstrates that athletes can compete at the international level, and even win an Olympic gold medal, despite having exercise-induced asthma.

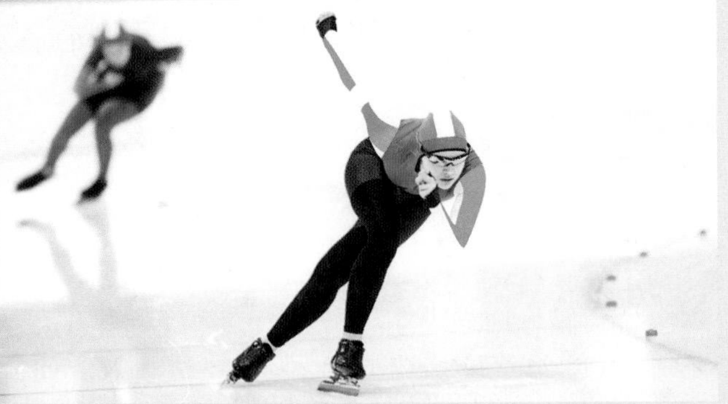

Dmitry Kalinovsky/Shutterstock.com

United States speed skating team. Winter sport athletes often have higher rates of EIB.

Research Notes Pulmonary Rehabilitation

Most patients who have lung resection surgery experience pulmonary complications such as respiratory muscle weakness, decreased pulmonary function, and dyspnea. A recent study published in the *Journal of Physical Therapy Science* investigated whether educating the in-home caregivers of lung resection patients on pulmonary rehabilitation would improve respiratory muscle strength and lessen dyspnea (difficulty breathing) after surgery. Pulmonary rehabilitation has been shown to help patients experiencing these complications. However, many lung resection patients are unable to attend hospital-based pulmonary rehabilitation, so researching the efficacy of a home-based pulmonary rehabilitation program was warranted.

In the study, caregivers in the experimental group received four weeks of training that included information on splinted coughing (holding a pillow over the incision when coughing), stretching and strengthening exercises, and airway clearance. Then, those caregivers practiced these pulmonary rehabilitation techniques at home with the people they were caring for.

Results of the study showed that respiratory muscle strength and dyspnea improved significantly in patients whose caregivers received pulmonary rehabilitation education. Those in the control group, whose caregivers did not receive this education, experienced less improvement after surgery. These findings may help improve the lives of post-surgical lung resection patients.

Lung Cancer

More people in the United States die from lung cancer than any other form of cancer. This statistic is particularly tragic because lung cancer is highly preventable. In about 90% of cases, smoking is the cause of lung cancer. Exposure to secondhand smoke, radon, asbestos, and other toxins are also risk factors for lung cancer.

The majority of people with lung cancer die within a year of diagnosis because the cancer was not diagnosed at a treatable stage. Lung cancer metastasizes (spreads) quickly to lymph nodes and other organs, such as the brain and the breasts, making it harder to treat.

Lung cancer is classified as *non-small cell* or *small cell* lung cancer. Non-small cell lung cancer is the more common, and it is prevalent in smokers. Non-small cell lung cancer spreads more slowly than small cell lung cancer. Small cell lung cancer develops and spreads quickly in the early stage of the disease, often before a detectable tumor forms on one of the lungs. Because a tumor is usually the identifying element of lung cancer, small cell cancer has ample time to spread before it is detected.

Treatment options for both non-small cell and small cell lung cancer include radiation therapy and chemotherapy. Unfortunately, radiation therapy and chemotherapy are often not effective because lung cancer tends to metastasize, or spread quickly throughout the body. In some cases, if the diagnosis is made before the cancer has metastasized, surgery called *lung resection* is performed to remove the cancerous growth.

Alternative treatment options have been developed, including an inhalable, dry chemotherapy drug. One promising treatment option involves creating personalized chemotherapy drugs based on a patient's unique biological response to treatment methods.

SECTION 10.3 REVIEW

Mini-Glossary

acute bronchitis a condition characterized by a temporary inflammation of the mucous membranes that line the trachea and bronchial passageways; causes a cough that may produce mucus

asthma a disease of the lungs characterized by recurring episodes of airway inflammation that causes bronchospasms and increases mucus production

bronchospasms spasmodic contractions of the bronchial muscles that constrict the airways during an asthma attack

chronic bronchitis a long-lasting respiratory condition in which the airways of the lungs become obstructed due to inflammation of the bronchi and excessive mucus production

(continued)

chronic obstructive pulmonary disease (COPD) any lung disorder characterized by a long-term airway obstruction that makes it difficult to breathe; the two most common forms are emphysema and chronic bronchitis

emphysema a form of COPD that leads to chronic inflammation of the lungs, which damages the alveoli and causes an accumulation of carbon dioxide in the lungs

hyperventilation excessive breathing that leads to increased oxygen and expulsion of a larger amount of carbon dioxide

influenza a viral infection that affects the respiratory system; also known as the *flu*

laryngitis inflammation of the larynx, or voice box

nasopharyngitis inflammation of the nasal passages and pharynx

pharyngitis inflammation of the pharynx, or throat

pneumonia an infection of the lungs that causes inflammation; caused by a virus, bacterium, fungus, or—in rare cases—parasite

sinusitis inflammation of the sinuses

tonsillitis inflammation of the tonsils

tuberculosis (TB) a highly contagious bacterial infection caused by *Mycobacterium tuberculosis*

Review Questions

1. What is the difference between pharyngitis and nasopharyngitis?
2. Which upper respiratory tract illness can lead to voice loss?
3. What common illness is caused by group A streptococcus?
4. List some ways in which upper respiratory tract illnesses can be prevented.
5. What are the symptoms of influenza?
6. Name three lower respiratory tract illnesses.
7. How is pneumonia treated?
8. What is COPD?
9. Montee has not been feeling well for a few weeks. He has been coughing frequently. His cough regularly produces mucus, but sometimes it also contains blood. Montee has been very tired and feverish, often waking in the middle of the night because he is warm and sweating profusely. After considering his symptoms, which disease do you think Montee has?
10. Explain the difference between pulmonary function for a person with healthy lungs and for someone with emphysema or chronic bronchitis.
11. Why are people with a family history of allergies at a higher risk for asthma?
12. In what way can purse-lipped breathing help people who have COPD?

Medical Terminology: The Respiratory System

By understanding the word parts that make up medical words, you can extend your medical vocabulary. This chapter includes many of the word parts listed below. Review these word parts to be sure you understand their meanings.

-al	pertaining to
-ary	pertaining to
alveol/o	alveolus
bronchi/o	bronchial tube
chem/o	chemical
intra-	within, into
-itis	inflammation
mechan/o	mechanical
nas/o	nose
or/o	mouth
pharyng/o	pharynx
-plasty	surgical repair
pleur/o	pleura
pneum/o	lung, air, gas
pulmon/o	lung
rhin/o	nose
sept/o	septum of the nose

Now use these word parts to form valid medical words that fit the following definitions. Some of the words are included in this chapter. Others are not. When you finish, use a medical dictionary to check your work.

1. inflammation of the pleura
2. receptor site on a cell that responds to chemical stimuli
3. within the nasal cavity
4. surgical repair of the alveoli
5. surgical repair of the nasal septum
6. pertaining to the mouth and nose
7. pertaining to the mouth and pharynx
8. therapy that involves a mechanical machine
9. surgical repair of the pharynx
10. pertaining to the bronchi and lungs

11. spasm of the pharynx
12. agent that dilates the bronchi
13. inflammation of the nose
14. inflammation of the bronchioles
15. prophylaxis (prevention) of disease using chemicals

Chapter 10 Summary

- The main structures of the upper respiratory tract are the nose, mouth, nasal cavity, pharynx, and larynx.
- The lower respiratory tract includes the trachea, bronchi, bronchioles, alveoli, and lungs.
- The four main tasks involved in respiration are pulmonary ventilation, external respiration, respiratory gas transport, and internal respiration.
- The main function of the respiratory system is gas exchange. Gas exchange supplies the body with fresh oxygen while removing harmful carbon dioxide.
- Nonrespiratory air maneuvers include coughing, sneezing, hiccupping, and yawning, which often occur as a reflexive response to a stimulus within the respiratory passages.
- Neural, chemical, and mechanical factors, as well as emotions and conscious control, play key roles in controlling respiration.
- Lung volume varies based on age, height, weight, gender, and race.
- Common upper respiratory tract illnesses include pharyngitis, nasopharyngitis, sinusitis, laryngitis, tonsillitis, and influenza.
- Bronchitis, pneumonia, and tuberculosis are among the most common lower respiratory tract illnesses.
- Chronic obstructive pulmonary disease (COPD) is any lung disorder that causes long-term airway obstruction and difficulty breathing; the two most common forms are emphysema and chronic bronchitis.
- Asthma causes the airways to become narrow and inflamed; it is generally treated by limiting exposure to irritants that can trigger an asthma attack and using prescription medications such as bronchodilators, anti-inflammatory drugs, and steroids.
- The two types of lung cancer are non-small cell and small cell lung cancer; of these, small cell lung cancer develops and spreads quickly, making it difficult to detect at an early stage.

Chapter 10 Review

Understanding Key Concepts

1. The main purpose of the respiratory system is to provide a constant supply of oxygen while eliminating ______.
2. Which of the following is *not* part of the respiratory system?
   A. nose
   B. lungs
   C. duodenum
   D. trachea
3. The nasal cavity contains oily, coated hairs called ______ that trap particles and prevent them from entering the nose.
4. *True or False?* The palate is the roof of the mouth.
5. ______ are air-filled cavities that surround the nose.
6. *True or False?* The pharynx is part of both the respiratory system and the digestive system.
7. The nonmedical term for the larynx is the ______.
8. The flap of cartilage that covers the opening of the larynx during swallowing to prevent food or liquids from entering the trachea is called the ______.
   A. uvula
   B. tonsils
   C. epiglottis
   D. pharynx
9. *True or False?* The trachea is commonly called the *voice box.*
10. The trachea divides into right and left ______.
11. The air-filled sacs in the lungs are called ______.
12. *True or False?* The left lung is wider than the right lung.
13. The main function of the respiratory system is to conduct ______.

14. Another name for breathing is _____.
15. _____ is the respiratory process by which air is continuously moved into and out of the lungs.
    A. Pulmonary ventilation
    B. External respiration
    C. Respiratory gas transport
    D. Internal respiration
16. _____, also called *inhalation*, is the process by which air flows into the lungs.
17. *True or False?* Normal expiration is an active process.
18. Biological factors that influence breathing rate include _____.
    A. hair color
    B. gender
    C. height
    D. hygiene
19. *True or False?* Your postural position affects your breathing rate.
20. The _____ monitor cerebrospinal fluid pH to detect high levels of carbon dioxide in the body.
    A. stretch receptors
    B. central chemoreceptors
    C. peripheral chemoreceptors
    D. mechanoreceptors
21. Lung volume varies according to _____.
    A. time of day
    B. red blood cell count
    C. body hydration
    D. weight
22. Explain in your own words the difference between each of the following pairs of lung capacity measurements.
    A. tidal volume and inspiratory reserve volume
    B. expiratory volume and vital capacity
    C. FEV_1 and ERV
23. *True or False?* Lung volume cannot predict the average athlete's performance.
24. During maximal exercise, the average person uses only about _____ of the lungs' vital capacity.
    A. 30%
    B. 50%
    C. 65%
    D. 85%
25. Inflammation of the throat is called _____.
26. Laryngitis is inflammation of the _____.
27. Which disorder has symptoms that include white or yellow patches in the throat, swollen neck glands, and painful, difficult swallowing?
    A. sinusitis
    B. tonsillitis
    C. laryngitis
    D. nasopharyngitis
28. *True or False?* Influenza causes white or yellow patches to form on the tonsils.
29. Acute bronchitis usually develops in response to an ongoing _____ infection.
30. *True or False?* People with tuberculosis must be quarantined at home or in the hospital for two to four years to avoid spreading this highly contagious disease.
31. The two most common forms of COPD are emphysema and _____.
32. Bronchitis is considered chronic when a person has a cough that has lasted _____.
    A. two to three weeks
    B. five or six days
    C. three months to two years or longer
    D. ten years or longer
33. What factors, other than smoking, may result in COPD?
34. About 8% of adults and _____ of children in the United States have asthma.
    A. 3%
    B. 10%
    C. 9%
    D. 14%
35. *True or False?* Emotional stress can trigger an asthma attack.

36. *True or False?* Non-small cell lung cancer is prevalent among smokers.
37. Surgery, radiation therapy, and ______ are treatment options for lung cancer.

Thinking Critically

38. Explain in your own words how the nasal conchae filter inspired air. Why is this filtering method so effective?
39. The anterior part of the trachea is supported by cartilaginous, C-shaped rings that prevent it from collapsing. On the posterior side, the C-shaped rings are open and contain no cartilage. Why is this beneficial?
40. Explain the following formula: VC + RV = TLC. What does each abbreviation mean? Why do these two elements equal TLC?
41. Recall what you have learned about neural and chemical factors that control breathing rate. Why is it not possible to hold your breath for long periods of time?
42. Imagine that you are a doctor and a female patient visits your office with a complaint of headache, fatigue, sinus pain, nasal stuffiness, body aches, and chills. You check her temperature and discover that she has a fever of 102°F (38.9°C). She tells you that she felt fine the night before but woke up that morning feeling terrible. Based on the patient's symptoms, what disease do you think this patient has, and why?
43. Identify the respiratory diseases associated with the terms *pink puffers* and *blue bloaters*. Why are these terms appropriate for each disease?

Clinical Case Study

Read again the Clinical Case Study at the beginning of this chapter. Use the information provided in the chapter to answer the questions at the end of the scenario.

44. Among the conditions discussed in this chapter, what may be happening to Jenna?
45. Which diagnosis is most likely?
46. What types of tests would help evaluate Jenna's condition?

Analyzing and Evaluating Data

Imagine that you are a physician and one of your patients is an active, 15-year-old boy named Toua. Toua complains of tightness in his chest, wheezing, and breathlessness. Using a spirometer, you test Toua's lung volume. His test results (shown below) confirm your suspicion—Toua has asthma. Review Toua's test results, and then answer the questions that follow.

Tidal Volume (TV) = 200 ml
(normal = 500 ml)
Residual Volume (RV) = 600 ml
(normal = 1,200 ml)
Total Lung Capacity (TLC) = 4,400 ml
(normal = 4,400–6,400 ml)
Vital Capacity (VC) = 3,000 ml
(normal = 4,500–5,500 ml)
Inspiratory Reserve Volume (IRV) = 1,500 ml
(normal = 3,000 ml)

47. Explain why Toua's symptoms indicate asthma.
48. Review Toua's tidal volume. What explains this low level?
49. What does Toua's vital capacity indicate? Why does a below-average VC suggest asthma?
50. Why is Toua's TLC in the normal range even though he has asthma?

Investigating Further

51. List the most common symptoms of pharyngitis and nasopharyngitis. Do research to find out why each symptoms occurs. For example, a sore throat is caused by mucus dripping into the pharynx and producing irritation and inflammation.
52. Investigate breathing recovery rates after exercise. First, determine your resting breathing rate by counting your breaths for 1 minute. Do this three times, find the average, and record your resting breathing rate. Then run in place for 2 minutes. Immediately afterward, count your breaths for 1 minute. Wait 1 minute and count your breaths again. Continue until your breathing returns to its resting rate. Consider the amount of time it took your breathing to return to normal. What might this information tell you about your level of fitness?

11 The Blood

Clinical Case Study

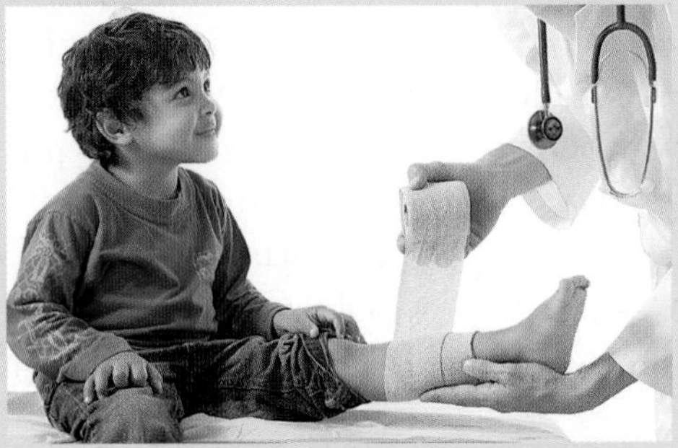
JPC-PROD/Shutterstock.com

Donya, a pre-med student, was excited to be accepted into the summer abroad program that would provide medical services to underserved people in South America. After a thorough medical exam, including the proper immunizations, she was cleared to go. In addition to making a positive impact on the lives of others, she wanted to immerse herself in the culture as much as possible and was eager to try the foods and customs.

After weeks of working long hours assisting the doctors and PAs in treating a wide range of medical disorders, Donya and her classmates helped build a staircase that bridged an impoverished low-lying area to a more affluent area on a hill. The workers accrued many scrapes and bruises, but the staircase was completed, and everyone feasted on the local cuisine. Donya and the others arrived home exhausted but gratified.

In the month that followed, Donya's exhaustion intensified. She lost weight and developed abdominal discomfort. Her parents insisted that she be evaluated by the family physician. Among the medical conditions and disorders discussed in this chapter, what are the possible causes of Donya's ailment, and which one is the most likely diagnosis? What types of tests would help evaluate Donya's condition?

Chapter 11 Outline

People have not always had a clear understanding of the life-giving functions of blood. As early as ancient Greece, physicians thought that draining blood from the body, a procedure known as *bloodletting*, would cure the sick and restore health to the body. This practice continued into the late 1800s.

As you may suspect, some individuals did not fare well from bloodletting. Bloodletting contributed to the death of President George Washington. During a brief illness that began with a sore throat and fever, Washington's physicians bled him. Over the course of 16 hours, physicians drained 5 to 7 pints of Washington's blood. That is equivalent to 40% to 60% of the body's supply of blood! Not surprisingly, President Washington died shortly thereafter.

Today, people understand the important role that blood plays in maintaining health and sustaining life. For this reason, many people donate their blood to organizations such as the American Red Cross, which maintains blood banks. One pint of donated whole blood can be separated into four different components: erythrocytes (red blood cells), leukocytes (white blood cells), thrombocytes (platelets), and plasma. Each component can be used for different people. This process of using blood, called *component therapy*, allows more than one individual to benefit from a single blood donation. According to the American Red Cross, every two seconds someone in the United States will need blood, so blood donations truly do give the gift of life!

This chapter describes the functions and composition of blood. It also discusses blood types and common blood disorders and diseases.

SECTION 11.1

Functions and Composition of Blood

Objectives

- Explain the major functions of the blood.
- Describe the physical properties and functions of the solid and liquid components of blood.
- Describe how the body manufactures blood cells.

Key Terms

buffy coat
coagulation
diapedesis
endothelial cells
erythrocytes
erythropoiesis
erythropoietin (EPO)
fibrin
fibrinolysis
formed elements
hematocrit
hematopoietic cells
hemoglobin
hemolysis
hemostasis
hypoxia
leukocytes
mesenchymal cells
phagocytosis
plasma
platelet plug
platelets
prothrombin
prothrombin activator (PTA)
red blood cells (RBCs)
thrombocytes
white blood cells (WBCs)

Every day, the human body undergoes so many changes that it would be hard to quantify them. Even with all of these changes, however, the body maintains homeostasis through many dynamic regulatory systems. Blood is one of the body's most comprehensive regulatory and transport systems. The blood plays a vital role in gas exchange; body temperature maintenance; and acid-base, fluid, and electrolyte balance. **Figure 11.1** summarizes the different roles that blood plays in maintaining homeostasis.

Functions of the Blood	
Transports	oxygen and carbon dioxide
	waste products of metabolism (urea and lactic acid)
	hormones
	enzymes
	nutrients (glucose, fats, amino acids, vitamins, and minerals)
	blood cells (white and red)
	plasma proteins (fibrinogen, albumin, globulin)
Regulates	body temperature
	acid-base balance (pH)
	fluid and electrolyte balance
Protects	white blood cells protect against infection
	antibodies detect foreign material
	clotting factors prevent excessive bleeding

Figure 11.1 *Goodheart-Willcox Publisher*

Functions of Blood

The blood is a liquid connective tissue. It is responsible for providing transportation, regulation, and protection throughout the body.

Transportation

Blood is a major transport system. It transports oxygen from the lungs to cells throughout the body and removes carbon dioxide from the body cells by carrying it to the lungs where it can be exhaled. Blood also carries nutrients from the gastrointestinal tract and hormones from the endocrine glands to their target organs. In addition, blood transports waste products produced by the body cells by carrying them to the kidneys for elimination.

Regulation

Blood plays a key role in maintaining body temperature by absorbing heat produced by active muscles. The blood redistributes the heat and transports it to the skin's surface to promote cooling. The many buffers found in circulating blood also help the body maintain a relatively constant and appropriate pH. In addition, the osmotic pressure of the blood helps to regulate the water balance of cells.

Protection

The blood's clotting ability helps protect the body from excessive blood loss after an injury. In addition, the blood helps the body fight infection through the action of white blood cells in a process known as *phagocytosis*. Circulating blood also carries antibodies and proteins that attack foreign bodies to help protect against disease.

SELF CHECK

1. What two gases does the blood transport throughout the body?
2. In what ways does the blood help protect the body?

Composition of Blood

The blood has two basic types of components: the liquid component, called ***plasma***, and the solid components, collectively referred to as the ***formed elements*** (**Figure 11.2**). The formed elements consist of red blood cells (erythrocytes), white blood cells (leukocytes), and platelets (thrombocytes). Red blood cells carry oxygen to tissue, white blood cells protect the body from infection, and platelets play a vital role in blood clotting. The formed elements make up approximately 45% of the blood in adults, and plasma comprises the remaining 55%.

The components of blood can be separated by spinning a tube containing a blood specimen in a centrifuge. A centrifuge is a machine that spins rapidly, generating a centrifugal force that separates elements in the blood by weight. The centrifugal force separates the blood into three layers: liquid plasma rises to the top of the tube, red blood cells settle at the bottom of the tube, and a thin layer called the ***buffy coat*** settles between the red blood cells and plasma. The buffy coat contains white blood cells and platelets (**Figure 11.3**).

Separating these blood elements allows health professionals to determine a person's ***hematocrit***: the proportion of the total blood volume that is composed of red blood cells. This proportion is expressed as a percentage of total blood volume.

Hematocrit values range from 42% to 54% of total blood volume in men and from 38% to 46% of total blood volume in women. Each person's hematocrit value is fairly constant, but dehydration can cause hematocrit to increase due to loss of blood plasma, or decreased blood volume. It can also be lowered due to a decrease in red blood cells, which is common in people who are anemic. However, if a person lives at a high altitude, his or her hematocrit may increase to 60% or 65% of total blood volume because chronic altitude exposure increases red blood cell production. This is due to an increased secretion of the hormone erythropoietin by the kidneys.

Physical Properties

Blood is a thick fluid that makes up roughly 8% of total body weight. Generally, blood volume ranges from 5 to 6 liters (L) in men and from 4 to 5 L in women. However, blood volume depends on body size, muscle mass, and physical fitness. Athletes, for example, have higher blood volumes than other people.

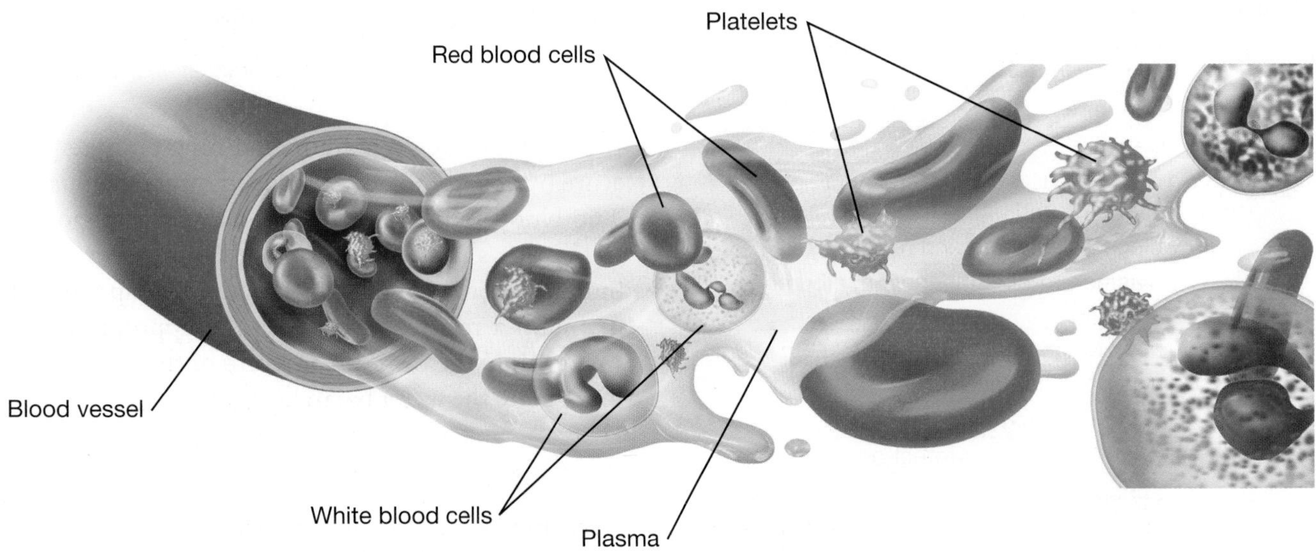

Figure 11.2 Blood has both liquid (plasma) and solid (formed) components.

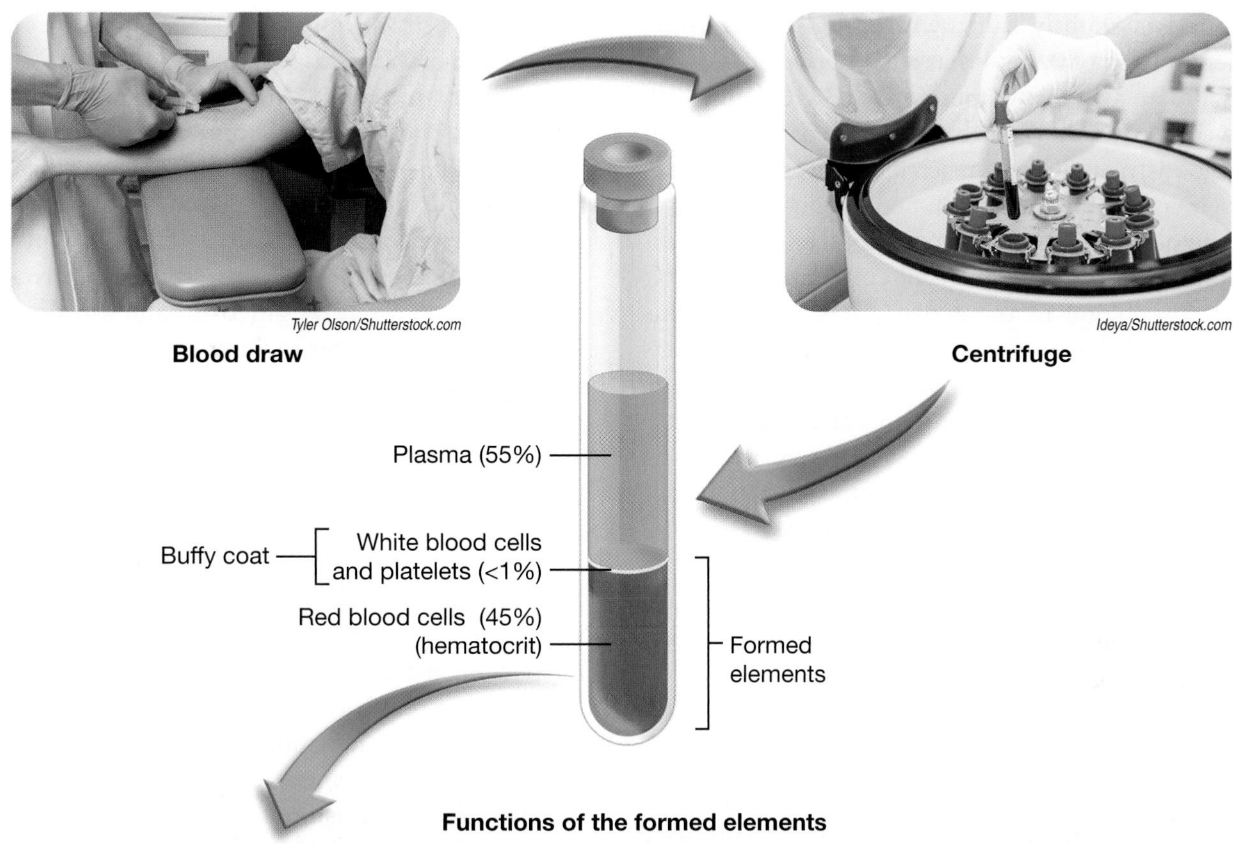

Functions of the formed elements

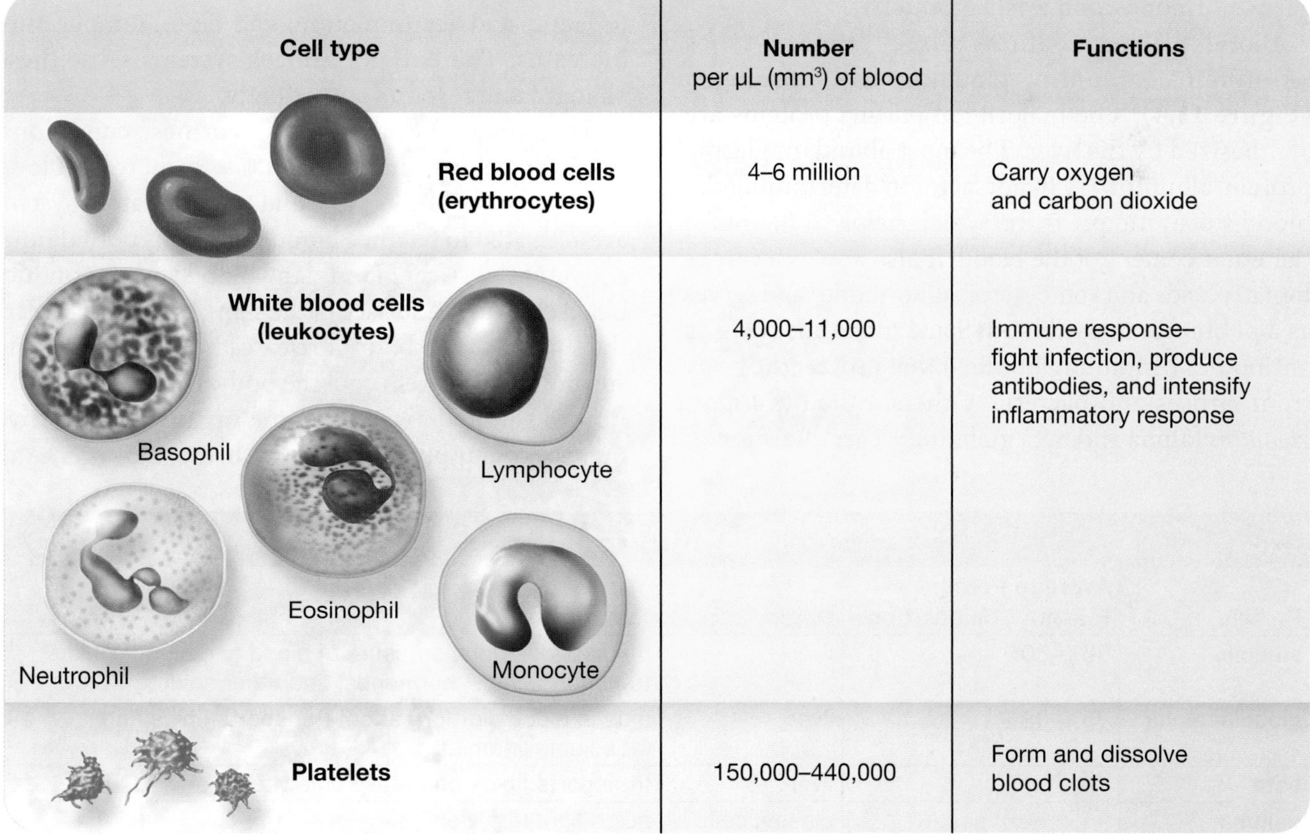

Cell type	Number per µL (mm^3) of blood	Functions
Red blood cells (erythrocytes)	4–6 million	Carry oxygen and carbon dioxide
White blood cells (leukocytes)	4,000–11,000	Immune response–fight infection, produce antibodies, and intensify inflammatory response
Platelets	150,000–440,000	Form and dissolve blood clots

© Body Scientific International

Figure 11.3 Blood is drawn into tubes that are then centrifuged to separate the formed elements from the liquid component of blood.

Blood is slightly salty, with a sodium chloride concentration of 0.9%. It has a pH between 7.35 and 7.45 and an average temperature of 38°C (100.4°F). The color of blood varies based on the oxygen level in the bloodstream. Oxygen-rich blood in the arteries is a brighter red than the oxygen-poor blood in the veins.

The old saying that "blood is thicker than water" is literally true. At its average temperature of 38°C (100.4°F), blood is about five times more viscous (thicker and more resistant to flow) than water. This is because blood contains components such as the formed elements, plasma proteins, and electrolytes.

Blood viscosity contributes to blood flow resistance. In general, the more viscous the blood, the harder the heart has to work to maintain blood flow. Factors that increase blood viscosity include dehydration, decreased blood temperature, prolonged exposure to a high altitude, and an elevated hematocrit level.

Plasma

Plasma is a pale yellow fluid composed of 90% water and 8% plasma proteins. The remaining 2% is a mixture of electrolytes, nutrients, ions, respiratory gases, hormones, and waste products.

Blood plasma contains three primary types of proteins: albumin, globulin, and fibrinogen (**Figure 11.4**). The majority of plasma proteins are synthesized by the liver. The most abundant plasma protein, albumin, is a major factor in determining the blood's osmotic pressure, which helps to maintain the water content of the blood. It also acts as a carrier for fatty acids and some steroidal hormones and serves as a pH buffer in the blood. Some globulins serve as antibodies (immunoglobulins) that protect the body from viruses and bacteria. Others, called *transport globulins* (alpha and beta globulins), carry hormones, electrolytes, iron, lipids, and fat-soluble vitamins. Fibrinogen plays a vital role in blood clotting.

Other organic compounds found in plasma include electrolytes, nutrients, regulatory substances, and waste products. The electrolytes include sodium, potassium, chloride, magnesium, and calcium, all of which help maintain fluid and electrolyte balance. Nutrients include lipids (cholesterol, fatty acids, glycerol), carbohydrates (mainly glucose), and amino acids. Regulatory substances include hormones, enzymes, and vitamins. Waste products such as urea, uric acid, creatinine, bilirubin, and ammonia are carried to various sites for disposal.

The composition of plasma is similar to that of interstitial fluid because water, electrolytes, and small solutes are constantly exchanged between the walls of the capillaries and the interstitial fluid in the tissues. Homeostatic mechanisms monitor and maintain relatively constant plasma composition. Maintaining homeostasis requires constant effort by many of the body's organs. Think about all the changes that take place in the body during a 30-minute run, for example. As the exercise session continues, blood glucose levels decline, blood pH becomes more acidic due to lactic acid accumulation, and blood temperature increases. The body's feedback systems sense these changes and respond accordingly.

To maintain homeostasis under these conditions, the liver begins gluconeogenesis to increase blood glucose levels. The kidneys and the respiratory system are activated to balance blood pH, the hypothalamus activates the sweat glands, and blood vessels conduct blood close to the surface of the skin. As the blood nears the surface of the body, it releases heat to the person's surroundings to help cool the body. In addition, blood flow is shunted away from the organs to the active muscle to supply the cells with more oxygen and

Plasma Proteins

Protein	Average Percent of Plasma Composition	Origin	Function
albumin	55%–60%	liver	regulates osmotic pressure of blood and blood volume; transports lipids, hormones, and other solutes
globulin alpha	35%–38%	liver	aids in blood clot formation; transports lipids and fat-soluble vitamins
beta		liver	transports lipids and fat-soluble vitamins
gamma		plasma cells	helps fight infection
fibrinogen	4%–6%	liver	aids in blood clot formation

Figure 11.4 *Goodheart-Willcox Publisher*

nutrients needed due to the increase in metabolism. Plasma plays an important role in each of these responses. It would be impossible to maintain the body's homeostasis without it.

Erythrocytes

Red blood cells (RBCs), also called ***erythrocytes***, are part of one of the most important functions in the body—gas exchange. They carry oxygen to every living cell in the body and carry carbon dioxide away.

RBCs are the most abundant cells in the blood, numbering between 4 and 6 million per cubic millimeter. A cubic millimeter is so small that it is almost invisible to the naked eye. Imagine how small RBCs must be to fit 4 to 6 million in a tiny, nearly invisible speck! Red blood cells measure only 7 or 8 micrometers in diameter. To put this measurement into perspective, 1 millimeter is equal to 1,000 micrometers.

Shape and Size

Mature red blood cells are biconcave disc-shaped cells that look like a disc with a flattened middle because mature red blood cells have no nucleus. As the RBC develops, its nucleus is forced out, causing the center of the cell to collapse. This mechanism of development serves three important functions:

- It increases the surface area of the cell, providing a larger area for oxygen and carbon dioxide diffusion.
- It increases the flexibility of the cell, allowing it to change shape so it can fit into capillary openings that are half its size.
- It limits the cell's life span to 120 days. Without a nucleus, the cell is unable to replicate.

Hemoglobin

The ***hemoglobin*** molecule is the functional part of the red blood cell because it carries out the important job of gas exchange. Approximately 98% of oxygen and 20%–30% of carbon dioxide in the body attach or bind to the hemoglobin molecules of the RBCs. As a result, hemoglobin is known as the *binding site* of a red blood cell.

Hemoglobin levels differ between men and women. In men, they range from 13.5 to 17.5 grams per deciliter (g/dL). In women, they range from 12 to 15 g/dL. One RBC contains approximately 280 million hemoglobin molecules. This means that one RBC can carry over 1 billion oxygen molecules.

Hemoglobin is actually composed of two molecules: a large protein called *globin* and an iron-containing molecule called *heme*. Oxygen binds to the heme molecule, and carbon dioxide binds to globin. Each hemoglobin molecule has four heme binding sites for oxygen (**Figure 11.5**).

In the capillaries of the lung, when oxygen binds to the heme molecule on hemoglobin, an oxyhemoglobin molecule is formed. These oxygen-rich RBCs travel to systemic tissue capillaries. Within these capillaries, the hemoglobin in the RBCs unloads its oxygen, and the oxygen diffuses from the blood into the oxygen-deprived tissues.

As carbon dioxide diffuses from the tissues into the RBCs, it binds to the globin protein of a hemoglobin molecule, and a carbaminohemoglobin molecule is formed. The carbaminohemoglobin molecule transports some of the carbon dioxide from the tissues back to the lungs for elimination.

Erythropoiesis

The kidneys regulate red blood cell production through a process called ***erythropoiesis***. When blood oxygen content decreases, a condition known as ***hypoxia***, the kidneys secrete a hormone called ***erythropoietin (EPO)***. Erythropoietin stimulates stem cell production of RBCs in the red bone marrow (**Figure 11.6**).

When additional RBCs are produced and blood oxygen levels rise, erythropoietin levels diminish, slowing RBC production. Any condition or factor, such as emphysema or high-altitude exposure, that results in hypoxia causes the kidneys to release erythropoietin

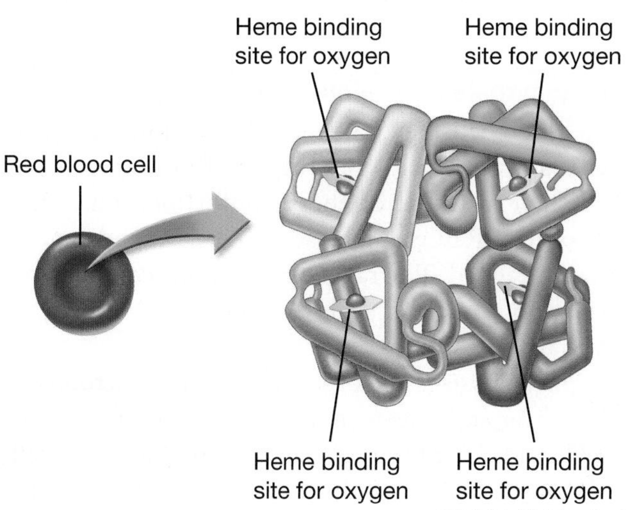

© Body Scientific International

Figure 11.5 During gas exchange, oxygen binds to hemoglobin at each of the four heme binding sites.

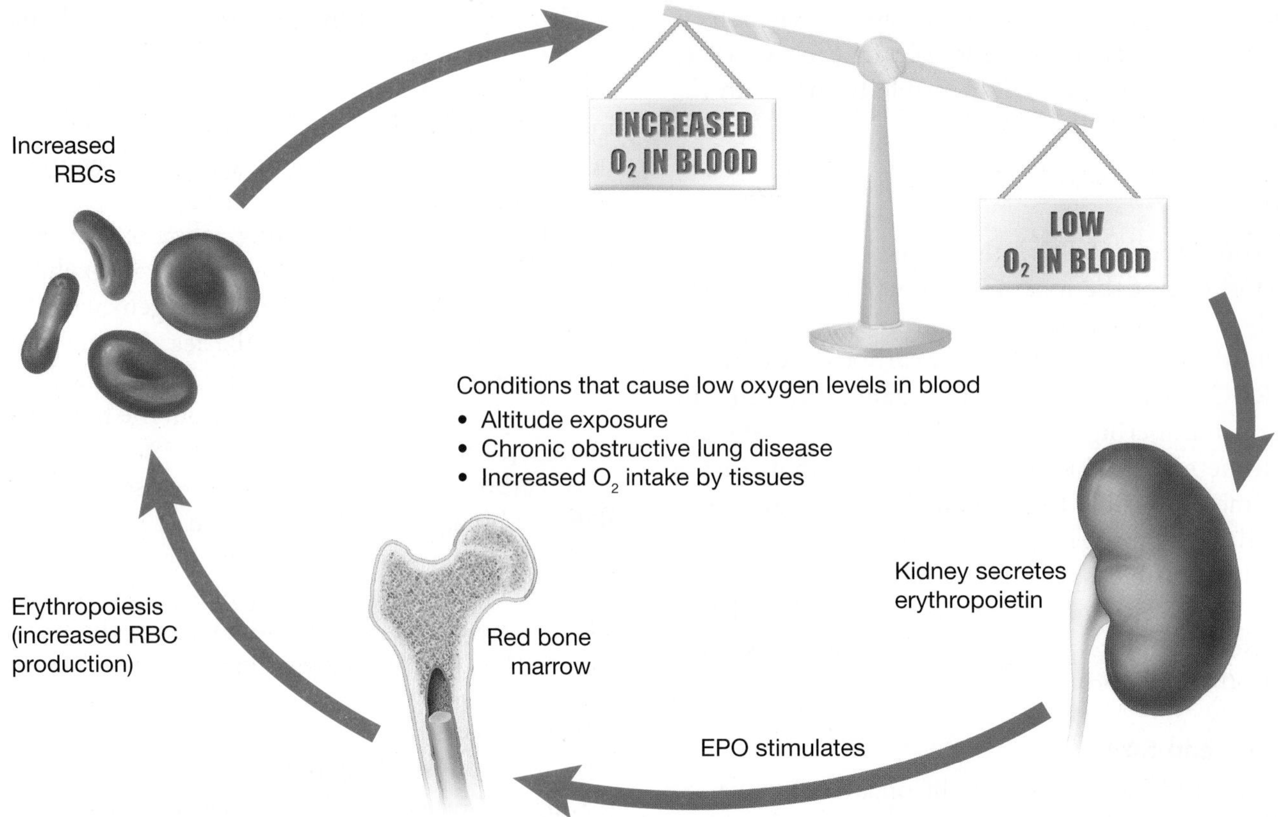

Figure 11.6 The blood works with the endocrine system to release erythropoietin, which stimulates red blood cell production.

and stimulate RBC production. If an excess of RBCs is produced, polycythemia can develop. Polycythemia is discussed later in this chapter.

Iron, folic acid, vitamin B_{12}, and protein are needed for RBC production, as well as for red bone marrow. People who are anemic, and potentially those who have an iron-deficient diet, lack enough iron to properly form the heme component of hemoglobin. The result is iron-deficient anemia, which is discussed later in this chapter.

Phagocytosis and Hemolysis

Red blood cells have the remarkable ability to bend, twist, and turn, allowing them to fit into capillaries half their size. All of these contortions take their toll on the RBC, quickly causing its membrane to become ragged. The ragged membrane, coupled with the lack of a nucleus, seals the fate of the RBC: death by phagocytosis.

Phagocytosis is the process by which macrophages in the liver and spleen envelop, digest, and recycle old RBCs and other types of cells. Macrophages are cells that play a major role in immune system function. Chapter 13 discusses macrophages, phagocytes, and phagocytosis in more detail.

Recycling also occurs through ***hemolysis***, or the rupture of RBCs. This occurs when RBCs approach the end of their 120-day life span. Hemolysis can also result from RBC disorders caused by antibodies, infections, or blood transfusion complications.

With the exception of the hemoglobin molecules, the RBC membrane breaks down easily. For a hemoglobin molecule to be recycled, it must first be separated into its two parts—globin and heme. The globin protein is further broken down into amino acids that are later used to make new proteins. The heme is broken down into iron and bilirubin, a waste product.

The iron is stored in the liver or spleen until the bone marrow needs it to manufacture new RBCs. The bilirubin is excreted by the liver into bile. Most of the bile is transported to the gallbladder, travels through the intestines, and is reabsorbed in the distal ileum. It then is transported to the liver through the portal circulation. Some bile is excreted in the feces.

Leukocytes

White blood cells (WBCs), or ***leukocytes***, serve as the body's infection fighters; they play an important role in immune response. At any given time, blood

Focus On Training at High Altitudes

Many athletes believe that training at high altitudes can improve their performance at sea level in endurance events. This belief stems from the increase in red blood cell production that occurs at high altitudes due to increased erythropoietin. A greater number of RBCs improves the blood's oxygen-carrying capability and the performance of muscle.

What athletes do not realize, however, is that living at high altitudes decreases the intensity at which they are able to train, thereby negating any of the beneficial effects of having more red blood cells. VO_2 max, the best test to measure cardiopulmonary (aerobic) fitness, is defined as the amount of oxygen consumed by the tissues during maximal intensity exercise. Most runners, cyclists, and other athletes who compete in endurance events strive to achieve the highest VO_2 max possible. For every 1,000 feet above about 4,920 feet (1,500 meters), VO_2 max decreases by 3%, so high-intensity training is impaired.

Instead, athletes should consider living at high altitudes and training at lower altitudes. This practice is known as "living high and training low." Research suggests that an athlete's sea-level performance can be improved by living at a moderately high altitude and engaging in high-intensity training at a lower altitude. Living at a moderately high altitude for a certain period of time causes the kidneys to secrete more erythropoietin, a hormone that causes bone marrow to increase red blood cell production.

A recent study on elite runners shows that four weeks of "living high" (at moderately high altitudes of 8,100 ft or 2,500 m) and "training low" (at altitudes of 4,100 ft or 1,250 m) can significantly improve the ability of muscles to utilize oxygen during maximal intensity exercise. Research shows that erythropoietin levels nearly doubled during the four-week altitude training program, which is thought to be the reason for the improved performance.

In fact, oxygen utilization improved by 3%, and the runners' 3,000-meter race times improved by 1.1%. These are significant improvements for athletes who were already considered to be the best runners in the United States.

contains about 4,300 to 10,800 white blood cells per cubic millimeter. For every 1 white blood cell in the blood, there are approximately 700 red blood cells.

Although RBCs far outnumber WBCs, the ratio of 1 WBC for every 700 RBCs is a bit misleading, because WBCs can leave the blood, but RBCs cannot. Through a process called ***diapedesis***, WBCs, primarily neutrophils and cytokines, pass through spaces in the capillary walls as they move from the blood to infection sites in body tissues. The ratio stated above does not include WBCs that are in the body but not in the blood, so it does not represent the true number of WBCs in the body.

As stated earlier, WBCs play an important role in the body's defense systems and immune response. When a foreign microorganism, such as a virus or bacterium, is detected, the body dramatically increases WBC production. Within a matter of hours, the number of WBCs doubles to battle the infection. Generally, WBCs have a lifetime of 13–20 days.

WBCs have an arsenal of weapons that they use to fight infection. Some WBCs, such as neutrophils, monocytes, and eosinophils, engulf and digest pathogens and other microorganisms through phagocytosis (**Figure 11.7**). Other WBCs produce antibodies, intensify the inflammatory response (which increases swelling and draws more white blood cells to the site of an injury or infection), play a role in allergic reactions, or destroy parasitic worms.

Classifying White Blood Cells

There are five different types of white blood cells. Each type varies by size, appearance, and function.

- neutrophils
- eosinophils
- basophils
- lymphocytes
- monocytes

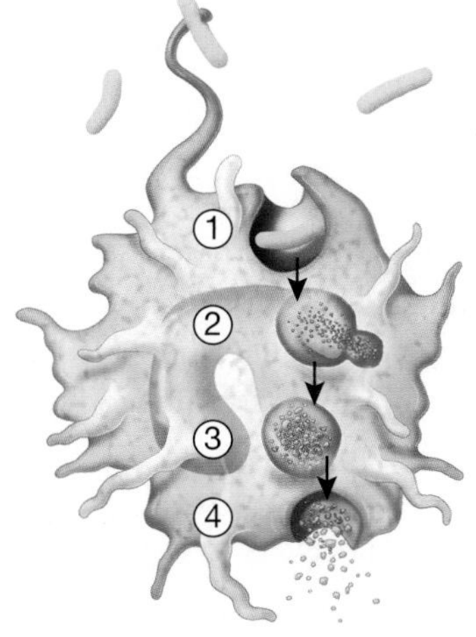

① White blood cell engulfs enemy cell (bacteria, dead cells)
② Enzymes start to destroy enemy cell
③ Enemy cell breaks down into small fragments
④ Indigestible fragments are discharged

Figure 11.7 Phagocytosis.

Research Notes Bioengineering Red Blood Cells

Since Roman times, scientists have been looking for viable substitutes for blood. Doctors and scientists have experimented with animal blood and animal milk. Even wine has been suggested as a possible alternative to blood.

Researchers at the Université Pierre et Marie Curie in Paris, France, have been studying the possibility of manufacturing red blood cells from stem cells. These researchers were able to generate billions of RBCs from a single stem cell. The RBCs were then injected into the stem cell donor. The stem cells were treated with several different growth factors to stimulate them to develop into mature RBCs.

After 5 days, the survival rate of the human-engineered RBCs was 94% to 100%. Of these RBCs, 41% to 63% were still alive after 26 days. This is similar to the survival rate of a normal RBC. This research is critical, especially when you consider how these engineered RBCs might be used.

Each year, the American Red Cross alone distributes about 6 million units of RBCs. According to the World Health Organization (WHO), each year more than 90 million blood donations are made at hospitals, clinics, blood banks, and donation centers around the world. However, some of these donations come from paid donors. In addition, the majority of blood donations are made in high-income countries.

Successful engineering of RBCs would limit dependence on paid donors, especially in low-income nations where voluntary donation is less common. Research continues, but this first successful attempt holds promise for a new way to achieve an unlimited blood supply.

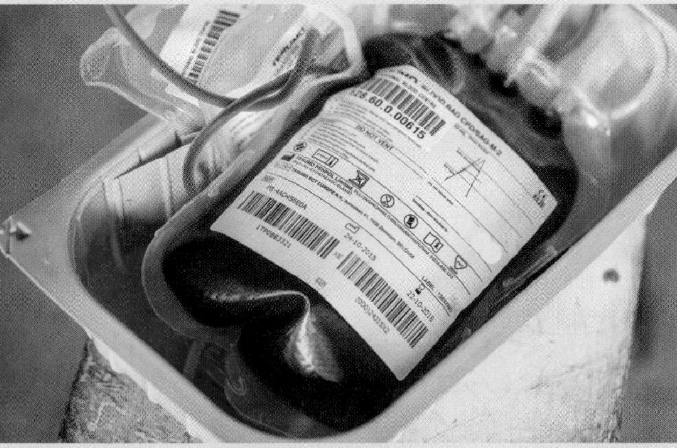

sit/Shutterstock.com

People who need blood replacement today are largely dependent on blood obtained from volunteers and paid donors.

Neutrophils, eosinophils, and basophils are classified as granulocytes because they have granules in their cytoplasm. Lymphocytes and monocytes are classified as agranulocytes because their cytoplasm lacks granules. Generally, WBCs have a lifetime of 13–20 days.

Unlike RBCs, WBCs have a nucleus. The nucleus of a WBC is visible under a microscope when exposed to Wright's stain, a staining solution that scientists use to differentiate blood cell types. Staining can also reveal the presence of any granules. WBCs are classified by size, nucleus shape and color, and the color of any granules (**Figure 11.8**).

Neutrophils

Neutrophils are the most abundant type of white blood cells. They are also the most important component of the body's immune system because they are the "first responders." Neutrophils are active phagocytes and kill foreign invaders such as bacteria, viruses, and fungi. Neutrophils are vital to fighting infection; therefore, a neutrophil deficiency is a potentially life-threatening condition.

Eosinophils

Eosinophils make up only a small portion of the white blood cell count—about 1% to 3%. Eosinophils participate in many inflammatory processes, especially allergic reactions, and are capable of phagocytosis. They are particularly active in the presence of parasites and worms.

Basophils

Basophils are the least abundant type of white blood cells. They produce histamine, which induces an inflammatory response and summons more infection-fighting WBCs to a site of injury or infection. Basophils also produce heparin, an anticoagulant that prevents blood clotting. Basophils are often associated with allergic reactions and asthma. They also play an important role in T cell adaptive immune responses.

Lymphocytes

Lymphocytes are the second most abundant type of white blood cells in the body. There are three types of lymphocytes: T cells, B cells, and natural killer cells. More than 80% of lymphocytes are T cells. T cells and B cells have special protein receptors on their surfaces that allow them to recognize and form antibodies specific to a particular type of antigen. Natural killer cells are capable of killing cells infected with a virus and some tumor cells. Lymphocytes play an important role in the immune response. Lymphocytes are also essential in fighting cancer cells.

Monocytes

Monocytes, the largest white blood cells, are produced in red bone marrow and then move to the blood, where they remain for one to three days before migrating into body tissues. Once they have arrived in the tissues, monocytes develop into macrophages that devour microorganisms.

Characteristics of White Blood Cells				
Granulocytes				
Type	**Microscopic appearance**	**Percentage of WBCs**	**Diameter**	**Function**
neutrophil	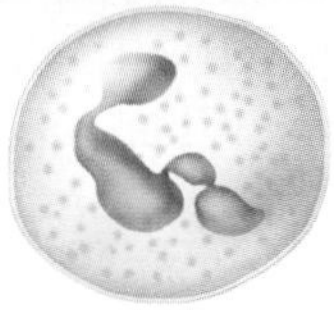 pale pink stain with fine granules in the cytoplasm; multi-lobed, deep purple nucleus	55%–77%	10–12 micrometers	"first responder"; performs phagocytosis
eosinophil	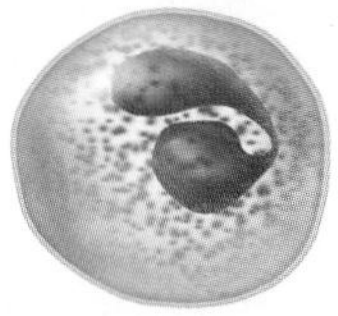 rose-colored stain with coarse granules in the cytoplasm; two blue-red, irregularly shaped nuclei	1%–3%	10–12 micrometers	destroys parasitic worms; controls allergic responses
basophil	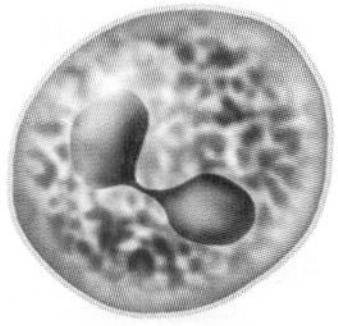 dark blue stain with large purple granules in the cytoplasm; nucleus with 2–3 lobes	<1%	8–10 micrometers	releases histamine; produces heparin; active in allergic reactions
Agranulocytes				
Type	**Microscopic appearance**	**Percentage of WBCs**	**Diameter**	**Function**
lymphocyte	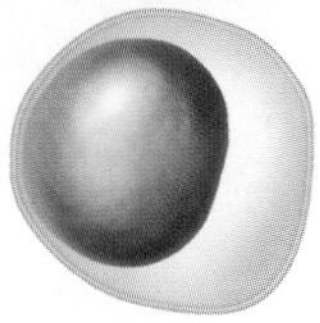 light blue-stained cytoplasm and dark blue, disc-shaped nucleus	25%–33%	7–8 micrometers	forms antibodies to fight antigens; fights cancer cells; T cells and B cells
monocyte	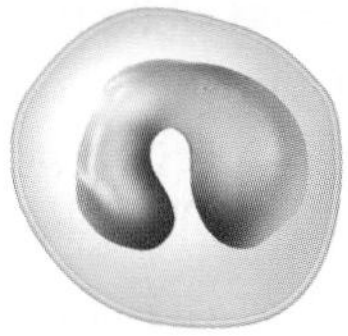 grayish-blue cytoplasm; blue-purple stained, kidney-shaped nucleus	2%–10%	7.5–10 micrometers	morphs into macrophage that removes dead cell debris and attacks microorganisms

Figure 11.8

© Body Scientific International; Goodheart-Willcox Publisher

Thrombocytes

Thrombocytes, also called ***platelets***, are part of the formed elements of the blood. They are small, irregularly shaped cell fragments and have a lifetime of 8–9 days. As cell fragments, platelets do not have a nucleus. Old platelets are removed from the body by phagocytosis in the spleen and liver.

Platelets are derived from multinucleated megakaryocytes, which are specialized bone marrow cells. Like red and white blood cells, megakaryocytes develop from a hematopoietic stem cell. The hormone thrombopoietin (thrahm-boh-POY-eh-tin) regulates platelet production from megakaryocytes. Thrombopoietin is produced by the liver and kidneys.

Platelets play an important role in ***hemostasis***, the sequence of events that causes blood clots to form and bleeding to stop (**Figure 11.9**). Hemostasis involves four key steps:

1. **Vessel wall injury and constriction.** When the endothelium, or inner lining of a blood vessel, is injured, it releases endothelin (ehn-doh-THEE-lin), a hormone that causes the blood vessel to constrict and spasm for several minutes. This constriction helps reduce blood loss at the site of the vessel wall injury. Under normal circumstances, platelets do not adhere to the blood vessel wall because the wall is coated with a platelet repellent called *prostacyclin*. When the blood vessel wall is injured, collagen fibers along the wall are exposed.

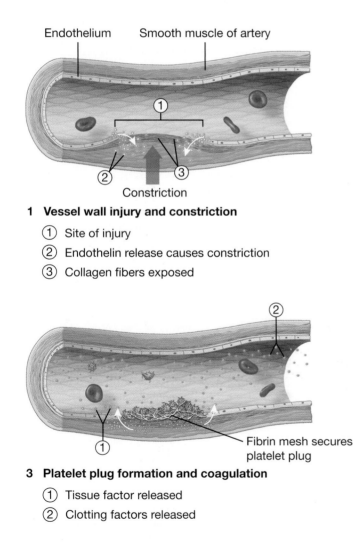

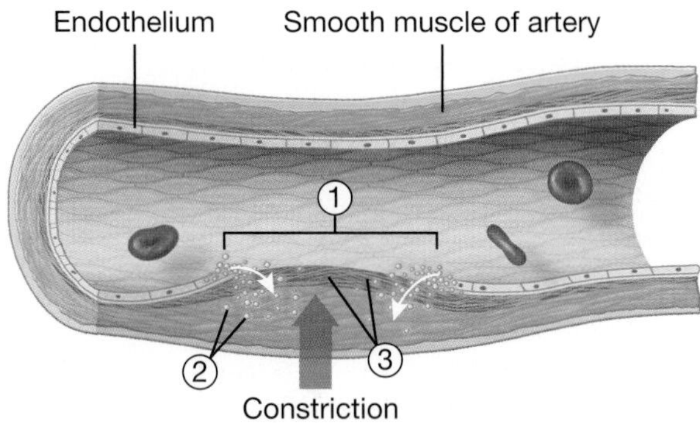

1 Vessel wall injury and constriction

① Site of injury
② Endothelin release causes constriction
③ Collagen fibers exposed

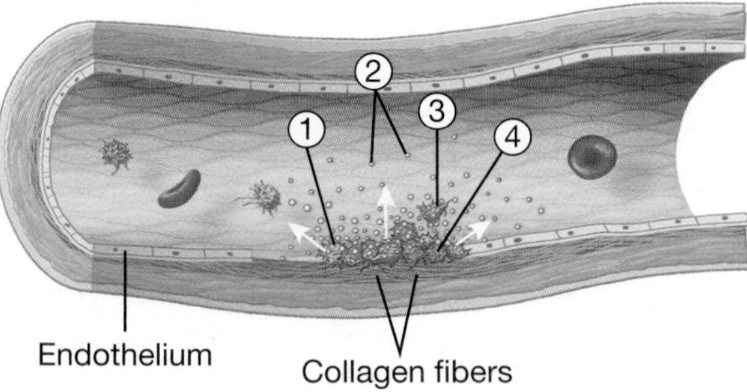

2 Platelet aggregation

① Platelet adhesion
② Chemicals released by platelets
③ Platelets gather
④ Platelets cluster to repair wall

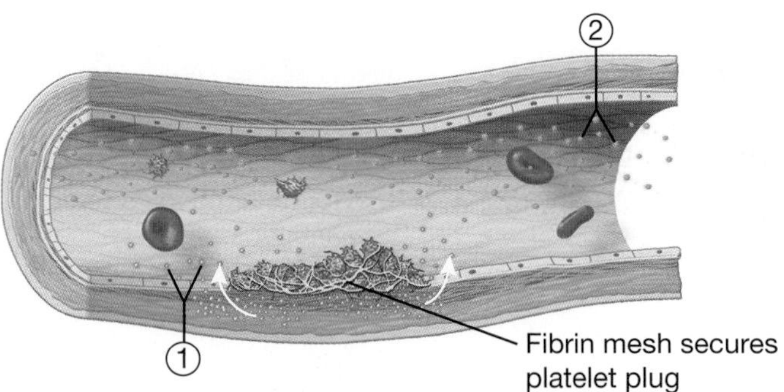

3 Platelet plug formation and coagulation

① Tissue factor released
② Clotting factors released

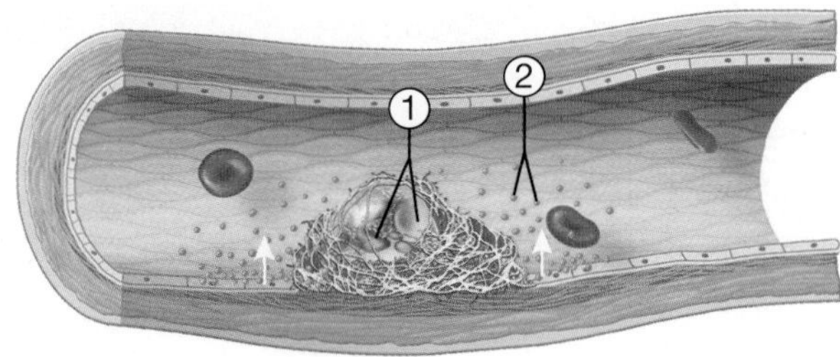

4 Blood clot formation

① Red and white blood cells are trapped in mesh
② Release of coagulation inhibitors and other chemicals

Figure 11.9 The four steps in the process of hemostasis.

2. **Platelet aggregation.** Platelets stick to the collagen fibers and to the rough edges of the blood vessel wall (platelet adhesion). The platelets act like a spackling compound to repair the hole or tear. In addition, the platelets release chemicals that maintain constriction of the blood vessel and attract more platelets to the damaged wall.
3. **Platelet plug formation and coagulation.** This gathering of platelets forms a small, loose mass called a ***platelet plug*** at the site of the injury. To initiate ***coagulation***, the injured blood vessel releases a chemical called *tissue factor*. Tissue factor activates eleven different clotting factors, or proteins, in the blood. These activated clotting factors produce ***prothrombin activator (PTA)***. In the presence of calcium and the platelet chemicals, ***prothrombin*** is activated to form thrombin. Thrombin activates the protein fibrinogen. The combination of thrombin and fibrinogen produces ***fibrin***, a long, sticky, threadlike fiber. The fibrin strands weave in and around the platelet plug, forming a strong, tightly woven fibrin mesh (**Figure 11.10**). The process can be compared to throwing a fishing net around the platelet plug.
4. **Blood clot formation and retraction.** Red and white blood cells become trapped in the fibrin mesh, giving the blood clot a red color. When coagulation is complete—after about 2 to 15 minutes—the blood clot has formed. Shortly after the fibrin mesh is in place, the blood clot begins to retract, or shrink in size. This process normally takes 30 to 60 minutes.

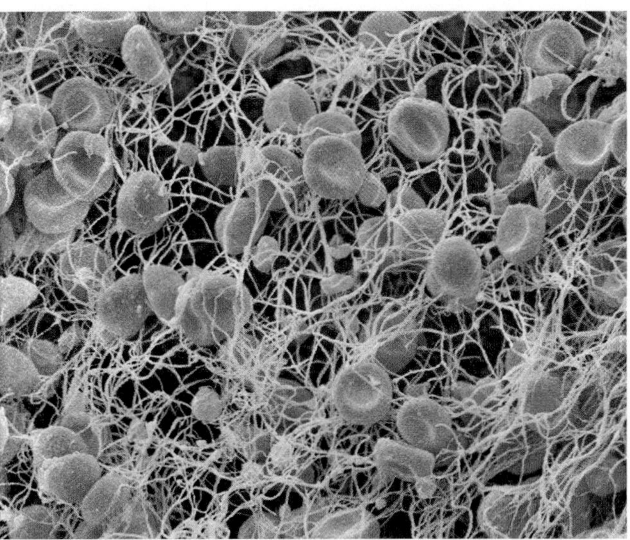

Susumu Nishinaga/Science Source

Figure 11.10 Scanning electron microscopic photo of a blood clot.

As the blood clot retracts, platelets pull the fibrin threads together. This, in turn, draws together the edges of the tear in the vessel. Meanwhile, the factors that started the hemostasis sequence are rapidly inactivated to prevent excessive clotting. In addition, coagulation inhibitors are released to prevent further clot formation. Eventually, other chemicals cut the fibrin strands and dissolve the blood clot completely. The blood clot is dissolved by a process called ***fibrinolysis***, which occurs when fibrin is broken down by enzymatic action of plasmin. Plasmin is formed from its inactive form, plasminogen, which is normally found in circulating blood. Plasminogen is activated when tissue plasminogen activator (TPA) is formed by the injured tissue.

Clinical Application Human Umbilical Cord Blood

Recent research shows that human umbilical cord blood (HUCB) contains ***hematopoietic cells***, ***mesenchymal cells***, and ***endothelial cells***, which were previously thought to exist only in bone marrow. This relatively new discovery has important clinical applications for the treatment of hematologic and metabolic diseases, immune deficiencies, and autoimmune disorders, as well as the creation of regenerative medical treatments.

Collecting HUCB involves a relatively quick and simple process that does not pose any danger to the baby or mother. One drawback to HUCB is that there is only a small quantity of blood to be harvested, but this is alleviated by invitro expansion procedures, which allow the generation of blood cells in a petri dish.

SELF CHECK

1. What are the two basic types of components in the blood?
2. Typically, approximately what percentage of the blood is plasma?
3. Which proteins are most abundant in the plasma?
4. Which organ regulates red blood cell production through the process of erythropoiesis?
5. What is the name of the process in which red blood cells rupture when they reach the end of their life span?
6. List the five different types of white blood cells.
7. What is the difference between a granulocyte and an agranulocyte?

Manufacturing Blood Cells

Each blood cell has a limited life span, so the body's ability to create new blood cells is important. New blood cells are created through a process called *hematopoiesis*. Refer to Chapter 5 for more information about this process.

Blood cells are manufactured in bone marrow, a soft, spongy substance found inside the bones. There are two types of bone marrow: yellow and red. Only red bone marrow, found in the vertebrae, ribs, hips, sternum, and skull, can produce stem cells for blood cell production.

Each of the formed elements in the blood starts as a hematopoietic stem cell, which develops into another type of stem cell by the process known as mitosis before it develops into a blast cell. Depending on which growth or stimulating factors and hormones influence the blast cell, it matures into a red blood cell, white blood cell, or platelet (**Figure 11.11**). As new blood cells develop in bone marrow, they enter the bloodstream as it flows through the bone.

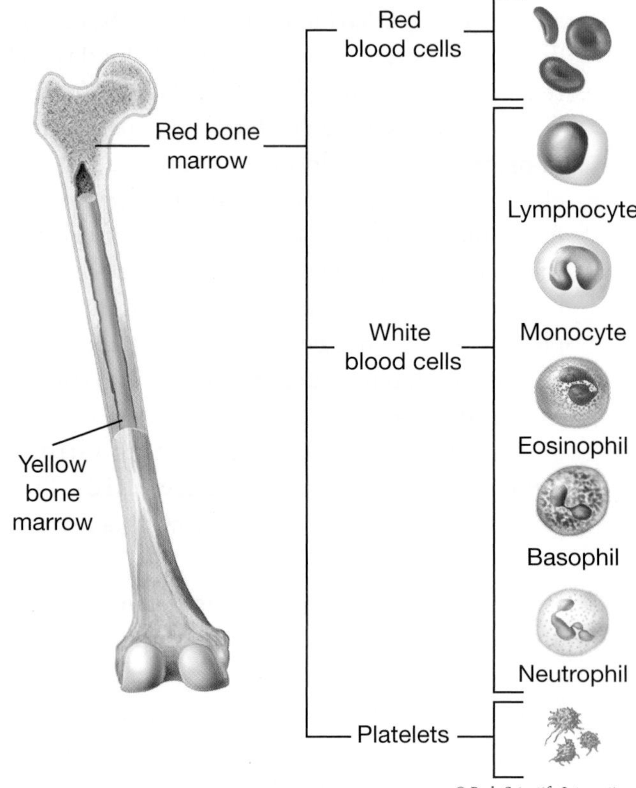

Figure 11.11 Red blood cells, white blood cells, and platelets develop from stem cells in bone marrow.

SECTION 11.1 REVIEW

Mini-Glossary

buffy coat a thin layer of white blood cells and platelets that lies between the red blood cells and plasma in a blood specimen that has gone through a centrifuge

coagulation the process by which the enzyme thrombin and the protein fibrinogen combine to form fibrin, a fiber that weaves around the platelet plug to form a blood clot

diapedesis the passage of blood, or any of its formed elements, through the blood vessel walls into body tissues

endothelial cells a thin layer of squamous cells that line all blood and lymphatic vessels

erythrocytes red blood cells

erythropoiesis the process by which red blood cells are produced

erythropoietin (EPO) a hormone secreted by the kidneys that stimulates the production of red blood cells

fibrin a long, threadlike fiber created by the combination of thrombin and fibrinogen

fibrinolysis the process of breaking down fibrin to dissolve a blood clot

(continued)

formed elements the solid components of blood; includes red blood cells, white blood cells, and platelets
hematocrit the percentage of total blood volume that is composed of red blood cells
hematopoietic cells the cells that are responsible for creating blood cells
hemoglobin an essential molecule of the red blood cell that serves as the binding site for oxygen and carbon dioxide; composed of globin and heme
hemolysis the rupture of red blood cells
hemostasis the sequence of events that causes a blood clot to form and bleeding to stop
hypoxia a condition of having too little oxygen in the blood
leukocytes white blood cells
mesenchymal cells stromal cells that can develop into tissues of the circulatory and lymphatic systems as well as connective tissues
phagocytosis the process by which macrophages in the liver and spleen envelop, digest, and recycle old RBCs and other types of cells
plasma the liquid component of blood
platelet plug a gathering of platelets that forms a small mass at the site of an injury
platelets cell fragments that play a vital role in blood clotting; also known as *thrombocytes*
prothrombin a protein in the blood that is activated to form thrombin during clot formation
prothrombin activator (PTA) a protein that activates the protein fibrinogen
red blood cells blood cells that contain hemoglobin, a protein responsible for oxygen and carbon dioxide transport; also known as *erythrocytes*
thrombocytes platelets
white blood cells blood cells that fight infection and protect the body through various mechanisms; also known as *leukocytes*

Review Questions

1. List at least six functions of blood, two in each of the three major categories described in this section.
2. A centrifuge is used to separate the elements of blood into three layers. Describe the components of each layer.
3. Name at least four physical properties of blood.
4. Where are blood cells manufactured?
5. What does hematocrit measure? List the normal ranges for males and females.
6. Compare and contrast the different functions of red blood cells, white blood cells, and platelets.
7. Explain the blood clotting process.

SECTION 11.2 Blood Types

Objectives

- Describe the ABO blood grouping system.
- Explain the Rh classification system and why it is important.

Key Terms

agglutination	Rh factor
antibody	RhoGAM
antigen	universal donor
erythroblastosis fetalis	universal recipient

Everyone's blood contains some similar elements: red blood cells, white blood cells, and platelets. However, not all blood is the same. Several typing systems are used to differentiate among the various types of blood.

ABO Blood Grouping System

In the ABO blood typing system, there are four distinct types of blood: A, B, AB, and O. Reagents can be used to detect the differences in a process known as *blood typing*. ABO blood typing was made possible by the groundbreaking work of Karl Landsteiner, an Austrian scientist who won the Nobel Prize for his discovery.

Do you know your blood type? Have you ever wondered what determines your blood type? Like eye or hair color, blood type is inherited. **Figure 11.12** provides a list of possible blood types that a person may have based on the blood types of his or her parents. The presence of antigen A on the red blood cell indicates type A blood, antigen B indicates type B blood, and the presence of both antigen A and B indicates type AB blood. Some people have neither antigen A nor B on their red blood cells. These people have type O blood. Blood types tend to vary among ethnic groups and regions of the world. Type O is the most common in the United States, and type AB is the rarest (**Figure 11.13**).

Antigens and Antibodies

Antigens are large, complex molecules, such as proteins and glycolipids, on the surface of red blood cells.

Inherited Blood Type											
	Parent 1	**AB**	**AB**	**AB**	**AB**	**B**	**A**	**A**	**O**	**O**	**O**
	Parent 2	**AB**	**B**	**A**	**O**	**B**	**B**	**A**	**B**	**A**	**O**
Possible blood type of child	**O**					X	X	X	X	X	X
	A	X	X	X	X		X	X		X	
	B	X	X	X	X	X	X		X		
	AB	X	X	X			X				

Figure 11.12 Goodheart-Willcox Publisher

Blood Type by Ethnicity					
	Prevalence (% of US Population)				
Blood Group	**Caucasian**	**African-American**	**Hispanic**	**Asian**	**Native American**
AB	3	4	2	5	1
B	9	20	10	27	4
A	41	27	31	28	16
O	47	49	57	40	79

Figure 11.13 Goodheart-Willcox Publisher

They identify cells as "self" or "nonself," making it possible for the body to tell the difference between its own cells and foreign cells. The presence of foreign cells causes the immune system to produce ***antibodies*** that mark the foreign cells for destruction. Antibodies circulate in plasma and bind to any cells that have antigens different from those found in the host's blood (or blood recipient during a transfusion). Chapter 13 describes antigens and antibodies in more detail.

Figure 11.14 shows the antigens and antibodies associated with each blood type. People with AB blood have A and B antigens on their RBCs, but neither A nor B antibodies in their plasma, making them a ***universal recipient***. A universal recipient can safely receive blood of any type. People with type A blood have RBCs with only A antigens on their RBCs and B antibodies in their plasma, and those with type B blood have only B antigens on their RBCs and A antibodies in their plasma. People with type O blood have neither A nor B antigens on their red blood cells, but both A and B antibodies in their plasma. Because type O blood has no antigens, anyone can receive type O blood. Thus, people with type O blood are ***universal donors***.

Blood Transfusions

Understanding blood types is critical for blood transfusions and surgery. The history of blood transfusions shows that the earliest outcomes of this technology were grim. In the fledgling days of medicine, physicians did not know about the different blood types. Some transfusions were successful due in large part to luck, but others resulted in serious complications or death.

When a person with type A blood is transfused with blood from a type B blood donor, the recipient's anti-B antibodies bind to the donor's red blood cells. This causes the donated red blood cells to clump together in a process called ***agglutination***. Agglutination creates blockages in smaller blood vessels and is potentially fatal.

Agglutination also causes hemolysis, or destruction, of the donated red blood cells. Hemolysis releases hemoglobin into the bloodstream. Hemoglobin may accumulate in the kidneys, causing kidney damage and failure, or even death. Blood transfusion reactions can also be milder, with symptoms ranging from fever and chills to vomiting. Regardless, it is *extremely important* that blood types be classified and matched *before* transfusion.

SELF CHECK

1. What determines a person's blood type?
2. Name the four blood types in the ABO blood grouping system.
3. Which blood type classifies someone as a universal recipient? a universal donor?

The ABO Blood Group System				
Blood Type	**Erythrocyte (Red Blood Cell) Antigens**	**RBC Antigens**	**Antibodies**	**Blood That Can Be Received**
AB	A and B	A B	neither anti-A nor anti-B antibodies	A, B, AB, O (universal recipient)
B	B		anti-A	B, O
A	A		anti-B	A, O
O	Neither A nor B	No antigens	anti-A and anti-B	O (universal donor)

Figure 11.14

© Body Scientific International; Goodheart-Willcox Publisher

Rh Classification System

Besides the antigens that determine blood type, there are other antigens on the surface of the red blood cells that determine the ***Rh factor***. It is called the *Rh factor* because it was originally discovered in the rhesus monkey.

Not everyone possesses the Rh factor. Those who have the Rh factor on the surface of their red blood cells are classified as Rh-positive (Rh^+); those who lack it are classified as Rh-negative (Rh^-). The majority of people (approximately 85%) are Rh-positive.

When writing out an ABO blood type with the Rh factor, drop the "Rh" and simply add a positive or negative superscript to the blood type. For example, a person who has the Rh factor and type AB blood would be described as AB^+.

Clinical Application Determining Blood Type

Blood typing is a simple procedure performed in a laboratory or even as part of a classroom activity. The procedure can be performed in a matter of minutes.

Blood typing involves a forward and a reverse typing. In the forward typing process, a person's RBCs are mixed with a known chemical reagent containing only anti-A antibodies or only anti-B antibodies. If the blood cells clump together (agglutinate) in the sample with only anti-A antibodies, then it is type A blood. If it agglutinates in the sample containing only anti-B antibodies, then it is type B blood. If the blood agglutinates in both reagents then the blood is type AB. If no agglutination occurs, it is type O blood.

The reverse typing involves a similar procedure. However, the person's serum or plasma, rather than whole blood, is tested for agglutination.

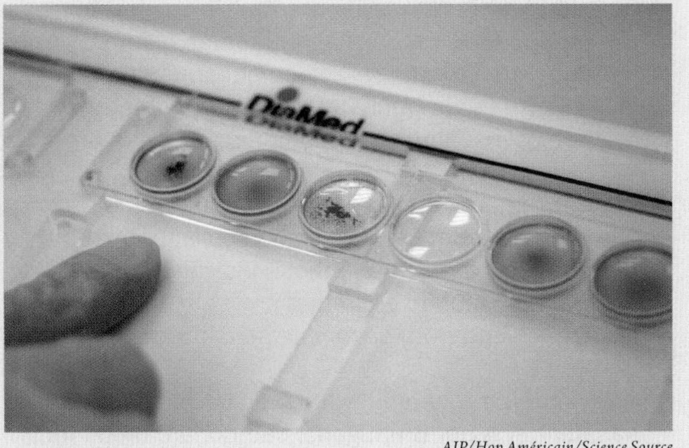

AJP/Hop Américain/Science Source

In the ABO blood grouping system, the reaction of a blood specimen to various reagents determines its type.

Transfusion Reactions

Plasma does not naturally contain an antibody for the Rh factor. However, antibodies to the Rh factor will develop if a person with Rh^- blood is transfused with Rh^+ blood. After exposure to the Rh^+ blood, antibodies begin to form against the positive Rh antigen. If the person is exposed to Rh^+ blood again, the antibodies will cause agglutination and hemolysis.

Pregnancy Complications

Any woman considering pregnancy should know her blood type and seek early prenatal healthcare. It is essential for the health of the woman and her baby because women can become sensitized to the Rh factor during pregnancy. If a woman who is Rh^- has a baby who is Rh^+, her first pregnancy will not cause a problem because her blood has not yet developed antibodies, or sensitivity to the Rh^+ blood. However, during childbirth, some of the baby's Rh^+ blood may come in contact with the woman's Rh^- blood through the placenta, the organ that transports nutrients from the woman to her child. Once the woman's blood has been exposed to the Rh^+ blood, she will develop anti-Rh^+ antibodies.

If the woman becomes pregnant with another child who is Rh^+, the woman's anti-Rh^+ antibodies will attack the red blood cells of the fetus, causing agglutination and hemolysis. This condition causes anemia and an elevated plasma bilirubin level leading to jaundice. The action by the antibodies also depletes the number of mature RBCs in the fetus. As a result, erythroblasts (immature RBCs) leave the bone marrow of the fetus before they are mature. If this condition is left untreated, the baby will develop ***erythroblastosis fetalis***, or hemolytic disease of the newborn (HDN). Erythroblastosis fetalis can be fatal.

Fortunately, erythroblastosis fetalis is rare in developed countries due to good pre- and post-natal care as well as the development of the immune serum ***RhoGAM***. RhoGAM prevents the mother's immune system from developing antibodies against Rh+ blood, which could affect a future Rh+ fetus. RhoGAM is administered to the Rh^- woman shortly after she has given birth to an Rh+ baby.

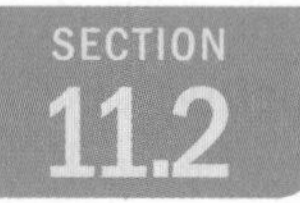

REVIEW

Mini-Glossary

agglutination the process by which red blood cells clump together, usually in response to an antibody

antibodies immune proteins that react with the antigen that caused its synthesis

antigen a protein on the surface of RBCs that is used to identify blood type by identifying cells as "self" or "nonself" (foreign) cells

erythroblastosis fetalis a severe hemolytic disease found in fetuses or newborns that is caused by the production of maternal antibodies against the antigens on fetal red blood cells; usually involves Rh incompatibility between the mother and fetus; also known as hemolytic disease of the newborn (HDN)

Rh factor the antigen of the Rh blood group that is found on the surface of red blood cells; people with the Rh factor are Rh^+ and those lacking it are Rh^-

RhoGAM an immune serum that prevents a Rh^- pregnant woman's blood from becoming sensitized to her Rh+ fetus

universal donor a person with type O blood, which has neither A nor B antigens; can donate blood for transfusion to people of all blood types

universal recipient a person with type AB blood, which has neither A nor B antibodies; can safely receive a transfusion of any blood type

Review Questions

1. What is an antigen?
2. Explain the process of agglutination.
3. Besides the antigens that determine blood type, what other antigen is sometimes found on the surface of red blood cells?
4. Define *RhoGAM* and explain its use.
5. If a person's parents both have type B blood, what blood types might that person have?
6. If you have type B blood, what kind of antibodies do you have?
7. *True or False?* If you are Rh-positive, you have a higher than normal amount of Rh factor.
8. What is the difference between an antigen and an antibody?
9. Explain why a person with type AB blood is a universal recipient.
10. Explain why a person with type O blood is a universal donor.

SECTION 11.3

Blood Disorders and Diseases

Objectives

- Identify the measurements performed in a complete blood count.
- Describe the various types of anemia.
- Identify common blood disorders and diseases.

Key Terms

acute lymphocytic leukemia (ALL)
acute myeloid leukemia (AML)
anemia
aplastic anemia
chelation therapy
chronic lymphocytic leukemia (CLL)
chronic myeloid leukemia (CML)
complete blood count (CBC)
embolus
hemophilia
iron-deficient anemia
jaundice
leukemia
multiple myeloma
pernicious anemia
phlebotomy
polycythemia
sickle cell anemia
thalassemia
thrombus

Blood disorders and diseases can be diagnosed in a variety of ways, including a complete blood count test. What causes a disorder or disease of the blood? Many health problems affecting the blood are inherited, but some are caused by environmental factors, poor diet, or even old age. This section explains the measurements made during a complete blood count and explores some of the most common disorders and diseases of the blood, as well as their causes, symptoms, and treatments or management strategies.

Complete Blood Count

A ***complete blood count (CBC)*** is a test that helps detect blood disorders or diseases such as anemia, infection, abnormal blood cell counts, clotting problems, immune system disorders, and cancers of the blood. The test measures the number of RBCs, WBCs, and platelets, and determines hemoglobin, hematocrit, and other RBC parameters. **Figure 11.15** illustrates the results of a complete blood count test. Values that are higher or lower than the normal range appear in red.

A low RBC count may indicate anemia, bleeding, or dehydration. In addition, the number of each of the five different types of WBCs is measured for signs of infection, blood cancers, or immune disorders. A reduced platelet count may indicate a bleeding or a thrombotic (clotting) disorder. Hemoglobin and hematocrit levels are also measured for signs of any anemias.

SELF CHECK

1. What does a complete blood count measure?
2. What diseases and disorders may be indicated if a person's red blood cell count is low?

Anemia

Anemia is a condition characterized by a decreased concentration of erythrocytes (RBCs), hemoglobin, or hematocrit due to a decreased production or an increased destruction of RBCs or excessive blood loss. In all cases, the oxygen-carrying capacity of the blood is reduced.

Anemia can be acquired or inherited. Acquired anemia means a person was not born with a condition that could cause anemia; inherited means that a person was born with a gene that results in anemia. Symptoms of anemia include pallor, headache, dizziness, weakness, fatigue, and difficulty breathing or shortness of breath.

There are several types of anemia. Some forms are mild and easily treated by adopting a healthful diet; others can be severe, debilitating, and even life-threatening if they remain undiagnosed or untreated. For milder forms of anemia, a healthful diet provides the building blocks for RBC production: iron, folic acid, and vitamin B.

Low red blood count, hemoglobin, and hematocrit signal anemia.

Elevated white blood count may signal disease or infection.

Complete Blood Count Example Test Results				
Test	**Results**	**Low/High**	**Units**	**Normal Ranges**
CBC with Differential				
Red Blood Count		3.5 (L)	× 10-6/µl	4.1–5.1 (F) / 4.70–6.10 (M)
Hemoglobin		10.8 (L)	g/dl	12.0–16.0 (F) / 14.0–18.0 (M)
Hematocrit		31.1 (L)	%	37.0–48.0 (F) / 42.0–52.0 (M)
Platelets	302		× 10-3/µl	140–415
White Blood Count	7.2		× 10-3/µl	4.5–11
Lymphocytes		48 (H)	%	17–44
Monocytes	7.0		%	3–10
Neutrophils		43 (L)	%	45–76
Eosinophils	2.0		%	0–4
Basophils	0		%	0–2

M = Male F = Female

Goodheart-Willcox Publisher

Figure 11.15 The results of a CBC can be used to determine the presence of a disease or disorder. The Low/High column shows counts lower (L) or higher (H) than normal.

Acquired Anemias

Many conditions and factors may cause an acquired anemia. Examples include a dietary deficiency, blood loss, hormones, exposure to parasitic worms, chronic diseases, pregnancy, or damage to a specific part of the body.

Iron-Deficient Anemia

The most common type of anemia, ***iron-deficient anemia***, accounts for nearly 50% of all anemias worldwide. Iron-deficient anemia typically results from an insufficient dietary intake of iron or loss of iron from intestinal bleeding.

Parasitic worms that result in intestinal bleeding are the main cause of iron-deficient anemia worldwide. Parasitic worms are most commonly found in developing or low-income countries.

Pregnant women may also suffer from iron-deficient anemia. This happens because their bodies must supply the fetus with hemoglobin, depleting the woman's own iron levels. (Recall that the heme molecule in hemoglobin is composed of iron.)

If iron-deficient anemia is caused by a poor diet, an iron supplement can be prescribed. Foods rich in iron, such as leafy, green vegetables, are also recommended (**Figure 11.16**).

Aplastic Anemia

A rare but serious condition known as ***aplastic anemia*** is caused by damage to the stem cells in the bone marrow. When bone marrow stem cells are damaged, they cannot produce a sufficient number of RBCs, WBCs, and platelets. The small number of blood cells that are manufactured in the bone marrow have difficulty developing into mature blood cells, resulting in aplastic anemia. Bone marrow stem cell damage may be caused by:

- toxins (such as those found in pesticides)
- radiation therapy or chemotherapy
- infectious diseases (for example, hepatitis, Epstein-Barr virus, human immunodeficiency virus (HIV), and autoimmune disorders such as rheumatoid arthritis and lupus)
- cancer in another part of the body that affects the bone marrow
- idiopathic causes (unknown causes)

Treatments for aplastic anemia are aimed at reducing the factors that are damaging bone marrow stem

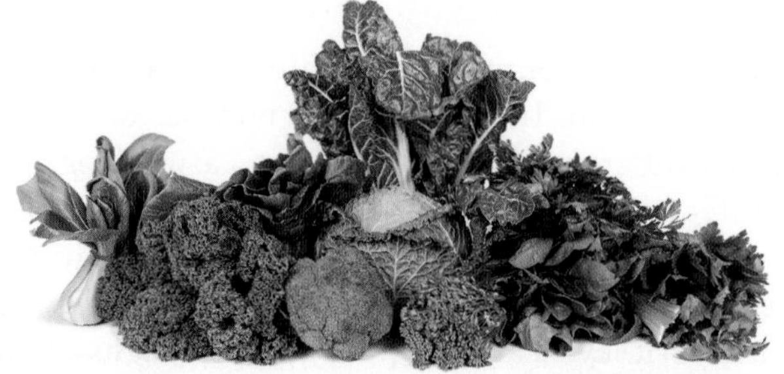

Robyn Mackenzie/Shutterstock.com

Figure 11.16 One way to help fight iron-deficient anemia is to adopt a diet rich in leafy green vegetables like those shown here.

cells. This includes removing toxins or discontinuing radiation or chemotherapy. Blood transfusions may also be indicated to help improve the RBC count. In severe cases, bone marrow stem cell transplants can be performed.

Pernicious Anemia

When the intestines are unable to absorb B_{12}, a vitamin essential for RBC production, the result is ***pernicious anemia***. This condition develops when the stomach stops producing intrinsic factor, a key protein in vitamin B_{12} absorption. The body may also attack intrinsic factor as a result of a weakened stomach lining or an autoimmune disorder.

Pernicious anemia usually develops later in life. On average, diagnosis occurs in patients around 60 years of age. Certain diseases, such as type I diabetes mellitus, Addison's disease, and chronic thyroiditis, can increase the risk of developing pernicious anemia.

Common signs and symptoms of pernicious anemia include a red, swollen tongue; pale skin; fatigue; and shortness of breath. Other symptoms include diarrhea or constipation. Treatment usually consists of vitamin B_{12} supplements or injections.

Anemias Caused by Chronic Disease

Chronic illnesses such as rheumatoid arthritis or kidney disease can cause anemia. For example, kidney disease may lower production of the hormone erythropoietin, which regulates RBC production. Inflammatory conditions associated with diseases such as rheumatoid arthritis can affect the bone marrow's response to erythropoietin, resulting in decreased RBC production. Diseases characterized by chronic infections, such as HIV, tuberculosis, cirrhosis of the liver, and certain cancers, can also cause anemia.

Treatment of anemia caused by chronic disease involves diagnosing and resolving the underlying disease. In the short term, blood transfusions may be used as part of the treatment plan for managing anemia.

Inherited Anemias

Inherited anemias are determined by genetic makeup. In commonly inherited anemias such as sickle cell anemia and thalassemia, a child must receive an anemia gene from both parents to experience symptoms of an inherited anemia. If an anemia gene is received from only one parent, the child will be a carrier but will not experience symptoms.

Sickle Cell Anemia

Recall that normal RBCs are disc-shaped. However, the RBCs of a person with ***sickle cell anemia*** are shaped like a crescent or sickle, a large cutting instrument with a curved metal blade (**Figure 11.17**). The hemoglobin molecules in the RBCs of a patient with sickle cell anemia are misshaped, causing the RBCs to take on the abnormal shape.

Sickle-shaped hemoglobin molecules carry less oxygen than normal hemoglobin molecules. Because of their shape and sticky texture, sickle-shaped RBCs easily become stuck in small blood vessels, disrupting normal blood flow. **Figure 11.17** illustrates how the sickle-shaped RBCs become lodged in blood vessels.

Symptoms of sickle cell anemia include excruciatingly painful episodes called *crises*. Crises can last anywhere from a few hours to several days, and these episodes require hospitalization. The pain associated with crises usually occurs in the back and around long bones, such as the femur, where tissues can be damaged from oxygen deprivation. Other symptoms include bacterial infection, fatigue, shortness of breath, rapid heart rate, and jaundice, a yellowing of the skin and eyes. Strokes may also occur if RBCs become lodged in the small vessels of the brain.

Treatment of sickle cell anemia may require daily doses of antibiotics to prevent bacterial infection, especially in small children who have the disease. Blood transfusions are given frequently to increase RBC count. Folic acid supplements are also recommended. In the event of a crisis, patients are given blood transfusions, pain medications, and fluids.

Individuals who inherit the sickle cell gene from only one parent have the sickle cell trait, which means they are a carrier but will not develop any of the symptoms of the disease. Sickle cell anemia is most common in African-Americans and individuals of Mediterranean descent. In the past, sickle cell anemia resulted in death at an early age, but medical advances are helping people with this disease live to 50 years of age and beyond.

Thalassemia

Thalassemia, also called *Cooley's anemia*, is a type of anemia that affects hemoglobin. This condition limits the body's ability to produce fully developed hemoglobin and the proper number of RBCs. As a result, the blood's oxygen-carrying capability is reduced.

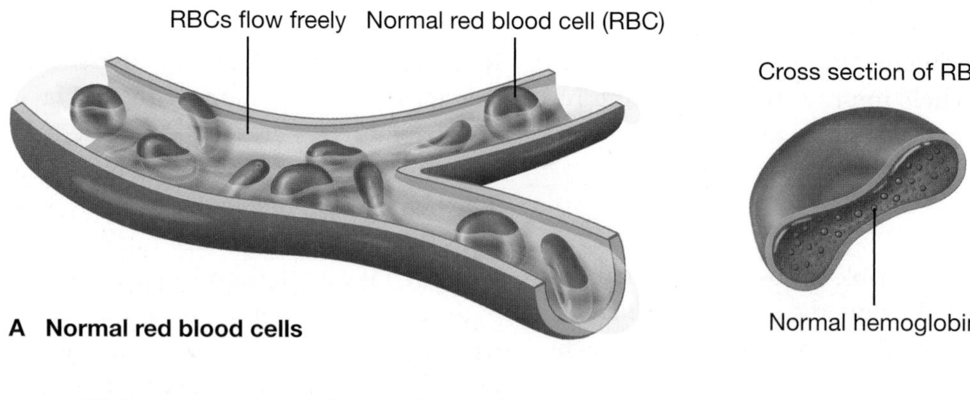

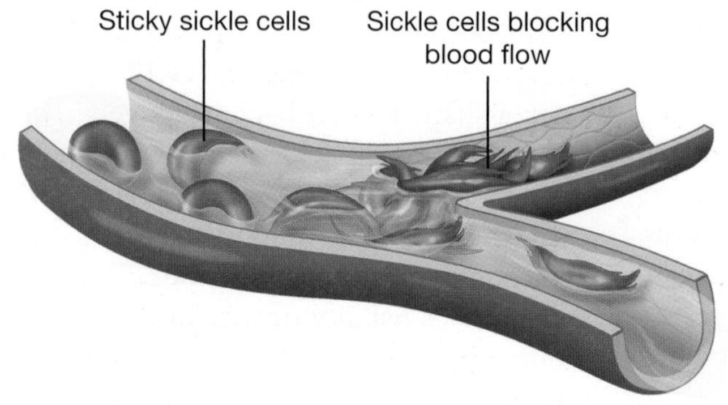

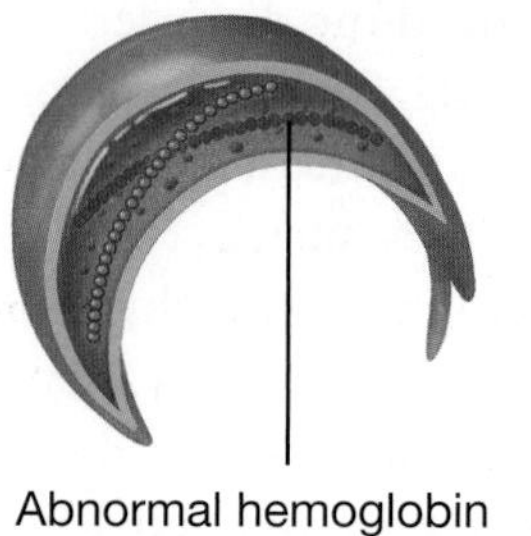

Figure 11.17 Sickle-shaped red blood cells get stuck more easily in smaller blood vessels, causing painful episodes called *crises*.

People with thalassemia require frequent blood transfusions to increase their RBC counts. However, these transfusions can be dangerous because they can increase the iron in the blood to toxic levels. Excessive amounts of iron are especially harmful to the heart, liver, and endocrine organs. Iron accumulation leads to heart attack and death in 50% of people with thalassemia before they reach 35 years of age.

Chelation therapy is a procedure that removes excess metals, such as iron, from the blood. In many cases, chelation therapy is essential for preventing organ damage and failure in patients with thalassemia. During this therapy, the chelating drug is pumped into the body either intravenously (through an IV) or subcutaneously (by injection). It then binds with whatever metal is present in excess amounts.

Research Notes: Extending Life Expectancy of Patients with Sickle Cell Anemia

People with sickle cell anemia are prone to life-threatening infections, fatigue, and painful crises. Historically, this has meant that people with sickle cell anemia have a shortened life span. In the 1960s, 15% of children born with sickle cell anemia died before two years of age, and many more died as teenagers. Since that time, research funded by the National Heart, Lung, and Blood Institute (NHLBI) has shown that infants with sickle cell anemia who are given daily doses of penicillin have an 84% reduction in infections, which greatly improves their life expectancy.

Because sickle-shaped RBCs can become lodged in the blood vessels of the brain, people with sickle cell anemia are prone to stroke. NHLBI-funded research has led to the development of the Transcranial Doppler (TCD) screening test, which can identify whether or not a patient with sickle cell anemia is at risk for stroke. Frequent blood transfusions have proven to lower these patients' risk of stroke and increase their life expectancy.

In another effort to increase the life expectancy of patients with sickle cell anemia, NHLBI researchers performed a partial stem cell transplant on ten individuals with severe sickle cell disease; nine of them were cured.

Research continues with the goal of finding a permanent cure for sickle cell anemia. Meanwhile, a disease that was once associated with an early death is now a manageable condition, with life expectancies ranging from 40 to 50 years of age and beyond.

In the case of iron poisoning, the chelating drug binds with the iron and prepares it for elimination from the body via the urine. The drug is usually administered at night and is infused slowly over an eight-hour period, four to six nights a week.

SELF CHECK

1. What are the three main causes of anemia?
2. Which type of anemia is the most common worldwide?
3. Which type of anemia is caused by the inability of the intestines to absorb vitamin B_{12}?
4. Why might a person with rheumatoid arthritis be more likely to develop anemia than someone without rheumatoid arthritis?

Other Common Blood Disorders and Diseases

Anemia is not the only disorder that affects the blood. Many other diseases, disorders, and conditions are possible as well.

Jaundice

Jaundice is a condition that is actually a symptom caused by several disorders. Characterized by yellowing of the skin and whites of the eyes, it can be caused by an excess of bilirubin—a by-product of RBC breakdown—in the bloodstream. Bilirubin is typically converted to bile in the liver, so jaundice can result either from liver damage or from disease.

Jaundice may also occur in newborns as the result of an immature liver. In addition, a newborn is more likely to be jaundiced when his or her Rh antigen is different from the mother's. For example, if the mother is Rh-negative and the baby is Rh-positive, the mother's antibodies may attack the baby's red blood cells and release excess bilirubin, causing jaundice. This severe form of jaundice is not the usual cause of mild jaundice in newborns.

Mild forms of infant jaundice are treated with phototherapy using ultraviolet light, which lowers the bilirubin levels in the baby's blood (**Figure 11.18**). Infant jaundice is usually resolved within two to four weeks of birth.

Hemophilia

Hemophilia is a disorder in which the blood does not clot properly because one of the clotting factors responsible for coagulation is missing. There are 13 clotting factors involved in the coagulation process. As discussed earlier in this chapter, platelets and clotting factors form a blood clot to stop an injured blood vessel from bleeding. People with hemophilia typically lack either clotting factor VIII or IX.

Hemophilia is usually inherited but, in very rare cases, may be acquired if the body forms antibodies that attack one of the clotting factors. Cases of hemophilia can range from mild to severe depending on which clotting factor is missing. This disease is more common in males, and it occurs in one out of every 5,000 births each year. Treatments include blood transfusions, transfusions of the deficient clotting factors themselves, or administration of drugs that increase the lacking clotting factors.

Polycythemia

Polycythemia, also known as *polycythemia primary* or *polycythemia vera*, is a condition in which the bone marrow manufactures too many red blood cells. Living at a high altitude contributes to polycythemia because long-term exposure to high altitude causes the kidneys to produce more erythropoietin. Erythropoietin stimulates stem cell production in the bone marrow, and more erythropoietin leads to increased RBC production. However, people who live at a high altitude do not develop polycythemia unless they also have a rare genetic mutation that increases bone

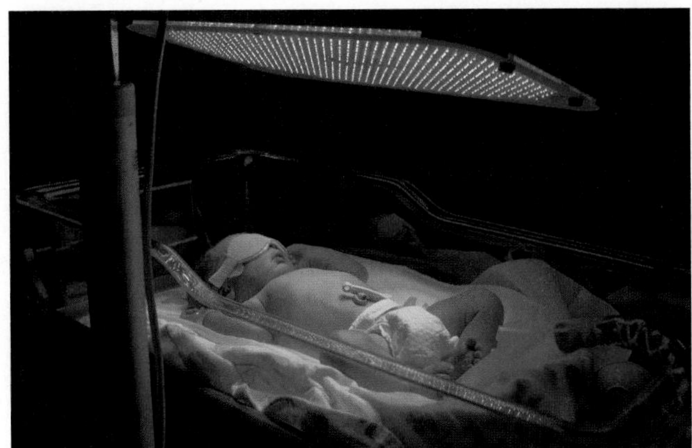

phakimata/iStock.com

Figure 11.18 Phototherapy employs ultraviolet light to help break down excess bilirubin so that it can be excreted in the urine and feces.

marrow sensitivity to erythropoietin, causing even more RBCs to be produced. High RBC counts cause blood to become more viscous, increasing the likelihood of blood clot formation.

Polycythemia is diagnosed by testing hemoglobin or hematocrit levels. Unusually high levels of hemoglobin or hematocrit indicate excessive RBC production.

Phlebotomy, the process of drawing or removing blood from the body, is the standard treatment for polycythemia. Phlebotomy reduces the number of RBCs circulating in the body. This helps correct hematocrit levels. Aspirin has also been used to treat polycythemia because it prevents excess clotting, but aspirin therapy is not advised for anyone with a history of spontaneous bleeding or stroke.

Intravascular Clotting

Normally, due to the body's anticoagulating and fibrinolytic mechanisms, blood clots do not form in an unbroken vessel. However, sometimes blood clots do form in an intact blood vessel, usually a vein. This intravascular clot is called a ***thrombus***. The clot may dissolve on its own, but if it remains in the vessel and becomes large enough, it may cause a blockage that results in damage to or death of the tissue supplied by that vessel. For instance, a blockage in a coronary artery could result in a heart attack. If the clot becomes dislodged from the vessel wall and is transported in the bloodstream it is called an ***embolus***. An embolus floating in the bloodstream that enters a smaller diameter artery could cut off blood flow to an organ. When an embolism blocks blood flow to the lungs, it is called a *pulmonary embolism*, and it is potentially fatal.

Intravascular clots may develop due to a roughening of the endothelium of the vessel resulting from trauma, atherosclerosis, severe burns, or infection. The roughened endothelial lining leads to platelet aggregation and clot formation. Clots may also occur when blood flows too slowly and clotting factors accumulate, allowing clot formation. Risk factors for clot formation include pregnancy, individuals over 60 years of age, or sitting for long periods of time like on a flight or after surgery. Therapy for intravascular clots includes aspirin or use of an anticoagulant such as heparin or Coumadin.

Leukemia

Leukemia is a cancer of the blood that causes the bone marrow to produce abnormal, cancerous white blood cells. These cancerous WBCs multiply uncontrollably and grow larger than normal WBCs, but they lack the infection-fighting ability of normal WBCs. Cancerous white blood cells have a negative impact on bone marrow, which leads to decreased production of RBCs, WBCs, and platelets.

Leukemia is classified as either acute or chronic. Acute leukemia worsens quickly, while chronic leukemia progresses more slowly. Children with leukemia usually have acute leukemia. Adults may contract either acute or chronic leukemia. There are four types of leukemia. Two types are acute and two are chronic.

- ***Acute lymphocytic leukemia (ALL)***: ALL is characterized by an overproduction of lymphocytes. It is most common in children under the age of 15 years but may also occur in adults over age 45. ALL is the most common type of cancer in children.
- ***Acute myeloid leukemia (AML)***: AML develops when the bone marrow produces too many myeloblasts, or immature WBCs. Myeloblasts ultimately develop into neutrophils, eosinophils, and basophils. It is the most common form of leukemia in adults.
- ***Chronic lymphocytic leukemia (CLL)***: Like acute lymphocytic leukemia, CLL is characterized by extremely high levels of lymphocytes. CLL is rare in children and most often affects middle-aged adults.
- ***Chronic myeloid leukemia (CML)***: In CML, the bone marrow manufactures too many granulocytes (neutrophils, eosinophils, and basophils).

People with chronic leukemia may not experience any symptoms, sometimes even for years after they develop the disease. By comparison, people with acute leukemia often seek medical care because they feel sick. Symptoms of both chronic and acute leukemia include weakness, fever, bone and joint pain, and stomach swelling and pain from an enlarged spleen or liver. People with leukemia also have frequent infections because their abnormal WBCs are unable to aid in the immune response.

A complete blood count is often used to help diagnose leukemia. This disease increases the number of WBCs and decreases platelet and hemoglobin counts. A physical examination is done to check for swelling in the lymph nodes, spleen, or liver. In addition, doctors may perform a biopsy (removal and examination of body tissues or bone marrow) and other tests to look for cancerous cells (**Figure 11.19**).

Treatment options for leukemia vary but often include chemotherapy, radiation therapy, and stem cell transplants. The five-year survival rate for acute myeloid leukemia varies with age. Those *younger* than 50 years of age at the time of diagnosis have a survival rate of 25% over a five-year period, while those *older* than 50 years of age have a survival rate of 50% over a five-year period. New drug treatments for chronic myeloid leukemia have led to a promising 90% survival rate over the course of five years.

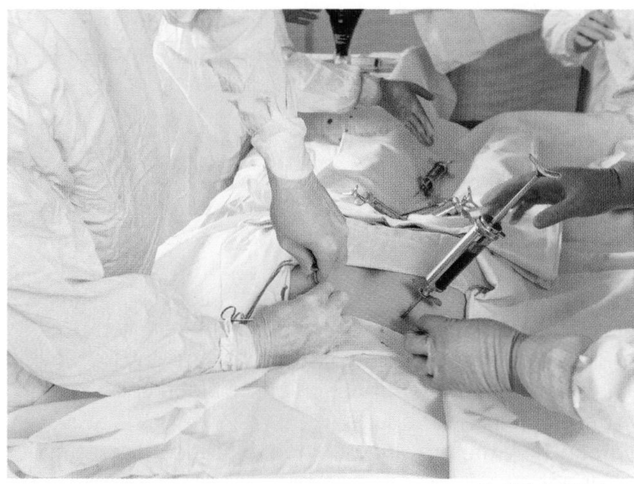

OlegMalyshev/iStock.com

Figure 11.19 Bone marrow is harvested from a healthy individual in preparation for a stem cell transplant. Transplanted bone marrow replaces the diseased bone marrow of a person with leukemia or multiple myeloma and produces healthy WBCs, RBCs, and platelets.

Multiple Myeloma

Multiple myeloma is a cancer of the plasma cells in bone marrow. The plasma cells of a person with this disease divide many times, creating even more plasma cells that are cancerous. Cancerous plasma cells are called *myelomas*.

Myeloma cells deposit in the bone marrow, forming tumors that can damage the bone. As a result, people with multiple myeloma are prone to bone fractures and bone pain, particularly in the back and ribs. Other symptoms of this disease include excess blood calcium levels, kidney damage, and frequent infections.

Multiple myeloma is a treatable but incurable condition. Treatment methods include steroid drugs, chemotherapy, and stem cell transplants.

Multiple myeloma is the second most common blood cancer in the United States, accounting for 15% of all blood cancer cases. Each year, this disease affects between 1 and 4 out of every 100,000 people. African-Americans are twice as likely as Caucasians to develop multiple myeloma. Survival rates continue to improve as a result of new drug therapies and stem cell transplant techniques.

SECTION 11.3 REVIEW

Mini-Glossary

acute lymphocytic leukemia (ALL) the most common form of leukemia in children under 15 years of age characterized by overproduction of lymphocytes

acute myeloid leukemia (AML) the most common form of leukemia in adults; develops when the bone marrow produces too many myeloblasts

anemia a condition characterized by a decrease in the number of red blood cells or an insufficient amount of hemoglobin in the red blood cells

aplastic anemia a rare but serious condition in which the bone marrow stem cells are incapable of making new red blood cells

chelation therapy a procedure in which excess metals, such as iron, are removed from the blood

chronic lymphocytic leukemia (CLL) a form of leukemia characterized by extremely high levels of lymphocytes; most often found in middle-aged adults

chronic myeloid leukemia (CML) a form of leukemia characterized by overproduction of granulocytes

complete blood count (CBC) a blood test that helps detect blood disorders or diseases, such as anemia, infection, abnormal blood cell counts, clotting problems, immune system disorders, and cancers of the blood

embolus a clot that has become dislodged from the wall of a blood vessel and travels through the bloodstream

hemophilia a condition in which blood does not clot properly due to the absence of a clotting factor

(continued)

iron-deficient anemia the most common type of anemia; caused by an insufficient dietary intake of iron, loss of iron from intestinal bleeding, or iron-level depletion during pregnancy

jaundice a blood disorder characterized by yellow-colored skin and whites of the eyes

leukemia a cancer of the blood that causes the bone marrow to produce cancerous white blood cells

multiple myeloma a cancer of the plasma cells in bone marrow

pernicious anemia a severe anemia caused by the inability of the intestines to absorb vitamin B_{12}, which is essential for the formation of red blood cells; usually develops in older adults

phlebotomy the drawing of blood; a standard treatment for polycythemia

polycythemia a condition in which the bone marrow manufactures too many red blood cells; caused by prolonged altitude exposure and a genetic mutation

sickle cell anemia a disease in which the red blood cells are shaped like a sickle, or crescent, rather than a disk; caused by irregularly shaped hemoglobin molecules in the red blood cells

thalassemia a condition that limits the body's ability to produce fully developed hemoglobin and red blood cells; also known as *Cooley's anemia*.

thrombus a clot that forms in an intact blood vessel, usually a vein

Review Questions

1. What conditions may be indicated by an abnormal number of white blood cells?
2. Which condition is characterized by a decreased number of red blood cells, fatigue, shortness of breath, and dizziness?
3. What type of food and mineral supplement are recommended for a person with iron-deficient anemia?
4. What is another name for Cooley's anemia?
5. Which condition results from damage to bone marrow stem cells, making them unable to produce mature blood cells?
6. Diseases such as type I diabetes mellitus, Addison's disease, and chronic thyroiditis increase the risk of developing which type of anemia?
7. What factor might increase the likelihood that a newborn will develop jaundice?
8. Which disease includes a symptom known as a *crisis*? How would you describe a crisis?
9. What are the most common treatments for sickle cell anemia?
10. Which disease requires people to be more concerned than normal about skin punctures and cuts?
11. Describe the number and condition of white blood cells in leukemia.
12. Why would a bone marrow stem cell transplant help a person with multiple myeloma?

Medical Terminology: The Blood

By understanding the word parts that make up medical words, you can extend your medical vocabulary. This chapter includes many of the word parts listed below. Review these word parts to be sure you understand their meanings.

a-, an-	no, not, without
-crit	to separate
cyt/o	cell
-emesis	vomiting
-emia	blood condition
erythr/o	red
hem/o, hemat/o	blood
-ic	pertaining to
leuk/o	white
-lysis	breakdown, destruction
-penia	deficiency
-poiesis	formation
-stasis	stop

Now use these word parts to form valid medical words that fit the following definitions. Some of the words are included in this chapter. Others are not. When you finish, use a medical dictionary to check your work.

1. condition of not having enough blood
2. to stop the flow of blood
3. destruction of blood cells
4. low white blood cell count
5. creation of blood cells
6. pertaining to white blood cells
7. formation of red blood cells
8. deficient number of red blood cells
9. vomiting blood
10. blood separation

Chapter 11 Summary

- The blood is a liquid connective tissue that provides transportation, regulation, and protection throughout the body.
- Blood has two types of components: liquid (plasma) and solid (formed elements).
- The formed elements include erythrocytes (RBCs), five types of leukocytes (WBCs), and thrombocytes (platelets).
- Blood cells are manufactured by stem cells in the red bone marrow through a process called *hematopoiesis*.
- The ABO blood grouping system includes four blood types: A, B, AB, and O; a person's blood type depends on the antigens and antibodies his or her blood contains.
- The Rh factor is an antigen on the surface of red blood cells. People with the Rh antigen are Rh-positive (Rh^+), and people without it are Rh-negative (Rh^-).
- A complete blood count is a test that measures the number of red blood cells, white blood cells, and platelets, as well as hemoglobin, hematocrit, and other RBC characteristics.
- Anemia is characterized by a decreased number of red blood cells or an insufficient amount of hemoglobin in red blood cells; its three main causes are decreased production of red blood cells, excessive blood loss, and a high rate of red blood cell destruction.
- Other blood disorders and diseases include jaundice, hemophilia, polycythemia, intravascular clotting, leukemia, and multiple myeloma.

Chapter 11 Review

Understanding Key Concepts

1. *True or False?* Blood is considered a regulatory system.
2. Which of the following is *not* a basic component of blood?
   A. myocytes
   B. plasma
   C. thrombocytes
   D. leukocytes
3. Approximately what percentage of blood is composed of plasma?
4. Blood makes up approximately _____ of total body weight.
   A. 3%
   B. 8%
   C. 12%
   D. 15%
5. Which of the following is *not* a protein found in blood plasma?
   A. fibrinogen
   B. globulin
   C. albumin
   D. casein
6. *True or False?* Red blood cells have an unlimited life span.
7. Only _____ bone marrow is capable of producing blood cells and new stem cells.
8. The kidneys regulate red blood cell production through a process called _____.
9. _____ are the most abundant type of white blood cells in the body.
10. Basophils are white blood cells that _____.
    A. attack invading microorganisms
    B. produce histamine
    C. give red blood cells their disk shape
    D. give blood its color
11. *True or False?* In the ABO blood grouping system, there are three major blood types.
12. _____ are molecules on the surface of cells that help the body distinguish between "self" and "nonself" cells.
13. A person who has _____ blood is considered to be a universal donor.
    A. type A
    B. type B
    C. type AB
    D. type O
14. *True or False?* The term *Rh factor* was inspired by the rhesus monkey.
15. The potentially fatal process that causes blood to clump and create blockages is called _____.
    A. coagulation
    B. agglutination
    C. erythroblastosis fetalis
    D. hemolysis

16. *True or False?* Blood was first classified according to type by an Austrian scientist named Karl Landsteiner in 1901.
17. Which of the following is *not* measured in a CBC?
    A. hematocrit
    B. number of white blood cells
    C. myoglobin
    D. hemoglobin
18. Agglutination can cause ______ of donated red blood cells.
19. A person who has ______ blood is considered to be a universal recipient.
    A. type A
    B. type B
    C. type AB
    D. type O
20. Which of the following is one of the three main causes of anemia?
    A. increased production of white blood cells
    B. platelet destruction
    C. decreased production of red blood cells
    D. blood vessel injury
21. *True or False?* Iron-deficient anemia accounts for almost 50% of all anemias.
22. Aplastic anemia is characterized by the inability of the bone marrow stem cells to make new ______.
    A. white blood cells
    B. plasma
    C. hemoglobin
    D. proteins
23. Pernicious anemia is caused by the inability of the intestines to absorb vitamin ______.
24. *True or False?* It is possible to inherit an anemic condition.
25. To develop sickle cell anemia, you must inherit the sickle cell gene from ______.
    A. your mother
    B. your father
    C. both parents
    D. your grandfather
26. ______ is a disease that affects proteins in hemoglobin and prevents the body from producing fully developed hemoglobin.
27. Which type of therapy is used to remove excess iron from the blood?
    A. chemotherapy
    B. radiation therapy
    C. chelation therapy
    D. vitamin B_{12} injection therapy

Thinking Critically

28. Explain the process of hemostasis that occurs when a blood vessel wall has been injured.
29. Explain the characteristic that is used to distinguish among blood types in the ABO blood grouping system. Why is it dangerous to mix certain blood types for blood transfusions?
30. Identify the characteristic that makes blood types either positive (+) or negative (–). Explain the significance of these classifications.
31. Kelsey is a fifteen-year-old girl whose parents moved to Chicago from their native Sicily five years before she was born. When Kelsey was a baby, she was diagnosed with a blood disorder. As a result of this disorder, Kelsey experiences back and leg pain. She is often short of breath and tired. Which blood disorder is Kelsey experiencing? What can she do to manage her disease?
32. Rachael is a young mother with Rh-negative blood. Her first child, Hazel, was born two years ago and has Rh-positive blood. Rachael is now pregnant with her second child. What complications might arise if her second baby also has Rh-positive blood? What can Rachael's doctor do to avoid these complications?

Clinical Case Study

33. Among the topics discussed in the chapter, what may be happening to Donya?
34. Which diagnosis is most likely?
35. What types of tests might help evaluate Donya's condition?

Analyzing and Evaluating Data

The chart on the right shows survival rates for leukemia and multiple myeloma patients from 1960 to 2007. Use this chart to answer the following questions.

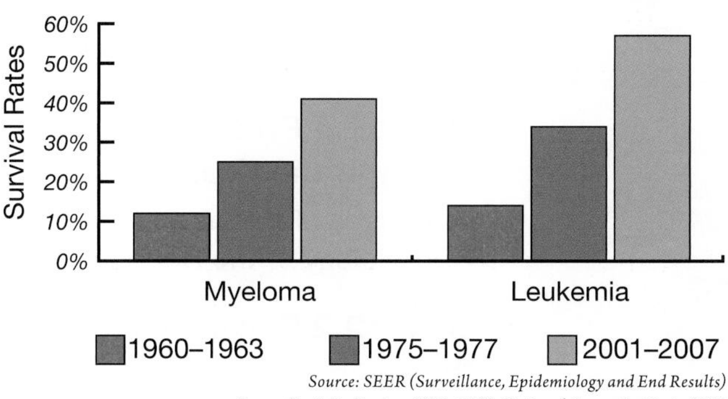

Source: SEER (Surveillance, Epidemiology and End Results) Cancer Statistics Review, 1975–2008. National Cancer Institute; 2011

36. By what percentage did survival rates for multiple myeloma cases improve between the 1960s and 2007?
37. If a person was diagnosed with leukemia in 1976, what survival rate could be expected?
38. If a person was diagnosed with multiple myeloma in 2003, what survival rate could be expected?
39. Survival rates for both multiple myeloma and leukemia have consistently risen since the 1960s. Why do you think this is?

Investigating Further

40. What are the current five-year survival rates for multiple myeloma and leukemia? Research the statistics online and determine the survival-rate percentage for both diseases.
41. In 1985, the United States established mandatory screenings of donated blood for blood-borne diseases, such as HIV. Research the blood donation process. For what other diseases must donated blood be screened to prevent transmission of diseases? Besides screening for blood-borne diseases, what steps must be taken to ensure that donors are healthy candidates for donation? Can people with tattoos donate blood? What about someone with a cold virus?
42. Hemophilia is a genetic blood disorder that is usually inherited. One of the most well-known carriers for hemophilia was Queen Victoria of England. Research the history of hemophilia in Queen Victoria's family. Did this disease affect royal families in other nations? If so, why? Also, look into which members of her family were carriers and which suffered from the disease. Create a family tree to organize the information.
43. Research the history of blood transfusions from the 1600s to the present. Why did some transfusion efforts fail? What technological developments improved transfusion success rates?

12 The Cardiovascular System

Clinical Case Study

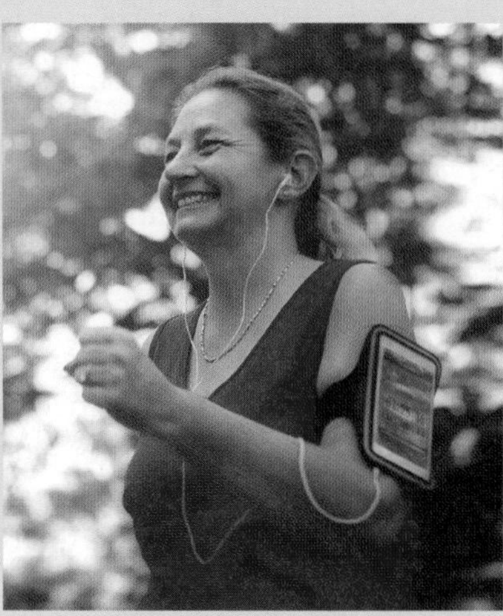
Rawpixel.com/Shutterstock.com

Ann was an apparently healthy 60-year-old, nonsmoking female with a history of hypertension. At her last office checkup, Ann's blood pressure was 150/90 mmHg, her total cholesterol was 260mg/dL and her body mass index was 29 kg/m^2. Her electrocardiogram (ECG) was normal. Her physician was concerned about her elevated blood pressure and cholesterol level, so he added a new blood pressure medication and told her to get a home blood pressure monitor. The physician also recommended that she lose weight and become more physically active.

Ann was determined to get her numbers down, so she started a walking program and began eating a low-fat, low-calorie diet. She also bought a blood pressure monitor, and her home recordings averaged in the 120/80 to 130/80 mmHg range. After three months on her new diet and exercise regime, Ann returned to her physician's office for a checkup. Her blood pressure was now 130/80 mmHg, and her total cholesterol was 220mg/dL. Ann had lost 15 pounds, and her fitness monitor showed she was walking an average of 3 miles per day. Ann's doctor was pleased with her progress, but became concerned when Ann said she was increasingly fatigued and sometimes short of breath during her daily walks.

What do Ann's blood pressure, BMI, and total cholesterol numbers tell you about her health? Among the medical conditions and disorders discussed in this chapter, what are the possible causes of Ann's shortness of breath, and which one is the most likely diagnosis?

Chapter 12 Outline

"You gotta have *heart*!"
"Follow your *heart*."
"Know it by *heart*."
"Let's get to the *heart* of the matter!"

Is there an organ in the human body that is referenced in everyday language more often than the heart? What does this say about the function and importance of the heart?

The beating heart is just one part of the complex cardiovascular system. The system—comprising the heart, blood, and blood vessels—has a major impact on every living cell in the body.

The heart beats 24 hours a day, 7 days a week. It pumps approximately 1.3 gallons (5 liters) of blood per minute, or approximately 2,000 gallons (7,571 liters) of blood each day. By comparison, a typical oil well pumps about 94 gallons of oil a day. The amount of blood pumped through the heart could fill 45 oil barrels a day and 2 oil supertankers in a lifetime. That is an extraordinary feat for a muscle that is about the size of a fist and weighs less than one pound! This chapter describes how the heart pumps blood through thousands of miles of passageways in the body to nourish every cell and remove waste products.

SECTION 12.1

Functional Anatomy of the Heart

Objectives

- Describe the location, size, and structures of the heart.
- Outline the flow of blood through the heart.

Key Terms

aorta
aortic valve
atrioventricular (AV) valves
cardiac output
cardiomyocytes
diastole
endocardium
epicardium
fibrous pericardium
inferior vena cava
interatrial septum
interventricular septum
mediastinum
mitral valve
myocardium
papillary muscle
parietal pericardium
pulmonary valve
semilunar valves
serous pericardium
stroke volume
superior vena cava
systole
tricuspid valve
vasoconstriction
vasodilation

The cardiovascular system, also called the *circulatory system*, consists of the heart, an extensive network of blood vessels, and blood. The system transports oxygen, hormones, and other nutrients to cells and rids the cells of carbon dioxide and other metabolic waste products.

Additionally, the cardiovascular system helps to regulate body temperature through vasodilation and vasoconstriction of blood vessels. ***Vasodilation*** is an expansion in the diameter of blood vessels, which increases blood flow. ***Vasoconstriction*** is a decrease in the diameter of blood vessels, which decreases blood flow. The cardiovascular system has many other functions as well, including maintaining the body's acid-base balance and assisting with immune function.

Anatomy of the Heart

The heart is the hardest-working organ in the human body. A normal adult heart rate is 72 to 82 beats per minute (bpm), or approximately 3 billion beats in a person's lifetime. This fatigue-resistant organ is about the size of a clenched fist. It weighs a little less than the combined weight of two baseballs, or about 8 to 10 ounces in women and 10 to 12 ounces in men.

Location and Size

The heart is located in the thoracic cavity directly under the sternum, or breastbone, centered in the chest with two thirds of it lying to the left of the sternum. It is located in the ***mediastinum*** (mee-dee-a-STIGH-nuhm), which is the anatomical region between the sternum and the vertebral column, from the first rib to the diaphragm, and between the two lungs. It is anchored in the mediastinum by its attachments to the diaphragm, sternum, and ribs. The broad base of the heart is positioned closer to the neck, at the second rib and is primarily formed by the atria. The pointed apex, or bottom, of the heart is formed by the left ventricle, lies at approximately the fifth rib and points down toward the left hip (**Figure 12.1**).

Chambers

The heart has an atrium and a ventricle on its right side and an atrium and a ventricle on its left side. The two atria (plural of *atrium*) act as low-pressure collecting chambers, while the two ventricles are powerful pumps. The atria are located superior to the ventricles. The atria and ventricles are lined with endothelial cells, which allow blood to flow smoothly within the chambers.

An ***interatrial septum*** separates the right and left atria, and the two ventricles are divided by a much thicker ***interventricular septum***. The septal walls prevent oxygen-rich blood on the left side of the heart from mixing with the oxygen-poor blood on the right side.

The wall of the left ventricle is approximately three times thicker than that of the right ventricle (**Figure 12.2**). This is because the left ventricle pumps against the greater resistance present in the high-pressure systemic circulatory system, while the right ventricle pumps to the relatively low-pressure pulmonary circulatory system.

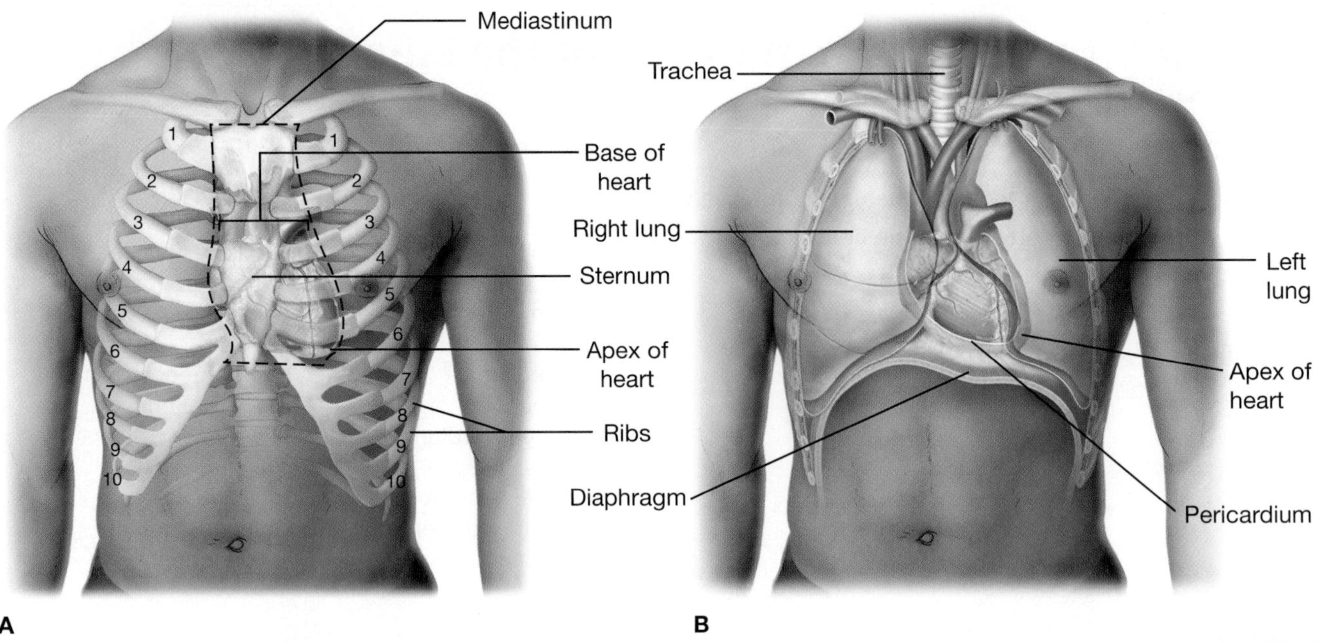

© Body Scientific International

Figure 12.1 Position of the heart. A—Position of the heart in the thoracic cavity. B—Position of the heart in relation to the lungs and diaphragm.

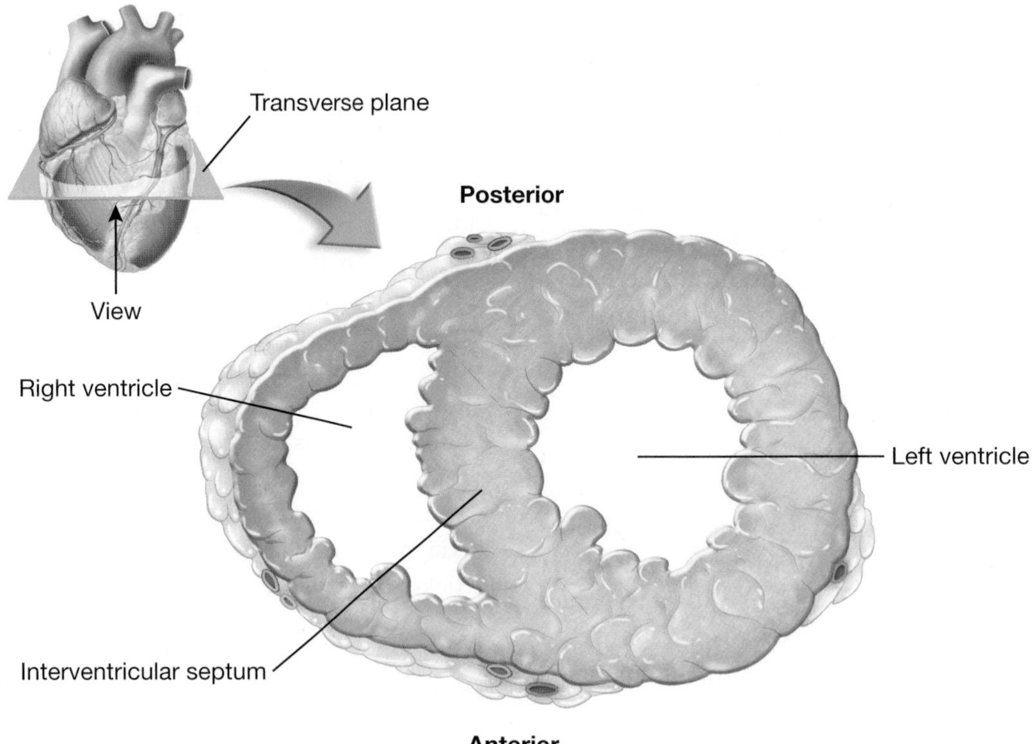

© Body Scientific International

Figure 12.2 The left ventricle has thicker walls than the right ventricle because it needs more power to push blood throughout the body in the high-pressure systemic system.

Clinical Application Why It Is Important to Know the Heart's Location

If you are studying to become a nurse, doctor, or any other type of healthcare worker, it is important for you to know the heart's location. This knowledge will enable you to properly apply electrodes when performing an electrocardiogram, position your stethoscope correctly when listening to heart sounds, or even position your hands correctly when performing CPR. The chest compressions delivered in CPR are effective in pumping blood from the heart because the heart is located between two firm structures—the sternum and the vertebral column.

Knowing the position and location of the heart is important even if you are not a healthcare worker. Bystanders often perform CPR when heart attacks and other cardiovascular emergencies occur in public. In 2015, the American Heart Association recommended that untrained bystanders should deliver hands-only chest compressions to the center of the chest, to a depth of two inches, at a rate of 100 to 120 compressions per minute. If you know where the heart is located, you can better deliver life-saving compressions until professional help arrives.

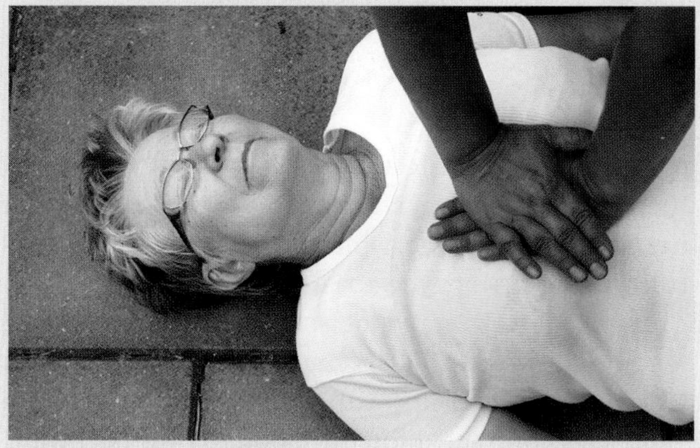

AnneMS/Shutterstock.com

Correct placement of the hands is critical when performing chest compressions in CPR.

Note: Call 911 first and put your phone on speaker so you can talk to the 911 operator while performing the chest compressions. If you are trained, you should perform 30 compressions followed by 2 breaths (ratio of 30:2) until paramedics arrive.

Heart Valves

The heart is outfitted with four valves, which permit blood to flow in only one direction. **Figure 12.3** shows the heart valves in open and closed states.

Atrioventricular Valves

The ***atrioventricular (AV) valves*** are the two valves located between the atria and the ventricles. When these valves are open, they allow blood to flow from the atria into the ventricles. When they are closed, the AV valves prevent blood from flowing from the ventricles backward into the atria as the ventricles contract.

The AV valve on the right side of the heart is called the ***tricuspid valve*** because it has three cusps, or flaps. The AV valve on the left side of the heart is called the *bicuspid valve*, or the ***mitral valve***, because it has two cusps.

Attached to these cusps are chordae tendineae (KOR-dee TEHN-di-nee), which are thin, fibrous

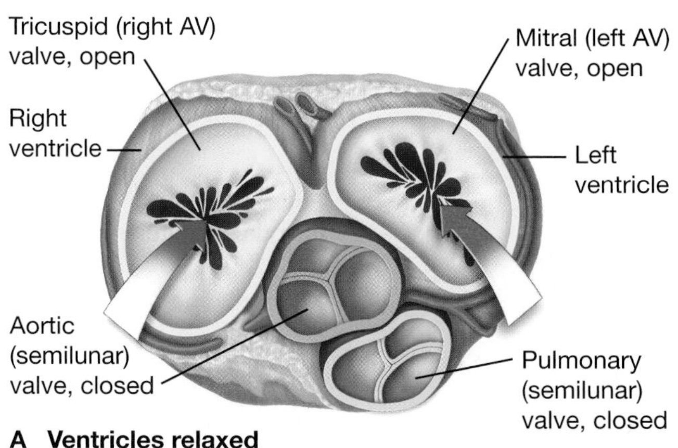

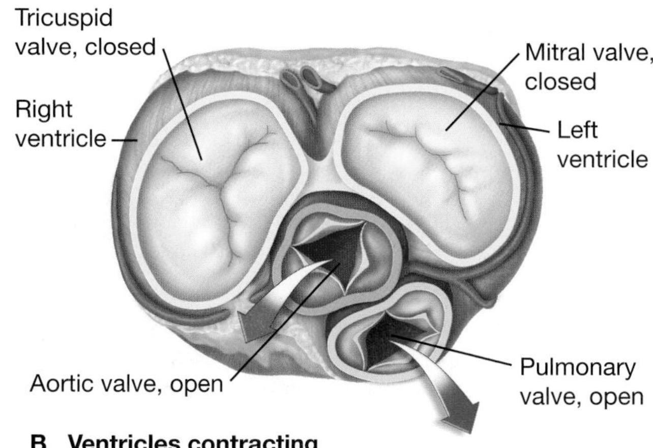

© Body Scientific International

Figure 12.3 Superior view of the heart valves. The red arrows indicate the flow of oxygenated blood. The blue arrows indicate the flow of deoxygenated blood.

Understanding Medical Terminology

These tips should help you remember the locations of the different heart valves. You can remember that the **T**ricuspid valve is on the **R**ight side of heart by noting that the letters **R** and **T** are close together in the alphabet. The **M**itral valve is on the **L**eft side of heart, so remember that **L** and **M** are side by side in the alphabet.

cords that connect to the ***papillary muscles***. When the ventricles contract, the papillary muscles pull on the chordae tendineae, which prevents the valve cusps from swinging into the atria.

If the valves were not secured by the chordae tendineae and the papillary muscles, the AV valve cusps would be pushed upward into the atria when the ventricles contract, allowing blood to flow backward into the atria. This backward blood flow is what happens when a person has a heart murmur.

Semilunar Valves

The ***semilunar valves*** allow blood to flow from the ventricles to the lungs and the rest of the body. The ***pulmonary valve*** and ***aortic valve*** each have three semilunar (half-moon) cusps that do not need to be anchored. When they close, these cusps are strong enough to brace each other, similar to the three legs of a stool. The pulmonary valve lies between the right atrium and the pulmonary trunk, which transports the blood to the lungs for oxygenation. The aortic valve lies between the left ventricle and the ***aorta***, which conducts blood to the rest of the body.

Pericardium

The heart is a hollow organ enclosed in a fluid-filled sac called the *pericardium*. This protective sac consists of three layers (**Figure 12.4**).

The tough, fibrous, nonelastic outer wall of the sac is called the ***fibrous pericardium***. This outer layer protects the heart, prevents it from being over-stretched, and anchors it to surrounding structures within the mediastinum, such as the diaphragm and sternum. The top part of the fibrous pericardium is also connected to the connective tissues of the blood vessels that enter and leave the heart, such as the pulmonary trunk.

The inner wall of the sac is called the ***serous pericardium***. The serous pericardium is divided into two layers (parietal and visceral), which are separated by the fluid-filled pericardial cavity that allows the heart to beat in a frictionless environment.

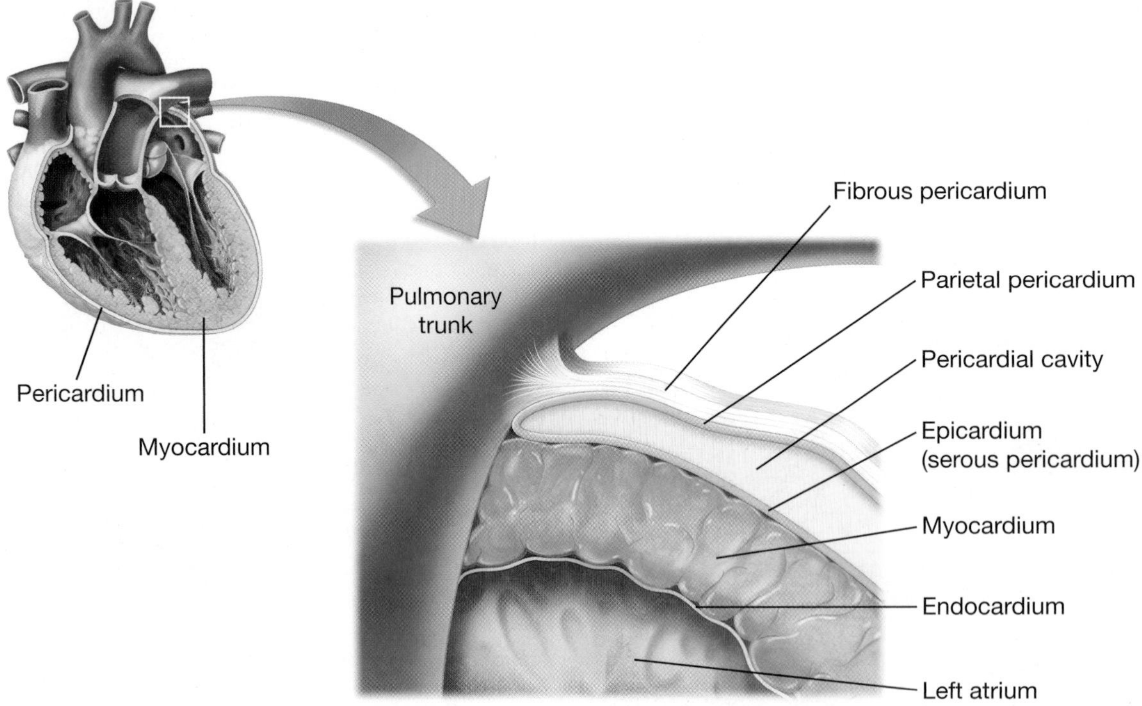

Figure 12.4 Layers of pericardium.

The parietal layer, also known as the ***parietal pericardium***, is located between the fibrous and serous layers of the pericardium. It secretes the slippery serous fluid found in the pericardial cavity. The visceral layer, also called the *epicardium*, is both the innermost layer of the pericardium and the outermost layer of the heart. It also secretes serous pericardial fluid.

Layers of the Heart

The heart has three layers of tissue. They are the epicardium (*epi* = "outside, on top of"), the myocardium (*myo* = "muscle"), and the endocardium (*endo* = "inner").

The ***epicardium*** is the outermost layer of the heart, and it is also the visceral layer of the serous pericardium. It is composed primarily of connective tissue and fat, which provides an additional layer of protection for the heart. The epicardium is fused directly to the myocardium, and the coronary arteries lie on its surface.

The ***myocardium***, the middle layer of the heart, is composed of cardiac muscle cells called ***cardiomyocytes*** that contract and relax like skeletal muscle cells, but they have very different properties. Although they are striated like skeletal muscle cells, they are controlled involuntarily and are capable of conducting an electrical impulse through the intercalated discs that connect them (**Figure 12.5**). This is the reason that all cardiac cells contract almost simultaneously, causing the heart to be an impressively effective pump. The myocardium makes up about 95% of the heart muscle. It is the "workhorse" of the heart, contracting with enough force to pump blood through the 60,000 miles of vessels and back to the heart.

The innermost layer, the ***endocardium***, is a smooth, thin layer of endothelial cells. This layer lines the interior of the heart chambers and covers the valves of the heart. The endocardium connects to the great vessels that are attached to the heart. The endothelial cells in the endocardium help blood flow smoothly throughout the heart and into the great vessels.

Blood Flow through the Heart

Figure 12.6 shows the flow of blood through the heart in a numbered, step-by-step view. Remember that the right and left sides of the heart contract and relax almost simultaneously, with the atria contracting slightly before the ventricles.

1. Deoxygenated blood enters the right atrium from both the ***inferior vena cava*** and the ***superior vena cava***. The blood collects in the right atrium.
2. The collecting blood increases the pressure against the tricuspid valve, causing the valve to open. At this stage, with the tricuspid valve open, the right ventricle fills passively. The right atrium then contracts, forcing the remaining blood into the ventricle.
3. The right ventricle contracts, and pressure increases in the chamber. This causes the tricuspid valve to close and the pulmonary valve to open, forcing blood into the pulmonary trunk.
4. The pulmonary trunk branches to the pulmonary arteries, which carry the blood to the lungs, where it becomes oxygenated in the capillary network of the lungs.
5. The newly oxygenated blood enters the left atrium via the pulmonary veins. Blood collects in the left atrium.
6. The collecting blood increases pressure in the chamber, forcing the mitral (bicuspid) valve to open.
7. At this stage, with the mitral valve open, the left ventricle fills passively.
8. The left ventricle contracts, forcing the remaining blood from the left atrium into the left ventricle, and the pressure increases in the chamber. The increased pressure in the chamber causes the mitral valve to close and the aortic valve to open. The blood is forced into the aorta.
9. Oxygenated blood begins its journey of supplying oxygen to all parts of the body.

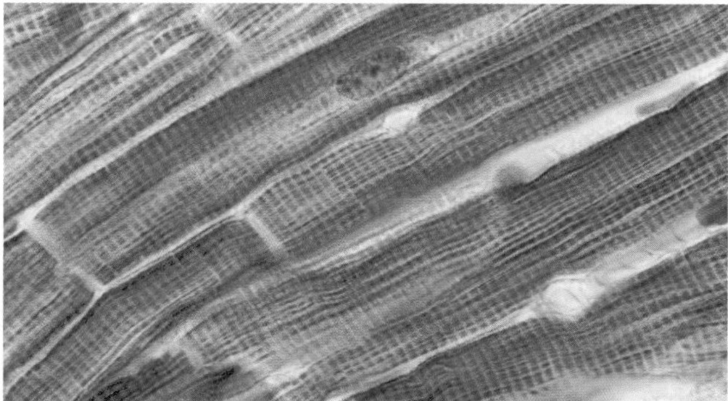

Jose Luis Calvo/Shutterstock.com

Figure 12.5 Cardiomyocytes are connected by intercalated disks that help ensure that the cells contract in a coordinated manner to pump blood through the heart and throughout the body.

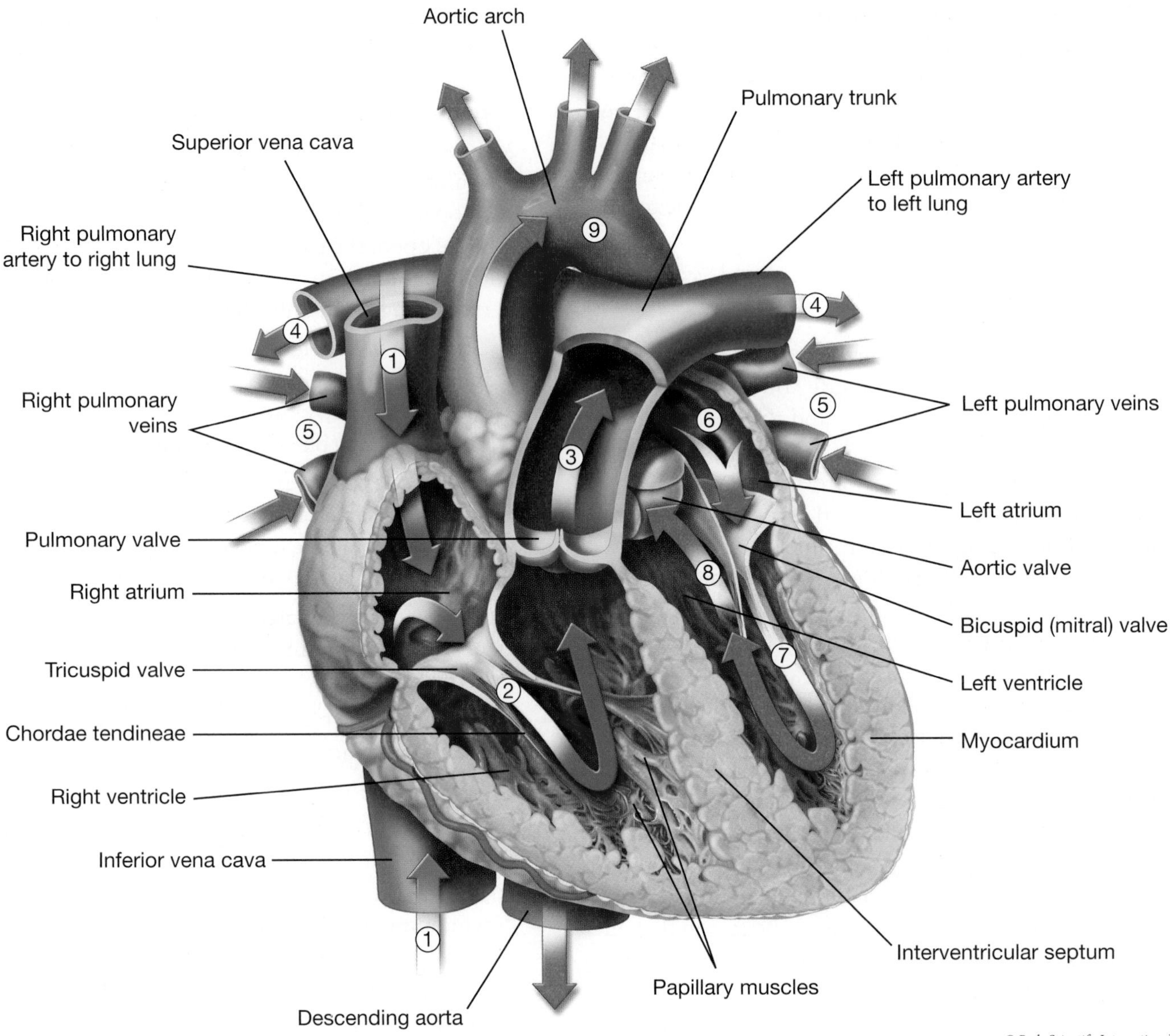

Figure 12.6 Heart chambers and valves, great vessels, and blood flow through the heart. The arrows indicate the direction of blood flow through the heart. The blue arrows indicate deoxygenated blood. The red arrows indicate oxygenated blood.

SELF CHECK

1. When a pulmonary valve opens, blood is forced into which artery and which main respiratory organ?
2. Which valve does blood move through as it goes from the right atrium to the right ventricle?
3. What is the name of the sac that encases the heart?
4. Name the three layers of the heart.

Physiology of the Heart

The beating of the heart is a complex event that requires great coordination not only among the individual cells, but also among the various parts of the heart. This section describes the cardiac cycle—the events included in a "heartbeat"—and explains the results in terms of cardiac output and stroke volume.

Cardiac Cycle

The cardiac cycle consists of two phases: contraction and relaxation. During one complete cardiac cycle, the four chambers of the heart undergo a period of relaxation called ***diastole*** when the chambers fill with blood. Each cycle also includes a period of contraction called ***systole***, when the chambers pump blood out of the heart.

The terms *systole* and *diastole* usually refer to what is happening in the ventricles because they are the major pumps of the heart. In a healthy heart, contraction times are slightly offset when the atria contract, the ventricles are relaxed. When the ventricles contract, the atria are relaxed.

One cardiac cycle lasts approximately 0.81 second. In general, for an individual who has a resting heart rate of 72 to 82 bpm, approximately two-thirds of the cardiac cycle is spent in diastole, and one-third is spent in systole. This ratio is the basis for the formula for mean arterial pressure:

$$\text{Mean Arterial Pressure (MAP)} = \text{2/3 Diastolic Blood Pressure} + \text{1/3 Systolic Blood Pressure}$$

The mean arterial pressure is a measure of the overall pressure within the cardiovascular system, which determines blood flow to various organs. If this pressure falls below 60 mmHG (millimeters of mercury), the organs of the body will become damaged from lack of oxygen. A lower blood pressure also means that the body will not receive the nutrient-rich blood flow that it needs.

At a typical physical examination, the physician may use a stethoscope to listen to the patient's heart. During the cardiac cycle, the AV valves and the semilunar valves make sounds when they close. The doctor is listening for those sounds, which are referred to as "lub-dub" sounds. The "lub" sound is produced when the AV valves close, and the "dub" sound is produced when the semilunar valves close. If the valves do not close properly, there may be an additional sound called a *heart murmur*. Many children are told by their doctors that they have a heart murmur. Most of these murmurs are harmless and are caused by a rapid growth spurt rather than a heart abnormality.

Stroke Volume and Cardiac Output

Stroke volume is the amount of blood pumped from the heart per beat, and the unit of measurement is milliliters per beat (mL/beat). Stroke volume is determined by four factors:

- amount of blood that returns to the heart during diastole (venous return or preload)
- degree of stretch in the myocardial muscle fibers when they are maximally extended (myocardial stretch)
- strength of the left ventricle (LV) contraction
- resistance to the blood being ejected from the heart (afterload)

Research Notes How the Heart Adapts to Exercise

An echocardiogram is an ultrasound test that allows healthcare professionals to examine the structures of the heart and determine whether the heart valves are opening and closing properly. This test can also measure the pumping capacity of the heart.

Echocardiogram studies have shown that athletes who train aerobically (by running, cycling, or swimming, for example) have larger left ventricular chambers and thicker left ventricular walls than the average person. By contrast, athletes who train using resistive exercise (weight lifting) have thicker left ventricular walls but average-sized ventricular chambers.

Stroke volume among athletes is almost twice that of untrained individuals. This occurs due to increased parasympathetic tone, which causes athletes' resting heart rate to fall below 60 beats per minute. Maximal parasympathetic stimulation can decrease heart rate to 20–30 beats per minute. The parasympathetic branch of the autonomic nervous system is the dominant branch at rest, and it causes a reduced resting heart rate.

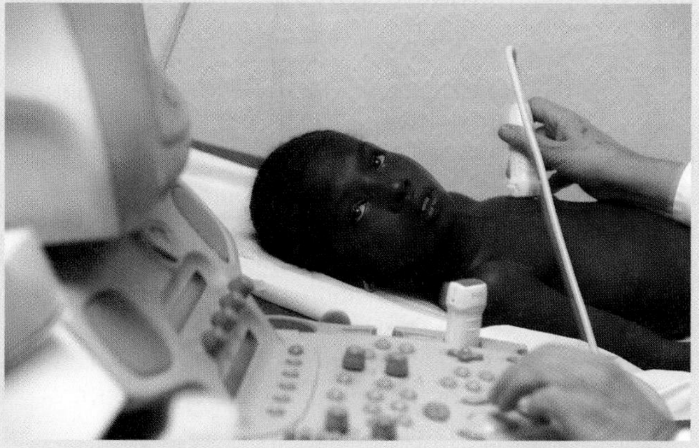

GODONG/Science Source

A cardiovascular technologist performs an echocardiogram on a pediatric patient.

A reduced resting heart rate increases filling time for the ventricles during the relaxation phase of the cardiac cycle, which results in an increased stroke volume.

As the amount of blood that returns to the heart increases, the amount of blood in the LV before it contracts (preload) increases as well. A large preload increases stroke volume. When more blood returns to the left ventricle, the myocardial muscle fibers are stretched more. Increased myocardial stretch will also increase stroke volume. When the myocardial fibers are stretched, the number of cross bridges between the actin and myosin filaments in the cardiac muscle fibers increases. This, in turn, increases the force of left ventricular contraction, thereby increasing stroke volume. The relationship between increased myocardial stretch and increased strength of left ventricular contraction is known as the *Frank Starling mechanism*. An increase in sympathetic nervous system activity can also increase the strength of left ventricular contraction.

As the afterload decreases, a greater amount of blood can leave the heart. Therefore, a low afterload increases stroke volume. Afterload is determined by the mean arterial pressure against which the heart must contract.

The amount of blood pumped from the heart per minute is called ***cardiac output*** (Q). Cardiac output is important because it has an effect on blood pressure, cardiovascular fitness level, and body temperature.

The unit of measurement for cardiac output is liters per minute (L/min). Cardiac output is determined by multiplying the heart rate (HR) by the stroke volume (SV). Heart rate, and the mechanisms that control it, will be discussed in more detail in the next section.

The average cardiac output for an adult is between 5 and 6 L/min. Cardiac output is influenced by many factors, such as body size, exercise, emotions, diet, and physical activity.

The average heart rate and stroke volume for a typical 154-pound male are approximately 72 beats/min and 70 mL/beat, which means that the cardiac output is 5,040 milliliters per minute (mL/min), or 5.0 L/min. Women, because of their generally shorter stature and smaller size, have lower cardiac outputs than men.

Cardiac output is calculated in the following way:

$$\text{SV (mL/beat)} \times \text{HR (beats/min)} = \text{Q (cardiac output)}$$

$$70 \text{ mL/beat} \times 72 \text{ beats/min} = 5,040 \text{ mL/min or } 5.0 \text{ L/min}$$

SECTION 12.1 REVIEW

Mini-Glossary

aorta a large arterial trunk that arises from the base of the left ventricle and channels blood from the heart into other arteries throughout the body

aortic valve the semilunar valve between the left ventricle and the aorta that prevents blood from flowing back into the left ventricle

atrioventricular (AV) valves the two valves (tricuspid and mitral/bicuspid) situated between the atria and the ventricles

cardiac output the amount of blood pumped from the heart per minute; also known as *cardiac volume*

cardiomyocytes cardiac muscle cells

diastole the period of relaxation in the heart when the chambers fill with blood

endocardium the innermost layer of the heart, which lines the interior of the heart chambers and covers the valves of the heart

epicardium the outermost layer of the heart and the visceral layer of the serous pericardium

fibrous pericardium the tough, nonelastic outer wall of the pericardium

inferior vena cava the largest vein in the human body, which returns deoxygenated blood to the right atrium of the heart from body regions below the diaphragm

interatrial septum the wall that separates the right and left atria in the heart

interventricular septum the thick wall between the two ventricles in the heart

mediastinum the anatomical region between the sternum and the vertebral column, and between the lungs

mitral valve the atrioventricular valve that closes the orifice between the left atrium and left ventricle of the heart; also known as the *bicuspid valve*

myocardium the middle layer of the heart, which makes up about 95% of the heart

papillary muscle one of the small muscular bundles attached at one end to the chordae tendineae and to the endocardial wall of the ventricles at the other; maintains tension on the chordae tendineae as the ventricle contracts

parietal pericardium the parietal layer of the serous pericardium; secretes the serous fluid found in the pericardial cavity

pulmonary valve the semilunar valve that lies between the right atrium and the pulmonary trunk

semilunar valves the valves situated at the opening between the heart and the aorta, and at the opening between the heart and the pulmonary artery; prevent backflow of blood into the ventricles

(continued)

serous pericardium the inner wall of the pericardium; divided into the parietal layer (parietal pericardium) and the visceral layer (epicardium)
stroke volume the volume of blood pumped from the heart per beat
superior vena cava the second largest vein in the body, which returns deoxygenated blood to the right atrium of the heart from the upper half of the body
systole a period of contraction when the chambers pump blood out of the heart
tricuspid valve the atrioventricular valve that closes the orifice between the right atrium and right ventricle of the heart; composed of three cusps
vasoconstriction narrowing of the blood vessels, which decreases blood flow
vasodilation widening of the blood vessels, which increases blood flow

Review Questions

1. Name the large blood vessels that bring blood back to the heart and empty it into the right atrium.
2. Which muscles control the AV valves?
3. What blood vessels carry blood to the lungs?
4. What are the main differences between the AV valves and the semilunar valves?
5. What does the name *chordae tendineae* tell you about the characteristics of these structures?
6. What have echocardiogram studies revealed about the different effects of exercise on the hearts of aerobic athletes (runners, for example) and anaerobic athletes (weight lifters)?
7. Calculate cardiac output for a person whose heart rate is 40 beats/min, and whose stroke volume is 93 mL/beat.

SECTION 12.2 Regulation of the Heart

Objectives

- Describe the internal mechanisms that regulate the heart.
- Explain how external mechanisms help regulate the heart.
- Identify the components of the heart's conduction system.

Key Terms

atrioventricular (AV) node
Bachmann's bundle
baroreceptors
bundle branches
bundle of His
chemoreceptors
depolarize
mechanoreceptors
Purkinje fibers
repolarize
sinoatrial (SA) node

The heart is regulated by several different mechanisms. One mechanism is inside the heart, and the others are outside of the heart.

Internal Control

When a heart is transplanted from one individual to another, it will still beat on its own. How is this possible? The heart will continue to beat on its own because of a very important internal control mechanism called the ***sinoatrial (SA) node***, which is often called the *pacemaker* of the heart because it generates electrical impulses that cause the cardiomyocytes to contract at a regular rate. The SA node is located at the top of the right atrium, slightly lateral and inferior to the opening of the superior vena cava.

In a normal heart, the SA node initiates electrical impulses at a rate between 60 and 100 bpm. If the SA node fails to fire, the ***atrioventricular (AV) node*** will fire as a backup mechanism, but at a slower rate of 40–60 bpm. If the AV node also fails, the ventricles may pace the heart, but their intrinsic rate is even slower, between 15 and 40 bpm. This slower heart rate reduces cardiac output. If cardiac output becomes too low, it may cause dizziness, lightheadedness, or even syncope (fainting).

SELF CHECK

1. Which structure is known as the *pacemaker* of the heart?
2. What is the difference between the impulses generated by the SA node and those generated by the AV node?

External Control

The heart is also regulated by several external mechanisms. The cardiac center, located in the medulla oblongata, can be affected by higher brain centers, sensory receptors, some of the hormones secreted by the endocrine system, and other factors (**Figure 12.7**).

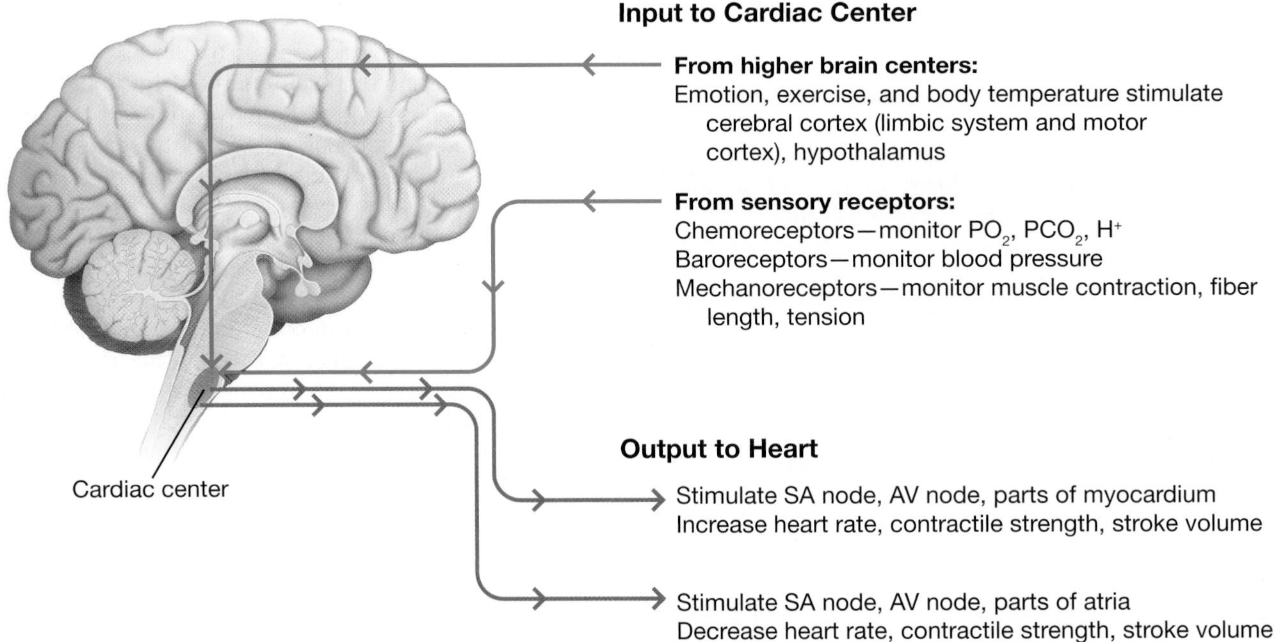

Figure 12.7 Location of the cardiac center in the medulla oblongata of the brain.

Cardiac Center

The portion of the medulla oblongata that controls heart rate and strength of contraction is sometimes referred to as the *cardiac center* of the brain. The cardiac center accepts input from both the sympathetic and parasympathetic branches of the autonomic nervous system (ANS). The sympathetic nerve fibers stimulate the SA node, AV node, and other parts of the myocardium. Parasympathetic nerve impulses, which come from the right and left vagus nerves, innervate the SA node, AV node, and parts of the atria (**Figure 12.7**).

The sympathetic nerves release norepinephrine, which activates the beta-1 adrenergic receptors in the heart. These receptors stimulate ventricular contractility, so activating them causes an increase in heart rate. Acetylcholine, released by the parasympathetic nerve fibers, has the opposite effect, slowing the heart rate.

The cardiac center continually monitors and adjusts heart rate, contraction strength, stroke volume, and degrees of vasodilation/vasoconstriction in the blood vessels. It stimulates the sympathetic branch of the ANS when the body requires an increase in heart rate, force of contraction, or stroke volume. It stimulates the parasympathetic branch when a decrease in heart rate, contractile strength, or stroke volume is needed.

As you can see, the two branches of the ANS work together to balance the heart rate. Neither could achieve balance alone. Maximal stimulation by the parasympathetic branch would result in heart rates between 20 and 30 bpm. Maximal stimulation by the sympathetic nervous system would result in a heart rate close to 200 bpm in a 20-year-old individual.

At rest, the parasympathetic nerves control the cardiac center, which is why the resting heart rate is lower than the intrinsic firing rate of the SA node. Without parasympathetic stimulation of the heart, resting heart rate would be approximately 90 bpm. During exercise, in heated environments, or in stressful conditions, the sympathetic branch takes over.

As you can see, the two branches of the cardiac center work together to balance the heart rate. Neither could achieve balance alone. Maximal stimulation by the parasympathetic branch would result in heart rates between 20 and 30 bpm. Maximal stimulation by the sympathetic nervous system would result in a heart rate close to 200 bpm in a 20-year-old individual.

Higher Brain Centers

Earlier chapters in this book discussed the fight-or-flight response; when faced with a dangerous situation, the body has to prepare itself to fight or run from the danger at hand. In such a situation, a set of brain structures within the cerebral cortex, called the *limbic system*, stimulates the sympathetic branch in the cardiac center.

The motor cortex, also part of the cerebral cortex, acts through the hypothalamus during exercise to increase heart rate and cause vasodilation in the active tissue. The hypothalamus itself can also alter heart rate, cardiac output, and blood flow to the tissues in response to changes in body temperature. During exercise, when body temperature increases, the hypothalamus causes an increase in heart rate, cardiac output, and vasodilation. Conversely, if body temperature drops, the hypothalamus causes a decrease in heart rate, cardiac output, and vasodilation.

Sensory Receptors

Three types of receptors in the nervous system send impulses to the cardiac center in the medulla oblongata: baroreceptors, chemoreceptors, and mechanoreceptors. These receptors act to influence heart rate, cardiac output, and vasodilation and vasoconstriction in the vessels.

Baroreceptors are sensitive to blood pressure. They are located in the atrium of the heart, the aortic arch, and the carotid arteries. The baroreceptors constantly monitor blood pressure and send sensory information back to the cardiac center, stimulating either the parasympathetic or sympathetic branches of the ANS.

Understanding Medical Terminology

Barometers measure the atmospheric pressure. Baroreceptors measure blood pressure.

Chemoreceptors are located near the baroreceptors in the aortic arch and carotid arteries. These receptors are sensitive to pH levels, decreased partial pressure of oxygen (P_{O_2}), increased partial pressure of carbon dioxide (P_{CO_2}), and increased levels of hydrogen ion (H^+) in the arterial blood. During exercise, when P_{CO_2} and H^+ increase or P_{O_2} decreases, there is an increase in cardiac output and vasoconstriction of most arterioles.

Mechanoreceptors are sensitive to mechanical stretch in tissues such as the heart and other muscles. Mechanoreceptors are activated during exercise due to muscular contraction, changes in muscle fiber length, and tension. Activation of the mechanoreceptors stimulates the cardiac center to adjust autonomic output to the SA node, increasing heart rate.

Hormonal Regulation

As described in Chapter 9, the endocrine system is composed of many glands that secrete hormones, which can cause many changes that affect other body systems. The adrenal medulla and the thyroid glands, for example, can affect the cardiovascular system. When the adrenal medulla secretes epinephrine and norepinephrine, heart rate increases. Similarly, when the thyroid gland releases thyroxine, heart rate increases.

Other Factors

Heart rate can also be affected by factors such as exercise, age, gender, and fitness level. Exercise activates the sympathetic branch of the ANS, which releases hormones such as epinephrine, norepinephrine, and thyroxine. These hormones cause increases in heart rate, strength of myocardial contraction, stroke volume, and cardiac output.

Babies have resting heart rates above 120 bpm. As people age, their heart rate declines. Maximal heart rate can be estimated by subtracting a person's age from 220. Women usually have higher resting heart rates than men, if they have similar fitness levels. Exercise results in an increased parasympathetic tone in both men and women, which results in a lower resting heart rate (**Figure 12.8**).

Clinical Application Beta Blockers

Beta-adrenergic blocking agents, commonly referred to as *beta blockers*, are commonly used cardiac medications that block the effects of the sympathetic nervous system on the beta-1 adrenergic receptors in the heart. If these receptors are not being stimulated, heart rate decreases. Therefore, individuals taking beta blockers typically have resting heart rates in the 50s and 60s and maximal heart rates of 100 to 110 bpm, depending on how well the beta-1 adrenergic receptors in the heart are blocked by the drugs.

Beta blockers are used to treat many cardiovascular disorders, such as hypertension, heart failure, cardiac dysrhythmias, and angina (chest pain caused by lack of oxygen supply to the heart). They are also used to control anxiety disorders, migraines, and tremors.

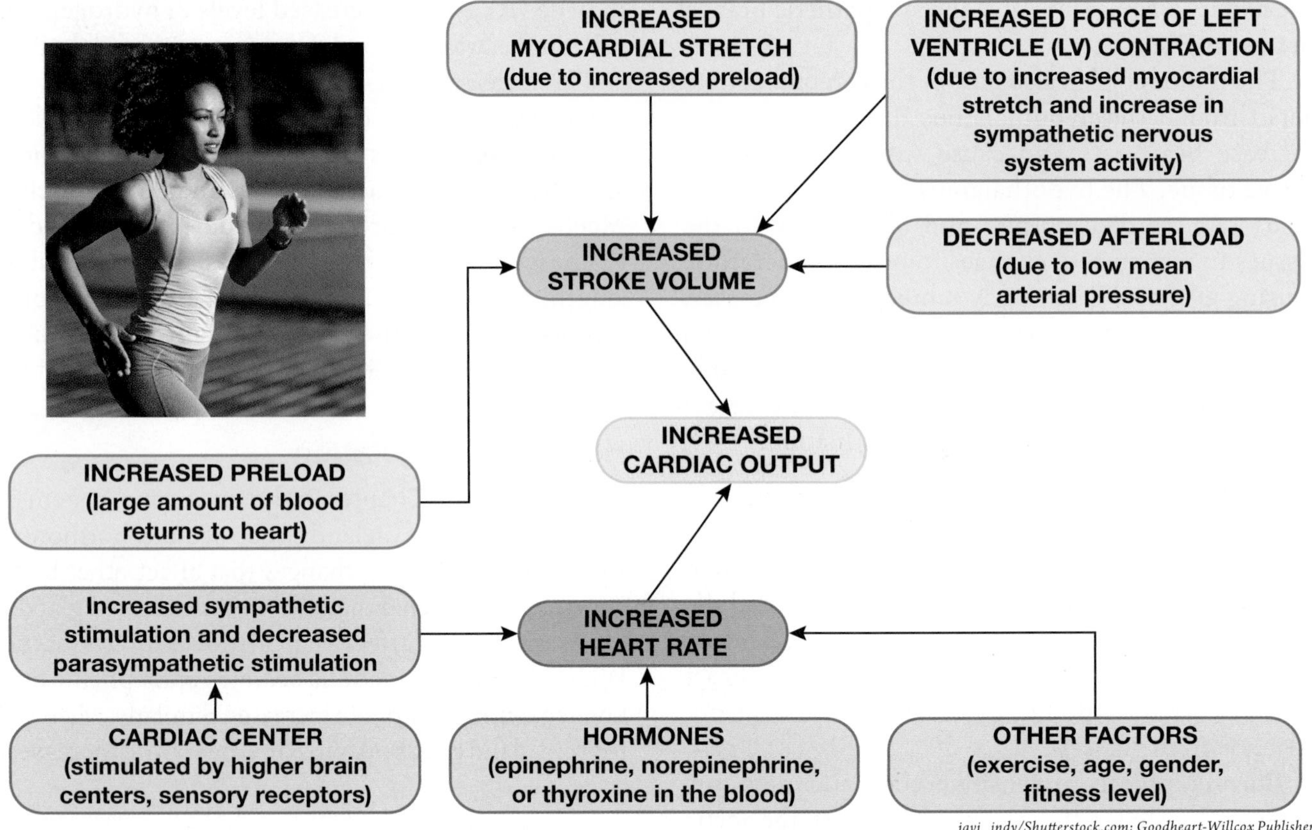

javi_indy/Shutterstock.com; Goodheart-Willcox Publisher

Figure 12.8 Factors that increase heart rate, stroke volume, and cardiac output.

SELF CHECK

1. Which part of the brain contains a region known as the "cardiac center"?
2. Name three hormones released by the endocrine system that affect heart rate.

Conduction System

Conduction is the process of conveying or transmitting various types of energy, such as electrical impulses. The conduction system in the heart transmits signals that control both heart rate and contraction strength of the muscle tissues. The conduction system of the heart includes two areas of nodal tissue and a network of nerve fibers that conduct the electrical impulses generated by the SA node throughout the heart.

The fibers in the conduction system have a resting potential energy that results from the concentration of charged particles inside and outside the cells. This resting potential energy is called *polarization*. The impulses initiated by the SA node cause the cells to electrically ***depolarize***, which results in contraction of the cardiomyocytes. After the impulse passes, the cells ***repolarize***, or return to their initial polarization.

Figure 12.9 shows the pathway of an electrical impulse generated by the SA node. Once the SA node fires, the right atrium contracts and simultaneously the electrical impulse is carried to the left atrium via ***Bachmann's bundle***, causing the left atrium to contract as well. The impulse also travels to the atrioventricular (AV) node via three internodal pathways. The AV node is a dense network of fibers, which delays the electrical impulse for approximately a tenth of a second. This small delay allows for a phenomenon known as *atrial kick*, in which the atria fill more completely before contracting.

Once the impulse leaves the AV node, it is carried through conducting fibers called the ***bundle of His***, or the *common bundle*, in the interventricular septum. (The bundle of His is alternately known in scientific circles as the *atrioventricular bundle*.) The bundle of His then divides into left and right ***bundle branches***, and the electrical impulse travels down the bundle branches to millions of ***Purkinje fibers*** in both ventricles. The Purkinje fibers stimulate the ventricular cells to contract, starting at the apex and forcing the blood upward through the remainder of the ventricles into the semilunar valves.

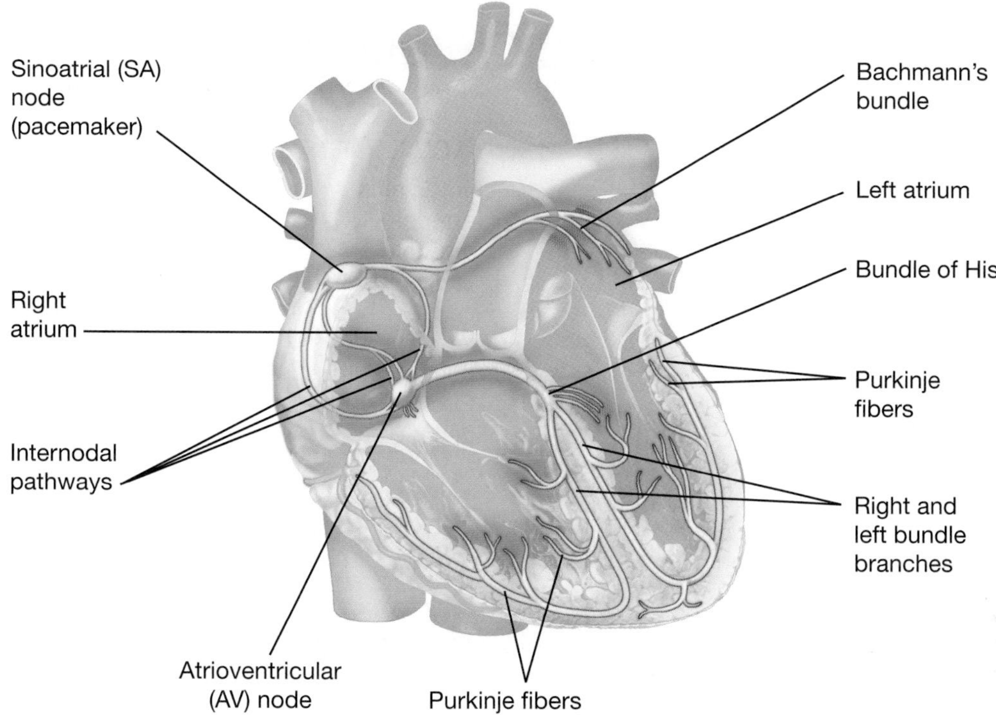

Figure 12.9 Conduction system of the heart.

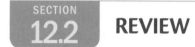

SECTION 12.2 REVIEW

Mini-Glossary

atrioventricular (AV) node a small mass of tissue that transmits impulses received from the sinoatrial node to the ventricles via the bundle of His

Bachmann's bundle a tract that runs from the left atrium to the right atrium, carrying the impulse generated by the SA node; also called the *interatrial tract*

baroreceptors receptors located in the atrium, aortic arch, and carotid arteries that are sensitive to changes in blood pressure

bundle branches the left and right branches that extend from the bundle of His to transport electrical impulses to the Purkinje fibers in the ventricles

bundle of His a slender bundle of modified cardiac muscle fibers that conducts electrical impulses from the AV node, through the left and right bundle branches, to Purkinje fibers in the ventricles

chemoreceptors receptors located in the aortic arch and carotid arteries that are sensitive to pH levels, decreased partial pressure of oxygen, increased partial pressure of carbon dioxide, and increased concentration of hydrogen ions

depolarize to change the electrical polarity of cells from their normal resting polarity, causing contraction of the heart muscle

mechanoreceptors receptors that are sensitive to mechanical stretch in tissues

Purkinje fibers special fibers that rapidly transmit impulses throughout the ventricles, causing ventricular contraction

repolarize to restore the original electrical polarity of cells that have been depolarized to their normal resting polarity, causing the heart muscle to relax

sinoatrial (SA) node a small mass of specialized tissue located in the right atrium that normally acts as the pacemaker of the heart, causing it to beat at a rate between 60 and 100 bpm

Review Questions

1. How does the nervous system help regulate heart rate?
2. What do baroreceptors monitor and where do they send messages?
3. What type of receptor monitors the pH of the blood?
4. Which two endocrine system glands release hormones that affect heart rate?
5. What is the estimated maximal heart rate for a 68-year-old individual? For a 21-year-old individual?
6. What happens to an electrical impulse when it reaches the AV node in the conduction system of a normally functioning heart?
7. List in order the structures through which an electrical impulse travels on its way to the muscle fibers of the ventricles.

SECTION 12.3

Blood Vessels and Circulation

Objectives

- Identify the differences among the three types of vessels.
- Describe the various types of circulation of blood through the body.

Key Terms

aortic arch
arteries
arterioles
capillaries
capillary beds
coronary sinus
ductus arteriosus
foramen ovale
hepatic portal system
precapillary sphincter
pulmonary circulation
systemic circulation
tunica externa
tunica intima
tunica media
veins
venules

The human body has three main types of blood vessels. Each type has different characteristics and performs a slightly different function in circulating blood throughout the body.

Blood Vessels

Three main types of blood vessels form a closed loop of tubes that carry blood from the heart to the rest of the body, and then back to the heart. These vessels are the ***arteries***, ***capillaries***, and ***veins***. Arteries branch into smaller ***arterioles***, which in turn branch to form capillaries, where gas exchange takes place. Then the capillaries combine to form ***venules***, or small veins, which combine to form the veins that transport the blood back to the heart. **Figure 12.10** summarizes the structure and function of each of these types of blood vessels.

Blood Vessel Walls

All blood vessels, with the exception of capillaries, are composed of three layers that surround the blood-filled opening called the *lumen* (**Figure 12.11**). ***Tunica intima***, the innermost layer, is composed of a single layer of squamous (flattened) epithelial cells over a sheet of connective tissue. The tunica intima provides a smooth, frictionless surface that allows blood to flow smoothly through the vessel.

Tunica media, the middle layer of a blood vessel, is a thicker layer containing smooth muscle cells, elastic fibers, and collagen. The smooth muscle cells in this layer are directed by the sympathetic nervous system to vasodilate and vasoconstrict, allowing blood flow to be increased to certain tissues and decreased to other tissues as needed.

Vasodilation and vasoconstriction of the vessels also play a major role in regulating and determining

Structure and Function of Vessels		
Vessel Type	**Structure**	**Function**
Artery	three-layered vessel (intima, media, adventitia); thick, elastic, muscular walls	transports oxygen-rich blood away from heart to arterioles*; influenced by the sympathetic nervous system (contraction/dilation)
Arteriole	thinner, three-walled vessel; mostly smooth muscle cells	transports blood from arteries to capillaries; influenced more by the sympathetic nervous system; directs blood flow in the body
Capillary	single layer of epithelial cells	gas/nutrient and waste-product exchange between blood and tissues
Venule	thin-walled vessel; multiple venules typically bundled together to form a vein	transports blood from capillary to vein
Vein	three-layered (intima, media, externa), thin-walled vessel with one-way valves	transports oxygen-poor blood back to the heart

*Exception: Pulmonary arteries carry deoxygenated blood.

Figure 12.10

Goodheart-Willcox Publisher

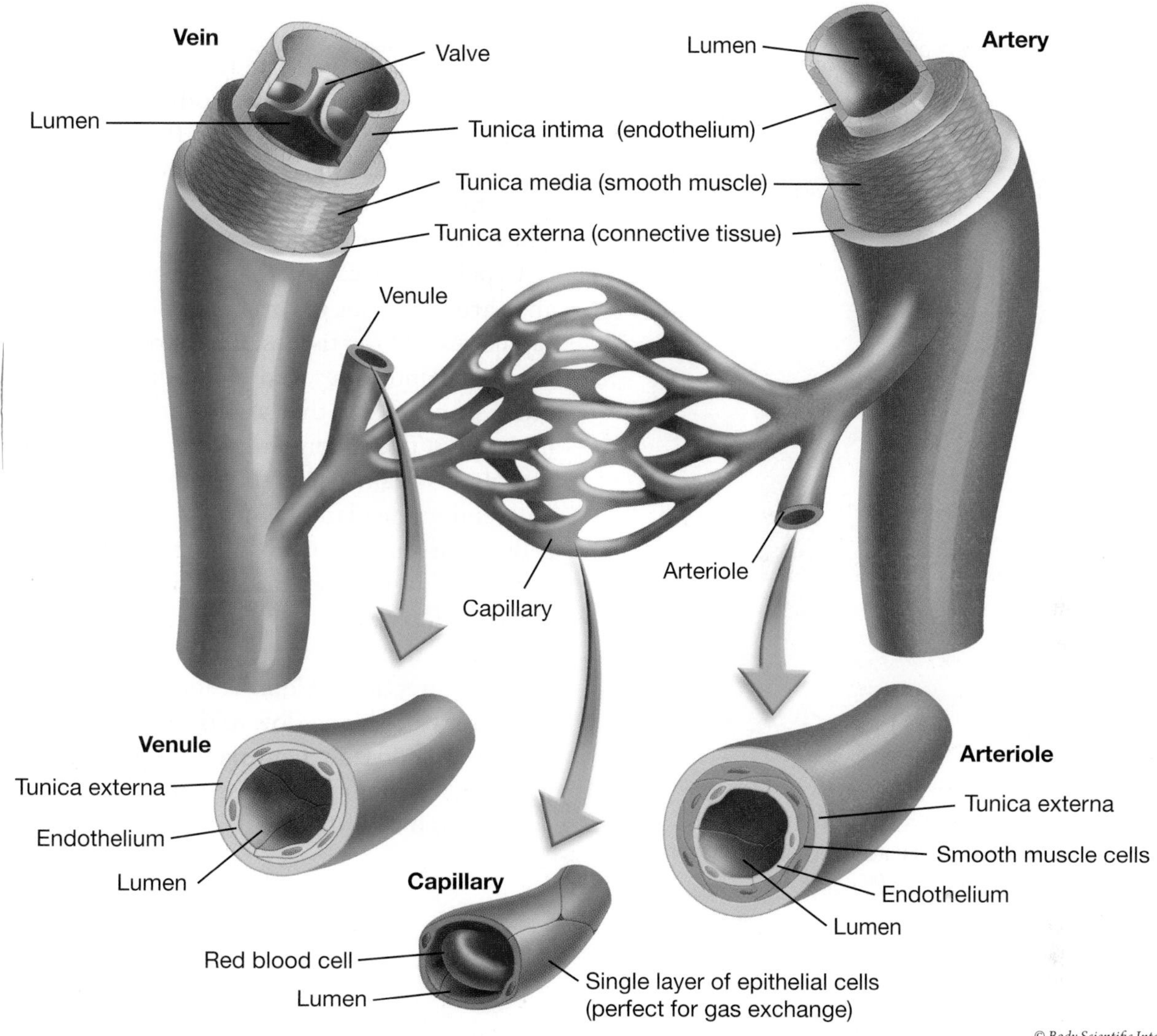

Figure 12.11 Types of blood vessels. Traditionally, venous vessels (veins and venules) are shown in blue to indicate lack of oxygenation, whereas arteries and arterioles are shown in red to indicate a high level of oxygen.

blood pressure. When a vessel vasodilates, blood pressure is lowered. When the vessel vasoconstricts, blood pressure is increased.

Tunica externa is the outermost layer of a blood vessel. It is composed mostly of fibrous connective tissue, which serves to support and protect the vessels.

Arteries and Veins

Although arteries and veins each have three layers, the relative thickness and composition of the layers differ, as does the size of the lumen. These differences exist because the two vessels have very different functions in the cardiovascular system. **Figure 12.12** details the structural differences between arteries and veins.

The arterial vessels carry blood away from the heart, so they must be able to withstand large increases in pressure when the heart contracts. Therefore, arteries have the thickest, strongest, most elastic walls. The aorta, the largest artery in the body, leaves the heart and branches into progressively smaller arteries that eventually become arterioles (**Figure 12.13**).

Differences between Arteries and Veins		
Structures	**Arteries**	**Veins**
walls	strong, thick, elastic	thin, less elastic
pressure	high	low
lumen	small	large
valves	no	yes

Figure 12.12 Goodheart-Willcox Publisher

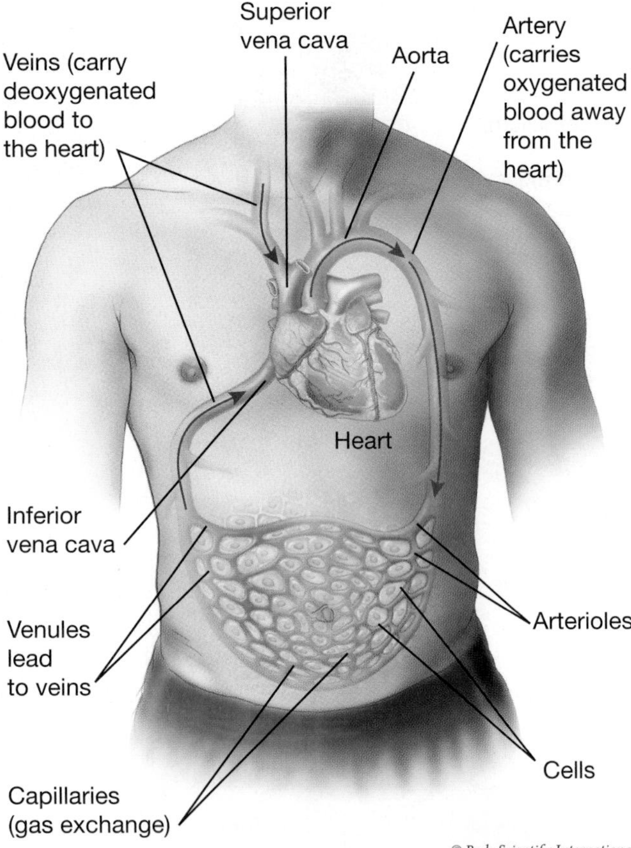

Figure 12.13 Relationships among the various types of blood vessels in the cardiovascular system.

The venous system carries blood back to the heart. Unlike arteries, veins do not have to deal with large increases in pressure. Thus, the walls of the veins are thinner and less elastic than the walls of the arteries. The venous system acts as a reservoir, housing 65% of the blood in the body.

As explained earlier, the blood enters the venules from the capillaries. The venules merge together to form progressively larger veins until they reach the largest veins, the inferior and superior venae cavae. These two veins empty into the right atrium of the heart.

In spite of being a low-pressure system, the venous system is able to pump blood back to the heart because it has one-way valves that allow blood to flow only toward the heart. In addition, when the muscles that surround the veins contract, they "milk" the blood toward the heart (**Figure 12.14**).

Venous return of blood is also assisted by the pump-like action of the respiratory system. Changes in abdominal and thoracic pressure that occur with breathing help to pump blood back to the heart.

Capillaries

Arterioles connect with the smallest and most numerous vessels in the body—the capillaries. Capillaries range in size from 0.0025 to 0.25 cm. Capillaries are so narrow that red blood cells must pass through them in a single line, one at a time. They are also the thinnest of the blood vessels.

Capillaries are called *exchange vessels* because oxygen and carbon dioxide gas exchange occurs between the capillaries and the tissues. Capillaries in the kidneys, liver, small intestines, and endocrine glands also have microscopic pores that allow the passage of small molecules. These pores allow hormones to pass into the bloodstream when the pores come in contact with endocrine glands. They also allow white blood cells to pass into tissue to kill harmful bacteria.

Blood flow through the capillaries is controlled by a ***precapillary sphincter***, a band of smooth muscle fibers that encircles the capillaries at the arteriole-capillary junctions. Contraction of the precapillary sphincter stops blood flow to the capillary; relaxation increases blood flow. Contraction or relaxation of the precapillary sphincter is based on the local chemical conditions in the tissue (pH, oxygen, carbon dioxide,

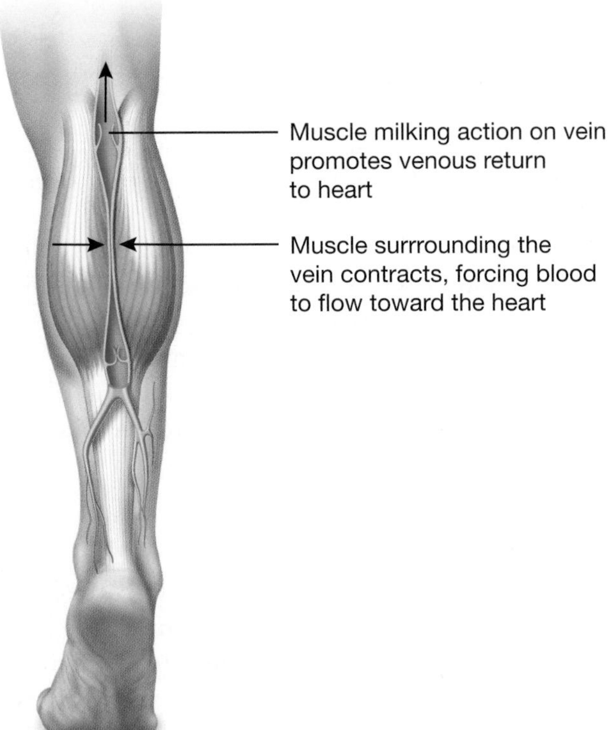

Figure 12.14 When muscles contract, they squeeze the blood vessels, achieving a "milking" action that assists in the flow of blood through the veins and back to the heart.

temperature). For instance, approximately 15% of blood flow goes to your muscles at rest. During exercise, however, when the metabolic needs of the muscles dramatically increase, approximately 85% of the blood flow goes to the working muscles.

Capillaries do not operate separately; they form an expansive network of intertwined vessels called ***capillary beds***. Blood begins its journey back to the heart when the capillaries merge with venules. The venules then merge with larger, thicker-walled veins that eventually lead back to the heart.

SELF CHECK

1. All blood vessels, with the exception of capillaries, consist of what three layers?
2. What is the name of the smallest type of artery?
3. What types of vessels carry blood back to the heart?
4. What is the purpose of the precapillary sphincters?

Circulation

As mentioned earlier, the cardiovascular system is an extensive network of blood vessels that stretches 60,000 miles within the body. It includes several different types of circulation. The two major circuits are circulation between the heart and lungs, and circulation between the heart and the rest of the body (**Figure 12.15**). Several other types of circulation occur as well, such as circulation within the heart itself and circulation through the liver for nutrient loading. When a woman is pregnant, a fetal circulatory system also develops. This section describes each type of circulation.

Pulmonary Circulation

The movement of blood from the right side of the heart, through the lungs, and back to the left side of the heart is called ***pulmonary circulation***, or *cardiopulmonary circulation*. As explained earlier, this process involves several steps:

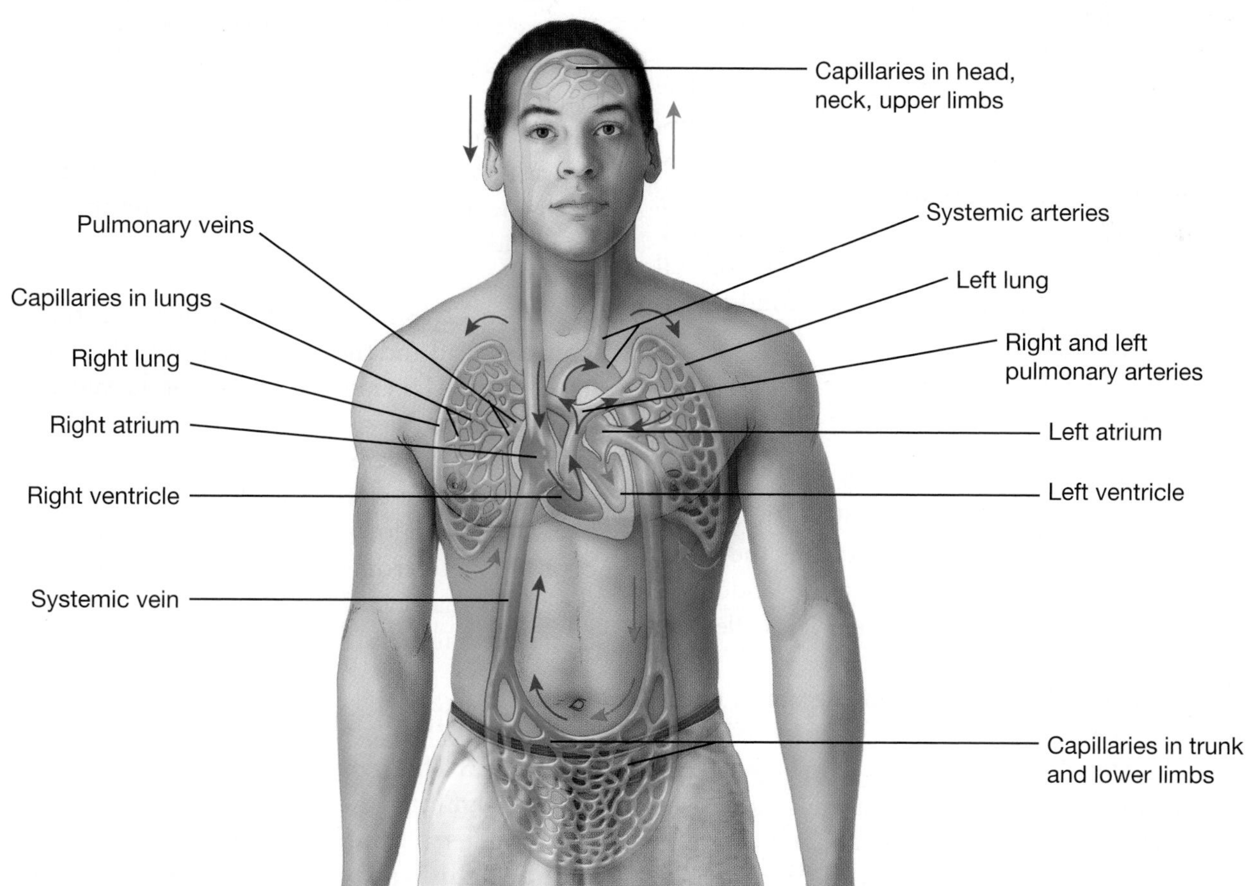

Figure 12.15 The heart pumps blood through two major circuits: the pulmonary circuit and the systemic circuit. The right side of the heart pumps blood to the lungs (pulmonary circulation), and the left side of the heart pumps blood throughout the body (systemic circulation).

1. Deoxygenated blood enters the right atrium from the inferior and superior venae cavae.
2. Deoxygenated blood flows through the tricuspid valve into the right ventricle.
3. The right ventricle contracts, and deoxygenated blood is ejected through the pulmonary valve into the pulmonary trunk.
4. The deoxygenated blood flows from the pulmonary trunk into the right and left pulmonary arteries.
5. Blood travels through the pulmonary arteries that branch further into arterioles, which merge with the capillary network in the lungs.
6. The blood becomes oxygenated in the lungs, and then flows through the venules, which merge with the four pulmonary veins that carry the oxygenated blood back to the heart.
7. The pulmonary veins empty oxygenated blood into the left atrium.

Systemic Circulation

Systemic circulation is the movement of oxygen-rich blood from left side of the heart throughout the body. The systemic circulatory system consists of the closed-loop network of arteries, arterioles, capillaries, venules, and veins that circulate oxygen, hormones, water, and other nutrients to tissues, and then carry carbon dioxide and waste products back to the heart.

This section traces the journey of a red blood cell through systemic circulation. Keep in mind that it has 60,000 miles to go!

The journey begins when the left ventricle pumps blood through the aorta, which is the largest artery in the body. The ascending branch of the aorta rises up from the heart, arches to the left (thus the term ***aortic arch***), and then proceeds downward (called the *descending aorta*), into the thorax along the spine, through the diaphragm, and into the abdomen. Once this vessel reaches the abdomen, it is called the *abdominal aorta*.

Many other arteries arise from the aorta, and a red blood cell may take any of these potential paths (**Figure 12.16**). The right and left coronary arteries branch from the ascending aorta and supply the heart with blood. The brachiocephalic, left common carotid, and left subclavian arteries branch from the aortic arch and supply the head, neck, and arms with blood. These arteries subdivide into many more arteries, including the right subclavian and right

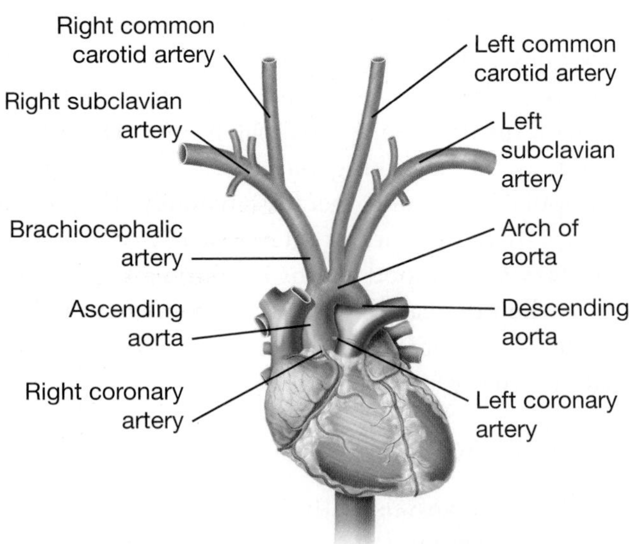

© Body Scientific International

Figure 12.16 Arteries arising from the aorta.

common carotid arteries. Many arteries branch from the descending aorta to supply blood to various organs, including the liver, spleen, kidneys, stomach, and the rest of the lower body.

The major arteries of the body are shown in **Figure 12.17**. Recall that these arteries branch into smaller and smaller vessels, eventually becoming arterioles. The arterioles merge with capillaries, where the blood distributes nutrients to the tissues and picks up waste materials. The red blood cell's journey back to the heart begins with blood moving through the capillaries and draining into the venules, which merge to form veins.

Figure 12.18 illustrates the major veins that drain from the head and the trunk, as well as the upper and lower limbs. Generally, the names of the veins are the same as their arterial counterparts (for example, *renal* artery and *renal* vein).

The systemic circulatory journey ends when the blood from the lower veins enters the inferior vena cava and blood from the upper veins empties into the superior vena cava. The inferior and superior venae cavae drain into the right atrium.

Cardiac Circulation

How does the heart receive its oxygen supply? Although it may seem that the blood that circulates through the chambers of the heart would provide oxygen to the heart, this is not true. The oxygen-rich blood that nourishes the heart is supplied by the right and left coronary arteries that lie on the epicardial (outermost) surface of the heart (**Figure 12.19**).

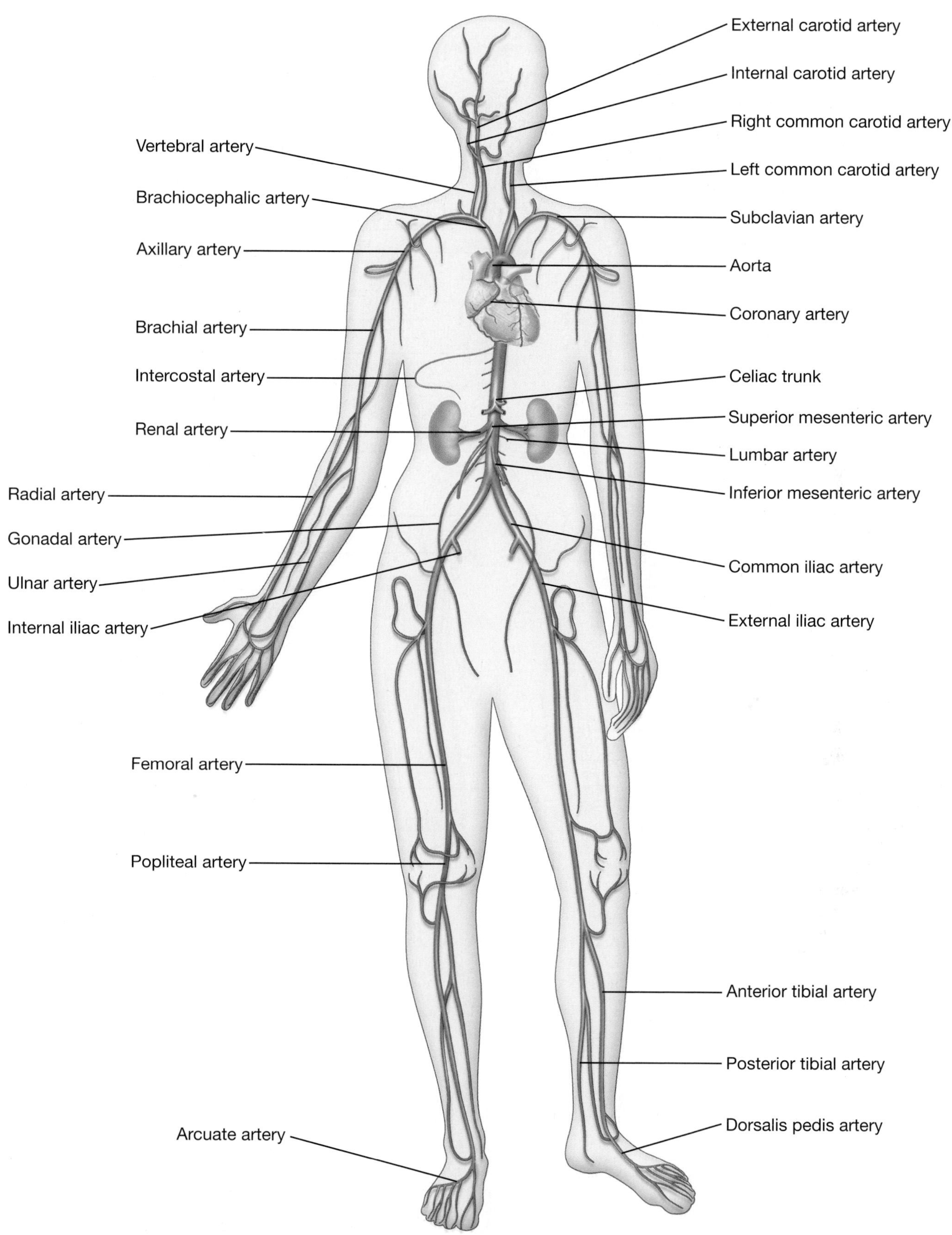

Figure 12.17 Major arteries of the body.

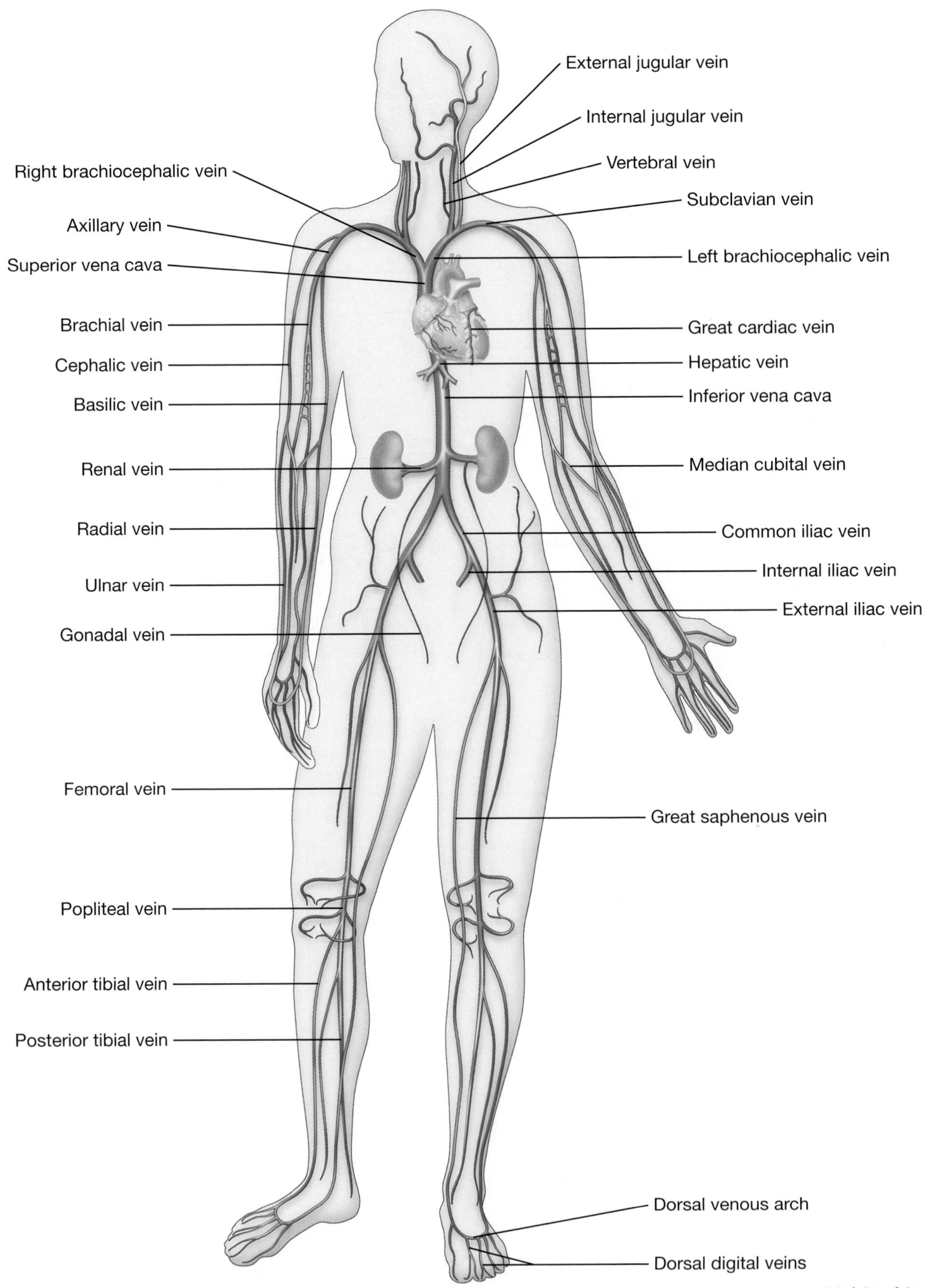
External jugular vein
Internal jugular vein
Vertebral vein
Subclavian vein
Right brachiocephalic vein
Axillary vein
Superior vena cava
Left brachiocephalic vein
Brachial vein
Cephalic vein
Basilic vein
Great cardiac vein
Hepatic vein
Inferior vena cava
Renal vein
Median cubital vein
Radial vein
Ulnar vein
Gonadal vein
Common iliac vein
Internal iliac vein
External iliac vein
Femoral vein
Great saphenous vein
Popliteal vein
Anterior tibial vein
Posterior tibial vein
Dorsal venous arch
Dorsal digital veins
© Body Scientific International

Figure 12.18 Major veins of the body.

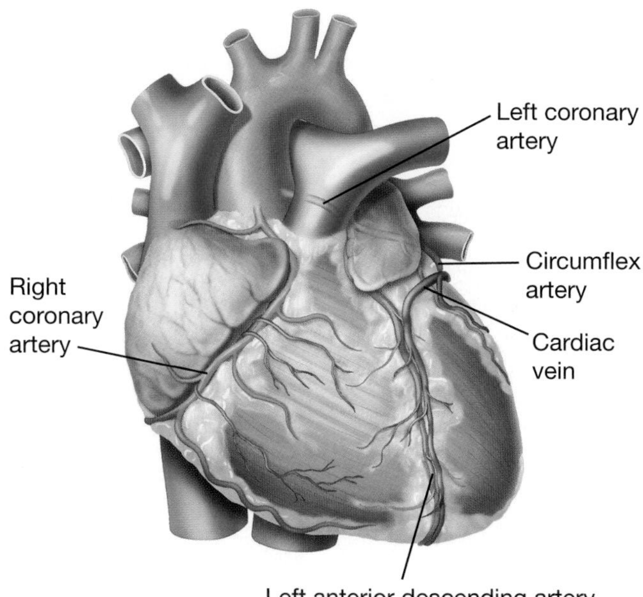

© Body Scientific International

Figure 12.19 Anterior view of the coronary arteries.

The right coronary artery has two main branches, which supply blood to the inferior and posterior walls of the heart. The left coronary artery divides into two arteries, the left anterior descending artery and the circumflex artery, which supply oxygen-rich blood to the anterior, lateral, and posterior walls of the heart.

The coronary arteries arise from the ascending aorta and fill when the ventricles are relaxed. The coronary arteries are closed when the ventricles contract, so they are protected from the high pressure that is generated during contraction. Blood from the coronary arteries flows into capillaries that carry it to the cardiac tissues, which require oxygen and other nutrients from the blood, just like all other body cells.

The blood distributes nutrients and collects carbon dioxide and waste products from the tissues before emptying into several cardiac veins. The main cardiac veins are the great cardiac, middle cardiac, small cardiac, and anterior cardiac veins. All cardiac veins drain into a large vessel called the ***coronary sinus***, which is located in the posterior wall of the heart. The coronary sinus drains into the right atrium.

Understanding Medical Terminology

Keep in mind that the names of the arteries and veins often refer to the organ or location that they supply with blood. For example, the *femoral* artery supplies blood to the femoral region of the leg, which is parallel to the femur. The *lumbar* artery supplies blood to the lumbar area of the back.

Research Notes Why Records Are Not Broken on Hot, Humid Days

Marathoners will not soon forget the environmental conditions at the 2012 Boston Marathon: direct sunlight, temperatures in the mid-80s, and high humidity. This was a recipe for slow race times and heat-related mishaps. Geoffrey Mutai, the 2011 winner, dropped out with heat-related cramps at mile 18, and the 2012 winner was 10 minutes slower than Mutai's 2011 time. Why do you think this occurred?

Research indicates that exercise performed in a heated environment causes internal competition for blood supply. As body temperature increases, a greater percentage of blood goes to the skin to cool the body. In addition, increased sweat rates cause blood volume to decrease. The result of these conditions is that less blood goes back to the heart. When less blood travels to the heart, the stroke volume must decrease.

How does the heart react to a decrease in stroke volume? For sufficient cardiac output to be maintained, heart rate must increase. This means that the heart has to work harder, causing the body to use fuel more quickly. Over time, performance declines.

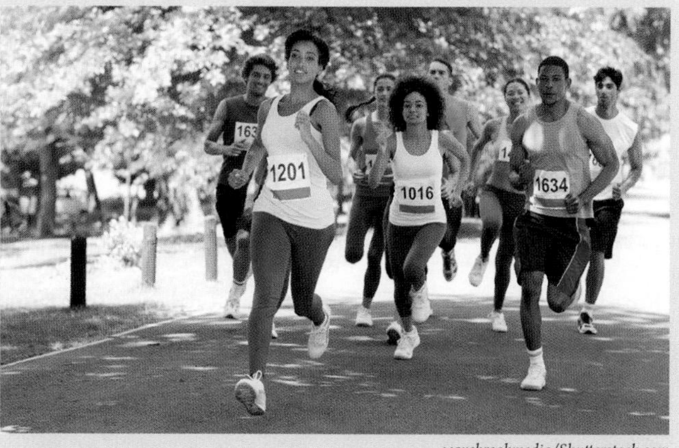

wavebreakmedia/Shutterstock.com

These runners are attempting to complete a marathon, which is just over 26 miles.

Therefore, to minimize performance declines during severe heat conditions, it is important to stay hydrated by drinking plenty of plain water or water that contains a mixture of carbohydrates and sodium.

Hepatic Portal Circulation

In order to supply body cells with nutrients, the blood has to have a source where it can obtain them. This section describes the way in which nutrients, such as carbohydrates, fats, and proteins, are stored in or released into the bloodstream. Storage and circulation of these valuable nutrients is critical for providing the energy needed to perform daily activities.

The ***hepatic portal system*** plays a vital role in maintaining proper carbohydrate, fat, and protein levels in the blood. Whereas the arteries of the systemic circulatory system deliver blood to different parts of the body, the veins of the hepatic portal circulation system supply blood only to the liver.

The veins that drain the stomach, spleen, and pancreas (splenic vein), and the small intestine and colon (superior and inferior mesenteric veins) deliver blood to the liver through the hepatic portal vein (**Figure 12.20**). This blood is rich with nutrients such as carbohydrates and fats. As the blood percolates through the liver, some of the nutrients are removed, stored, or repackaged for another use.

The best example of this process is the storage of glucose. After a meal, the blood that drains into the liver may be high in glucose. The liver, which plays a role in regulating blood glucose levels, stores glucose as glycogen until the body needs the glucose for energy. Suppose that a person is exercising and her blood glucose level starts to drop. As this happens, the liver breaks down its stored glycogen and releases it into the bloodstream as glucose, thereby maintaining blood glucose levels. Once blood has been filtered by the liver, it returns to the inferior vena cava through the hepatic veins. You will learn more about this process in Chapter 14.

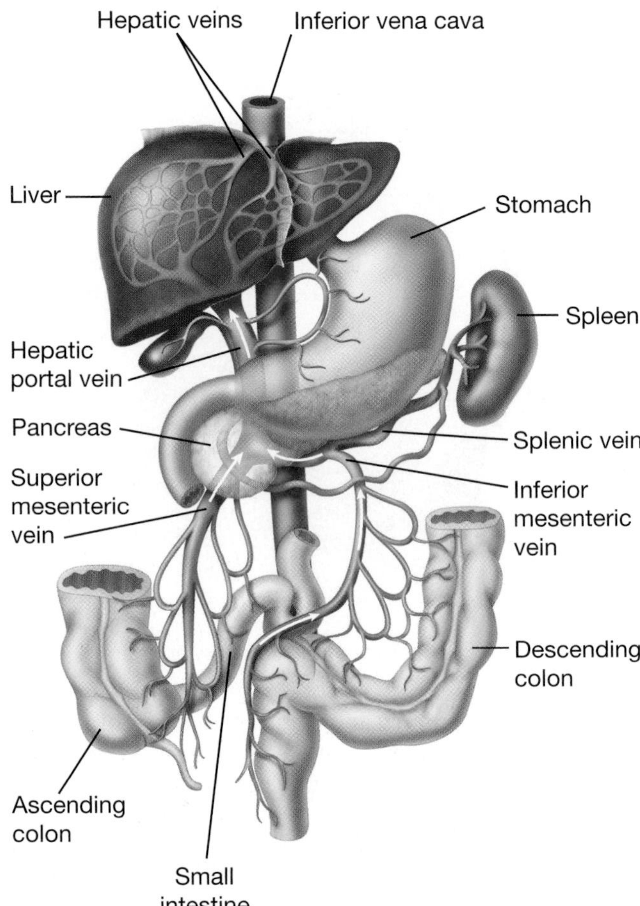

Figure 12.20 Hepatic portal circulation. Veins from the stomach, spleen, pancreas, small intestine, and colon drain into the hepatic portal vein. The liver filters the blood before the blood empties into the inferior vena cava.

Fetal Circulation

Fetal circulation is the process by which an unborn infant receives oxygen and nutrients and disposes of waste products. One large umbilical vein carries oxygen and nutrients from the mother's blood to the infant. Waste products are cleared through the two umbilical arteries in the placenta that pass through the umbilical cord to the fetus (**Figure 12.21**). This process is necessary because the lungs and digestive system of the fetus are underdeveloped and not yet functioning.

Most blood enters the fetal heart through the ductus venosus vein, bypassing the liver and going directly to the right atrium by way of the inferior vena cava. Blood bypasses the right ventricle and is shunted to the left atrium through an opening in the septal wall, between the atria, called the ***foramen ovale***. A small amount of blood does go to the right ventricle, but it is drained through the ***ductus arteriosus***, a vessel that connects the pulmonary artery to the aorta.

Once the blood is pumped from the left ventricle, the oxygenated blood flows through the infant's body. Deoxygenated blood returns to the placenta via the umbilical arteries. Shortly after birth, the ductus arteriosus and ductus venosus close, as does the foramen ovale.

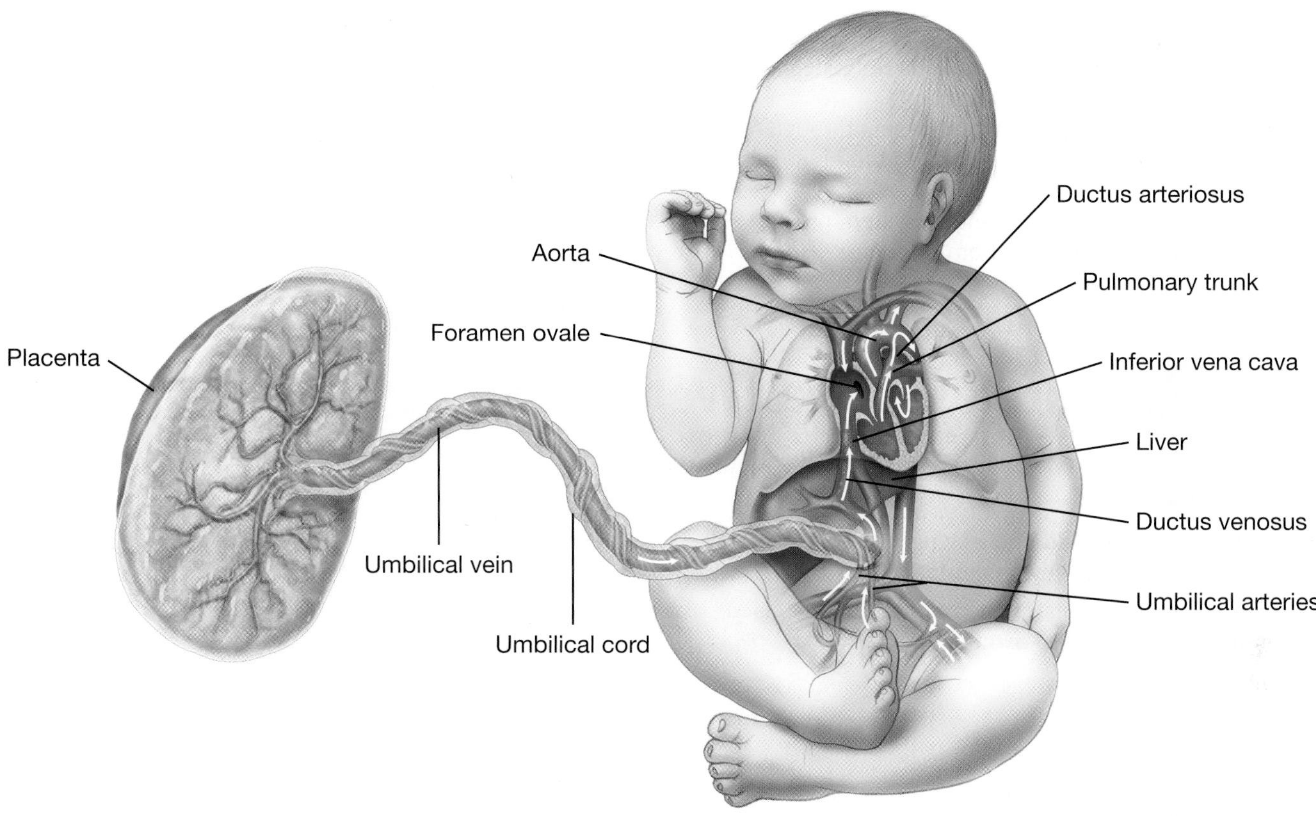

Figure 12.21 Fetal circulation. Here you see the circulation of blood in a full-term fetus (before birth).

SECTION 12.3

REVIEW

Mini-Glossary

aortic arch the curved portion of the aorta; located between the ascending and descending parts of the aorta

arteries blood vessels that carry blood away from the heart

arterioles microscopic arteries that connect with capillaries

capillaries small, thin-walled blood vessels in which oxygen and carbon dioxide gas exchange occurs

capillary bed a network of intertwined capillaries

coronary sinus the large venous channel between the left atrium and left ventricle on the posterior side of the heart that empties into the right atrium at the junction of the four chambers

ductus arteriosus a short, broad vessel in the fetus that connects the left pulmonary artery with the descending aorta, allowing most of the blood to bypass the infant's lungs

foramen ovale an opening in the septal wall between the atria; normally present only in the fetus

hepatic portal system the circulatory system through which blood picks up nutrients for distribution throughout the body

precapillary sphincter a band of smooth muscle fibers that encircles each capillary at the arteriole-capillary junction and controls blood flow to the tissues

pulmonary circulation the circulation of oxygen-poor blood from the right ventricle and through the lungs, returning to the left atrium with oxygen-rich blood

systemic circulation the circulation of oxygenated blood from the left ventricle, through the arteries, capillaries, and veins of the circulatory system, returning to the right atrium

tunica externa the outermost layer of a blood vessel, composed mostly of fibrous connective tissue that supports and protects the vessel

tunica intima the innermost layer of a blood vessel, composed of a single layer of squamous epithelial cells over a sheet of connective tissue

tunica media the thicker middle layer of a blood vessel that contains smooth muscle cells, elastic fibers, and collagen

veins blood vessels that carry blood to the heart

venules the smallest veins; connect the capillaries with the larger systemic veins

(continued)

Review Questions

1. Which layer of the blood vessel is responsible for vasodilation and vasoconstriction?
2. Starting at the heart, list the vessels through which blood travels and returns to the heart during systemic circulation.
3. Which structures in the venous system prevent blood from flowing away from the heart? How is this accomplished?
4. How many pulmonary veins take blood back to the heart? Is the blood oxygenated or deoxygenated? Explain your answer.
5. Explain why capillaries are called *exchange vessels*.
6. A fetus has several structures, such as openings and shunts, that close shortly after birth. Why do you think these structures are necessary for the unborn fetus before but not after birth?

SECTION 12.4 Cardiovascular Wellness and Disease

Objectives

- Demonstrate methods of checking heart rate, blood pressure, and other key health factors.
- Identify several common types of heart diseases and disorders and their symptoms.

Key Terms

aneurysm
angina pectoris
atherosclerosis
atrial fibrillation
brachial artery
bradycardia
cardiomyopathy
carotid arteries
cerebrovascular accident (CVA, stroke)
coronary artery disease (CAD)
dysrhythmia
endocarditis
heart block
heart murmur
hypertension
ischemia
mitral valve prolapse
myocardial infarction (MI)
myocarditis
palpitations
pericarditis
peripheral vascular disease (PVD)
premature atrial contraction (PAC)
premature ventricular contraction (PVC)
radial artery
tachycardia
transient ischemic attack (TIA)
valvular stenosis
ventricular fibrillation (VF)
ventricular tachycardia (VT)

Cardiovascular health and wellness is monitored routinely during wellness checkups. Like all body systems, the cardiovascular system is subject to several disorders and diseases. This section describes ways to monitor heart health, as well as potential cardiovascular diseases and disorders.

Monitoring Heart Health

For those who are interested in—and proactive about—their health, pulse monitoring and blood pressure measurement are important skills to acquire. These skills are even more important for those who are interested in pursuing a healthcare career.

Pulse monitoring is essential if a person wants to ensure that he or she is exercising at an intensity level that will improve cardiovascular fitness. Blood pressure measurement is a simple procedure that can provide lifesaving information about one's physical condition.

Checking a Pulse

The pulse is a rhythmic, throbbing sensation that can be felt when the heart contracts and blood is forced through the arteries. To measure your pulse, use your index and middle fingertips to apply light pressure to any point where an artery comes close to your skin. The most common anatomic locations for measuring your pulse include the following:

- ***Radial artery***: With your palm facing upward, feel for your pulse on the thumb side of your wrist (**Figure 12.22A**).
- ***Carotid artery***: On the side of your neck, feel for your pulse to the right or left of your trachea, or windpipe (**Figure 12.22B**).
- ***Brachial artery***: At the fold of your elbow, feel for your pulse along the inner portion of your arm.

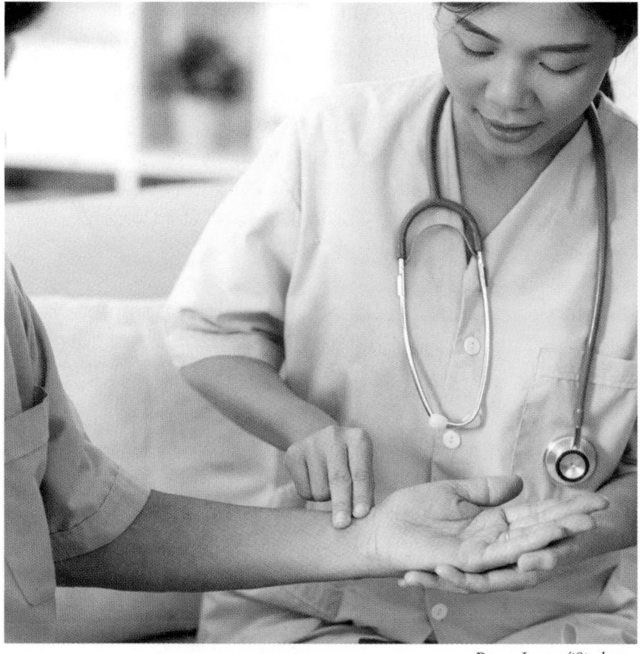
A DragonImages/iStock.com

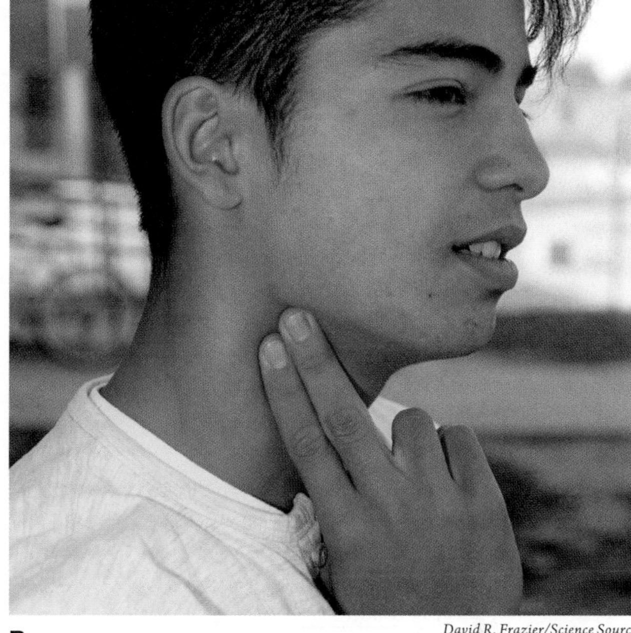
B David R. Frazier/Science Source

Figure 12.22 Measuring pulse. A—Radial artery. B—Carotid artery.

For most purposes, you can count the number of beats for 15 seconds and multiply that number by 4. In a healthcare setting, however, or if the pulse seems irregular, count the number of beats for a full minute.

Understanding Medical Terminology

What makes your body healthy? With the right lifestyle, your body **MENDS** itself!

Make sure that your weight, blood pressure, cholesterol, and glucose are normal.

Exercise most days for 30 minutes at a moderate intensity level.

No smoking or use of tobacco products.

Diet should be rich in fruits and vegetables and low in saturated fat and sodium.

Stress less, laugh more. Recent research shows that laughter may lower disease risk!

Measuring Blood Pressure

Blood pressure is measured at the brachial artery using a stethoscope and a sphygmomanometer, or blood pressure cuff. Inflating the cuff causes the brachial artery to collapse. As the cuff is deflated, the brachial artery gradually reopens, and the pulse can be heard in the form of a tapping sound. When the artery is completely open, the tapping sound disappears.

Use the following steps to measure blood pressure (**Figure 12.23**):

1. Place two fingertips above the fold of the elbow, and use this as a guide for placing the blood pressure cuff. The bottom edge of the blood pressure cuff should be positioned just above the two fingers. Place the blood pressure cuff around the arm, with the arrow on the cuff pointed toward the brachial artery.
2. Make sure that the stethoscope is in the "on" position by gently tapping the diaphragm of the chest piece.
3. Place the head of the stethoscope over the brachial artery.
4. Squeeze the bulb of the sphygmomanometer repeatedly while listening for a "tapping" sound.
5. After the tapping sound stops, pump up the cuff 30 millimeters of mercury (mmHg) more. This would be approximately 150 mmHg for someone with a normal blood pressure of less than 120/80 mmHg. **Figure 12.24** shows the current guidelines from the American Heart Association (AHA).
6. Open the release valve so that the cuff deflates at a rate of about 2 mmHg/second.
7. The first "tap" that you hear is the systolic blood pressure. The last muffled sound that you hear is the diastolic blood pressure.

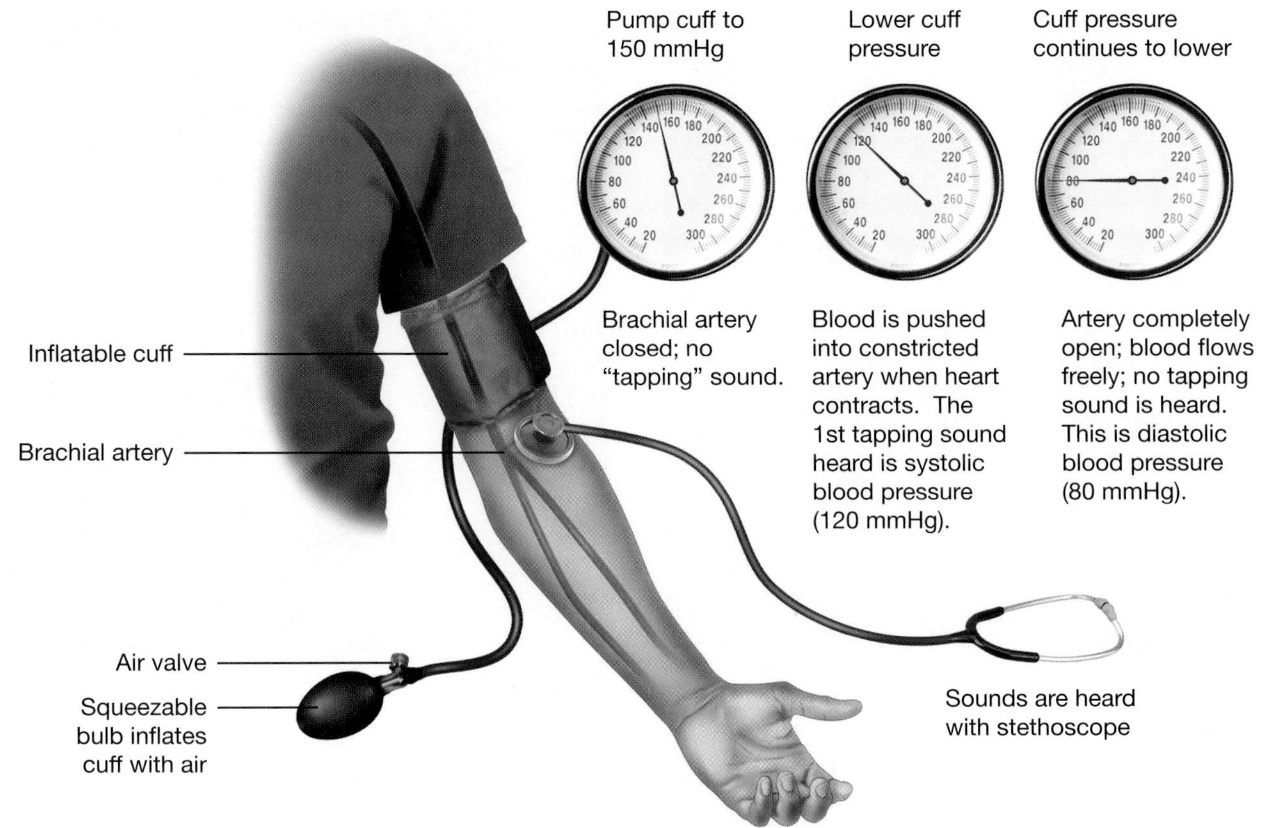
Pump cuff to 150 mmHg
Lower cuff pressure
Cuff pressure continues to lower
Inflatable cuff
Brachial artery
Brachial artery closed; no "tapping" sound.
Blood is pushed into constricted artery when heart contracts. The 1st tapping sound heard is systolic blood pressure (120 mmHg).
Artery completely open; blood flows freely; no tapping sound is heard. This is diastolic blood pressure (80 mmHg).
Air valve
Squeezable bulb inflates cuff with air
Sounds are heard with stethoscope
© Body Scientific International

Figure 12.23 Blood pressure measurement.

Blood Pressure Classification			
Normal	**Elevated**	**Stage 1 Hypertension**	**Stage 2 Hypertension**
<120/80 mmHg	Systolic: 120–129 mmHg AND Diastolic: < 80 mmHg	Systolic: 130–139 OR Diastolic 80–89	Systolic: 140 mmHg or greater OR Diastolic at least 90 mmHg

Figure 12.24 Goodheart-Willcox Publisher

The systolic blood pressure is the pressure in the artery when the left ventricle contracts. The diastolic blood pressure is the pressure in the artery when the left ventricle is relaxed and filling with blood.

Optimal blood pressure for an adult is 110/70 mmHg. Generally, lower blood pressure is not a problem, but it could cause dizziness when standing up too quickly. Adults whose blood pressure is greater than 140/90 mmHg should consult their physician.

Other Important Numbers

In addition to knowing how to measure pulse and blood pressure, you should know and monitor some other key body-related numbers. These numbers will give you an indication of how healthy you are compared to the general population.

Weight

Body mass index is an indication of healthy weight for a person's individual stature. An adult's body mass index (BMI) should range from 18.0 to 24.9, which represents a healthy weight. People with BMIs less than 18 are classified as thin. Those with BMIs equal to or greater than 25 are considered overweight. People with BMIs greater than 30 are classified as obese.

To calculate your body mass index, divide your weight (in kilograms) by your height (in meters) squared.

$$\text{BMI} = \frac{\text{wt (kg)}}{\text{ht (m)}^2}$$

This BMI calculation method is a general guideline only. It may incorrectly classify athletes or people who have a lot of muscle mass as overweight or obese.

This could happen because the formula does not take body composition into account. The same incorrect result could occur if you used height and weight tables, whether or not you were in the normal range for your age and size.

Body composition is another way of determining whether a person's weight is healthy. This measurement identifies the body's proportion of lean tissue to fat tissue. Body composition can be measured with a weight scale that has bioelectric impedance technology. These special scales are available in many pharmacies and schools. Yet another way to measure body composition is to use a caliper to do a skinfold test.

Cholesterol

Recall from Chapter 2 that cholesterol is a steroid found in blood. Cholesterol is essential for cell function and for absorption of fat-soluble vitamins. It is also a precursor to the development of steroid hormones. Cholesterol is carried in the blood by lipids.

Cholesterol level can be determined by having blood drawn and tested. Knowing your total cholesterol level is helpful. It is more helpful, however, to know how much of the total cholesterol consists of high-density lipoprotein (HDL) and how much of it consists of low-density lipoprotein (LDL). HDL is "good" cholesterol, and LDL is "bad."

LDL carries fat to the arterial walls and deposits it there. Over time, these fatty deposits can cause buildup of plaque, leading to blockages in the arteries. By contrast, HDL removes fat from the arterial walls and brings it back to the liver, where it is broken down. Triglycerides are another form of fat that can increase the risk of cardiovascular disease.

The following are desirable levels for each of these substances:

- Total cholesterol: less than 200 mg/dL
- LDL: less than 100 mg/dL
- HDL: more than 40 mg/dL, preferably more than 60 mg/dL
- Triglycerides: less than 150 mg/dL

Understanding Medical Terminology

To remember the differences between HDL (the good type of cholesterol) and LDL (the bad type), keep in mind the following hint: HDL is healthy, and LDL is lousy.

Diagnostic Tests

Several types of tests are performed to help diagnose suspected heart disorders. Depending on the severity of a patient's symptoms, blood tests, an echocardiogram, and even a cardiac catheterization may be performed. But the most common of all tests is the electrocardiogram.

An electrocardiogram, commonly called an *ECG* or *EKG*, is a recording of the electrical activity of the heart (**Figure 12.25** and **Figure 12.26**). In a sense, an ECG speaks the language of the heart. It illustrates what is happening electrically when the atria and ventricles depolarize and repolarize, as well as what happens mechanically when they contract and relax. By studying the tracings obtained from an ECG, healthcare professionals can learn much about the patient's heart health. Therefore, in addition to its use as a diagnostic tool when a problem is noted, ECGs are commonly performed as part of a routine wellness exam.

Cardiovascular Disorders and Diseases

Cardiovascular diseases account for one in six deaths in the United States, or approximately 2,200 deaths per day, according to the American Heart Association. To put this statistic into perspective, someone will have a coronary event—a heart attack or chest pain, for example—approximately every 25 seconds.

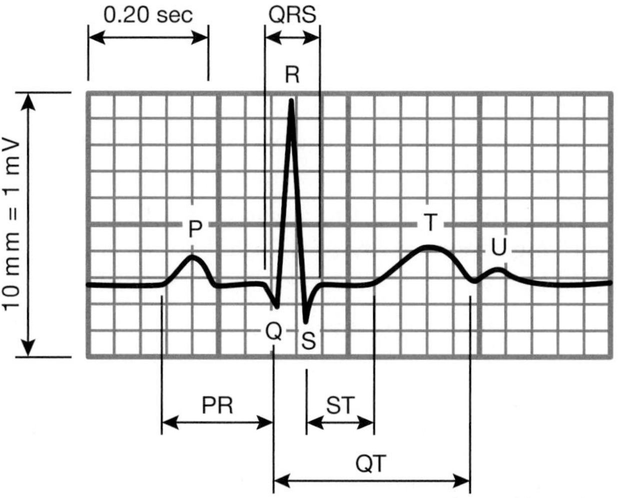

chromatos/Shutterstock.com

Figure 12.25 An ECG is a piece of graph paper containing a tracing, or record of the electrical events in the heart. The placement of the electrodes on the body surface affects the size and shape of the waves recorded. This example shows a normal ECG tracing.

Electrical and Mechanical Events on an ECG Tracing		
ECG Recording	**Electrical Event**	**Mechanical Event**
P wave	SA node fires and atrial depolarization occurs	atrial contraction
QRS complex	impulse travels to the Purkinje fibers and ventricular depolarization occurs	ventricular contraction
T wave	ventricular repolarization occurs	ventricular relaxation
U wave (not always seen)	repolarization of the bundle of His and Purkinje fibers	relaxation of the bundle of His and Purkinje fibers

Figure 12.26

Goodheart-Willcox Publisher

In addition, someone will die from a coronary event every minute. Heart disease is not only epidemic but also costly: the direct and indirect costs of heart disease in the United States are estimated at $300 billion annually.

Cardiac Dysrhythmias

Usually the heart follows a sequence of events at regular intervals. In a normal, healthy heart, the rhythm is regular, and the rate is between 60 and 100 beats per minute. **Figure 12.27A** shows an ECG of a normal sinus rhythm.

Sometimes, however, a beat comes too soon, or the conduction system does not work properly, and an abnormal rhythm occurs. This irregularity is called a ***dysrhythmia***. Generally, dysrhythmias that originate in the ventricle are more dangerous than those that originate in the atria or AV node and can be life threatening.

Dysrhythmias have many causes, including damage to the heart muscle (such as from a heart attack), coronary artery disease, hypertension, smoking, excessive alcohol consumption, excessive caffeine ingestion from coffee or soft drinks, electrolyte imbalances, illicit drug use, stress, medications, and dietary supplements that contain stimulants.

As stated earlier, the ECG is the best tool for detecting abnormal rhythms. Listed below, and shown in **Figure 12.27**, are several types of arrhythmias.

A. (Normal sinus rhythm)

B. ***Bradycardia***—a normal heart rhythm but with a rate below 60 bpm. This condition is common in athletes.

C. ***Tachycardia***—a normal rhythm but with a rate above 100 bpm.

D. ***Premature atrial contractions (PACs)***—a condition in which an irritable piece of atrial heart tissue fires before the SA node. This causes the contraction to occur too early in the rhythm. Usually PACs are harmless. Caffeine ingestion, other types of stimulants, and stress can increase their likelihood.

E. ***Atrial fibrillation***—a condition in which the atrial tissue is very irritated, causing the atria to beat at a rate greater than 350 bpm. The atria do not beat in a coordinated manner; they simply quiver. On an electrocardiogram, the baseline for atrial fibrillation is a wavy line, and the ventricular response is irregular. Atrial fibrillation is the most common type of arrhythmia worldwide. In fact, many people with atrial fibrillation go about their daily routine without any symptoms. However, if the ventricular rate is too low or too high, pharmacological intervention or a pacemaker may be needed.

Research Notes: How Transplanted Hearts Function

Research on heart-transplant patients has found that their resting heart rates are higher than normal, at approximately 90 bpm. According to exercise stress-test studies, increases in heart rates occur more slowly in transplant patients, and recovery heart rates remain elevated for longer periods of time.

This is because the parasympathetic and sympathetic systems do not regulate heart rate in a transplanted heart. This means that heart rate is higher at rest, and it only begins to rise during exercise due to an increase in hormones such as epinephrine and norepinephrine.

F. ***Premature ventricular contractions (PVCs)***—a condition in which the Purkinje fibers fire before the SA node, causing the ventricles to contract prematurely. Single PVCs are not dangerous. However, frequent PVCs (more than six per minute) or multifocal PVCs (those that occur at multiple sites in the ventricle) may be dangerous and therefore require treatment.

G. ***Ventricular tachycardia (VT)***—a life-threatening dysrhythmia in which the ventricles initiate the beat rather than the SA node. The heart rate is between 150 and 250 bpm, requiring immediate medical intervention such as intravenous lidocaine or cardioversion.

H. ***Ventricular fibrillation (VF)***—a life-threatening condition in which the ventricles quiver instead of contracting in an organized manner, so the heart does not beat and there is no cardiac output. Immediate steps to defibrillate the heart must be undertaken. Defibrillation is the delivery of a measured electric shock with the hope that the system will reset and regain a normal, healthy rhythm.

I. ***Heart block***—a condition in which the impulses traveling from the SA node to the ventricles are delayed, blocked intermittently, or completely blocked by the AV node. These are commonly called *first-degree* (impulse-delayed), *second-degree* (intermittently blocked), and *third-degree* (completely blocked) *heart blocks*. Third-degree heart block is a dangerous dysrhythmia because there is no electrical communication between the atria and the ventricles. The atria fire at the rate of the SA node, between 60 and 100 bpm, but the ventricles beat at their own rate, between 15 and 40 bpm. Because the ventricles fire at such a slow rate, cardiac output is too low to adequately supply blood to the rest of the body. A pacemaker is usually inserted into the heart to remedy this condition.

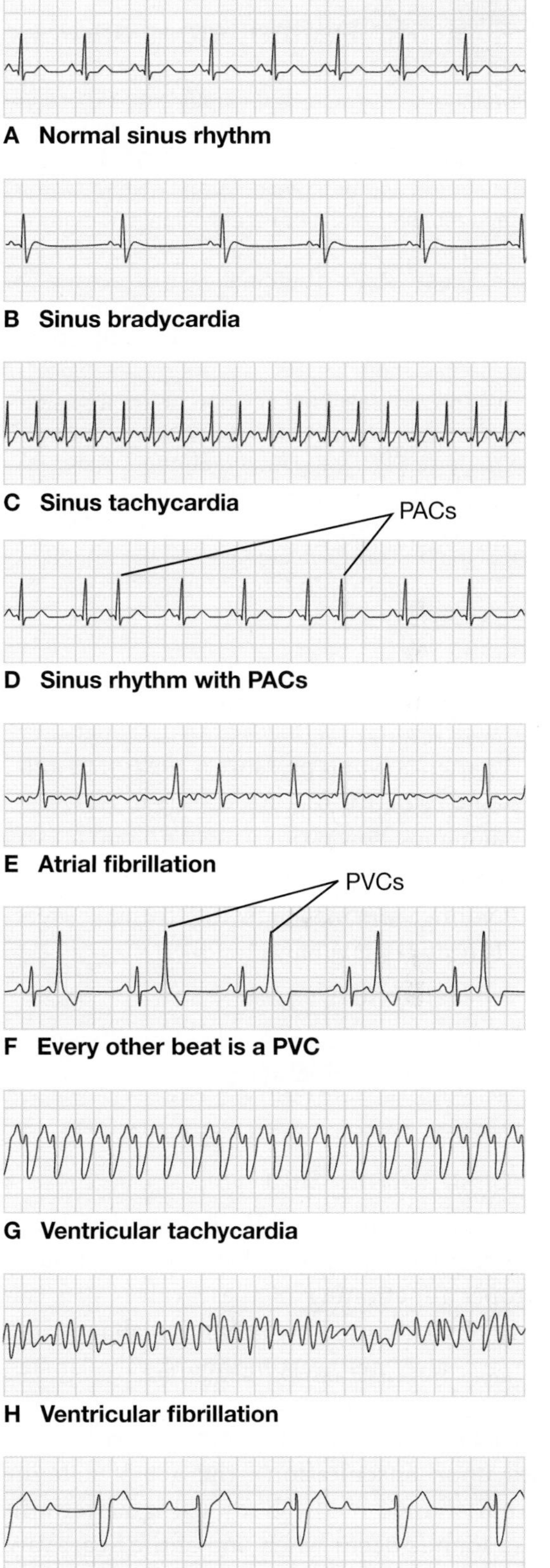

Figure 12.27 A—A normal ECG. B through I—Different types of arrhythmias.

Focus On Defibrillators and Life-Threatening Dysrhythmias

A defibrillator is a device that can deliver a therapeutic dose of electric current that momentarily stops the heart, allowing its built-in pacemaker, the SA node, to assume control and produce a normal rhythm. Automated external defibrillators (AEDs) are available in many public gathering places, such as airports, shopping malls, and schools. These devices automatically detect the type of dysrhythmia present and deliver an electrical shock if appropriate, thus allowing people with little or no training to use them.

The American Heart Association offers a basic cardiopulmonary resuscitation (CPR) course that can train you to perform CPR and use an automatic external defibrillator. This course is recommended for everyone. If, however, you are involved in a rescue, and you have not taken such a course, you can still use the AED. With its foolproof, two- to three-step process, it is simple to use.

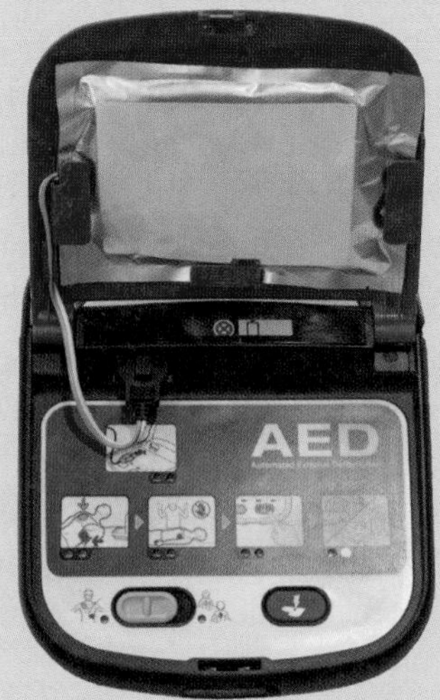

Baloncici/Shutterstock.com

An automated external defibrillator, or AED.

SELF CHECK

1. A patient's blood pressure is measured and found to be 132/84. According to AHA guidelines, how is this patient's blood pressure classified?
2. A young woman weighs 187 lb and is 5 feet 11 inches tall. What is her BMI?
3. What are PACs?
4. Which type of heart block is considered life-threatening? Why?

Valve Abnormalities

Recall from earlier in this chapter that the heart valves regulate the flow of blood through the heart. Improper functioning of these valves can cause a variety of problems. Three common abnormalities of the heart valves are heart murmurs, valvular stenosis, and mitral valve prolapse.

Heart murmurs are whooshing or swishing sounds heard upon auscultation—the act of listening to internal sounds of the body using a stethoscope. These sounds occur when one of the heart valves is not closing properly. They can be caused by congenital heart defects, which are present at birth, or by valvular disease as a result of aging, infection, rheumatic fever, or other condition. Heart murmurs are common in young children and usually do not require any special treatment.

Valvular stenosis is a narrowing of the heart valve due to stiff or fused valve cusps (**Figure 12.28**). Valvular stenosis can occur in one or more of the valves, making the heart work very hard to pump blood through the smaller-than-normal valve opening. People with a mild case of stenosis may be symptom-free. Those with a moderate form, however, may have to restrict their physical activity, and those with a severe case may need surgery to replace the valve.

Mitral valve prolapse is an incomplete closing of the mitral valve. Mitral valve prolapse is fairly common, occurring in up to 10% of the population. It is usually benign and does not require any restrictions.

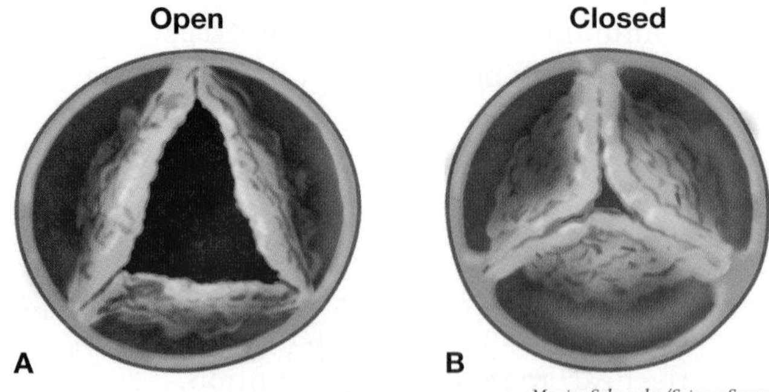

Monica Schroeder/Science Source

Figure 12.28 Valvular stenosis. A—When a stenotic aortic valve is open, the opening is a little smaller than in a normal valve due to stiffness and irregularities. The white areas show calcification of the valve leaflets (flaps), which makes them stiff and unable to open properly. B—A stenotic aortic valve is unable to close all the way, so blood can leak through when the valve is closed.

In a small number of cases, mitral regurgitation occurs. This is a disorder in which blood flows backward through the mitral valve into the left atrium when the ventricle contracts (hence the term *prolapse*). Symptoms may include shortness of breath, ***palpitations***, fatigue, and chest pain. In some instances, the valve has to be repaired or replaced.

Inflammatory Diseases

As you may recall from earlier chapters, the suffix *-itis* means "inflammation." Inflammation can affect several different parts of the heart:

- ***Pericarditis*** is an inflammation of the pericardial sac that surrounds the heart. This condition causes the heart to rub against the pericardial sac as the heart contracts, producing friction that causes a stabbing pain in the chest. Shortness of breath, fatigue, and rapid pulse may also occur. Medications are usually prescribed to fight any infection that may be present and to decrease inflammation and pain.
- ***Myocarditis*** is an inflammation of the myocardium, the middle layer of the heart. Myocarditis can cause symptoms similar to those of pericarditis.
- ***Endocarditis*** is an inflammation of the innermost lining of the heart, including the inner surfaces of the chambers and valves, usually caused by an infection. This condition can destroy the heart valves and cause life-threatening complications if left untreated. Treatment consists of treating the underlying infection.

Heart Failure

Heart failure is a condition in which the heart cannot adequately pump blood to meet the oxygen needs of the body, or the heart muscle becomes stiff and has difficulty filling with blood. Heart failure can occur in the right or left ventricle.

When the heart's pumping ability diminishes, fluid backs up in the lungs, liver, arms, legs, and gastro-intestinal tract. This causes symptoms including shortness of breath, cough, edema (excessive fluid) in the ankles, weight gain, and frequent waking at night to urinate.

The most common cause of heart failure is coronary artery disease, but heart failure can also be caused by infection that weakens the heart muscle. This condition is called ***cardiomyopathy***. Heart failure usually happens gradually, but it can develop quickly after a heart attack has damaged the heart muscle.

Heart failure is not curable, but several different medications are used to treat heart failure with good outcomes. These include diuretics that prevent water retention, vasodilators, and cardiostimulatory and cardioinhibitory drugs as needed. Cardiostimulatory drugs enhance heart function by increasing heart rate; cardioinhibitory drugs decrease heart rate.

Heart transplants are often performed on individuals with end-stage heart failure and, in some rare cases, on children with congenital heart defects. Open-heart surgery is performed, and the patient's diseased heart is replaced with the donor's heart while the patient is connected to a heart-lung machine.

The first-year survival rate among heart transplant patients (81%) has greatly improved with the advent of immunosuppressant drugs, which help reduce the risk of organ rejection. Five-year survival rates are 75%, and most individuals are able to return to their normal activities of daily living. However, they need to stay on a lifelong regimen of multiple medications to prevent rejection of the donated heart.

Diseases of the Arteries

Arteries play the vital roles of transporting blood containing oxygen and nutrients throughout the body and removing wastes from the body cells. This section describes some of the common problems and diseases that can inhibit or prevent these vital functions.

Aneurysms

An ***aneurysm*** is the abnormal ballooning of a blood vessel—usually an artery—due to a weakness in the wall of the vessel (**Figure 12.29**). Although the causes of an aneurysm are often unclear, hypertension, high cholesterol, and cigarette smoking increase the risk of developing an aneurysm.

Pain and swelling are common symptoms of an aneurysm, but some individuals have no symptoms. Common locations for aneurysms include the aorta, the brain, the artery behind the knee, and the intestines. Imaging techniques such as computed tomography (CT), ultrasound, and magnetic resonance angiography (MRA) are used to diagnose an aneurysm.

Aneurysms can rupture, causing sudden death or life-threatening side effects. This condition requires immediate surgical attention to repair the ruptured wall of the artery.

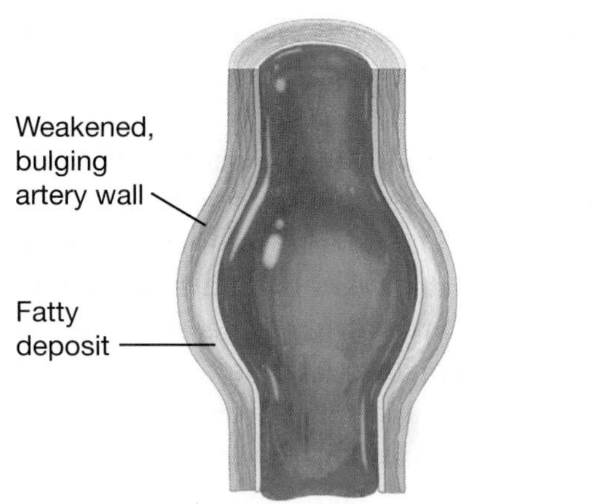

Figure 12.29 Aneurysm.

Coronary Artery Disease

Coronary artery disease (CAD) is caused by a narrowing of one or more of the coronary arteries due to a buildup of plaque. This plaque hardens over the course of many years, developing into the disease known as ***atherosclerosis***.

A buildup of arterial plaque often starts with an injury to the tunica intima, the innermost lining of the artery. The injury can be caused by high blood pressure, smoking, high blood glucose levels from insulin resistance or diabetes, or high levels of fats and cholesterol in the blood.

Once an artery has been injured, the body tries to repair it by applying its version of a spackling compound, which consists of certain fats, cholesterol, calcium, and other substances in the blood. The accumulation of these substances creates the plaque buildup (**Figure 12.30**).

LDL cholesterol is one of the main culprits in the formation of plaque because it enters the intimal wall through the injury and starts to accumulate. White blood cells digest the LDL particles, become engorged with fat, and create a foamy substance, which is why they are called *foam cells*. In addition, smooth muscle cells migrate from the tunica media of the vessel wall into the intimal lining where they ingest fats, multiply, and deposit collagen and elastin fibers.

The arterial plaque grows gradually, narrowing the channel through which blood flows. When the vessel opening is decreased by 50% or more, the heart may not receive a sufficient amount of blood at certain times, such as during exercise or stressful situations.

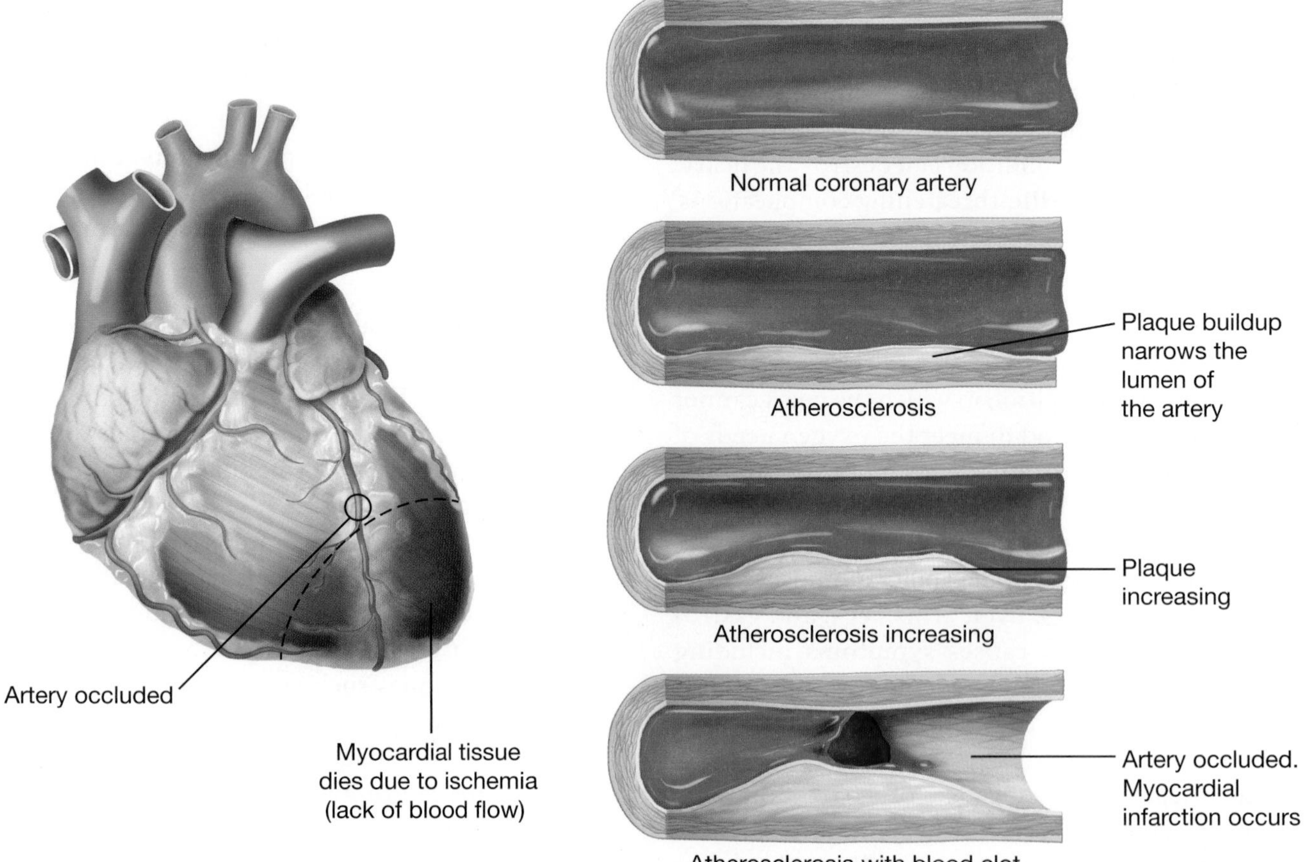

Figure 12.30 Progression of atherosclerosis and development of blockage.

This insufficient blood supply may cause ***angina pectoris***, or heart-related chest pain. Patients can take the drug nitroglycerine to dilate the coronary arteries, which helps to alleviate the pain.

Chest pain is the most common symptom that arises from lack of oxygen and ***ischemia***, or lack of blood flow to the heart. Other symptoms include throat dryness, jaw pain, pain going down the left arm, nausea, increased perspiration, shortness of breath, and fainting. These are all "classic" symptoms because they are the symptoms that men typically experience. It was long thought, mistakenly, that heart disease was primarily a problem for men. Women do experience heart disease, but they often do not have any of the classic symptoms. Instead, they may feel unusually fatigued, have flu-like symptoms, or experience no pain at all. Nevertheless, cardiac ischemia and angina are just as serious for women as for men.

Myocardial Infarction

If an artery becomes completely blocked, a ***myocardial infarction (MI)***, or heart attack, occurs. This can happen suddenly when a piece of arterial plaque ruptures and occludes (closes) the artery. Many people who have had an MI remark that they "felt like an elephant was sitting on [their] chest" or that "the pain was crushing." Morphine and/or other pain medications are administered to diminish the pain.

You may not think that people who have symptoms such as chest pain or shortness of breath before a heart attack are lucky, but in a way, they are. These symptoms are early warnings, which give the people a chance at survival. Others are not so lucky: in approximately one-third of all heart attacks, the first symptom is death.

People with cardiac symptoms should take an aspirin and call 911 within five minutes of onset of the symptoms. Time is of the essence. The first two phases of a heart attack—ischemia and injury to the heart tissue—are reversible with proper intervention. But there is only a 20- to 60-minute window before the death of cardiac tissue, which is irreversible.

A goal of the American College of Cardiology (ACC) is to ensure that MI patients receive treatment within 90 minutes of their arrival at a hospital. Within 30 minutes of their arrival in the emergency room, patients should receive fibrinolytic therapy, which entails the use of special drugs to dissolve the clot. This therapy minimizes the threat of permanent damage to the heart. The ACC also recommends that MI patients receive a balloon angioplasty to open the blocked vessel, and that a stent (a circular, hollow, wire mesh tube) be inserted within 90 minutes of arrival in the ER (**Figure 12.31**).

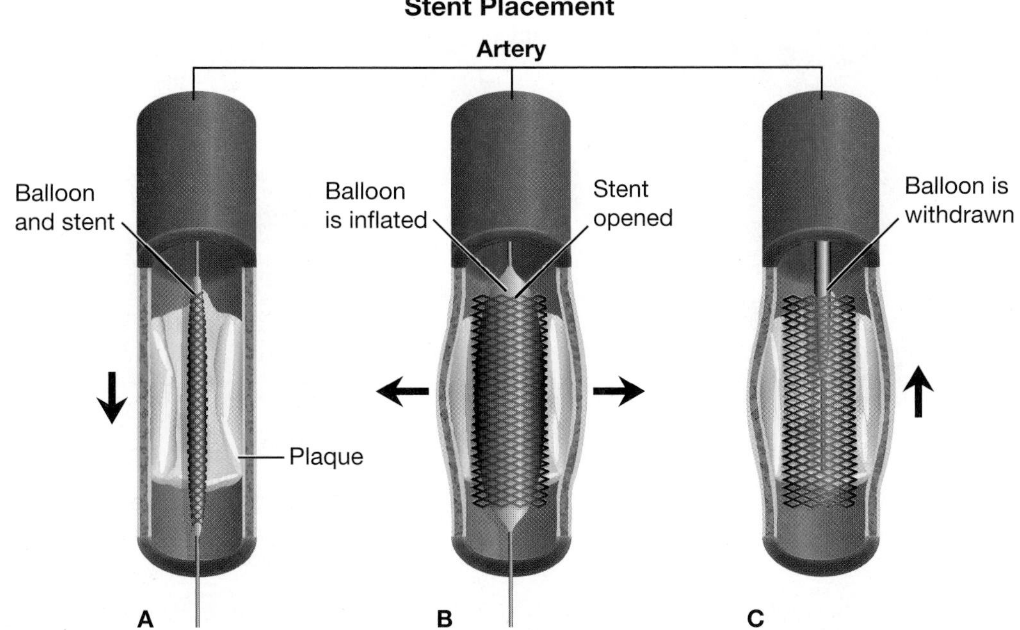

Figure 12.31 Balloon angioplasty and stent placement. A—A hollow wire is threaded through the blood vessel to the location of the blockage. B—An expandable balloon is inflated to press the plaque against the walls of the blood vessel, opening the lumen. C—A wire mesh stent is placed at the location to hold the vessel open after the balloon is removed.

Focus On Sudden Death in Athletes

Flo Hyman, Pete Maravich, Sergei Grinkov, Korey Stringer...what do all of these famous athletes have in common? They all died of cardiac-related complications due to congenital abnormalities, cardiac arrhythmias, or heatstroke.

Leading Cause of Sudden Death: Congenital Heart Abnormalities

The most common reason for sudden death in athletes is congenital abnormalities of the heart, valves, or blood vessels. It is estimated that 2 to 4 of every 100,000 people die as a result of congenital heart abnormalities. This means 100 to 150 deaths each year. These disorders are most prevalent in African-American athletes, and they occur most often in the sport of basketball.

The most common congenital abnormality is hypertrophic cardiomyopathy, which is characterized by an extensive enlargement of the left ventricular wall. This condition can cause ventricular fibrillation, which can be fatal. Many athletes have died from this abnormality.

Marfan syndrome, another common congenital abnormality, is a connective tissue disorder that weakens blood vessels, heart valves, and other tissues. Flo Hyman, a 1986 Olympic volleyball standout, died of Marfan syndrome. Individuals with Marfan syndrome are usually tall and lanky with loose joints.

"Pistol" Pete Maravich, often described as the best and most creative offensive player in basketball history, played for three NBA teams and was the youngest inductee to the basketball hall of fame. He died suddenly during a "pickup" game at age 40. Autopsy results revealed that he had a rare congenital heart defect in which only one coronary artery supplied blood to the four walls of the heart.

Sergei Grinkov, two-time Russian Olympic gold medalist, died at age 28 during a practice session. It was later discovered that two of his coronary arteries were almost completely occluded.

Taking certain precautions can help reduce the incidence of sudden death among athletes with congenital heart abnormalities. Pre-participation physicals, preferrably with a baseline ECG, are suggested and

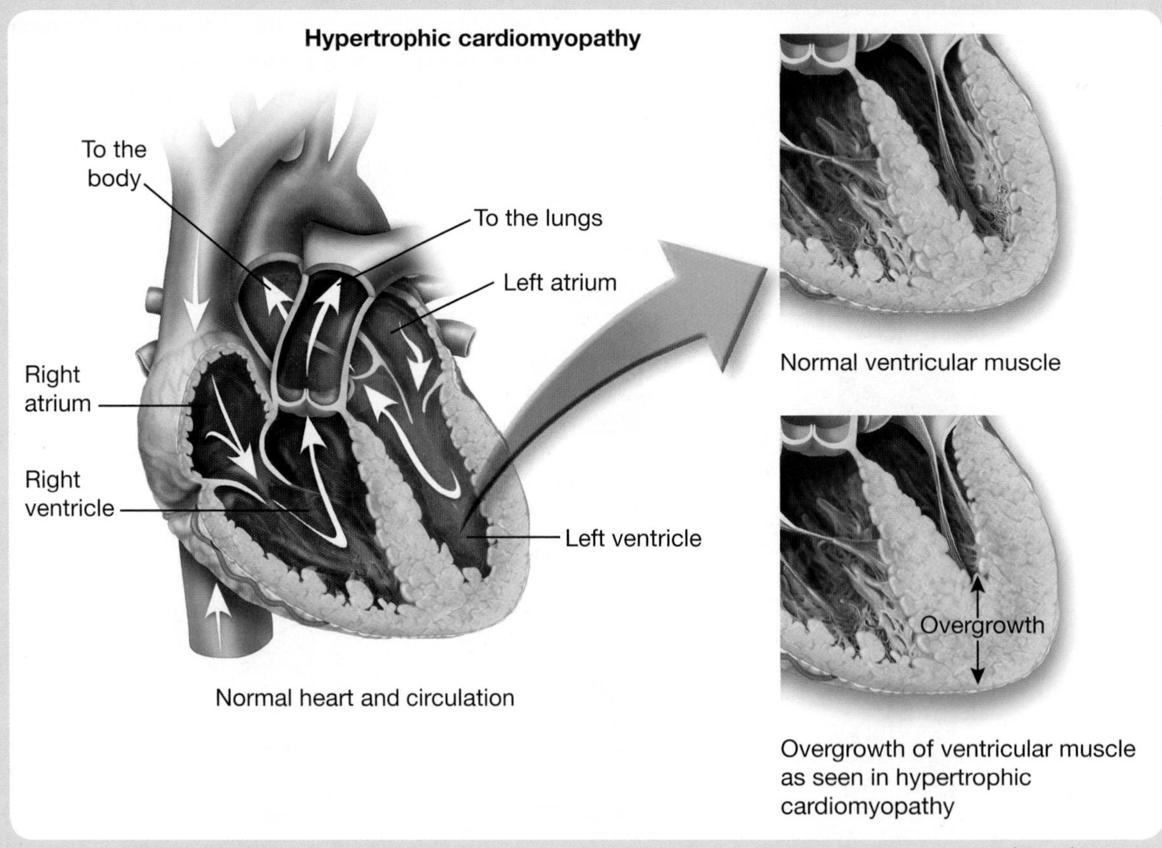

Hypertrophic cardiomyopathy.

(continued)

highly recommended if an athlete experiences lightheadedness, fainting, or other cardiac symptoms. In addition, each athletic facility should be equipped with an AED.

Other Causes of Death in Athletes

Korey Stringer, Minnesota Vikings offensive tackle, died of heatstroke during a practice session. People rarely think of heatstroke as cardiac related, but heat exhastion and heatstroke are the result of the cardiovascular system's inability to cool the body by transporting blood from the core to the skin, where evaporative cooling occurs. This is why increased heart rate is one of the symptoms of heat exhastion. When this occurs, body temperature rises, the hypothalamus stops working, and death will result unless the body is cooled within a few minutes by immersion in an ice bath. The Korey Stringer Institute, founded in the wake of Stringer's death, undertakes research, education, and lobby efforts to decrease the number of heat-related illnesses.

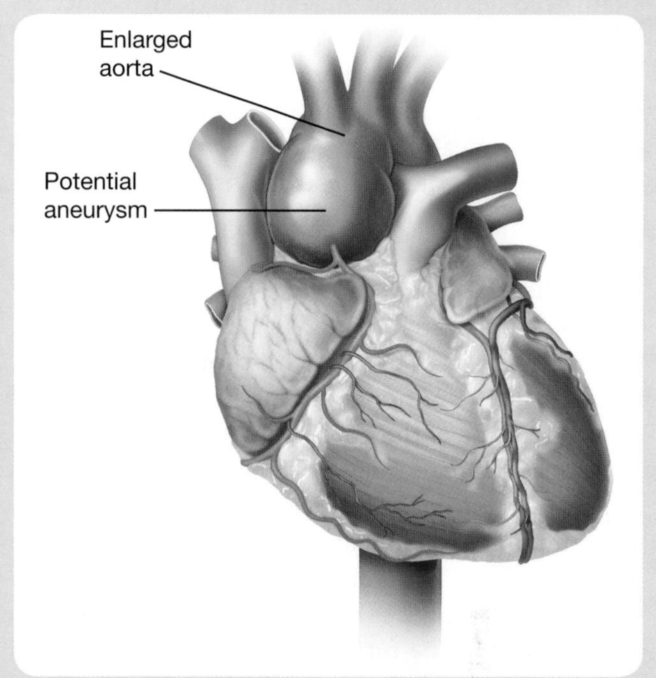

Marfan syndrome can cause the aorta to enlarge and bulge, sometimes causing an aortic aneurysm.

Hypertension

Hypertension is the medical term for high blood pressure. This condition occurs when the force of blood against the arterial wall remains elevated for an extended period of time. Individuals with a blood pressure reading greater than 140/90 mmHg on three separate occasions are considered to have high blood pressure. In many cases, physicians are unable to determine what causes hypertension. Hypertension with no known cause is called *essential hypertension*.

Many people do not know that they have high blood pressure because there are often no symptoms. This is why hypertension is called the *silent killer*. In fact, the Centers for Disease Control (CDC) estimates that one in five US adults has high blood pressure without knowing it. Approximately one-third of the people in the United States have high blood pressure, and the risk of developing it increases substantially with age. Risk factors for developing hypertension include obesity, smoking, physical inactivity, sensitivity to salt, and a family history of hypertension.

When energy intake exceeds the body's energy needs, the excess energy is stored for future use in the form of triglycerides or glycogen. Because the body's glycogen storage capacity is limited, chronic energy excess leads to fat formation and obesity. In turn, obesity increases the risk of hypertension, stroke, and coronary artery disease.

Peripheral Vascular Disease (PVD)

Peripheral vascular disease (PVD) is a condition characterized by a narrowing of the arteries in the legs. PVD usually results in a lack of blood flow to the thighs, calf muscles, and feet. Symptoms generally include pain, fatigue in the lower extremities, and a burning sensation in the calf muscle. Initially, these symptoms may be apparent only while walking, but they may also occur at rest as the condition worsens.

PVD strikes both men and women, but African-Americans are at greater risk. Smoking greatly increases a person's risk of developing PVD. Exercise lowers the risk of PVD and lessens its symptoms. Medications that dilate the arteries and prevent blood clots help control the disease. In severe cases, surgery or the placement of a stent to open the narrowed artery may be required.

Cerebrovascular Accident

A ***cerebrovascular accident (CVA, stroke)***, is a medical emergency that occurs when blood flow to the brain stops. There are two different types of strokes. An ischemic stroke occurs when one of the arteries in the brain becomes blocked. A hemorrhagic stroke occurs when one of the arteries ruptures, causing bleeding in the brain. In both types, the brain is deprived of oxygen within minutes, causing many complications and possibly death.

According to the CDC, stroke is the fourth leading cause of death in the United States and is the leading cause of long-term, severe disability. The CDC estimates that the cost of care for stroke survivors in the United States is approximately $20 billion each year.

Paralysis, loss of speech, problems walking, uncontrolled emotional outbursts, depression, and coma are some of the potential side effects of stroke. These side effects may be temporary if a person experiences a ***transient ischemic attack (TIA)***, which is a temporary lack of blood flow to the brain. In the case of a TIA, symptoms usually disappear within one to two hours. A TIA is a warning sign that stroke could occur in the future, so steps should be taken to correct the underlying condition and risk factors.

Risk factors for stroke include high blood pressure, diabetes, high cholesterol, use of birth control pills, family history of stroke, and race (specifically, African-American ancestry). Smoking, excessive alcohol consumption, illicit drug use, overweight or obese conditions, and physical inactivity also increase the risk of stroke.

Understanding Medical Terminology

Signs of a stroke are easy to remember if you use the F.A.S.T. tip developed by Methodist Health Systems.

F—Face Is one side drooping?
A—Arms Is one arm weak or numb?
S—Speech Is speech slurred?
T—Time Time is critical. Call 911 or get to the hospital quickly.

SECTION 12.4 REVIEW

Mini-Glossary

aneurysm the abnormal ballooning of a blood vessel, usually an artery, due to a weakness in the wall of the vessel

angina pectoris a condition characterized by severe, constricting pain or a sensation of pressure in the chest, often radiating to the left arm; caused by an insufficient supply of blood to the heart

atherosclerosis hardening of the arteries

atrial fibrillation a condition in which the atria contract in an uncoordinated, rapid manner (rate above 350 bpm), causing an irregular ventricular response

brachial artery the artery located at the fold of the elbow

bradycardia a normal heart rhythm but with a rate below 60 bpm

cardiomyopathy a disease such as an infection that weakens the myocardium and causes heart failure

carotid arteries the arteries located on either side of the windpipe; where the carotid pulse is felt

cerebrovascular accident (CVA, stroke) a sudden blockage of blood flow, or the rupture of an artery in the brain, that causes brain cells to die from lack of oxygen

coronary artery disease (CAD) a condition characterized by narrowing of one or more of the coronary arteries due to a buildup of plaque

dysrhythmia an irregular heartbeat or rhythm

endocarditis inflammation of the innermost lining of the heart, including the inner surfaces of the chambers and valves

heart block a condition in which the impulses traveling from the SA node to the ventricles are delayed, intermittently blocked, or completely blocked before they reach the ventricles

heart murmurs extra or unusual sounds during a heartbeat that can be heard by a stethoscope; may be harmless or indicative of a problem with one of the heart valves

hypertension high blood pressure; a condition that occurs when the force of blood against the arterial wall remains elevated for an extended period of time

ischemia a lack of blood flow, usually due to the narrowing of a blood vessel

mitral valve prolapse an incomplete closing of the mitral valve, which causes blood to flow backward into the left atrium when the left ventricle contracts

myocardial infarction (MI) a condition characterized by blockage of a coronary artery; also known as a *heart attack*

myocarditis inflammation of the middle layer of the heart, or myocardium

palpitations sensations of a rapid heartbeat

pericarditis inflammation of the pericardial sac that surrounds the heart

peripheral vascular disease (PVD) a condition characterized by a narrowing of the arteries in the legs

(continued)

premature atrial contractions (PACs) a condition in which an irritable piece of atrial heart tissue fires before the SA node, causing the atria to contract too soon

premature ventricular contractions (PVCs) a condition in which Purkinje fibers fire before the SA node, causing the ventricles to contract prematurely

radial artery the artery located on the thumb side of the wrist; where the radial pulse is detected

tachycardia a normal heart rhythm but with a rate above 100 bpm

transient ischemic attack (TIA) a temporary lack of blood flow to the brain

valvular stenosis a narrowing of the heart valve due to stiff or fused valve cusps

ventricular fibrillation (VF) a life-threatening condition in which the heart ventricles quiver at a rate greater than 350 bpm

ventricular tachycardia (VT) a life-threatening arrhythmia in which the ventricles, rather than the SA node, initiate the heartbeat; the heart rate is between 150 and 250 bpm, requiring swift medical attention

Review Questions

1. Which blood vessel is used when pulse is measured on a person's neck?
2. According to the American Heart Association, what are the criteria for stage 2 hypertension?
3. What level of cholesterol is considered "normal" in the human body?
4. For what two purposes are ECGs routinely used?
5. What are the differences between atrial fibrillation and ventricular fibrillation?
6. What surgical method can be used to remedy some valve abnormalities?
7. What is the medical term for *heart attack*?
8. What disease is known as the *silent killer*?
9. Explain why the body's attempt at repairing an injury to an artery can become a problem.

Medical Terminology: The Cardiovascular System

By understanding the word parts that make up medical words, you can extend your medical vocabulary. This chapter includes many of the word parts listed below. Review these word parts to be sure you understand their meanings.

cardi/o	heart
vascul/o	vessels
-ar	pertaining to
inter-	between
-al	pertaining to
atri/o	atrium
ventricul/o	ventricle
my/o	muscle
-id	like, similar to
tri-	three
vas/o	vessel, duct
-pathy	disease
-plasty	surgical repair
-plegia	paralysis
pulmon/o	lung

Now use these word parts to form valid medical words that fit the following definitions. Some of the words are included in this chapter. Others are not. When you finish, use a medical dictionary to check your work.

1. pertaining to the blood vessels
2. septum that separates the atria
3. pertaining to the heart muscle
4. valve that has three cusp-like leaflets
5. constriction of a blood vessel
6. disease of the heart muscle
7. pertaining to both the ventricles and the atria
8. surgical repair of a ventricle
9. paralysis of the heart
10. pertaining to the heart and lungs

Chapter 12 Summary

- The heart is located in the center of the thoracic cavity, is encased in the pericardium, and is made up of three layers: the epicardium, myocardium, and endocardium.
- Blood flows from the right atrium to the right ventricle, then to the lungs, back to the left atrium and left ventricle, which pumps the blood to the rest of the body; the blood then returns to the right atrium and the cycle repeats.

- The heart is regulated internally by the sinoatrial node (SA node), which sends an impulse through the atrioventricular node (AV node) to the bundle of His and down the left and right bundle branches to the Purkinje fibers.
- Externally, the heart is controlled by the cardiac center in the medulla oblongata and by higher brain centers, sensory receptors, some hormones, and other factors.
- In a normal heart, cardiac impulses originate in the SA node and are conducted through the AV node, the bundle of His, and the bundle branches to the Purkinje fibers, causing a coordinated depolarization of the cells.
- Arteries carry blood away from the heart and have thick, strong, elastic walls; veins carry blood back toward the heart and have thin, less elastic walls and one-way valves; capillaries are the site of gas exchange.
- The two main types of circulation are pulmonary and systemic circulation.
- Understanding how to check a pulse and measure blood pressure, and knowing what other numbers are important, can help people maintain good health.
- There are many different types of dysrhythmias, many of which can be detected with an ECG.

Chapter 12 Review

Understanding Key Concepts

1. The myocardium is the ______.
   A. sac surrounding the heart
   B. thick, muscular wall of the heart
   C. inner lining of the heart
   D. septum between the chambers of the heart
2. The bicuspid (mitral) valve is located between the ______.
   A. right and left ventricles
   B. left atrium and left ventricle
   C. left and right atria
   D. left ventricle and the aorta
3. The fluid-filled sac that surrounds the heart is called the ______.
   A. pericardium
   B. endocardium
   C. myocardium
   D. epicardium
4. The heart is flanked on either side by the ______.
   A. diaphragm
   B. lungs
   C. hips
   D. sternum
5. The "lub" of the heart's "lub-dub" sound is caused by the closing of the ______ valves.
6. The wall that separates the atria from each other is called the ______.
7. Attached to the cusps of heart valves are thin, fibrous cords called ______, which are connected to ______ muscles.
8. The "pacemaker" of the heart is the ______.
   A. mitral valve
   B. atrioventricular node
   C. sinoatrial node
   D. bundle of His
9. Which of the following statements about the SA node is true?
   A. It is located at the top of the right atrium.
   B. It is the pacemaker.
   C. It is located near the bundle of His.
   D. It is the origin of Purkinje fibers.
10. Sympathetic nerve fibers stimulate the SA node, which ______.
    A. increases the heart rate
    B. decreases the heart rate
    C. causes the ventricles to contract
    D. makes the heart rate irregular
11. Which of the following is *not* considered a component of the heart's conduction system?
    A. sinoatrial (SA) node
    B. epicardium
    C. Purkinje fibers
    D. atrioventricular (AV) node
12. The cardiac center of the brain works with the ______ and ______ branches of the autonomic nervous system to help control heart activity.
13. The ______, which are sensitive to pressure, are located in the aortic arch and carotid arteries.

14. Which layer of the heart provides a smooth, frictionless surface for the flow of blood in a vessel?
    A. tunica media
    B. tunica intima
    C. tunica externa
    D. medulla oblongata
15. Which vessel has the thickest, strongest, and most elastic walls?
    A. artery
    B. capillary
    C. exchange vessel
    D. vein
16. Blood is carried to the lungs by the ______.
    A. pulmonary vein
    B. pulmonary artery
    C. aorta
    D. inferior vena cava
17. The smallest, most numerous vessels in the body are the ______.
    A. venules
    B. arterioles
    C. capillaries
    D. veins
18. Blood returning to the heart via the inferior vena cava and the superior vena cava collects in the ______.
    A. left ventricle
    B. right ventricle
    C. right atrium
    D. left atrium
19. Blood pressure measured when the left ventricle contracts is called ______ pressure.
    A. diastolic
    B. stroke
    C. systolic
    D. mean
20. The artery located on the side of your neck, where you can clearly feel your pulse, is called the ______.
21. Inflammation of the middle layer of the heart is called ______.
22. The most common cause of heart failure is ______.
23. A disease, such as an infection, that weakens the heart muscle is called ______.
24. Listening to heart sounds using a stethoscope is called ______.
25. The ______ is one common location for an aneurysm.
    A. carotid artery
    B. aorta
    C. jugular vein
    D. brachial artery
26. Atherosclerosis is a hardening of the ______.
    A. veins
    B. blood vessels
    C. arteries
    D. athero valve
27. Which term describes a narrowing of the heart valve due to stiff or fused valve cusps?
    A. valve prolapse
    B. valvular stenosis
    C. palpitations
    D. heart murmurs

Thinking Critically

28. What do you think would happen if the interventricular septum had a hole in it?
29. Arteries carry only oxygenated blood and veins carry only deoxygenated blood. Is this a correct statement? Explain and defend your answer.
30. What would happen if a person's parasympathetic nervous system did not function?
31. How do the endocrine and nervous systems work together to help a person escape from a dangerous situation?
32. Why is blood considered a connective tissue?
33. Drawing on the information in the first three sections of this chapter, explain why low blood pressure is considered a potentially dangerous condition.
34. How is the function of the heart affected by a myocardial infarction?
35. Compare and contrast a TIA and a hemorrhagic stroke.
36. How would having too much LDL cholesterol in your blood vessels increase your risk of having a myocardial infarction?

Clinical Case Study

Read again the Clinical Case Study at the beginning of this chapter. Use the information provided in the chapter to answer the questions at the end of the scenario.

37. What do Ann's blood pressure, BMI, and total cholesterol numbers tell you about her health?
38. Among the topics discussed in this chapter, what may be happening to Ann?
39. Based on the information in this chapter, which diagnosis is most likely?

Analyzing and Evaluating Data

This bar graph shows the number of deaths from heart disease for selected years. Use the graph to answer the following questions.

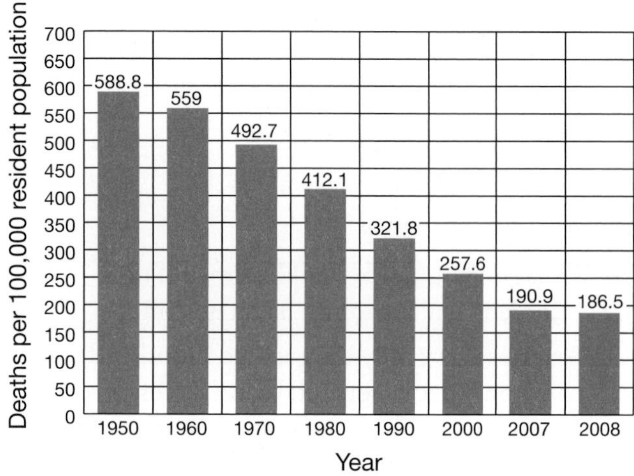

40. How many people died from heart disease in 1980?
41. Between which years is the greatest reduction in the number of heart disease-related fatalities?
42. Between which 10-year periods is the smallest reduction in the number of heart disease-related fatalities? How might this be interpreted in a positive way?
43. What is the difference in the number of heart disease-related fatalities between 1950 and 2008?

Investigating Further

44. Conduct research to discover more about the "nontraditional" symptoms of cardiac ischemia and myocardial infarction in women. For what symptoms should women watch? What other groups typically have nontraditional symptoms of heart disease? Why?
45. The American Heart Association (AHA) publishes guidelines describing normal blood pressure and various stages of high blood pressure. These guidelines are updated from time to time based on current research and other factors. Look up the current AHA guidelines. Then have your blood pressure checked by a healthcare professional or use the blood pressure machine at a local pharmacy. How does your blood pressure compare to the guidelines?
46. There are significant differences in both the causes and the symptoms of left heart failure and right heart failure. Conduct research to find out more about the two types of heart failure. What are their causes? Their symptoms? How does treatment of the two types differ?

13 The Lymphatic and Immune Systems

Clinical Case Study

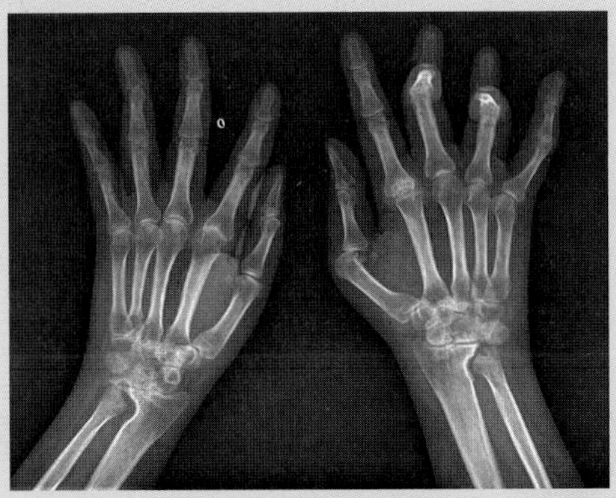
ZEPHYR/Science Source

Nina, 42 years old, is an elementary school teacher who enjoys her job. She does yoga on Wednesdays and Saturdays, and she is a nonsmoker. She takes over-the-counter allergy medicine as needed.

Nina's hands have been increasingly sore for about 4 months, and lately her shoulders have also been bothering her when she tries to raise her arms fully. She has been taking one 200 mg ibuprofen tablet two to three times a day for the last several weeks. She made an appointment with her doctor because she read that one should not take ibuprofen for more than 10 days for pain unless directed by a physician.

When asked, Nina reports that she feels stiff all over for about an hour when she wakes up. She says she has not had a fever and has not felt ill since well before the present symptoms surfaced. When asked about her usual physical activity, she says her sole outdoor activity is walking her dog daily in the park near her apartment. She stays on the paved path and says she has never found a tick on her dog.

Physical examination shows that several of her metacarpophalangeal joints are slightly swollen and tender. Her wrists are also slightly swollen and tender, and they have less than normal range of motion. Her shoulder range of motion is limited. The metatarsophalangeal joints are also tender, although not swollen. Her skin appears normal, with no evidence of a rash.

Where are the metacarpophalangeal (MCP) and metatarsophalangeal (MTP) joints? What are some possible causes of Nina's symptoms? How do her history and presentation help distinguish between possible diagnoses?

Chapter 13 Outline

Section 13.1 The Lymphatic System

- Organization of the Lymphatic System
- Functional Anatomy of the Lymphatic System

Section 13.2 Nonspecific Defenses

- Physical Barriers
- Cellular and Chemical Defenses
- Inflammatory Response
- Fever

Section 13.3 The Immune System: Specific Defenses

- Antigens
- Immune System Cells
- Antibody-Mediated Immunity
- Primary and Secondary Immune Responses
- Cell-Mediated Immunity

Section 13.4 Disorders of the Lymphatic and Immune Systems

- Cancer and Lymph Nodes
- Allergies
- Organ Transplantation and Rejection
- Autoimmune Disorders
- HIV and AIDS

The world can be a dangerous place full of bacteria, viruses, fungi, and toxins. Because the human body is an attractive host for these and other infectious agents, it must continuously defend itself against assault from disease-producing microbes. People are usually unaware of this battle, which takes place on a microscopic level. Like a medieval town protected by walls, pots of burning oil, and guards, the body is protected by physical and chemical barriers, as well as a cellular defense system.

This chapter explores the lymphatic system and the body's defenses against infection and disease. First, it discusses the anatomy and basic physiology of the lymphatic system and related lymphatic tissues. Next, it describes the nonspecific defense system, which works without regard for the specific identity of an infectious agent. Finally, the chapter examines the body's specific defense system, which generates cells and antibodies that are custom-made for targeting invading organisms. It also discusses disorders and diseases that commonly affect the lymphatic and immune systems.

SECTION 13.1

The Lymphatic System

Objectives

- Explain the organization of the lymphatic system, including paths of lymph flow and drainage.
- Describe anatomy and functions of the cells, tissues, and organs that make up the lymphatic system.

Key Terms

B lymphocytes (B cells)
endothelial cells
interstitial fluid
lingual tonsils
lymph
lymph nodes
lymphatic nodules
lymphatic trunks
lymphatic valves
lymphatic vessels
lymphocytes
macrophages
mucosa-associated lymphatic tissue (MALT)
natural killer (NK) cells
palatine tonsils
pathogens
pharyngeal tonsil
spleen
T lymphocytes (T cells)

The lymphatic system performs three vital functions in the human body: it solves a "plumbing" problem, it provides the main pathway for fat absorption, and it constantly remains on the lookout for foreign invaders that may cause infection and disease.

The plumbing problem is caused by capillaries that naturally leak. As blood travels through the capillaries, a small amount of blood plasma leaks out of the capillaries and into the surrounding tissue. The normal leakage rate, across the entire body, is 2 to 3 mL per minute, which is a tiny amount compared to the 5,000 mL of blood that pass through the capillaries each minute. How could such a small leak (about one twentieth of one percent) possibly be a problem? The answer is found by considering how a small leak leads to accumulating losses over time: 2 mL per minute times 1,440 minutes in a day adds up to about 3 liters a day. That is roughly equal to the total amount of plasma in the average human body. Therefore, this "small leak" would cause a potentially fatal loss of blood volume in less than a day if the excess fluid were not returned to the cardiovascular system by the lymphatic system.

Lymphatic structures in the small intestine provide the main pathway for absorption of fats from food during digestion, and for the absorption of vitamins A, D, E, and K, which are fat soluble. This process will be explained in more detail in Chapter 14.

The lymphatic system also plays a vital role in the body's immune system, which provides protection against disease. It enables the body to meet the challenge of quickly recognizing and mounting a counterattack against infectious agents. As the lymphatic system reabsorbs fluid from the leaking capillaries, it removes bacteria and virus-infected cells from body tissues. It also activates specific immune defenses.

Organization of the Lymphatic System

The lymphatic system includes lymphatic vessels, lymphatic fluid (called *lymph*), and lymphatic organs, such as lymph nodes and the spleen (**Figure 13.1**). The cells that fight infection develop, reside, and travel through the organs and vessels of the lymphatic system.

The lymphatic system resembles the cardiovascular system in that both extend throughout almost all parts of the body. Both systems also have a network of vessels that vary in size from microscopic capillaries to large vessels. However, the lymphatic and cardiovascular systems differ in terms of overall architecture and pressure. The lymphatic system has an open architecture: lymph enters at one end and exits at the other end. The cardiovascular system, on the other hand, has a closed architecture: blood flows around and around in a closed, but slightly leaky, loop (**Figure 13.2**). Pressure throughout the lymphatic system is much lower than the pressure found in arteries.

Understanding Medical Terminology

The word *lymph* comes from the Latin word *lympha*, which means "water." Most of the time, lymph is a clear fluid that resembles water. However, its composition, produced by a combination of chemical substances, differs throughout the body. When lymph drains from the small intestine, for example, it takes on a milky appearance from the lipids (fats) that it collects as it travels through the small intestine.

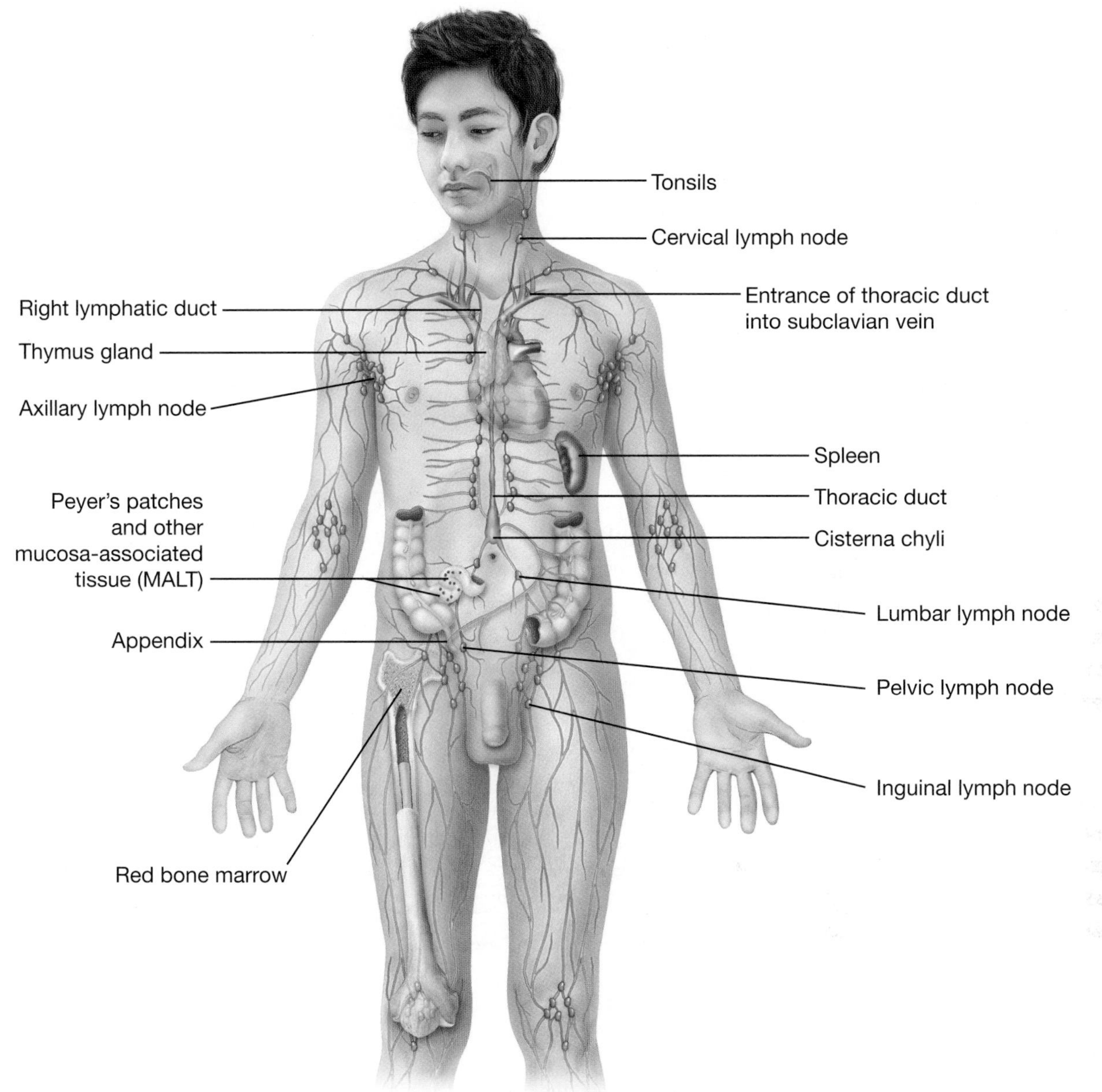

Figure 13.1 The lymphatic system includes lymph, lymphatic vessels, lymphatic cells and tissues, and lymphatic organs.

Lymph Formation and Flow

Normal ***lymph*** is similar in composition to blood plasma, but it contains less protein. Lymph consists mostly of water and dissolved molecules, such as sodium and chloride. Lymph is transparent or sometimes slightly yellow in color, and it contains few cells. Lymph formation begins with fluid that leaks out of blood vessel capillaries (**Figure 13.3**). When this fluid is inside the blood vessels, it is called *blood plasma*. When it leaks out and enters the spaces between cells, it is called ***interstitial fluid***. Capillaries are permeable to blood plasma and interstitial fluid, meaning that these substances can move in and out of capillaries.

Pressure is slightly greater inside the "upstream end" of capillaries (the end closer to the arteries) than in the interstitial fluid. This pressure difference causes some of the plasma in the capillaries to move into the surrounding spaces. Pressure is lower at the "downstream end" of capillaries (closer to the veins), so interstitial fluid tends to enter the capillaries there. Slightly more blood plasma leaves the capillaries at the upstream end than enters at the downstream end. This disparity leads to the slow but steady loss of 2 to 3 mL of plasma per minute mentioned in this section's introduction.

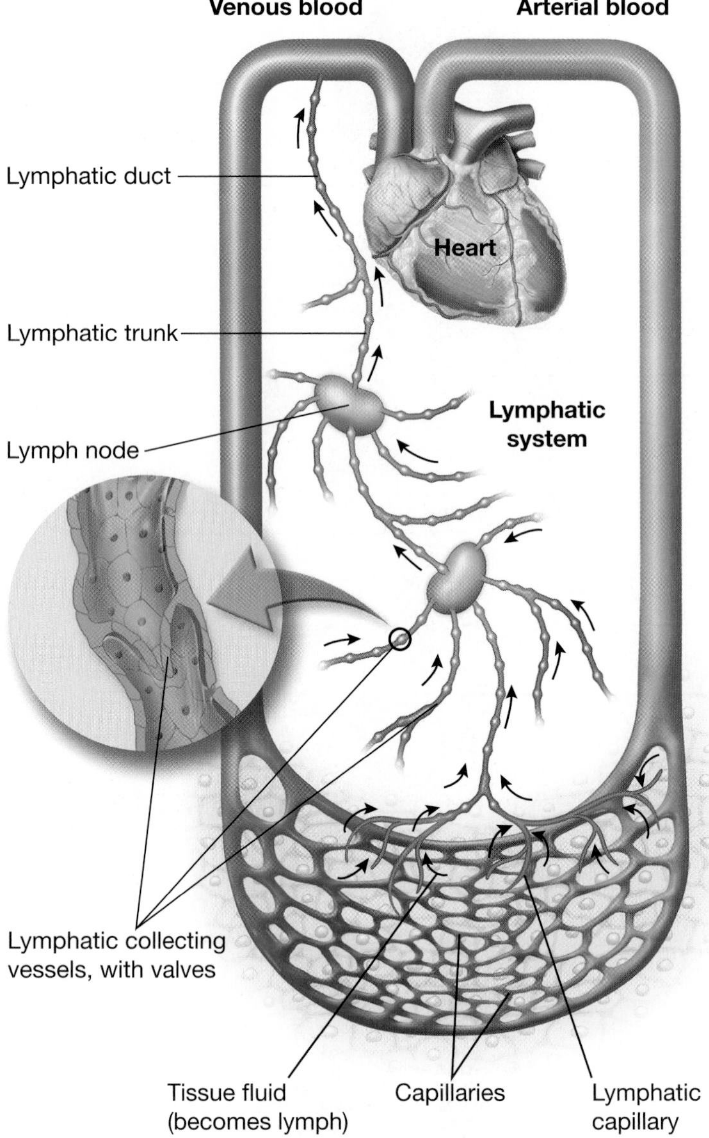

Figure 13.2 Relationship between the lymphatic system and the cardiovascular system.

As fluid from the upstream end of capillaries builds up in the interstitial space, some of it enters the lymphatic capillaries through small gaps between the ***endothelial cells,*** which form the walls of the lymphatic capillaries. The endothelial cells overlap and are tethered to one another in a way that makes it easy for fluid to enter the lymphatic capillaries but hard for it to leave. Once the fluid enters the lymphatic capillaries or the larger ***lymphatic vessels,*** it is called *lymph*. The lymphatic capillaries join together to form collecting vessels, which in turn link together to form even larger vessels called *lymphatic trunks*. The ***lymphatic trunks*** drain lymph from different parts of the body.

The human body does not have a pump similar to the heart to help propel lymph through this network of vessels. However, muscular contractions and the movement of organs compress the lymphatic vessels, advancing the lymph along its route. This process is aided by ***lymphatic valves,*** which are tissue flaps that act as one-way gates inside the lymphatic vessels. When a lymphatic vessel is compressed by surrounding tissue, the valves allow the lymph to go only in one direction—away from the lymphatic capillaries.

Lymph Drainage

Each lymphatic trunk is named for its location and the part of the body it drains. These include the left

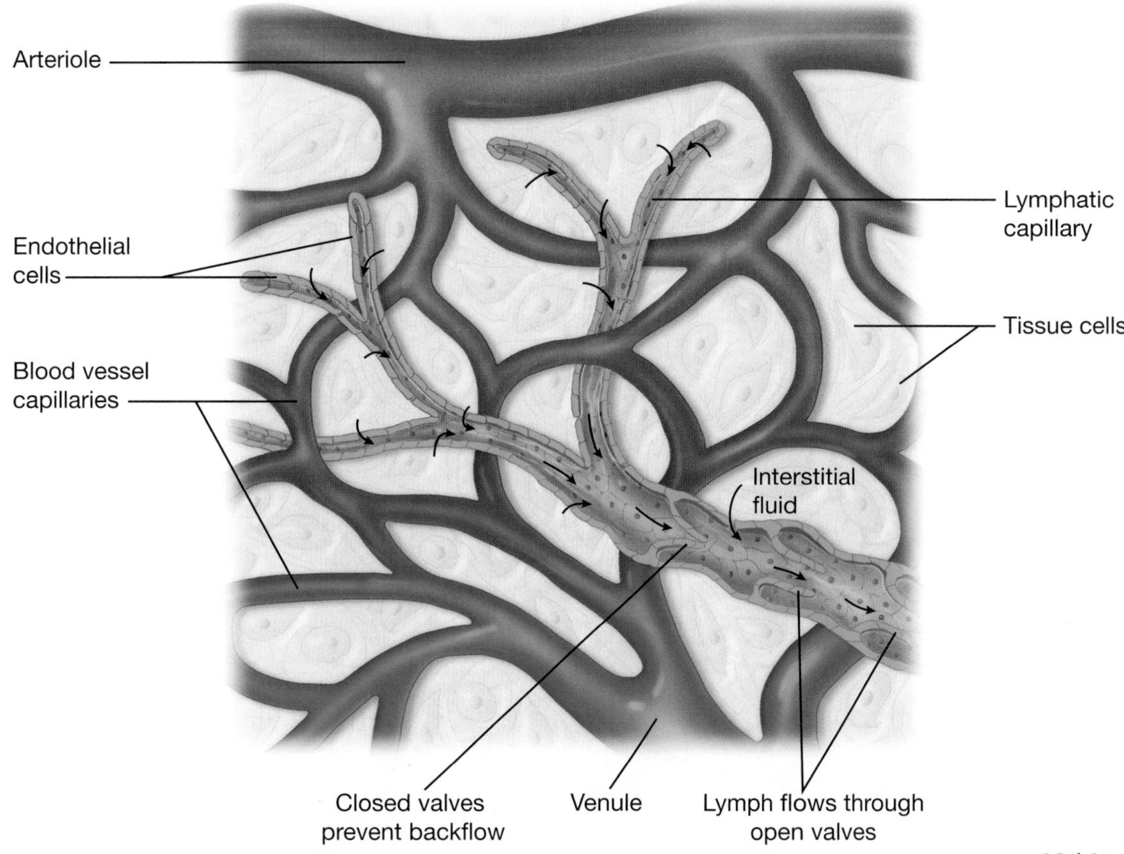

© Body Scientific International

Figure 13.3 Lymph formation and flow. Blood plasma leaks out of blood capillaries and mixes with the interstitial fluid. It then enters lymphatic capillaries. The overlapping endothelial cells of the lymphatic capillaries make it easy for fluid to enter the capillaries but hard for it to leave. Lymph flows from lymphatic capillaries to progressively larger lymphatic vessels. Lymphatic vessels have internal flaps that act as one-way valves, which prevent lymph from flowing backward to the capillaries.

and right jugular trunks, the left and right subclavian trunks, the left and right bronchomediastinal trunks, the intestinal trunk, and the left and right lumbar trunks. The two lumbar trunks and the intestinal trunk converge at the cisterna chyli (KIGH-ligh), an enlarged chamber located just in front of the vertebral column, at the diaphragm level (**Figure 13.4A**).

Lymphatic ducts are generally larger and less numerous than lymphatic trunks. Lymph moves from the trunks to the ducts as it makes its way back toward

Clinical Application Lymphedema

Lymphedema is the accumulation of lymph in the extracellular space due to blockage of the lymphatic vessels. It results in swelling of the affected area. In western countries, including the United States, lymphedema usually develops as a result of damage to lymph vessels and nodes during surgery and/or radiation therapy to treat cancer.

For example, axillary (underarm) lymph nodes may be removed in breast cancer surgery if it is suspected that the cancer may have spread to those nodes. This compromises the lymphatic drainage from the arm, and the patient is at risk for lymphedema of the arm. The patient may wear a tight-fitting sleeve on the affected arm to prevent lymph accumulation.

In poor areas of tropical countries, a parasitic infection with roundworms, known as *lymphatic filariasis*, is the most common cause of lymphedema. The roundworms may lodge in and damage lymphatic vessels, leading to lymphedema. If this lymphedema goes untreated, the affected tissue gradually changes: the skin becomes thick and rough, and significant disfigurement known as *elephantiasis* may result. More than a hundred million people suffer from lymphatic filariasis, and tens of millions of those are disfigured and disabled by elephantiasis. The 2015 Nobel Prize in Chemistry was given to Satoshi Omura and William Campbell for discovering ivermectin, a drug that cures roundworm and other parasitic infections.

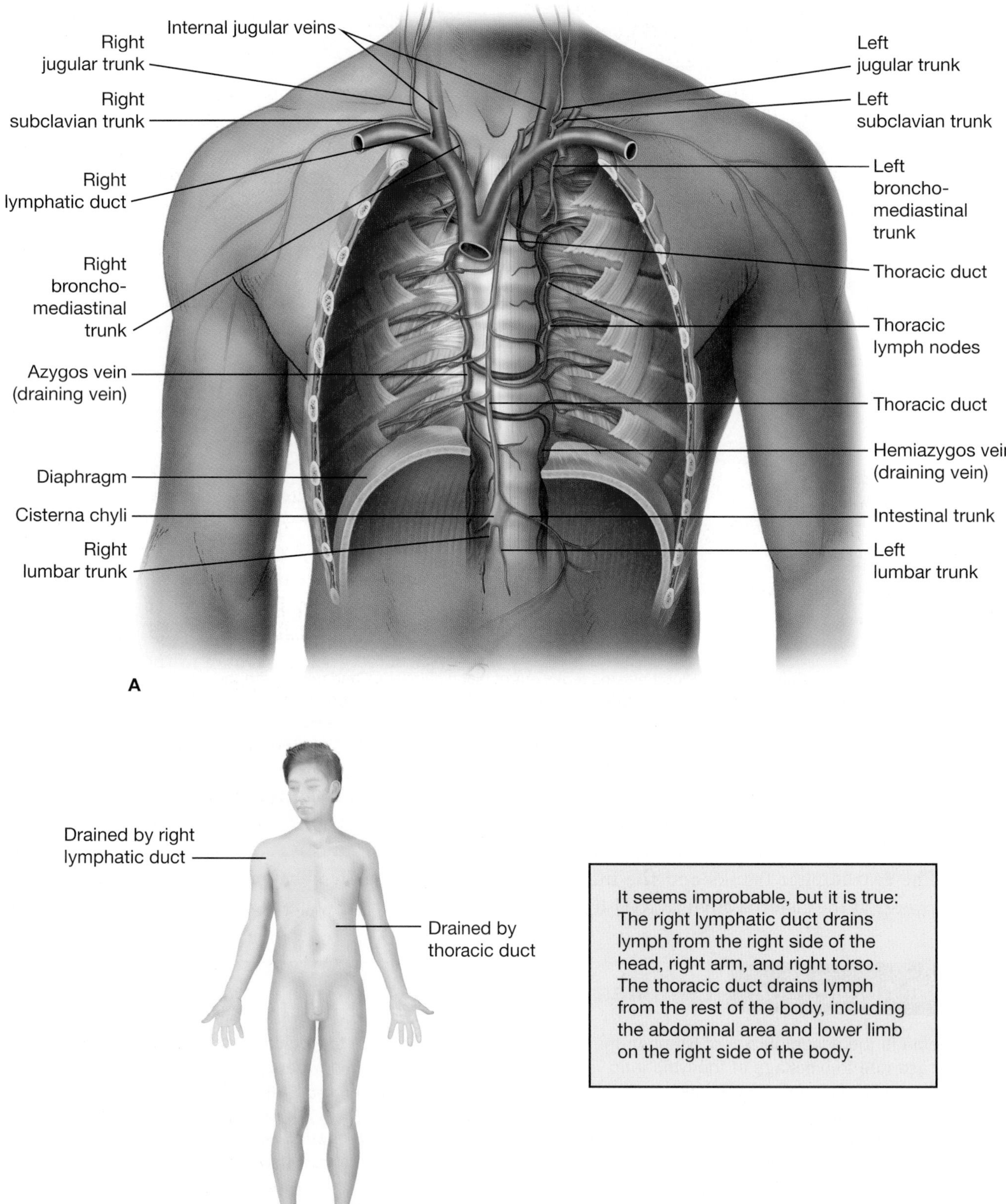

Figure 13.4 A—Locations of the lymphatic ducts and vessels. B—The right lymphatic duct collects lymph from the right jugular, subclavian, and bronchomediastinal trunks and drains into the right subclavian vein. The thoracic duct collects lymph from the left jugular, subclavian, and bronchomediastinal trunks and drains into the left subclavian vein.

the circulatory system. The thoracic duct carries lymph upward from the cisterna chyli. At its superior end, the thoracic duct receives lymph from the left jugular, subclavian, and bronchomediastinal trunks. These trunks drain lymph from the left side of the head, left arm, and chest and lower neck, respectively (**Figure 13.4B**). The thoracic duct also carries lymph coming from the small intestine and lower limbs. This lymph is milky white due to the presence of microscopic fat particles, which are absorbed from food during digestion. This fat-rich lymph is called *chyle*.

The right lymphatic duct receives lymph from the right jugular, subclavian, and bronchomediastinal trunks. These trunks drain lymph from the right arm and the right side of the thorax and head (**Figure 13.3B**).

Lymph rejoins the circulation at the subclavian veins: the right lymphatic duct drains into the right subclavian vein, and the left lymphatic duct drains into the left subclavian vein. Once lymph enters the veins, it mixes with, and is indistinguishable from, the blood plasma.

SELF CHECK

1. What three vital functions does the lymphatic system perform in the body?
2. What other body system does the lymphatic system most resemble? Explain.
3. How does lymph formation begin?
4. How is lymph moved throughout the lymphatic vessels?

Functional Anatomy of the Lymphatic System

The lymphatic system is a complex network of cells, tissues, and organs that play vital roles in the body's nonstop battle against invasion by disease-causing agents. This section discusses the structure and function of the lymphatic system.

Lymphatic Cells

Lymphocytes are the distinctive cells of the lymphatic system. Lymphocytes make up about 20% to 30% of the white blood cells in whole blood (blood that contains all of its components). Lymphocytes are abundant in lymphatic tissues, such as lymph nodes and the spleen.

All lymphocytes, along with other white and red blood cells, are generated in the bone marrow. Some lymphocytes migrate to the thymus, an organ in the thoracic cavity, where they complete their maturation before moving out to the blood and the rest of the body. These lymphocytes are called ***T lymphocytes (T cells)***. (The *T* stands for "thymus.") The lymphocytes that remain in the bone marrow become either ***B lymphocytes (B cells)*** or ***natural killer (NK) cells***.

Natural killer cells play an important role in the body's nonspecific defense system. They recognize and destroy virus-infected cells and cancer cells. By contrast, B and T cells are the main "soldiers" in the specific defense system. For example, B cells provide antibody-mediated immunity. This means that when they are activated, B cells divide to make plasma cells, which produce antibodies, or proteins involved in immune function. Antibodies circulate

Understanding Medical Terminology

The term *interstitial* comes from the Latin root word *stit/o* ("standing") and the prefix *inter-* ("between" or "among"). Thus, interstitial fluid occupies the spaces between cells, or the *interstitial space*. Interstitial fluid is also sometimes called *extracellular fluid*, which simply means "fluid outside of cells."

The bronchomediastinal trunks are so named because they receive lymph from the lungs and from the mediastinum, which is the collection of thoracic organs and tissues between the lungs, including the heart, trachea, esophagus, and thymus. The root word *bronch/o-* means "airway" (into the lungs). The word *mediastinum* comes from the Latin word meaning "middle." The organs and tissues that make up the mediastinum lie in the middle of the chest cavity, between the lungs.

The subclavian trunks, veins, and arteries all lay beneath the clavicle, or collarbone. The word *subclavian* comes from the Latin prefix *sub-* ("under") and the Latin word *clavicula* ("little key"). Ancient Roman physicians thought the clavicle resembled a small door key.

as free proteins in the bloodstream. T cells include cytotoxic T cells, which provide cell-mediated immunity. They also include helper and regulatory T cells, which regulate the activity of B and T cells.

Although they are not lymphocytes, ***macrophages*** are important cells in lymphatic tissues. Macrophages start out as white blood cells called *monocytes*. When a monocyte migrates out of lymphatic circulation into the surrounding tissue, it develops into a macrophage. Macrophages phagocytize (surround and destroy) foreign cells and substances, and they help to activate T lymphocytes.

Lymphatic Tissue

Lymphatic tissue is loose connective tissue that contains many lymphocytes. Lymphatic tissue is present in mucous membranes and certain organs throughout the body. Mucous membranes, which line passageways open to the outside world (such as the respiratory, gastrointestinal, urinary, and reproductive tracts), are potential routes of entry for infectious agents. Inside these passageways, ***mucosa-associated lymphatic tissue (MALT)*** keeps lymphocytes ready and waiting to stop the invaders.

Clusters of MALT in the small intestine are called *Peyer's patches*. MALT also protects the appendix, a small, worm-shaped tube at the junction of the large and small intestines.

The tonsils—small, almond-shaped masses of lymphatic tissue—form a ring of MALT around the pharynx. A single ***pharyngeal tonsil*** (often called the *adenoids*, even though it is typically a single small mass of tissue) lies at the back of the nasopharynx, the part of the throat located above the palate that opens into the nasal cavity. The left and right ***palatine tonsils*** lay at the back of the mouth. The palatine tonsils are the largest and the most commonly infected tonsils. The ***lingual tonsils*** are located on either side of the base of the tongue.

In some parts of the body, lymphocytes and macrophages form small, localized clusters of dense tissue called ***lymphatic nodules***. These nodules develop in areas often exposed to foreign microorganisms and help protect those areas from invasion.

Lymphatic Organs

The three organs of the lymphatic system are the lymph nodes, the spleen, and the thymus. This section describes these organs in more detail.

Lymph Nodes

Small, bean-shaped organs called ***lymph nodes*** are located along the lymphatic vessels throughout the body (**Figure 13.5**). Lymph nodes serve a dual purpose. They cleanse the lymph by trapping bacteria, viruses, and other harmful substances, which in turn are destroyed by white blood cells. Lymph nodes

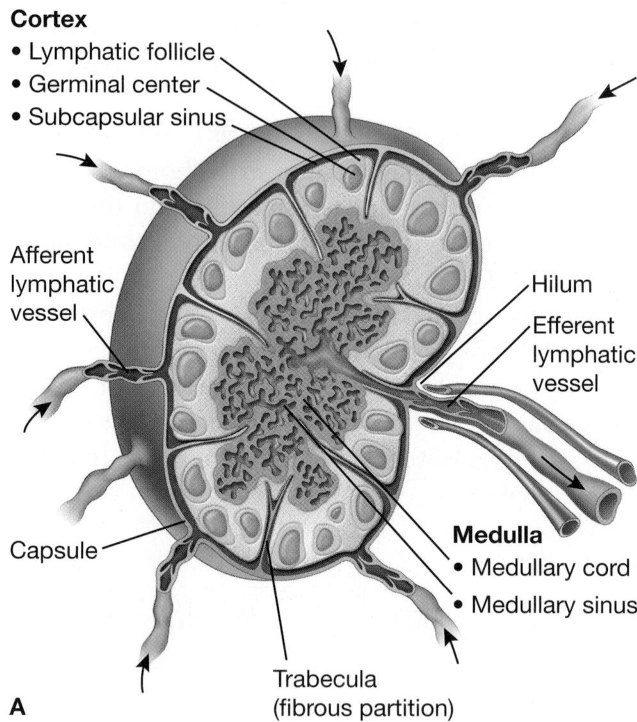

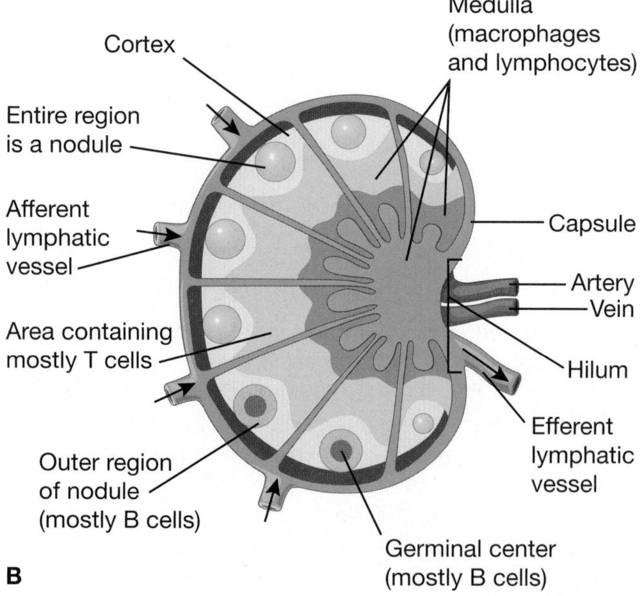

Figure 13.5 Lymph nodes. A—Cross section through a lymph node and associated lymphatic vessels. B—Simplified diagram distinguishing the cortex and medulla of a lymph node.

also store and produce T cells and B cells that help fight infection.

Lymph nodes vary in size from smaller than a pea (.04 inch or 1 mm in diameter) to the size of a lima bean (1 inch or 25 mm in diameter). They have a fibrous capsule and a spongy interior that is packed with lymphocytes and macrophages.

Afferent lymphatic vessels carry lymph into the lymph nodes from the lymphatic capillaries. After lymph enters a node, it spreads out in the subcapsular sinus, the space just inside the capsule of the node. The lymph then moves slowly through the cortex, or outer portion of the lymph node, to the deeper medulla. The cortex is divided into lymphatic follicles, which contain mostly B cells. When the immune system is actively fighting an infection, the germinal centers of the follicles, which are full of dividing B cells, are prominent. The medulla of the lymph node contains many macrophages as well as B and T cells.

One or two efferent lymphatic vessels emerge from the hilum, a small indentation on one side of the node, and carry lymph to the next node. Efferent lymphatic vessels carry lymph *away from* the lymph nodes.

Most lymph passes through several lymph nodes on its way from a lymphatic capillary to the subclavian vein. Because lymph flows slowly, there is ample time for lymphocytes to detect foreign particles such as bacteria or viruses, and for macrophages to engulf foreign particles by phagocytosis. If a lymphocyte does detect a foreign particle, it can activate an immune response.

When an immune response is activated, lymphocytes quickly multiply, causing the lymph nodes to enlarge. When you have a throat infection, for example, the lymph nodes in your neck may become swollen. If you see a physician to treat a cold, he or she will probably examine your neck for "swollen glands"—a common description for enlarged lymph nodes.

Spleen

The ***spleen***, located in the abdomen below the diaphragm, is the largest lymphatic organ in the human body (**Figure 13.6**). It measures 4 to 5 inches (10 to 12 cm) long and weighs 5 to 7 ounces (150 to 200 g). However, its size can vary considerably, even among healthy people. The spleen is located in the upper-left quadrant of the abdomen, lateral to the stomach and below the diaphragm.

Until the advent of "modern" medicine, most physicians in the Western world believed that the spleen was the source of and reservoir for "black bile," the alleged cause of melancholy. The Greek word roots *melan-* and *choly* mean "black" and "bile." These roots appear in other medical terms, such as *melanin* and *cholesterol.* In ancient times, laughing was a sign that the spleen was successfully keeping the black bile from escaping to the rest of the body.

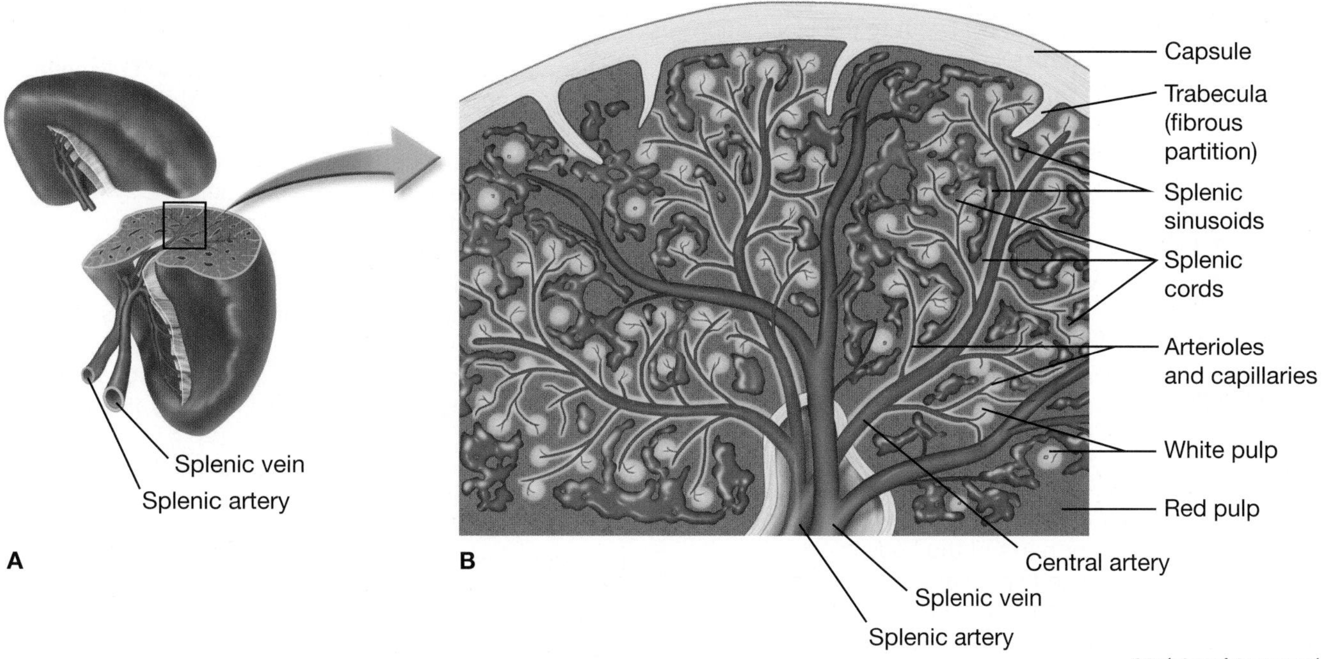

Figure 13.6 A—Diagram of the spleen, anterior view. B—Simplified diagram of the histology (tissue structure) of the spleen.

Of course, black bile does not exist, and scientists know a lot more about what the spleen actually does. One could say that the lymph nodes filter lymph, and the spleen filters blood. There is some truth to this simple statement, but a more accurate description of the spleen's functions include scanning, cleaning, and, if necessary, activating the immune response.

Like a lymph node, the spleen has a thin outer capsule and a spongy interior. This organ is dark red due to its large blood supply, which enters and leaves via the splenic artery and vein. The functional tissue inside the spleen contains red pulp and white pulp. The white pulp is rich in lymphocytes, which monitor blood flowing through the spleen for infectious cells and viruses. When the spleen detects an infectious agent, an immune response is activated, and lymphocytes begin to multiply.

Within the red pulp of the spleen, macrophages destroy old, worn-out red blood cells. The macrophages also remove old blood platelets and ***pathogens***, or disease-causing agents, from the blood. Like lymph nodes, the spleen often becomes enlarged during an infection.

Because the spleen consists of a soft interior enclosed by a thin capsule, the organ may sustain damage during a traumatic blow to the abdomen. This can happen during contact sports or a motor vehicle accident, for example. A person whose spleen has been surgically removed (that is, a splenectomized person) can lead a normal life but has increased susceptibility to infection.

Thymus

The thymus is a lymphatic organ that extends from the base of the neck downward into the thoracic cavity. It lies behind the sternum and in front of the heart, trachea, and esophagus. The thymus is also an endocrine gland, as described in Chapter 9. When compared to body size, the thymus is largest during childhood. It slowly shrinks after puberty.

After first developing in the bone marrow from lymphatic stem cells, some lymphocytes then migrate to the thymus, where they complete their maturation into T cells. Unlike lymph nodes, MALT, and the spleen, the thymus is not a site where lymphocytes lie in wait to ambush infectious agents. Rather, the thymus functions as a nursery for T cells.

SECTION 13.1 REVIEW

Mini-Glossary

B lymphocytes (B cells) lymphatic cells that mature in the bone marrow before moving out to the blood and the rest of the body; also known as *B cells*

endothelial cells the cells that form the walls of lymphatic and blood capillaries, and which form the inner lining of larger blood vessels

interstitial fluid the fluid located in the spaces between cells

lingual tonsils two masses of lymphatic tissue that lie on either side of the base of the tongue

lymph a clear, transparent, sometimes faintly yellow fluid that is collected from tissues throughout the body and flows in the lymphatic vessels

lymph nodes small, bean-shaped structures found along the lymphatic vessels throughout the body

lymphatic nodules small, localized clusters of dense tissue formed by lymphocytes and macrophages

lymphatic trunks large lymphatic vessels that drain lymph from different parts of the body

lymphatic valves tissue flaps that act as one-way gates inside the lymphatic vessels

lymphatic vessels the vessels that carry lymph

lymphocytes the distinctive cells of the lymphatic system

macrophages cells that engulf and destroy foreign cells, such as bacteria and viruses

mucosa-associated lymphatic tissue (MALT) lymphatic tissue found in mucous membranes that line passageways open to the outside world

natural killer (NK) cells lymphocytes that play an important role in the nonspecific defense system by killing virus-infected cells and cancer cells

palatine tonsils two masses of lymphatic tissue that lie at the back of the mouth, on the left and right sides; the largest and most commonly infected tonsils

pathogens disease-causing agents

pharyngeal tonsil lymphatic tissue that lies at the back of the nasopharynx; commonly known as the *adenoid* or *adenoids*

spleen the largest lymphatic organ in the body, located in the abdomen below the diaphragm; filters blood and activates an immune response when necessary

T lymphocytes (T cells) lymphatic cells that complete their maturation in the thymus before they move out to the blood and the rest of the body

(continued)

Review Questions

1. List the differences among lymphatic fluid, blood plasma, and interstitial fluid.
2. Explain the role the lymphatic system plays in maintaining blood pressure.
3. Identify the type of cell that forms the walls of the lymphatic capillaries.
4. Identify the point at which blood plasma becomes lymphatic fluid.
5. List the lymphatic trunks and identify the parts of the body in which they are located.
6. Distinguish between T cells and B cells.
7. Explain why lymphatic fluid, which is usually clear, takes on a milky white appearance when it has drained from the small intestine.
8. Summarize the process by which lymphatic fluid moves through the lymphatic system.

SECTION 13.2 Nonspecific Defenses

Objectives

- Describe the role of physical barriers in protecting the body against infectious agents.
- Understand the body's cellular and chemical defenses against infectious agents.
- Describe the inflammatory response and explain its purpose.
- Explain what happens during a fever.

Key Terms

alternative pathway
classical pathway
complement proteins
complement system
exocytosis
fever
inflammatory response
interferons
lectin pathway
mast cells
monocytes
neutrophils
opsonins
phagocytes
phagocytosis
prostaglandins
pyrogens

You have already seen how the lymphatic system works to keep fluids in balance and activate immune responses against foreign substances. This section examines the body's arsenal of defenses against diseases that do *not* require recognition of the precise identity of a pathogen. These *nonspecific* defenses include physical barriers, cellular and chemical defenses, inflammation, and fever.

The nonspecific defenses discussed in this section and the specific defenses described in the next section work closely together. For example, the complement system, which is considered a nonspecific defense, can be activated by cells of the specific defense system.

Physical Barriers

The body's defense against infectious agents begins with physical barriers to their entry. The skin is quite effective as a barrier, as long as it is intact (**Figure 13.7**). Its outer layer, the epidermis, is a stratified squamous epithelium. That is, the epithelial (surface) cells of the skin are flattened (squamous) and arranged in layers (stratified). The protein keratin, a major constituent of hair and nails, fills the flattened keratinocytes (keratinized cells) in the top layer of the epidermis. This keratin layer is flexible, strong, and hard to penetrate, due in part to the desmosomes that bind the deeper epithelial cells together.

Hair on the skin provides additional protection from chafing, sunburn, and insects. The acidic secretions of sweat glands and sebaceous glands (which produce sebum, a fatty lubricating substance) contain toxic chemicals that prevent bacteria from growing. When the skin is breached—by cuts or punctures, for example—the human body is at a much greater risk for infection. Burns also compromise, or even destroy, the protective function of the skin. For this reason, patients with serious burns are at a high risk for infection.

As stated in the previous section, protective mucous membranes line the respiratory, digestive, urinary, and reproductive tracts. Such protective linings are important because these tracts are open to the outside world and, therefore, are vulnerable to invasion. The mucus secreted by these linings forms a sticky layer that can trap microorganisms. Underlying MALT in the membranes increases the chance that microorganisms will be quickly recognized and destroyed.

The cells in the mucous membranes of the respiratory tract contain cilia. These tiny hair-like structures continually sweep mucus upward to the

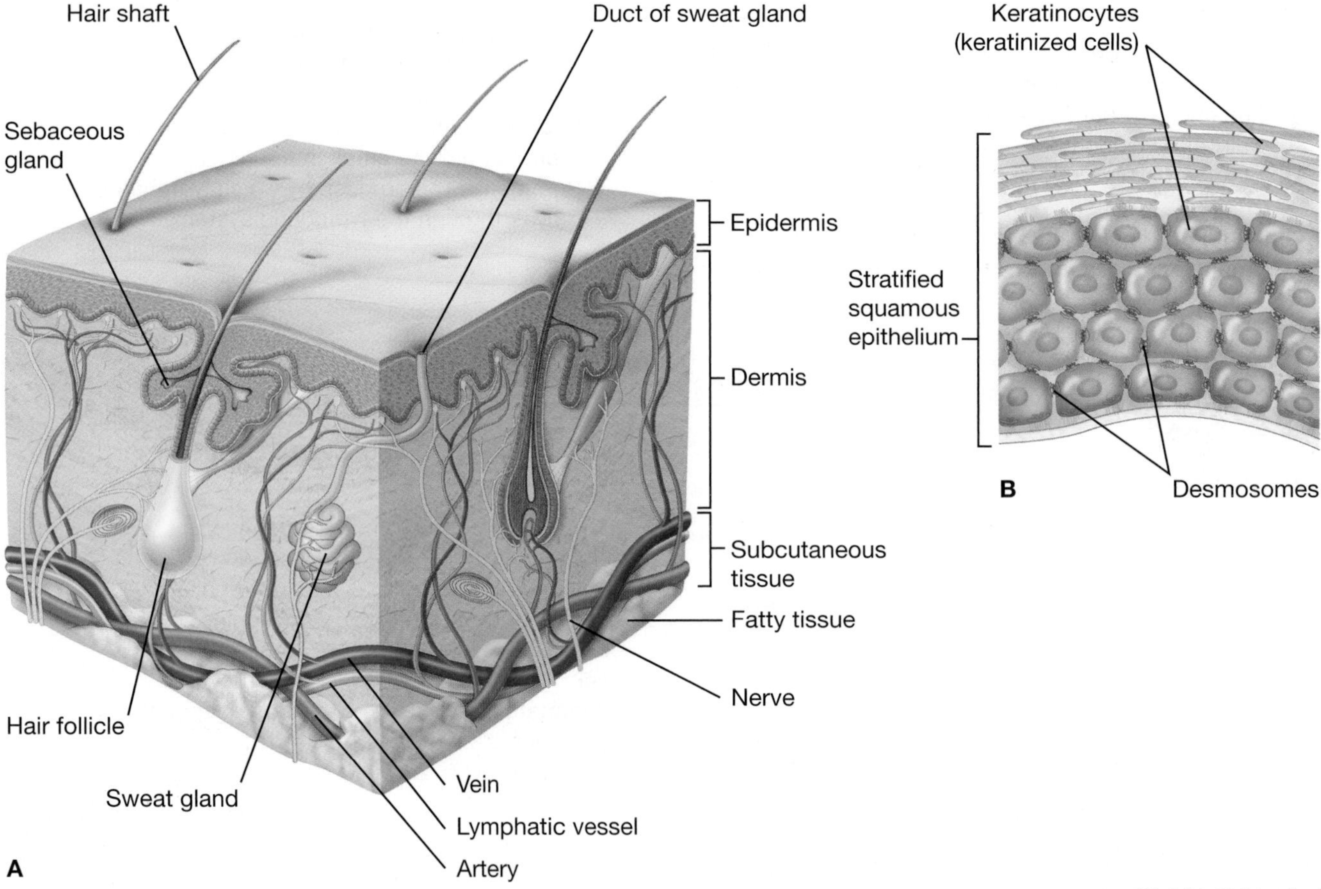

© Body Scientific International

Figure 13.7 A—The skin and its structures help protect the body by serving as physical barriers against infectious agents. B—A layer of flattened cells filled with keratin, and deeper cells connected by desmosomes, make the skin strong and tough. Hair and the secretions of sweat glands and sebaceous glands provide additional protection.

throat, where it is swallowed. Bacteria caught in the respiratory mucus are then likely to be destroyed in the acidic environment of the stomach.

SELF CHECK

1. Where does the body's defense against infectious agents begin?
2. Which protein makes the epidermis flexible, strong, and hard to penetrate?

Cellular and Chemical Defenses

When pathogens penetrate the body's physical barriers, they face an array of cellular and chemical defenses. Within these defense systems, cells such as ***phagocytes*** and natural killer (NK) cells help protect the body against foreign invaders. In addition, interferons and antimicrobial proteins in the form of ***complement proteins*** act as chemical defenders against pathogens.

Each of these defense mechanisms prevents or fights infection in its own way. These mechanisms also interact to produce an inflammatory response, which is important because it speeds up tissue repair and boosts the body's ability to fight infection.

Phagocytosis

The process by which cells engulf and destroy foreign matter and cellular debris is called ***phagocytosis***. Phagocytosis begins when a phagocyte recognizes its target and binds to it. A phagocyte is any cell that has the ability to carry out phagocytosis. Various types of phagocytes have different specialized roles in immune defense and tissue maintenance.

For example, ***neutrophils***, the most common type of leukocytes, can slip out of capillaries and into surrounding tissue. In the tissue, neutrophils phagocytize bacteria and cellular debris. Some ***monocytes***, another class of leukocytes, develop into macrophages when they leave the bloodstream. From there, macrophages enter tissues to phagocytize pathogens.

How does phagocytosis work? When the phagocyte contacts a foreign target, such as a virus or bacterium, it extends one or more pseudopods (extensions of the cytoplasm). These pseudopods wrap around the target, engulf it, and pull it back to the main body of the cell (**Figure 13.8A**). The target, now inside the cell, is enclosed in a phagosome, or phagocytic vesicle (**Figure 13.8B**). The phagocytic vesicle protects the phagocyte from damaging itself with the chemicals that it uses to destroy the engulfed target.

A lysosome, an organelle that contains acid and lysosomal enzymes, fuses with the phagocytic vesicle. The lysosomal enzymes and acid usually destroy the target, leaving behind debris that is released from the cell through ***exocytosis***. In exocytosis, the membrane of the phagocytic vesicle fuses with the phagocyte's membrane, pushing the debris outside the cell.

Natural Killer Cells

Natural killer (NK) cells are lymphocytes that recognize and destroy abnormal body cells, such as those infected with a virus or those that are cancerous. Virus-infected cells and cancer cells often display unusual proteins on their surface, or they fail to display the usual proteins. In either case, they attract NK cells.

Based on this attraction, NK cells bind to abnormal cells. The NK cells then use exocytosis to release perforins—proteins that destroy foreign cells—into the narrow space between the NK cell and the abnormal cell. The perforins embed themselves in the abnormal cell's membrane and self-assemble into doughnut-shaped pores. This process creates perforations in the abnormal cell. The abnormal cell, now full of holes, soon dies.

Complement System

The ***complement system*** is a set of more than 30 proteins that circulate in the blood plasma throughout the body and work together to destroy foreign substances. The complement system is so named because it complements, or adds to and enhances, the effects of antibodies.

The proteins of the complement system circulate in an inactive form. The system can be activated in three primary ways: via the classical pathway, the lectin pathway, or the alternative pathway. All three pathways lead to the production of molecules that help the body destroy pathogens.

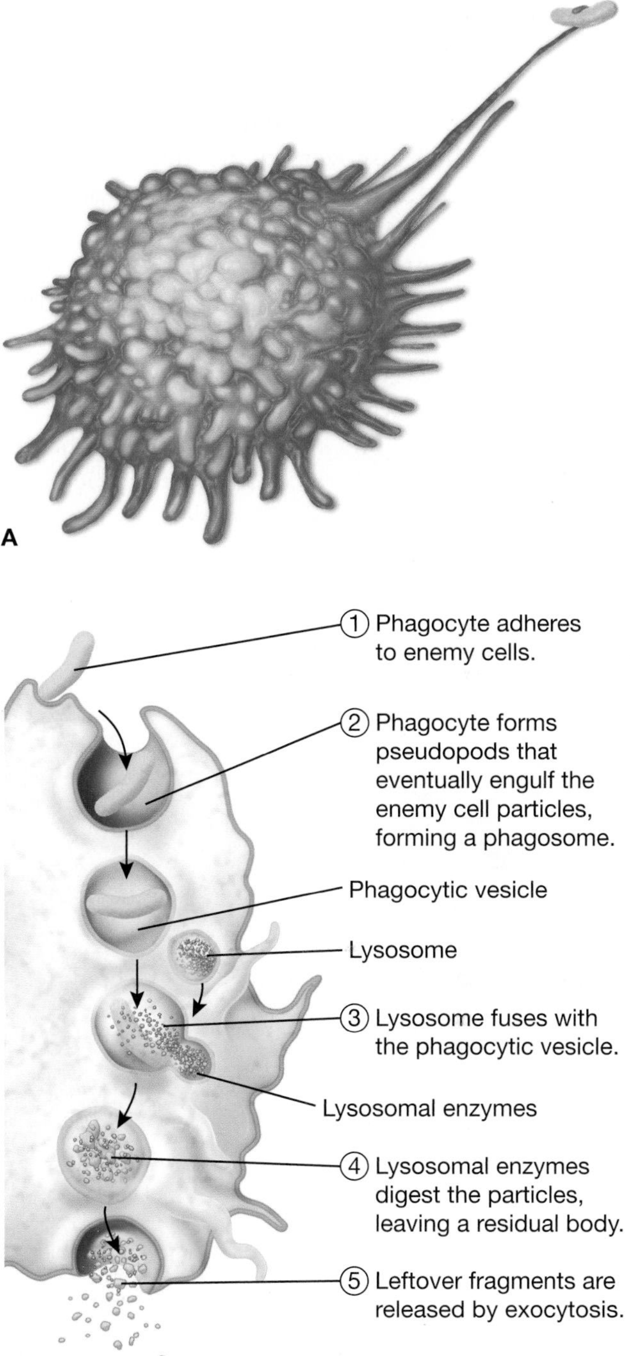
A
(1) Phagocyte adheres to enemy cells.
(2) Phagocyte forms pseudopods that eventually engulf the enemy cell particles, forming a phagosome.
Phagocytic vesicle
Lysosome
(3) Lysosome fuses with the phagocytic vesicle.
Lysosomal enzymes
(4) Lysosomal enzymes digest the particles, leaving a residual body.
(5) Leftover fragments are released by exocytosis.
B
© Body Scientific International

Figure 13.8 A—A phagocyte (purple) extending its cytoplasm to engulf a bacterium (yellow). B—The events of phagocytosis.

The ***classical pathway*** begins when complement protein C1 recognizes an antibody that is bound to a target, such as a bacterium. Antibodies are proteins of the specific immune defense system. You will learn more about antibodies in the next section. Interacting with the antibody causes C1 to change its conformation, or shape, from inactive to active. The activated C1 protein splits the C4 molecule, and then the C2 molecule. Parts of the split C4 and C2 molecules combine to form a protein that splits the inactive complement protein C3 into C3a and C3b. Note that complement proteins are numbered in the order of their discovery, which does not always correspond with the order in which they are activated or split.

The ***lectin pathway*** begins when a circulating protein called *lectin* binds to a sugar molecule that is present on the surfaces of bacteria. Lectin that is bound to the sugar on a bacterium causes activation of other proteins, which lead to the splitting of C3 into C3a and C3b. The ***alternative pathway*** begins when C3 binds directly to certain bacteria, becomes active, and converts other C3 molecules into C3a and C3b.

All three pathways lead to the production of proteins C3a and C3b, which then perform functions that help the body destroy pathogens (**Figure 13.9**). C3a and another complement protein, C5a, cause ***mast cells***, a type of cell found in connective tissue, to release histamine. Histamine is a compound that activates an inflammatory response. Mast cells and the inflammatory response are discussed in more detail later in this chapter. C3a also attracts macrophages, which phagocytize foreign cells.

C3b coats the surfaces of pathogens, making them attractive targets for phagocytes. Proteins that make cells more attractive to phagocytes are called ***opsonins***. The process of making cells attractive to phagocytes is called *opsonization*. When antibodies are bound to a target cell, they can also act as opsonins.

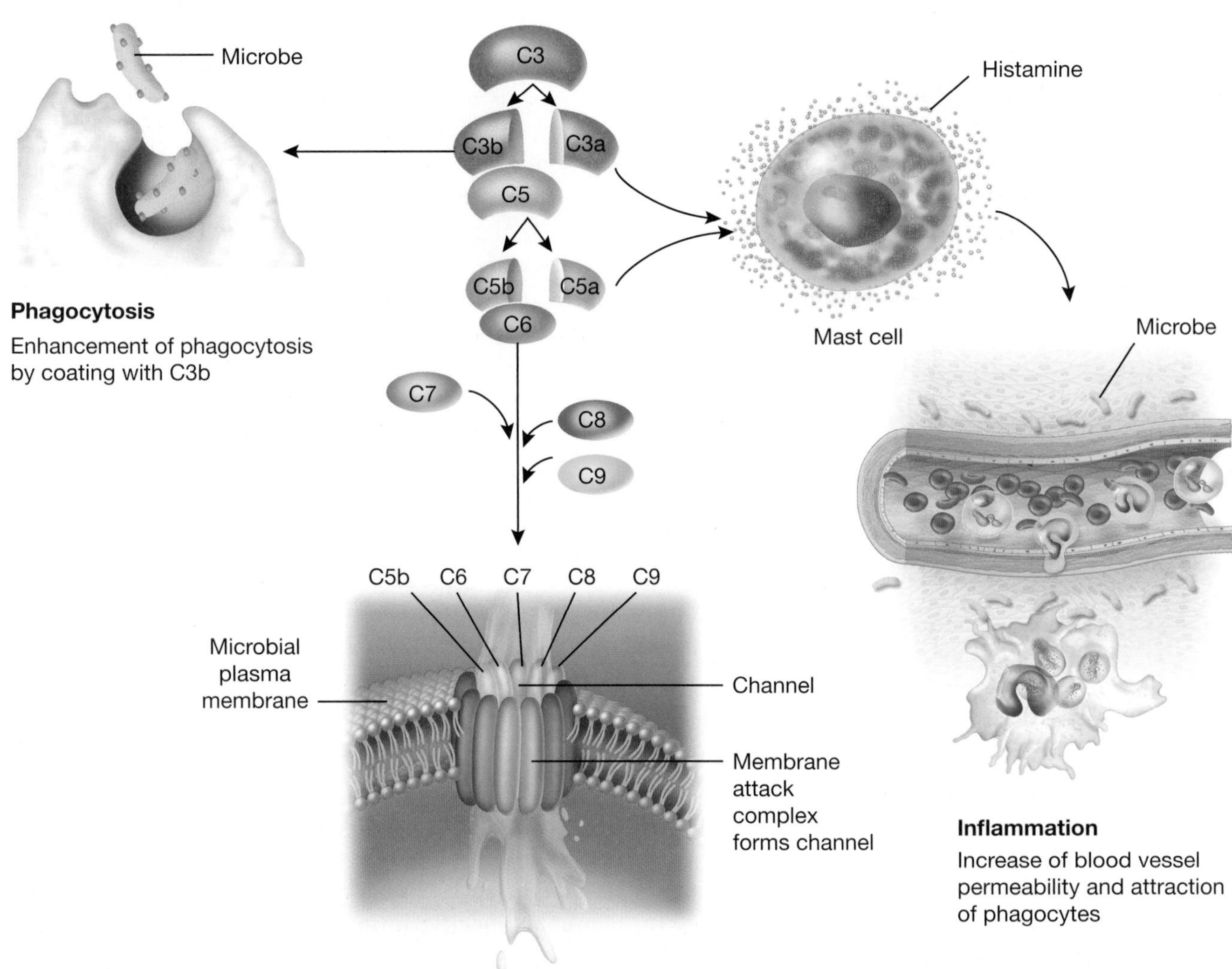

Figure 13.9 The classical, lectin, and alternative pathways converge at the complement protein identified as *C3*. Activation of any of the pathways causes the protein to split into C3a and C3b. These proteins then assist in the destruction of pathogens in several ways.

C3b also activates other complement proteins that lead to the creation of complement protein complexes on the surfaces of bacteria. Together, several of these protein complexes form a membrane attack complex (MAC), which creates a large, lethal hole in the cell membranes of bacteria. The process by which complement proteins penetrate the cell membrane of a bacterium is similar to the way in which perforin molecules, produced by NK cells, make holes in their targets.

Interferons

A virus, unlike a bacterium, is not a cell. A virus is a tiny assembly of nucleic acids with a protein coat. A virus cannot reproduce by itself. To reproduce, a virus must enter a cell and take over the intracellular machinery. This process enables the virus to make many copies of itself. When the newly reproduced copies of the virus are released, they invade nearby cells. Thus, a viral infection begins and spreads.

Interferons are proteins released by cells that have been infected with viruses. Interferons are so named because they interfere with the replication and spreading of viruses. These proteins cannot help cells that are already infected. They do, however, help neighboring cells to resist viral infection.

There are several classes of interferons, including alpha, beta, and gamma interferons. Alpha interferons are produced by virus-infected leukocytes. Beta interferons are produced by virus-infected fibroblasts (connective tissue cells). Both alpha and beta interferons can bind to receptors on neighboring cells, causing those cells to make proteins that slow down protein synthesis and therefore hinder the reproduction of viral particles. Gamma interferons are produced by NK cells and T cells that have been activated by detection of foreign materials. Gamma interferons help activate macrophages, enabling them to attack virus-infected cells more quickly and vigorously.

Because interferons help to block protein synthesis, they tend to hinder the growth and division of cells, including cancer cells. When interferons were first discovered, the scientific community held high hopes that these antiviral proteins would be able to halt or cure many types of cancer. Although these hopes have not been fully realized, interferons have been useful in treating certain diseases, including hepatitis C, some forms of leukemia (a cancerous disease of the white blood cells), and certain types of lymphoma (cancer that affects lymphatic tissue).

SELF CHECK

1. What is the name for the process by which cells engulf and destroy foreign matter and cellular debris?
2. What do NK cells and MACs have in common?
3. Name three classes of interferons.

Inflammatory Response

The ***inflammatory response***, also called *inflammation*, occurs when tissues have been damaged by bacteria, toxins, or trauma. Although inflammation is often uncomfortable, its purpose is to promote the repair of damaged tissue.

Key steps in the inflammatory response are illustrated in **Figure 13.10**. When cells are damaged, proteins and chemicals that they usually store are released. The appearance of these unusual substances in the interstitial fluid causes mast cells in the area to degranulate. This means that the mast cells release their intracellular stores of histamine granules, ***prostaglandins***, and other chemicals.

Histamine and the other chemicals in mast cells attract phagocytes and lymphocytes to the injured or diseased area. The phagocytes consume cellular debris and pathogens, making the capillaries more permeable and causing the arterioles to dilate (increase their diameter). Increased capillary permeability results in more leakage of fluid from the capillaries, which causes the interstitial fluid to increase in volume. The result is swelling of tissues in the injured or diseased area.

The increased permeability inside the capillaries also allows clotting proteins to move from the blood into the tissues, where they are activated to form a clot. The stretching of tissue related to swelling, and the direct effect of histamine on nerve fibers, causes pain. The dilation of arterioles in the affected region causes more blood to flow to that region, which produces redness and localized warming, or heat.

The localized warming associated with the inflammatory response boosts the metabolic rate of cells in the injured area. The accompanying increase in blood flow ensures that plenty of nutrients will be available for repair processes. Heat, redness, swelling, and pain are the four signs of inflammation. Taken together, the events of inflammation lead to faster tissue cleanup and repair.

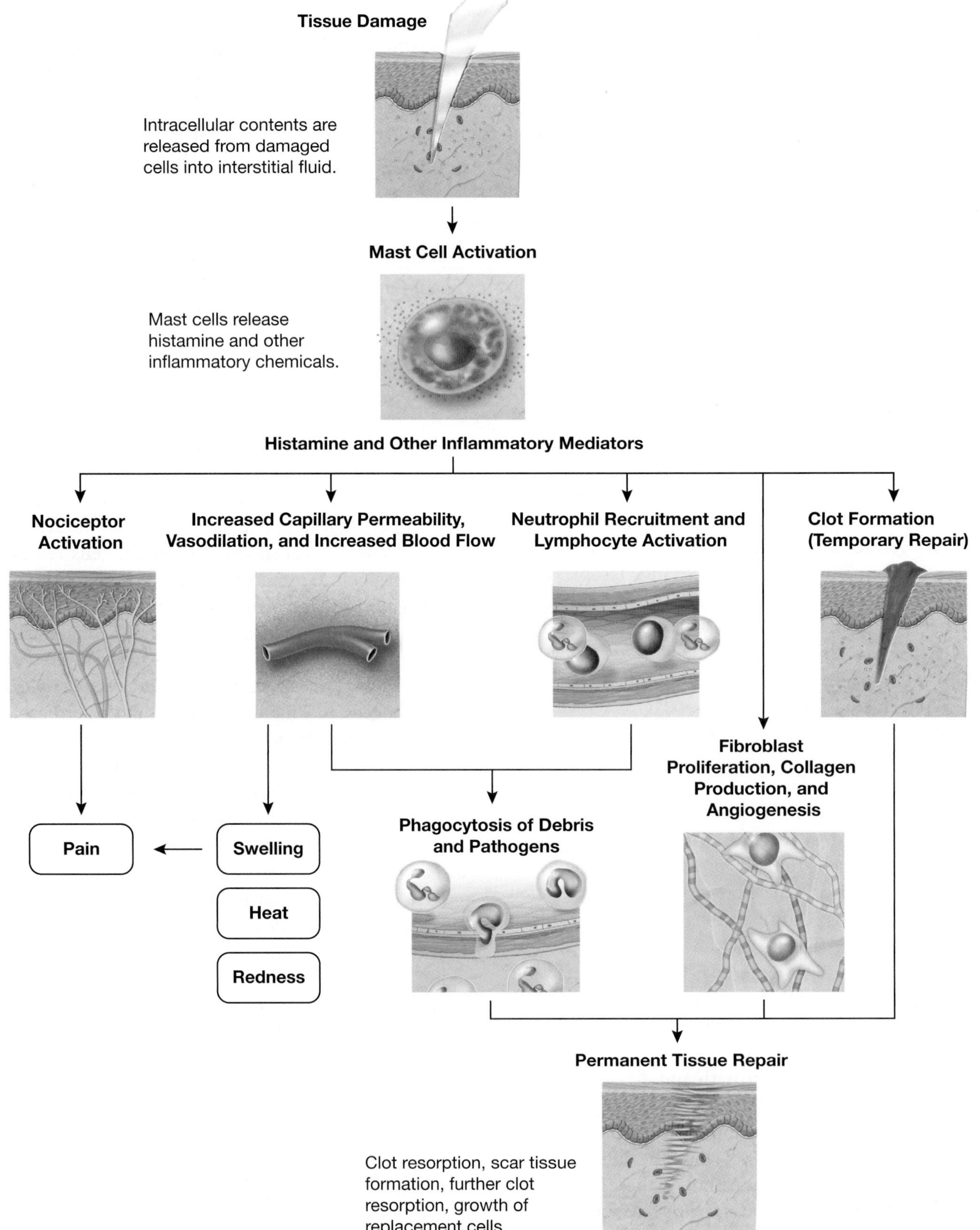

Figure 13.10 The development of inflammation. The hallmarks of inflammation are heat, redness, swelling, and pain.

A very mild example of an inflammatory response is the skin's reaction to a mosquito bite. When a mosquito bites the skin, physical tissue damage occurs and the mosquito injects anti-coagulant chemicals to promote easier withdrawal of blood. These injuries provoke a reaction from mast cells, lymphocytes, and macrophages in the area. Mast cells respond by releasing their stores of histamine. The histamine causes greater permeability of capillaries (swelling) and greater blood flow to the area (redness). Perhaps the most bothersome effect of histamine is that it activates nerve fibers that cause itching.

Acute inflammation in a limited area, such as the response to a mosquito bite, may be annoying, but it is useful. However, prolonged (chronic) inflammation is a different story. In the last decade, researchers have learned that long-lasting, low-level inflammation that is spread throughout the body plays a key role in cancer, heart disease, obesity, type 2 diabetes, and other illnesses associated with aging. People who experience chronic inflammation may be more likely to develop these diseases, and the diseases themselves can cause further inflammation. This creates an unwanted and unhealthy self-perpetuating cycle. Fortunately, simple measures such as regular moderate exercise can reduce chronic inflammation.

SELF CHECK

1. What causes the pain associated with an inflammatory response?
2. What are the four signs of inflammation?

Fever

Fever is the maintenance of body temperature at a higher-than-normal level. Neurons in the hypothalamus of the brain work to regulate body temperature. The neurons in this area compare the body's actual temperature to its "set point," which is the ideal or desired body temperature. If the actual temperature is higher or lower than the set point, the hypothalamic neurons fire commands throughout the body to make adjustments that will bring the temperature to the desired level.

If the body is warmer than the desired temperature, sweat glands are activated and blood flow is redirected toward the skin to help heat dissipate. If the body is cooler than the desired temperature, blood flow to the skin and extremities is reduced to minimize heat loss. If the reduction in blood flow does not fix the problem, shivering begins.

As you probably know, the normal set point for body temperature is about 98.6°F (37°C). The normal set point often deviates when infection occurs in the body. Infection activates leukocytes and macrophages, which can cause the cells to release ***pyrogens***. These chemicals increase the set-point temperature of the hypothalamic neurons. Those neurons then cause reflex adjustments that increase body temperature.

For every 1.8°F (1°C) increase in temperature, there is a 10% increase in the rate of biochemical reactions in the cells. This can have both helpful and harmful effects. Faster reaction rates speed up the body's disease-fighting processes, but the higher temperature also allows bacteria and viruses to reproduce more quickly. A severe fever is dangerous because it can cause proteins to denature, or partially unfold, and can cause abnormal heart rhythms and seizures.

SECTION 13.2 REVIEW

Mini-Glossary

alternative pathway one of the primary ways in which the complement system can be activated; this pathway is triggered when the C3b complement protein binds to foreign material

classical pathway one of the primary ways in which the complement system can be activated; this pathway is triggered when complement protein C1 recognizes an antibody bound to foreign material

complement proteins the proteins in the blood that work with immune system cells and antibodies to defend the body against infection

complement system a system of more than 30 proteins that circulate in the blood plasma and work together to destroy foreign substances

exocytosis a process in which the cell membranes of a vesicle and a cell fuse together and push debris from the vesicle outside of the cell

(continued)

fever the maintenance of body temperature at a higher-than-normal level

inflammatory response a physiological response to tissue injury or infection that is characterized by heat, redness, swelling, and pain; also called *inflammation*

interferons proteins released by cells that have been infected with viruses; interfere with virus reproduction

lectin pathway one of the primary ways in which the complement system can be activated; this pathway is triggered when lectin binds to a sugar molecule present on the surfaces of bacteria

mast cells connective tissue cells that contain stores of histamine

monocytes leukocytes that develop into phagocytizing macrophages when they migrate out of lymphatic circulation into surrounding tissue

neutrophil the most common type of white blood cell; can slip out of capillaries and into surrounding tissue to destroy bacteria and cellular debris

opsonins proteins that make cells more attractive to phagocytes

phagocytes cells that engulf and consume bacteria, foreign material, and cellular debris

phagocytosis the process by which a cell engulfs and destroys foreign matter and cellular debris

prostaglandins fatty acids involved in the control of inflammation and body temperature

pyrogens chemicals that cause fever by increasing the set-point temperature of hypothalamic neurons

Review Questions

1. Describe how the skin acts as a physical barrier against infectious agents.
2. Explain how the skin thwarts bacterial growth and reduces the risk of infection.
3. Identify the structures of the respiratory tract that are responsible for sweeping bacteria into the stomach to be destroyed.
4. Summarize the process of phagocytosis.
5. Describe the role of histamine in the inflammatory response.
6. Describe in detail the three ways in which the complement system can be activated.
7. Describe the characteristics of a virus and explain how an infection caused by a virus develops and spreads.
8. Explain why someone with an injury or illness might say that the affected part of his or her body feels as though it is "on fire."

SECTION 13.3

The Immune System: Specific Defenses

Objectives

- Explain how antigens enable the body to distinguish cells as either "self" or "nonself."
- Describe the roles of various types of cells in the immune system.
- Understand the role of antibodies in the specific defense system of the body.
- Explain the difference between the primary and secondary immune responses.
- Describe the process of cell-mediated immunity.

Key Terms

active immunity
antibody-mediated immunity
antigen-presenting cells (APCs)
apoptosis
cell-mediated immunity
clonal selection
immune system
immunoglobulins
major histocompatibility complex glycoproteins (MHCs)
memory cells
passive immunity
precipitation
primary immune response
secondary immune response

The specific defense systems are the most remarkable and complicated of the human body's defenses against diseases. The cells and chemicals that contribute to these defenses make up the ***immune system***. The immune system is also called the *specific immune system*, or the *adaptive immune system,* because the immune system is highly specific in its responses to foreign substances. It is able to recognize new challenges, adapt to those challenges, and "remember" what it has learned. The lymphatic organs and tissues are the physical components of the immune system.

As with many body functions, people do not notice or appreciate the immune system as it works. The immune system is constantly finding, targeting, and eliminating bacteria and viruses. It even kills the body's own cells when they show signs of infection or cancerous development.

Patients with a compromised immune system are susceptible to diseases that never trouble those with a normal immune system. For example, babies born with severe combined immune deficiency (SCID), a genetic immune system deficiency, have a tragically poor prognosis unless they receive a successful bone marrow transplant, or gene therapy. SCID, also known as the *bubble boy disease*, gained global attention in the 1970s with news reports of David Vetter, a boy with SCID who had to live in a sterile, plastic bubble to avoid contact with bacteria and viruses (**Figure 13.11**). An infection that is minor for a person with a healthy immune system is potentially fatal for a person with SCID.

The many cells and chemicals of the immune system interact with one another in complex ways that are still not completely understood. This complexity makes the immune system challenging to study.

Antigens

As you may recall from Chapter 11, antigens are large molecules such as proteins, polysaccharides, glycolipids, or nucleic acids that are located on the surfaces of cells. Antigens identify cells as either "self" or "nonself," thereby making it possible for the body to distinguish between its own cells and any foreign cells. This also allows the immune system to recognize foreign cells and respond to them, which it does by producing antibodies that bind to and mark the foreign antigens. Foreign antigens may be parts of bacteria, viruses, or abnormal cells, but they are not necessarily pathogens. For example, substances that people are allergic to are foreign antigens, but they are not pathogens.

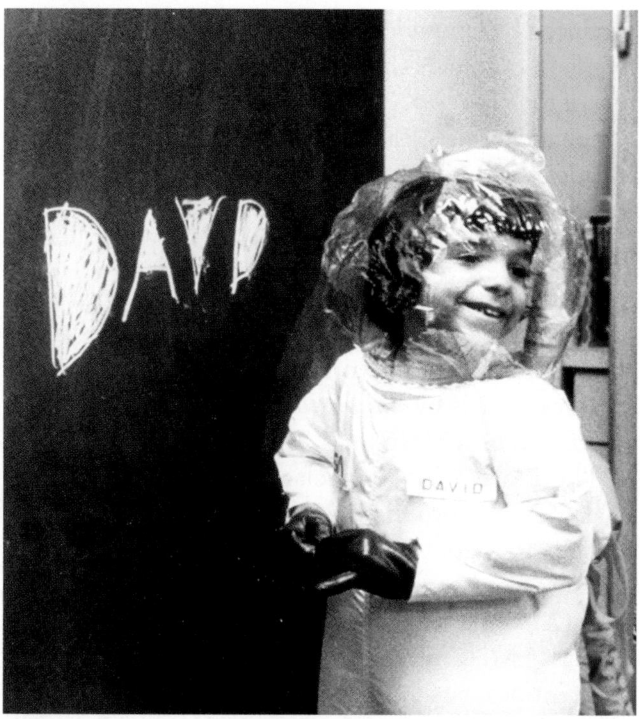

NASA/Science Source

Figure 13.11 David Vetter was a highly publicized victim of severe combined immune deficiency (SCID), also known as *bubble boy disease*. SCID results in a poor prognosis unless the patient receives a successful bone marrow transplant.

A single complex antigen molecule can have multiple foreign parts, or antigenic determinants. Larger molecules, especially proteins, are more likely to provoke an immune response than small ones because they have more antigenic determinants.

The antigens on the surfaces of a person's own cells (the "self" antigens described earlier) do *not* provoke an immune response. Any immature lymphocytes that *do* respond to "self" molecules are killed off early in the development process.

SELF CHECK

1. What is an antigen?
2. Why is the immune system also called the *specific immune system*?

Immune System Cells

As stated earlier in this chapter, lymphocytes are the signature cells of the lymphatic system. However, other cells, such as ***antigen-presenting cells (APCs)***, are also essential for proper immune function. These cells process protein antigens and present them on their surfaces in a form that can be recognized by lymphocytes. Macrophages, dendritic cells (immune system cells in the skin and lymphatic organs), and B cells can all act as APCs (**Figure 13.12**).

Lymphocytes

Recall that lymphocytes initially develop from stem cells in red bone marrow. Some lymphocytes travel to the thymus to complete their maturation; these are called *T* (for *thymus*) *lymphocytes*, or *T cells*. Other lymphocytes complete their maturation in bone marrow; these are called *B lymphocytes*, or *B cells*.

All lymphocytes go through a screening process. If, during the screening process, a lymphocyte responds to the body's self-antigens as foreign matter, it undergoes ***apoptosis***, a programmed process of cellular self-destruction. This selective apoptosis ensures that the lymphocytes that reach maturity will not attack the body's own tissues. This process does not always work with 100% success. When it does not work perfectly, the result is often autoimmune disease, in which the immune system attacks the body's own tissue. Autoimmune diseases are described later in this chapter.

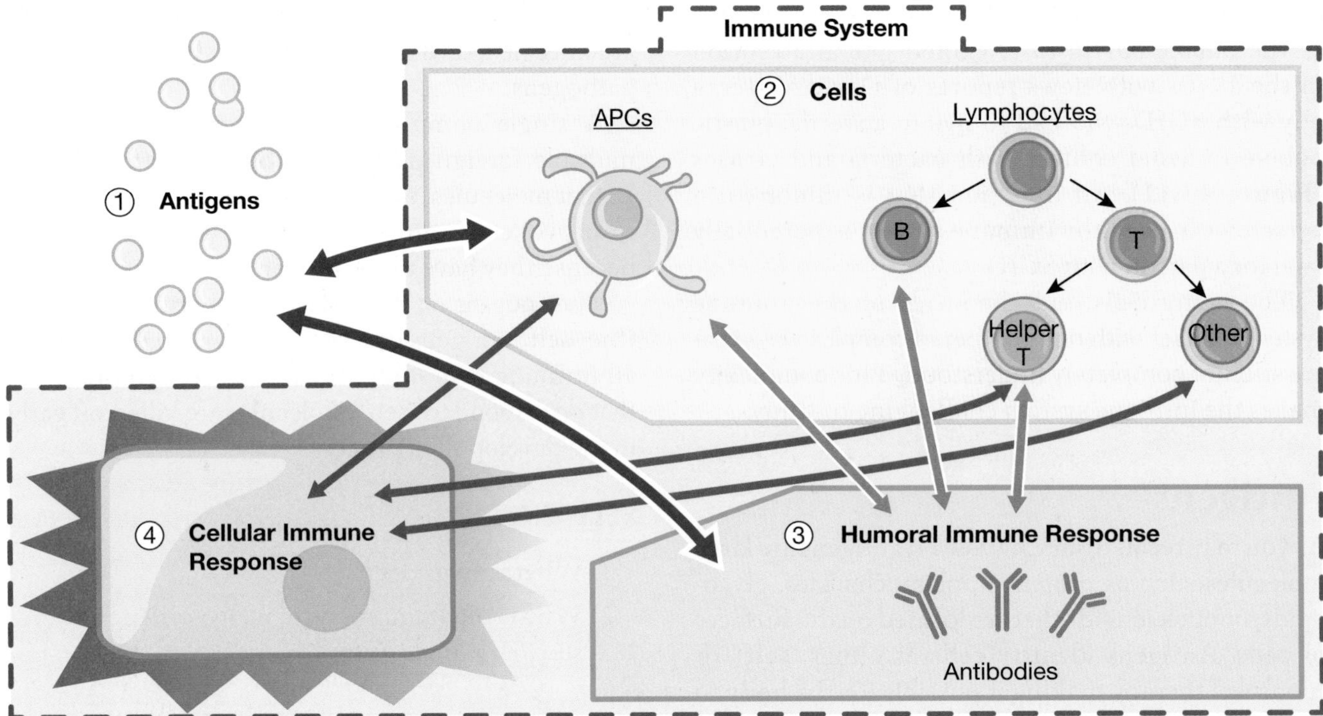

© Body Scientific International

Figure 13.12 Diagram of the immune system. Helper T cells play a significant role in both humoral and cellular immune responses. Other T cells are associated mainly with the cellular response. B cells are associated with the humoral response. Antigen-presenting cells (APCs) are involved in both types of responses.

Once lymphocytes have matured, they travel throughout the blood to all parts of the body. Some lymphocytes circulate continuously, while others settle in lymph nodes, the spleen, or other lymphatic tissues.

Each lymphocyte has many antigen receptors in its membrane. Each receptor in a given lymphocyte membrane recognizes one—and only one—antigen. The human body has millions of populations of lymphocytes, and each population recognizes a particular antigen. It is the great specificity of these cells that makes them the key players in specific defenses.

Over the course of a lifetime, only a fraction of the lymphocytes ever encounter the antigen that binds to their particular antigen receptors. Lymphocytes that do not meet their antigen remain quiescent, or inactive.

When a lymphocyte does encounter its antigen, antigen receptor binds to the antigen, stimulating the lymphocyte to differentiate. This means that the lymphocyte divides repeatedly, making many copies of itself. Each copy is an exact genetic duplicate, or clone, of the original cell that was stimulated. This process is called ***clonal selection***. Most of the clones produced by lymphocytic differentiation become short-lived effector cells that fight an infectious invader. A few of the clones become ***memory cells*** that reside in lymphatic tissues, ready to respond if the same antigen invades the body again.

MHC Proteins

The presence of antigens is not enough to activate an immune response. The antigens must be presented in a particular way. Antigens are displayed on the surfaces of cells by ***major histocompatibility complex glycoproteins (MHCs)***.

There are two main classes of MHC proteins. Class I MHC proteins are found on the surfaces of all cells that contain nuclei. Class II MHC proteins are found only on the surfaces of antigen-presenting cells (APCs) and lymphocytes.

Class I MHC proteins display fragments of the many different proteins found inside the cells on which they are present. This means that a normal body cell displays normal protein fragments (self-antigens) on its surface. When the immune system is working properly, passing lymphocytes ignore self-antigens.

Class I MHC proteins also display fragments of any abnormal, undesirable proteins that are inside their cells. Therefore, if a cell is infected or cancerous, it displays parts of the infectious agent or cancer-related proteins on its surface.

As **Figure 13.13** shows, an antigen-presenting cell, such as a macrophage or a dendritic cell, can internalize and break down a foreign particle. Then it displays the fragments of this "digested" foreign particle on class II MHC proteins on its surface.

SELF CHECK

1. Name at least three types of antigen-presenting cells (APCs).
2. What are MHC proteins?

Antibody-Mediated Immunity

Antibody-mediated immunity, also called *humoral immunity*, is effective against extracellular pathogens, or those located outside of cells. Humoral immunity begins when a B cell encounters the antigen that binds to its antigen receptors. During this encounter, the B cell undergoes clonal selection, as described previously. The B cell divides repeatedly, making many copies of itself.

B cell reproduction is most strongly activated when the B cell, with an antigen bound to it, presents the antigen to a helper T cell that also has a receptor for that antigen. When the helper T cell detects presentation of an antigen by a B cell, it releases interleukins, which are chemicals that stimulate an immune response. The interleukins fully activate the B cell by binding to it.

Plasma Cells

Some of the daughter cells produced by clonal selection become memory B cells, but most become plasma cells. Each plasma cell has a cytoplasm full of rough endoplasmic reticulum (RER), a membranous network that is involved in protein synthesis.

The RER in plasma cells produces large quantities of antibodies that are secreted into the interstitial fluid. These antibodies recognize and bind to the same antigen that stimulated the original B cell. Thus, the

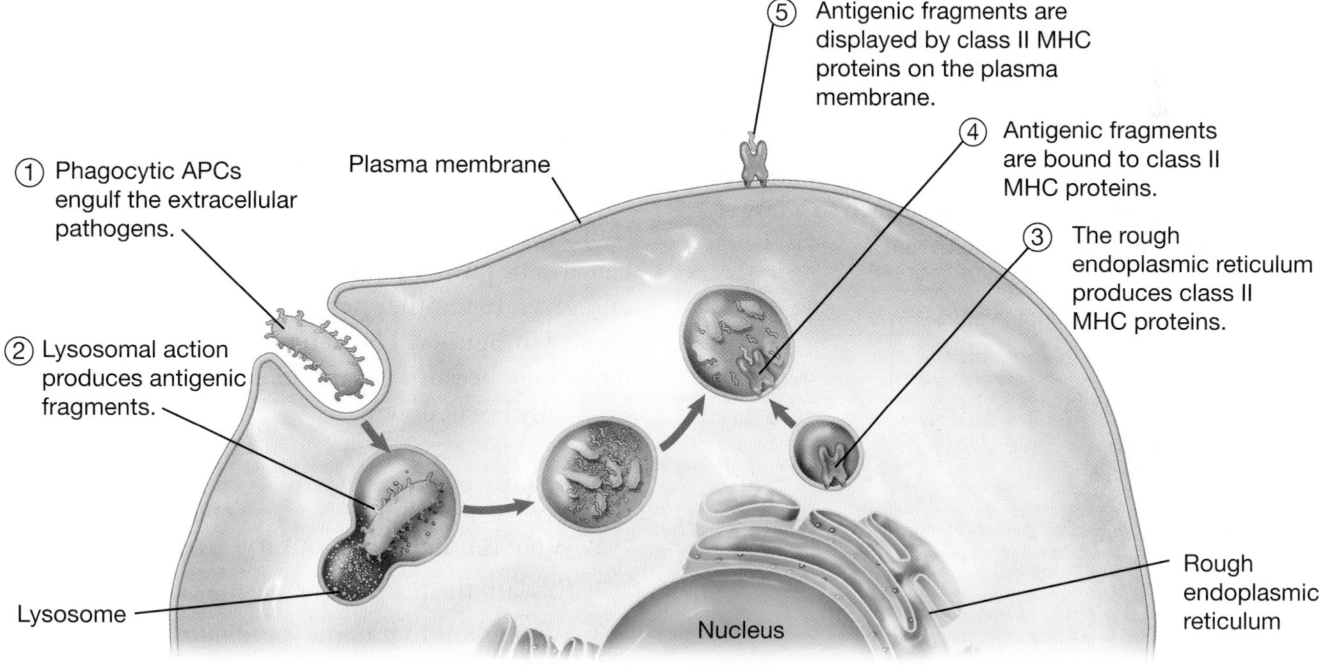

Figure 13.13 Diagram of antigen presentation by an antigen-presenting cell (APC). APCs use class II MHC proteins to display fragments of foreign molecules (antigens) on their surface. (1) The process begins when the APC phagocytizes the foreign object, such as a bacterium. (2) A lysosome, which contains digestive enzymes, fuses with the engulfed object and breaks it down into many pieces. (3) Meanwhile, the cell also produces class II MHC proteins packaged in vesicles. (4) A vesicle containing class II MHC proteins fuses with the vesicle containing digested antigenic fragments. (5) These digested fragments bind to the class II MHC proteins, which are then displayed on the cell membrane.

clonal selection process for B cells produces an army of plasma cells, each of which makes antibodies that bind specifically to the invading antigen the original B cell encountered.

Antibodies

Antibodies are proteins that recognize particular antigens with great specificity. Antibodies are also called ***immunoglobulins*** because they are involved with immune function, and they were originally thought of as globular in shape.

An antibody is a Y-shaped protein made up of four polypeptide chains (**Figure 13.14**). The antigen-binding sites at the tips of the Y have amino acid sequences that vary among antibodies. This variation allows different antibodies to bind to different antigens. The variable regions on the two arms of the Y match each other, so that both arms will bind to the same antigen. The stem and the lower parts of the arms do not vary; they are the same for all antibodies of a given class.

Figure 13.15 describes the five classes of antibodies. Antibodies do not directly destroy antigens. However, they interfere with antigen function and mark antigens for destruction. The formation of an antigen-antibody complex can eliminate the threat of an antigen through multiple mechanisms:

- An antibody can neutralize a virus or bacterial toxin (a toxic chemical secreted by a bacterium) by occupying the binding site that the virus or toxin would normally use to attach to a target cell, thus eliminating the threat.

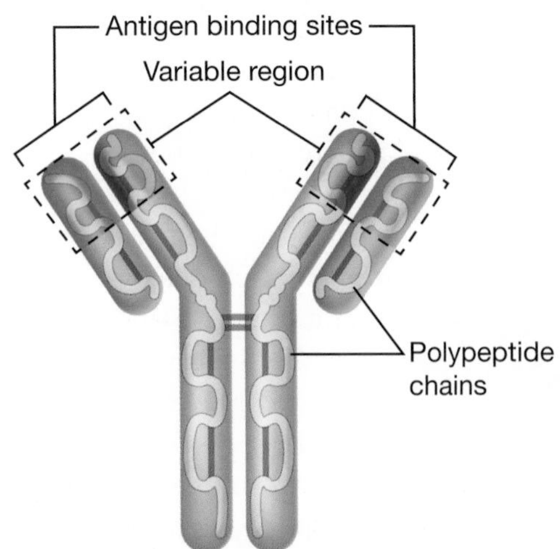

Figure 13.14 An antibody is a Y-shaped protein composed of four polypeptide chains. This type of protein recognizes certain pathogens and targets them specifically. The tips of the arms of the Y contain a variable amino acid sequence where antigens bind.

- ***Precipitation*** causes small, soluble antigen molecules, rather than whole cells, to clump together. The resulting antigen complexes are so big that they are insoluble. Phagocytic cells dispose of the insoluble clumps.
- Agglutination is similar to precipitation, except that it occurs with antigens that lie on the surface of a cell or virus. Thus, the clumping process involves cells, viruses, or bacteria rather than small molecules. As in the case of precipitated antibody-antigen complexes, the agglutinated clumps of material are disposed of through phagocytosis.
- The binding of an antibody to its target pathogen causes a slight change in shape along the stem of the Y. Binding sites on the antigen are then exposed, activating the complement system described earlier. The presence of antibodies and complement proteins on a pathogen make it more appealing to phagocytes, which can destroy it.
- Antibody-antigen complexes also stimulate inflammation by causing mast cells and basophils to release histamine and other chemicals. These chemicals eliminate antigens.

Normal antibody-mediated immunity is also called ***active immunity*** because the antibodies are made by the body's own cells as a result of previous exposure to a disease or a vaccine. ***Passive immunity***, by contrast, is antibody-mediated immunity that comes from antibodies received from an outside source. For example, breast-fed infants have passive immunity because they receive antibodies in breast milk. Antibodies can also be purified from the plasma of a blood donor and given to another person by injection, providing passive immunity. The benefit of a single injection is temporary, because the antibodies, like other proteins, gradually break down.

SELF CHECK

1. What is humoral immunity?
2. Explain the purpose of plasma cells.
3. What is another name for *immunoglobulin*?

Primary and Secondary Immune Responses

A ***primary immune response*** occurs when the body is first exposed to a foreign invader, such as a virus

IgG		Immunoglobulin G (IgG), the most common type of circulating antibody, provides resistance against many infectious agents.
IgD		Immunoglobulin D (IgD) is found in the membranes of B cells, where it forms the antigen receptors on the cell surface.
IgE		The stem of immunoglobulin E (IgE) binds to mast cells and basophils and causes them to release histamine and other chemicals that play roles in inflammation and allergy.
IgA		Immunoglobulin A (IgA) is a dimer (made of two subunits) that is found in secretions, such as mucus, saliva, tears, and semen. It binds to antigens when they are still outside of the body and prevents them from crossing the epithelium and entering the body tissue.
IgM		Immunoglobulin M (IgM), a pentamer (made of five subunits), is the first class of antibody secreted by activated B cells. It activates the complement system. Because it has 10 binding sites, it is good at causing agglutination, or clumping up, of antigens.

Figure 13.15 The five classes of antibodies.

or bacterium. When an antigen enters the body for the first time, the immune system response is neither fast nor widespread. Because memory cells for the new antigen do not yet exist in the body, detection of the threat may take a while. When the threat is detected, the immune system response is limited.

A ***secondary immune response*** occurs when a virus or bacterium enters the body for a second or subsequent time. The secondary immune response involves the memory cells that developed during the body's initial exposure to the potentially harmful invader. The memory cells "remember" the pathogen, providing a faster, stronger response to a smaller amount of antigen.

The difference in intensity between the primary and secondary immune responses, shown in **Figure 13.16**, is the reason that vaccination works. The word *vaccine* comes in part from the Latin word *vacca*, which means "cow." In the mid- and late 1700s, English physician Edward Jenner heard that milkmaids were much less likely than other people to contract smallpox, a disease characterized by a rash and raised blisters on the skin. At the time, it was known that the disease cowpox, which could infect people as well as cows, was similar to smallpox but less severe.

Jenner, and others before him, believed that the exposure of milkmaids to cowpox made them resistant to smallpox. He tested his idea by exposing healthy individuals to pus from the blisters of people infected with cowpox. He then tried to give those healthy individuals smallpox by injecting them with pus from patients infected with smallpox. (Such experiments would be prohibited, with good reason, by the human subjects protection board of a modern hospital.) Jenner's series of careful experiments showed that a substance in the cowpox pus gave people a long-lasting immunity to smallpox.

Exposure to cowpox provided protection against smallpox because the viruses that cause the diseases are very similar. A person exposed to cowpox will have a primary immune response to the illness. As a result, the person's lymphoid tissues become seeded with memory B cells that recognize and respond to the cowpox virus. Subsequent exposure to the smallpox virus causes a secondary immune response because the lymphocytes that respond to cowpox also respond to smallpox.

Today, vaccines expose people to a harmless form of a pathogen, which allows them to have a primary

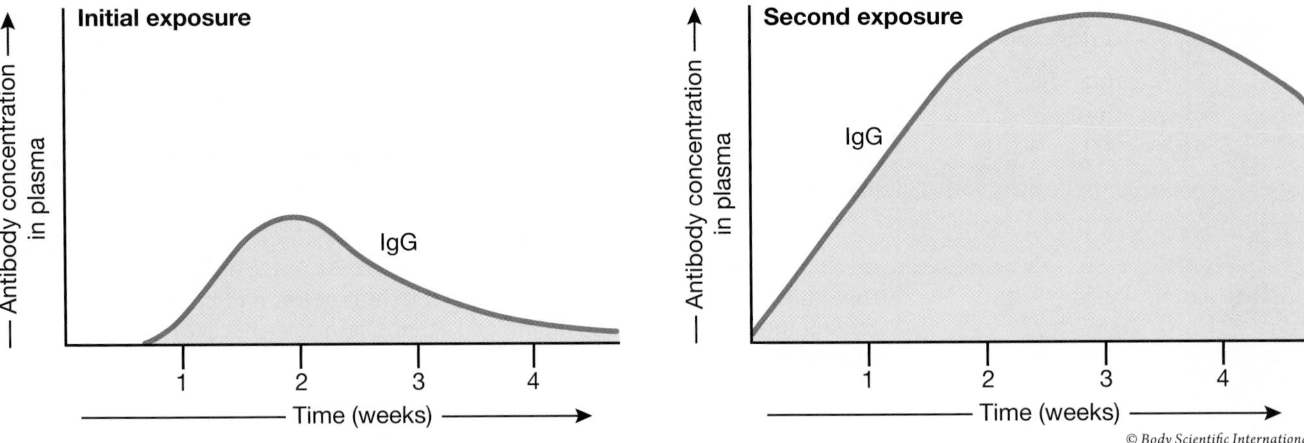

Figure 13.16 Primary and secondary immune responses. These graphs show the levels of immunoglobulin G (the most common antibody) in the blood plasma during an initial infection (left) and during a second infection (right). The response to the second exposure is larger and faster than the response to the first exposure.

immune response. This provides them with memory lymphocytes that respond specifically to that pathogen. Then, if a person is exposed to the real pathogen later, the secondary immune response will react strongly and quickly, usually preventing the person from becoming ill.

SELF CHECK

1. Why is a secondary immune response faster and stronger than a primary immune response?
2. Briefly explain the principle behind vaccination.

Cell-Mediated Immunity

Cellular immunity, or ***cell-mediated immunity***, is facilitated (mediated) by T cells. Cell-mediated immunity is not only *mediated by* cells, it is also *directed at* cells.

As mentioned earlier, viruses enter the body cells and reproduce inside them. A number of bacteria, including salmonella and tuberculosis, also enter body cells and reproduce inside them. When an infectious organism is inside a host cell, the antibodies of humoral immunity cannot attack it. However, cell-mediated immunity can recognize and destroy infected cells.

When body cells are infected by a bacterium or virus, or when they become cancerous or precancerous, they display abnormal proteins on their surfaces that cause a cell-mediated immune response. Cells of transplanted tissue also display foreign antigens. If the tissue from the donor is not well matched to the recipient, it will provoke a cell-mediated immune response that leads to organ rejection.

T cells play a key role in cellular immunity. Different types of T cells have different roles and different molecules on their cell membranes. The two most common types of T cells are those with CD4 glycoproteins on their surfaces ($CD4^+$ T cells, pronounced "CD four positive T cells") and those with CD8 glycoproteins on their surfaces ($CD8^+$ T cells, pronounced "CD eight positive T cells"). The CD4 glycoprotein can bind to class II MHC proteins. (Recall that class II MHC proteins are found on antigen-presenting cells and on B lymphocytes.) The CD8 glycoprotein can bind to class I MHC proteins, which are found on almost all body cells.

The cellular immune response begins when an antigen-presenting cell (APC), such as a macrophage or a dendritic cell, engulfs an antigen and displays fragments of it on its surface with a class II major histocompatibility (MHC) protein (**Figure 13.17A**). The APC can activate a T cell by supplying two signals. The first signal, antigen binding, has two parts: binding of the antigen to a complementary "pocket" on the T cell's receptor, and binding of the T cell's CD4 glycoprotein to the class II MHC molecule on the APC (**Figure 13.17B**). The second signal is called *co-stimulation*. This is the binding of specific molecules in the T cell membrane to corresponding co-stimulatory molecules in the APC membrane.

The combined effects of antigen binding and co-stimulation cause the $CD4^+$ T cell to divide and become helper T cells, memory helper T cells, or less commonly, regulatory T cells. This selection process, like the specific selection of B cells is called *clonal selection* because the daughter cells are exact genetic copies, or clones, of the original activated lymphocyte. This means their T cell receptors specifically recognize the same antigen as the original cell.

Clonal selection of a CD4$^+$ T cell generates helper T cells, memory helper T cells, and regulatory T cells (**Figure 13.17C**). Helper T cells help activate CD8$^+$ T cells. Memory helper T cells take up residence in lymphoid tissues throughout the body, so that the immune system can respond more rapidly and forcefully if the same pathogen returns. Regulatory T cells secrete chemicals that prevent over-activation of cell-mediated immunity. Without regulatory T cells, the cell-mediated response could cause collateral damage to normal cells.

Activation and clonal selection of CD8$^+$ T cells is similar to the corresponding process for CD4$^+$ cells, except CD8 binds to class I MHC molecules, whereas CD4 binds to class II MHC molecules, and CD8$^+$ activation is facilitated by the release of interleukins.

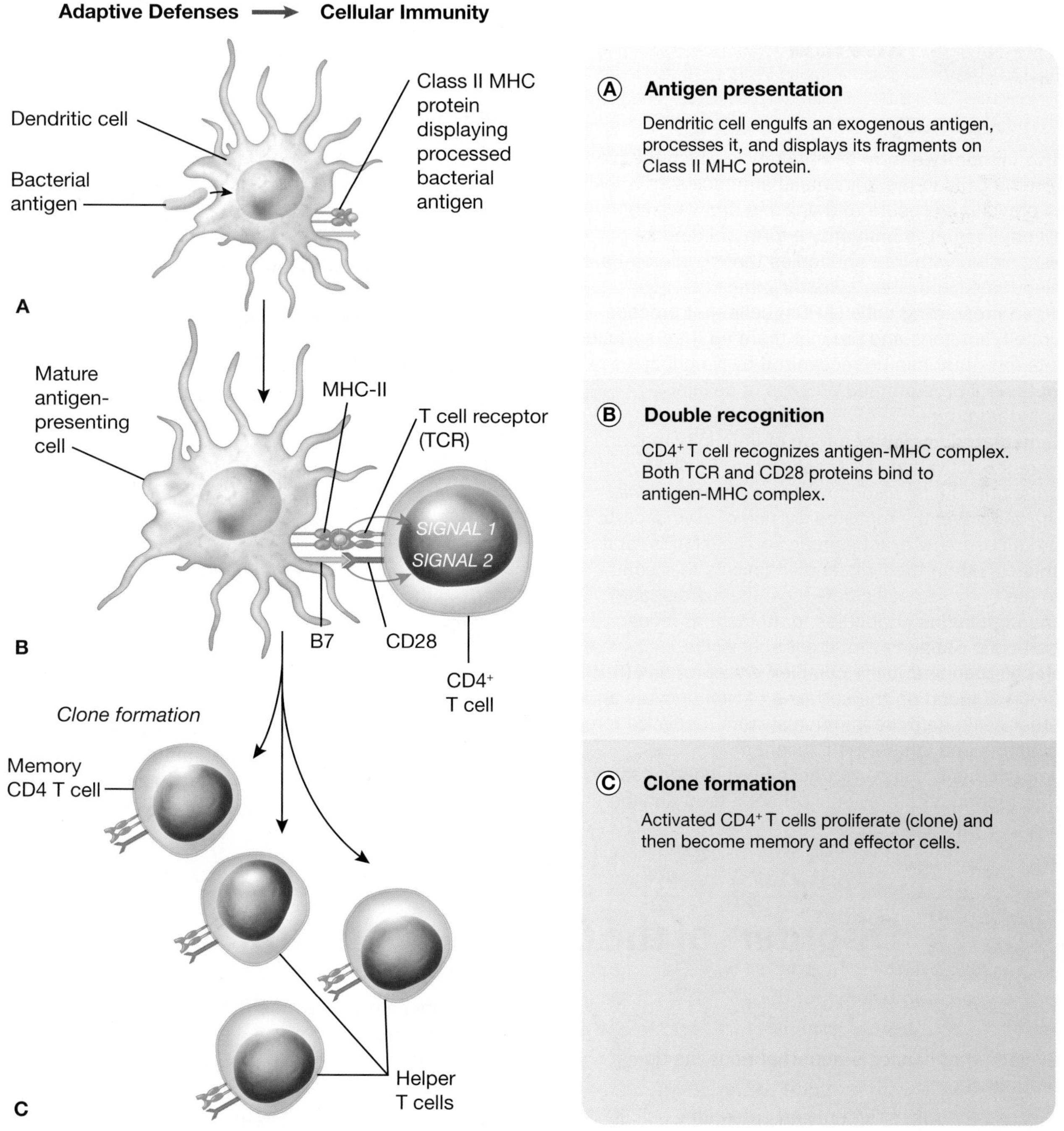
Adaptive Defenses → Cellular Immunity
Dendritic cell
Bacterial antigen
Class II MHC protein displaying processed bacterial antigen
A
Ⓐ Antigen presentation
Dendritic cell engulfs an exogenous antigen, processes it, and displays its fragments on Class II MHC protein.
Mature antigen-presenting cell
MHC-II
T cell receptor (TCR)
SIGNAL 1
SIGNAL 2
B7
CD28
CD4+ T cell
B
Ⓑ Double recognition
CD4+ T cell recognizes antigen-MHC complex. Both TCR and CD28 proteins bind to antigen-MHC complex.
Clone formation
Memory CD4 T cell
Helper T cells
C
Ⓒ Clone formation
Activated CD4+ T cells proliferate (clone) and then become memory and effector cells.

Figure 13.17 Activation and clonal selection of T cells. A—Antigen presentation. B—Double recognition. C—Clone formation.

An activated $CD8^+$ cell can differentiate into a cytotoxic T cell. The cytotoxic T cell binds to a cell displaying the foreign antigen recognized by that T cell. Once the T cell binds to the target cell, it attempts to kill the target cell using one of several mechanisms. It may stimulate intracellular pathways in the target that lead to apoptosis (programmed cell destruction). The cytotoxic T cell may also release perforin molecules to kill its target. Perforin molecules insert themselves into the target cell's membrane and assemble to form a relatively large opening, or perforation, in the cell. This large hole is lethal to the target cell.

As you may recall, natural killer (NK) cells also use this technique to kill their targets. The difference between cytotoxic T cells and NK cells is in what provokes them to "attack." NK cells attack cells that do not display type I major histocompatibility complex (MHC) proteins on their surface. Cytotoxic T cells attack cells that display abnormal type I MHC proteins.

SECTION 13.3 REVIEW

Mini-Glossary

active immunity a form of immunity in which the blood plasma cells in the body make antibodies as a result of previous exposure to a disease or a vaccine

antibody-mediated immunity a form of immunity associated with free antibodies that circulate in the blood; also known as *humoral immunity*

antigen-presenting cells (APCs) cells that process protein antigens and present them on their surfaces in a form that can be recognized by lymphocytes

apoptosis a programmed process of cellular self-destruction

cell-mediated immunity a form of immunity that arises from the activation of T lymphocytes (T cells) by antigen-presenting cells; also known as *cellular immunity*

clonal selection the repeated division of a lymphocyte that produces many exact genetic copies (clones) of itself

immune system the cells and chemicals that contribute to the body's specific defenses against disease

immunoglobulins antibodies; proteins that recognize particular antigens with great specificity

major histocompatibility complex glycoproteins (MHCs) proteins found on the surfaces of lymphocytes and other cells; help the immune system recognize foreign antigens and ignore "self" tissues

memory cells B cells and T cells in lymphatic tissues that respond if a previously encountered antigen invades the body again

passive immunity a form of immunity that comes from antibodies received from an outside source, such as breast milk

precipitation the formation of an insoluble complex, such as a clump of antigen molecules joined together by antibodies

primary immune response the initial immune response to a foreign invader, such as a virus or bacterium

secondary immune response the response of the immune system to an infectious agent that it has encountered before

Review Questions

1. Describe the genetic immune system deficiency that is more commonly known as *bubble boy disease*.
2. Identify the types of cells that can act as antigen-presenting cells (APCs).
3. Explain the importance of the thymus to the body's immune system.
4. What two types of cells have antigen receptors, making humoral immunity possible?
5. Explain why T lymphocytes and B lymphocytes are so named.
6. Describe the sequence of events that occurs when a lymphocyte encounters an antigen.
7. Using what you have learned about humoral immunity, list the steps that occur when a B cell undergoes clonal selection.

SECTION 13.4 Disorders of the Lymphatic and Immune Systems

Objectives

- Explain what cancer is and what happens during metastasis.
- Discuss the role of an antigen-presenting cell (APC) in an allergic response.
- Identify potential issues that may occur during organ transplantation.
- Explain what an autoimmune disorder is and give one example.
- Explain how HIV is related to AIDS.

(continued)

Key Terms

acquired immunodeficiency syndrome (AIDS)
allergen
allergen immunotherapy
anaphylaxis
autoimmune disorder
human immunodeficiency virus (HIV)
immunosuppression
lymphedema
metastasis
opportunistic infection
tolerance

From allergies to AIDS, many health problems can be linked to a compromised immune system. This section explores some common disorders and diseases of the body's defense systems.

Cancer and Lymph Nodes

Cancer is a disease in which the normal control of cell division (mitosis) fails, and a cell divides too quickly and without limit. As a solid tumor grows, cancerous cells sometimes break free from the tumor and migrate to other areas of the body. The process of cancer spreading from its initial location to another part of the body is called ***metastasis***. A cancer that has spread is said to be metastatic.

Metastatic cells can spread by entering a lymphatic vessel and traveling in the lymph to the nearest lymph node. When the cells reach the lymph node, they may become caught in the node's reticular tissue and continue growing. When some types of cancer have been diagnosed, it is standard for an oncologist to obtain a sample of nearby lymph node tissue to determine whether the cancer has spread. The sample may be obtained by surgically removing one or more lymph nodes or by performing a needle biopsy using a syringe.

If cancer has metastasized to lymph nodes, then more lymph nodes may be removed to reduce the chance of further metastasis. Although this may help reduce cancer development, lymph node removal has risks. The biggest issue is that removing lymph nodes disrupts the lymphatic drainage in the affected area of the body. As a result, fluid that leaks out of blood capillaries builds up in the interstitial space, causing tissue swelling and damage. This buildup of extracellular fluid is called ***lymphedema***.

Breast cancer often metastasizes to axillary (underarm) lymph nodes. Removal of axillary lymph nodes increases the risk of lymphedema of the arm, the most common type of lymphedema. Treatment options for lymphedema include a compression sleeve, physical therapy, and carefully designed light exercise.

SELF CHECK

1. How does cancer spread?
2. What is the cause of lymphedema?

Allergies

Do you sneeze, cough, or suffer from itchy, watery eyes when you are exposed to dust, pollen, or animal dander? If so, you are not alone. Approximately 55% of Americans have an allergy to one or more substances in the environment.

An allergy is an inappropriately strong immune response to an environmental antigen, such as dust mites, pet dander, pollen, or certain foods (**Figure 13.18**). In such cases, the antigen is not really a threat; the problem is an over-reactive immune system.

Allergies arise when an antigen-presenting cell (APC) presents the antigen—an ***allergen***—to a helper T cell in a person susceptible to allergies. This allergen presentation activates the helper T cell, which in turn activates B cells, causing them to produce IgE antibodies. The IgE antibodies interact with mast cells and basophils, which become sensitive to the allergen. The next time the allergen is encountered, basophils and mast cells respond by secreting large amounts of histamine.

Histamine causes an inflammatory response, which can lead to symptoms, such as a runny nose and watery, itchy eyes. In severe cases, such as with bee-sting allergies and certain nut allergies, exposure to the antigen causes large quantities of histamine to be released throughout the body. Excessive histamine in the body can lead to life-threatening symptoms. These include pulmonary obstruction due to inflammation and swelling of the airways and low blood pressure due to leakage of blood plasma into the interstitial space from excessively leaky capillaries. Such a severe allergic reaction is called ***anaphylaxis***.

Anaphylaxis can be treated with an injection of epinephrine, a hormone that opens up the airways and constricts (narrows) the blood vessels. Antihistamine drugs, which block the effects of histamine, can

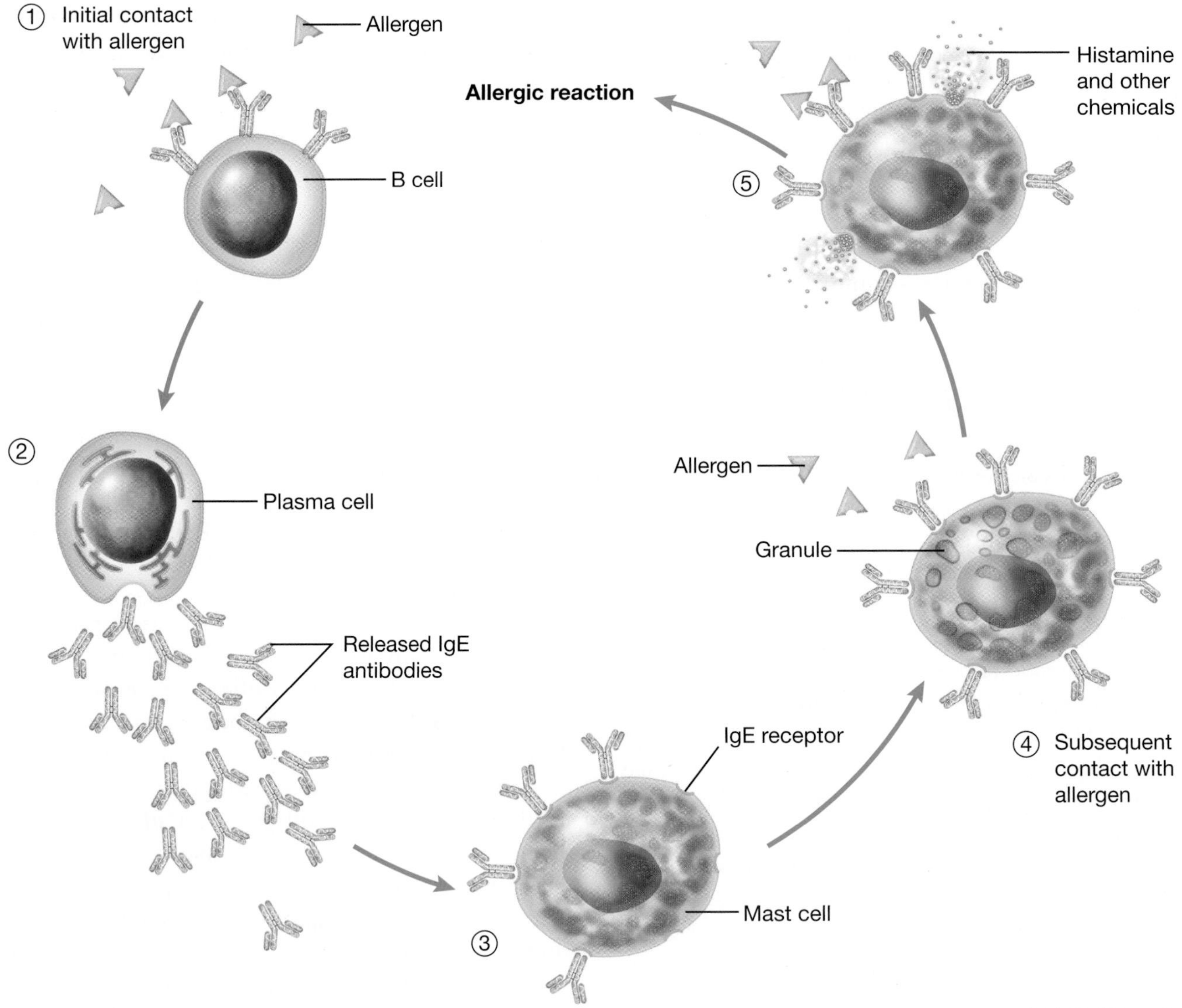

Figure 13.18 Diagram of an allergic reaction.

be used to treat anaphylaxis as well as less severe allergic reactions.

Allergy shots, or ***allergen immunotherapy***, are a longer-term treatment aimed at preventing allergic reactions before they occur. In allergy-shot treatment, a specific allergen is injected underneath the skin, starting with tiny amounts and gradually building up to larger amounts. This gradual approach often leads to the development of immune system ***tolerance*** of the antigen. As a result, the allergic response may be reduced or eliminated.

Asthma is a reaction to the presence of inhaled allergens in the airways of the lungs. During an asthma attack, mast cells release histamine in the walls of the airways. The resulting swelling and edema in the airway wall reduces the diameter of the opening in the center of the airway, restricting airflow. A person experiencing an asthma attack feels like she or he is breathing through a thin straw.

SELF CHECK

1. What causes itchy, watery eyes from exposure to dust, pollen, or animal dander?
2. What is the effect of excessive amounts of histamine in the body?
3. Name two treatments for anaphylaxis.

Organ Transplantation and Rejection

When a patient needs an organ transplant, potential donors are screened to find a "match." A good match is one in which the donor has MHC proteins that are highly similar to those of the recipient. The only source of a perfect match would be an identical twin.

Even when the match is good, the T cells of the recipient could still react to the slightly unfamiliar class I MHC proteins on the cells of the transplanted organ. This can lead to an attack by cytotoxic T cells on the "foreign" tissue, causing the transplanted organ to be rejected.

To reduce the likelihood of rejection, transplant recipients are usually given drugs that cause ***immunosuppression***, or a reduction in the activity and sensitivity of the immune system. However, immunosuppression is potentially dangerous in itself because the immunosuppressed patient is more vulnerable to infection.

SELF CHECK

1. What causes a transplanted organ to be rejected by the recipient's body?
2. Name a disadvantage of administering immunosuppressive medications to a transplant recipient.

Autoimmune Disorders

An ***autoimmune disorder***, like an allergy, is a condition in which the immune system overreacts to an antigen that ordinarily does not pose an actual threat. In an allergy, the antigen is a substance from the external environment. In an autoimmune disorder, the antigen is part of the body's own tissue. When the immune system perceives the body's own tissue as foreign, it attacks that tissue as it would attack an invading pathogen.

The cause of an autoimmune disorder is often unclear. An autoimmune disorder sometimes develops when a genetically susceptible person is exposed to an environmental antigen that resembles one of the body's own molecules. Due to the resemblance, the body responds to its own cells while responding to that environmental antigen.

More than 80 different types of autoimmune disorders have been identified. Examples include rheumatoid arthritis, in which the immune system attacks the synovial membrane that lines joint cavities (see Chapter 8); multiple sclerosis, in which the immune system attacks the myelin sheath that surrounds nerve cells (see Chapter 7); and type I diabetes mellitus (see Chapter 9).

In type I diabetes mellitus, cytotoxic T cells attack the cells in the pancreas that manufacture insulin, a hormone that metabolizes carbohydrates and fats and regulates blood glucose levels. Without a regular supply of insulin, blood glucose levels can become dangerously high. Unfortunately, the cytotoxic T cell attacks are usually very effective, and all or most of the insulin-producing cells are destroyed. Once the insulin-producing cells are gone, they do not replenish. Type I diabetes is also called *insulin-dependent diabetes* because individuals with this autoimmune disease require regular insulin injections from an outside source.

SELF CHECK

1. How is an autoimmune disorder different from an allergy?
2. What are some common autoimmune disorders?

HIV and AIDS

As its name indicates, ***human immunodeficiency virus (HIV)*** is a virus that causes immune deficiency in humans. HIV is the virus that can lead to ***acquired immunodeficiency syndrome (AIDS)***. HIV is commonly transmitted sexually; through sharing of needles during illegal drug use; or from mother to child during pregnancy, birth, or breast-feeding. Less common modes of transmission include blood transfusions or being accidentally "stuck" with a contaminated needle. The latter is a risk for health-care workers.

Within a few weeks of infection, a person with HIV may develop flu-like symptoms that last one or two weeks. Others may not experience any symptoms at all. Although individuals infected with HIV may feel perfectly healthy, the virus is at work inside their bodies.

HIV damages the immune system and compromises the body's ability to fight disease-causing organisms. As shown in **Figure 13.19**, HIV infects lymphocytes that have the CD4 protein on their surface ($CD4^+$ cells).

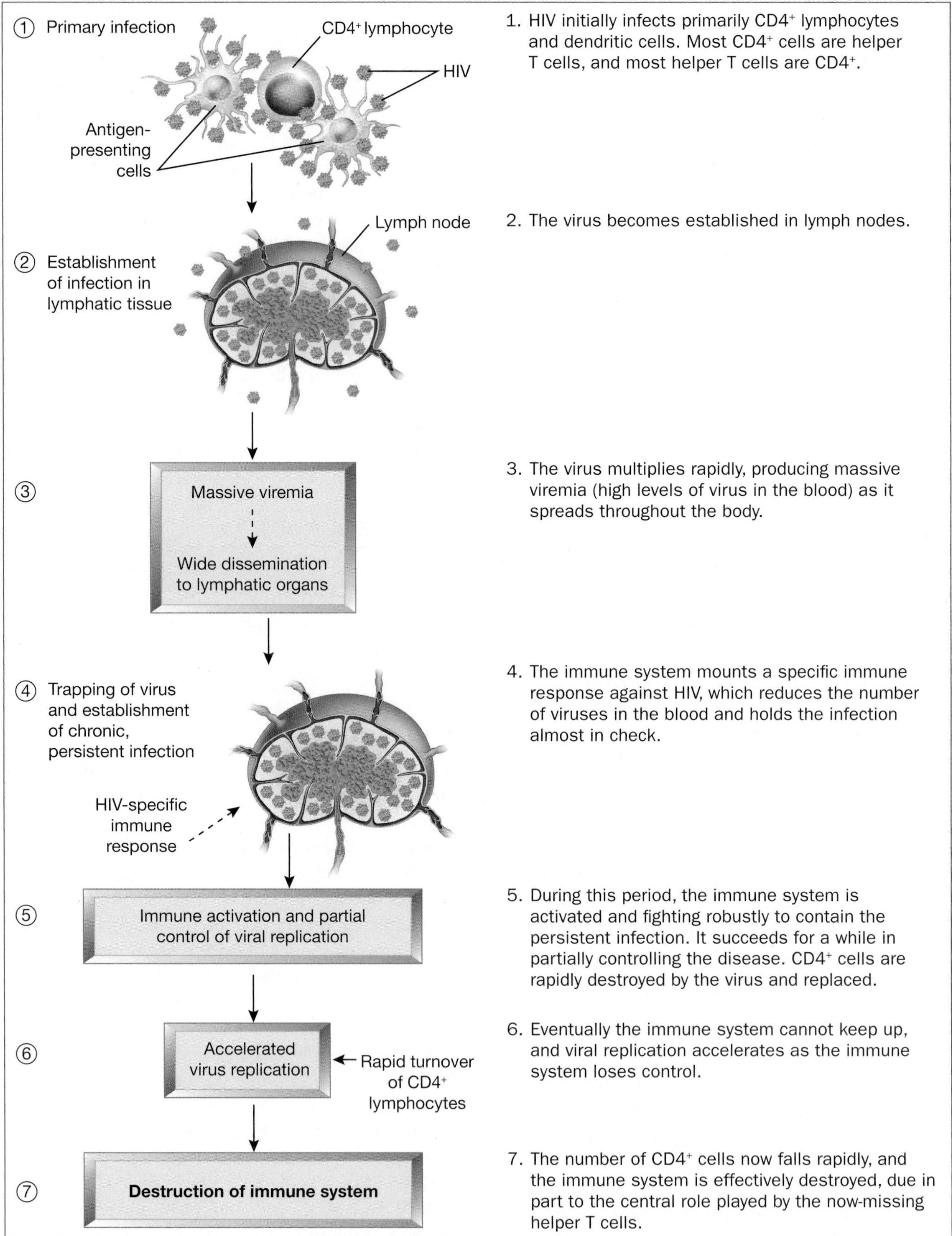

① Primary infection
CD4+ lymphocyte
HIV
Antigen-presenting cells
1. HIV initially infects primarily CD4+ lymphocytes and dendritic cells. Most CD4+ cells are helper T cells, and most helper T cells are CD4+.
Lymph node
② Establishment of infection in lymphatic tissue
2. The virus becomes established in lymph nodes.
③
Massive viremia
Wide dissemination to lymphatic organs
3. The virus multiplies rapidly, producing massive viremia (high levels of virus in the blood) as it spreads throughout the body.
④ Trapping of virus and establishment of chronic, persistent infection
HIV-specific immune response
4. The immune system mounts a specific immune response against HIV, which reduces the number of viruses in the blood and holds the infection almost in check.
⑤
Immune activation and partial control of viral replication
5. During this period, the immune system is activated and fighting robustly to contain the persistent infection. It succeeds for a while in partially controlling the disease. CD4+ cells are rapidly destroyed by the virus and replaced.
⑥
Accelerated virus replication
Rapid turnover of CD4+ lymphocytes
6. Eventually the immune system cannot keep up, and viral replication accelerates as the immune system loses control.
⑦
Destruction of immune system
7. The number of CD4+ cells now falls rapidly, and the immune system is effectively destroyed, due in part to the central role played by the now-missing helper T cells.

Figure 13.19 HIV infection and the development of AIDS.

Research Notes Antibody-Based Drugs

Many drugs have side effects that limit their usefulness by affecting processes other than the specific disease mechanisms that the drugs intended to affect. Because antibodies bind very specifically, it has long been thought that they could make better, more specifically focused drugs.

In recent years, many antibody-based drugs have made it to market. These drugs are made by fusing a B lymphocyte with a cultured cell derived from a cancerous lymph cell. The resulting cell can divide without limit because it is derived from a cancer cell, and it makes one specific antibody because it is also derived from a B lymphocyte.

This cell is allowed to divide and grow. The cells that result from these divisions are genetic copies of the original fused cell, so they are called *clones*. The antibodies secreted by these cells are called *monoclonal antibodies* because they come from a single clone. These antibodies are harvested and packaged as a drug. You can recognize many drugs that are made of monoclonal antibodies because they usually have the word segment *-mab* (for "monoclonal antibody") in their generic name.

Infliximab (brand name Remicade®) is an antibody to tumor necrosis factor, a protein that plays an important role in rheumatoid arthritis, the disease for which it is most often prescribed. Trastuzamab (brand name Herceptin®) is an antibody to the human epidermal growth factor receptor 2 (HER2), which is found on the surface of some kinds of breast cancer cells. This antibody is given as a chemotherapeutic agent to patients with HER2-positive breast cancer. Many other monoclonal antibody drugs exist, and the list continues to grow with advances in research.

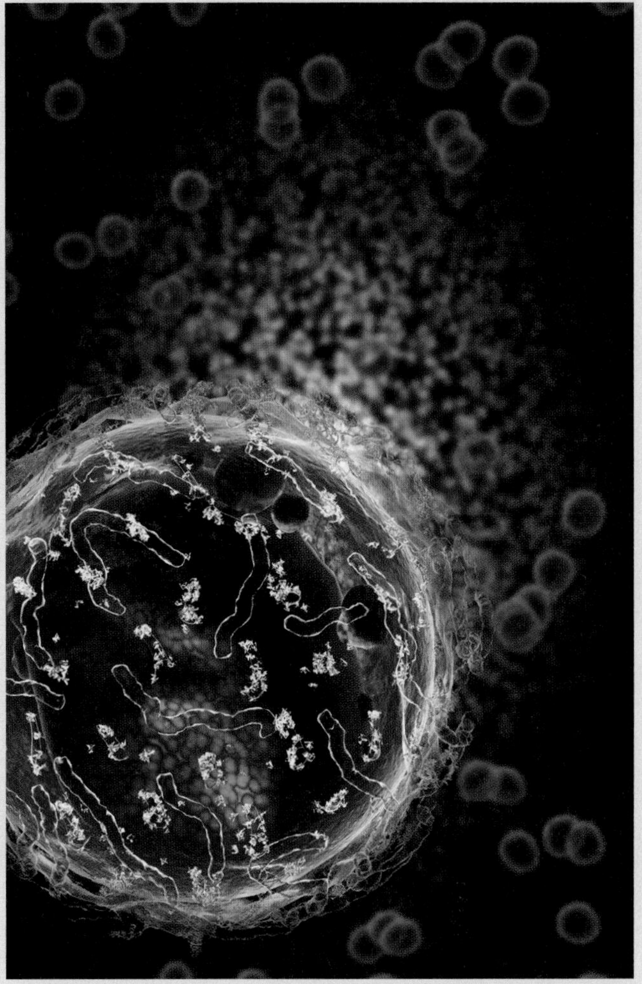

3D4Medical/Science Source

B lymphocyte.

Most CD4⁺ cells are helper T cells, and most helper T cells have the CD4⁺ protein. After the virus uses the intracellular machinery to make copies of itself, it breaks open the cell, killing the cell and releasing new, infectious virus particles.

Of all the immune cells, the helper T cells are probably the cells that the body can least afford to lose. The helper T cells are essential for strong activation of the humoral and cellular immune responses. In a person infected with HIV, the helper T cells are eventually overwhelmed by the influx of virus particles. As the body's concentration of helper T cells drops, the immune system is seriously weakened.

A patient with a low level of helper T cells is highly susceptible to developing rare forms of cancer and ***opportunistic infections***—unusual infections that are rarely seen in people with healthy immune systems. A patient is diagnosed with AIDS if he or she has one of these rare diseases, and if his or her number of CD4⁺ T cells is less than 200 per cubic milliliter of blood. Multidrug treatments for HIV are effective at suppressing viral reproduction for many years. However, these drugs can have serious side effects, such as nausea, vomiting, weight loss, and fatigue. Also, AIDS antiviral drugs are expensive and must be taken for life. Therefore, the scientific community continues its effort to create an HIV vaccine.

SECTION 13.4
REVIEW

Mini-Glossary

acquired immunodeficiency syndrome (AIDS) a disease in which the immune system is greatly weakened due to infection with HIV, making a person more susceptible to rare cancers and opportunistic infections

allergen an antigen that causes an inappropriately strong immune system response

allergen immunotherapy a long-term, preventive treatment for allergies; also known as *allergy shots*

anaphylaxis a severe and potentially life-threatening allergic reaction that may include airway obstruction and very low blood pressure

autoimmune disorder a condition in which the immune system attacks the body's own tissue

human immunodeficiency virus (HIV) the virus that causes immune deficiency in humans and leads to AIDS

immunosuppression a reduction in the activity and sensitivity of the immune system

lymphedema a buildup of extracellular fluid in the body because of disruption in lymphatic drainage

metastasis the spreading of cancerous cells from their original location to another part of the body

opportunistic infection an infection that rarely occurs in people with a healthy immune system but may occur in a person with a damaged immune system, such as someone with AIDS

tolerance a reduction or elimination of the allergic response, which may occur after immunotherapy

Review Questions

1. What surgical procedures may be used to determine whether cancer has spread from its initial location to another part of the body?
2. List the potential risks associated with having a lymph node removed.
3. State the treatment options for a patient with lymphedema of the arm as a result of having axillary lymph nodes removed.
4. How are IgE antibodies produced?
5. Identify the two cells responsible for secreting large amounts of histamine in response to an allergen.
6. Summarize the purpose of allergen immunotherapy.
7. Explain the difference between HIV and AIDS.
8. Describe the process by which an antibody-based drug is made.
9. Identify the area of the body where breast cancer often metastasizes.
10. Based on what you have learned about severe allergies, describe two ways in which histamine could cause life-threatening symptoms.
11. Imagine that you are a physician who has just seen the following patients. What diagnosis might you make for each patient? Use information that you learned in this section as well as information from previous chapters to make your diagnoses.

    Patient A: tests show very high cell counts in certain lymph nodes; the patient is not currently experiencing any pain or fatigue

    Patient B: severe pain in the hands and feet; severe inflammation and swelling in the hands; fatigue

    Patient C: excessive sneezing, coughing, and watery eyes; symptoms began during a recent hiking trip

    Patient D: has two different infections; standard tests have failed to identify the cause of either infection; patient reports that she has been very healthy for the past two years

Medical Terminology:
The Lymphatic and Immune Systems

By understanding the word parts that make up medical words, you can extend your medical vocabulary. This chapter includes many of the word parts listed below. Review these word parts to be sure you understand their meanings.

agglutin/o	clumping, sticking together
-al	pertaining to
-ation	process, condition
bronch/o	bronchial tube, lung
cyt/o	cell
-ectomy	removal, excision
-edema	swelling
-gen	substance that produces
lymph/o	lymph
lymphangia/o	lymph vessel
macro-	large
melan/o	black
-oma	tumor
path/o	disease
phag/o	eat, swallow
pyr/o	fever, fire
splen/o	spleen

Now use these word parts to form valid medical words that fit the following definitions. Some of the words are included in this chapter. Others are not. When you finish, use a medical dictionary to check your work.

1. large cell that devours pathogens (macrophage)
2. pertaining to the middle of the chest cavity, between the lungs (bronchomediastinal)
3. something that produces disease (pathogen)
4. excision of a lymph vessel (lymphangiectomy)
5. black cell (melanocyte)
6. removal of the spleen (splenectomy)
7. something that produces fever (pyrogens)
8. process of clumping (agglutination)
9. swelling due to fluid buildup caused by disrupted lymph drainage (lymphedema)
10. tumor in the lymphatic system (lymphangioma)

Chapter 13 Summary

- The lymphatic system performs three vital functions in the human body: (a) it reabsorbs fluid from leaking capillaries and returns it to the cardiovascular system; (b) it provides the main pathway for fat absorption; and (c) it provides protection against disease.
- The lymphatic system includes lymphocytes, lymphatic vessels, lymphatic fluid, and lymphatic organs (lymph nodes, the spleen, and the thymus).
- The skin functions as a physical barrier against infectious agents, so when the skin is breached, the risk for infection is much greater.
- The body's cellular and chemical defenses include phagocytosis, natural killer cells, the complement system, and interferons.
- The purpose of the inflammatory response is to promote the repair of damaged tissue.
- Fever occurs when infection activates leukocytes and macrophages, which cause the body cells to release pyrogens.
- Antigens allow the body to recognize cells as "self" or "nonself."
- Key types of cells within the immune system include antigen-presenting cells (APCs), lymphocytes, and MHC proteins.
- Antibody-mediated immunity (humoral immunity) eliminates antigen threats with mechanisms such as neutralization, precipitation, agglutination, binding, and inflammation.
- A primary immune response occurs when the body is first exposed to a foreign invader. A secondary response occurs when the invader enters the body a second or subsequent time.
- Cell-mediated immunity begins when an antigen-presenting cell (APC) presents an antigen on its surface with a class II major histocompatibility (MHC) protein.
- The process by which cancer spreads from its initial location to another part of the body via the lymphatic system is called *metastasis*.
- Allergies are caused by an inappropriately strong immune response.
- Organ transplant rejections can occur if the transplant recipient's T cells fail to recognize the class I MHC proteins on the cells of the transplanted organ.
- Common autoimmune disorders include rheumatoid arthritis, multiple sclerosis, and type I diabetes.
- Human immunodeficiency virus (HIV) damages the immune system and compromises the body's ability to fight disease-causing organisms.

Chapter 13 Review

Understanding Key Concepts

1. What three vital functions does the lymphatic system perform in the human body?
2. *True or False?* The normal leakage rate of blood plasma across the entire body is 2 to 3 mL per minute.
3. *True or False?* Lymph formation begins with fluid that leaks out of blood vessel capillaries.
4. *True or False?* The human body has a pump similar to the heart that helps propel lymph through the network of lymph vessels.
5. Lymph from the thoracic duct drains into the ______ vein.
6. *True or False?* During the process of lymph drainage, lymphatic fluid never rejoins the blood to once again become blood plasma.

7. *True or False?* When skin has been cut or punctured, the body is at a much greater risk for infection.
8. The process by which cells engulf and destroy foreign matter and cellular debris is called _____.
   A. exocytosis
   B. phagocytosis
   C. inflammation
   D. opsonization
9. _____ develop into macrophages when they leave the bloodstream and enter tissues.
10. The process by which cell membranes fuse together and push debris from the cell vesicles to the outside of the cell is called _____.
11. The _____ is a set of more than 30 proteins that circulate in the blood plasma and work together to destroy bacteria.
12. The process by which complement proteins make cells more attractive to phagocytes is called _____.
   A. opsonization
   B. activation
   C. phagocytosis
   D. precipitation
13. *True or False?* A virus spreads by reproducing itself.
14. Where is the physical "home" of the immune system?
15. A(n) _____ is a large molecule on the surface of a cell that helps the body distinguish between "self" and "nonself" cells.
16. Which of the following *cannot* act as an antigen-presenting cell (APC)?
   A. macrophage
   B. histamine
   C. dendritic cell
   D. B cell
17. Where do T lymphocytes travel to complete their maturation?
18. The programmed process of cellular self-destruction is called _____.
   A. differentiation
   B. clonal selection
   C. apoptosis
   D. metastasis
19. *True or False?* Antibodies, also known as *immunoglobulins*, are Y-shaped.
20. How many classes of antibodies exist?
21. What do body cells display on their surfaces when they are infected by viruses or bacteria?
22. A cancer that has spread is said to be _____.
23. Approximately what percentage of Americans has an allergy to one or more substances in the environment?
24. _____ is a hormone that opens up the airways and constricts the blood vessels.
   A. Antihistamine
   B. Anaphylaxis
   C. Immunoglobulin
   D. Epinephrine
25. A(n) _____ is a condition in which the immune system overreacts to an antigen that, in and of itself, does not pose an actual threat
26. Which virus can lead to the development of AIDS?
27. Development of an immune system _____ of an antigen may reduce or eliminate an allergic response.
28. A severe allergic reaction that may include pulmonary obstruction and low blood pressure is called _____.

Thinking Critically

29. Assume that you are a physician talking to the parents of a high-school football player with a ruptured spleen. Evaluate the causes and effects of this trauma in an explanation they could understand.
30. Explain the process that causes your lymph nodes to become swollen in response to exposure to an infection.
31. The complement system can be activated in three ways. Identify the three pathways and describe how each one is initiated.
32. Explain how the immune system uses a vaccine to build a defense through the primary and secondary immune response.
33. Explain how clonal selection, or cloning of lymphocytes, works and what becomes of the clones.
34. Describe the process by which a patient transitions from HIV-positive status to a diagnosis of AIDS.

Clinical Case Study

Read again the Clinical Case Study at the beginning of this chapter. Use the information provided in the chapter to answer the questions at the end of the scenario.

35. Where are the metacarpophalangeal (MCP) and metatarsophalangeal (MTP) joints?
36. What are some possible causes of Nina's symptoms? How do her history and presentation help distinguish between possible diagnoses?

Analyzing and Evaluating Data

The chart shown here gives the percentages of the population (between 15 and 49 years of age) infected with HIV in selected countries. Use the chart and your knowledge of geography (do some research if necessary) to answer the following questions.

Percentages of Age 15 to 49 Population with HIV in Select Countries			
Country	**%**	**Country**	**%**
Argentina	0.5	Japan	0.1
Canada	0.2	Mexico	0.3
Chile	0.4	Mozambique	11.5
China	0.1	Nigeria	3.6
Colombia	0.5	South Africa	17.8
France	0.4	United Kingdom	0.2
Germany	0.1	United States	0.6
India	0.3		

37. What percentage of people between 15 and 49 years of age in the United States have contracted HIV? (Round your answer to the nearest whole number.)
38. List, in descending order, the six countries in the Western Hemisphere with the highest incidence of HIV, based on percentage of HIV infections.
39. Of the countries listed in the chart, is the average incidence of HIV greater in Asia or Europe?
40. What is the ratio of people in South Africa who have HIV compared to those in Japan, Germany, or China who have HIV?
    A. 64 to 1
    B. 18 to 1
    C. 180 to 1
    D. 22 to 1

Investigating Further

41. Perform further research on vaccinations. What are the standard vaccination schedules for children born in the United States? How do these schedules vary from those in other developed countries? In underdeveloped countries?
42. Using the Centers for Disease Control (CDC) website as a source, research anaphylaxis. What are the proper steps to follow when you encounter someone who may be in anaphylactic shock?

14 The Digestive System and Metabolism

Clinical Case Study

Kyra is 23 years old and works as an online customer support agent for a software company. She comes to the emergency department complaining of nausea, vomiting, and diarrhea. She says her symptoms came on rapidly, starting about 12 hours ago. Kyra's physical examination indicates that her heart rate and blood pressure and temperature are normal. Palpation of her abdomen causes discomfort, but there is not one specific area of her abdomen that is most tender. She is somewhat dehydrated.

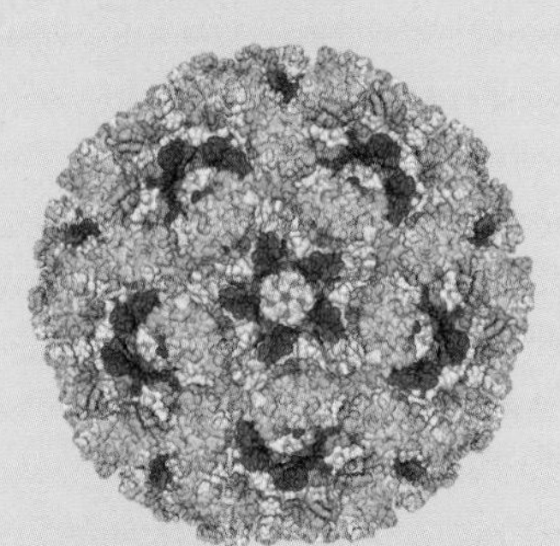

Image created with NGL Viewer using Norovirus structure from the Protein Data Bank, www.rcsb.org. PDB ID: 1IHM. Prasad BV, Hardy ME, Dokland T, Bella J, Rossmann MG, Estes MK (1999) Science 286:287–290. Rose AS, Hildebrand PW (2015) Nucleic Acids Res. 43:W576–579.

The physician asks questions to learn about Kyra's past medical history and other information that could help in the diagnosis. Kyra says she hardly ever has vomiting or diarrhea. She has never traveled abroad, and she has not been around anyone sick for the last week. She says that she has no history of sexually transmitted infection or other significant illness. She says she texted her boyfriend while on the way to the ER. He texted back that he too is experiencing nausea and vomiting which started recently. The last time she saw her boyfriend was when they went to a wedding two nights ago. She had the chicken at the dinner, and he had the fish. They both had salad and cake and fresh strawberries. She does not know if other people who were at the wedding got sick. The physician calls the local department of public health. The health department says others who attended the wedding have also reported illness. Almost all of those affected are reporting diarrhea and vomiting. The health department requests that the physician send a stool sample from Kyra for analysis.

What are possible causes of Kyra's symptoms? How do Kyra's physical examination and history help narrow down the likely diagnosis?

Chapter 14 Outline

Section 14.1 Metabolism

- Energy
- Metabolic Processes

Section 14.2 Nutrition

- Macronutrients
- Micronutrients

Section 14.3 Anatomy and Physiology of the Digestive System

- Overview of the GI Tract
- Functions of the Digestive Organs

Section 14.4 Disorders and Diseases of the Digestive System

- Diseases and Disorders of the GI Tract
- Diseases and Disorders of the Accessory Organs
- Cancer

Life requires energy. The source of that energy is about 93 million miles away, at the center of the solar system. Plants here on Earth convert the energy from sunlight into chemicals. The chemical energy is stored in covalent bonds (see Chapter 2) in molecules of plant cells. These molecules include sugars such as fructose and sucrose, oils such as oleic and linoleic acid, and proteins such as glycinin in soybeans. By eating plants and animals (that also eat plants), humans obtain the fuel they need.

However, people need more than just energy to survive and thrive. They also need certain molecular building blocks that are essential for growth and maintenance. The digestive system brings all the needed molecules into the body—including the molecules that provide energy.

Eating is only the first step of the digestive process. Many more steps are involved in breaking down bite-sized fragments of food into microscopic pieces. These microscopic pieces are eventually absorbed into the blood. The digestive system also disposes of the parts of food that cannot be absorbed by the body This chapter explains how the structures and functions of the digestive system work together to process and store the energy and nutrients needed for a healthy body.

SECTION 14.1

Metabolism

Objectives

- Describe the different forms of energy and how energy is measured.
- Explain metabolic processes, including anabolism and catabolism, and the major metabolic pathways.

Key Terms

anabolism
basal metabolic rate (BMR)
Calorie
catabolism
energy
metabolism

Why might a chapter about the digestive system begin with sections about metabolism and nutrition? The answer is that the digestive system exists to provide nutrients to the body, and these nutrients are essential for metabolism. In earlier chapters, you read about the composition and function of blood before you studied the cardiovascular system. This chapter takes a similar approach, studying metabolism and the nutrients found in food before examining the digestive system itself.

Energy

As you read this paragraph, your body is growing, moving, breathing, pumping blood, and staying warm. To perform these activities and many others, the body needs ***energy***, which is the ability of a physical system to do work.

Types of Energy

Energy takes many forms. Chemical energy is the energy stored in the bonds of atoms and molecules. Chemical energy may be stored or released during chemical reactions. Kinetic energy is the energy of motion present in a moving object. Potential energy is stored energy, such as the energy stored in a stretched spring.

Energy is conserved—that is, the total amount of energy in a closed system does not change. However, although the total *amount* of energy does not change, the energy may change from one type to another. A car engine converts the chemical energy in gasoline into kinetic energy. Muscle cells (Chapter 6) convert chemical energy into kinetic and potential mechanical energy. Nerve cells (Chapter 7) convert chemical energy into electrical energy. In all three cases, the conversion of chemical energy to another form is not 100% efficient, and the "lost" energy is not really lost—it just turns into heat energy.

Measuring the Body's Energy Use

Just as there are many forms of energy, there are many ways to measure energy. For example, electric companies use a unit of measure called the *kilowatt hour (kWh)* to calculate the amount of energy used by their customers.

Food scientists are interested in the potential energy found in foods. Food energy is often measured in terms of an item's capacity to produce heat. Heat energy is measured in Calories or (in the metric system) joules.

The term *calorie* is used in many contexts, but the type of calorie used by food scientists is written with a capital C. The ***Calorie***, also called the *kilocalorie (kcal)*, is used to measure the potential energy in foods. A single Calorie is equal to the amount of heat required to raise the temperature of 1 kilogram of water by 1°C.

SELF CHECK

1. How is kinetic energy different from potential energy?
2. What unit is used to count and measure energy in nutrition science?

Metabolic Processes

At any moment, there are thousands of different types of chemical reactions occurring in the human body. Some reactions are simple, such as the combination of carbon dioxide (CO_2) and water (H_2O) to make carbonic acid (H_2CO_3). Other reactions are complicated, such as the synthesis of a new DNA molecule in a cell that is about to divide.

Metabolism refers to all of the chemical reactions, or changes, that occur within the body cells. Metabolism includes two basic processes: catabolism and anabolism.

Anabolism and Catabolism

Catabolism is the process of breaking down large molecules into smaller ones. Catabolic reactions generally break chemical bonds to release the energy that is stored in those bonds. Catabolic reactions serve two major purposes in cells: to produce the small molecular building blocks needed to create new large molecules, and to create ATP. ATP is the energy-carrying molecule, discussed in Chapter 2, that is used in many cellular processes, especially anabolic processes.

Anabolism is the process of assembling small molecules into larger ones. Anabolic reactions generally require a source of energy to assemble large molecules. Anabolic reactions create the molecules needed for cell maintenance and for growth, and they create energy storage molecules, such as glycogen and fats, for future use. Testosterone and its chemical cousins are called *anabolic steroids* because they stimulate "building up," or *anabolic*, reactions that produce more muscle tissue, and because they are members of the steroid chemical family.

Understanding Medical Terminology

The word *metabolism* comes from a similar Greek word that means "to change." Metabolism is all about molecular changes. The Greek word has two parts: *meta*, meaning "beyond," and *bola*, meaning "to throw." So, the Greek word *meta-bola*, literally "to throw beyond," meant "to change."

The root words *cata-* and *ana-* mean "down" and "up," respectively. Therefore, *catabolism* means breaking down molecules to smaller constituents, and *anabolism* means building up large molecules. (No, anabolism is not a synonym for throwing up.) Meanwhile, *meta* has caught on as a standalone word of its own. It is generally used to mean "way out there."

Major Metabolic Pathways

Carbohydrates, fats, and proteins are the major sources of energy in the human diet. This section discusses the process by which cells make ATP from carbohydrates in moderate detail, and provides an overview of some other key metabolic processes. You may find it helpful to review the structures of these classes of molecules, which were presented in Chapter 2, before continuing.

Breakdown of Carbohydrates and Production of ATP

Carbohydrates include simple carbohydrates, which consist of one or two sugar molecules, and complex carbohydrates, which consist of many connected sugar molecules. Simple carbohydrates can be absorbed directly from the digestive tract into the blood. Complex carbohydrates must be broken down into simple carbohydrates in the digestive tract before being absorbed into the blood. This is the first stage of carbohydrate catabolism (**Figure 14.1**).

Glucose, the most abundant simple sugar in the body, is carried throughout the body by the blood, and enters the cells, where enzymes in the cytoplasm break down each glucose molecule into two pyruvate molecules. This process is called *glycolysis*. Glycolysis produces a net yield of two ATP molecules and two molecules of NADH (an energy-carrying molecule that will be used later) from every glucose molecule.

If sufficient oxygen is available, and it usually is except during periods of intense exertion or in certain illnesses, the pyruvate molecules and the NADH molecules enter mitochondria, where the remaining chemical energy is harvested. In the central region of each mitochondrion, known as the *mitochondrial matrix*, the pyruvate is first converted to acetyl coenzyme A, referred to as *acetyl-CoA*. Acetyl-CoA sits at the intersection of multiple metabolic pathways.

Acetyl-CoA is broken down in a set of reactions called the *citric acid cycle*. These reactions are also referred to as the *Krebs cycle*, or the *tricarboxylic acid cycle*. The citric acid cycle produces NADH and $FADH_2$. It also consumes oxygen and produces CO_2. The CO_2 leaves the cell, and the blood carries it to the lungs, where it is exhaled.

The NADH and $FADH_2$ from the citric acid cycle, and the NADH from glycolysis, all carry significant chemical energy in their bonds. Enzymes on the inner mitochondrial membrane use the energy from NADH and $FADH_2$ to pump hydrogen ions (H^+) into the space between the inner and outer mitochondrial membranes. These reactions are called the *electron transport chain* because electrons from NADH and $FADH_2$ are passed from one molecule to another, ultimately producing water (H_2O). Due to their high concentration and the mutual repulsion of their positive charges, the hydrogen ions in the intermembrane space have a large amount of potential energy.

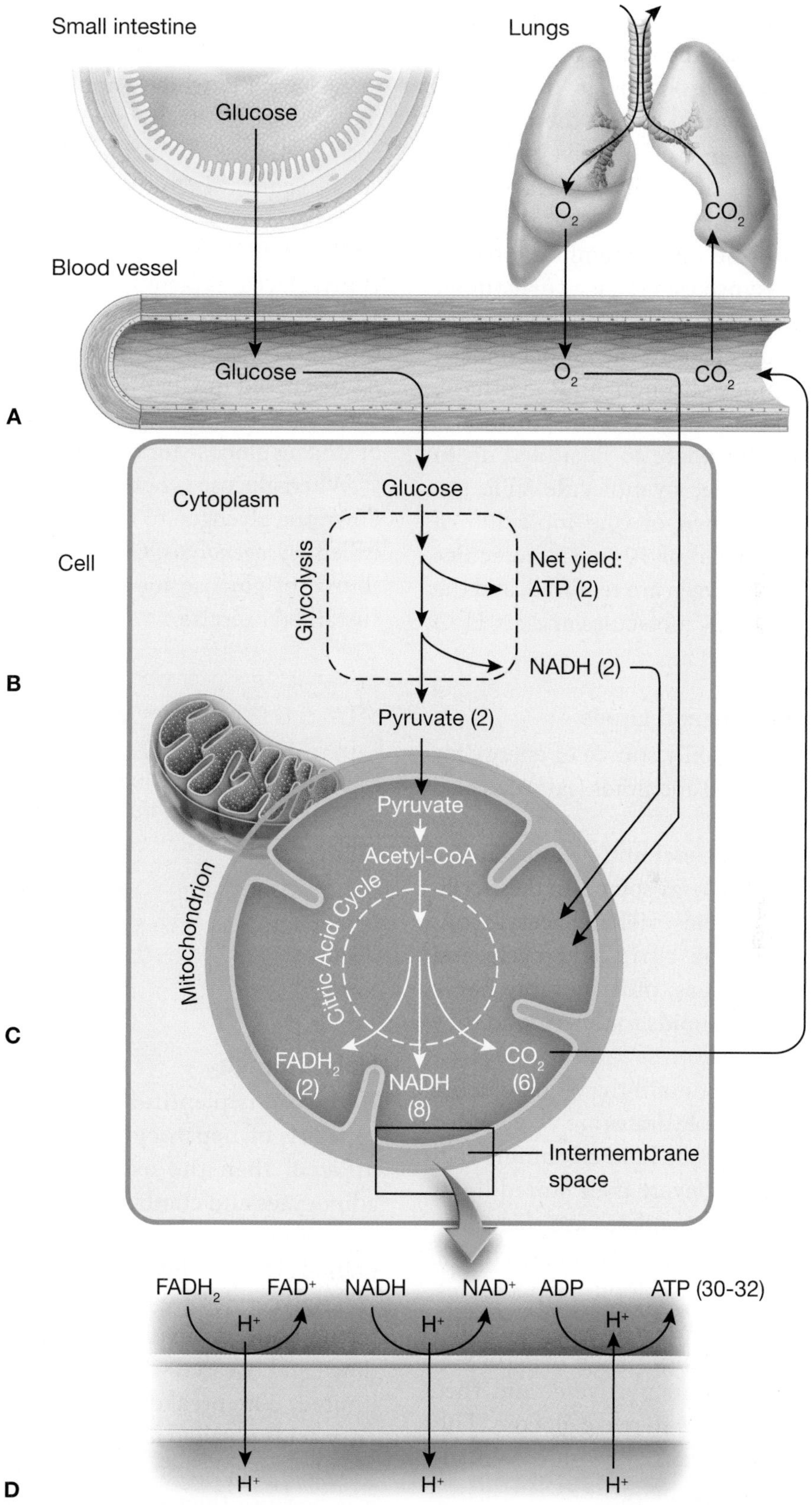

Figure 14.1 ATP production. (A) Glucose in the small intestine enters blood vessels from the small intestine and travels to the body cells. (B) Glucose enters the cytoplasm and is broken down through glycolysis, producing two pyruvate molecules, and the net yield is two ATP molecules and two NADH molecules. (C) The pyruvate and NADH molecules enter the mitochondrion, where the pyruvate molecule is converted into acetyl-CoA. Acetyl-CoA is broken down through the citric acid cycle. The resulting NADH and $FADH_2$ molecules are used to power the pumping of hydrogen ions into the intermembrane space of the mitochondrion. (D) Hydrogen ions leave the intermembrane space through ATP synthase, which produces ATP from ADP.

The high potential energy of the concentrated hydrogen ions is used in the final step of ATP production. This step is made possible by the enzyme ATP synthase. This enzyme captures the potential energy of the hydrogen ions as they leave the intermembrane space and uses that energy to make ATP. Like the electron transport chain enzymes, ATP synthase is located on the inner membrane of the mitochondrion. ATP synthase is like a turnstile: it allows hydrogen ions to pass through as they move from the intermembrane space to the mitochondrial matrix. As the ions move through ATP synthase, they force part of the synthase enzyme to rotate. This rotation causes phosphate to be added on to ADP, producing the high-energy molecule ATP.

The complete breakdown of one molecule of glucose produces a net yield of 30 to 32 molecules of ATP. Six molecules of oxygen are required, and the by-products include six CO_2 molecules and six H_2O molecules.

Energy from Amino Acids and Lipids

Carbohydrates are not the only source of energy for cells. Proteins (amino acids) and lipids (fats) can also serve as energy sources.

Some tissues, such as skeletal muscle and cardiac muscle, can use lipids as an energy source. In these cells, enzymes break down the lipids, yielding acetyl-CoA. The acetyl-CoA enters the citric acid cycle and produces ATP. Other tissues, most notably nerve tissue, cannot directly use lipids for energy, so they rely on glucose in the blood.

The body attempts to maintain the blood glucose level even when dietary carbohydrates are very limited or absent. Adipocytes, which are lipid-containing cells better known as *fat cells*, convert their stored lipids into glycerol and fatty acids, and release them into the blood. Protein in muscle cells also breaks down, releasing amino acids into the blood. Hepatocytes, or liver cells, take up amino acids, glycerol, and fatty acids from the blood. Enzymes in the hepatocytes convert the amino acids into pyruvate, and then combine glycerol and pyruvate to make glucose. This process is called *gluconeogenesis*. The glucose made in hepatocytes through gluconeogenesis is released into the blood and is carried to tissues that require it, such as the brain. In this manner, the liver keeps the glucose level normal, even during fasting.

Other enzymes in hepatocytes convert fatty acids into acetyl-CoA. Some of the acetyl-CoA is used to make ATP, which supplies the energy needs of the hepatocyte itself. The remaining acetyl-CoA is converted into chemicals that are collectively called *ketone bodies*, which enter the blood.

Carbohydrate Storage

When glucose is plentiful, the enzymes in hepatocytes and muscle cells link glucose molecules together to form glycogen. This process is called *glycogenesis*. As discussed in Chapter 2, a glycogen molecule can contain thousands of glucose molecules. This is a way of storing glucose for future use.

When glucose is not plentiful, other enzymes break down the glycogen to release glucose. This process is called *glycogenolysis*. Glycogenolysis is an important source of glucose for muscular contraction during sustained exercise.

Understanding Medical Terminology

The processes of gluconeogenesis, glycogenesis, and glycogenolysis have to do with creating and breaking down substances. The word root *gluco-* means "glucose" and *glyco-* means "glycogen." The suffix *-genesis* means "generation" or "creation," whereas the suffix *-lysis* means "breakdown." Therefore, *gluconeogenesis* is the creation of glucose, *glycogenesis* is the creation of glycogen, and *glycogenolysis* is the breakdown of glycogen.

Lipid Storage

If glucose is plentiful, and if the glycogen storage capacity of hepatocytes and muscle cells is fully utilized, then the excess glucose is taken up by adipocytes and combined with fatty acids to make a type of lipid known as *triglycerides*. This generation of lipids is called *lipogenesis*.

Triglycerides are the most abundant form of lipid in the body. As explained earlier, lipids are broken down and released when dietary sources of energy are limited. The breakdown of lipids into glycerol and fatty acids is called *lipolysis*.

When people lose fat mass by dieting or exercising, it is because they are using more energy than they are taking in through their diet. The body meets its energy needs in this situation by activating lipolysis in adipocytes.

Focus On Metabolism

You might hear someone say, "My cousin has a high metabolism, so she can eat whatever she wants, and she never gets fat." Does this statement make any physiological sense?

Well, it could be correct. The speaker is using the word *metabolism* to refer to the cousin's supposedly high basal metabolic rate (BMR). If the cousin really does have a high BMR, she would be able to consume a few more calories each day than someone with a lower BMR, without gaining weight.

If there were a drug that could increase a person's BMR, would it help the person lose weight? Yes, in fact, there are a number of drugs that increase BMR. One infamous drug is dinitrophenol, or DNP. This drug is extremely dangerous and has been illegal for human use in the United States since 1938. DNP is a mitochondrial uncoupler. It works by severing the link that normally couples pyruvate breakdown to ATP production in mitochondria. As a result, carbohydrates and fats are broken down in cells in an unsuccessful attempt to make ATP. The "wasted" energy is released as heat. Even very small doses of the drug can be fatal, due to the extremely high body temperature that results from the unproductive breakdown of cellular fuel.

It was once thought that overweight people might be overweight because their BMRs are lower than normal, which would mean they do not use as much energy as others. However, recent research suggests that overweight individuals have relatively high BMRs. Unfortunately, research on weight loss also indicates that when an overweight person loses significant weight, his or her BMR decreases, even when adjusted for the lower body mass. This is unfortunate because the decrease in BMR, or calories consumed at rest, makes it even harder to keep weight off once it is lost.

Basal Metabolic Rate

To perform metabolic activities—especially anabolic activities—the body needs energy. The amount of energy needed varies. Not surprisingly, people require more energy when they are physically active than when they are sleeping, reading, or texting (**Figure 14.2**).

Scientists use a measure called the ***basal metabolic rate (BMR)*** to identify the amount of energy required to sustain a person for one day if he or she is at complete rest. BMR is expressed as Calories per day. For example, an average adult who weighs 150 pounds (68 kg) and has a body fat percentage of 25% has a BMR of just under 1,500 Calories per day. If this

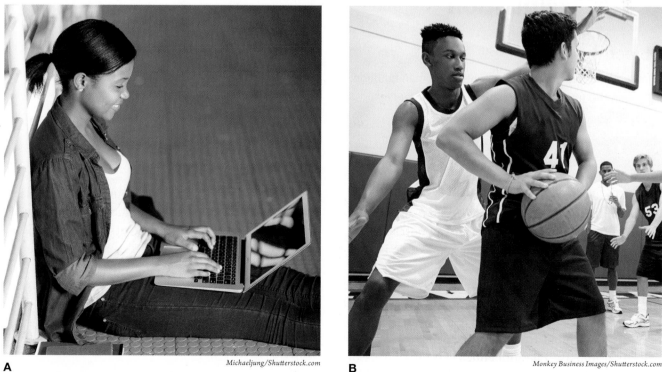

A Michaeljung/Shutterstock.com

B Monkey Business Images/Shutterstock.com

Figure 14.2 One of the factors in BMR is activity level. A—At rest, the body needs less energy, or fewer Calories. B—The body needs more energy as activity level increases.

person introduced any amount of activity into his or her day, the BMR would become higher.

BMR can differ significantly from one individual to the next. Factors that influence BMR include age, gender, height, body mass, and body fat percentage. Because few people are inactive all day, they generally require 20% to 70% more calories than indicated by the BMR. The more active they are, the more energy and calories they need. For example, the average person needs about 50 Calories more than his or her BMR to walk a mile.

SECTION 14.1 REVIEW

Mini-Glossary

anabolism process by which small molecules are assembled into larger ones

basal metabolic rate (BMR) the amount of energy required to sustain a person's metabolism for one day if he or she is at complete rest

Calorie the unit food scientists use to measure the potential energy in foods; the amount of heat required to raise the temperature of 1 kilogram of water by 1°C; also called a *kilocalorie*

catabolism process by which large molecules are broken down into smaller ones

energy the capacity of a physical system to do work

metabolism term that describes all of the chemical reactions that occur within the body's cells

Review Questions

1. List three different forms of energy.
2. What happens to the "lost" energy when energy is converted from one form to another?
3. What is the definition of *Calorie* as it pertains to food science?
4. What is the difference between anabolism and catabolism?
5. Explain what must happen to complex carbohydrates before they can be absorbed into the blood.
6. How many ATP molecules can be produced by breaking down a single molecule of glucose?
7. What is the difference between glycogenesis and glycogenolysis?
8. List the factors that affect a person's basal metabolic rate (BMR).

SECTION 14.2 Nutrition

Objectives

- Identify the roles of macronutrients on human nutrition.
- Explain the functions of vitamins and minerals in the body.

Key Terms

coenzymes
enzyme
lipids
macronutrients
micronutrients
minerals
monounsaturated fats
nutrients
polyunsaturated fats
trans-unsaturated fats
vitamin deficiency
vitamins

The human body requires many different ***nutrients*** for energy, growth, and maintenance. The two main classifications of nutrients are macronutrients and micronutrients. Water is also considered a nutrient.

The *Dietary Guidelines for Americans* is published by the United States Department of Agriculture (USDA) and the US Department of Health and Human Services, with input from advisory panels of doctors and nutritionists. The guidelines state the levels of nutrients people need to achieve a healthy diet. The 2015–2020 *Dietary Guidelines for Americans* is available online. You can also find nutrition information by visiting the USDA's Food and Nutrition Information Center online.

Macronutrients

Macronutrients are nutrients the body needs in relatively large quantities. They include carbohydrates, proteins, and lipids.

Carbohydrates

Sugars and starches are foods, or ingredients in foods, that are classified as carbohydrates. Examples of sugar include fructose, which is found in fruits, and sucrose, more commonly known as *table sugar*. Sugars occur naturally in many foods, and they are often added to food and beverages in processing and preparation. Sources of starches include pasta, bread, and cereal (**Figure 14.3**). Once it has been fully digested, 1 gram of carbohydrate provides about 4 Calories of energy.

The 2015–2020 *Dietary Guidelines for Americans* recommend that people get 45%–65% of their calories from carbohydrates. For example, a person consuming a total of 2,000 Calories a day should get about 900–1,300 Calories from carbohydrates. This would equal about 225 to 325 grams (8 to 11 ounces) of carbohydrates per day. This does not mean that you should eat only 8 to 11 ounces of food. Remember that the 8 to 11 ounces is the weight of the carbohydrates alone. This measurement does not include, for example, the food's water weight, which is a significant part of the weight of most foods.

The source of the carbohydrates is also important. Less than 10% of total calories should come from added sugars such as those found in soft drinks.

Proteins

The 2015–2020 *Dietary Guidelines for Americans* recommend that 10%–30% of Calories be derived from proteins. In a diet of 2,000 Calories per day, that translates to 50–150 grams (about two to six ounces) of protein per day. Each gram of protein provides about 4 Calories of energy.

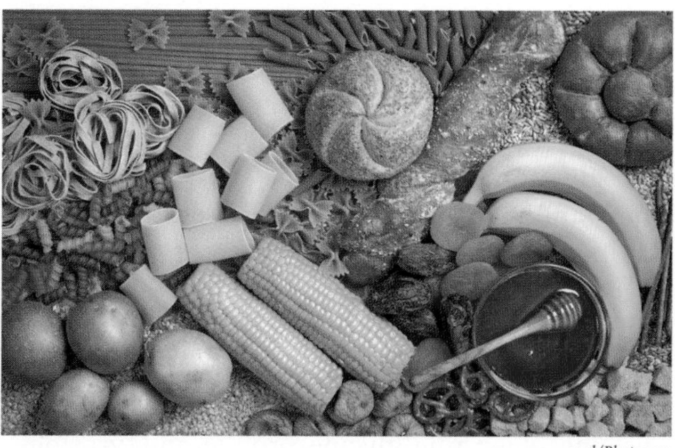

egal/Photo.com

Figure 14.3 Breads, pastas, and many vegetables are significant sources of carbohydrates.

As explained in Chapter 2, proteins are made of amino acids. Twenty amino acids are used to synthesize the proteins in the body. These amino acids are commonly classified as essential or nonessential.

Nine of the amino acids are considered essential, because the human body cannot make them in sufficient amounts, even if the other amino acids are present. These include histidine, isoleucine, leucine, lysine, methionine, phenylalanine, threonine, tryptophan, and valine. It is important to include foods that contain these amino acids in your daily intake.

Research Notes Dietary Advice

Few subjects are more contentious than dietary advice. Many people want to know the best diet for losing weight. Others want to know which diet is best for maintaining good health. From vegan to paleo, there are many different diets to choose from.

Many studies have been done comparing weight-loss diets, but the majority of these studies are not of high quality. A high-quality study has a control group, or it compares two or more alternatives, and it assigns participants randomly to different test and control groups. A high-quality dietary study follows subjects for at least 12 months and preferably more, since weight lost early in the study usually returns later. The authors, funders, and publishers of a valid study have no vested interest in the outcome.

An article in the November 2014 issue of the journal *Circulation: Cardiovascular Quality and Outcomes* reviewed 12 studies that met the above criteria and focused on four then-popular diet plans: Atkins, South Beach, Zone, and Weight Watchers. The journal concluded, "Our results suggest that all four diets are modestly efficacious for short-term weight loss, but that these benefits are not sustained long-term." They also stated, "Although North Americans spend millions of dollars in the weight loss industry, available data are conflicting and insufficient to identify one popular diet as being more beneficial than the others."

Upon hearing such results, some people decide they will just eat as much as they want of whatever foods they want. That would be a mistake, however. An editorial in the same issue of *Circulation* reviews this and other broad studies, and it concludes that although no one diet is "best," there are a few common dietary themes that correlate with longevity and relatively low incidence of chronic disease: foods direct from nature, high in fiber, and low in refined sugar, with a lot of vegetables. The influential food writer Michael Pollan summarized it succinctly: "eat food, not too much, mostly plants."

Nonessential amino acids are those that the body can produce in sufficient amounts, if the essential amino acids are present. These include alanine, arginine, asparagine, aspartic acid, cysteine, glutamic acid, glutamine, glycine, proline, serine, and tyrosine. Some amino acids that are nonessential in healthy adults may be conditionally essential in infancy (because the biosynthetic pathways are not yet sufficient to meet the high demands of rapid growth) or during certain illnesses. Those amino acids that may become conditionally essential include arginine, cysteine, glutamine, glycine, proline, and tyrosine.

Meat, which is composed mostly of protein, includes significant quantities of all 20 amino acids. However, meat is not required in order to obtain all of the essential amino acids, as long as the sources of dietary protein are varied (**Figure 14.4**). Different types of vegetables contain different amounts of essential amino acids. Combining vegetable choices judiciously allows a person eating a vegetarian diet to obtain sufficient protein, with all of the essential amino acids.

In 2015, the Dietary Guidelines Advisory Committee of the USDA reported that "higher intake of red and processed meats was identified as detrimental compared to lower intake." This does not mean people need to eliminate meat from the diet, but it does mean that most Americans eat more meat than is ideal.

Lipids

Lipids, or fats, include oils and solid fats. Fats contain combinations of different types of fatty acids, both saturated and unsaturated. Most saturated fatty acids come from animal sources, such as meats and dairy products. In addition, some oils that come from plants, such as coconut oil and palm oil, are high in saturated fatty acids.

Most unsaturated fatty acids come from plant sources. Unsaturated fatty acids are classified as ***monounsaturated fats***, ***polyunsaturated fats***, or ***trans-unsaturated fats***. Corn and soybean oils are high in polyunsaturated fatty acids (**Figure 14.5**). Canola oil and olive oil are high in monounsaturated fatty acids. The majority of trans-unsaturated fats, often called *trans fats*, are artificially produced.

Most fats that contain a high percentage of saturated and trans fats are solid at room temperature. Fats that contain a high percentage of monounsaturated and polyunsaturated fatty acids tend to be liquid at room temperature.

Many scientific studies have shown that diets high in saturated fatty acids and trans fats are unhealthy, especially for the cardiovascular system. Several studies have established the benefits of replacing saturated fats and trans fats in the diet with naturally unsaturated fats, especially monounsaturated fats.

Each gram of fat delivers about 9 Calories of energy, which is about twice as much energy per gram as

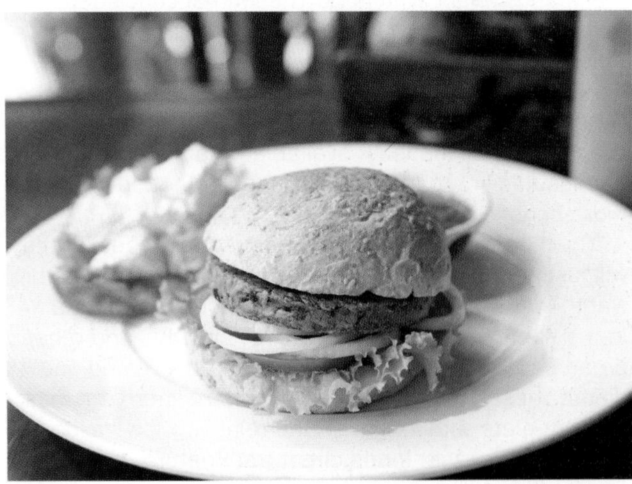

Piyato/Shutterstock.com

Figure 14.4 Although meat is a major source of dietary protein for many Americans, complete protein can also be obtained from plant sources, as in this veggie burger.

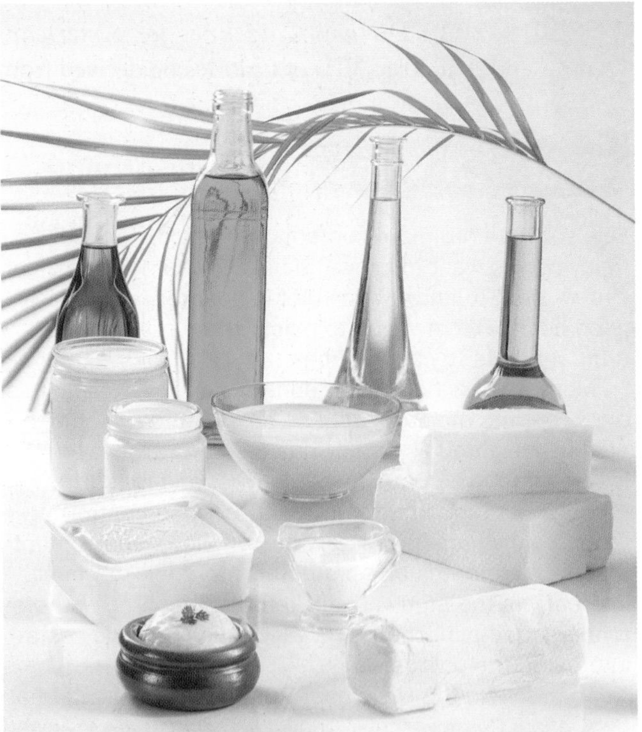

JPC-PROD/Photo.com

Figure 14.5 Oils and fats are a necessary part of a healthy diet, but they should be used sparingly.

carbohydrates or protein. The 2015–2020 *Dietary Guidelines for Americans* recommend that adults obtain 20%–35% of their total calories in the form of fats. This corresponds to about 2 to 3 ounces of fats and oils per day for a person consuming 2,000 Calories a day. The guidelines also recommend that people limit saturated fats to less than 10% of calories per day, and that they consume no trans fats, or as few as possible.

Understanding Medical Terminology

Saturated fats are called *saturated* because their hydrocarbon chains are fully loaded, or saturated, with hydrogen atoms. Unsaturated fats are not fully saturated with hydrogen atoms.

SELF CHECK

1. Which nutrients are classified as macronutrients?
2. Identify a food or ingredient that is a carbohydrate.
3. What are the building blocks of proteins?
4. What are sources of saturated fatty acids?

Micronutrients

Elements that the body needs in relatively small amounts, but are essential for the proper functioning of the body, are classified as ***micronutrients***. Two important classes of micronutrients are vitamins and minerals. Vitamins are organic compounds (carbon-based chemicals) that the body needs in small amounts to help regulate its processes. Minerals are elements, such as calcium and iron, that are required to maintain good health.

Vitamins

Vitamins are organic chemicals that are needed for metabolism to function normally. The body needs only small amounts of vitamins to achieve good health. However, the body itself produces an insufficient amount of most vitamins, so vitamins must be obtained from food (**Figure 14.6**).

Vitamins are classified as either fat-soluble or water-soluble based on substance—fat or water—in which they dissolve. A vitamin's solubility determines how the body absorbs, stores, and transports it. Fat-soluble vitamins enter the body with fats and can be stored in adipose tissue. Excess fat-soluble vitamins are not easily excreted from the body; they can be toxic, causing infection or disease.

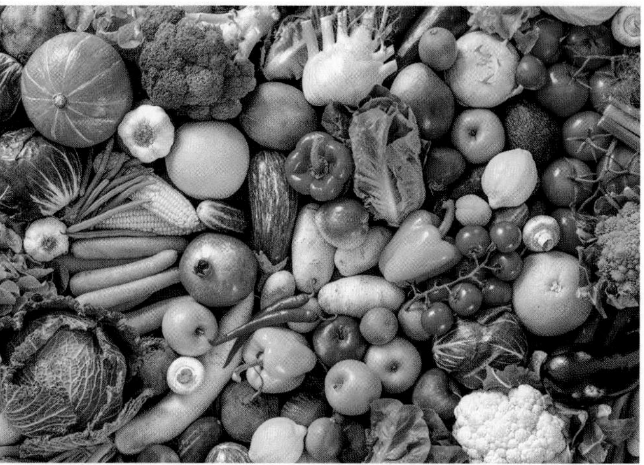

AlexRaths/Photo.com

Figure 14.6 Fruits and vegetables contain many of the vitamins and minerals that the body needs.

By contrast, fat does not play a role in the absorption of water-soluble vitamins. Water-soluble vitamins are generally not stored in the body. If a person consumes more water-soluble vitamins than are needed, the excess is expelled from the body in urine.

Most water-soluble vitamins are ***coenzymes***. A coenzyme is a molecule that combines with a protein to make a working ***enzyme*** that can catalyze a chemical reaction.

Figure 14.7 lists and describes the functions of some of the vitamins the body needs. Each person's recommended daily vitamin intake depends on age, gender, and health status. Long-term lack of a particular vitamin is called a ***vitamin deficiency***. Certain health problems are related to vitamin deficiencies. For example, a vitamin D deficiency can cause osteoporosis, muscle weakness, or high blood pressure.

Minerals

Minerals that are vital for good health include potassium, sodium, calcium, phosphorus, and iron. Potassium and sodium are key dissolved constituents in intracellular and extracellular fluids, respectively, throughout the body. Calcium and phosphorus are major components of bone. Iron is a key component of hemoglobin, the protein that transports oxygen in the blood.

The average daily recommended intake of the various minerals varies greatly. For example, about 4,700 mg of potassium is recommended each day, but only 0.0015 mg of manganese is recommended.

Micronutrients and Their Functions	
Water-Soluble Vitamins	
Thiamine (B_1)	Coenzyme that works in multiple body systems; needed for many biochemical reactions, including ATP-generating reactions; needed for the synthesis of acetylcholine, a chemical used by nervous system cells
Riboflavin (B_2)	Coenzyme that works in multiple body systems; needed for cellular reactions in eyes, skin, intestinal epithelia, and blood cells
Niacin (B_3)	Coenzyme that works in multiple body systems; needed for breakdown of fats and for skin cell metabolism
Pantothenic acid (B_5)	Coenzyme that works in multiple body systems; used in the creation of several hormones; needed for biochemical processing of carbohydrates, lipids, and amino acids
B_6	Coenzyme that works in multiple body systems; needed for chemical reactions involving amino acids (the building blocks of proteins)
Folate (Folic acid, B_9)	Needed for chemical reactions involving amino acids and nucleic acids
B_{12}	Plays a role in the formation of red blood cells and in chemical reactions involving nucleic acids (the building blocks of DNA and RNA)
Ascorbic acid (C)	Promotes protein synthesis, including collagen formation; an antioxidant that neutralizes free radicals, highly reactive chemicals that could otherwise cause damage
Fat-Soluble Vitamins	
A	Helps form a light-sensitive chemical in the eyes; helps epithelial cells grow normally
D	Aids calcium and phosphorous absorption in the intestine, and prevents loss of those elements in the urine; needed for bone growth
E	Inhibits the breakdown of cell membranes; needed for red blood cell formation and for formation of DNA and RNA; an antioxidant that neutralizes free radicals
K	Plays a major role in blood clotting
Minerals	
Calcium (Ca)	Helps form and maintain healthy bones and teeth; decreases the risk of developing some cancers; plays a role in regulation of blood pressure and immune system function
Fluoride (F)	Supports the deposition of calcium and phosphorus in bones and teeth; helps prevent cavities
Iodine (I)	A component of thyroid hormones that controls the regulation of body temperature, BMR, growth, and reproduction
Iron (Fe)	Part of hemoglobin and myoglobin, which transport oxygen in the body; component of many enzymes; essential for brain growth and function
Phosphorus (Ph)	An essential component of ATP; helps form and maintain healthy bones; helps activate and deactivate enzymes; a component of DNA and RNA
Potassium (K)	Plays a role in muscle contractions and the transmission of nerve impulses; helps regulate blood pressure
Sodium (Na)	Helps regulate water distribution and blood pressure; involved in nerve transmission and muscle function; aids in the absorption of some nutrients

Figure 14.7 *Goodheart-Willcox Publisher*

The amount of sodium that the body needs is a subject of debate in the medical and public health community. People mostly consume sodium through salt, or sodium chloride. Government health organizations recommend that most people keep their sodium intake below 1,500 mg per day. However, most Americans have diets high in salt, consuming an average of 3,400 mg of sodium each day. Many Americans frequently eat high-sodium foods, such as processed foods and meals from fast-food restaurants.

There is strong evidence that people who consume a high-sodium diet are more likely to have high blood pressure. People with high blood pressure have an increased risk of developing cardiovascular disease and having heart attacks and strokes. The scientific debate around sodium intake concerns how low sodium intake should be and whether reducing sodium intake has health benefits for people who do not have high blood pressure. The American Heart Association recommends reducing sodium intake.

SECTION 14.2 REVIEW

Mini-Glossary

coenzymes molecules that are necessary for enzyme action

enzyme a substance that catalyzes a chemical reaction

lipids substances found in foods that include oils and solid fats; can be classified as saturated or unsaturated; also called *fats*

macronutrients substances such as carbohydrates, proteins, and fats that the body requires in relatively large quantities

micronutrients substances such as vitamins and minerals that are essential to the body in small amounts

minerals elements that the body needs in relatively small amounts

monounsaturated fats one category of unsaturated fatty acids; sources include canola oil and olive oil

nutrients chemicals that the body needs for energy, growth, and maintenance

polyunsaturated fats one category of unsaturated fatty acids; sources include corn oil and soybean oil

trans-unsaturated fats one category of unsaturated fatty acids; artificially produced; also called *trans fats*

vitamin deficiency the long-term lack of a particular vitamin in one's diet; may result in certain health problems

vitamins organic chemicals needed by the body for normal functioning and good health

Review Questions

1. According to current dietary recommendations, how much of a person's energy should be obtained from protein?
2. Compare and contrast saturated and unsaturated fats.
3. What are the three classifications of unsaturated fatty acids?
4. Explain why some nutrients are called *micronutrients*.
5. Name the two classifications of vitamins.
6. List five minerals that are essential to good health.
7. Why should people limit their intake of sodium?
8. Suppose that you are a dietitian and one of your patients recently suffered a heart attack. Tests show that the patient has significant plaque buildup in his arteries. What might you recommend for this patient?

SECTION 14.3 Anatomy and Physiology of the Digestive System

Objectives

- Describe the GI tract, including the processes involved in digestion.
- Explain the functions of each organ in the digestive system.

Key Terms

absorption
alimentary canal
chemical breakdown
chyme
colon
defecation
emulsification
esophagus
gallbladder
gastrointestinal (GI) tract
gingiva
ingestion
large intestine
mechanical breakdown
propulsion
rectum
small intestine
stomach

The digestive system consists of a set of connected canals and cavities running through the body, with organs alongside it to help with the digestive process. The connected canals and cavities are collectively known as the ***alimentary canal***, or the ***gastrointestinal (GI) tract***.

Overview of the GI Tract

The GI tract begins with the mouth and ends with the anus. The primary organs of the digestive system are the structures that make up the GI tract: the mouth, pharynx, esophagus, stomach, small intestine, and large intestine.

Besides these primary organs, the digestive system includes accessory organs, such as the salivary glands, pancreas, liver, and gallbladder. These accessory organs are connected to the GI tract by ducts. The accessory organs secrete substances through the ducts that aid in chemical breakdown and absorption of food. **Figure 14.8** shows an overview of the GI tract and accessory organs of digestion.

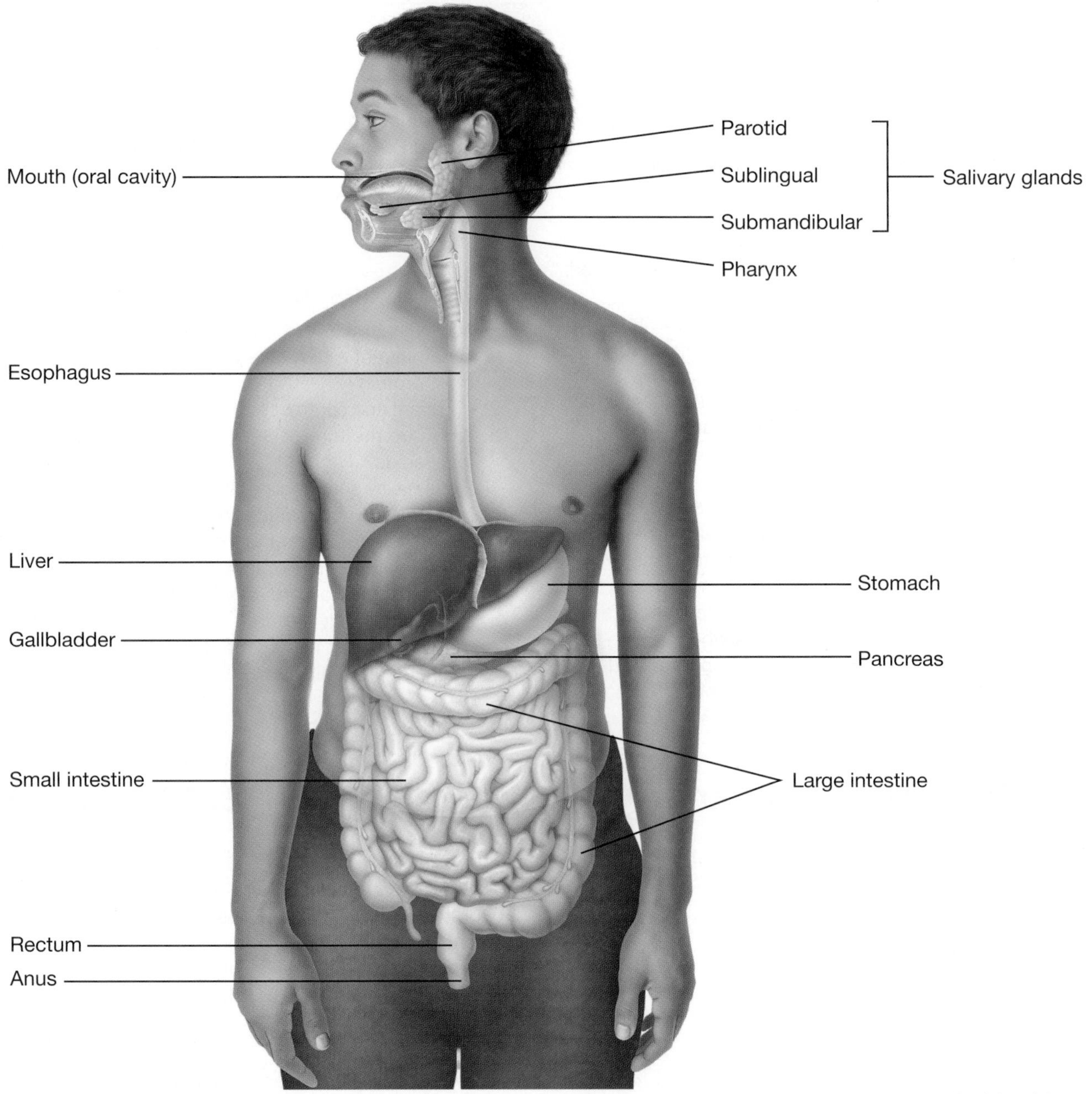

© Body Scientific International

Figure 14.8 The organs of the digestive system include those that are part of the GI tract as well as accessory organs that aid in digestion and nutrient absorption.

Layers of the GI Tract

The walls of the GI tract have four basic layers. From the inside out, the layers are the mucosa, submucosa, muscularis externa, and serosa. These layers are shown in **Figure 14.9**.

Mucosa

The mucosa, or mucous membrane, is layered as well. The mucosa has an inner layer of epithelial tissue, the surface of which is covered by mucus secreted by unicellular and multicellular glands. The mucosa also has a slightly deeper layer of areolar connective tissue. This tissue contains blood vessels, lymphatic vessels, nerves, and, in some parts of the alimentary canal, multicellular mucus-secreting glands.

Submucosa

Below the mucosa lies the submucosa, a layer of irregular, dense connective tissue that contains blood vessels, lymphatic vessels, and nerves. Lymphatic tissue and glands in some parts of the submucosa in the alimentary canal secrete substances that aid in digestion and absorption.

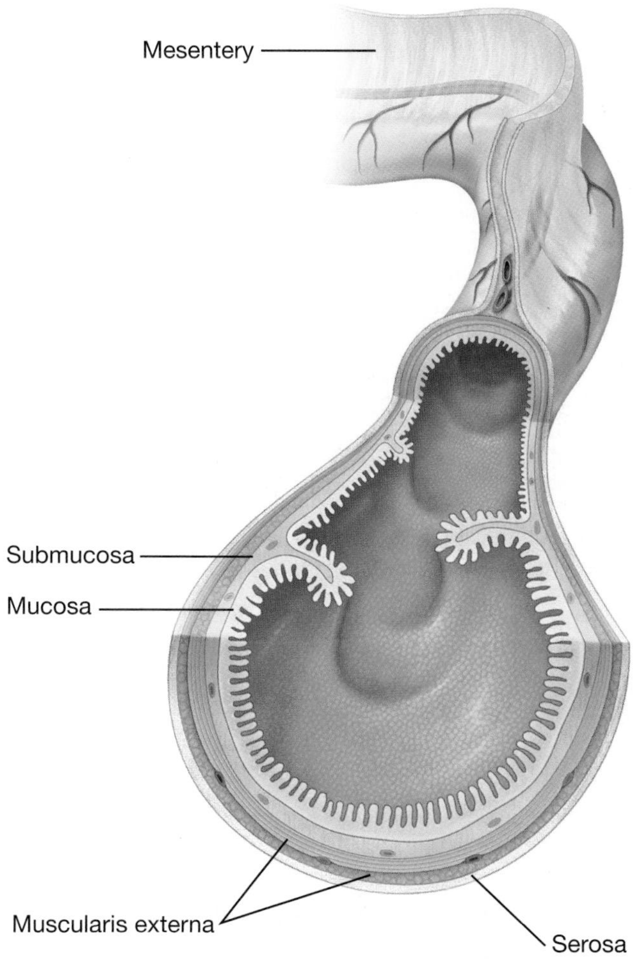

Figure 14.9 The layers of the walls of the GI tract, as seen in the small intestine. The mesentery helps ensure that the small intestine maintains its proper position as the body twists and moves.

Muscularis Externa

The muscularis externa surrounds the submucosal layer. The muscularis externa propels food through the GI tract by means of peristalsis. Mechanical breakdown of the food also occurs as the muscularis externa churns and segments the food.

In most of the GI tract, the muscularis externa has two layers of smooth muscle. The inner layer (closer to the lumen) contains fibers that run in a circular manner around the lumen of the canal. The outer layer contains fibers that run longitudinally, or lengthwise, along the canal. A layer of nerve fibers between the two muscle layers regulates the activity of each layer.

Serosa

The outermost layer of the alimentary canal is the serosa, so named because it is a serous membrane. Serous membranes are thin, slippery membranes that help minimize friction between organs and between organs and the body cavity wall.

In the abdominopelvic cavity, which contains most of the organs of digestion, the serous membrane is also known as the *peritoneum* (**Figure 14.10**). The peritoneum is divided into two layers: the parietal peritoneum and the visceral peritoneum. The parietal peritoneum is the part of the peritoneum that lines the body wall. The visceral peritoneum wraps around the organs and forms the outer layer of those organs.

The parietal and visceral peritonea are connected to each other by the mesentery, a double layer of serous membrane. Blood and lymphatic vessels and nerves travel in the mesentery between the dorsal body wall and the organs of digestion. The mesentery also helps hold the abdominopelvic organs in their proper place, particularly the small intestine.

The space between the parietal and visceral peritonea is called the *peritoneal cavity*. It is filled with a watery fluid that allows the organs to move with minimal friction. Some organs—the kidneys and pancreas, for example—lie against the dorsal wall of the abdominopelvic cavity. These organs are said to be *retroperitoneal* ("behind the peritoneum").

Activities of Digestion

The digestive process includes six different activities (**Figure 14.11**). The first activity in the process of digestion is ***ingestion***—getting the food into the body. Ingestion involves the mouth, including the teeth, lips, and tongue.

Propulsion begins after ingestion and continues all the way along the GI tract. Propulsion is initiated by swallowing at the pharynx. It continues with

Understanding Medical Terminology

When used to describe the layers of the alimentary canal walls, the word *deeper* means farther away from the lumen. The submucosa, which means "under the mucosa," is deeper than the mucosa. Thus, the submucosa is farther from the lumen than the mucosa.

A surgeon who has entered the abdominal cavity and is cutting into the GI tract first slices into the serosa, then the muscularis externa, followed by the submucosa, and finally the mucosa. After cutting the mucosa, the surgeon will have reached the lumen.

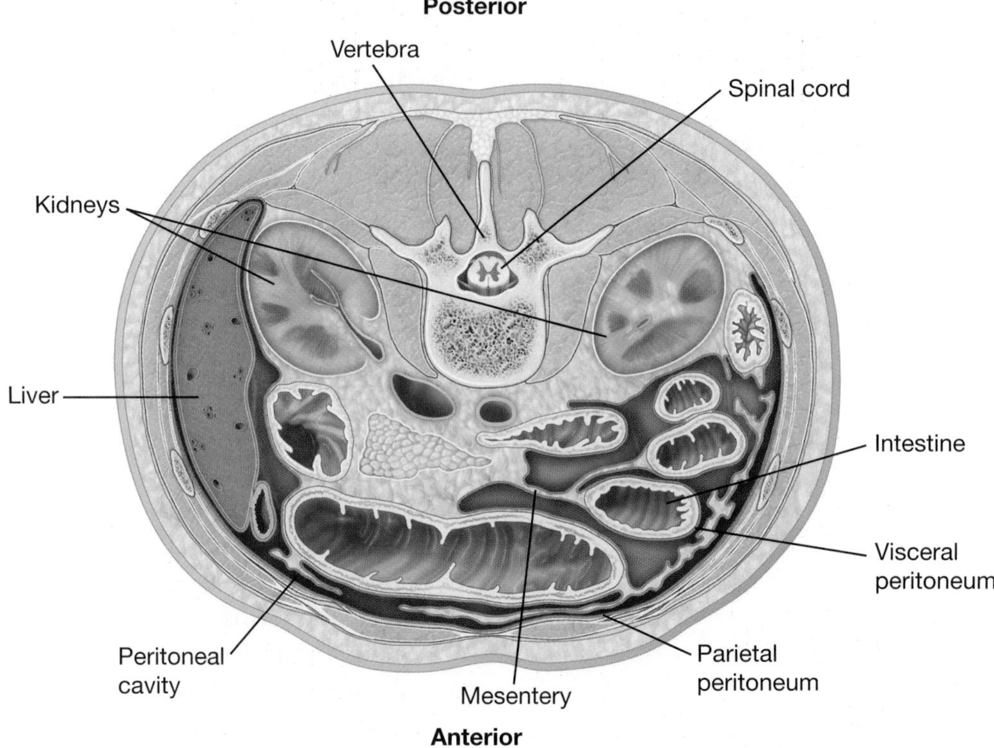

Figure 14.10 Transverse view of the abdominopelvic cavity. Some abdominal organs, such as the kidneys and pancreas, are retroperitoneal; that is, they lie behind the peritoneum.

peristalsis, the rhythmic contractions of muscles that move food along the remainder of the GI tract.

The actual digesting, or breaking down of the food particles, occurs in two ways: mechanical breakdown and chemical breakdown. ***Mechanical breakdown*** reduces food into smaller pieces and increases the surface area of the food. Chewing, churning in the stomach, and further churning by muscular contraction in the small intestine all contribute to the mechanical breakdown of food.

The ***chemical breakdown*** of food is the part of the process that has historically been referred to as *digestion*. Enzymes in the lumen—the central opening of the alimentary canal—and on the walls of the GI tract break large food molecules into smaller molecules of nutrients.

Absorption, the fifth step in digestion, involves the movement of small nutrient molecules from the lumen of the small intestine into the blood. Once absorption has occurred, the blood carries the nutrients to other parts of the body.

The final activity in the process of digestion is ***defecation***—the expulsion of the food that was not absorbed. This waste matter, known as *feces*, exits the body via the rectum and anus.

SELF CHECK

1. Starting with the innermost layer, identify the layers of the GI tract.
2. List the organs or structures of the GI tract, beginning with the mouth and ending with the anus.
3. List the accessory organs of digestion.

Understanding Medical Terminology

When used in an anatomical sense, the word *lumen* means "the open space inside a hollow tubular structure," such as an intestine or a blood vessel. At the hardware store, you will see the word *lumens* listed on a light bulb package. In this context, the number of lumens indicates the brightness of the bulb. *Lumen* is Latin for "light." If the alimentary canal is a tunnel, then it could be said that there is light at the end of the tunnel—the lumens at the end of the lumen!

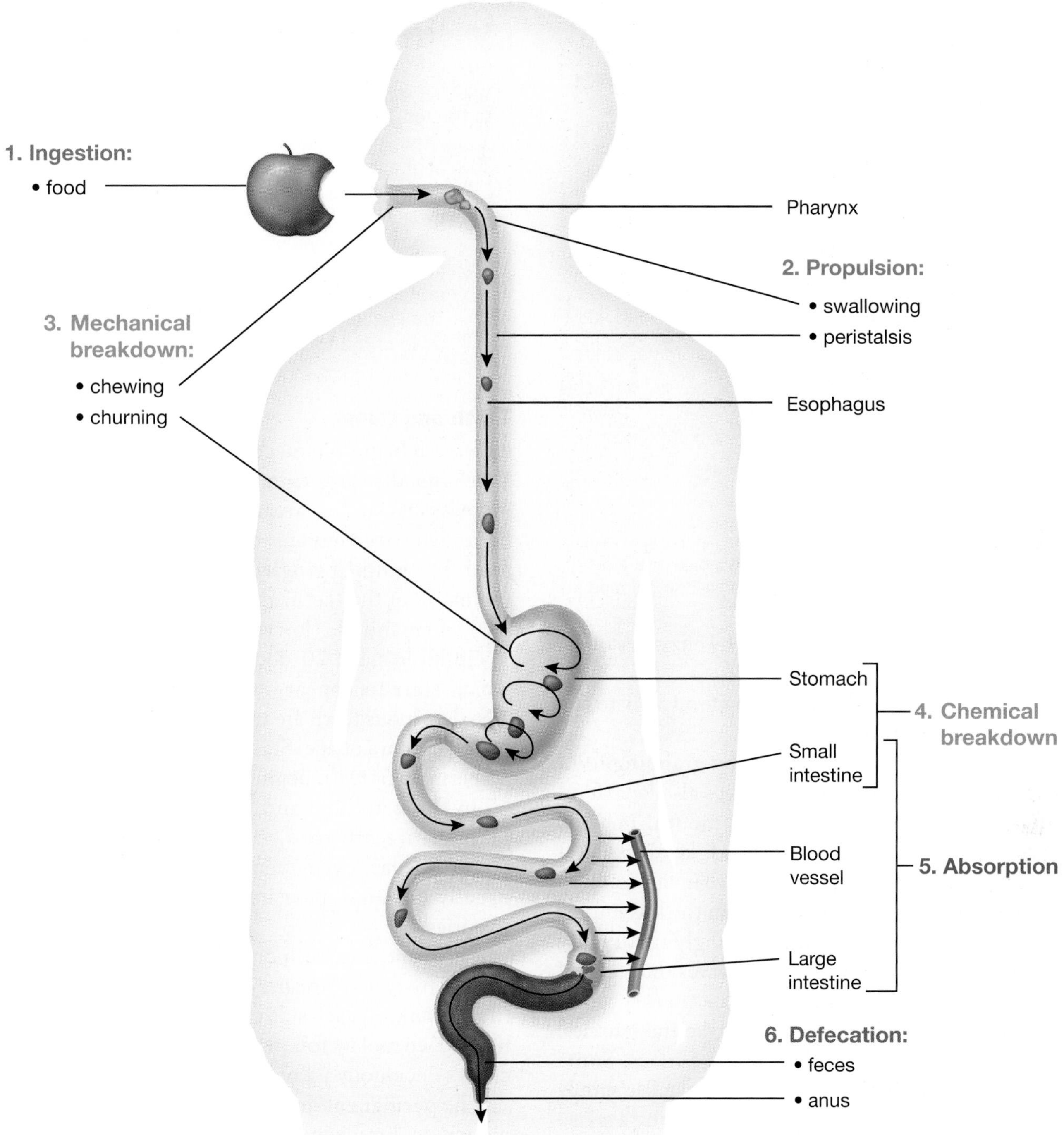

© Body Scientific International

Figure 14.11 From ingestion to defecation, digestion involves six processes.

Functions of the Digestive Organs

The digestive process involves several organs throughout the body. Some organs play a major role, while others aid in the process of digesting and absorbing nutrients.

The Oral Cavity

The mouth is also called the *oral cavity* (**Figure 14.12**). The mouth helps accomplish four of the six key activities of digestion:

- ingestion of food
- mechanical breakdown of food (by chewing)

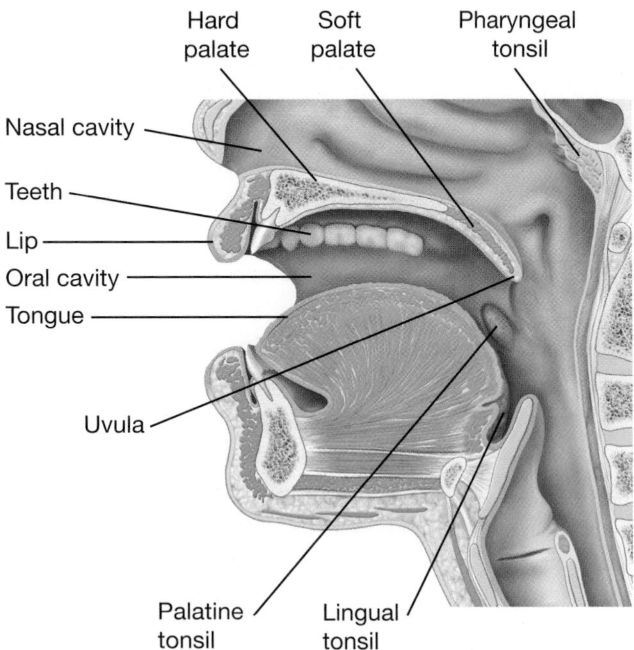

Figure 14.12 The oral cavity houses many digestive tools that begin the chemical and mechanical breakdown of food.

- chemical breakdown of food (by enzymes in the saliva)
- propulsion of food (by pushing food back to the pharynx for swallowing)

The lips assist with ingestion by grabbing food and pulling it into the mouth. The lips also keep food and liquids from leaking out of the mouth. The lips contain the *orbicularis oris* muscle. Like all skeletal muscles, the orbicularis oris is under voluntary control. Anyone who has ever lost function in the lips understands the importance of this seemingly small body part. Strokes sometimes affect the nerves that control the lip muscles, causing loss of lip function.

The tongue, like the lips, contains skeletal muscles. It also has bumps, or papillae, on its surface. Some papillae house taste buds, whereas other papillae simply help the tongue grip food. Besides providing a sense of taste, the tongue aids digestion by manipulating food in the mouth and by moving chewed food to the back of the mouth for swallowing.

The cheeks form the lateral borders of the oral cavity. The palate is the roof of the oral cavity. The front part of the palate, which is formed from parts of the maxillae and palatine bones, is called the *hard palate.* The posterior portion of the palate is called the *soft palate.* The soft palate is formed from a fold of mucous membrane. The uvula hangs from the soft palate in the back of the mouth and helps prevent food from entering the nasal cavity when you swallow.

Understanding Medical Terminology

Many structures in and around the mouth contain the root word *-glosso-* or *-lingua-*, both of which refer to the tongue:

- The hypoglossal and glossopharyngeal nerves connect to the tongue region.
- The genioglossus (JEH-nee-oh-GLAHS-us) and hyoglossus muscles form part of the tongue.
- The lingual frenulum is the thin band of tissue under the tongue that helps anchor it in the oral cavity.
- The lingual tonsil is located at the back of the base of the tongue.

Teeth and Gums

The teeth begin the mechanical breakdown of food. Mechanically breaking food into smaller pieces increases its surface area. The enlarged surface area helps digestive enzymes chemically break down the food. The gum, or ***gingiva,*** is a soft tissue that covers the necks of the teeth, as well as the maxilla (upper jaw) and mandible (lower jaw).

Children have 20 deciduous (temporary) teeth, which start to appear at around 6 months of age. The deciduous teeth are usually all visible by approximately 2 years of age. Starting around 6 years of age, 32 permanent teeth begin to form in the jawbones—16 in the mandible and 16 in the maxilla. As the permanent teeth grow, they push out the deciduous teeth. The last permanent teeth, the wisdom teeth, usually do not appear until the late teens or early twenties.

The front four teeth on the top and bottom of the mouth are called *incisors.* Just lateral and posterior to the incisors, on each side of the mouth, are the canine teeth. Two molars follow each canine and complete a child's deciduous set of teeth, or dentition.

The permanent dentition adds two premolars, or bicuspids, between the canines and the molars. A third molar (wisdom tooth) is also added to each side of the mouth (**Figure 14.13**).

The incisors are shaped to be good at cutting. The molars are good at crushing and grinding. The canines and premolars are intermediate, with the canines more adapted for cutting and the premolars more adapted for grinding and crushing.

The part of the tooth that projects out of the jawbone is called the *crown.* The part embedded in the jawbone is the *root.* The middle part, located between the crown and the root, is the *neck* (**Figure 14.14**).

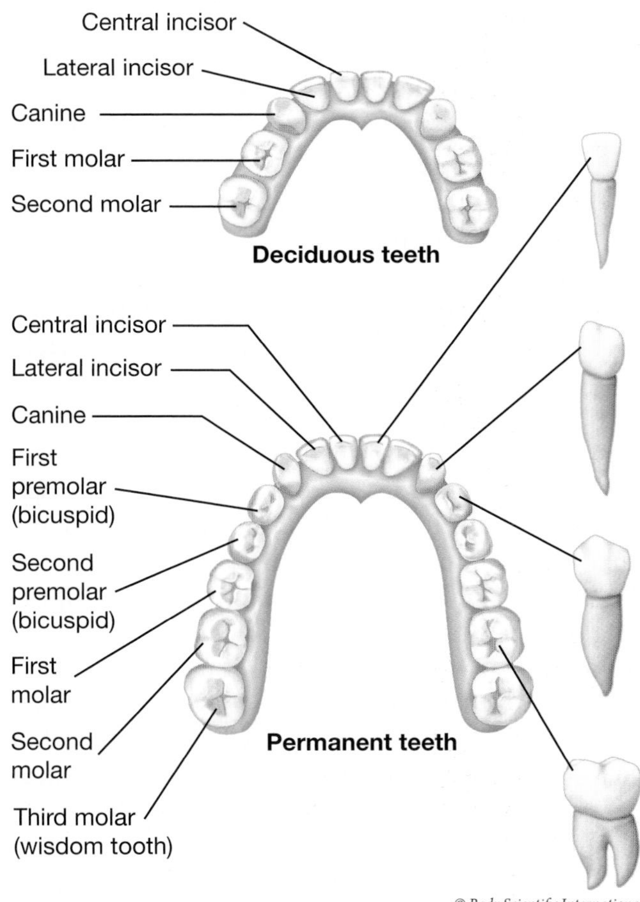

Figure 14.13 Deciduous teeth are eventually replaced by permanent teeth. The same permanent teeth appear on both the maxilla and mandible.

The crown of each tooth has a coating of enamel. Enamel is the hardest material in the body, considerably harder than bone. The body of the tooth is made of dentin, a material that is similar to, but harder and denser than, bone. The pulp cavity is a hollow central region in the tooth that contains soft tissue, nerves, and blood vessels. The hollow root canal provides a passageway for nerves and blood vessels to reach the pulp cavity from the mandible or maxilla. The nerves that occupy the pulp cavity alert you to oral pain or sensitivity by sending signals via the nervous system.

Each tooth is securely anchored in its bony socket by the periodontal ligament, a meshwork of collagen fibers surrounding the root. Each incisor and canine has a single root; each premolar has one or two roots; and each molar has two or three roots.

Salivary Glands

The first accessory organs of digestion that contribute to the chemical breakdown of food are the three pairs of salivary glands (refer again to **Figure 14.8**). The salivary glands are located within the tissues surrounding the oral cavity. They secrete saliva into the mouth via connecting ducts.

The parotid glands, the largest salivary glands, lie under the skin just below and in front of the ears. The submandibular salivary glands lie on the medial

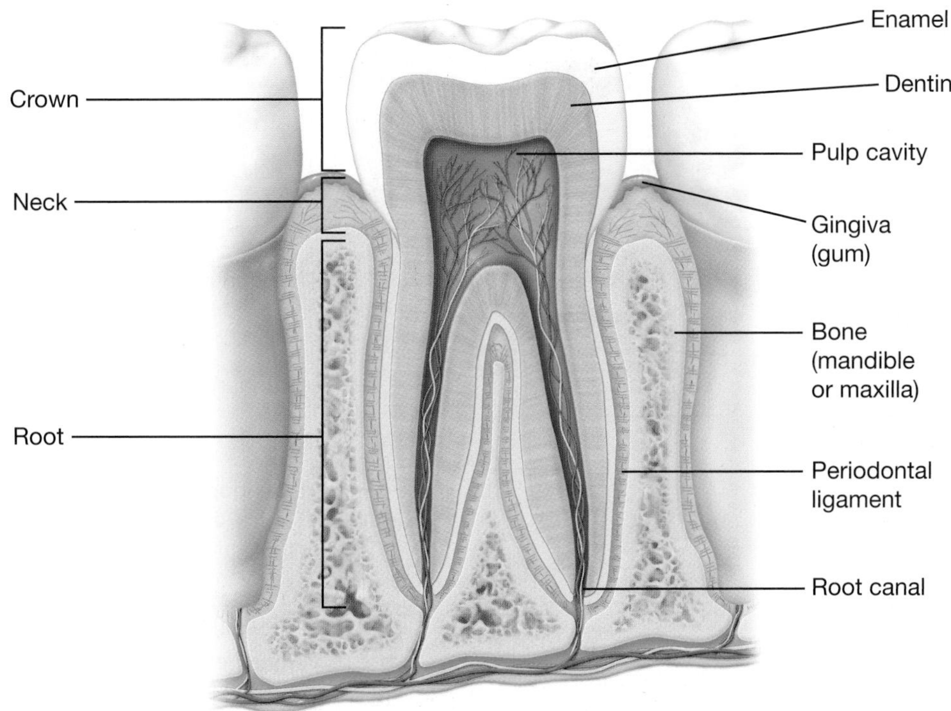

Figure 14.14 The structure of a tooth.

side of the lower back part of the mandible. The sublingual salivary glands are located under each side of the tongue.

Saliva is composed mostly of water. It also contains mucus, antibodies, and several enzymes, including salivary amylase and lingual lipase. The water and mucus help moisten and lubricate food, while the antibodies protect the mouth against bacterial infection. Salivary amylase breaks down complex carbohydrates into shorter chains of sugar subunits. Lingual lipase initiates the chemical breakdown of fats.

Understanding Medical Terminology

Many enzymes have names that end with the suffix *-ase*. These enzymes usually break down a molecule into smaller parts. *Proteases* break down proteins (long chains of amino acids) into short amino acid chains. *Lipases* break down lipids into free fatty acids and glycerol. *Amylases* break down complex carbohydrates into progressively shorter chains of sugar subunits, ultimately producing chains that are two or three subunits long.

Pharynx

The pharynx is the region that connects the mouth and nasal cavity to the trachea and the esophagus (**Figure 14.15**). The pharynx plays an important role in respiration as well as digestion. From top to bottom, the pharynx is composed of three main parts:

- The nasopharynx connects the nasal cavity to the oropharynx. Only air passes through the nasopharynx.
- The oropharynx lies at the back of the mouth. Food, liquids, and air pass through the oropharynx.
- The laryngopharynx includes the glottis—the opening to the larynx and trachea—and extends down to the top of the esophagus.

The epiglottis is a fold of tissue on the front side of the oropharynx and laryngopharynx. During the act of swallowing, coordinated contractions of the longitudinal and circular muscle layers in the walls of the pharynx push food through the pharynx and on to the esophagus. As food or liquid is swallowed, the epiglottis contracts downward to cover the glottis so that neither the food nor the liquid enters the trachea.

Figure 14.12 shows the tonsils, which are small bundles of lymphatic tissue. Like fortresses full of guards, the tonsils are full of lymphocytes that protect the body from infection. The pharyngeal tonsil, located on the posterior wall of the nasopharynx, is often referred to as the *adenoid*. A palatine tonsil lies on each side of the entrance to the oropharynx. The lingual tonsil is located at the base of the tongue, in the oropharynx.

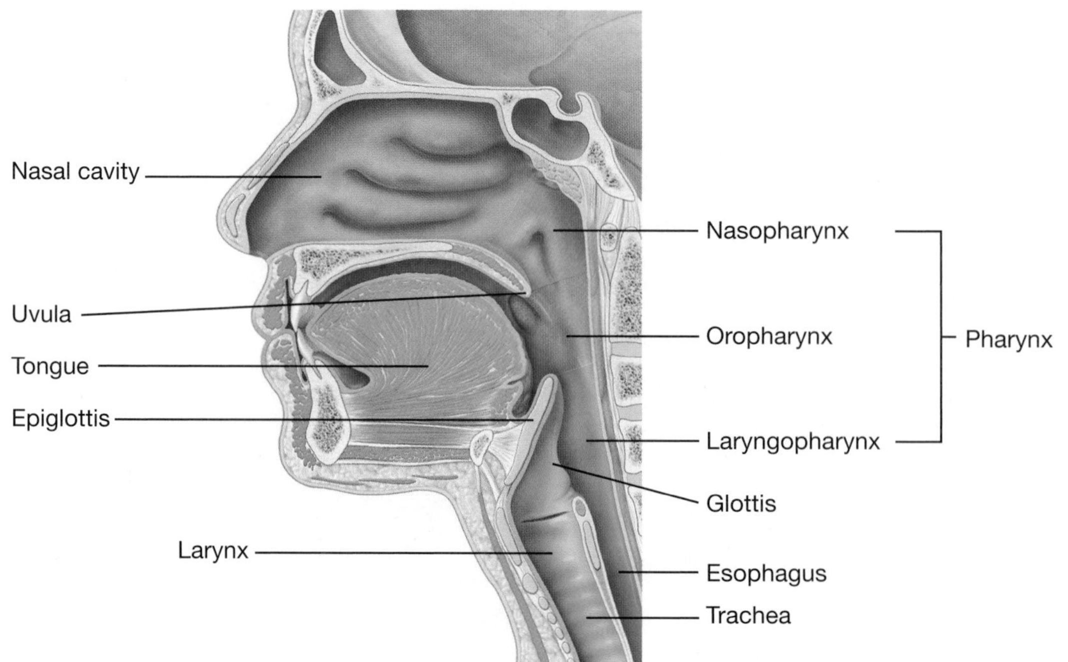

Figure 14.15 The pharynx is divided into three sections: the nasopharynx, oropharynx, and laryngopharynx.

Esophagus

The ***esophagus*** is a muscular tube that connects the pharynx to the stomach. It lies posterior to the trachea and heart and passes through an opening in the diaphragm, which is the muscle that separates the thoracic (chest) and abdominal cavities.

Just below the diaphragm, the esophagus reaches the stomach. When food enters the top of the esophagus during the act of swallowing, a wave of peristalsis begins. This wave of muscular contraction pushes food downward and into the stomach.

Stomach

The ***stomach*** is a reservoir in which food is further broken down both mechanically and chemically before it enters the small intestine (**Figure 14.16**). Major regions of the stomach include the cardia, the fundus, the body, and the pyloric region.

The cardia (a term meaning "near the heart") is the region closest to the opening of the esophagus. The fundus is the upper end of the stomach, the body is the middle part, and the pyloric region is at the lower end.

The empty stomach has an internal volume of about 50 mL (1 2/3 oz). However, the folds of the inside wall, called *rugae*, can flatten. As the stomach stretches, the rugae flatten, increasing the stomach's volume. When the rugae flatten until they almost disappear, the stomach can hold two liters or more.

Unlike most of the GI tract, which has only longitudinal and circular muscle, the wall of the stomach consists of three layers of muscle. The extra layer, called the *oblique* muscle layer because its fibers run diagonally, sits beneath the circular and longitudinal muscle layers of the stomach. The oblique muscle layer helps the stomach churn food and remains strong even when stretched.

The pylorus is the opening from the stomach into the small intestine. The wall of the pylorus contains the pyloric sphincter, a ring of circular, smooth muscle that must relax to allow food to pass into the small intestine.

Stomach Lining

The lining of the stomach is a simple columnar epithelium made of mucus-secreting cells. (For a review of columnar epithelial tissue, see Chapter 2.) A microscopic view of the stomach lining reveals millions of tiny openings called *gastric pits* (**Figure 14.17**). Each opening leads to a tubular gastric gland that secretes gastric juice. Gastric juice is also secreted as part of a parasympathetic nervous system response—seeing,

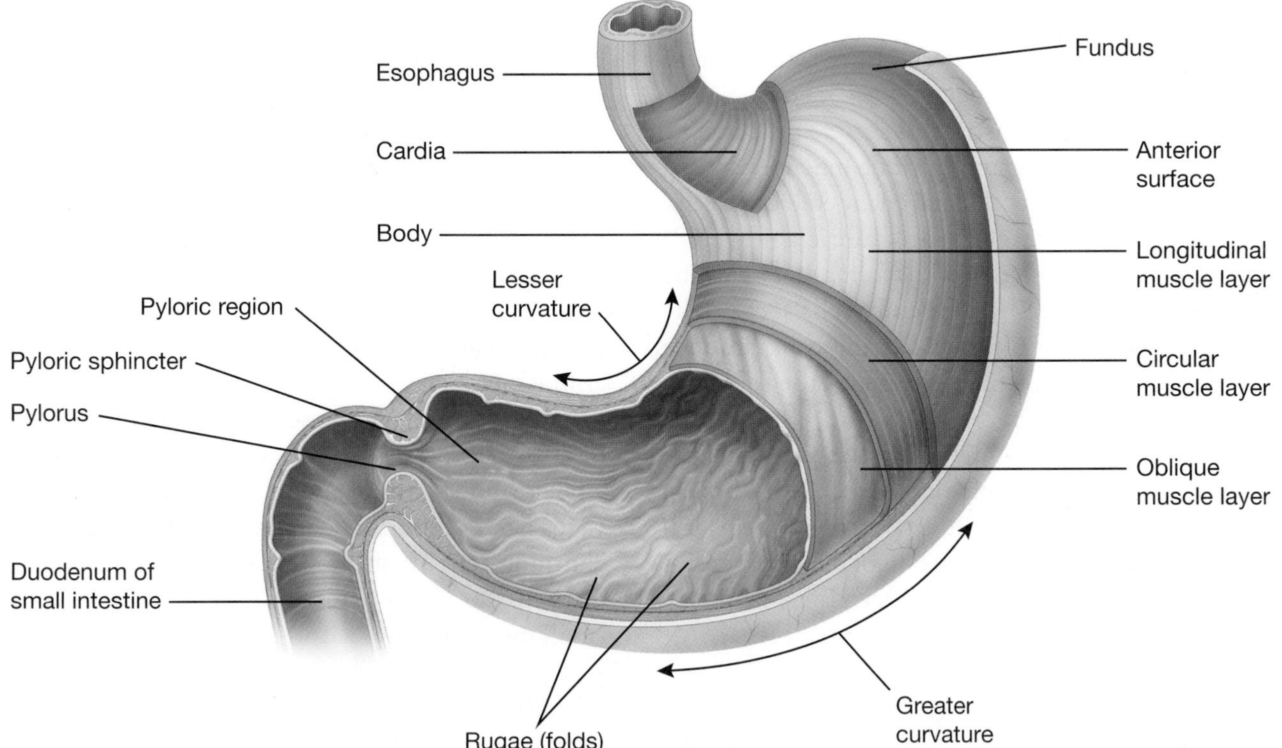

Figure 14.16 The stomach contains three layers of muscle, unlike most of the GI tract, which only has two layers.

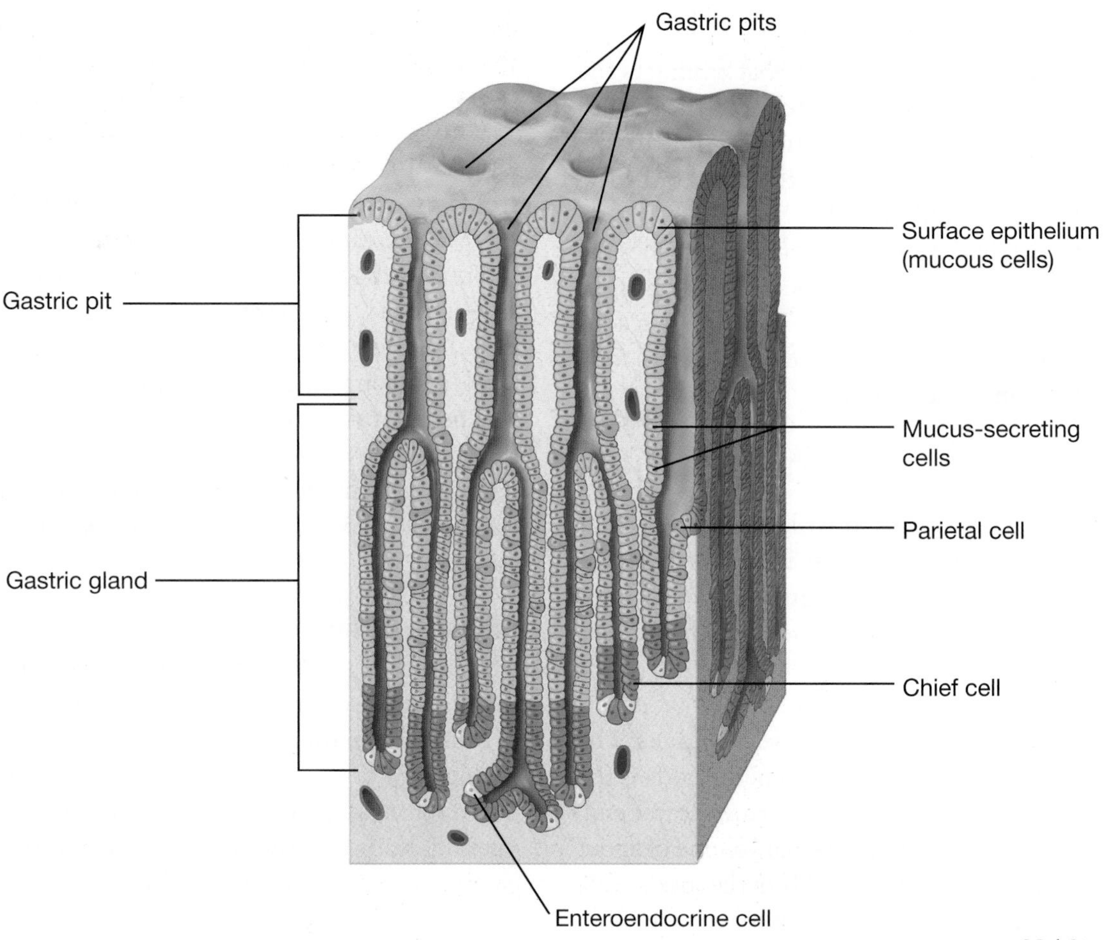

Figure 14.17 The lining of the stomach contains gastric pits and gastric glands. A gastric pit is a tubular opening in the stomach lining that connects to a deeper, tubular gastric gland.

smelling, and tasting food alerts the nervous system that digestion is about to begin.

The cells lining the gastric pits secrete mucus. The cells lining the gastric glands include mucus-secreting cells, parietal cells, chief cells, and enteroendocrine cells. The parietal cells secrete hydrochloric acid (HCl) and a glycoprotein called *intrinsic factor* that helps the body absorb vitamin B_{12}. The chief cells secrete the protein pepsinogen. Enteroendocrine cells produce the hormone gastrin, which stimulates the secretion of more gastric juice.

Hydrochloric acid secreted by the parietal cells makes the stomach contents very acidic, with a typical pH of 1.5 to 2.5. This acidic environment helps kill bacteria and aids in the conversion of inactive pepsinogen to active pepsin, a protein-digesting enzyme.

Chemical Reactions

The secretion of protein-digesting enzymes in the GI tract creates a potentially dangerous situation: the enzymes could start digesting, or breaking down, the body's own tissues. The body is able to avoid this dangerous situation as long as adequate mucus is produced. The mucus lines the stomach wall and protects it from the eroding effects of hydrochloric acid and the protein-digesting enzymes such as pepsin.

When food enters the stomach, it mixes with the acidic gastric juice to form ***chyme***. Active contractions of the muscular wall keep the mixture well stirred. Pepsin breaks down proteins in the food into shorter amino acid chains. Intrinsic factor binds to any vitamin B_{12} molecules present, enabling the vitamin to be absorbed later when it reaches the small intestine. The hormone gastrin and nerve impulses sent to the vagus nerve stimulate secretion of gastric juice and the churning activity of the stomach muscles. Relaxation of the pyloric sphincter allows chyme to enter the small intestine.

Small Intestine

The ***small intestine*** gets its name from its average diameter, which is much smaller than that of the large intestine. If intestines were named for their length, the small intestine would be called the *long* intestine. The small intestine is the longest segment of the GI tract, with a length of 4 to 6 meters (about 13–20 feet) in live patients. Most chemical breakdown of food occurs in the small intestine. It is also the site of all food absorption and most water absorption.

Segments of the Small Intestine

The small intestine has three segments: the duodenum, the jejunum, and the ileum, all shown in **Figure 14.18**. The duodenum is the first and shortest segment. It begins at the pyloric sphincter and continues for about 10 inches (about 25 centimeters).

The secretions of the liver, gallbladder, and pancreas enter the duodenum via the duodenal ampulla, a small chamber in the wall of the duodenum. The duodenal papilla, a small cone of tissue on the wall of the duodenum, contains the opening of the duodenal ampulla.

The jejunum follows the duodenum and is about 8 feet (about 2.5 meters) long. The ileum is the last and longest segment of the small intestine, measuring between 12 to 13 feet (3.5 and 4 meters) long. Chemical digestion, absorption, and propulsion by peristalsis occur in all three segments of the small intestine.

Lining of the Small Intestine

The surface area of the lining of the small intestine is greatly increased by several structural features. The inner surface of the small intestine has circular folds that are large enough to see with the unaided eye (**Figure 14.19A**). The surface of each fold is covered with finger-like projections called *villi*, and with tubular indentations called *intestinal crypts*, which are similar to the gastric pits in the stomach (**Figure 14.19B**).

Each villus (the singular form of *villi*) contains a lymphatic capillary called a *lacteal*, as well as blood capillaries. The epithelial cells of the villi have tiny, fingerlike projections on the exposed surfaces of the cells, which face the lumen of the intestine. These microscopic projections are called *microvilli* (**Figure 14.19C**). The microvilli are collectively called the *brush border* because, when viewed with a microscope, they resemble a fuzzy edge on one side of the cell.

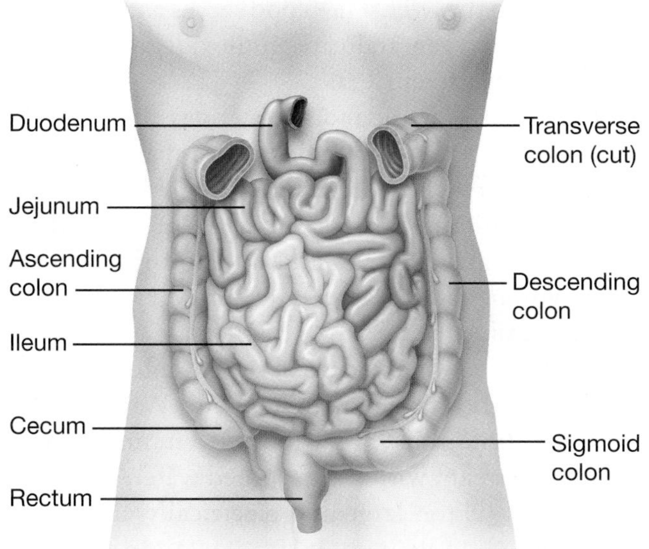

Figure 14.18 The small intestine is divided into three segments: the duodenum, jejunum, and ileum.

> **Understanding Medical Terminology**
>
> Recall that a villus is made up of many cells and has lacteal and blood capillaries in its core. A microvillus, on the other hand, is much smaller than a single cell. It contains little more than cytoplasm and a few protein filaments for stiffening. The basic cellular information in Chapter 2 may also help you remember the difference between villi and microvilli.

Chemical Breakdown in the Small Intestine

Chyme moves from the stomach into the duodenum, where it mixes with bile and pancreatic juice. Bile plays an important role in ***emulsification***, the breakdown of large fat particles into smaller, more evenly distributed particles.

Pancreatic juice contains several chemicals, including bicarbonate, pancreatic amylase, pancreatic lipase, and inactive pancreatic proteases. These chemicals break down the chyme and food particles in the duodenum. Bicarbonate is an alkaline molecule that neutralizes acidic chyme. Pancreatic amylase breaks down starches into chains that are as short as two sugar molecules (disaccharides). Pancreatic lipase breaks down lipids into their constituent fatty acids and monoglycerides. This breakdown process is facilitated by the emulsification of lipids by bile salts, which greatly increases the surface area of the lipids.

When inactive pancreatic proteases reach the duodenum, they are converted into their active forms. This happens because the pancreas, like the stomach, must avoid being digested by its own proteases. The pancreas protects itself by secreting proteases in an inactive form.

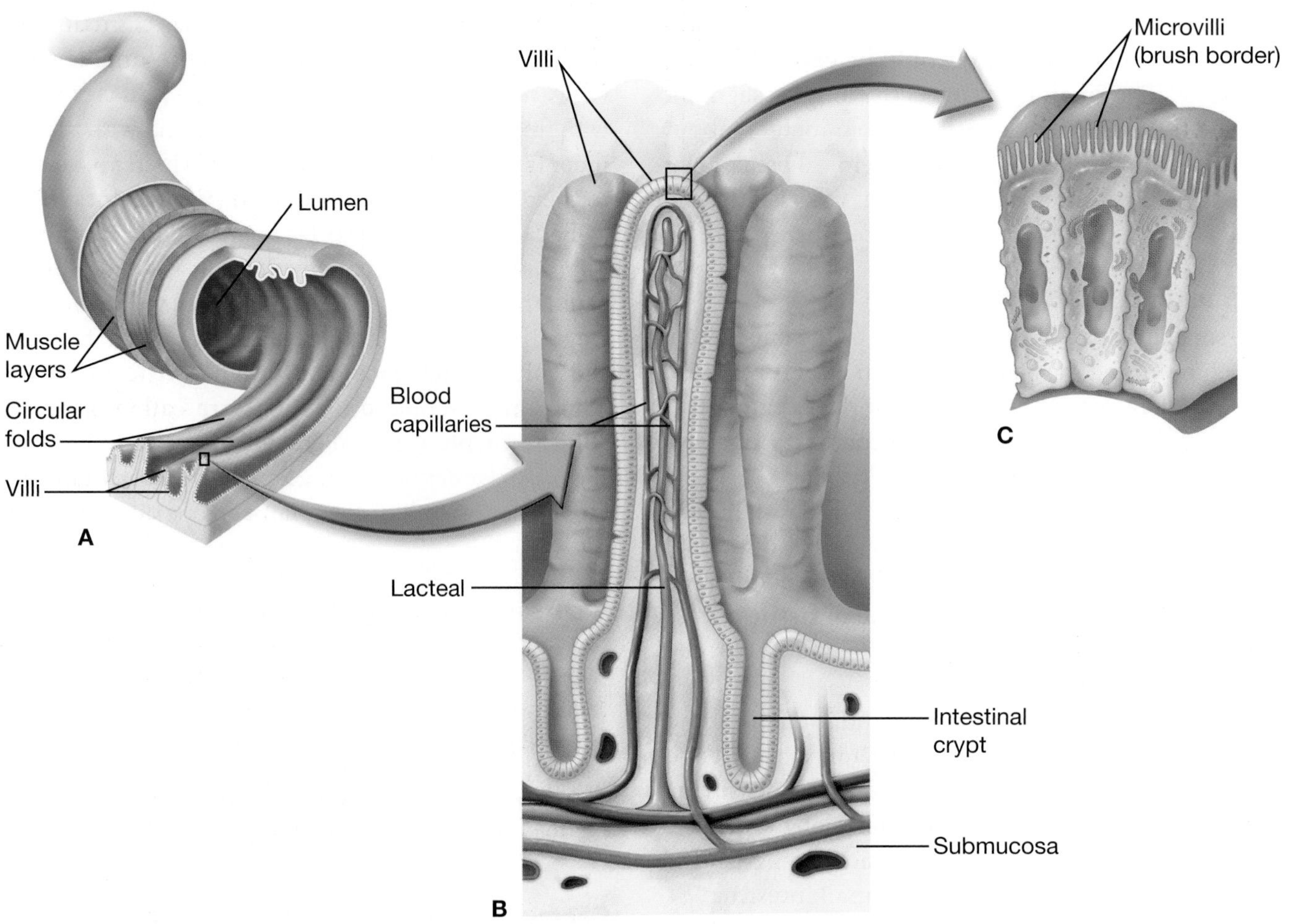

Figure 14.19 The wall of the small intestine. A—The lining of the small intestine contains circular folds. B—The surfaces of the folds are covered with villi and intestinal crypts. C—The epithelial cells covering the villi have microvilli on the part of the cell membrane that faces the lumen of the intestine.

By the time carbohydrates and proteins approach the end of the small intestine, their chemical breakdown is nearly complete. The final stage of carbohydrate and protein breakdown is performed by brush border enzymes attached to the surfaces of the microvilli. Sucrase, for example, is a brush border enzyme that breaks sucrose (table sugar) into the single sugar molecules glucose and fructose.

Absorption from the Small Intestine into the Blood

Absorption of food molecules into the blood occurs in all three segments of the small intestine. This process is enhanced by the large surface area created by the intestinal folds, villi, and microvilli.

Monosaccharides, such as glucose, and most amino acids are actively transported into the epithelial cells of the small intestine. The monosaccharides move from the epithelial cells into the blood capillaries within each villus. The blood in these capillaries, now rich in nutrients, is collected by the portal vein, which delivers the blood to the liver. The blood serves as a transport system for oxygen and carbon dioxide, and it helps the body absorb nutrients.

Free fatty acids and monoglycerides also enter the epithelial cells. The epithelial cells repackage these lipid subunits with proteins to form chylomicrons. The chylomicrons are too large to enter the blood capillaries, but they can and do enter the lacteals. The lymph in the lacteals eventually enters the bloodstream.

Most of the water that is absorbed into the blood is also absorbed in the small intestine. Water-soluble vitamins (vitamin C and most B vitamins) enter the bloodstream with the absorbed water. However, vitamin B_{12} is too large and electrically charged to be absorbed on its own. Instead, vitamin B_{12} binds to intrinsic factor, which is produced by the parietal cells of the stomach. Epithelial cells in the ileum have receptors for intrinsic factor, which enable them to actively take in the intrinsic factor-B_{12} combination. Fat-soluble vitamins (A, D, E, and K) are absorbed with lipids.

Liver and Gallbladder

The liver and the gallbladder are accessory organs of digestion. The ***gallbladder*** is the digestive organ that stores bile and delivers it to the duodenum when needed.

You can live without a gallbladder (many people do), but you cannot live without a liver. The digestive functions of the liver and gallbladder are to make bile, store it, and deliver it to the duodenum in a timely manner. The duodenum uses bile to aid in the chemical breakdown of lipids.

Figure 14.20 shows the shape and position of both the liver and the gallbladder. The liver is the largest organ, by weight, in the abdominopelvic or thoracic cavity. It lies just under the diaphragm, primarily on the right side of the body.

Functions of the Liver

Most of the liver's many functions are metabolic, which means that they are related to the synthesis and processing of various chemicals. These functions fall under the general category of maintaining a stable, healthy internal body environment—in other words, maintaining homeostasis. The specific metabolic functions of the liver include:

- maintenance of normal blood concentrations of glucose, lipids, and amino acids
- conversion of one nutrient type to another; for example, conversion of carbohydrates into lipids or amino acids into glucose
- synthesis and storage of glycogen
- secretion of cholesterol, plasma proteins (such as albumin), and clotting factors
- storage of iron, lipids, and fat-soluble vitamins
- absorption and inactivation of toxins, hormones, immunoglobulins, and drugs

Blood Supply for the Liver

The liver has an unusual blood supply. It receives oxygenated blood from the hepatic artery, which branches off the aorta. Blood leaves the liver via the hepatic vein, which drains into the inferior vena cava. These aspects of circulatory anatomy are not unusual.

What *is* unusual is that the liver also receives deoxygenated, nutrient-rich blood from the stomach

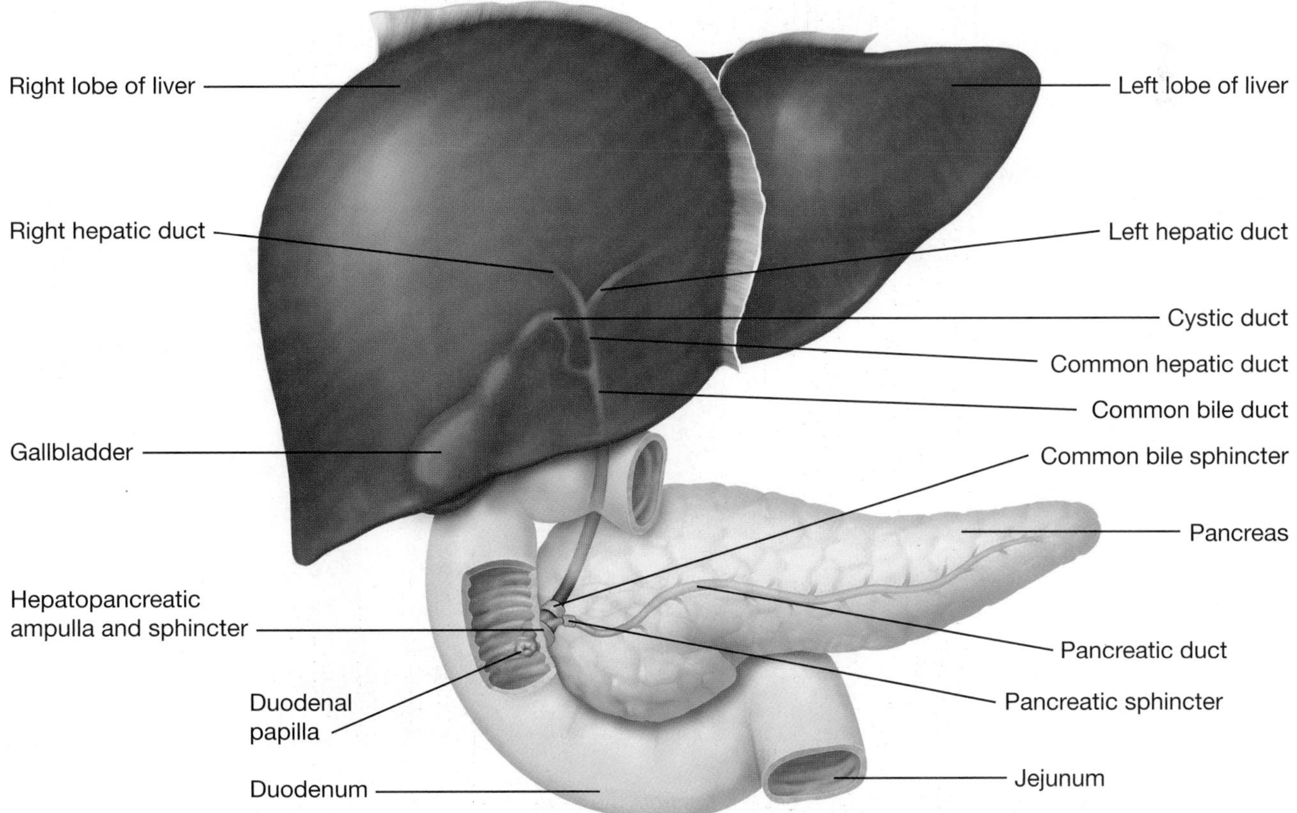

Figure 14.20 Anterior view of the liver, gallbladder, pancreas, and duodenum.

and intestines via the hepatic portal vein. This blood makes its way through the capillaries of the stomach, the small intestine, or the large intestine. In these organs, the blood loses its oxygen and absorbs whatever nutrients are present. Then it travels to the liver via the hepatic portal vein, and on through the liver capillaries.

Usually, blood goes through only one set of capillaries on its way from the arterial side of the cardiovascular system to the venous side. In this case, however, the blood goes through two sets of capillaries.

The liver capillaries, called *sinusoids,* are "leakier" than most capillaries (**Figure 14.21**). Sinusoids contain fenestrations, or holes, in their walls, and they lack a surrounding basement membrane, which is present in most capillaries. The resulting leakiness makes it easy for nutrients to diffuse from the sinusoids to the hepatocytes, and for proteins secreted by the hepatocytes to enter the sinusoids.

Hepatic portal circulation serves an important function: to deliver concentrated nutrients to the liver. Without this system, the nutrients from the stomach and intestines would be diluted, mixing with blood from the rest of the body. This would make the liver's job of processing and storing nutrients much harder.

Understanding Medical Terminology

The root word *hepato-* means "liver." *Hepatocytes* are liver cells. *Hepatitis* is an inflammation of the liver. *Hepatic* blood vessels go to and from the liver.

Portare is a Latin word meaning "to carry." *Portal* veins *carry* blood from one capillary bed to another. The hepatic portal system is by far the largest portal system in the body. There is also a tiny, but important, portal circulation system between the hypothalamus and the pituitary gland in the brain.

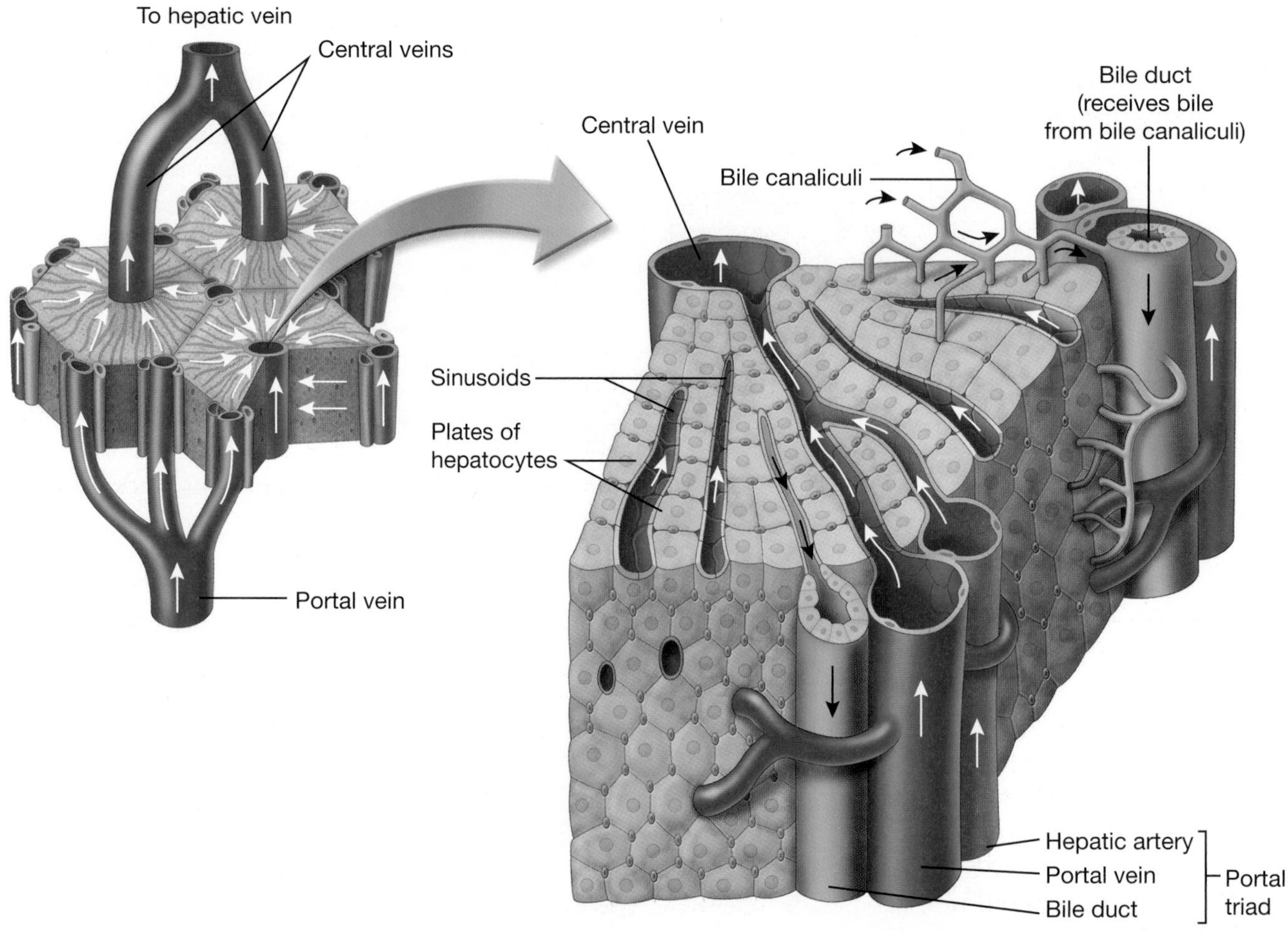

Figure 14.21 Detailed anatomy of a liver lobule. Blood flows from the triads through the sinusoids toward the central vein, as indicated by the solid white arrows. Bile produced by hepatocytes is collected in bile canaliculi and flows to the bile duct branches at the triads.

Liver Lobules

At a microscopic level, the liver is made up of a million or so functional units called *liver lobules* (**Figure 14.21**). A lobule is a fraction of an inch (about one millimeter) across. Each lobule includes hepatocytes, blood vessels, bile canaliculi ("little canals"), and ducts that collect bile.

At each corner of each liver lobule is a portal triad that consists of a bile duct, a small hepatic artery, and a small portal vein. Blood enters the lobule through the portal vein and the hepatic artery. The blood flows through the sinusoids, exchanging nutrients, oxygen, and other substances with the hepatocytes. The blood is collected in the central vein, and from there it flows to the hepatic vein. The hepatic vein carries the blood from the liver to the vena cava.

Bile

While blood is flowing rapidly from the portal triads to the central vein, bile is moving slowly in the opposite direction. Bile is a watery solution containing bile salts, which are derived from cholesterol. When bile salts combine with fat droplets in chyme, the bile salts emulsify, or break apart, the fats. Emulsification greatly increases the total surface area of fats, thus aiding their breakdown by lipases.

Bile is made and secreted by hepatocytes and then moves into the bile canaliculi, which carry it to the bile ducts at the portal triads. Small bile ducts join together to form the right and left hepatic ducts, which travel from the right and left lobes of the liver. These two ducts merge to form the common hepatic duct (**Figure 14.20**).

The common hepatic duct then joins with the cystic duct, coming from the gallbladder, to form the common bile duct. The common bile duct and the pancreatic duct meet at the wall of the duodenum to form a small chamber, the duodenal ampulla, which opens into the duodenum at the duodenal papilla.

Gallbladder

The liver makes bile at a fairly steady rate of about 1 liter per day. However, the body does not need bile at a steady rate. Bile is needed only after a meal, when there is chyme in the duodenum.

This mismatch between the liver's steady supply of bile and the body's intermittent demand for it is the reason for the gallbladder. The gallbladder stores bile and releases it after a meal that contains fat. Several sphincters work together to control bile outflow. These include the common bile sphincter, the pancreatic sphincter, and the hepatopancreatic sphincter, which encircles the duodenal papilla.

When the body's demand for bile is low, bile coming down the hepatic duct travels up the cystic duct to be stored in the hollow gallbladder. Bile stored in the gallbladder becomes somewhat more concentrated because some of its water is absorbed. When chyme—especially chyme containing a lot of fat—enters the duodenum, the muscular wall of the gallbladder contracts, squeezing out stored bile. At the same time, the common bile duct and hepatopancreatic sphincter relax, so that the bile can flow into the duodenum to emulsify the fat.

People with gallstones may have their gallbladder removed surgically. A person without a gallbladder still produces and secretes bile at a modest rate but does not get the surge of bile that is needed to help digest a particularly fatty meal. Therefore, a person without a gallbladder should avoid large, fatty meals to prevent steatorrhea, or the presence of excess fat in feces, which can cause fecal incontinence.

Pancreas

Like the liver and the gallbladder, the pancreas is an accessory organ of digestion. As **Figure 14.8** shows, the pancreas is nestled behind and underneath the stomach.

The pancreas is also part of the endocrine system, and it functions as both an endocrine and an exocrine gland. It secretes products into the blood (endocrine function) and into the lumen of the small intestine (exocrine function).

Like the liver, the pancreas has both digestive and metabolic functions. Its digestive function is to make and secrete pancreatic juices into the duodenum. Its metabolic function is to make the hormones insulin and glucagon and secrete them into the bloodstream.

Pancreatic Juices

Pancreatic juices contain digestive enzymes that break down all the major classes of nutrients: proteases, amylases, and lipases. The pancreas produces and secretes proteases in an inactive form to prevent self-digestion of the pancreas and its ducts. In the duodenum, these inactive proteases are converted into the active proteases trypsin, chymotrypsin, and carboxypeptidase. The active proteases break down proteins. Pancreatic juices also contain pancreatic amylases that break down starches and pancreatic lipases that break down lipids.

Pancreatic juices are alkaline due to the presence of bicarbonate. The bicarbonate neutralizes the hydrochloric acid in the chyme that comes from the stomach.

Glucose Regulation

The metabolic function of the pancreas is to secrete hormones that regulate the concentration of glucose in the blood. This is a classic example of hormonal regulation of the internal environment, for the purpose of maintaining homeostasis.

A high concentration of glucose in the blood causes beta cells in the pancreas to produce insulin and secrete it into the blood. The blood transports the insulin, which binds to receptors on cells throughout the body. In the liver, insulin causes hepatocytes to extract more glucose from the blood and store it by converting it to glycogen (glycogenesis). The binding of insulin to adipocytes causes greater glucose uptake and conversion of glucose into fat for storage (lipogenesis). These actions cause the concentration of glucose in the blood to fall.

Glucagon is a hormone that is made and secreted by alpha cells in the pancreas when blood glucose levels are low. Like insulin, glucagon binds to receptors on cells throughout the body. However, its effects are opposite those of insulin. Glucagon promotes conversion of glycogen to glucose (glycogenolysis) and conversion of amino acids to glucose (gluconeogenesis) in liver cells. The actions of glucagon have the overall effect of increasing the concentration of glucose in the blood.

> **Understanding Medical Terminology**
>
> To distinguish *glucagon* from terms such as *glucose* and *glycogen*, remember that "glucagon is secreted when glucose is gone."

Large Intestine and Anus

The ***large intestine*** has a larger diameter than the small intestine, but a shorter length; it measures about 5 feet (1.5 meters) when relaxed. The main functions of the large intestine are propulsion and elimination of waste. Absorption of water, electrolytes, and some vitamins are additional, but limited, functions.

A distinctive feature of the large intestine is the presence of large colonies of bacteria. These bacteria perform some helpful tasks, including synthesis of some B vitamins and vitamin K. These bacteria are usually harmless, although the smelly gas they produce, which is occasionally expelled through the anus, may be annoying.

The major segments of the large intestine are the cecum, colon, rectum, and anal canal. The anal canal terminates at the anus.

Cecum

The cecum is the first part of the large intestine to receive food from the small intestine. The end of the ileum connects to the cecum at the ileocecal valve. This valve is usually closed, but it opens in response to gastrin released by the stomach. It is also partially controlled by the nervous system. When the ileocecal valve opens, digested remnants of food travel from the ileum into the cecum.

The appendix hangs off the lowest part of the cecum and contains lymphocytes that help protect the body from infectious organisms in digested food. Unfortunately, these lymphocytes do not protect the appendix itself from blockage, inflammation, and infection—appendicitis. The treatment for appendicitis is surgical removal of the appendix.

Colon

The ***colon*** is the longest section of the large intestine. It has four major segments: the ascending, transverse, descending, and sigmoid colons. The ascending colon extends upward from the cecum to the right kidney, where it takes a 90-degree turn. Here the transverse colon begins. It crosses from right to left, and when it reaches the left edge of the abdominopelvic cavity, it turns down and becomes the descending colon. The descending colon leads to the sigmoid colon, which twists around and ends at the rectum (**Figure 14.22**).

When the digested remnants of food reach the large intestine, almost all of the extractable nutrients have been harvested. During the 12 to 24 hours that the remnants spend in the colon, additional water, some electrolytes (sodium and chloride), and water-soluble vitamins are absorbed. The colon absorbs fewer of these substances than the small intestine does.

> **Understanding Medical Terminology**
>
> *Sigma* is the name for the Greek letter S. The sigmoid colon is shaped like an S.

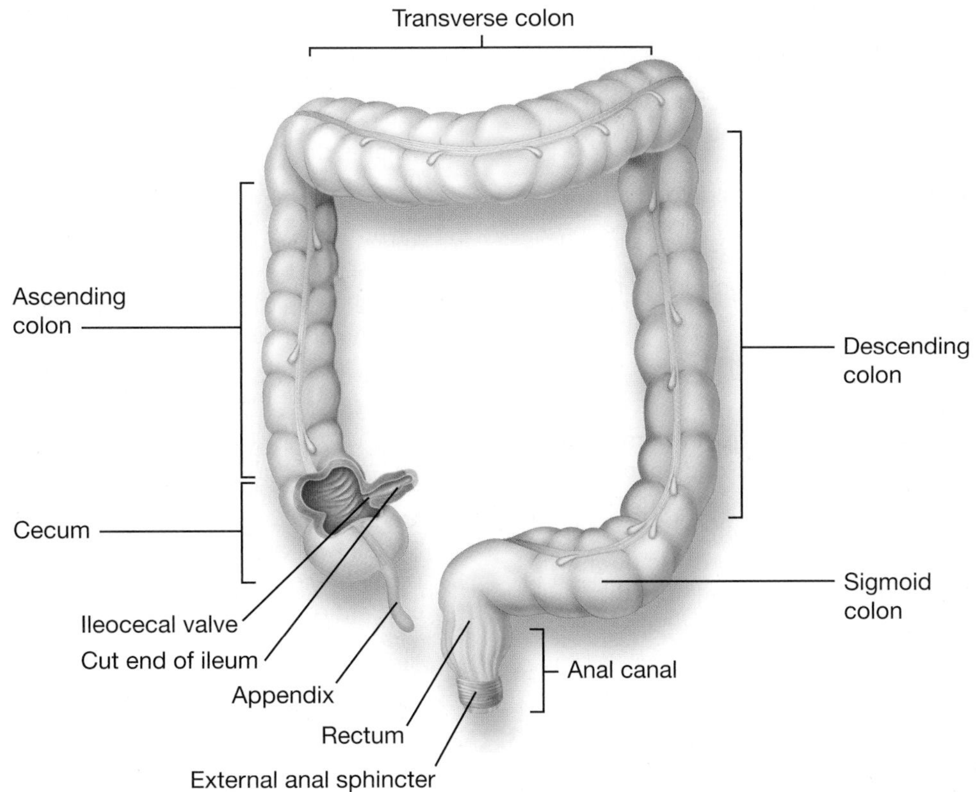

© Body Scientific International

Figure 14.22 Anterior view of the large intestine. (The small intestine has been removed for clarity in this image.)

Rectum, Anal Canal, and Anus

The final parts of the alimentary canal are the rectum and anal canal, which empties into the anus. The ***rectum*** is a short segment at the end of the sigmoid colon whose lower end comprises the anal canal. The anus is the opening to the outside world and is usually closed due to constriction of the internal and external anal sphincters. The internal anal sphincter is made of smooth muscle. The external anal sphincter is composed of skeletal muscle.

Defecation, the elimination of solid waste, begins when waste reaches the rectum. The waste stretches the rectal wall, initiating reflex contractions of muscles in the sigmoid colon and rectum. These reflex contractions push the waste toward the anus, causing the internal anal sphincter to relax. As a skeletal muscle, the external anal sphincter is under voluntary control. It relaxes when the time is appropriate, allowing defecation to occur.

SECTION 14.3 REVIEW

Mini-Glossary

absorption the movement of nutrient molecules from the small intestine into the blood

alimentary canal the connected canals and cavities that run from the mouth to the anus through the pharynx, esophagus, stomach, and intestine; also known as the *gastrointestinal tract*

chemical breakdown the breakdown of large food molecules into smaller molecules by enzymes

chyme the mixture of food and digestive juices in the stomach and duodenum

colon the longest segment of the large intestine

defecation the discharge of feces from the anus

emulsification the breakdown of large fat particles into much smaller particles, aided by bile

esophagus the muscular tube that connects the pharynx and stomach

gallbladder the digestive accessory organ that stores bile and delivers it to the duodenum when needed

gastrointestinal tract the connected canals and cavities that run from the mouth to the anus through the pharynx, esophagus, stomach, and intestine; also known as the *alimentary canal*

(continued)

gingiva the soft tissue that covers the necks of the teeth, the mandible, and the maxilla; also called the *gum*
ingestion the intake of food and liquids via the mouth
large intestine the portion of the GI tract between the small intestine and the anus; includes the cecum, colon, rectum, and anal canal
mechanical breakdown the breakdown of food into smaller pieces, thus increasing its surface area
propulsion the movement of food through the GI tract; stimulated by swallowing at the pharynx and peristalsis, muscular contractions that move food through the rest of the GI tract
rectum the short, final segment of the GI tract whose lower end is the anal canal
small intestine the portion of the GI tract where most of the chemical breakdown of food, food absorption, and water absorption occurs; the longest segment of the GI tract
stomach the reservoir in which food is broken down mechanically and chemically before it enters the small intestine

Review Questions

1. List the six activities of digestion.
2. Which four activities of digestion does the oral cavity help to accomplish?
3. What is the difference between the hard palate and the soft palate?
4. Through what structures do the salivary glands secrete saliva into the mouth?
5. What substances combine to form saliva?
6. Where in the GI tract is the pyloric sphincter located?
7. List the chemicals found in pancreatic juices.
8. What does the root word *hepato-* mean?
9. What are the main functions of the large intestine?
10. Explain the functions of the water, mucus, antibodies, and enzymes found in saliva.
11. Describe the purpose of the acidic environment in the stomach.
12. Explain why a person cannot live without a liver.
13. Describe how the pancreas regulates the concentration of glucose in the blood.

SECTION 14.4 Disorders and Diseases of the Digestive System

Objectives

- Describe common diseases of the digestive system.
- Explain how diseases and disorders of the accessory organs can affect digestion.
- Identify types of cancer that affect the GI tract.

Key Terms

cholecystectomy
constipation
Crohn's disease
diarrhea
gallstones
gastroenteritis
gastroesophageal reflux
gastroesophageal reflux disease (GERD)
hepatitis
inflammatory bowel disease
pancreatitis
peptic ulcer
periodontal disease
ulcerative colitis

Digestive ailments are some of the most common reasons that people of all ages seek medical attention. Each time you eat, you ingest nonsterile foreign material, some of which contains potential pathogens. The digestive environment itself is harsh, with strong acids and enzymes that can be very damaging. Considering the state of the digestive environment, you might expect digestive illnesses to be even more common than they are.

Diseases and Disorders of the GI Tract

Diseases of the digestive system are not limited to stomachaches. Every part of the GI tract, from the oral cavity to the anus, can be affected.

Periodontal Disease and Gingivitis

The health of the oral cavity can affect the entire body. ***Periodontal disease*** is any disease that affects the supporting structure of the teeth. Gingivitis is the most common form of periodontal disease.

Gingivitis is an inflammation of the gingiva, or gum tissue (**Figure 14.23**). Gingivitis is caused by long-term plaque accumulation on the teeth. Plaque is a sticky mixture of bacteria, food particles, and mucus that hardens to form tartar if it is not regularly removed by brushing and flossing. Buildup of plaque and bacteria activates an inflammatory response from the immune system. If not treated, gingivitis can cause damage to the jawbone around the tooth and weaken the periodontal ligament that holds the tooth in its socket. Untreated gingivitis can eventually lead to tooth loss.

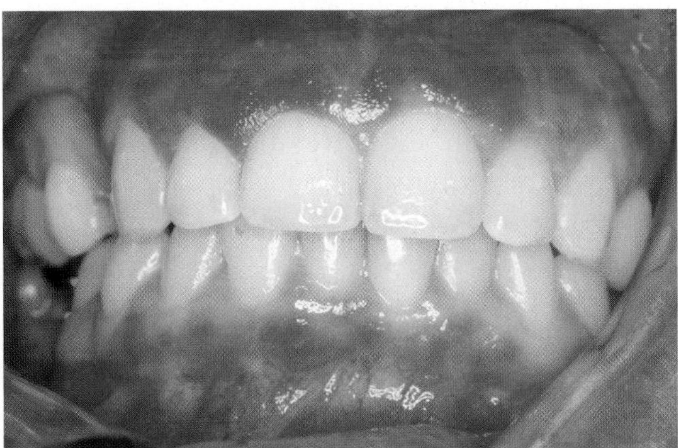

Clinical Photography, Central Manchester University Hospitals NHS Foundation Trust, UK/Science Source

Figure 14.23 Gingivitis is an inflammation of the gum tissues.

People with gingivitis are at an increased risk of developing cardiovascular disease. The inflammation of oral tissue is thought to shift the entire body into a pro-inflammatory state, increasing the likelihood of atherosclerosis, or hardening of the arteries. Gingivitis can usually be treated through professional teeth cleaning and improved oral hygiene.

Gastroesophageal Reflux Disease

Gastroesophageal reflux is the movement of chyme from the stomach into the lower esophagus. The stomach wall is protected from the harmful effects of the acids in chyme by a thick layer of mucus, but the esophagus is unprotected. As a result, gastroesophageal reflux can cause a painful burning sensation commonly known as *heartburn*, due to its location in the esophagus near the heart.

If heartburn occurs regularly, the lower esophagus can become chronically inflamed. This condition is called ***gastroesophageal reflux disease (GERD)***. Pregnancy can cause GERD because the growing uterus pushes other abdominal organs up and out of their usual positions. GERD can also be caused by a hiatal hernia, in which part of the stomach protrudes through the hiatus, or opening in the diaphragm that normally accommodates the esophagus. Obesity can also contribute to GERD.

Treatment for GERD includes eating smaller, more frequent meals. It is also wise to avoid eating before bedtime because lying down after a meal worsens symptoms. If a hiatal hernia is the cause, surgery can be performed to fix the hernia, thereby reducing GERD symptoms.

Peptic Ulcer

A ***peptic ulcer*** is a break in the protective lining of the stomach, duodenum, or lower esophagus. Ulcers can be extremely painful because the break in the lining causes the deeper structures of the body to be exposed to, and damaged by, the acidic chyme and protein-digesting enzymes.

Most cases of peptic ulcer are caused by infection from the bacterium *Helicobacter pylori*, or *H. pylori*. The name of this bacterium reflects its helical shape and its discovery in tissue samples from the pyloric region of the stomach.

The long-held belief that stress or spicy food can cause ulcers is not supported by scientific evidence. Some evidence does suggest, however, that stress or spicy food can make an existing ulcer worse. Ulcer treatment includes antibiotics to kill the infectious bacterium. Drugs that slow down the release of acid in the stomach are often prescribed to reduce the painful symptoms.

Gastroenteritis

Gastroenteritis is an inflammation of the stomach or intestine that produces some combination of nausea, vomiting, diarrhea, and abdominal pain. Gastroenteritis is often contagious and is sometimes called *stomach flu*, although it is unrelated to influenza. The most common cause of gastroenteritis in children is infection with rotavirus. The goal of treatment is to reduce symptoms through restoration of lost fluid and electrolytes, preferably through oral rehydration therapy.

Inflammatory Bowel Disease

Inflammatory bowel disease is a condition in which the walls of either the small or large intestine become chronically inflamed. Inflammatory bowel disease often results in diarrhea and pain. The cause of this condition is not clear. ***Ulcerative colitis*** is a form of inflammatory bowel disease that usually affects only the colon and the mucosal layer of the intestinal wall.

Another type of inflammatory bowel disease, ***Crohn's disease***, can affect all four layers of the digestive tract wall. Inflammation from Crohn's disease usually affects the small intestine or colon. Patients with Crohn's disease and ulcerative colitis also suffer from malabsorption of nutrients through the intestinal wall. This can result in weight loss when the illness flares up, and it may require high-calorie supplements.

Each of these inflammatory diseases is often characterized by alternating periods of pain and remission during which symptoms are mild. Treatment may include steroids to reduce inflammation during flare-ups. Lifestyle changes such as reduction of fiber in the diet also help.

Constipation and Diarrhea

Constipation and diarrhea are digestive ailments that are often symptoms of other diseases. ***Constipation***, or difficulty with defecation, usually occurs when waste spends too much time in the colon. So much water is absorbed from the waste that the remaining waste becomes nearly solid and more difficult to pass. Causes of constipation include weakness of the bowel muscle, lack of fiber in the diet, lack of exercise, and some prescription drugs.

Diarrhea is characterized by abnormally frequent, watery bowel movements. It occurs when waste does not spend enough time in the colon, where excess water would be absorbed. As a result, the waste contains more water than usual. Diarrhea also occurs when unusually large amounts of water are left in the waste despite normal travel time through the intestine.

Causes of diarrhea include dysentery (an infection of the intestines or stomach by a bacterium, virus, or parasites), food poisoning, inflammatory bowel disease, and milk consumption by a person with lactase deficiency. Lactase deficiency is the inability to break down lactose, or milk sugar. This condition is common in people who are not of European descent. Lactase deficiency causes no problems if milk and other dairy products are avoided.

Treatment for diarrhea and constipation depends on the cause. In cases of diarrhea, lost water and electrolytes may be replaced orally or by intravenous infusion.

SELF CHECK

1. What is gingivitis?
2. Which bacterium causes most peptic ulcers?
3. What effect does malabsorption have on patients with Crohn's disease?
4. What is usually the cause of constipation?

Diseases and Disorders of the Accessory Organs

Several common digestive disorders affect the digestive accessory organs. Examples include hepatitis, pancreatitis, and gallstones.

Hepatitis

Hepatitis is a disease characterized by inflammation of and damage to the liver. Hepatitis has many possible causes, treatments, and prognoses (likely outcomes). Liver damage is the common feature among all types of hepatitis.

Causes of hepatitis include viral infection, excessive use of alcohol or drugs (prescription, over-the-counter, or illegal), and poisoning (such as from certain mushrooms). Acute hepatitis, which lasts for less than six months, may allow for healing of the liver and a return to normal liver function. Unfortunately, acute hepatitis may also lead to progressive liver damage and death. Chronic hepatitis lasts longer than six months, and its symptoms are usually less severe.

At least five viruses are known to cause acute hepatitis; these are labeled *A* through *E*. Hepatitis viruses vary in severity and ease of spread. Proper hygiene is essential for preventing the spread of viral hepatitis. Vaccines are available for hepatitis A and B. New anti-viral medications can cure more than 95% of cases of hepatitis C.

Because the liver is the site of many biological and chemical processes, damage to this vital organ can cause a wide variety of symptoms. One common symptom of hepatitis is jaundice, or yellowed skin and whites of the eyes. A damaged liver is unable to discharge bilirubin, a product of red blood cell destruction, into the bile. As a result, people with hepatitis sometimes develop jaundice as bilirubin accumulates in the body.

Another symptom of hepatitis is the inability of blood to clot normally. The liver produces the clotting proteins that circulate in the blood, but a damaged liver does not produce enough of these proteins. One sign of hepatitis that is visible during laboratory analysis of blood samples is the presence of liver enzymes in the blood. These enzymes are released from dying liver cells.

Pancreatitis

Pancreatitis is an inflammation of the pancreas. It occurs when the pancreatic enzymes, especially proteases, become active while they are still in the pancreas. When this occurs, the pancreas starts to break down its own tissues, resulting in severe abdominal pain.

In the United States, most cases of pancreatitis are linked to alcoholism. There is no cure for pancreatitis. Treatment includes prescribing medication to reduce pain and replenishing lost fluids.

Occasionally, pancreatitis is caused by a gallstone that lodges in the common outflow tract of the pancreas and gallbladder. This blockage prevents the release of pancreatic juice. Eventually, the enzymes in the juice become active and start damaging the tissue.

Gallstones

Gallstones are solid crystals that form from substances in bile (**Figure 14.24**). Gallstones are usually created in the gallbladder and then become stuck in the cystic duct or common bile duct. This blockage prevents further secretion of bile, resulting in pain and an inability to digest fat.

Medications may be used to dissolve gallstones, but usually the gallbladder is removed in a procedure called a ***cholecystectomy***. This surgical procedure is often done laparoscopically (through a few small openings). After a person's gallbladder is removed, he or she should eat smaller, more frequent, and less fatty meals.

SELF CHECK

1. Why do people who have hepatitis often appear jaundiced?
2. What causes most cases of pancreatitis in the United States?
3. Which procedure is performed to remove gallstones?

Cancer

Cancers of the digestive system are among the most common forms of cancer. They can also be among the deadliest. In the United States, for example, colon cancer is the third most common cancer in men and women and the second leading cause of cancer-related deaths. Only lung cancer causes more deaths than cancers of the digestive system.

Typically, cancers of the digestive system grow slowly. In some cases, they are not detected until they have entered nearby body tissues. These cancers usually originate in the epithelial cells of the GI tract or the accessory organs of digestion. Primary tumors (tumors that are new and did not spread from another site) can arise anywhere in the digestive system. Besides colon cancer, cancers of the rectum, the mouth, and the tissues surrounding the mouth are the most common types. Cancers of the esophagus, stomach, pancreas, and liver are less common, but they have high mortality rates.

Cancers of the digestive system can be serious, but screening and early detection play a big role in improving treatment outcomes. Currently, the intestines are the only organ in the digestive system that can be screened for cancer or precancerous growths (polyps).

Colonoscopy is a common screening test for cancers of the colon and rectum. During a colonoscopy, a physician examines the entire length of the large intestine and rectum with a long, flexible scope called a *colonoscope*. A small video camera attached to the colonoscope enables the physician to take pictures or video of the colon. Instruments can be passed through the colonoscope to biopsy tissue samples, if necessary. Colonoscopies are typically done in a hospital outpatient department, clinic, or physician's office.

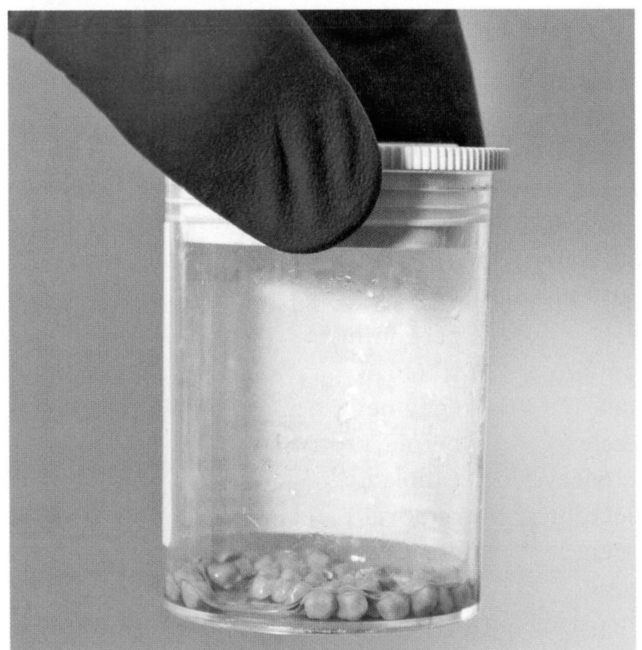

fotojog/Photo.com

Figure 14.24 Gallstones affect the ability of the gallbladder to secrete bile.

SECTION 14.4

REVIEW

Mini-Glossary

cholecystectomy surgical removal of the gallbladder
constipation a condition characterized by difficulty in defecating
Crohn's disease a chronic inflammatory bowel disease that usually affects the small intestine or colon
diarrhea the occurrence of frequent, watery bowel movements
gallstones solid crystals that form from substances in the bile of the gallbladder
gastroenteritis an inflammation of the stomach or intestine that produces some combination of nausea, vomiting, diarrhea, and abdominal pain
gastroesophageal reflux the movement of chyme from the stomach into the lower esophagus
gastroesophageal reflux disease (GERD) chronic inflammation of the esophagus caused by the regular upward flow of gastric juice from the stomach into the lower esophagus
hepatitis a disease characterized by inflammation of and damage to the liver
inflammatory bowel disease a condition in which the walls of the small and/or large intestine become chronically inflamed
pancreatitis inflammation of the pancreas
peptic ulcer a break in the lining of the stomach, duodenum, or lower esophagus
periodontal disease a disease that affects the supporting structure of the teeth and the gums
ulcerative colitis an inflammatory bowel disease that usually affects the colon and the mucosal layer of the intestinal wall

Review Questions

1. What causes gingivitis?
2. Explain why the buildup of plaque on the teeth and gums can be dangerous and potentially lead to heart disease.
3. Explain why GERD is common during pregnancy.
4. What is a hiatal hernia?
5. Why are ulcers commonly treated with antibiotics?
6. Which digestive disorder is often called *stomach flu*, although it is unrelated to influenza?
7. Explain the relationship between constipation and water absorption in the large intestine.
8. Why is pancreatitis so painful?
9. Why do people with gallstones have a difficult time digesting fat?
10. Where do most cancers of the digestive system originate?

Medical Terminology
The Digestive System

By understanding the word parts that make up medical words, you can extend your medical vocabulary. This chapter includes many of the word parts listed below. Review these word parts to be sure you understand their meanings.

-al	pertaining to
amyl/o	starch
-ase	enzyme
-cele	hernia, protrusion
cholecyst/o	gallbladder
-ectomy	removal
-genesis	creation, generation
gluc/o	glucose
hepat/o	liver
-ia	condition
-itis	inflammation
lip/o	fat, lipid
-lysis	breakdown, destruction
peri-	around, surrounding
prote/o	protein
-stalsis	contraction
ur/o	urine

Now use these word parts to form valid medical words that fit the following definitions. Some of the words are included in this chapter. Others are not. When you finish, use a medical dictionary to check your work.

1. breakdown of fats
2. condition of having sugar in the urine
3. muscular contraction around a canal such as the digestive tract
4. generation of lipids
5. enzyme that breaks down proteins
6. inflammation of the pancreas

7. enzyme that breaks down glucose and starch
8. hernia of the liver
9. pertaining to the stomach and esophagus
10. removal of the gallbladder

Chapter 14 Summary

- Energy is the ability of a physical system to do work.
- Various metabolic processes in the body provide energy using mechanisms such as anabolism and catabolism.
- Macronutrients needed by the body include carbohydrates, proteins, and fats.
- Micronutrients include vitamins and minerals and are needed in very small amounts.
- The alimentary canal, or GI tract, is a continuous series of canals and hollow organs that stretches from the oral cavity to the anus; the digestive accessory organs aid in digestion but are not part of the GI tract.
- The activities of digestion include ingestion, propulsion, mechanical breakdown, chemical breakdown, absorption, and defecation; these activities are performed at various points during the movement of food through the GI tract.
- Disorders of the GI tract include periodontal disease, gastroesophageal reflux disease, peptic ulcers, gastroenteritis, inflammatory bowel disease, constipation, and diarrhea.
- Diseases and disorders of the accessory organs include hepatitis, pancreatitis, and gallstones.
- Cancers of the digestive system organs usually originate in the epithelial cells of the GI tract or accessory digestive organs.

Chapter 14 Review

Understanding Key Concepts

1. Growing, moving, and breathing are activities that require the body to use _____.
2. Food scientists use the kilocalorie, or _____, to measure the potential energy in food.
3. The sum of all the chemical and physical reactions that occur in the body is called _____.
4. *True or False?* Catabolism refers to reactions in which small molecules are assembled into larger ones
5. In the _____ of cells, the pyruvate is converted to acetyl coenzyme A, or *acetyl-CoA.*
6. Through the process of _____, the enzymes in hepatocytes and muscle cells link glucose molecules together to form glycogen.
7. If a person's daily routine changed from an inactive to an active lifestyle, his or her BMR would _____.
   A. go up
   B. go down
   C. remain the same
   D. fluctuate
8. Which of the following foods is classified as a carbohydrate?
   A. chicken breast
   B. rice
   C. olive oil
   D. butter
9. Proteins are made up of varying amounts of 20 different _____.
   A. vitamins
   B. lipids
   C. chromosomes
   D. amino acids
10. _____ fatty acids are derived mainly from animal sources.
11. Unsaturated fatty acids may be either _____ or _____.
12. *True or False?* Fat-soluble vitamins can be stored in the body.
13. *True or False?* Water-soluble vitamins can be stored in the body.
14. The alimentary canal is also called the _____.
15. The _____ breakdown of food reduces food into smaller pieces through chewing and stomach churning.
16. The process of muscles contracting for the purpose of moving food particles along the GI tract is called _____.
    A. absorption
    B. peristalsis
    C. ingestion
    D. churning

17. Which of the following accurately lists the layers of the walls of the alimentary canal, starting from the innermost layer?
    A. submucosa, mucosa, serosa, and muscularis externa
    B. mucosa, submucosa, muscularis externa, and serosa
    C. serosa, submucosa, mucosa, and muscularis externa
    D. mucosa, serosa, submucosa, and muscularis externa
18. The mouth is also called the ______.
19. There are ______ pairs of salivary glands in the mouth.
    A. three
    B. five
    C. seven
    D. nine
20. The muscular tube that connects the pharynx to the stomach is called the ______.
    A. trachea
    B. small intestine
    C. esophagus
    D. colon
21. *True or False?* The folds in the wall of the stomach are called *rugae.*
22. The three segments of the small intestine, beginning with the segment closest to the stomach, are the ______.
    A. ileum, jejunum, and cecum
    B. duodenum, jejunum, and ileum
    C. cecum, colon, and ileum
    D. jejunum, ileum, and duodenum
23. Bile is made by the ______ in the liver and stored in the ______.
24. The purpose of bile is to emulsify ______ found in chyme.
25. The pancreas produces two hormones, insulin and ______, and secretes them into the bloodstream.
26. The four major segments of the large intestine, starting with the segment closest to the small intestine, are the ______.
    A. cecum, rectum, colon, and anal canal
    B. cecum, anal canal, rectum, and colon
    C. anal canal, rectum, colon, and cecum
    D. cecum, colon, rectum, and anal canal
27. Gingivitis is an inflammation of the ______, or gum tissue.
28. Gingivitis results from long-term buildup of ______ on the teeth.
29. Plaque is a sticky mix of bacteria, food particles, and ______ that hardens to form tartar if not removed by brushing and flossing.
30. Because of its location, GERD is commonly called ______.
31. Which bacterium causes most peptic ulcers?
32. Gastroenteritis in children is commonly caused by infection with ______.
    A. salmonella
    B. hepatitis
    C. rotavirus
    D. staphylococcus
33. ______ is a digestive disease that affects all four layers of the digestive tract wall.
    A. Inflammatory bowel disease
    B. Gastroesophageal reflux disease
    C. Crohn's disease
    D. Ulcerative colitis
34. ______ can be caused by waste spending too much time in the colon.
    A. Constipation
    B. GERD
    C. Diarrhea
    D. Ulcers
35. ______ occurs when waste does not spend enough time in the colon.
    A. Constipation
    B. GERD
    C. Diarrhea
    D. Ulcers

36. ______ is an inflammation of the pancreas.
37. ______ are solid crystals that form from bile and can block the secretion of bile into the small intestine.
38. Cancer of the digestive system organs usually originates in ______ cells of the GI tract.
    A. squamous
    B. blood
    C. nerve
    D. epithelial

Thinking Critically

39. Describe three ways in which energy can change from one type to another.
40. Explain the final step of ATP production.
41. Using what you have learned about the different kinds of fats—saturated, unsaturated, and trans fats—explain which are healthy and which are unhealthy.
42. Using what you have learned about propulsion and peristalsis in the GI tract, explain what reverse peristalsis is and what might cause it.
43. Recalling what you learned about the layers of the GI tract, why would it be important for a surgeon to know and understand these layers, particularly their order?
44. Evaluate the effect of periodontal disease on the structure and function of the cardiovascular system.
45. Why might chyme harm the esophagus but not the stomach?

Clinical Case Study

Read again the Clinical Case Study at the beginning of this chapter. Use the information provided in the chapter to answer the questions at the end of the scenario.

46. What are possible causes of Kyra's symptoms?
47. How do Kyra's physical examination and history help narrow down the likely diagnosis?
48. What treatment might the physician recommend for Kyra?

Analyzing and Evaluating Data

This bar graph from the Centers for Disease Control shows the incidence of colon cancer, by race/ethnicity and gender, in the United States in a particular year. Use the graph to answer the following questions.

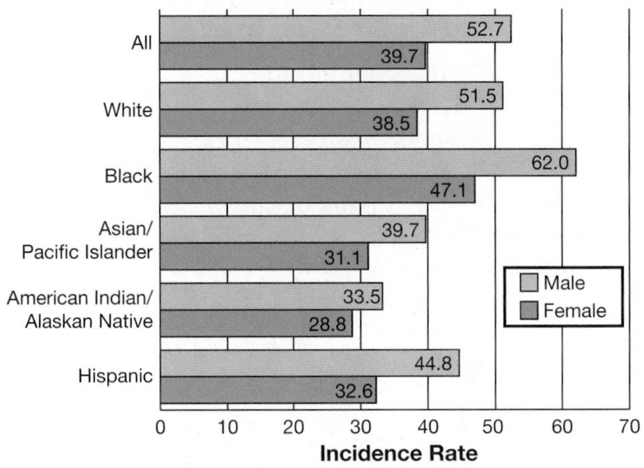

*Per 100,000 persons; age-adjusted to 2000 U.S. standard population. Not mutually exclusive from the other groups.

49. How many black females per 100,000 had colon cancer?
50. Which group had the highest incidence of colon cancer?
51. What is the difference in the number of cases of colon cancer between Hispanic males and white males per 100,000?
52. Which group had the lowest number of colon cancer diagnoses? Do some research to find out why this particular group has the lowest incidence of this disease.

Investigating Further

53. Research one of the following disorders or diseases: gingivitis, GERD, hiatal hernia, Crohn's disease, pancreatitis, or peptic ulcer. What research has been performed in the last 5 years regarding this disease, its diagnosis, or its cure?
54. Choose a disorder or disease that affects any part of the digestive system. Research special diets that may help ease the symptoms of the disease, including foods to choose or avoid, and explain why.

15 The Urinary System

Clinical Case Study

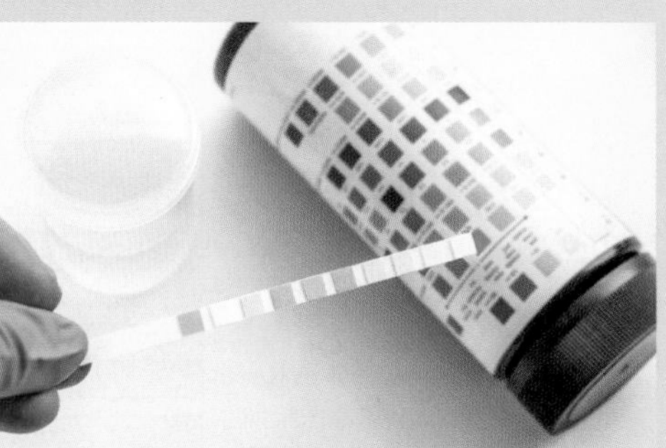
Sirirat/Shutterstock.com

Test strips are an important tool for urinalysis. The strip is dipped into the urine sample for a specified time. Separate pads on the strip indicate specific gravity, pH, protein, glucose, ketones, and other quantities. The strip is read by comparing the color of each pad to a reference chart, or by inserting it into a machine for automated evaluation.

John, age 54, has not seen a doctor in many years due to a lack of health insurance. He now has insurance, so he has come in for an initial office visit. Three days before the initial office visit, he provided blood and urine samples. Notable results from his blood and urine analyses include: fasting plasma glucose, 140 mg/dL; serum creatinine, 1.5 mg/dL; urinary albumin-to-creatinine ratio (ACR), 100 mg/g. His glomerular filtration rate (GFR), estimated from his serum creatinine level, is 50 mL/minute. Physical examination shows that John is 69 inches tall and weighs 195 pounds. His blood pressure is 168/114 and his heart rate is 75 beats per minute. He reports that he urinates eight to ten times daily. He takes Tylenol for headaches occasionally. He says he drinks beer in moderation and does not smoke.

What are some possible causes of John's test results and the findings on his physical exam? What might you conclude about John's kidney health? How do his different medical conditions relate to one another?

Chapter 15 Outline

"The urinary system eliminates chemical wastes from the body by producing and excreting urine." This statement is true, but it is impossible to capture the complexity and importance of the urinary system in a single sentence. A stable chemical environment inside the human body is essential for life and health. Just as a city must have a good waste disposal system to function effectively, the body must have a functioning urinary system. The biochemical reactions of life require watery surroundings and a stable level of salt in the body fluids. Proteins will not fold properly—and enzymes will not work—if the fluid that bathes, or surrounds, them is too salty or not salty enough.

The urinary system adapts to changing conditions so that the body's internal environment remains constant. The key organs in the urinary system are the kidneys. These two organs are remarkable for the number of tasks they accomplish. The other organs of the urinary system—two ureters, the bladder, and the urethra—are also essential, but their functions are much simpler than those of the kidneys.

This chapter explores the anatomy and physiology of each organ in the urinary system. It also covers urine formation, storage, and excretion, as well as tests of kidney function and disorders and diseases that affect the urinary system.

SECTION 15.1

The Kidney

Objectives

- Describe the basic anatomy of the kidney.
- Trace the flow of blood through the kidney.

Key Terms

collecting duct
distal convoluted tubule
glomerulus
nephron
nephron loop
proximal convoluted tubule (PCT)
renal corpuscle
renal cortex
renal medulla
renal pelvis
renal tubule
urinary system
vasa recta

In Chapter 1, homeostasis was introduced as a key concept for understanding physiology. Homeostasis is the essential ability of the body to keep various internal parameters, such as temperature, blood pressure, and pH, within their normal bounds.

The ***urinary system*** regulates the body's internal environment by controlling what leaves the body. The kidneys help maintain homeostasis more than any other organ. For example, if there is a surplus or shortage of calcium in the body, the kidneys excrete a higher or lower amount of calcium to bring the body's calcium level back to normal. The kidneys also maintain levels of many other compounds, including sodium, chloride, hydrogen ions, bicarbonate, potassium, magnesium, and phosphate. In addition, the kidneys regulate the molecule that makes up 70% of human body weight: water.

When primitive animals left the salty ocean to live on dry land hundreds of millions of years ago, they faced the threat of drying out. They also had to adapt to an environment in which they no longer had easy access to unlimited sodium and chloride. The kidneys play an important role in meeting these challenges. In a typical healthy adult, the kidneys remove wastes from about 7 liters (about 2 gallons) of blood plasma every hour. The kidneys eliminate these wastes while preventing excessive water loss, and at the same time regulate and minimize the loss of sodium and chloride in the waste fluid.

By controlling the volume of water in the body, the kidneys also control blood volume and blood pressure. They make the hormones erythropoietin and renin. They convert vitamin D to its active form. In short, no human-engineered device comes close to doing what a kidney does, especially in such a small package.

Anatomy of the Kidney

The kidneys are located on either side of the spinal column, high in the lumbar region (**Figure 15.1**). They are retroperitoneal; that is, they lie behind the peritoneum. (The prefix *retro-* means "back" or "located behind.") The two lowest ribs offer some protection to the kidneys against physical blows from behind.

Each kidney is about 4 to 5 inches (10 to 12 cm) long, 2 to 3 inches (5 to 7 cm) wide, and 3/4 to 1 inch (2 to 3 cm) thick—somewhat larger than a deck of cards. A normal, healthy kidney weighs about one-third of a pound (about 150 grams). The right kidney is usually slightly lower than the left due to the presence of the right lobe of the liver just above it. Each kidney has a convex lateral edge and a concave medial surface. The indentation on the medial surface, where blood vessels and nerves enter the kidney, is called the *renal hilum*. The kidney is usually cushioned by some fat. A small adrenal gland, an organ of the endocrine system, sits on top of each kidney.

The frontal section through the kidney shown in **Figure 15.2** shows its internal components. The lighter-colored, outer part of the kidney is called the ***renal cortex***. The darker inner part, the ***renal medulla***, is divided into renal pyramids. The "base" of each pyramid faces outward, toward the cortex. The rounded tip of the pyramid, the papilla, faces the center of the kidney. The pyramids are separated by renal columns, inward extensions of cortex-like tissue. The ***renal pelvis*** is a hollow space in the deepest part of the kidney, next to the hilum. Urine produced in the cortex and medulla seeps into the renal pelvis, which drains into the ureter, a tube that leads from the kidney to the bladder.

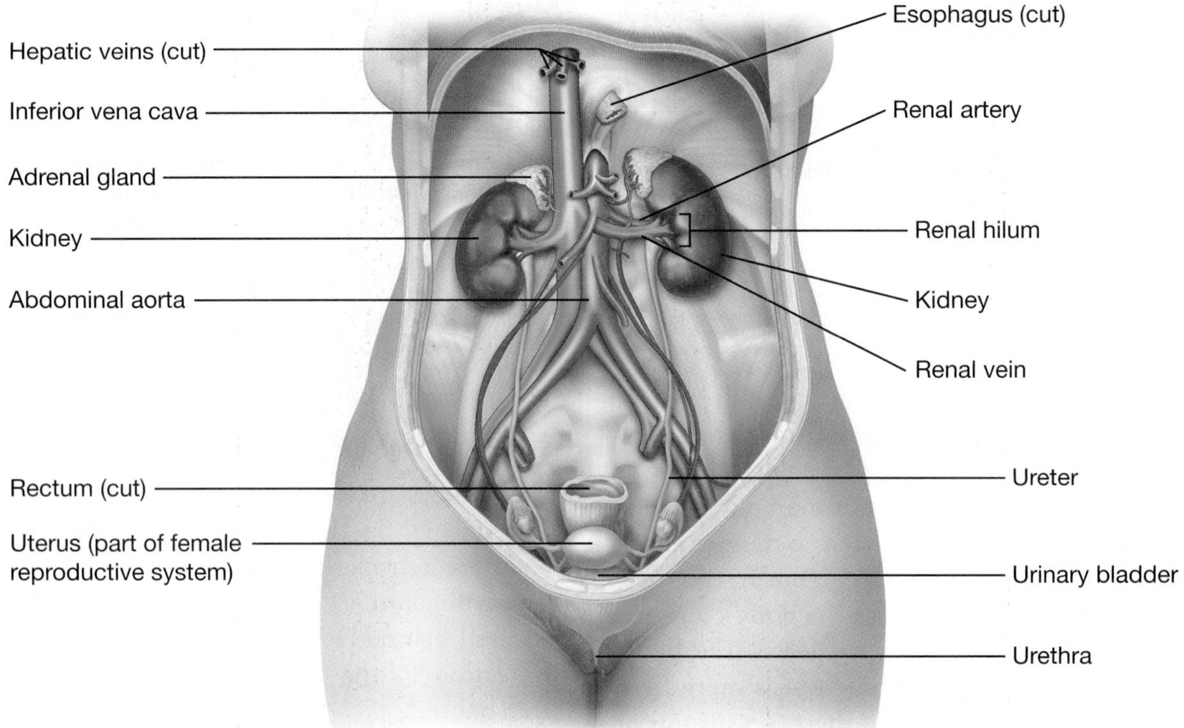

Figure 15.1 Urinary system anatomy. The kidneys lie against the posterior body wall, on either side of the spinal column.

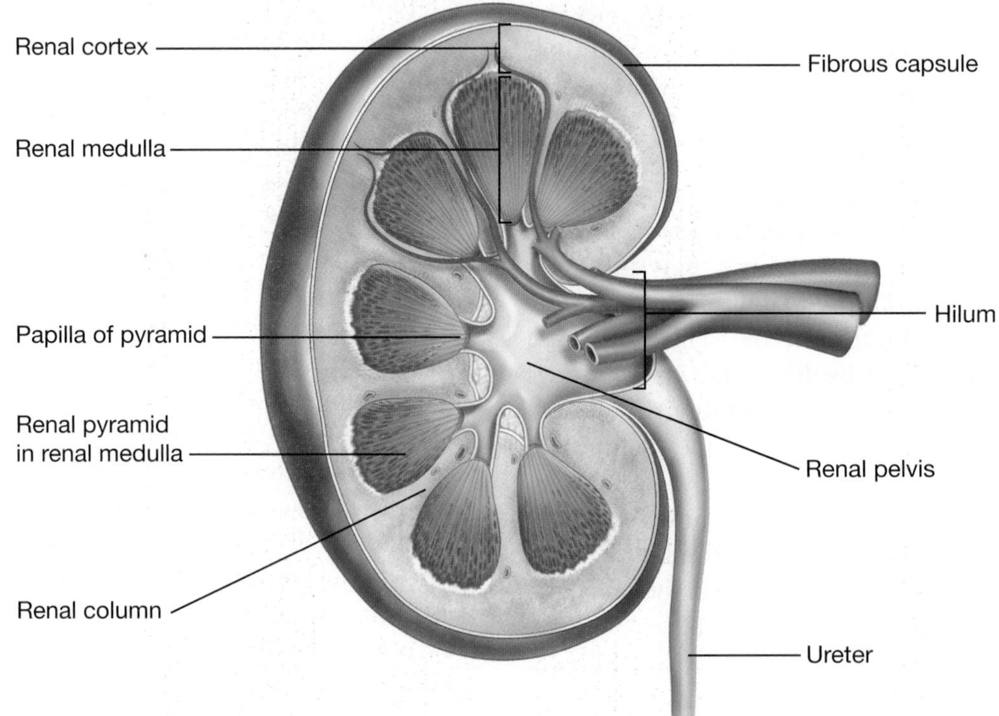

Figure 15.2 Frontal section through the right kidney. The kidney has a light-colored renal cortex around the outside and a darker renal medulla inside.

Nerve and Blood Supply

The kidneys make up about 0.5% of total body weight, but they receive 20% to 25% of the blood pumped by the heart, under resting conditions. Therefore, the kidneys have a large blood supply. The renal arteries branch off the abdominal aorta and transport blood to the kidneys. The renal veins bring blood back from the kidneys to the inferior vena cava. These blood vessels are shown in **Figure 15.1** and **Figure 15.2**.

The renal nerve fibers, which are mostly from the sympathetic division of the autonomic nervous system (Chapter 7), form an irregular mesh on the outside of the renal artery. The renal artery, vein, nerves, and ureter all connect to the kidney at the hilum.

The Nephron

The basic working unit of each kidney is the ***nephron***, shown in **Figure 15.3**. Each kidney contains about one million nephrons. Each nephron has its own blood supply and creates urine, which passes through a collecting duct to the renal pelvis. A nephron has two main parts: the ***renal corpuscle***, shown in **Figure 15.3A**, and the ***renal tubule***, shown in **Figure 15.3B**.

Focus On Normal and Abnormal Renal Anatomy

It is most common for each kidney to have one renal artery and one renal vein, as shown in **Figure 15.1** and **Figure 15.2**. However, some people have additional renal arteries or veins. About 30% of individuals have more than one renal artery for one or both kidneys, and the majority of these people never know it. It never causes any health problems. However, if a person with multiple renal arteries or veins needs surgery on or near the kidney, or an invasive kidney procedure, the abnormal renal blood vessel anatomy must be taken into account.

This illustrates an important and often neglected fact: anatomy textbooks present "typical" anatomy, but "atypical" anatomy is not uncommon. High-quality medical imaging, including CT, MRI, and ultrasound, is revealing more and more cases of abnormal anatomy. Sometimes the abnormality creates a risk; in these cases, it is prudent to treat or correct the abnormality, or institute a program of careful watching, to reduce the risk. For example, a patient who is found to have an atrial septal defect (see Chapter 12) is at higher risk of having a stroke, so the caregiver might consider putting the patient on anticoagulant drugs, or fixing the hole. Both of those approaches have risks of their own. In other cases, such as having an extra renal artery, there is no known added risk, and no treatment is necessary.

Sometimes it is not clear whether or not an abnormal finding requires further investigation and treatment. In such cases, the care provider must decide whether the expense and risk to the patient of further testing and treatment is justified. It is understandable that care providers are likely to err on the side of overtreatment, because they want to ensure patient safety, because they underestimate the risks associated with additional treatment, and sometimes because they do not want to get sued for "not doing enough."

The "horseshoe kidney" and the solitary kidney are other interesting examples of renal anatomical abnormalities. A horseshoe kidney, which forms during embryonic development, is two kidneys connected at their lower ends to form a single U-shaped organ. This developmental abnormality, whose estimated prevalence is 1 in every 400 to 800 live births, is associated with increased risk of blockage of the ureters and other problems. About one person in five hundred is born with only one functioning kidney: the solitary kidney. Regular testing is recommended for patients with a horseshoe kidney or a solitary kidney, even if they are not experiencing symptoms, since both conditions are associated with increased risk of renal disorders.

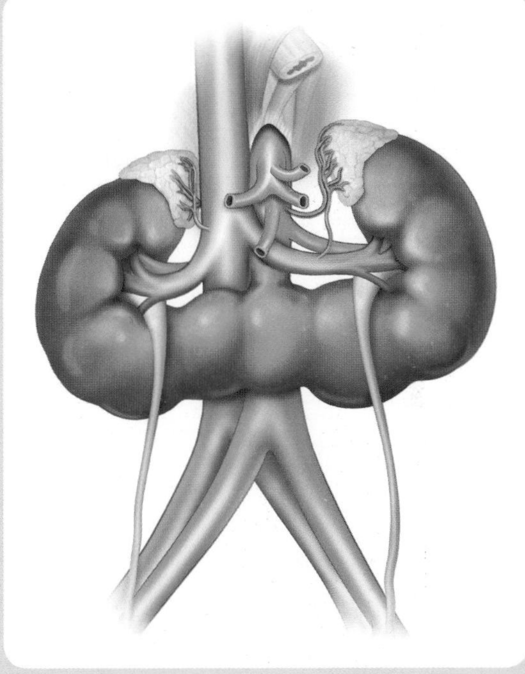

A horseshoe kidney consists of two kidneys connected at their lower ends.

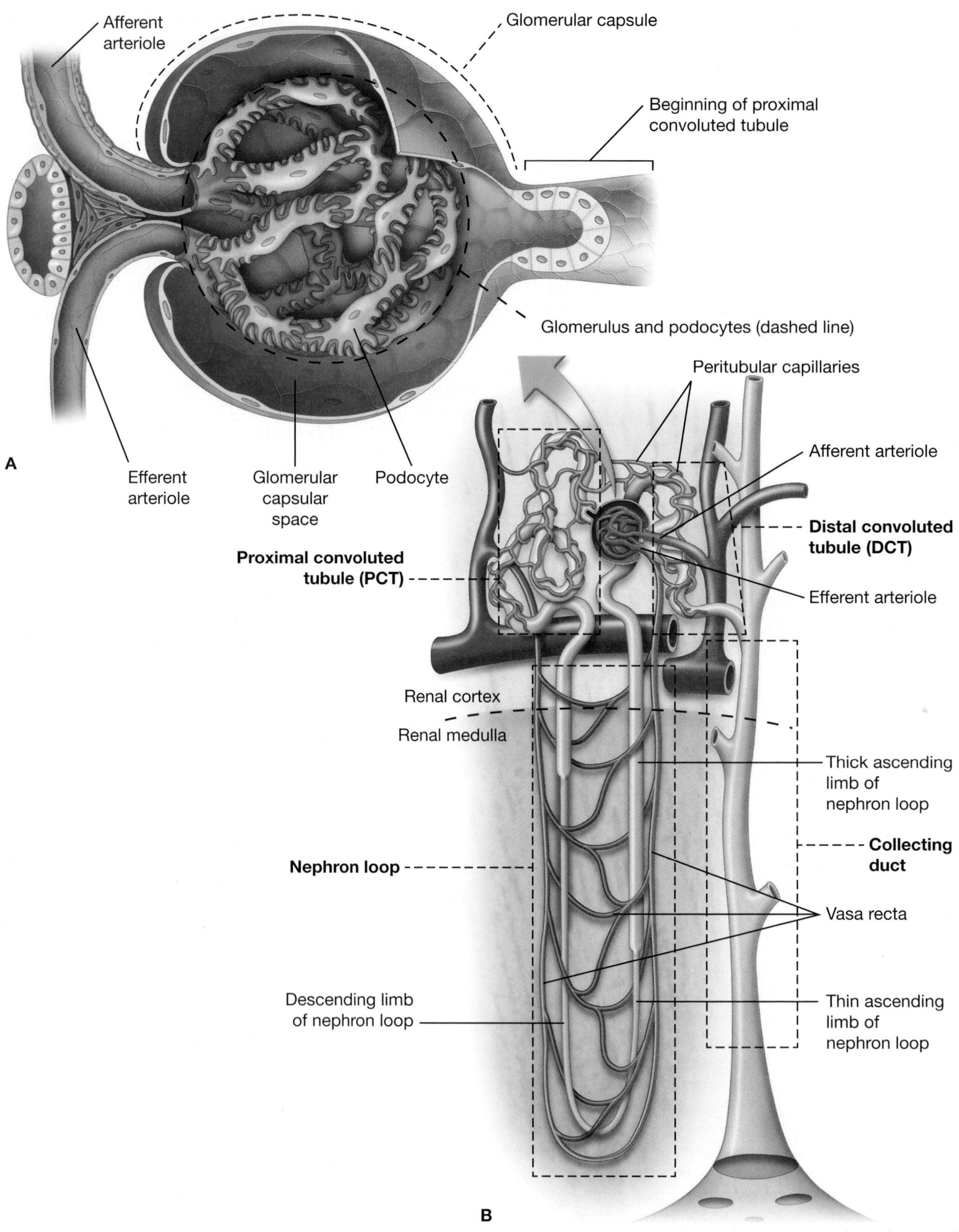

Figure 15.3 Structure of a nephron. A—Renal corpuscle. B—Renal tubule and surrounding capillaries. The renal tubule includes the proximal convoluted tubule, the nephron loop, and the distal convoluted tubule.

The renal corpuscle has a cluster of capillaries called the ***glomerulus*** and a surrounding, cuplike glomerular capsule. Blood enters the glomerulus through an afferent arteriole, passes through the "ball" of capillaries, and exits via the efferent arteriole.

Understanding Medical Terminology

Afferent comes from the Latin verb phrase *ad ferro*, which means "to carry toward." *Efferent* comes from the Latin *ex ferro*, which means "to carry away." The word *ferry* has the same origin.

The glomerular capsule has an outer surface and an inner surface, and a hollow space in between called the *glomerular capsular space*. The inner surface of this space is formed by podocytes—literally, "foot cells"—that wrap around the capillaries. The podocytes have finger-like processes that interdigitate (interlock) with one another. Between the processes of the podocytes are tiny filtration slits.

The glomerular filtration membrane refers to the structures that separate the blood from the glomerular capsular space. The filtration membrane is made up of capillary endothelial cells, a basement membrane (which is composed of extracellular proteins), and podocytes.

To understand the relationship between the glomerulus and the glomerular capsule, imagine punching your fist into a big water balloon softly enough that you do not pop the balloon. Your fist is like the ball of capillaries, and the balloon, now wrapped around your fist, is the capsule. The layer of the balloon touching your fist is like the podocytes, and the space inside the balloon is like the glomerular capsular space.

As blood passes through the glomerular capillaries, some of the blood plasma passes through the endothelial cells of the capillaries, through the filtration slits of the surrounding podocytes, and into the glomerular capsule. After much processing, which will be discussed in the next section, some of this filtered fluid will be excreted as urine. The formed elements in blood (red blood cells, white blood cells, and platelets) and proteins in the plasma do *not* cross the filtration membrane in a healthy kidney.

The renal tubule and the capillaries that surround the tubule are shown in **Figure 15.3B**. The renal tubule has three main parts: the proximal convoluted tubule, the nephron loop, and the distal convoluted tubule.

The ***proximal convoluted tubule (PCT)*** begins at the glomerular capsule. The fluid in the glomerular capsular space passes into the PCT. The fluid then enters the ***nephron loop*** (also called the *loop of Henle*), first through the descending limb and then through the ascending limb. The descending limb and the lower part of the ascending limb have much thinner walls than the rest of the ascending limb and the proximal and distal convoluted tubules.

After the fluid reaches the end of the thick part of the ascending limb of the nephron loop, it enters the ***distal convoluted tubule***. The fluid that reaches the end of the distal convoluted tubule enters the ***collecting duct***. Each collecting duct receives fluid from the distal convoluted tubules of several nephrons. The collecting ducts merge into larger ducts, which ultimately drain into the hollow renal pelvis.

The renal corpuscle and the proximal and distal convoluted tubules lie in the renal cortex. The nephron loops enter the renal medulla. The parallel nephron loops and surrounding capillaries give the renal medulla a striated (finely striped) appearance. Some nephrons, called *cortical nephrons*, have short nephron loops that penetrate only slightly into the medulla. Other nephrons, called *juxtamedullary nephrons*, have long nephron loops that penetrate deeply into the renal medulla. The juxtamedullary nephrons are the only nephrons that can produce highly concentrated urine.

The efferent arteriole, which carries blood out of the glomerulus, connects to a second set of capillaries called the *peritubular capillaries*. The peritubular capillaries surround the proximal and distal convoluted tubules. Many efferent arterioles from juxtamedullary nephrons give rise to capillaries that run parallel—first down and then up—with the long nephron loops. These capillaries are called ***vasa recta*** (Latin for "straight vessels").

Understanding Medical Terminology

The word *juxtamedullary* is made up of the prefix *juxta-* (which means "next to" or "nearby") and the word *medullary*. The corpuscles of juxtamedullary nephrons lie *next to* the adrenal medulla.

SELF CHECK

1. Where are the kidneys located in the abdominopelvic cavity?
2. What is the name of the outer part of the kidney, which is lighter in color than other parts?
3. What are the two main parts of a nephron?
4. What are the three main parts of the renal tubule?

Blood Flow through the Kidney

This section describes the path blood takes as it flows through the kidney. First, blood enters the kidney via the abdominal aorta and the renal artery. After passing through a series of progressively smaller arteries, the blood reaches the afferent arteriole at the entrance to the glomerulus.

The blood then flows through the glomerular capillaries. As it does, about 20% of the blood plasma enters the glomerular capsular space by crossing the filtration membrane, described earlier. The 20% plasma filtration rate of the glomerular capillaries is higher, by a factor of about 300, than the percent of plasma that leaves the capillaries elsewhere in the body. This high filtration rate enables the kidneys to eliminate wastes relatively quickly.

The blood then exits the glomerulus, passes through the efferent arteriole, and enters a second set of capillaries—either the peritubular capillaries or the vasa recta. Finally, as the blood passes through the second set of capillaries, it reabsorbs most of the fluid—but not the waste—that it lost in the glomerulus. The blood, now largely free of waste, collects into venules, which merge to form larger veins, and exits the kidney via the renal vein.

In most parts of the body, blood passes from arteriole to capillary to venule, and then into larger veins. The kidney's circulation does not follow this pattern. In the kidney, blood passes from afferent arterioles to capillaries, and then to efferent arterioles and another set of capillaries. Only then does the blood reach a venule and larger veins.

SECTION 15.1 REVIEW

Mini-Glossary

collecting duct a tube that collects urine from several nephrons and carries it to the renal pelvis

distal convoluted tubule the last part of a nephron through which urine flows before reaching the collecting duct

glomerulus a cluster of capillaries in a cup-like capsule at the end of a renal corpuscle

nephron the fundamental excretory unit of the kidney

nephron loop the U-shaped part of the nephron that is located between the proximal convoluted tubule and the distal convoluted tubule; has a descending limb and ascending limb; also known as the *loop of Henle*

proximal convoluted tubule (PCT) the part of the nephron between the glomerular capsule and the nephron loop; minerals, nutrients, and water are reabsorbed from the filtrate here

renal corpuscle the part of a nephron that consists of a glomerulus and its surrounding glomerular capsule

renal cortex the lighter-colored, outer layer of the kidney that contains the glomeruli and convoluted tubules

renal medulla the darker, innermost part of the kidney

renal pelvis a hollow, funnel-shaped cavity in the center of the kidney where urine collects before it flows into the ureter

renal tubule the part of a nephron that leads away from a glomerulus and empties into a collecting tubule; consists of a proximal convoluted tubule, nephron loop, and distal convoluted tubule

urinary system the organs involved in the formation, storage, and excretion of urine; includes the kidneys, ureters, bladder, and urethra

vasa recta thin-walled blood vessels that begin and end near the boundary between the renal cortex and the renal medulla, and which extend deep into the renal medulla, running parallel to the nephron loops; play a role in the formation of concentrated urine

Review Questions

1. What does it mean to say that the kidneys are *retroperitoneal*?
2. What happens to urine that is produced in the renal cortex and the renal medulla?
3. Where do the renal artery, renal vein, nerves, and ureter connect to the kidney?
4. What is the basic working unit of the kidney?
5. What are the names of the arteries that lead into and out of the glomerulus?
6. Which part of the renal tubule begins at the glomerular capsule?

(continued)

7. Which type of nephron has long nephron loops that penetrate deeply into the renal medulla?
8. What happens to blood as it passes through the peritubular capillaries or the vasa recta?
9. The kidneys, which make up about 0.5% of total body weight, receive 20% to 25% of the blood pumped by the heart (under resting conditions). What can you conclude about the kidneys based on this fact?
10. How does the flow of blood through the kidneys differ from the flow of blood through other parts of the body?

SECTION 15.2 Urine Formation, Storage, and Excretion

Objectives

- Explain how the kidneys produce urine.
- Describe how urine is stored and excreted from the body.
- List the steps in micturition.

Key Terms

aldosterone
angiotensin
antidiuretic hormone (ADH)
atrial natriuretic peptide (ANP)
detrusor
diuresis
external urethral sphincter
glomerular filtration
glomerular filtration rate (GFR)
hydrostatic pressure
internal urethral sphincter
micturition
osmosis
osmotic pressure
reabsorption
renin
secretion
trigone
ureter
urethra
urinary bladder

To better understand how the body disposes of wastes, consider two different ways to design a system for removing chemical wastes and toxins from fluid. The first approach is to design a filter that allows wastes and toxins to pass through, but does not allow anything "good" to pass through. This filter lets the "bad" substances escape and keeps the "good" substances within the system.

The second approach is to make a leaky filter with pores large enough to allow large quantities of water and other substances to pass through. Many good substances, as well as wastes, will pass through this nonselective filter. Therefore, the filtrate (fluid that has crossed a filter) must pass through another stage of processing, in which the good substances, and most of the water, are pumped back into the system. After that stage, only wastes, toxins, and a small amount of water remain in the filtrate. At that point, the filtrate is excreted.

The first approach sounds simpler and more efficient than the second. However, the kidney uses the second approach to remove chemical wastes and toxins. Why?

It is impossible to predict all the different kinds of wastes and toxins that an individual might need to excrete during his or her lifetime. Even if you did know ahead of time exactly what the body would need to excrete, it probably would be impossible to make the hypothetical filter described in the first approach. Sometimes, wastes and toxins are not very different from "good" molecules in terms of size, electrical charge, and other properties. Designing a filter to eliminate substances with certain properties might still eliminate "good," necessary substances.

The second approach works well even when the wastes and toxins are not known ahead of time. The filter simply "throws out everything" and then selectively reclaims the known "good" molecules.

Urine Formation

The first step in removing wastes and toxins from the body is the formation of urine. Three processes are involved in urine formation: ***glomerular filtration***, ***reabsorption***, and ***secretion***. **Figure 15.4** shows a simplified view of where these processes occur in the nephron. Notice the renal corpuscle with a capillary in its glomerular capsule, and the renal tubule and collecting duct with a capillary running next to it.

Filtration occurs at the corpuscle, where water and small, dissolved molecules pass from the capillary into the glomerular capsule. Water, ions (such as sodium and chloride), glucose, and other "good" substances are later reabsorbed into the capillary from the tubule.

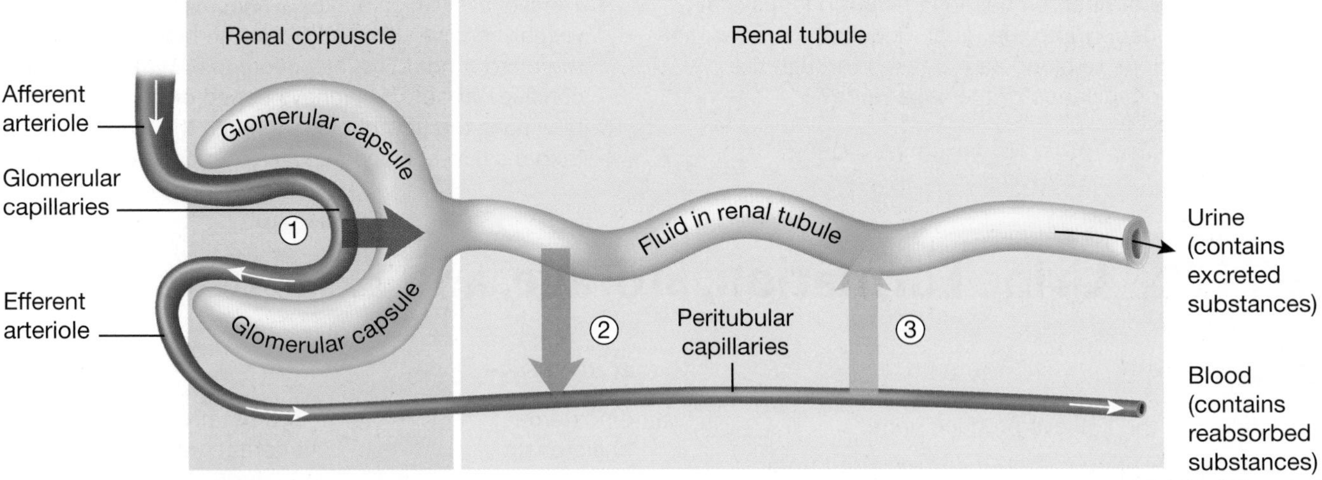

Figure 15.4 A functional view of formation of urine in the nephron. 1. Filtration from the glomerular capillaries into the glomerular capsule (brown arrow) occurs in the renal corpuscle. 2. Reabsorption is the movement of water, ions, glucose, and other substances back into the capillaries (pink arrow). 3. Wastes and some ions, drugs, and toxins are secreted from the capillaries into the tubule (orange arrow).

Some waste molecules, ions, and other molecules are secreted from the capillaries into the tubule and collecting duct.

Glomerular Filtration

Glomerular filtration, which occurs in the renal corpuscle, is the first step in urine formation. Glomerular filtration is the movement of water and solutes (dissolved substances) from the capillaries into the glomerular capsular space. The water that reaches the capsule is called *glomerular filtrate*. To reach the glomerular capsular space, water and solutes must cross the capillary endothelial cells, the basement membrane (a layer of extracellular protein), and the podocytes of the glomerular capsule. These three structures are collectively known as the *filtration membrane*.

Red and white blood cells and platelets are too large to cross the filtration membrane. Large and medium-size proteins, such as albumin—the most common protein in blood plasma—are also too large to cross the filtration membrane. However, water and small molecules and ions *can* cross this membrane. Substances that cross the filtration membrane include water, glucose, sodium, potassium, chloride, amino acids, urea (a waste product of metabolism), many kinds of prescription and over-the-counter drugs, and other molecules smaller than about 3 nanometers in diameter.

The total amount of water filtered in a unit of time is called the ***glomerular filtration rate (GFR)***. Laboratory tests are used to estimate GFR, which is one of the most important benchmarks for assessing kidney health. A normal GFR value is about 125 milliliters (mL) per minute in males and 105 mL per minute in females. If you multiply the normal GFR (the amount filtered per minute) by the number of minutes in a day, you get about 150 to 180 liters (L) of glomerular filtrate per day! The majority of the filtrate is eventually reclaimed by the body, so that typical urine output is (fortunately) nowhere close to 180 L per day. The driving force for glomerular filtration is pressure: hydrostatic pressure and osmotic pressure.

Hydrostatic Pressure

Hydrostatic pressure can be described as "regular" pressure. It is the pressure of water in a balloon that makes the balloon swell. It is the pressure in pipes that makes water come out when you turn on a faucet. It is the pressure you feel in the carotid artery in the neck or in the radial artery at the wrist. Hydrostatic pressure pushes water from areas of high pressure to areas of low pressure.

In a glomerulus, the hydrostatic pressure in the capillaries is the blood pressure there—about 55 mmHg (millimeters of mercury). This is considerably higher than the pressure of about 20 to 25 mmHg found in most capillaries. The pressure in the glomerular capsular space is only 15 mmHg, so the hydrostatic pressure difference of 40 mmHg pushes water from the capillaries into the capsule.

Osmotic Pressure

Unlike hydrostatic pressure, ***osmotic pressure*** is not apparent in everyday life. Osmotic pressure is created by the presence of dissolved substances in water. High osmotic pressure "pulls in" water from areas of low osmotic pressure. Hydrostatic pressure, by contrast, "pushes" water from areas of high to low pressure.

As the amount of dissolved substances in a fluid rises, the fluid's osmotic pressure also rises. Therefore, water is drawn into areas that are full of dissolved substances from areas that have fewer dissolved substances. The movement of water from an area of low osmotic pressure to an area of high osmotic pressure is called ***osmosis***.

In the renal corpuscle, the blood has a higher osmotic pressure than the filtrate because the proteins, which are too big to cross the filtration membrane, are present only on the blood side of the membrane. The molecules that are small enough to cross the membrane are present in equal concentrations on both sides, so they do not create an osmotic pressure difference. The osmotic pressure is about 30 mmHg higher in blood than in filtrate.

The size and direction of the pressure differences can be compared to determine the net amount and direction of pressure across the filtration membrane. Recall that the hydrostatic pressure is 40 mmHg higher in the capillary than in the glomerular capsular space, and the osmotic pressure is 30 mmHg higher in the capillary than in the capsular space. These pressures partially cancel each other out because they act in opposite directions: High hydrostatic pressure *pushes*, and high osmotic pressure *pulls*. Thus, there is a net filtration pressure of 10 mmHg pushing water from the capillary into the capsule (**Figure 15.5**).

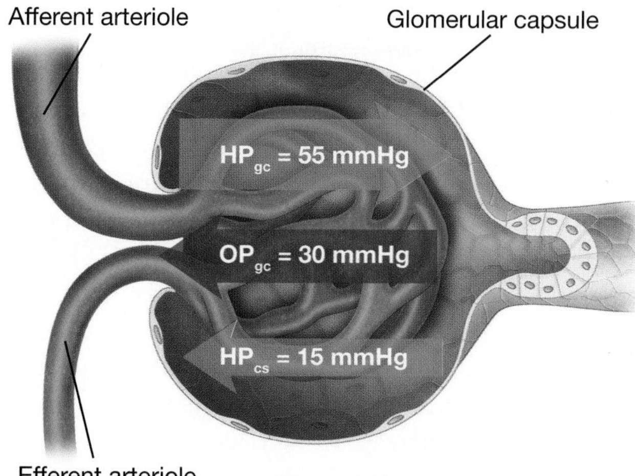

© Body Scientific International

Figure 15.5 Pressures driving filtration. Hydrostatic pressure in the glomerular capillary (HPgc) pushes water out of the capillary. Hydrostatic pressure in the capsule space (HPcs) pushes back from the capsule to the capillary. Osmotic pressure in the glomerular capillary (OPgc) pulls water into the capillary.

Control of Glomerular Filtration Rate

It is important that the body be able to control GFR. If GFR is too low, wastes and excess water will start to build up in the body. If GFR is too high, too much water may be lost, leading to dehydration. High GFR also means that other desirable substances, such as sodium, potassium, glucose, and calcium, may be lost, which can cause a variety of problems.

The main way in which the body controls glomerular filtration rate is by controlling the blood pressure in the glomerular capillaries. This is done by regulating the renal arterioles. Hormones and sympathetic nerves to the kidney both have this regulatory ability.

The high blood pressure in the glomerular capillaries is due in large part to the efferent arteriole, which is the "exit tube" from the glomerulus. The relatively small diameter of the efferent arteriole makes it somewhat difficult for blood to leave the glomerulus. This causes blood pressure to build up in the glomerulus. Constriction of the efferent arteriole causes glomerular pressure and the glomerular filtration rate to increase because blood cannot exit the glomerulus. By contrast, constriction of the afferent arteriole, which lies upstream of the glomerulus, limits inflow of blood to the glomerulus and causes glomerular pressure—and therefore glomerular filtration—to drop. The presence of both an afferent and an efferent arteriole provide the body with the ability to control glomerular pressure and glomerular filtration.

The sympathetic nerves have a greater effect on the afferent arterioles than on the efferent arterioles. Sympathetic nerve activity increases during exercise and during stressful situations that evoke a fight-or-flight response. When sympathetic nerve activity increases, the afferent arterioles constrict more than the efferent arterioles. This constriction causes glomerular capillary pressure and glomerular filtration rate to drop. The decrease in glomerular capillary pressure and GFR helps the body reduce urine output and keeps blood volume high, which is useful during exercise. These physiological effects probably gave people an advantage in surviving some fight-or-flight situations in the past.

Reabsorption

The filtrate from the glomerular capsule flows into the renal tubule. As it flows through the tubule and into the collecting duct, most of the water and dissolved substances are reabsorbed into the blood in the capillaries surrounding the tubule. Most reabsorption occurs in the proximal convoluted tubule (PCT). The remainder occurs in the distal convoluted tubule and the collecting duct.

The epithelial cells that form the wall of the PCT have microvilli on their luminal (lumen-facing) side. These microvilli increase the surface area of the PCT, enhancing its reabsorptive ability. The major steps involved in reabsorption are shown in **Figure 15.6**.

Sodium

Sodium is the most abundant ion in the filtrate. As the PCT reabsorbs substances from the filtrate, the sodium is actively pumped out of the tubular epithelial cells by sodium-potassium pump proteins. These carrier proteins use ATP to move sodium from the cells into the interstitial space that surrounds the peritubular capillary.

The active excretion of sodium from the cells by the sodium-potassium pump leaves the cytoplasm with little sodium. Since there is now a high concentration of sodium in the tubular fluid, sodium spreads into the cell from the tubule. The sodium that has been pumped out of the cells and into the space surrounding the capillaries then diffuses into the capillaries.

Cotransport proteins in the part of the cell membrane that faces the tubule bring sodium into the cells. Using the energy from this sodium entry, the cotransport proteins pump various desirable substances from the lumen into the cells. This is an example of secondary active transport.

Secondary Active Transport

In secondary active transport, the energy of one substance going "downhill" is used by a protein to pump another substance "uphill." Glucose, amino acids, some ions, and vitamins enter the cells from the tubule by means of secondary active transport with sodium. These valuable substances then spread out of the cells on the other side and diffuse into the peritubular capillary.

Osmotic Pressure

The positive charge on the sodium ions tends to draw negatively charged chloride out of the tubule and into the peritubular capillaries. The active pumping of sodium into the interstitial space, and its diffusion into the peritubular capillaries, creates a relatively high osmotic pressure in the capillaries and in the interstitial space.

The high osmotic pressure draws water out of the tubule, through the cells, and into the interstitial space and the capillary. Aquaporin channels in both sides of the cells give water an easy way to enter and exit the cells. Thus, the active pumping of sodium provides the driving force for reabsorption of glucose, amino acids, vitamins, chloride, and some other ions, as well as water.

Secretion

At the same time as the "good" substances are being reabsorbed by the blood, wastes still present in the blood are being secreted from the capillaries. Waste products that were not fully removed during filtration are actively pumped out of the capillaries and into the renal tubule by the cells that form the walls of the tubules. This active pumping of wastes from capillary blood into the tubules is called *secretion*. Unlike filtration, which is a passive process, secretion is active; that is, it uses chemical energy, often in the form of ATP, to move molecules.

The tubular epithelial cells actively push certain molecules into the lumen, or hollow central part, of the renal tubule. The lumen of the tubule contains the fluid that will eventually be eliminated from the body as urine. Pushing unwanted molecules into the lumen of the renal tubule is the body's way of getting rid of them. The active pushing of molecules into the lumen is called *tubular secretion*.

Two of the molecules that are actively secreted are urea and uric acid. *Urea* received its name because it was first discovered in urine. *Uric acid*, which is made of two urea molecules and a few linking atoms, was first discovered in kidney stones. Urea and uric acid are the primary forms of nitrogen-containing (nitrogenous) wastes.

Normal protein breakdown produces amino acids. The amine group ($-NH_2$) on each amino acid can react with hydrogen, which is plentiful in the body, to form ammonia (NH_4). Ammonia is a highly toxic molecule. Fortunately, the liver converts amine groups into urea and uric acid, which are much less toxic. Because these molecules are secreted into the filtrate, and because most of the water in the filtrate is reabsorbed, urea and uric acid are considerably more concentrated in the urine than in the blood.

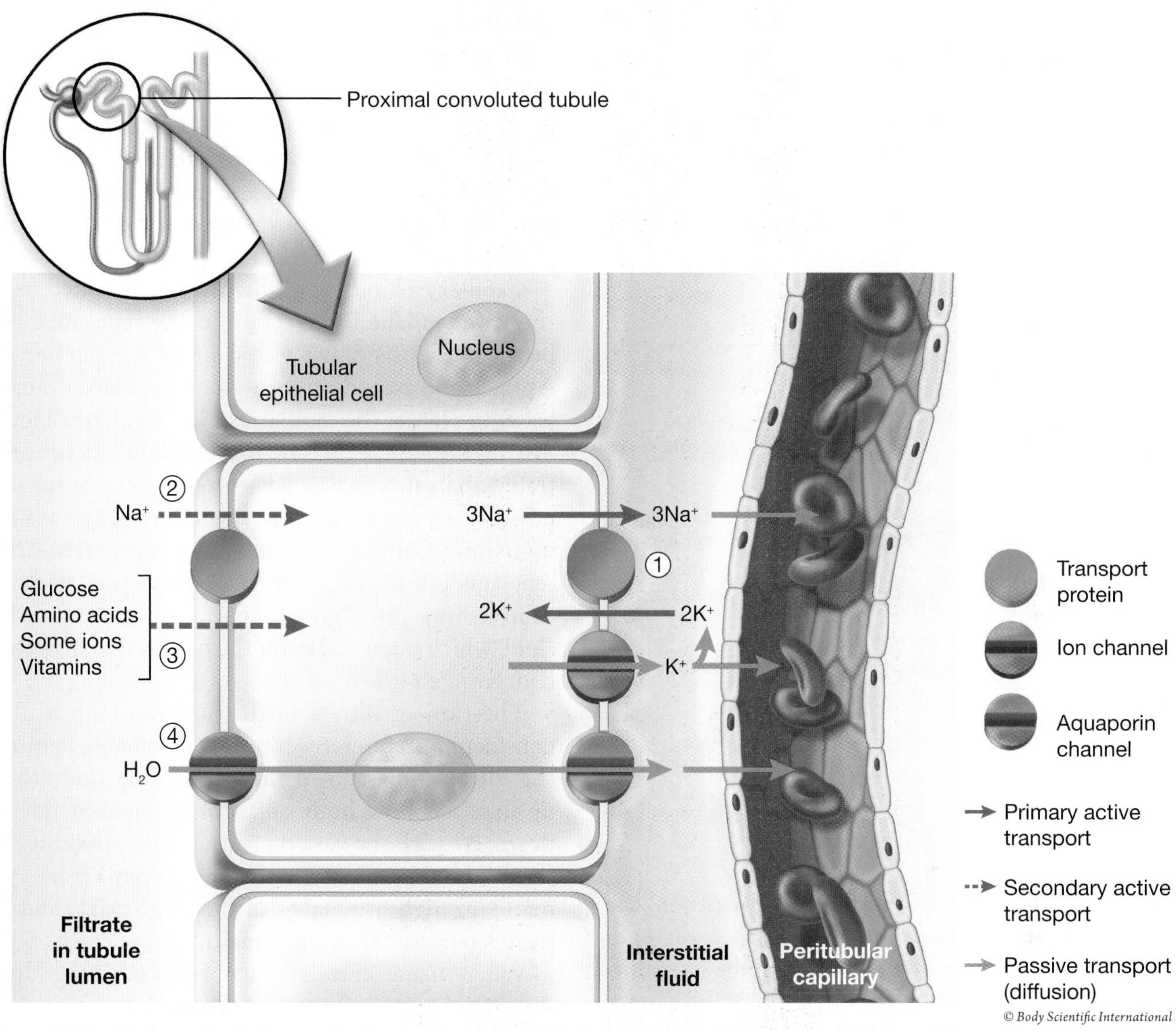

Figure 15.6 Reabsorption in the proximal convoluted tubule. The lumen of the tubule is at the far left, and the peritubular capillary is at the right. The cells lining the tubule have been enlarged to show details, and the microvilli on the luminal side of the cell have been omitted for clarity. 1. Sodium-potassium pumps (the green transport proteins shown above) actively pump sodium (Na^+) out of the tubule cell and potassium ions (K^+) into the cell. 2. Sodium flows down its energy gradient into the cell. 3. Glucose and amino acids are cotransported into the cell with sodium by secondary active transport. 4. Water enters the cell from the tubule through aquaporin channels and leaves the cell on the capillary side through aquaporin channels.

The tubular epithelial cells can also secrete hydrogen ions (acid, H^+) or bicarbonate ions (base, HCO_3) to maintain the pH of arterial blood at about 7.4. The renal tubule's epithelial cells also secrete, or push out, some drugs, if they are present in the blood. Penicillin and aspirin, for example, are eliminated from the body by the kidneys in this manner.

The Renal Medulla

From the renal cortex, the filtrate enters the renal medulla (**Figure 15.7**). The descending limb of the nephron loop is thin because the epithelial cells that form the wall of the tube lack the active pumping capability or intracellular machinery (such as mitochondria) of the PCT cells. Thus, no active reabsorption or secretion occurs in either the descending limb or the thin ascending limb of the nephron loop. Water can leave the filtrate in the descending limb, but not in the ascending limb, whose cells lack aquaporin channels. The thick portion of the ascending limb, which *does* have pumping capability, actively reabsorbs sodium, but water cannot follow, due to the lack of aquaporin channels in the ascending limb.

The reabsorption of sodium in the thick, ascending limb of the nephron loop, where water cannot be

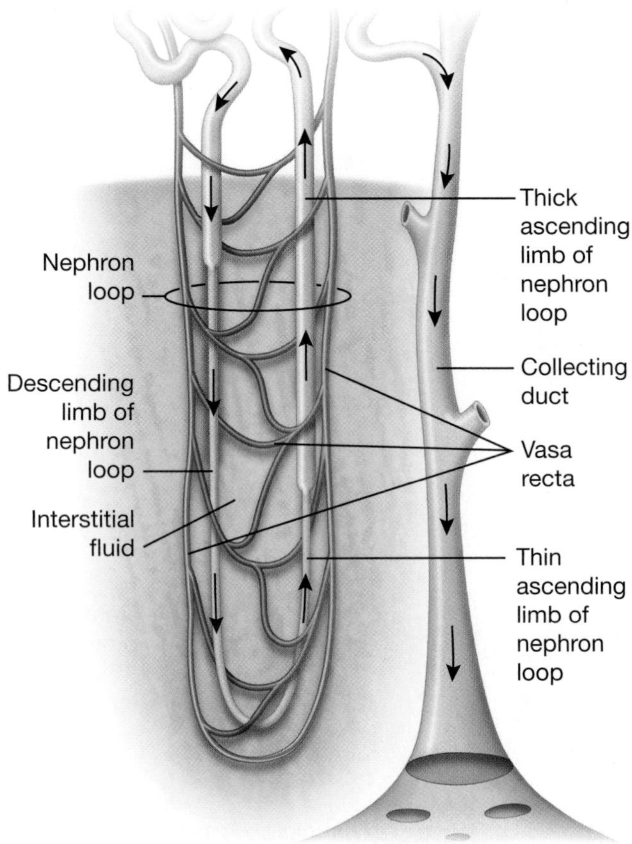

Figure 15.7 The renal medulla. Notice the change in thickness of the descending and ascending limbs.

reabsorbed, and the permeability to water of the descending limb of the nephron loop work together to create a high concentration of sodium in the interstitial fluid in the renal medulla.

Limited amounts of urea are intentionally allowed to reenter the interstitial space as urine travels down the collecting duct. Reentry of urea into the interstitial space contributes to the high osmolality of the interstitial fluid in the renal medulla. Osmolality is a measure of the number of dissolved molecules (in this case sodium molecules) per unit volume of fluid. The net result of these processes is that the deepest parts of the renal medulla can have an interstitial osmolality of about 1,200 milliosmoles (mOsm), approximately four times higher than normal interstitial fluid osmolality. (Milliosmoles are a measure of the number of ions, or particles, that contribute to the osmotic pressure of a solution. A milliosmole is equal to one-thousandth of an osmole per unit volume of fluid.)

The Countercurrent Mechanism

A key to maintaining the state of affairs just described is the geometric arrangement of the nephron loop and the parallel vasa recta capillaries. This arrangement, known as a *countercurrent mechanism*, is shown in **Figure 15.8**. It is called *countercurrent* because the blood flows "down" the vasa recta, then back past itself in the opposite direction.

Capillary blood grows highly concentrated as it travels down the vasa recta into the renal medulla because osmosis draws water out of the capillaries. As the blood ascends in the vasa recta, osmosis causes water to reenter the capillaries. As a result, the blood leaving the vasa recta is no more and no less concentrated than it was when it entered, despite having passed through an area of very highly concentrated interstitial fluid. This allows the deep parts of the renal medulla to get the blood flow they need without diminishing the high concentration of interstitial fluid, which is necessary for the production of highly concentrated urine.

The flow of filtrate in the nephron loop is also considered a countercurrent arrangement, because the filtrate flows down the descending limb, then up the ascending limb, adjacent to where it travels down. As with the vasa recta, the close proximity of these parallel pathways helps the kidney create and maintain high osmolality of the interstitial fluid in the deep parts of the renal medulla.

When urine travels down the collecting duct through the deepest parts of the medulla, water can be reabsorbed from the collecting duct by osmosis into the highly concentrated interstitial fluid. When this occurs maximally, the urine can reach, as stated previously, an osmolality of 1,200 milliosmoles because the water in the collecting duct reaches osmotic equilibrium with the interstitial space.

Hormonal Regulation of Urine

By the time the filtrate reaches the distal convoluted tubule, about 80% of the water and 90% of the sodium and chloride that entered the glomerular capsular space have been reabsorbed. The amount of reabsorption in the proximal convoluted tubule and nephron loop is relatively constant. The reabsorption in the distal convoluted tubule and collecting duct, however, is adjusted by hormones to maintain homeostasis.

In other words, the "fine tuning" of urine volume and composition occurs in the distal convoluted tubule

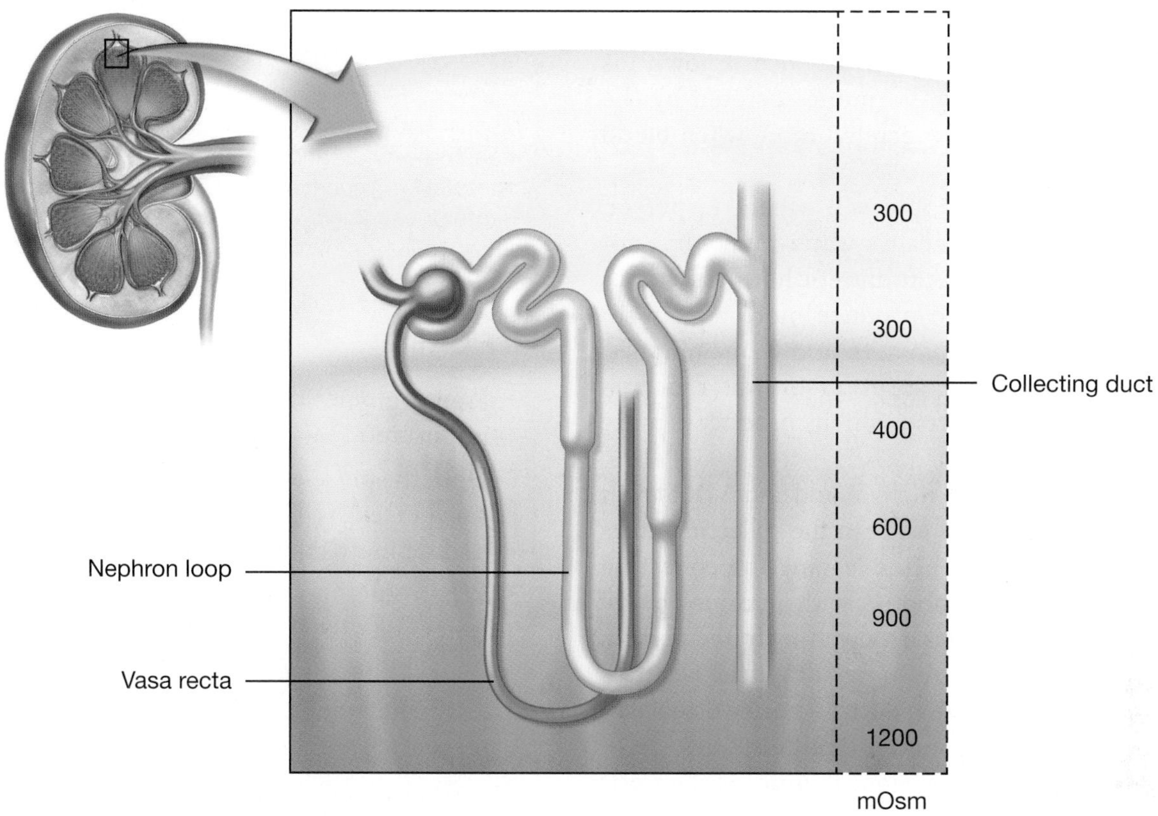

© Body Scientific International

Figure 15.8 Water permeability of the descending limb of the nephron loop, and active sodium reabsorption from the ascending limb, establish the high osmolality of the deep renal medulla. The countercurrent mechanism shown here helps maintain that high osmolality. The numbers on the right show the osmolality of the interstitial fluid in the renal medulla, represented in milliosmoles (mOsm).

and collecting duct. Three key hormones that control this fine tuning are aldosterone, atrial natriuretic peptide, and antidiuretic hormone.

Aldosterone

A steroid hormone called ***aldosterone*** is produced in the adrenal cortex. A drop in blood sodium concentration, or a rise in blood potassium concentration, directly stimulates the secretion of more aldosterone. A decrease in blood pressure also stimulates more aldosterone secretion, but by an indirect mechanism: decreased blood pressure causes greater secretion of the hormone ***renin***, an enzyme, by the kidney.

Renin circulates in the blood and binds to the circulating protein angiotensinogen to produce ***angiotensin***, a polypeptide hormone in the blood that constricts blood vessels and increases blood pressure. After binding to angiotensinogen, renin cuts the angiotensinogen into two fragments, one of which is angiotensin I. An enzyme in the lungs, appropriately named *angiotensin-converting enzyme*, converts angiotensin I into angiotensin II by removing two amino acids. Angiotensin II stimulates adrenal cortical cells to secrete more aldosterone.

Aldosterone acts on the distal convoluted tubule cells and the collecting duct to increase sodium reabsorption and potassium secretion. More sodium is reabsorbed than potassium is secreted, and water follows the sodium, so more aldosterone means greater water absorption. As a result, aldosterone causes a decrease in the volume and sodium content of urine, and an increase in its potassium content. The decreased urine volume means that more water is retained in the circulation, which causes blood pressure to rise, correcting the decrease in blood pressure that led—via the renin-angiotensin mechanism—to more aldosterone secretion.

Atrial Natriuretic Peptide

A hormone made by the atria of the heart, ***atrial natriuretic peptide (ANP)***, is released in response to increased stretching of the atria, which occurs when blood volume is high. ANP inhibits sodium reabsorption in the collecting ducts, which causes decreased water reabsorption due to osmotic pressure effects. As a result, urine volume and sodium excretion increase, which tends to correct the high blood volume that stimulated ANP production.

Antidiuretic Hormone

Antidiuretic hormone (ADH), also known as *vasopressin*, is a peptide hormone secreted by the pituitary gland. ADH is secreted more when blood osmolality increases.

Blood osmolality increases when a person becomes dehydrated because water intake has not kept up with water loss. Antidiuretic hormone causes collecting duct cells to produce more aquaporin molecules and insert them in their own membranes. As a result, more reabsorption of water occurs in the collecting ducts, which produces more concentrated urine.

When a person is very dehydrated and ADH levels are high, reabsorption of water in the collecting ducts is so effective that the urine leaving the collecting duct is extremely concentrated, with an osmolality of about 1,200 milliosmoles. In a well-hydrated person, ADH levels are low. As a result, little water is reabsorbed in the collecting duct, and urine osmolality can drop to between 50 and 100 milliosmoles.

Antidiuretic hormone reduces ***diuresis***. Diuretic drugs, which increase diuresis, are widely prescribed to reduce blood pressure and to reduce the buildup of fluid in the body that occurs in patients with weak or failing hearts.

Loop diuretics, such as furosemide (trade name Lasix®), reduce sodium reabsorption in the ascending limb of the nephron loop. Other blood pressure-lowering agents work by inhibiting angiotensin-converting enzyme, by blocking the receptors for angiotensin, or by other mechanisms.

Understanding Medical Terminology

The word *diuresis* is made up of the prefix *di/a-* meaning "through," the combining form *-ur/o-* meaning "urine," and the suffix *-sis*, which means "state of" or "condition." *Diuresis* literally means "state or condition of urine passing through"—in short, "urine production."

SELF CHECK

1. Why is glomerular filtration rate (GFR) important?
2. Does the presence of more dissolved substances in a fluid mean that fluid has a high or low osmotic pressure?
3. Where does most of the reabsorption of water and dissolved substances take place in the kidneys?
4. Active pumping of which ion provides the force for reabsorption of glucose and amino acids?
5. If you become dehydrated, will your body secrete more or less ADH?

Urine Storage

Urine is made continuously by the kidney. Unlike the respiratory system, which excretes waste (carbon dioxide) with every breath, the urinary system excretes waste only a few times a day. Therefore, a place is needed to store the urine until the time and place for elimination are appropriate. Plumbing is also

Research Notes Blood Pressure and the Kidneys

Hypertension, or high blood pressure, is a widespread condition. A large body of research in humans and animals shows that the kidneys play a key role in controlling blood pressure over the long term. Under normal conditions, if the blood pressure gets too high, the kidneys excrete slightly more urine for a period of hours or days. This reduces the volume of fluid in the body, which reduces blood volume and brings blood pressure back down to a normal level. If the blood pressure gets too low, the opposite happens: the kidneys excrete slightly less urine for a while, until the blood pressure gets back up to normal.

These slow but steady adjustments to maintain blood pressure require the participation of the autonomic nervous system and the endocrine system. The endocrine hormones that help regulate blood pressure are mentioned in this chapter: renin, angiotensin, aldosterone, and antidiuretic hormone all tend to cause urine retention and a rise in blood pressure. Atrial natriuretic peptide causes diuresis and a decrease in blood pressure.

Many drugs are used to treat hypertension, and most of them work by acting on the kidney. Thiazide diuretics are drugs that work by acting on the cells of the distal convoluted tubule to reduce the reuptake of sodium and water. This leads to more urine output. Angiotensin receptor blockers (ARBs) prevent angiotensin from binding to its cellular receptors. ACE inhibitors inhibit angiotensin-converting enzyme. Diuretics, ARBs, and ACE inhibitors are all effective in reducing blood pressure.

needed: structures to take the urine from where it is made to where it is stored, and from where it is stored to the outside environment.

Ureters

Each kidney is connected by a ***ureter*** to the bladder (**Figure 15.1**). The renal pelvis in each kidney connects to a hollow ureter, as shown in **Figure 15.2**. Each ureter is lined with epithelium and contains smooth muscle in its wall. The ureters connect to the bladder at the bladder's posterior wall.

Urinary Bladder

The ***urinary bladder*** is a hollow, muscular organ that stores urine. It sits on the floor of the pelvic cavity, under the peritoneum, and its superior surface is directly covered by the peritoneum. In men, the bladder is positioned directly in front of the rectum and above the prostate gland. In women, it is positioned in front of the vagina and uterus.

The bladder wall is made of smooth muscle, the ***detrusor***, with a layer of epithelial cells on its interior. When the bladder is empty, it collapses, causing folds to develop in the walls and lining. A moderately full bladder may contain 500 mL of urine. An extremely full bladder can contain as much as 1,000 mL.

The bladder has three openings: one ureteric orifice for each of the two ureters, plus the opening of the urethra. The urine enters at the ureteric orifices and exits through the urethra. The urethra connects to the bladder at the bladder neck. The imaginary triangle formed by the two ureteric openings and the urethra is the ***trigone*** of the bladder.

Urethra

The ***urethra*** is a thin tube that connects the urinary bladder to the outside environment (**Figure 15.9**). It begins at the neck of the bladder, at its midline. A layer of smooth muscle called the ***internal urethral sphincter*** encircles the urethra where it exits the bladder.

In men, the prostate gland lies directly below the bladder. The prostatic urethra is the portion of the urethra that passes right through the prostate gland.

The next part of the male urethra, the intermediate part, passes through the muscles of the pelvic floor, which make up the urogenital diaphragm. A ring of skeletal muscle, the ***external urethral sphincter***, surrounds the intermediate part of the urethra where it passes through the urogenital diaphragm.

The intermediate part of the urethra continues to the base of the penis and becomes the spongy urethra as it passes down the length of the penis, finally opening to the outside at the external urethral orifice. The total length of the male urethra is about 20 centimeters (8 inches).

The female urethra is only 1.5 inches (3 to 4 centimeters) long. Like the male urethra, it is surrounded by the external urethral sphincter as it passes through the urogenital diaphragm; its external opening is also called the *external urethral orifice*.

SELF CHECK

1. Why would the bladder be unnecessary if the urinary system functioned more like the respiratory system?
2. Where is urine stored?
3. Which tube in the urinary system leads to the outside of the body?

Urine Excretion

Thousands of collecting ducts in each kidney produce a steady trickle of urine into the renal pelvis. As fluid from the kidney enters the ureter, the ureter stretches. This stretching causes a wave of contractions to develop in the smooth muscle wall of the ureter. The wave of muscle contractions travels down the ureter, pushing the urine ahead of it. You may recognize this process of contractions pushing materials down a tube as peristalsis, which was presented in earlier chapters.

There are many words for the release of urine from the bladder, including *urination*, *voiding*, and ***micturition***. Micturition requires contraction of the detrusor to force urine out of the bladder, and simultaneous relaxation of both the internal and external sphincters to open the pathway for release.

Because the internal sphincter is made of smooth muscle, it is controlled subconsciously by the autonomic nervous system. By contrast, the external urethral sphincter is made of skeletal muscle, so it is consciously controlled by somatic motor nerve fibers. (The autonomic and somatic branches of the nervous system are described in Chapter 7.) In short, the autonomic reflexes of micturition occur in the spinal cord, while conscious control of the external urethral sphincter originates in the brain.

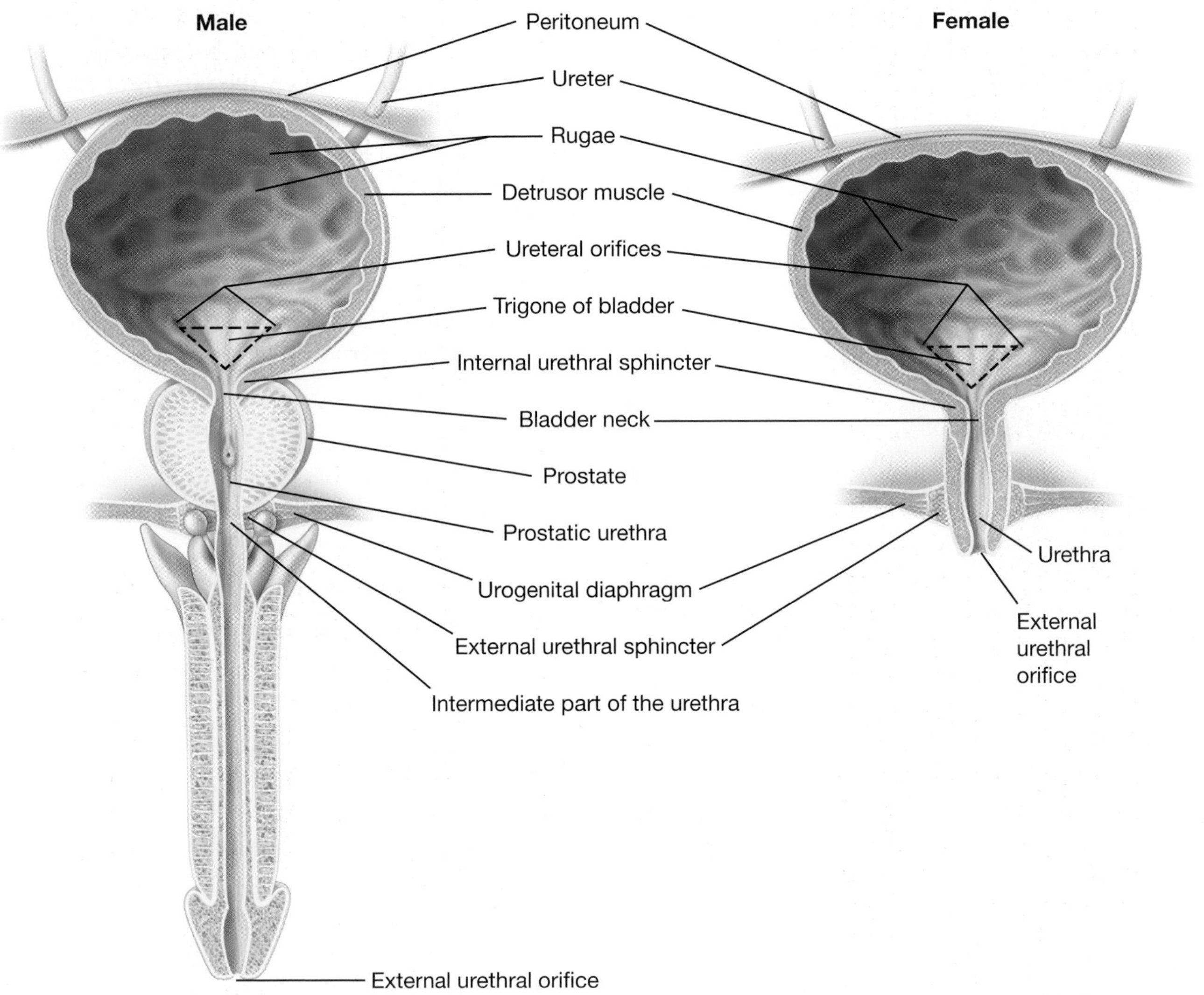

Figure 15.9 The male and female bladder and urethra.

Figure 15.10 shows the pathways and actions involved in micturition. The numbers in the following description correspond to the numbers in the figure.

1. As the bladder fills, it stretches. Stretch receptors in the wall generate action potentials that excite sensory neurons in the bladder wall. These neurons send impulses to the sacral portion of the spinal cord.
2. Interneurons in the spinal cord signal motor neurons in the sacral spinal cord that the bladder is stretched.
3. The sacral spinal cord neurons send impulses back out to the bladder via parasympathetic nerve fibers.
4. The impulses sent to the bladder through the parasympathetic nerve fibers cause the detrusor to contract and the internal urethral sphincter to relax.
5. While the detrusor is contracting and the internal urethral sphincter is relaxing, the spinal cord sends a signal to the brain, with the information that the bladder is stretched (from step 1).
6. The sensory message from the spinal cord activates the micturition reflex center in the brain stem, which sends impulses to the sacral spinal cord.

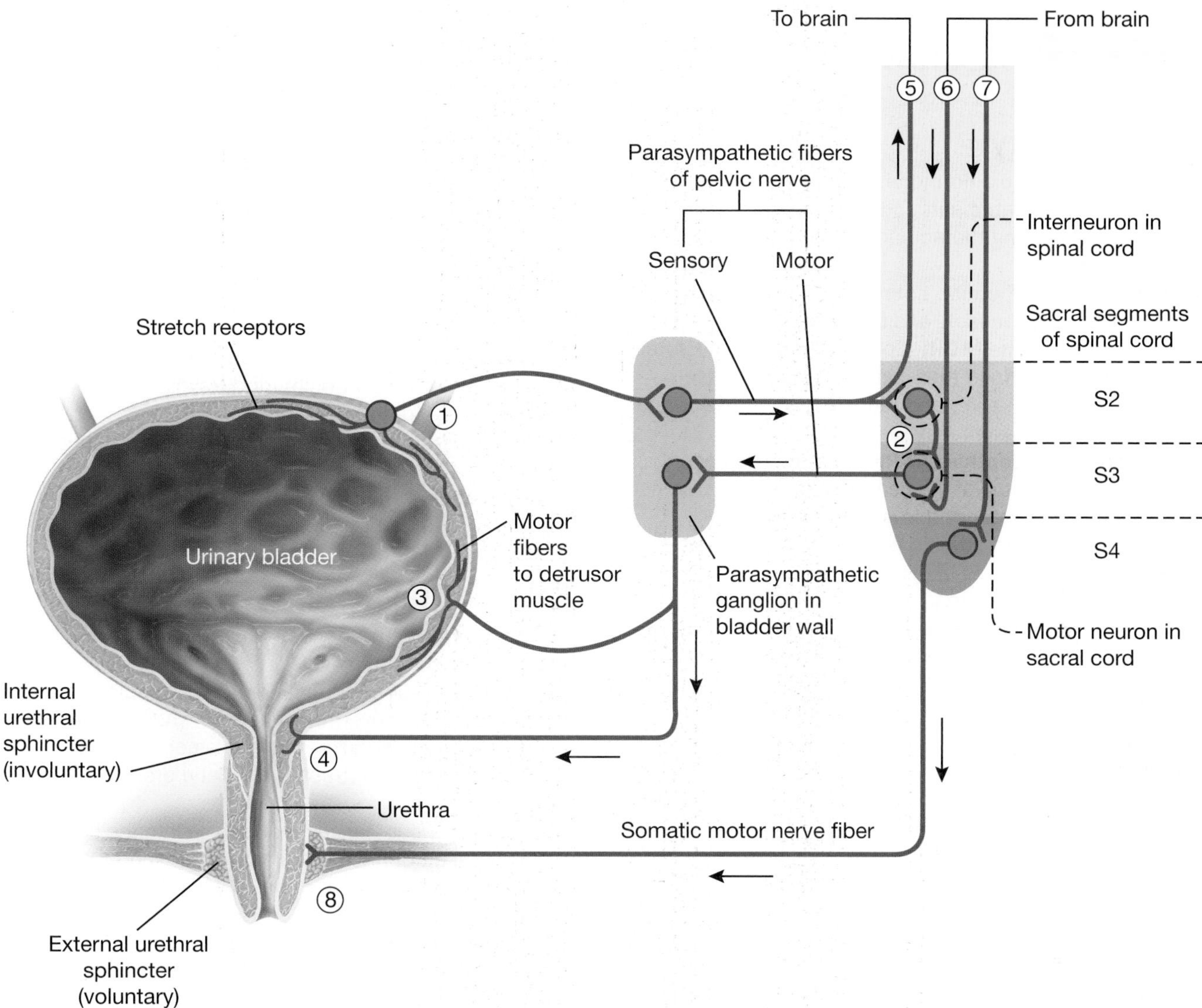

Figure 15.10 The pathways and actions involved in micturition.

7. As the detrusor contracts and the internal urethral sphincter relaxes, the person becomes consciously aware that the bladder is full. If the time is not right for urination, there is no change in the steady signal to the external urethral sphincter that causes it to stay contracted. If the time is right for urination, nerve impulses are sent from the brain stem to the sacral spinal cord.
8. From the sacral spinal cord, the nerve impulses travel to the external urethral sphincter, signaling it to relax. As a result, the pathway for micturition becomes fully open, the detrusor contracts, and the urine is expelled.

Early in childhood, people unconsciously learn that they can aid the expulsion of urine. They do this, without realizing it, by contracting the respiratory diaphragm and the skeletal muscles of the abdomen. This muscle contraction increases pressure in the abdominal cavity, which pushes down on the top of the bladder, thus helping to force out urine. This voluntary effort to raise intra-abdominal pressure is called the *Valsalva maneuver.* A Valsalva maneuver can also be useful in aiding defecation.

SECTION 15.2

REVIEW

Mini-Glossary

aldosterone a steroid hormone produced in the adrenal cortex that regulates salt and water balance in the body by increasing the amount of sodium reabsorbed from urine

angiotensin a polypeptide hormone in the blood that constricts blood vessels and increases blood pressure

antidiuretic hormone (ADH) a peptide hormone secreted by the pituitary gland that constricts blood vessels, raises blood pressure, and reduces excretion of urine; also known as *vasopressin*

atrial natriuretic peptide (ANP) a peptide hormone secreted by the atria of the heart that promotes excretion of sodium and water and lowers blood pressure

detrusor the smooth muscle that forms most of the bladder wall and aids in expelling urine

diuresis urine production

external urethral sphincter a ring of skeletal muscle that surrounds the intermediate part of the urethra where it passes through the urogenital diaphragm; this muscle is voluntarily controlled during release of urine from the body

glomerular filtration the movement of water and solutes from the capillaries into the glomerular capsular space

glomerular filtration rate (GFR) the total amount of water filtered from the glomerular capillaries into the glomerular capsule per unit of time; usually measured in milliliters per minute

hydrostatic pressure the pressure exerted by a liquid as a result of its potential energy

internal urethral sphincter a layer of smooth muscle located at the inferior end of the bladder and the proximal end of the urethra; this muscle, which prohibits release of urine, is under involuntary control

micturition urination

osmosis the movement of water molecules from a region of low osmotic pressure to a region of high osmotic pressure

osmotic pressure the pressure created by the presence of dissolved substances in water

reabsorption the movement of water and dissolved substances into the blood from the filtrate in a renal tubule

renin an enzyme made and secreted by the kidneys; aids in the production of angiotensin

secretion the active movement of substances from the blood into the filtrate, which will become urine

trigone the triangular region of the bladder formed by the two ureteric orifices and the internal urethral orifice

ureter a duct through which urine travels from the kidney to the bladder

urethra a thin tube that connects the urinary bladder to the outside environment

urinary bladder a hollow, muscular organ that stores urine; also called the *bladder*

Review Questions

1. What are the three major processes involved in urine formation?
2. During filtration in the glomerular capsule, water and solutes move from where to where? What is the water called after this movement?
3. Compare and contrast hydrostatic pressure and osmotic pressure.
4. Name four substances that diffuse into the capillaries as a result of secondary active transport.
5. For proper urine formation, should the osmolality levels of the interstitial fluid in the renal medulla be normal or higher or lower than normal?
6. List the three key hormones involved in fine-tuning urine volume and composition to maintain homeostasis.
7. Explain the relationship between antidiuretic hormone and dehydration.
8. How does the urinary system differ from the respiratory system in eliminating waste?
9. Which structure(s) contract during micturition and which structure(s) relax?
10. Explain how and why the nervous system is involved in excreting urine from the body.

SECTION 15.3

Diseases and Disorders of the Urinary System

Objectives

- Explain the various tests of renal function and what these tests tell us.
- Describe urinary system disorders, diseases, and treatment options.

Key Terms

chronic kidney disease
creatinine
hemodialysis
kidney stone
osmotic diuresis
peritoneal dialysis
renal dialysis
urinalysis
urinary tract infection (UTI)
urine specific gravity

Many illnesses, of both renal and nonrenal origin, cause changes in the urine. Therefore, the analysis of urine—***urinalysis***—is a standard part of a complete physical examination. This section describes some medical conditions of nonrenal origin that create abnormalities in the urine and eventually lead to kidney damage. It also identifies the causes and symptoms of several disorders and diseases of the urinary system, along with treatment options.

Assessing Renal Function

The amount, appearance, smell, and chemical content of urine can reveal clues about abnormalities in kidney function. Because the kidneys regulate the composition of blood, analysis of blood is also essential for evaluation of kidney function.

Physical Characteristics of Urine

Urine is normally clear and yellow (**Figure 15.11**). Cloudy urine may indicate a urinary tract infection. A color other than yellow may result from the presence of blood in the urine—which is never normal—or from the consumption of certain vitamin supplements, drugs, or foods.

The pH of urine varies from 4.5 to 8.0 under normal conditions. A urine pH of 6.0 is typical. ***Urine specific gravity*** is a measure of the density of urine (mass per unit volume), divided by the density of pure water. Normal urine has a specific gravity of 1.003 to 1.035, with higher numbers indicating more concentrated urine—that is, urine that contains more dissolved substances. A typical daily volume of urine is 1 pint to ½ gallon (0.5 to 2.0 L).

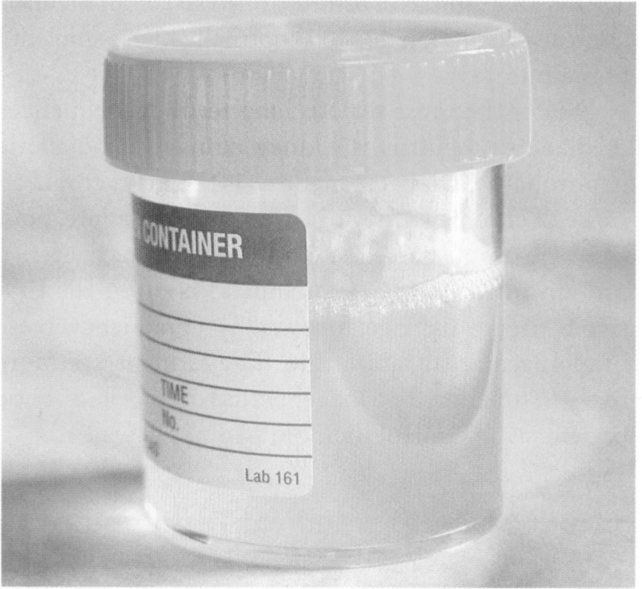

HSNphotography/Shutterstock.com

Figure 15.11 A sample of normal urine. Urine that is cloudy instead of clear indicates a possible urinary tract infection.

Chemical Composition of Urine

Urine is about 95% water. Urea is the most abundant solute in urine. As mentioned earlier, urea is a type of nitrogenous waste produced by the normal chemical breakdown of proteins. Potassium, chloride, sodium, and other ions are typically present in urine as well. The presence of red or white blood cells, protein, or glucose in urine is abnormal and usually leads to further testing to determine the cause.

Inexpensive test kits allow rapid measurement of many compounds in urine. The kits contain small plastic strips with chemicals that change color in response to the presence or concentration of various compounds in urine. A microscope is also essential for checking a urine sample for blood cells, bacteria, and other abnormalities.

Glomerular Filtration Rate

As mentioned earlier in the chapter, the measurement of glomerular filtration rate (GFR) is a key part of assessing kidney function. Recall that GFR is the total amount of water filtered in a unit of time. One approach to measuring GFR is based on the following idea: if a substance in blood plasma is easily filtered by the glomerulus, and the substance is neither reabsorbed nor secreted by the renal tubules, then the rate at which that substance collects in the urine should be an indicator of GFR. If one can measure the concentration of this substance in blood and in urine, one can estimate GFR using an equation.

Inulin, a nontoxic polysaccharide derived from plants, meets these requirements, and it has been used successfully by physiologists and clinicians to estimate GFR in research studies. Although inulin is considered an excellent way to measure GFR, it is not routinely used to measure GFR in humans because it requires an infusion of inulin into the patient's blood.

The most common way to estimate GFR is by measuring blood concentration of ***creatinine***, a normal byproduct of muscle metabolism that is produced at a steady rate. Creatinine is freely filtered by the glomerulus. To a small extent, creatinine is also secreted by the tubule, which means that it is not a perfect compound for measuring GFR, but it provides a good estimation. If the GFR is high, creatinine is removed rapidly from the blood by glomerular filtration, so the creatinine blood concentration is low. If the GFR is low, creatinine is not removed rapidly from the blood, so the creatinine blood concentration is high.

Equations have been developed and tested that allow one to estimate GFR based on a patient's blood creatinine level. The most widely used equation includes correction factors to adjust for the age, gender, and race of the patient.

SELF CHECK

1. Why is the analysis of urine a standard part of a complete physical examination?
2. What pH range is considered normal for urine?
3. When urine has a high specific gravity, what does this indicate?
4. What is the most common method of measuring glomerular filtration rate?

Common Diseases and Disorders

Although diabetes is an endocrine disorder, it affects the urinary system as well. Other diseases and disorders of the urinary system include several related specifically to the kidneys, as well as urinary incontinence and urinary tract infections.

Diabetes

Diabetes, which means "passing through" in Greek, refers to conditions in which urine output is abnormally elevated. In other words, too much water is passing through the body in these conditions. The two types of diabetes, as discussed in Chapter 9, are diabetes mellitus and diabetes insipidus. (When the term *diabetes* is used alone, it refers to diabetes mellitus.)

Diabetes Mellitus

Diabetes mellitus is characterized by the production of large amounts of urine that contains glucose, a sweet, colorless sugar. (The Latin word *mellitus* means "sweet.") Diabetes mellitus develops in one of two ways: when the body fails to produce insulin (a hormone produced in the pancreas), or when the body's cells fail to respond to insulin.

Diabetes mellitus can be considered a malabsorption disorder (inability to absorb nutrients) because cells do not absorb glucose across their membranes effectively. This results in the need for patients to match their caloric intake with their energy needs throughout the day. They need to choose calories carefully to avoid large peaks and valleys in blood glucose level.

Type I diabetes mellitus is an autoimmune disorder in which the body's immune system attacks and destroys the insulin-producing cells of the pancreas. Type II diabetes mellitus is less well understood. Both types of diabetes involve an inability to metabolize glucose properly after carbohydrate digestion. As a result, blood glucose levels can soar.

Figure 15.12 illustrates carbohydrate digestion and blood glucose regulation in a healthy person. Because a person with type I diabetes cannot make insulin, his or her blood glucose level soars after a carbohydrate-rich meal. The muscle cells and fat cells are not stimulated by insulin to take up and store glucose.

As explained earlier, glucose is normally filtered by the glomerulus and fully reabsorbed in the renal tubule due to cotransport with sodium in the tubule. In diabetes mellitus, so much glucose enters the filtrate from the glucose-rich plasma that the renal tubule cannot reabsorb it all. This is why the urine of patients with diabetes mellitus may have a sweet odor.

Excess glucose in the filtrate creates osmotic pressure, which interferes with normal water reabsorption in the tubule and collecting duct. The result is less water reabsorption and more urine production. This is an example of ***osmotic diuresis***, or an increase in urine production due to abnormally high osmolality of the filtrate.

One of the most serious long-term consequences of diabetes mellitus is kidney damage, or diabetic nephropathy. Diabetes mellitus is the most common cause of chronic kidney disease and renal failure, both of which are discussed later in this section. Excessive protein in the urine (proteinuria) is often the first sign of kidney damage, followed by a gradual decrease in glomerular filtration rate. The kidneys are more likely to function for a longer period of time in diabetic patients who control their blood glucose well.

Understanding Medical Terminology

The word *nephropathy* in the term *diabetic nephropathy* comes from the Greek words *nephros*, which means "kidney," and *pathos*, which means "disease" or "suffering."

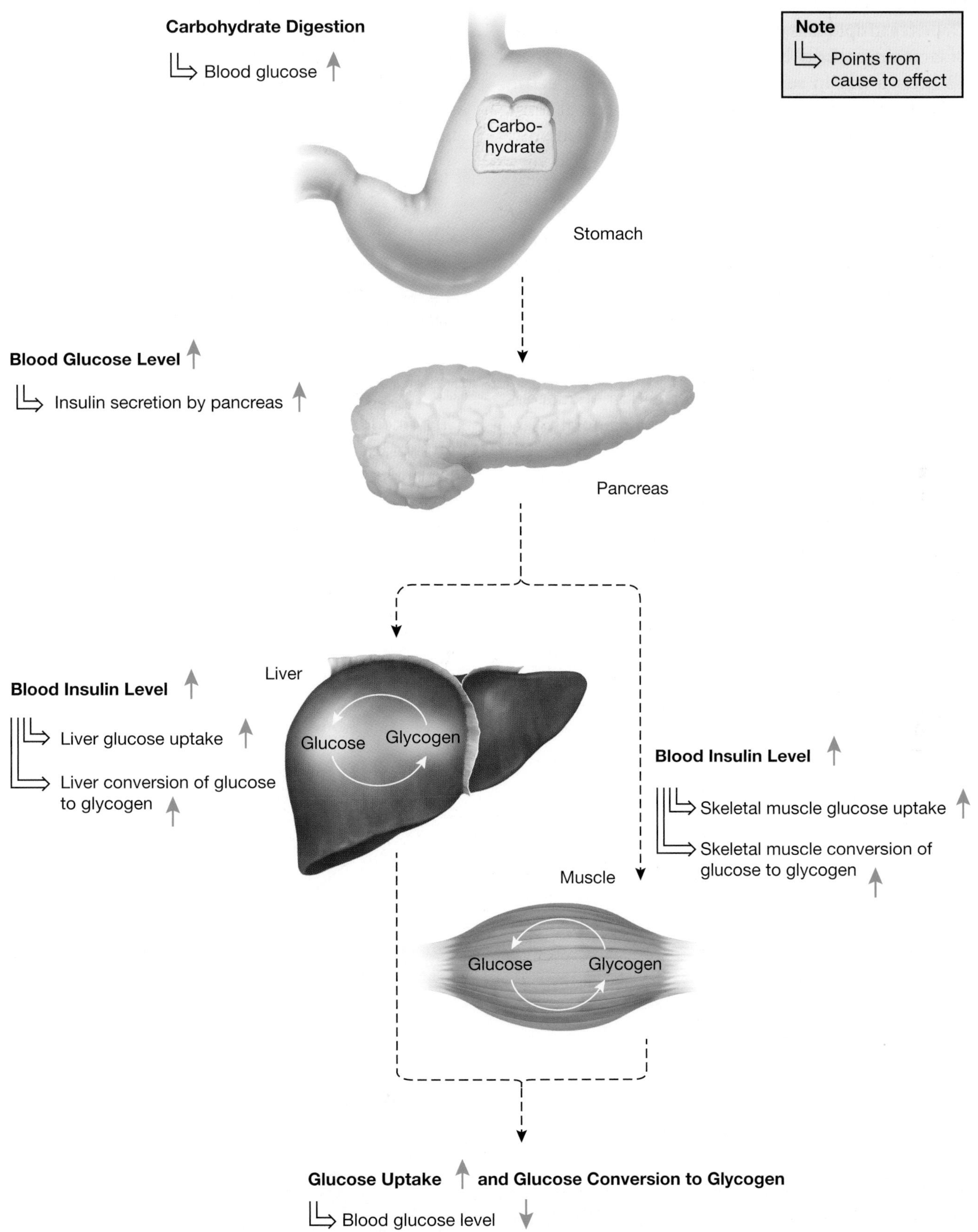

Figure 15.12 Effects of normal carbohydrate digestion on blood glucose and blood insulin levels.

Diabetes Insipidus

Diabetes insipidus is characterized by the production of large amounts of highly diluted urine (more than 12 liters a day in severe cases). The urine specific gravity is less than the normal lower normal limit of 1.002, and the urine osmolality is also low, indicating that the urine is mostly water with very few substances dissolved in it.

Diabetes insipidus is usually caused by failure of the pituitary gland to produce normal amounts of ADH. In a minority of cases, the disease is caused by unresponsiveness of the kidney to ADH.

ADH causes the collecting ducts to be permeable to water. The final stage of water reabsorption occurs in the collecting ducts; therefore, collecting duct reabsorption is critical for the formation of concentrated urine. The regulation of blood osmolality by ADH in a healthy person is shown in **Figure 15.13**. In the absence of ADH, or if the kidney cannot respond to ADH, little or no water is reabsorbed as the urine flows down the collecting duct.

In a person with diabetes insipidus, the brain does not make ADH (central diabetes insipidus), or the kidney does not respond to it (nephrogenic diabetes insipidus), so less water is reabsorbed than normal. As a result, urine output is much higher than normal, and the patient is always thirsty due to the constant loss of fluid. Patients whose diabetes insipidus is caused by a failure to produce ADH often can be helped with a prescription for a synthetic form of ADH.

Understanding Medical Terminology

In the term *diabetes insipidus*, the Latin word *insipidus* means "weak." The urine of a person with diabetes insipidus could be considered to be weak, because both its specific gravity and its osmolality are low.

Chronic Kidney Disease

Chronic kidney disease is diagnosed by evidence of kidney damage (usually proteinuria) or a glomerular filtration rate of less than 60 milliliters per minute for at least three months. Chronic kidney disease develops slowly. Diabetes mellitus is the most common cause, followed by hypertension. Careful management of diabetes and aggressive treatment of high blood pressure with drugs, such as angiotensin-converting

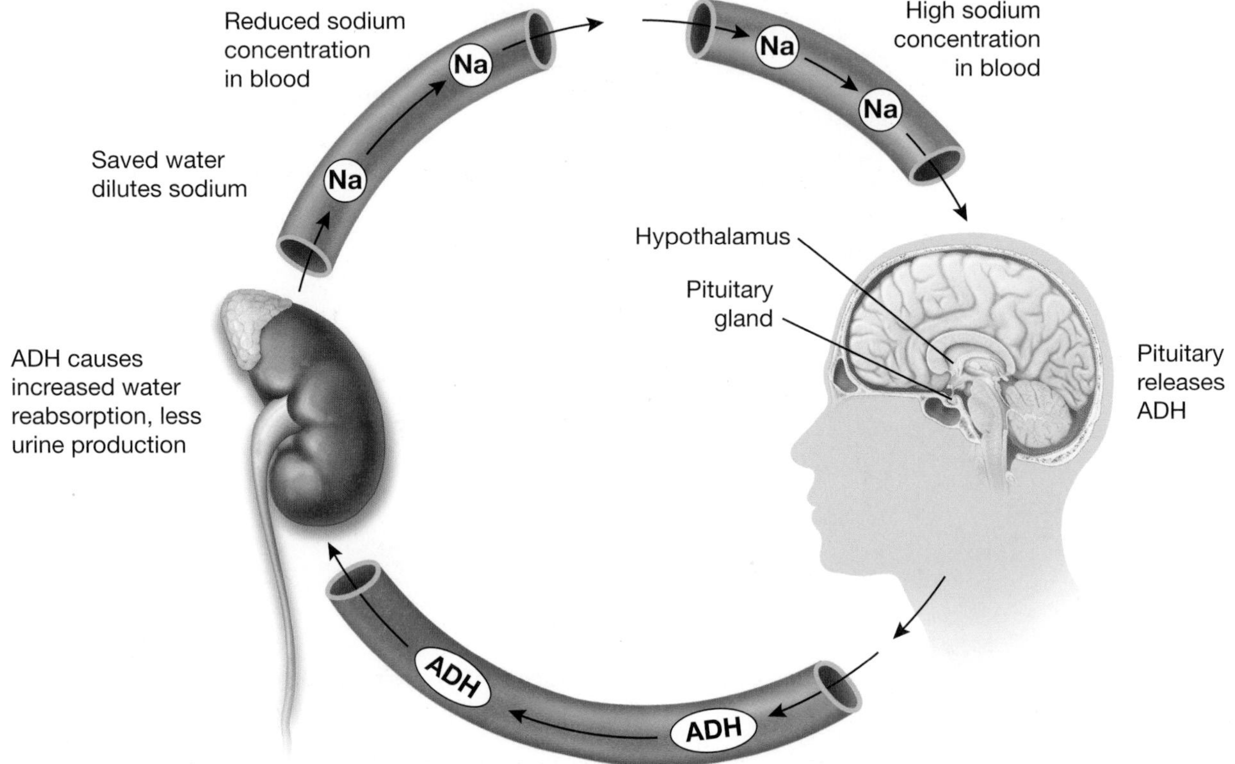

Figure 15.13 Regulation of blood osmolality by ADH. In a healthy person, regulation of both blood sodium concentration and blood osmolality is roughly equivalent because sodium is the biggest contributor to blood osmolality.

enzyme (ACE) inhibitors and angiotensin receptor blockers (ARBs), may slow the progression of chronic kidney disease.

Renal Failure

When GFR decreases to 15 mL per minute or less, a patient is said to have renal failure—the most severe stage of chronic kidney disease. In renal failure, the kidneys are unable to adequately perform their task of maintaining homeostasis. Without treatment, a person cannot survive very long in this state. Waste products accumulate in the blood, and levels of pH and various ions are no longer well controlled. At this stage, the patient must receive a kidney transplant or undergo renal dialysis, a medical technique in which the blood is filtered through a machine.

Because the supply of donor kidneys is very limited, most patients with renal failure undergo dialysis. However, the process of dialysis compromises a patient's health and lowers his or her life expectancy. In short, filtering the blood through a machine is not as good for one's health or life span as having a real kidney.

Renal Dialysis

Renal dialysis is the removal of wastes from the blood by artificial means. The two types of dialysis are hemodialysis and peritoneal dialysis. Both forms of dialysis remove water, urea, and some sodium from the body.

In ***hemodialysis***, blood is withdrawn from an artery, pumped through a dialyzer—a large blood filtering machine positioned next to the patient—and then returned to the patient through a vein. The dialyzer acts as an artificial kidney, although it does not perform all the functions of a real kidney (**Figure 15.14**).

In the dialyzer, the blood passes through thin tubes whose semipermeable walls make up the dialysis membrane. Dialysis fluid, known as *dialysate*, circulates around those tubes. Urea, other wastes, water, and some electrolytes diffuse out of the blood and into the dialysate. The dialysate is discarded, and the blood is returned to the body.

In ***peritoneal dialysis***, dialysate is added to the abdominopelvic cavity through a surgically implanted port in the abdomen. The dialysate remains in the

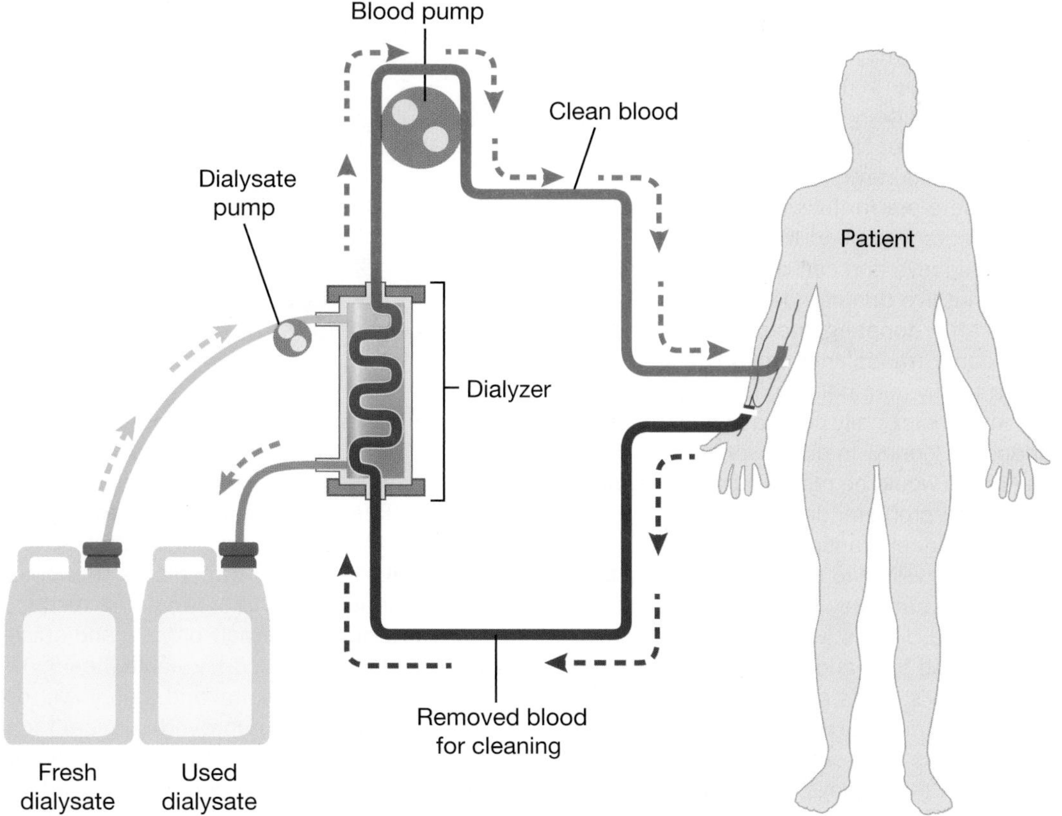

Figure 15.14 Hemodialysis is the most common treatment for renal failure. Blood is withdrawn from an artery, usually in the forearm, and is pumped through a dialyzer. In the dialyzer, a semipermeable membrane separates the blood from dialysate. Dialysate is a fluid with a chemical composition similar to blood plasma. Wastes, including urea, cross from the blood into the dialysate. The "cleaned" blood returns to the body and the used dialysate is discarded.

abdomen for an hour or more, absorbing water and wastes from capillaries in the mesentery (the membrane that attaches the intestines to the wall of the abdomen) and elsewhere in the abdominopelvic cavity. The peritoneum itself serves as the dialysis membrane that separates the blood from the dialysate.

Kidney Stones

A ***kidney stone*** is not really a stone. It is a solid crystalline mass that forms in the urine (**Figure 15.15**). Kidney stones are usually made of calcium-containing compounds, but they can also be composed of magnesium or uric acid.

Kidney stones usually form in the renal pelvis, but they may form in the ureter or bladder. Stones that are smaller than 5 millimeters in diameter may pass from the body in the urine without difficulty. If a larger stone develops in the kidney, it is carried by urine flow to the ureter, where it may become stuck. When a kidney stone becomes lodged in the ureter, it can cause intense pain.

Lithotripsy is the use of intense ultrasonic sound waves to break a kidney stone into pieces small enough to be passed from the body in the urine. The risk of additional kidney stone development can be reduced by drinking lots of fluids. Greater fluid intake increases the volume and flow rate of urine, reducing the likelihood of crystallization.

Urinary Incontinence

Urinary incontinence is the loss of bladder control, leading to release of urine at unintended times. This

Research Notes Paired Kidney Transplants

The human kidney is one of the most commonly transplanted organs in the body. A kidney transplant is performed when a person has end-stage renal failure. In the United States, the two leading causes of end-stage renal failure are diabetes and high blood pressure.

A transplanted kidney may come from a living donor or a recently deceased person. Research indicates that patients who receive a kidney from a live donor have better health and life expectancy outcomes than those who receive a cadaver kidney.

Unfortunately, there are far fewer kidneys available than there are patients who need them. Normally, everyone has two kidneys and can donate one of them. Research shows that live donors do not have shorter or less healthy lives after donating one of their kidneys.

However, live-donor transplants can be difficult to arrange. Often, a family member who is willing to donate a kidney is not immunologically compatible with the relative who needs a kidney. In other words, the kidney from the willing donor would be rejected by the recipient's body. To address this problem, doctors have sometimes performed "paired" kidney transplants.

For example, Bob is willing to donate a kidney to Mark, but Mark's blood type and body tissue are incompatible with Bob's. Meanwhile, Jody is willing to donate a kidney to Kim, but Kim's blood type and body tissue are incompatible with Jody's. Let's suppose that Bob is compatible with Kim, and Jody is compatible with Mark. If they all agree to make "crossed" donations, then both Mark and Kim will get the kidneys they need.

Paired kidney transplants can work in even larger circles of donors and recipients. In 2011, a chain of 30 linked kidney transplants was completed—the largest paired-kidney transplant chain ever. This "pay-it-forward" chain took four months to complete and involved hospitals throughout the United States. Such a large chain of linked kidney transplants was possible due to significant advances in organ donor technology.

For example, extremely precise and efficient methods were used to keep a kidney viable (healthy) while it was harvested at one hospital and then flown to a recipient in another location. Improved surgical techniques increased the odds of success for each operation. In addition, computer technology played a key role in the paired-kidney transplant chain. Before the operations were arranged, a special software program was used to identify possible matches between the patients and willing donors who had joined a national registry.

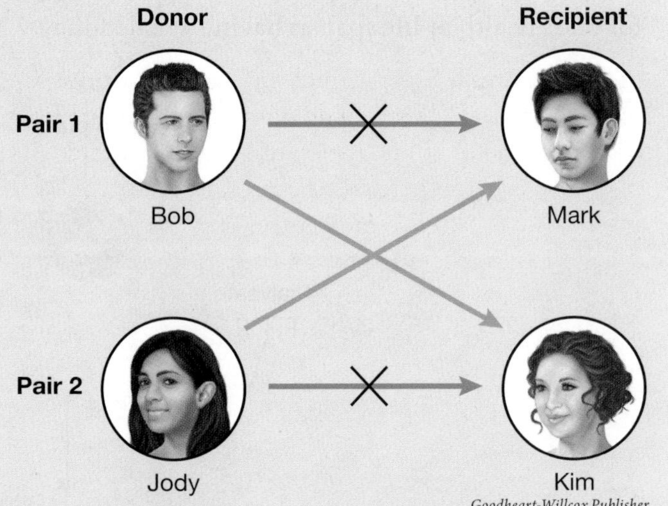

Paired kidney transplants with crossed kidney donation.

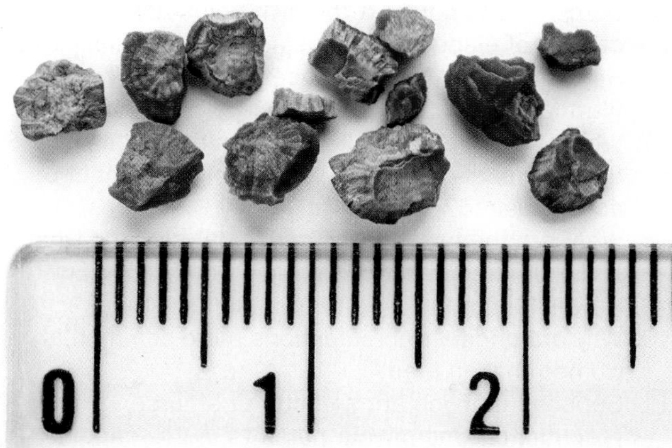

Piotr Malczyk/Shutterstock.com

Figure 15.15 Kidney stones.

is a common and embarrassing problem that affects women about twice as frequently as men. Two of the most common types of urinary incontinence are stress incontinence and urge incontinence.

Stress incontinence, the most common form of incontinence in women, is the release of urine during laughing, coughing, exercising, or heavy lifting. These activities all involve contraction of the muscles of the abdominal wall, which increases the pressure in the abdomen, pushing down on the bladder. This does not usually force urine out because the muscles of the internal and external urethral sphincters, and the pelvic floor muscles, keep the urethra closed. However, if the urethral sphincter muscles or pelvic floor muscles are weak, urine may leak out. Normal childbirth greatly stretches all of the tissues in this region, which increases the risk of stress incontinence. Treatment options include choosing to urinate more frequently so the bladder is never very full; performing exercises to strengthen the pelvic floor muscles; and taking drugs that relax the detrusor muscle, which forms the bladder wall, so that it will not contract as forcefully on the urine it contains.

Urge incontinence, sometimes referred to as *overactive bladder*, is the frequent and irresistible urge or need to urinate. The urge can come on quickly, and the patient may not have time to get to the bathroom. A urinary tract infection can cause urge incontinence. In men older than 50 years of age, the prostate gland often enlarges and squeezes on the ureter, which passes through it. This can result in an inability to fully empty the bladder during urination; as a result, the urge to go again may suddenly occur.

Urinary Tract Infections

A ***urinary tract infection (UTI)*** is usually caused by bacteria that enter the urethra at its outside opening. If the bacteria reach the bladder, the resulting infection can lead to cystitis, an inflammation of the bladder epithelium. Urinary tract infections are more common in women than in men because women have a shorter urethra, so bacteria can more easily reach the bladder.

UTI symptoms include pain during urination, increased urinary frequency, fever, and sometimes cloudy or dark urine. If the bacteria travel up the ureters to the kidneys, the kidneys themselves can become infected. The resulting condition is pyelonephritis. Besides the symptoms already described, patients with pyelonephritis often experience pain in the kidney region of the back.

SECTION 15.3 REVIEW

Mini-Glossary

chronic kidney disease a condition diagnosed by evidence of kidney damage or a glomerular filtration rate less than 60 mL per minute for at least three months

creatinine a normal byproduct of muscle metabolism; produced by the body at a fairly steady rate and freely filtered by the glomerulus

hemodialysis a procedure for removing metabolic waste products from the body; blood is withdrawn from an artery, pumped through a dialyzer, and then returned to the patient through a vein

kidney stone a solid crystalline mass that forms in the kidney, which may become stuck in the renal pelvis or ureter; usually made of calcium, phosphate, or uric acid

osmotic diuresis an increase in urine production caused by high osmotic pressure of the glomerular filtrate, which "pulls" more water into the filtrate

peritoneal dialysis a procedure for removing metabolic waste products from the body; the patient's peritoneum is used to filter fluids and dissolved substances from the blood

renal dialysis the removal of wastes from the blood by artificial means

(continued)

urine specific gravity the density of urine divided by the density of pure water

urinalysis laboratory analysis of urine to test for the presence of infection or disease

urinary tract infection (UTI) an infection of the urethra, bladder, ureters, and/or kidney, usually caused by bacteria that enter the urethra at its outside opening

Review Questions

1. Urine consists primarily of what substance? What is the most abundant solute in urine?
2. Why is blood creatinine concentration used to assess kidney function? Why is creatinine considered better than inulin for measuring GFR?
3. Why does the urine of many patients with diabetes mellitus have a sweet odor?
4. Why does the absence of antidiuretic hormone cause diabetes insipidus?
5. Compare and contrast the symptoms and the causes of diabetes mellitus and diabetes insipidus.
6. How is chronic kidney disease defined by glomerular filtration rate?
7. Which functions of the kidneys can be accomplished through renal dialysis? Which functions cannot be accomplished?
8. What are the two types of renal dialysis, and what is the difference between them?
9. How is lithotripsy used to treat kidney stones?
10. Why are urinary tract infections more common in women than in men?
11. Suppose that you are a doctor or a nurse practitioner. One of your patients, a 24-year-old woman, complains of frequent, painful urination. She has a slight temperature. You request a urine sample from her. Her urine is dark and cloudy. What do you think is causing her symptoms?

Medical Terminology: The Urinary System

By understanding the word parts that make up medical words, you can extend your medical vocabulary. This chapter includes many of the word parts listed below. Review these word parts to be sure you understand their meanings.

-al	pertaining to
-ary	pertaining to
cyst/o	urinary bladder
-ic	pertaining to
-itis	inflammation
juxta-	next to, nearby
lith/o	stone, calculus
natr/o	sodium
peritone/o	peritoneum
-plasty	surgery, plastic surgery
ren/o	kidney
retro-	behind
-rrhea	abnormal discharge, flow
-tripsy	to crush
ur/o	urine, urinary tract
ureter/o	ureter
urethr/o	urethra

Now use these word parts to form valid medical words that fit the following definitions. Some of the words are included in this chapter. Others are not. When you finish, use a medical dictionary to check your work.

1. pertaining to the kidney
2. pertaining to behind the peritoneum
3. inflammation of the urinary bladder
4. pertaining to near the medulla
5. pertaining to sodium and urine
6. inflammation of the urethra
7. relating to the ureter
8. plastic surgery of the ureters
9. procedure to crush stones
10. abnormal discharge from the urethra

Chapter 15 Summary

- A human kidney is about the size of a pack of cards and consists of an outer renal cortex, an inner renal medulla, and a central renal pelvis.
- In the kidney, blood passes from afferent arterioles to capillaries, and then to efferent arterioles and another set of capillaries. Only then does the blood reach a venule and larger veins.
- Three steps are involved in urine formation: glomerular filtration, reabsorption, and secretion.

- Urine is stored in the bladder, which stretches as it fills.
- When the bladder stretches, it generates actions in the nervous system that signal the detrusor muscle to contract and the internal urethral sphincter to relax. When the "time is right," the brain sends signals that cause the external urethral sphincter to relax, and the urine is expelled.
- The amount, color, pH, and specific gravity of urine are characteristics that can indicate abnormalities in kidney function.
- Diseases and disorders that affect the urinary system include diabetes, chronic kidney disease, kidney stones, urinary incontinence, and urinary tract infections.

Chapter 15 Review

Understanding Key Concepts

1. Which of the following names for the lighter-colored, outer part of the kidney is correct?
   A. renal cortex
   B. renal medulla
   C. renal pelvis
   D. renal pyramids
2. Which organs of the endocrine system sit on top of each kidney?
   A. adrenal glands
   B. pituitary glands
   C. thyroid glands
   D. pancreas
3. Approximately how many nephrons does each kidney contain?
   A. 1,000
   B. 100,000
   C. 1 million
   D. 10 million
4. Which blood vessel is connected to the kidney and carries blood into it?
   A. renal vein
   B. abdominal aorta
   C. glomerular capillaries
   D. renal artery
5. What is the name of the tube that leads from the kidney toward the bladder?
   A. PCT
   B. vasa recta
   C. ureter
   D. urethra
6. What are the three main parts of the renal tubule?
7. *True or False?* Cortical nephrons are the only nephrons that produce highly concentrated urine.
8. Where are the peritubular capillaries located?
9. Which of the following is *not* a step in the formation of urine?
   A. absorption
   B. reabsorption
   C. secretion
   D. filtration
10. The endothelial cells, basement membrane, and podocytes combine to form the ______.
11. Which of the following is an important benchmark in assessing kidney health?
    A. PCT
    B. ADP
    C. ADH
    D. GFR
12. *True or False?* Hydrostatic pressure is influenced by the amount of dissolved substances in water.
13. In the renal corpuscle, does the blood or the filtrate have a higher osmotic pressure?
14. What important purpose is served by the microvilli on the wall of the proximal convoluted tubule?
15. Which of the following structures allows water to easily enter and exit cells during reabsorption?
    A. sodium-potassium pump protein
    B. aquaporin channel
    C. cotransport protein
    D. renal tubule

16. Which of the following is *not* an accurate description of the interstitial fluid in the renal medulla?
    A. watery
    B. salty
    C. concentrated
    D. higher than normal osmolality
17. Which substances are reabsorbed from the renal tubule? Which substances are secreted into it?
18. A decrease in blood sodium or an increase in potassium results in secretion of ______.
19. *True or False?* The detrusor muscle must relax for urine to be excreted.
20. The external and internal sphincter muscles are controlled in different ways. Explain.
21. *True or False?* The brain plays a role in the excretion of urine.
22. Approximately what percentage of urine is water?
23. When GFR is high, creatinine concentration is ______; when GFR is low, creatinine concentration is ______.
24. Which of the following substances is normally present in urine?
    A. urea
    B. white blood cells
    C. glucose
    D. protein
25. *True or False?* In diabetes, too much water is passing through the body.
26. *True or False?* Diabetes is a kidney disease.
27. *True or False?* Creatinine is a normal byproduct of muscle metabolism.
28. An increase in urine production due to abnormally high osmolality of the filtrate is called ______.
29. A deficiency in the hormone ______ is linked to the development of diabetes mellitus.
30. What is often the first sign of kidney damage?
31. What are the two main causes of chronic kidney disease?
32. What are the two types of renal dialysis, and how does each one work?
33. What does dialysis remove from the blood?
34. What are kidney stones? How can they be treated and prevented?
35. Which organs of the urinary system may be affected by a urinary tract infection?

Thinking Critically

36. Compare and contrast the cortical nephrons and the juxtamedullary nephrons.
37. Why do the descending limb and the lower part of the ascending limb have thinner walls than the rest of the ascending limb and the proximal and distal convoluted tubules?
38. Explain why a GFR of 125 milliliters per minute indicates that the body reabsorbs most of the glomerular filtrate.
39. Compare and contrast the functions of the three key hormones involved in urine volume and composition.
40. Suppose that you are a patient with renal failure. Compare and contrast a kidney transplant with renal dialysis in terms of benefits and costs.

Clinical Case Study

Read again the Clinical Case Study at the beginning of this chapter. Use the information provided in the chapter to answer the questions at the end of the scenario.

41. Comment on John's blood and urine laboratory results. Refer to information in the chapter, and use online sources as necessary.
42. Comment on the results of John's physical examination.
43. What might you conclude about John's kidney health? How do his different medical conditions relate to one another?

Analyzing and Evaluating Data

This table shows selected urine measurements over a period of time for a 30-year-old adult male. Answer the questions using the data and what you have learned in this chapter.

Selected Urine Measurements				
Test	1	2	3	4
Specific gravity	1.023	1.031	1.027	1.046
Daily volume	1.25 L	1.20 L	1.15 L	1.0 L
GFR	125 mL/m	95 mL/m	80 mL/m	75 mL/m

44. Is the specific gravity of the patient's urine trending higher or lower?
45. Would the patient's urine be "saltier" in test 2 or test 4?
46. By what percentage did the patient's daily volume of urine production drop between test 1 and test 4?
    A. 80%
    B. 2%
    C. 8%
    D. 20%
47. How would you assess this patient's kidney health? Give specific reasons for your assessment.

Investigating Further

48. Conduct further research on renal failure. Compare and contrast acute and chronic renal failure, and describe the treatment options for each.
49. Find out more about the various elements included in a urinalysis. What is included in the physical examination of the urine? In the chemical examination? What information about general health do the various results provide?
50. Physicians often order a 24-hour urine collection for various diagnostic tests. A creatinine clearance test is one of these tests, but there are many others as well. Conduct research to find out what values can be determined and which tests can be performed on a 24-hour urine sample. What diseases might these tests help diagnose?

16 The Male and Female Reproductive Systems

Clinical Case Study

Anika, age 24, has come to her physician's office due to discomfort in the lower abdomen. She feels an uncomfortable sense of fullness in the right lower quadrant of the abdomen, which has developed over the last few weeks. She has also noticed the need to urinate more frequently. Her appetite has remained normal. She takes oral contraceptives, and her mother is a breast cancer survivor.

Physical examination shows that Anika's blood pressure, heart rate, respiration, and temperature are normal. Her weight is normal for her height. An unusual mass is palpable and tender in the lower right abdominal quadrant. She provides urine and blood samples, and her urinalysis and blood test results are within normal limits. Tests of the urine and blood for human chorionic gonadotropin are negative. Anika is referred to a gynecologist for follow-up. The gynecologist does a manual pelvic examination and an ultrasound examination of the abdomen and pelvis.

What features of pelvic anatomy and physiology are relevant to Anika's symptoms? How is her family history relevant? How do the physical examination and laboratory tests, paired with her symptoms, help clarify the possible diagnoses? What is the significance of the negative test results for human chorionic gonadotropin?

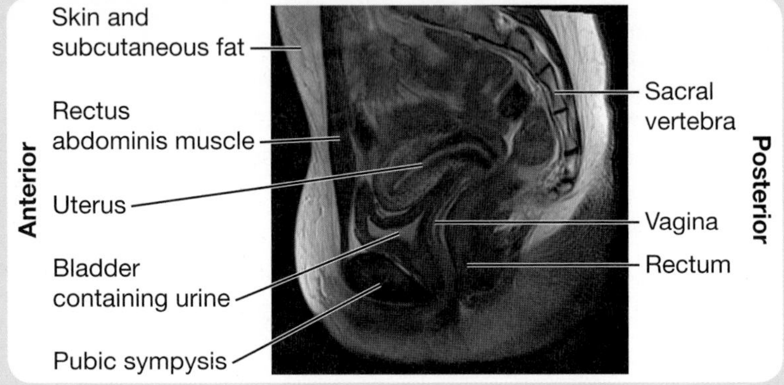

Steven Needell/Science Source

MRI of a normal female pelvis. This is a midsagittal view.

Chapter 16 Outline

The birth of a child is, for most parents, and for all children, the most significant life event. Viewed from a multigenerational perspective, all of the other physiological systems in the body exist to ensure that people live long enough to reproduce and care for their young until they can take care of themselves.

Most of the major body systems are similar between males and females. In the human reproductive system, however, major structural and functional differences exist between the sexes. For example, the male system has two principal functions, and the female reproductive system has five, as explained in this chapter.

The chapter begins by reviewing the differences between meiosis and mitosis—important information to have in mind when studying the generation of sperm and eggs. The chapter then explores the anatomy and physiology of the male reproductive system, followed by the anatomy and physiology of the more complicated and multifunctional female reproductive system. It discusses pregnancy, childbirth, and lactation. Finally, the chapter reviews some of the more common disorders and diseases of the male and female reproductive systems.

SECTION 16.1

The Human Reproductive Systems

Objectives

- Describe the main difference between sexual reproduction and asexual reproduction.
- Explain the differences between mitosis and meiosis.
- Describe the development of the reproductive systems from the embryonic and fetal stages through puberty.

Key Terms

centromere
chromatids
chromosomes
crossovers
diploid
fertilization
follicle-stimulating hormone (FSH)
gametes
haploid
luteinizing hormone (LH)
meiosis
menarche
zygote

This section examines both sexual and asexual reproduction and compares the two different processes involved in cell reproduction: mitosis and meiosis. It also explains the development of the male and female reproductive systems, both before birth and during puberty.

Reproduction

In most animals, including humans, both parents contribute genetic material to each of their offspring. This is called *sexual reproduction*. Another way of reproducing involves only one parent. In this case, the offspring are clones, or genetic copies, of the parent. This is called *asexual reproduction*.

Asexual reproduction is common in the plant kingdom. It occurs more rarely in a few primitive animal species, including flatworms. Asexual reproduction is simple because only one parent is required and combining genetic material is not necessary. Genetic diversity still occurs because of mutations that occasionally arise.

Sexual reproduction, which involves two parents, offers the advantage of producing individuals who are genetically different from their parents. However, sexual reproduction is more complicated than asexual reproduction, and the additional steps required provide more opportunities for things to go wrong.

Chromosomes are genetic material, the physical substance that contains the information necessary to make a unique human individual. you may recall from Chapter 2, each chromosome is a very long molecule of DNA and many associated proteins that bind to the DNA. Sexual reproduction requires that each parent produce ***gametes***, or cells for reproduction that contain half as many ***chromosomes*** as a normal cell.

Fertilization is the formation of a single cell containing the genetic material from two gametes—one gamete from each parent. The fertilized cell produced by the combining of gametes is called a ***zygote***. The zygote is the single cell from which a new human being will develop.

SELF CHECK

1. Explain why genetic diversity is possible in asexual reproduction.
2. Name an advantage of sexual reproduction over asexual reproduction.

Mitosis vs. Meiosis

Chapter 2 introduced the process of mitosis. This section describes a similar-sounding cell division process—***meiosis***. Mitosis occurs in all of the body's tissues, throughout the life span, as the body grows and renews itself. Meiosis, on the other hand, occurs only in the sex organs and produces a special kind of cell.

Mitosis

The development of a zygote into an infant requires that one cell give rise to trillions of cells. Mitosis is the process of cell division by which this growth occurs. In mitosis, one cell divides to make two "daughter" cells. The two daughter cells are genetically identical to the mother cell, except for the occasional mutation. The process of mitosis is shown in the left panel of **Figure 16.1**.

Before mitosis begins, the mother cell contains 23 pairs of chromosomes—22 pairs of autosomes, numbered 1 through 22, plus 2 sex chromosomes. The two members of a chromosomal pair are called *homologous*

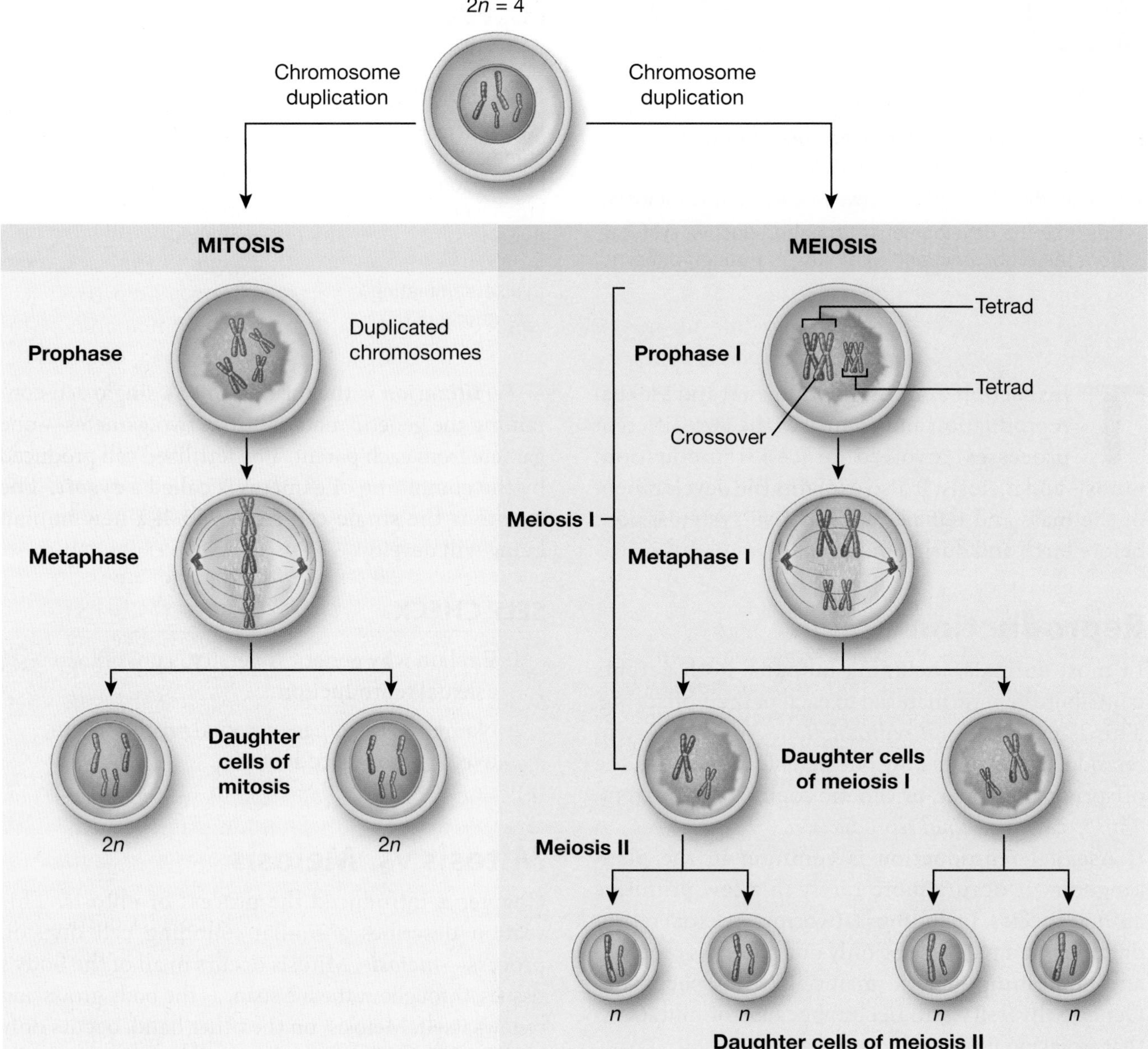

Figure 16.1 Comparison of mitosis with meiosis. An abbreviated look at mitosis is provided here. To more clearly illustrate the process, only 2 of the 23 pairs of chromosomes are shown. For a more complete look at the process, refer to Chapter 2.

chromosomes. For the purpose of explanation, only 2 of the 23 pairs are shown in **Figure 16.1**.

Homologous chromosomes are very similar, but they are not quite identical. The mother cell inherited 23 chromosomes from one parent and 23 chromosomes from the other parent. Therefore, you can think of the purple chromosomes shown in the mother cell in **Figure 16.1** as chromosomes from the mother, and you can think of the green chromosomes as being from the father—or vice versa. A complete diagram would depict 23 purple chromosomes and 23 green chromosomes.

Because humans have two homologous versions of each chromosome, they have two versions of each gene in their cells—one from each parent. The important exception to this general rule is that males have 22 homologous pairs, plus 1 pair that includes one X and one Y chromosome. The X and Y chromosomes are not homologous. This fact is important for understanding the inheritance patterns of certain genetic diseases that preferentially affect males. By contrast, females have 23 pairs of homologous chromosomes, including 1 pair with two X chromosomes.

In both mitosis and meiosis, DNA duplication occurs during the first stage of cell division, called *interphase* (refer to Chapter 2). Interphase is essentially the normal, resting state of a cell.

In prophase, the stage during which the cell prepares for mitotic division, the nuclear membrane dissolves. The DNA, which had been diffuse (scattered or spread out), condenses into chromosomes. The duplicated chromosomes, called sister ***chromatids***, remain attached to each other at a point along their length called the ***centromere***, as seen in **Figure 16.2**.

In metaphase, the chromosomes line up in the middle of the cell. A protein called *separase* splits the sister chromatids by cutting the centromeres in half.

In the remaining phases of mitosis (anaphase and telophase), each chromosome is pulled to one side of the cell or the other, and the cytoplasm divides. The result is two cells, each with 46 chromosomes that are identical to the 46 chromosomes in the mother cell.

Meiosis

A cell with two copies of each chromosome—in other words, a normal cell—is said to be ***diploid***. A cell with just one version of each chromosome is ***haploid***. Gametes, the cells for reproduction, are haploid cells.

In meiosis, the goal is to produce gametes, or haploid cells. This is done by duplicating the DNA once, and then dividing twice to produce four haploid cells.

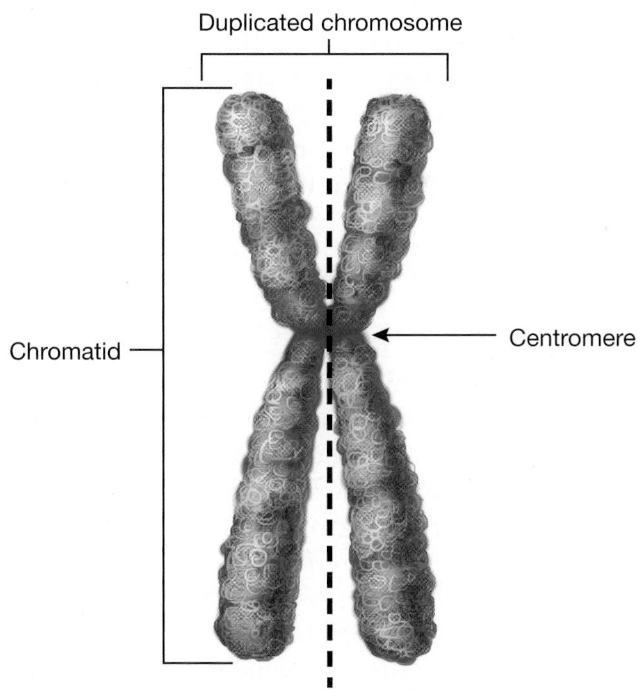

Figure 16.2 Sister chromatids.

Meiosis occurs only in the primary sex organs—the testes and the ovaries.

Chromosome duplication occurs before meiosis begins. This is followed by two phases of cell division: meiosis I and meiosis II. During prophase I of the first meiotic division ("Meiosis I" in **Figure 16.1**), duplicated pairs of homologous chromosomes come together to form tetrads, or clusters of four chromosomes. (The prefix *tetra-* comes from a Greek word meaning "four.")

The clustering of homologous chromosomes in tetrads allows ***crossovers*** to form. A crossover is a connection that forms between homologous chromosomes, resulting in the swapping of portions of chromosomes. Tetrads and crossovers form in meiosis but not in mitosis. Crossovers generate additional genetic diversity in the gametes. The right panel of **Figure 16.1** illustrates an example of a crossover event: in metaphase I, notice the small pieces of green and purple chromosomes that have switched to the homologous (different color) chromosome.

When chromosomes separate in the first meiotic division, the sister chromatids are not separated as they are in mitosis. The daughter cells of the first meiotic division contain 23 *duplicated* chromosomes. (Due to crossing over, these duplicates are not exactly identical.) By contrast, the daughter cells of mitosis contain 23 pairs of homologous chromosomes—in other words, 46 *different* chromosomes. Remember that a pair of homologous chromosomes consists of one from the father and one from the mother, whereas duplicated chromosomes are two copies of the same chromosome (two from the mother or two from the father).

In the first meiotic division, the segregation of chromosomes to one or the other daughter cell is random. It is as though the mother cell "flips a coin" to decide whether to send the purple or green version of chromosome 1 to the daughter cell on the left. (The homologous chromosome always goes to the other daughter cell.) Again, the mother cell "flips a coin" to determine whether the purple or green version of chromosome 2 goes to the cell on the left. This process continues for all 23 pairs of chromosomes.

When one flips a coin 23 times, more than 8 million possible outcomes can occur. Therefore, each mother cell that undergoes meiosis could produce any one of 8 million different possible daughter cells in the first meiotic division. That does not even take into account the additional genetic diversity generated by crossovers.

Focus On When Meiosis Goes Wrong

Occasionally the events of meiosis do not work as described in this chapter. This can result in a gamete (a sperm or oocyte) that has chromosomal abnormalities.

The daughter cells of meiosis I contain 23 duplicated chromosomes. If one of the duplicated chromosomes does not split apart normally during meiosis II, one of the daughter cells of meiosis II receives an extra copy of the chromosome, and the other daughter cell does not receive a copy of that chromosome. The failure of duplicated chromosomes to split apart normally is called *nondisjunction*. In most cases, a gamete with an extra or missing chromosome cannot produce a viable embryo. If such a cell combines with a normal sperm or oocyte to make a fertilized embryo, the embryo dies, resulting in miscarriage.

If the nondisjunction results in a gamete with an extra copy of chromosome 21, then the embryo may survive. This individual will have Down syndrome, also referred to as *trisomy 21*. The signs of Down syndrome include short stature and, often but not always, mental retardation. The probability of nondisjunction in the developing oocyte in meiosis II increases significantly with maternal age. As a result, the incidence of Down syndrome is considerably higher among older mothers.

Nondisjunction that involves the sex chromosomes X and Y also results in viable embryos. Nondisjunction of the sex chromosomes during meiosis of a sperm results in one sperm with an X chromosome and a Y chromosome, and a complementary sperm with neither an X nor a Y. If a sperm with no sex chromosome fertilizes a normal oocyte, a potentially viable embryo with one X chromosome and no Y results. Such an individual develops as a female but is infertile. This condition is called *Turner's syndrome*.

Similar combinations of oocytes and sperm that experienced nondisjunction of sex chromosomes may produce XXY, XXX, and XYY combinations. (An embryo with only a Y chromosome is not viable.) A person who has the XXY chromosome combination has Klinefelter syndrome, develops as a male, and has a significant likelihood of being infertile. People who have the XXX or XYY chromosome combinations develop normally with few, if any, symptoms. In most cases, they will never be aware of their chromosomal abnormality.

In the second meiotic division ("Meiosis II" in **Figure 16.1**), the two daughter cells of meiosis I divide without chromosome duplication. Sister chromatids are cut apart, and the four resulting cells each contain 23 chromosomes. These haploid cells are the final product of meiosis.

SELF CHECK

1. How is a gamete different from normal cells in the human body?
2. Is a haploid cell associated with mitosis or meiosis?
3. What is the goal of meiosis?

Development and Puberty

After the completion of meiosis, every oocyte contains one copy of each autosome (that is, chromosomes 1 through 22), plus an X chromosome. Every sperm contains one of each autosome, and either an X or a Y chromosome, in equal proportions. When an oocyte is fertilized by a sperm carrying an X chromosome, an XX embryo is created. It will develop into a female. Fertilization by a sperm carrying a Y chromosome results in an XY embryo, which will develop into a male. Therefore, the gamete from the father determines the sex of the offspring.

The Y chromosome contains a gene called SRY, which stands for "sex-determining region Y." The gene encodes a protein called a *transcription factor*, which controls when other genes are transcribed—in other words, when they are switched on or off. By regulating other genes, the protein from the SRY gene acts as a molecular switch that triggers a cascade of events leading to the development of male sex organs. A zygote *with* a normal Y chromosome, therefore, becomes a male. A zygote *without* a Y chromosome develops into a female.

Embryonic and Fetal Development

During the first six to seven weeks of development, male and female embryos are visually indistinguishable. Reproductive organs begin to develop in the fifth week, and they develop in the same way in both males and females for the next two weeks.

In the seventh week of development, the SRY gene begins to exert its effect in embryos that have a Y chromosome. Male sex organs begin to develop, starting with the testes. The cells in the developing testes secrete testosterone, which causes the penis, scrotum, and male accessory organs to develop.

Embryos that do not have an SRY gene will start to develop ovaries in the eighth week. In the absence of testosterone, female accessory organs and external genitals develop.

In the final two months of gestation, the testes descend from the pelvic cavity into the scrotum in males. In females, the ovaries descend somewhat, but they remain within the pelvic cavity.

The body's "default plan" is to develop female reproductive anatomy. The presence of the SRY gene on the Y chromosome, and the resulting production of testosterone, causes male anatomical structures to develop. Embryos that cannot produce testosterone—or whose cells do not recognize and respond to testosterone—develop the external genitalia of a female, even if they have a Y chromosome.

Unlike the other body systems, the male and female reproductive systems do not become functional until later in life. At the time of childbirth, the blood levels of ***follicle-stimulating hormone (FSH)*** and ***luteinizing hormone (LH)*** are high. However, these levels decline rapidly and remain low for 8 to 14 years, until the onset of puberty. Because FSH and LH are low, the testes do not produce testosterone, and the ovaries do not produce estrogen or progesterone. Thus, the reproductive organs remain nonfunctional for the first 8 to 14 years of life.

Puberty

Puberty is the final maturation of the reproductive system. Lasting several years, it marks the time when sexual reproduction becomes possible. Puberty normally begins between 8 and 13 years of age in females and between 9 and 14 years of age in males. *Adolescence* is defined as the period from the initial appearance of secondary sex characteristics to the time when adult height is reached.

The initial stimulus for puberty is elevated secretion of gonadotropin-releasing hormone, or GnRH. This hormone is secreted by the hypothalamus in the brain. GnRH causes the pituitary gland to produce more FSH and LH. In turn, FSH and LH stimulate production of gonadal hormones—testosterone in males, and estrogen and progesterone in females. The rising levels of gonadal hormones stimulate maturation of the reproductive organs and cause the appearance of secondary sex characteristics (**Figure 16.3**).

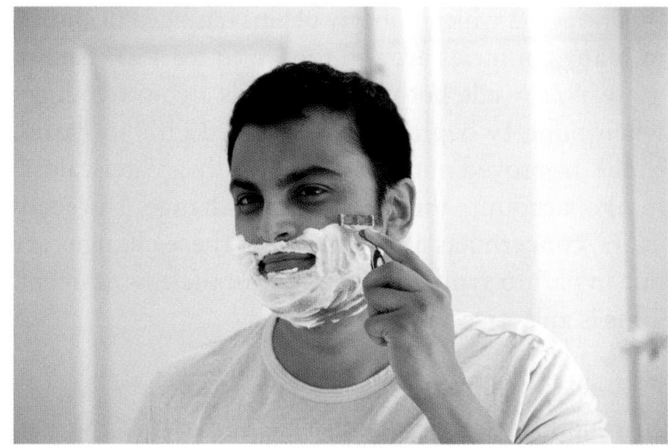

AshTProductions/Shutterstock.com

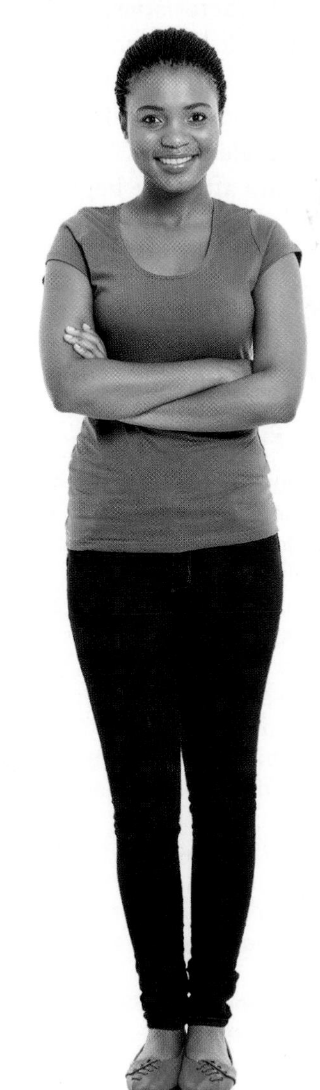

michaeljung/Shutterstock.com

Figure 16.3 Secondary sex characteristics appear at puberty. Both males and females develop underarm and pubic hair; males develop facial hair. Females develop breasts and a wider pelvis that eventually aids in pregnancy and childbirth.

The age at which puberty begins has been declining in many countries around the world for 150 years or more. As a result, both boys and girls are now younger when puberty begins than boys and girls in earlier times. Improved nutrition, specifically greater caloric intake, accounts for much of this change. In recent years, concern has also arisen that these changes are due in part to synthetic chemicals in the environment. This is an active area of research.

Female Development

In females, the first phase of puberty is marked by breast growth, followed by the development of secondary sex characteristics: growth of axillary (underarm) and pubic hair and a gradual increase in the width of the pelvis and the size of the pelvic outlet to facilitate pregnancy and childbirth. In addition, skeletal growth accelerates.

About two years after the beginning of puberty, ***menarche***—the first menstrual bleeding—occurs. Ovulation cycles are typically irregular for the first one or two years. They become more regular as puberty reaches its conclusion. At this time, the epiphyseal plates in the long bones close, causing height growth to stop.

Male Development

In males, the first visible phase of puberty is growth of the scrotum and testes. As in females, secondary sex characteristics appear, with a key difference: besides pubic and axillary hair growth, an increase in the size of the larynx and the length of the vocal folds causes the voice to deepen. The penis grows larger in proportion to body size.

During the early years of puberty, males typically experience erections at unexpected times, as well as an occasional nocturnal emission—the emission of semen during sleep. By the end of puberty, mature sperm are present in semen. As in females, the epiphyseal plates close, and the long bones in the body stop growing.

SECTION 16.1 REVIEW

Mini-Glossary

centromere the point on a chromosome that divides the chromosome into two arms; functions as the point of attachment for the sister chromatids; provides movement during cell division

chromatids paired strands of a duplicated chromosome that become visible during cell division and are joined by a centromere

chromosomes rod-shaped structures in the nuclei of body cells that contain individual DNA and genes

crossovers connections that form between homologous chromosomes during meiosis, resulting in the swapping of portions of chromosomes

diploid a cell containing two sets of chromosomes, one set from the mother and one set from the father

fertilization the formation of a single cell that contains the genetic material from two gametes, one from each parent

follicle-stimulating hormone (FSH) a hormone secreted by the anterior pituitary that stimulates the production of eggs in females and sperm in males

gametes mature haploid male or female cells that unite with cells of the opposite sex to form a zygote; known as eggs in females and *sperm* in males

haploid a cell containing a single set of unpaired chromosomes

luteinizing hormone (LH) a tropic hormone produced by the anterior pituitary that signals the egg's release from the follicle, stimulates the production of progesterone and small amounts of estrogen in women, and stimulates the interstitial cells of the testes to produce testosterone in men

meiosis a type of cell division that produces daughter cells with half the chromosomes of the parent cell; produces eggs in females and sperm in males

menarche the first menstrual bleeding

zygote a diploid cell produced by the fusion of a sperm with an egg; a fertilized egg

Review Questions

1. What are the offspring of asexual reproduction called?
2. Compare and contrast asexual and sexual reproduction, identifying and explaining as many differences as possible.
3. Which is simpler—sexual or asexual reproduction?
4. How many pairs of chromosomes are in a normal human cell?
5. How many pairs of homologous chromosomes do males have? How many do females have?
6. How many chromosomes are there in a mother cell as mitosis begins?
7. What is the difference between haploid and diploid cells?

(continued)

8. What role do crossovers play in genetic diversity?
9. What is the first major event of meiosis?
10. Compare and contrast mitosis and meiosis, explaining as many similarities and differences as possible.
11. Explain the differences between the embryonic and fetal development of the male and female sex organs.
12. What are the age ranges for the onset of puberty in males and in females? At what point does puberty end?

SECTION 16.2 The Male Reproductive System

Objectives

- Describe the anatomy of the male reproductive system.
- Explain male reproductive physiology.

Key Terms

bulbourethral glands
ductus deferens
ejaculation
epididymis
erection
gonads
penis
prostate gland
semen
seminal glands
seminiferous tubules
sperm

The male reproductive system has two primary functions. It is responsible for producing sperm and for delivering it to the female reproductive tract.

Male Reproductive Anatomy

For both males and females, the primary reproductive organs are the ***gonads***, the sites of gamete production. In males, the gonads are called *testes* (singular *testis*), or testicles, and the gametes are called *sperm*. ***Sperm*** are the male haploid cells that can fertilize an egg to make a zygote.

The accessory reproductive organs in the male reproductive system are the other structures needed for sperm maturation and delivery of sperm to the female. These include the external genitals—the penis and scrotum—and internal structures, including five accessory glands: the prostate, two seminal glands, and two bulbourethral glands.

Scrotum and Testes

The scrotum is a pouch of skin that hangs outside the body, below the pelvic cavity, in the midline, and anterior to the anus (**Figure 16.4**). The region between the scrotum and the anus is the perineum, not to be confused with the peritoneum, which was discussed elsewhere in this textbook. The scrotum contains the two testes and associated ducts.

The external location of the scrotum causes the temperature of the testes to be about 93.2°F (34°C), which is cooler than the core body temperature of 98.6°F (37°C). Sperm formation is most vigorous at this cooler temperature. Two muscles—the cremaster and the dartos—work together to maintain optimum temperature of the scrotum. The dartos is just beneath the surface of the skin of the scrotum. The cremaster is deeper and extends upward toward the abdomen. When the scrotum is cold, the cremaster and dartos muscles contract to pull the organ closer to the body and reduce the skin surface area. When the scrotum is warm, the cremaster and dartos relax to allow the scrotum more freedom and greater surface area for cooling.

The spermatic cord travels up the back of the scrotum to the abdomen. It contains the ***ductus deferens***, which transports sperm. An older name for the ductus deferens is *vas deferens*. A vasectomy (meaning "cutting of the vas") is a surgical sterilization procedure in which the ductus, or *vas*, deferens is tied and cut. The spermatic cord also contains the arteries, veins, and lymphatic vessels that supply and drain the testes and scrotum.

The testes are the two primary male reproductive organs inside the scrotum. **Figure 16.5** shows one testis and the ***epididymis***, a structure that curves over the superior and dorsal part of the testis. The testis contains a dense network of small tubes in which sperm forms. These are called ***seminiferous tubules***.

The seminiferous tubules converge and connect to the epididymis. The epididymis is composed of the duct of the epididymis and supporting connective tissue. The duct of the epididymis makes many folds as it travels down along the back of the testis. At the bottom of the testis, the duct bends back upward and becomes known as the *ductus deferens*.

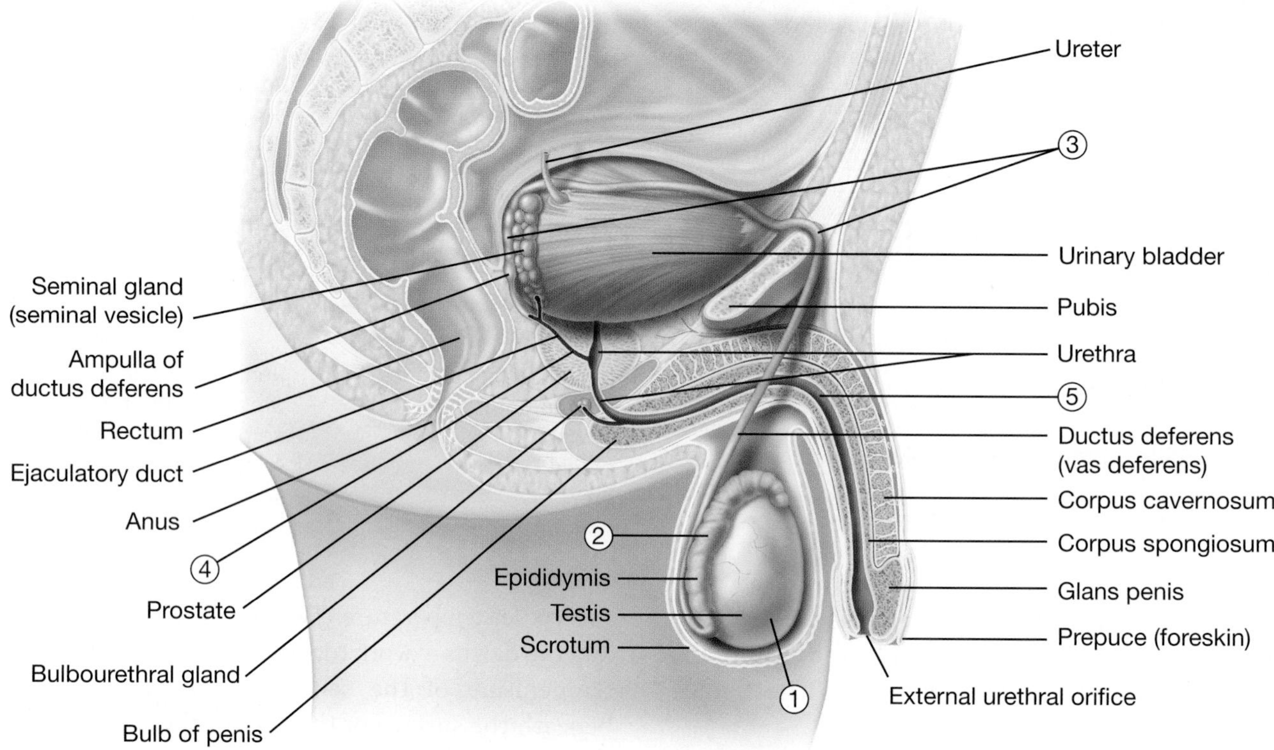

Figure 16.4 Sagittal view of the male reproductive organs. 1—Sperm form in the testes (one testis shown here). 2—Sperm spend 10 to 14 days in the epididymis before they reach full maturation. 3—Smooth muscle in the ductus deferens propels sperm toward the urethra. 4—Sperm from the ductus deferens and fluid from the seminal gland pass through the ejaculatory duct into the urethra. The prostate gland also secretes fluid into the urethra. 5—During ejaculation, semen moves through the urethra and out of the body.

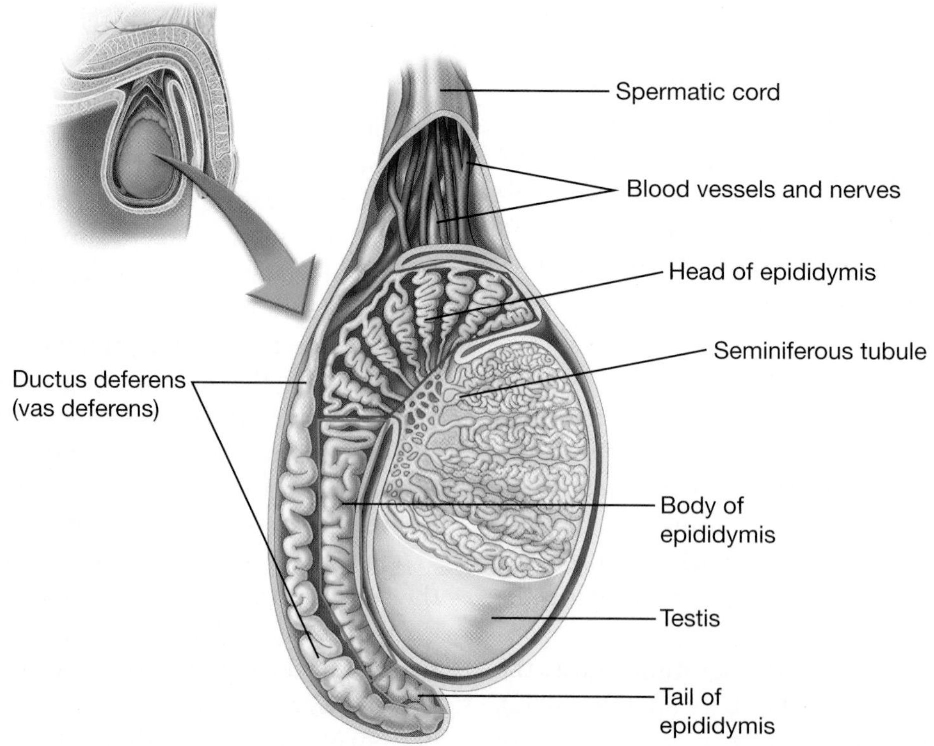

Figure 16.5 A testis and epididymis.

Clinical Application Hernias

A hernia is a condition in which an organ of the abdominopelvic cavity bulges outward through a weak spot in the cavity wall. Hernias that require treatment (usually surgery) occur much more often in men than in women. This is due to the differences in male and female reproductive system anatomy.

The opening at the base of the pelvic cavity, which allows the spermatic cord to pass through, is called the *inguinal canal*. There is one inguinal canal on each side of the midline. It is also the passageway for the descent of the testes from the pelvic cavity into the scrotum shortly after birth. The inguinal canal also exists in women, but it is much smaller because it carries only a nerve.

In men, the inguinal canal is a potential weak spot in the wall of the abdominopelvic cavity. In some individuals, a loop of the small intestine may enter the inguinal canal and protrude partially or fully into the scrotum. This is called an *inguinal hernia*, and it is the most common type of hernia. This condition is painful and dangerous because the loop of bowel is at risk of strangulation (having its blood supply cut off), which can have serious or even fatal consequences.

Inguinal hernias are most likely to occur when abdominal pressure is elevated, since the high pressure pushes out against the wall, forcing open potential weak spots. High abdominal pressure occurs during coughing, while lifting heavy objects or weights, or during forceful defecation or urination.

It is natural to subconsciously perform a Valsalva maneuver (closing the airway, discussed in Chapter 15) while lifting weights, since the Valsalva maneuver makes the trunk more rigid. However, maintaining an open airway while lifting, by breathing out during the lift, prevents extreme increases in intra-abdominal pressure, which in turn reduces the risk of an inguinal hernia occurring during such an activity.

Penis

The ***penis*** is designed to deliver sperm to the female reproductive tract. The shaft of the penis leads to the glans penis, the enlarged end. The prepuce, or foreskin, is a loose fold of skin that covers much of the glans penis.

Circumcision is the surgical removal of the prepuce. This practice may be done for religious, cultural, or hygienic reasons. Circumcision has been shown to reduce the risk of certain sexually transmitted infections. However, some cultures oppose infant circumcision as an unnecessary medical procedure.

The shaft of the penis contains erectile tissue and the urethra. The opening at the outer end of the urethra is the external urethral orifice. The erectile tissue in the shaft is separated into two corpora cavernosa (which lie parallel to each other and extend the length of the shaft) and one corpus spongiosum. These tissues contain spaces in which blood can pool. During sexual arousal, the erectile tissues become enlarged and rigid due to engorgement with blood.

Ducts of the Male Reproductive System

The male duct system (shown in **Figure 16.4** and **Figure 16.5**) transports sperm from the testes, where it is formed to the external urethral orifice at the tip of the penis. Sperm from the seminiferous tubules of each testis enter each epididymis. The duct of the epididymis carries sperm to the ductus deferens. The two ductus deferens carry sperm from the scrotum into the pelvic cavity, inside the body.

Each ductus deferens proceeds from front to back along the upper lateral border of the bladder. At the posterior side of the bladder, the ductus deferens turns downward and widens slightly to form a chamber called the *ampulla* of the ductus deferens. The outlet of the ampulla and the duct from the seminal gland merge to form the ejaculatory duct, which is much shorter than the ductus deferens. An ejaculatory duct enters the prostate from each side and, in the center of the prostate, joins the urethra. The urethra carries urine out of the body during micturition (urination), and it conveys sperm out of the body during sexual intercourse.

Accessory Glands and Semen

Semen is the sperm-containing fluid that is delivered to the female during intercourse. Sperm cells make up only about 10% of the volume of semen. Most seminal volume comes from the accessory glands.

The two ***seminal glands***, or seminal vesicles, produce up to 70% of the volume of semen. The ***prostate gland*** sits directly under the bladder. The urethra passes through the middle of the prostate gland as it descends from the bladder. The glandular tissue of the prostate secretes fluid that makes up one-quarter to one-third of seminal volume. Several ducts from the prostate join the urethra as it passes through the prostate. The two small ***bulbourethral glands*** lie below the prostate. Their ducts join the urethra and contribute a small amount of fluid to semen.

During ejaculation, the total volume of semen ejected typically is 2 to 5 mL. Semen contains 20 million to 150 million sperm cells per mL (**Figure 16.6**).

SELF CHECK

1. In what part of the testes do sperm form?
2. What percentage of the total volume of semen is sperm?

Male Reproductive Physiology

The male reproductive system has two principal functions. The first is to create sperm, and the second is to deliver those sperm to the site of fertilization.

Sperm Formation

Sperm formation, or spermatogenesis, occurs in the walls of the seminiferous tubules of the testes. Here, stem cells called *spermatogonia* undergo mitosis. One of the two daughter cells remains as a stem cell for future division, and the other daughter cell becomes a primary spermatocyte.

The primary spermatocyte is diploid—it has 46 chromosomes. The first meiotic division yields two secondary spermatocytes, and the second meiotic division produces four spermatids. The spermatids are gametes: they are haploid, with 23 chromosomes each.

Each immature spermatid develops a flagellum, or tail, which it will use to propel itself up the female reproductive tract. Once the spermatid has a flagellum, it is released into the lumen of the seminiferous tubule. At this stage, it is referred to as a *sperm*, although it is not yet mature.

It takes nine to ten weeks for a primary spermatocyte to develop into an immature sperm. Immature sperm move from the seminiferous tubules of the testes to the epididymis. The sperm complete their maturation over a period of about three weeks as they slowly progress through the epididymis.

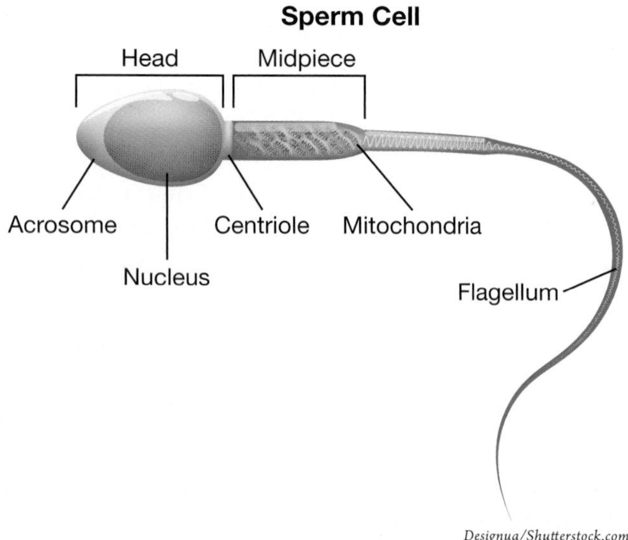

Figure 16.6 A sperm cell.

Sexual Response

The male sexual response can be divided into two major phases: erection and ejaculation. ***Erection*** permits the penis to gain entry to the female reproductive tract. ***Ejaculation*** is the discharge of sperm from the ejaculatory duct.

During erection, the penis enlarges and stiffens in response to sexual stimulation. Neural impulses travel along parasympathetic nerve fibers to the erectile tissues of the penis, triggering the production and release of nitric oxide (NO). This causes relaxation of the arterioles in the erectile tissues of the penis. As a result, more blood fills the tissues, and the penis becomes erect. At the same time, heart rate, blood pressure, and pulmonary ventilation increase.

Ejaculation is the ejection of semen from the body. When sexual stimulation is sufficient, a burst of nerve impulses occurs on sympathetic nerves leading to the male reproductive tract. These sympathetic nerve impulses cause peristaltic contractions of smooth muscle in the male duct system, and of smooth muscle in the male accessory glands.

The nerve impulses also cause contraction of the internal urethral sphincter at the base of the bladder, which prevents semen from entering the bladder. The smooth muscle contractions move semen from the base of the epididymis, ductus deferens, and ampulla to the urethra. Somatic nerve reflexes activate skeletal muscles at the base of the penis. The combination of sympathetic and skeletal muscle activation expels the semen from the urethra. The burst of nerve activity and ejaculation of semen, combined with a pleasurable sensation, are called an *orgasm*.

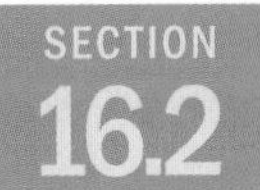

REVIEW

Mini-Glossary

bulbourethral glands two small glands at the base of the penis that secrete mucus into the urethra

ductus deferens the secretory duct of the testis, which extends from the epididymis and joins with the excretory duct of the seminal gland; also known as the *vas deferens*

ejaculation the discharge of sperm from the ejaculatory duct during the male sexual response

epididymis a system of small ducts in the testis in which sperm mature

erection the condition of erectile tissue when filled with blood, which permits the penis to gain entry to the female reproductive tract

gonads the organs that produce gametes (oocytes and sperm); the ovaries in females and the testes in males

penis the reproductive organ that delivers sperm to the female reproductive tract

prostate gland the gland that sits directly under the bladder and surrounds the beginning of the urethra in the male; produces about one-third of the fluid volume of semen

semen the fluid that contains sperm, which is delivered to the female during intercourse; also known as *penile ejaculate*

seminal glands the glands that produce up to 70% of the volume of semen; also known as *seminal vesicles*

seminiferous tubules small tubes in the testes in which sperm form

sperm (singular or plural) the male gamete; a haploid cell that can fertilize an egg to make a zygote

Review Questions

1. Where are gametes made?
2. From a reproductive standpoint, what is the penis designed to accomplish?
3. Trace the path of sperm from the testes to the external urethral orifice, naming each duct and organ through which the sperm travel.
4. What is the name of the fluid that contains sperm?
5. In which stem cells does the production of sperm cells begin?
6. Compare the structures and functions of spermatogonia, spermatocytes, and spermatids.
7. What is the purpose of the flagellum on a sperm?
8. Explain how the anatomy of the male reproductive system makes erection possible.
9. What is the role of sympathetic nerves in stimulating ejaculation?

SECTION 16.3 The Female Reproductive System

Objectives

- Identify the anatomy of the female reproductive system.
- Describe the physiology of the female reproductive system, including the changes that prepare a woman's body for fertilization and pregnancy.

Key Terms

cervix
clitoris
labia majora
labia minora
lactiferous duct
mammary glands
oocyte
oogenesis
ovarian cycle
ovulation
uterine cycle
uterine tubes
uterus
vagina

The female reproductive system has several functions. It not only produces ova, or eggs, for reproduction, but also receives sperm from the male and serves as a safe environment for the developing fetus until birth. In addition, the female reproductive system provides nutrition in the form of breast milk for newborn infants.

Female Reproductive Anatomy

In females, the primary reproductive organs are called *ovaries* and the gametes are called *oocytes*. Female accessory organs include uterine tubes, the uterus, the vagina, external genitalia, and mammary glands.

The Ovaries

The ovaries, shown in **Figure 16.7**, are the female gonads—the organs in which gametes are made. Just as the testes produce sperm and secrete the hormone testosterone, the ovaries produce ova (eggs) and secrete the hormones estrogen and progesterone.

The two oval-shaped ovaries, which are each about 3 centimeters long and 1.5 centimeters wide, are positioned against the posterior wall of the pelvic

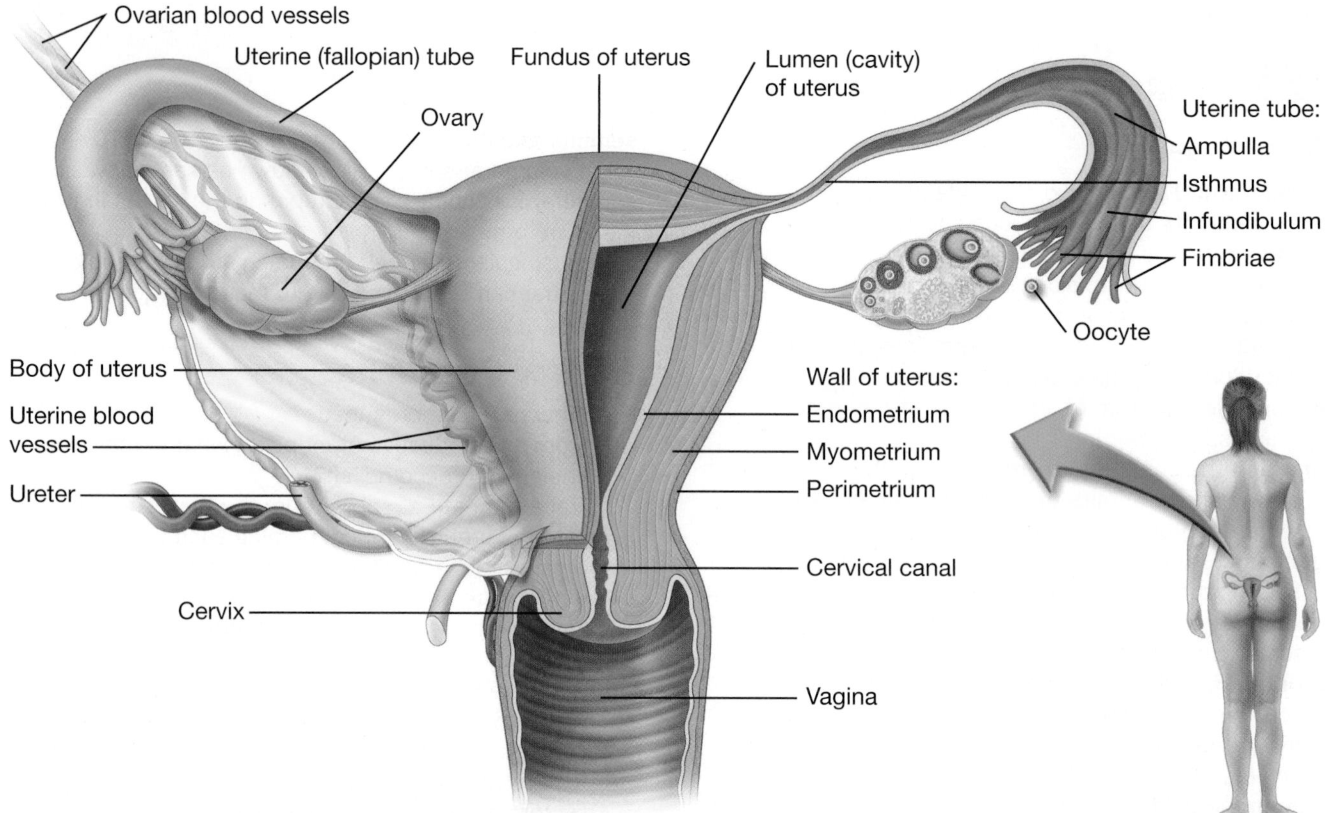

Figure 16.7 The female reproductive organs, posterior view. A cutaway view of one ovary shows development of an oocyte.

cavity. The ovaries, like the testes, have a fibrous outer covering, shown on the right ovary in **Figure 16.7**. Several ligaments help maintain the ovary in its normal position: the suspensory ligament on the lateral side; the ovarian ligament on the medial side; and the broad ligament, which is a sheet of connective tissue just in front of the ovary. The suspensory ligament also carries the ovarian artery, ovarian veins, and ovarian nerves.

Unlike the testes, the ovaries do not contain ducts. Instead, they contain many follicles. Each follicle inside the ovaries contains a single ***oocyte***, or egg cell, and multiple surrounding cells. At any given time, the ovaries of a woman in her reproductive years contain follicles in different stages of maturation. Primordial follicles are the most plentiful and least mature. They contain a single layer of cells surrounding the oocyte.

A primary follicle is slightly larger than a primordial follicle, but it still has only a single layer of cells surrounding the oocyte. Secondary and vesicular follicles are larger and have more cells surrounding the oocyte. Each month, one follicle reaches maturity, and the oocyte it contains is released from its ovary during ***ovulation***. Maturation of ovarian follicles and the details of ovulation are discussed later in this chapter.

Ducts of the Female Reproductive System

There are several differences between the female and male reproductive duct systems. One major difference is the open-ended design of the female system. In males, sperm are formed in the seminiferous tubules of the testes, which connect directly to the duct system that carries the sperm out of the body. In females, the duct system is open at the ovarian end.

Another significant difference is that the female reproductive system is completely separate from the urinary tract. The female urethra is not in any way a part of the reproductive tract. In males, by contrast, the urethra serves a dual purpose: it is both the outlet for the urinary system and the terminal portion of the reproductive tract.

A third major anatomical difference is the placement of the ovaries inside the pelvic cavity in women, while the testes are outside the pelvic cavity. This results in a weak spot in the male pelvic wall where the ducts enter, which creates a risk for hernias.

The biggest difference between the female and male duct system is that the female duct system provides

Focus On The Pelvic Floor

The term *pelvic floor* refers to the muscles at the lower part of the pelvis that support the organs in the pelvic cavity, including the urethra, bladder, and rectum. In women, these muscles also support the vagina, cervix, and uterus. The anal canal and the urethra cross the pelvic floor muscles in both women and men. In women, the vagina also crosses the pelvic floor muscles.

In both women and men, these muscles are essential for maintaining urinary and bowel continence (the ability to keep urine and stool inside the body when desired) because they compress the urethra and rectum. During childbirth, the muscles of the pelvic floor must relax and greatly stretch to allow the baby to pass through the vagina. Sometimes the muscles tear during childbirth, or they stretch so much that they never return to their original length, resulting in weakness.

The muscles of the pelvic floor can weaken with age, even in someone who has never given birth. This can cause weakness of the pelvic floor, also called *pelvic floor dysfunction*. This condition can cause urinary incontinence, bowel incontinence, or pelvic organ prolapse. In pelvic organ prolapse, the bladder, vagina, cervix, and/or uterus shift and bulge downward and outward. In some cases, surgery is recommended to treat pelvic organ prolapse.

the site of fertilization. It is the home in which the fertilized egg becomes first an embryo and then a fetus, and it is the outlet pathway for the fetus during childbirth.

Uterine Tubes

Each of the two ***uterine tubes*** begins at the lateral end of its ovary and curves up and around the ovary to terminate at the top lateral portion of the uterus (**Figure 16.7**). Each hollow uterine tube, also known as a *fallopian tube*, is open at the ovary. It has fringe-like projections called *fimbriae* that wrap part of the way around the ovary. The cells lining the uterine tube, including the fimbriae, have vibrating cilia, which are short, microscopic, hair-like structures.

At the time of ovulation, the vibrating cilia of the fimbriae sweep fluid and, usually, the ovulated oocyte into the uterine tube. Cilia in the tube, and peristaltic contractions of the smooth muscle in the wall of the tube, move the oocyte toward the uterus. The uterine tube passes through the wall of the uterus and opens into the lumen, or cavity, of the uterus.

The open-ended design of the female duct system has one great benefit and several drawbacks. The benefit is that it provides an ovulated oocyte with a means of entry into the reproductive tract. Once in the reproductive tract, the oocyte can be fertilized and develop into an embryo, and then a fetus. The fetus evolves into a newborn human being, which emerges through the cervix and vagina during childbirth.

On the other hand, because the female duct system is open at the ovaries, the oocyte released each month is not always captured by the fimbriae. The oocyte usually dies soon thereafter, but on rare occasions a sperm reaches the oocyte and fertilizes it while it sits in the pelvic cavity. If this happens, the fertilized egg may implant on the wall of the pelvic cavity. A fertilized egg that implants in the pelvic cavity, or in the uterine tube, rather than in the uterus results in an ectopic pregnancy.

The embryo in an ectopic pregnancy cannot survive because it is in an environment that is not designed to support development. Inevitably, a spontaneous abortion (naturally occurring premature termination of pregnancy) will end an ectopic pregnancy. This type of spontaneous abortion can be fatal for the mother. For this reason, an ectopic pregnancy is surgically terminated if it is detected before spontaneous abortion occurs.

The open-ended architecture of the female reproductive ducts also means that women are at risk for pelvic inflammatory disease, a condition that is discussed in more detail later in this chapter.

Uterus

The ***uterus***, also known as the *womb*, is a hollow, muscular organ located in front of the rectum and behind the bladder. It usually lies with its upper end tipped forward over the bladder, as **Figure 16.8** shows. Its purpose is to receive and nourish a fertilized egg, and to expel the fetus by forceful, muscular contractions during childbirth about nine months later.

The wall of the uterus has three layers, which are visible in **Figure 16.7**. The perimetrium is the thin, membranous outer layer. The myometrium, which comprises the bulk of the uterine wall, is made of smooth muscle. The endometrium is the mucosal tissue that forms the innermost layer of the uterus.

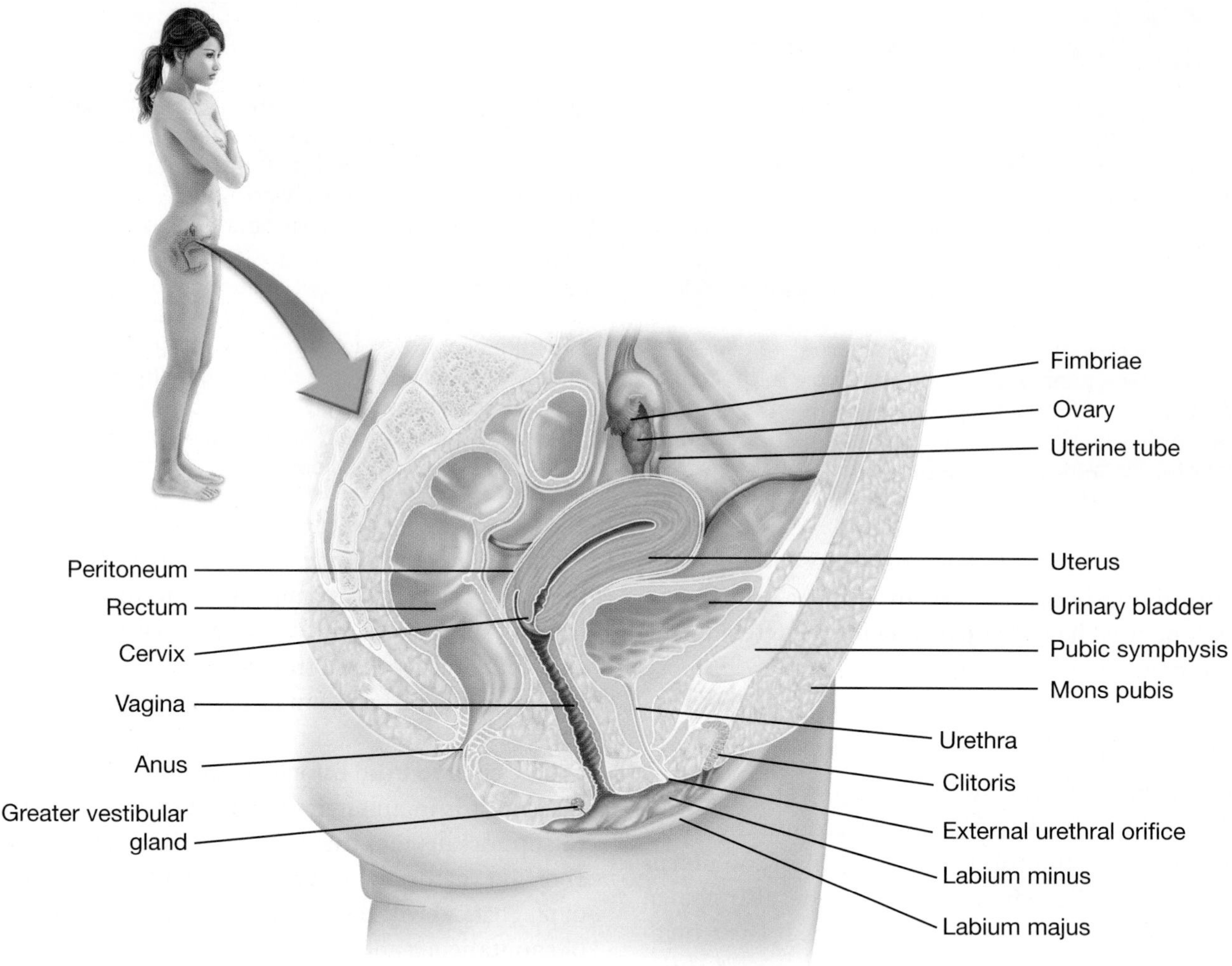

Figure 16.8 The female reproductive organs, midsagittal section.

The endometrium is perhaps the most fascinating layer of the uterus for a couple of reasons. First, it undergoes significant changes on a four-week cycle. Second, it is the layer that receives, envelops, and nourishes a fertilized egg.

The endometrium consists of two layers. The layer that is closer to the lumen is called the *functional layer.* It grows thicker under the influence of hormones and is shed during menstruation. The deeper layer, called the *basal layer,* is not shed during menstruation.

The narrow, lower end of the uterus is called the ***cervix***. The cervical canal is the narrow passageway that connects the lumen of the uterus to the lumen of the vagina.

Vagina

The ***vagina*** is a thin-walled tubular structure located below the uterus. It is sometimes called the *birth canal* because the infant passes through the vagina during

Understanding Medical Terminology

The word *uterus* comes from the Greek word *metra*, which means "womb." Ultimately, *metra* comes from the Greek word *meter*, which means "mother." The root word *metra* appears in the names for the walls of the uterus—*endometrium*, *myometrium*, and *perimetrium*.

The combining form *endo-* means "inside" or "within." Thus, the endometrium is the innermost layer of the uterine wall. The combining form *myo-* means "muscle." The myometrium, the middle layer of the uterine wall, is composed of muscle. Finally, the combining form *peri-* means "surrounding" or "enclosing." The perimetrium is the outer layer of the uterine wall—the layer that surrounds the myometrium and the endometrium.

birth. During intercourse, sperm are delivered to the lumen of the vagina. In normal, healthy adult women, the pH of the vagina is fairly acidic, which helps prevent bacterial infection. Except during childbirth or intercourse, the walls of the vagina usually touch each other. This means that the lumen of the vagina is a potentially open space rather than an actual open space.

External Genitalia

The reproductive structures on the outside of the body are the external genitalia. *Vulva* is another name for the external genitalia in females. The vulva includes the labia, mons pubis, clitoris, and vestibule. The female external genitalia are shown in **Figure 16.9**.

The mons pubis (pubic mound) is the region of skin and underlying fat in front of the vaginal opening on which pubic hair starts to grow during puberty. Just posterior to the mons pubis are the ***labia majora***, two skin folds that lie parallel on either side of the vaginal opening. *Labia majora* is plural for *labium majus*.

Inside the labia majora are the ***labia minora***, a smaller pair of skin folds. The labia majora and the labia minora (singular *labium minus*) limit entry of infectious material into the reproductive tract. Within the labia minora is the vestibule, the recessed area in which the vaginal and urethral openings lie. The two greater vestibular glands secrete lubricating mucus onto the epithelium of the vestibule.

The ***clitoris***, a small structure at the anterior end of the vestibule, is composed of erectile tissue. The clitoris is derived from the same embryologic precursor as the erectile tissue of the penis. The clitoris is covered anteriorly by a skinfold called the *prepuce*, and the exposed tip is called the *glans*. (As you can see, these terms echo the names of similar structures in the penis.) The clitoris is richly endowed with sensory nerve endings. The perineum is the region of skin from the posterior end of the vulva to the anus.

Mammary Glands

The female ***mammary glands*** produce milk for the newborn baby. Increased estrogen in females during puberty stimulates maturation of the mammary glands. A mature mammary gland is capable of lactation, or milk production, but does not produce milk unless stimulated to do so by the hormone prolactin, which is released after childbirth. **Figure 16.10** shows the structure of a lactating mammary gland.

The mammary glands are modified sweat glands. Like sweat glands, they are part of the skin. Each mammary gland lies on top of the *pectoralis major*, the most superficial muscle of the anterior chest wall. On the surface of the breast is the protruding nipple, which is surrounded by a ring of pigmented skin called the *areola*.

The mammary gland contains 15 to 20 lobes internally, each of which contains many smaller lobules

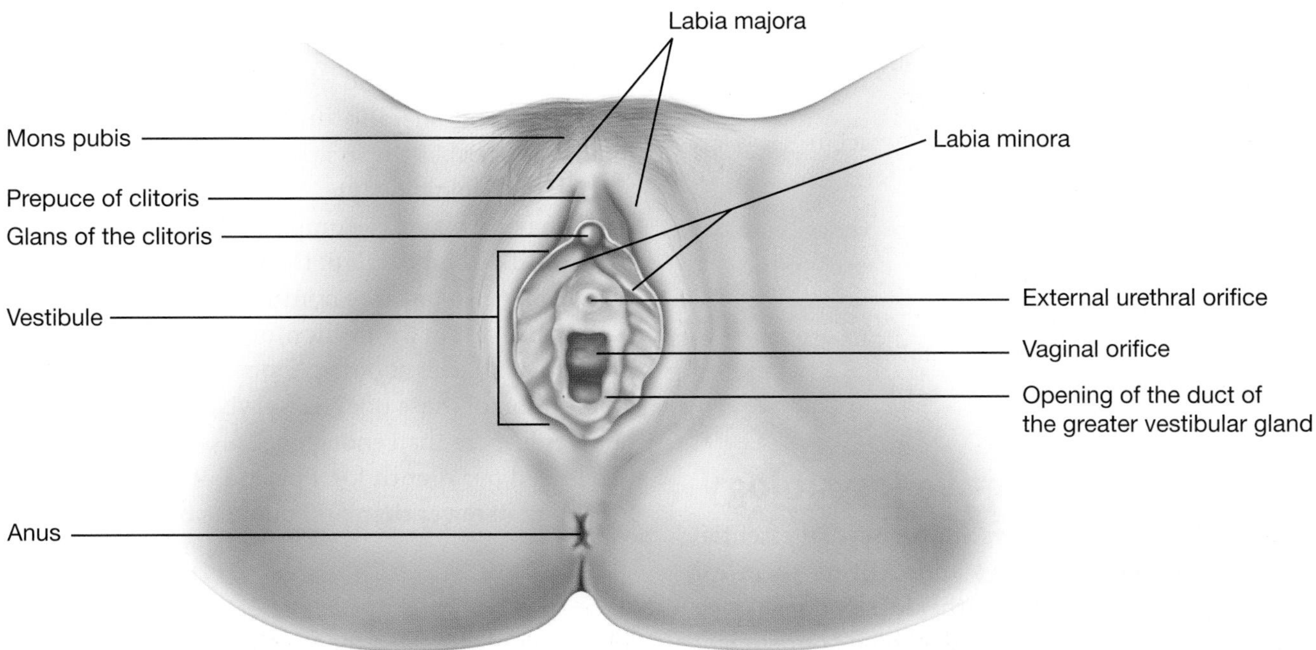

Figure 16.9 The female external genitalia.

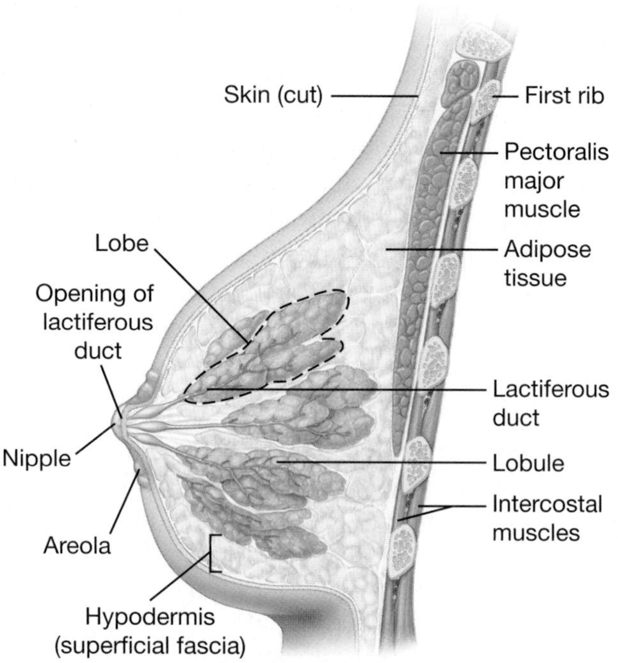

Figure 16.10 A lactating mammary gland.

capable of producing milk. Each lobe secretes its milk into a ***lactiferous duct*** that opens at the nipple. When the breast is not lactating, the glandular tissue remains undeveloped and occupies very little space. The size of the nonlactating breast is determined by the amount of adipose (fat) tissue and interspersed glandular tissue.

SELF CHECK

1. Which reproductive organs in the female are the counterparts to the testes in the male?
2. At ovulation, how does the oocyte move to the uterus?
3. How does an ectopic pregnancy occur?
4. Where is the uterus located?
5. What is the name of the narrow passageway that connects the lumen of the uterus to the lumen of the vagina?
6. Which gland of the female reproductive system is a modified sweat gland?

Female Reproductive Physiology

The female reproductive system has several essential functions. It generates eggs and delivers them for fertilization. It also nourishes the developing embryo and fetus, gives birth, and provides liquid nourishment after birth.

Oogenesis

Oogenesis is the process by which oocytes, or egg cells, are generated. Because gametes must be haploid, the oogenetic process involves meiosis. Oogenesis is similar to spermatogenesis, but also differs from it.

Oogenesis begins in the ovaries of the female fetus before birth. This means the cells of the next generation are being prepared when the present generation is not yet born. Oogonia, diploid stem cells that correspond to spermatogonia in males, undergo mitosis and produce primary oocytes, which correspond to primary spermatocytes. Each primary oocyte is surrounded by a single layer of follicle cells, thus forming a primordial follicle.

The oocyte in the primordial follicle starts the process of meiosis before the female fetus is born. However, meiosis stops partway through the first meiotic division. At puberty, the increased level of follicle-stimulating hormone triggers a small number of follicles to develop further each month. One of these follicles becomes the dominant follicle, and its oocyte completes the first meiotic division, producing two unequal daughter cells. One—the secondary oocyte—gets half of the chromosomes and almost all of the cytoplasm and organelles. The other cell—a polar body (nonfunctional cell)—gets half of the chromosomes and practically nothing more.

The secondary oocyte begins to undergo the second meiotic division, but meiosis stops partway through the division. The oocyte is released from the ovary—that is, ovulation occurs. The second meiotic division of the oocyte resumes and is completed after ovulation, but only if and when the oocyte is fertilized.

The second meiotic division follows the same unequal pattern as the first, yielding a tiny polar body and a large haploid oocyte. Meanwhile, the first polar body may or may not complete the second meiotic division. The end result of the process is one haploid oocyte and two or three nonfunctional polar bodies.

About one to two million oocytes are present as primordial follicles at birth. About one-quarter to one-half million of these oocytes survive to puberty. This number is more than enough because only one oocyte is released per month for a period of 30 to 40 years, for a total of fewer than 500 oocytes over a lifetime.

The Menstrual Cycle

The "monthly" cycle of the female reproductive system, commonly referred to as the *menstrual cycle*, spans

28 days on average, but the actual duration of the cycle varies from about 21 to 40 days. During this cycle, the ovaries and the uterus undergo changes, as do the levels of several key hormones (**Figure 16.11**).

This section looks first at what happens in the ovaries during one cycle. It then examines the changes taking place at the same time in the uterus. These changes are referred to as the *ovarian cycle* and the *uterine cycle*, but keep in mind that all of these changes are occurring at the same time, as part of one monthly cycle.

The Ovarian Cycle

The ***ovarian cycle*** is the sequence of events associated with maturation and release of an oocyte. The cycle has two main phases: the follicular phase, which lasts from day 1 to day 14, and the luteal phase (**Figure 16.11B**). Ovulation, or the release of the oocyte, marks the end of the follicular phase and the beginning of the luteal phase. These changes in the ovary are illustrated in **Figure 16.12**.

The Follicular Phase Each month, several primordial follicles from each of the two ovaries develop into primary follicles. Gradually, one of the primary follicles becomes dominant. This means that only one follicle, from one ovary, develops fully and is released (ovulated) each month.

The maturation of the primordial follicles into one dominant primary follicle marks the initial stage of follicular development. The cells of the primary follicle surrounding the oocyte divide. When these cells become more than one layer thick, they are called *granulosa cells*. At this stage, the follicle is called a secondary follicle.

The secondary follicle grows and the oocyte develops a clear, extracellular glycoprotein coat called the *zona pellucida*. Spaces filled with clear liquid begin to appear around the oocyte in the follicle. The follicle is now called a *late secondary follicle*. When the fluid-filled spaces in the follicle merge into a single, large, fluid-filled antrum (cavity), the follicle is called a *vesicular follicle*.

As the follicle develops first into a late secondary follicle, and then into a vesicular follicle, the growing number of granulosa cells are triggered by FSH to secrete greater amounts of estrogen. **Figure 16.11C** shows the steady rise of estrogen from day 5 to day 14. The rising estrogen level inhibits the release of FSH from the hypothalamus during this time, so the FSH level decreases slightly from about day 6 to day 12. The large vesicular follicle now bulges against the ovarian wall (**Figure 16.12**, step 4).

Near the end of the follicular phase, the rising level of estrogen stimulates the hypothalamus to secrete more GnRH and stimulates the anterior pituitary to release more LH. The increase in GnRH causes the release of more FSH from the anterior pituitary. This results in a surge in FSH and LH levels. The high level of LH causes the primary oocyte to complete its first meiotic division, and the secondary oocyte begins its second meiotic division.

The surge in LH then causes the bulging vesicular follicle to rupture the ovarian wall (**Figure 16.12**, step 5). The result is ovulation—the release of the secondary oocyte and a layer of surrounding cells, called the *corona radiata*, into the pelvic cavity. This release concludes the follicular phase of the ovarian cycle, and the luteal phase begins.

The Luteal Phase Once released, the oocyte is normally swept into the uterine tube by the vibrating cilia of the fimbriae. The remaining cells of the follicle, which are still in the ovary, form the *corpus luteum* (Latin for "yellow body"). Luteinizing hormone, which surged during ovulation, helps stimulate the formation of the corpus luteum (**Figure 16.12**, step 6). The disruption of the estrogen-secreting granulosa cells by ovulation causes blood estrogen levels to plummet after ovulation.

The cells of the corpus luteum begin to secrete progesterone, and the progesterone level in the blood rises steadily during the early part of the luteal phase, as the corpus luteum grows. The corpus luteum now secretes modest amounts of estrogen, leading to a slight rebound in estrogen levels during the early part of the luteal phase. These changes in progesterone and estrogen levels are shown in **Figure 16.11C**.

About 10 days after ovulation, if the oocyte has not been fertilized, the corpus luteum begins to disintegrate (**Figure 16.12**, step 7). This disintegration causes the progesterone and estrogen levels to drop in the late luteal phase. The corpus luteum turns into a small bundle of scar tissue called the *corpus albicans* (Latin for "white body"). If the oocyte is fertilized, hormones prevent atrophy of the corpus luteum, as will be discussed later in this chapter.

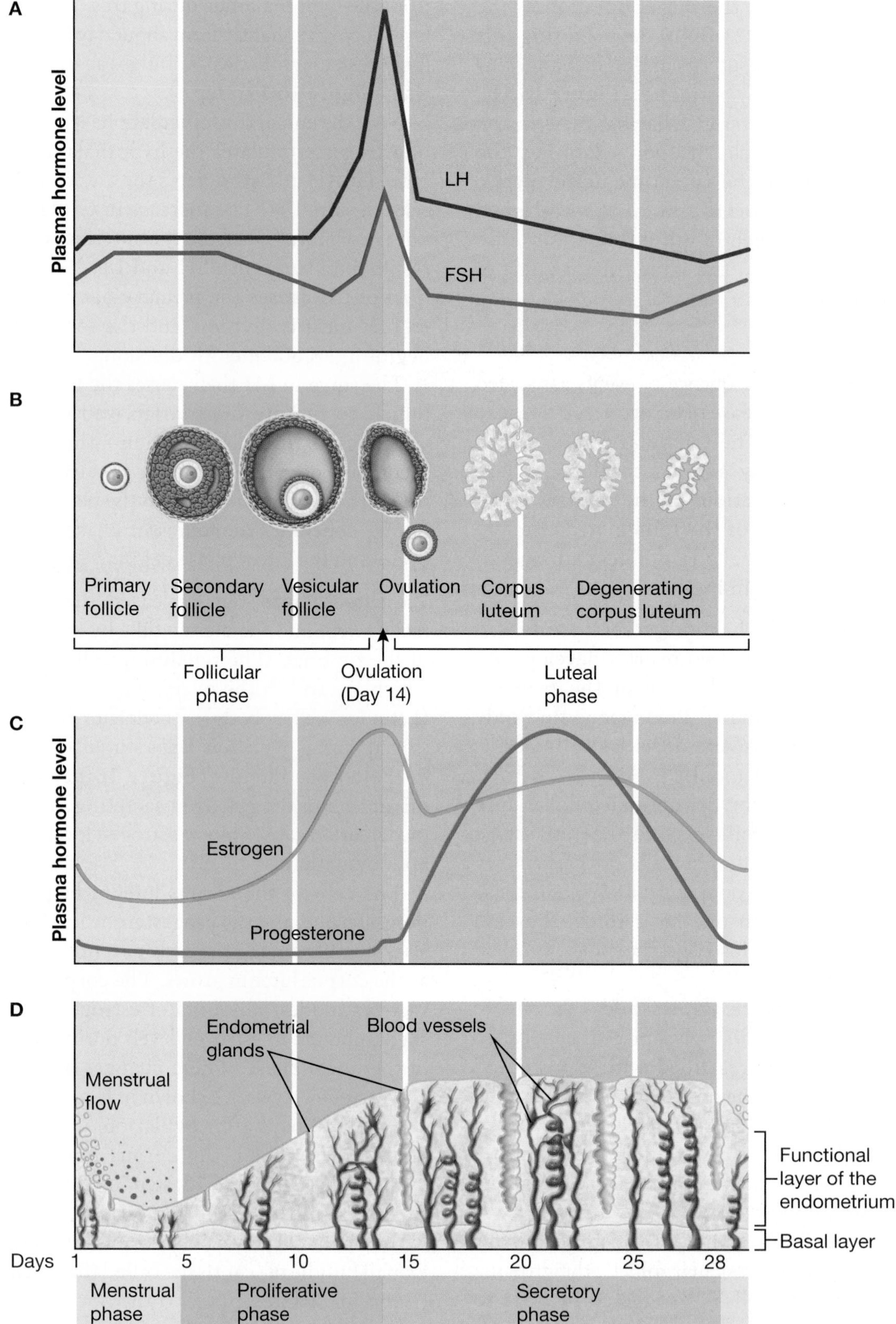

Figure 16.11 Hormonal and structural changes during the female menstrual cycle. The events of one complete 28-day cycle are shown. The time scale, shown horizontally at the bottom, applies to all four panels of the figure. These events apply only when the ovulated oocyte is not fertilized. If it were fertilized, the events of the second half of the cycle would be different in all four panels.

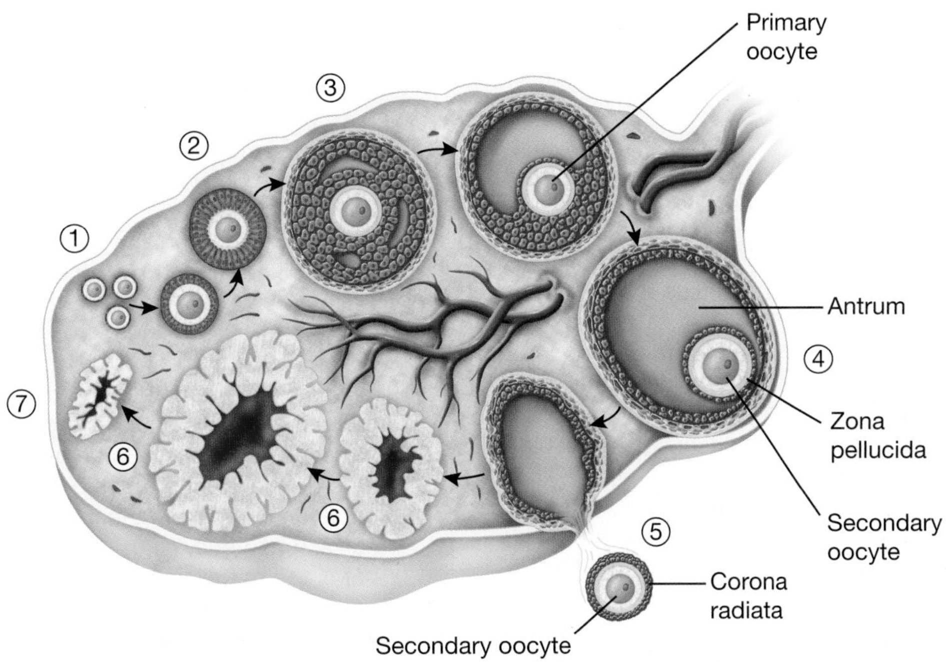

Figure 16.12 Changes in the ovary during the ovarian cycle. 1—Primary follicles. 2—Secondary follicle. 3—Late secondary follicle. 4—Vesicular follicle. 5—Ovulation. The secondary oocyte is released, along with surrounding corona radiata cells. 6—Remaining cells of the follicle turn into the corpus luteum (shown twice). 7—If fertilization does not occur, the corpus luteum turns into a small bundle of scar tissue.

The Uterine Cycle

While the ovaries are undergoing their changes, the uterus is also changing (**Figure 16.11D**). The three phases of the ***uterine cycle*** are the menstrual phase, the proliferative phase, and the secretory phase.

The menstrual phase lasts for the first four to five days of the cycle. During this time, the outer functional layer of the endometrium breaks down. The blood and tissue that are lost during this stage pass from the uterus, through the cervical canal, and out of the vagina, producing the menstrual discharge. By the end of the menstrual phase, the functional layer has been completely shed.

The proliferative phase begins as soon as the menstrual phase ends. The functional layer of the endometrium rapidly grows back, aided by the rising level of estrogen.

During ovulation, the rapid regrowth of the endometrium slows down. Now the rising level of progesterone, which is being made by the corpus luteum in the ovaries, causes the functional layer of the endometrium to develop a dense network of blood vessels. The endometrium also develops nutrient-secreting glands that will nourish an embryo, if one implants. These events take place in the secretory phase.

If fertilization does not occur, the corpus luteum begins to disintegrate, and the progesterone level in the blood falls. As a result, the blood vessels in the functional layer of the endometrium deteriorate, leading to tissue breakdown and bleeding. Thus, a new cycle begins.

Female Sexual Response

As in males, sexual excitement in females activates autonomic and somatic motor reflexes. Sexual stimulation, which can involve psychological and tactile (touch) stimuli, activates parasympathetic nerves to the erectile tissue of the clitoris, which becomes engorged with blood by the same mechanisms as in males. Heart rate, blood pressure, and respiratory rate rise. Increases in vestibular gland and vaginal wall secretions stimulate production of lubricating fluid that facilitates intercourse. The upper end of the vagina dilates, while the lower end constricts, increasing pressure on the penis and enhancing stimulation for both partners. In addition, autonomic nerves activate smooth muscle fibers in the nipples, causing them to become erect.

Orgasm is marked by intense pleasure and rhythmic contraction of smooth muscle in the reproductive tract that may help draw semen into the uterus from the vagina. In females, orgasm is not required for conception. In males, however, orgasm and associated ejaculation are required for successful delivery of sperm.

SECTION 16.3

REVIEW

Mini-Glossary

cervix the narrow, lower end of the uterus that includes the opening through which a baby passes during childbirth

clitoris a cylindrical body of erectile tissue that lies at the anterior end of the vulva

labia majora the two skin folds posterior to the mons pubis that lie parallel on either side of the vaginal opening

labia minora a smaller set of skin folds inside the labia majora

lactiferous duct the duct through which milk is secreted; opens at the nipple

mammary glands the milk-producing glands in the female

oocyte an egg cell

oogenesis the process by which oocytes are generated

ovarian cycle the sequence of events associated with maturation and release of an oocyte

ovulation the release of an oocyte from the ovarian follicle

uterine cycle the monthly cycle of changes that the uterus undergoes; includes the menstrual, proliferative, and secretory phases

uterine tubes the tubes in which the oocyte is fertilized; begin at the lateral end of the ovary and travel up and around the ovary to terminate at the top lateral portion of the uterus

uterus a hollow, muscular organ located in front of the rectum and behind the bladder; also known as the *womb*

vagina a thin-walled, tubular structure located below the uterus; also known as the *birth canal*

Review Questions

1. Explain how the female reproductive system is organized, including subdivisions of each component.
2. What does each follicle in an ovary contain?
3. Where do the uterine tubes begin and end?
4. What is an ectopic pregnancy, and why is it a medical emergency?
5. What is the narrow lower end of the uterus called?
6. Describe the anatomy of the vulva. What are the parts of the vulva called, and where are they located in relation to each other?
7. What is the function of the female mammary glands?
8. What sequence of events occurs during the ovarian cycle?
9. List the names of the uterine cycle phases, and describe what occurs during each phase.
10. Analyze the similarities and differences between the ovarian and uterine cycles.
11. Compare and contrast the three phases of the uterine cycle.

SECTION 16.4

Fertilization, Pregnancy, and Birth

Objectives

- Describe the sequence of events leading to oocyte fertilization.
- Describe the physiological changes that occur in the mother and developing child during pregnancy.
- Explain the sequence of events involved in childbirth.
- Explain how breast milk is produced and secreted.

Key Terms

amniotic fluid
blastocyst
delivery of the placenta
dilation
embryo
expulsion
fetus
human chorionic gonadotropin (hCG)
implantation
lactation
let-down reflex
oxytocin
placenta
prolactin
umbilical cord

For fertilization to occur, the sperm must fight almost overwhelming odds to reach and penetrate an oocyte. Only after this has occurred can the second meiosis be completed, beginning development of the zygote into what will eventually become a newborn.

Oocyte Fertilization

Fertilization occurs when the chromosomes of the oocyte and the sperm unite to produce a zygote, the first cell of a new individual. As you may recall, each gamete—the oocyte and the sperm—has 23 chromosomes. Thus, fusion of the gametes produces a zygote with a full set of 46 chromosomes.

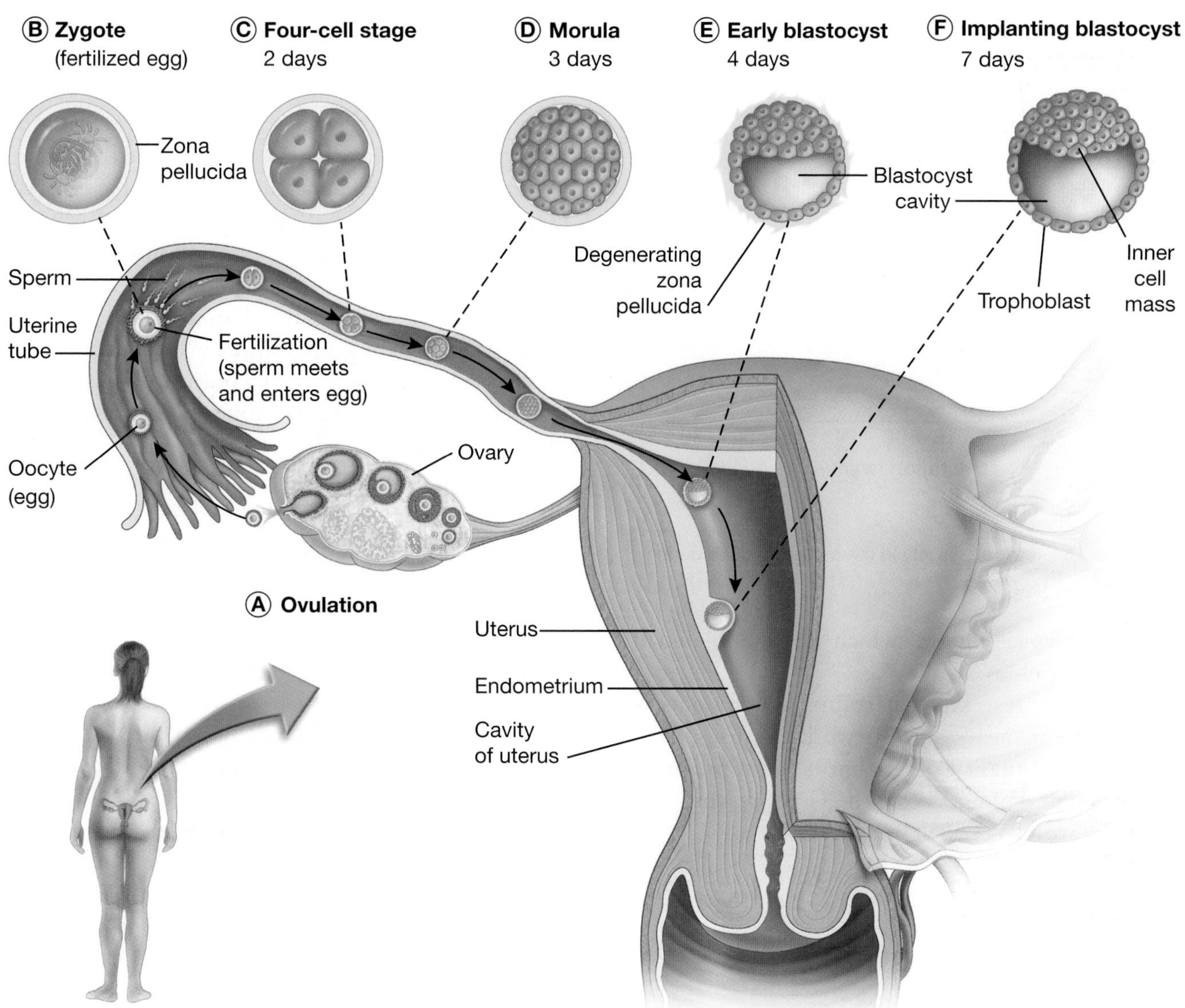

© Body Scientific International

Figure 16.14 Ovulation to fertilization to implantation. A—An oocyte is released from the ovary. B—The egg is fertilized by a sperm. The zygote divides by mitosis. C—The embryo reaches the four-cell stage. D—The embryo becomes a morula, a solid ball of cells. E—A fluid-filled cavity develops in the embryo, now called a blastocyst. F—The blastocyst implants on the endometrium.

Despite implantation, a potential problem awaits the blastocyst: the loss of the endometrial layer that is nourishing it. Recall that the endometrial layer begins to degenerate around day 27 or 28 of the monthly cycle. This would be 13 or 14 days after fertilization, just after the completion of implantation.

Recall that deterioration of the endometrium in a normal cycle (that is, a cycle without fertilization) results from a decline in the hormones estrogen and progesterone. The decline of estrogen and progesterone is due to the atrophy of the corpus luteum at the end of the month.

If the endometrial layer were to be shed during a cycle in which fertilization has occurred, as it usually is during this phase of the cycle, then the blastocyst would be lost. This does not happen, however, because the trophoblast cells surrounding the blastocyst secrete a hormone called ***human chorionic gonadotropin (hCG)***, which prevents atrophy of the corpus luteum, which continues to secrete progesterone and estrogen so that the endometrium is not shed.

The levels of hCG, estrogens, and progesterone in the blood during pregnancy are shown in **Figure 16.15**. The rise in estrogens and progesterone after week 12 occurs because the placenta (which is discussed in the next section) develops and starts to secrete these hormones. At the same time, hCG secretion diminishes

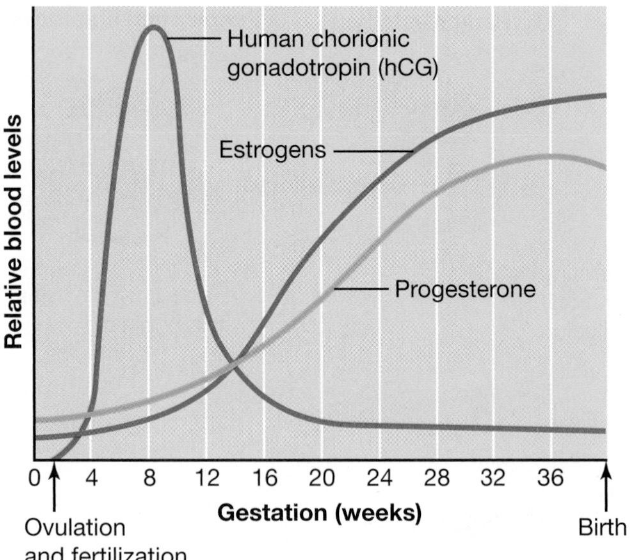

Figure 16.15 Hormone levels in the mother's blood during pregnancy.

and the corpus luteum, which has completed its mission, atrophies.

Pregnancy test kits determine the presence of hCG in the urine. Such tests work because hCG is present in pregnant women, but it is not present in nonpregnant women. When hCG is present, small amounts are also present in the urine.

Development of the Placenta, Embryo, and Fetus

As implantation progresses, the inner cell mass grows larger and more complex as its cells divide and rearrange. By the beginning of the third week, 15 to 16 days after fertilization, the inner cell mass has differentiated into an embryonic disk: a flattened mass of cells about 0.4 mm long, containing three layers: the ectoderm, the mesoderm, and the endoderm. As discussed in Chapter 3, these three layers give rise to all of the major tissues of the body.

When the ***embryo*** is tiny, it can get the nutrients it needs by simple diffusion from the tissue of the endometrium, which has a rich blood supply for this purpose. However, as the embryo grows, it needs more nutrients than the endometrium can supply. The ***placenta*** is the organ that grows in the uterus to meet the nutritional needs of the embryo, which is called a ***fetus*** after 8 weeks of development. The placenta of a 13-week-old fetus, shown in **Figure 16.16**, contains cells of the fetus and cells of the mother. The placenta spreads out like a pancake on the wall of the uterus.

The placenta contains intertwining blood vessels from the cardiovascular systems of the fetus and the mother. The cardiovascular system is the first organ system to function in a meaningful way in the embryo. Just three and one-half weeks after fertilization, when the embryo is only ¼ inch (6 mm) long, the immature heart begins to pump newly formed blood cells through newly formed blood vessels. Neither the embryo nor the fetus can receive oxygen (O_2) or expel carbon dioxide (CO_2) by breathing, and neither can obtain nourishment by eating. The placenta takes care of these needs.

Fetal vessels carry blood, pumped by the fetal heart, through the umbilical cord to and from the placenta. In the placenta, fetal capillaries are surrounded by cavities filled with maternal blood. The maternal and fetal blood do not actually mix; however, the thin layer of cells that separates them allows easy diffusion of nutrients from maternal blood to fetal blood, and diffusion of wastes in the reverse direction. Unfortunately, alcohol or drugs, if present in the mother's blood, can also reach the fetus by this pathway and affect its development.

As **Figure 16.16** shows, the fetus fills up the uterine cavity by week 13. It is surrounded by a set of membranes and bathed in clear ***amniotic fluid***. The inner membrane of its sac is called the *amnion*. Outside the amnion is the chorion, which, like the amnion, is derived from the fetal tissue. The outermost membrane is called the *decidua capsularis* (Latin for "capsule that falls off, or sheds"), which is derived from the mother's tissue. The ***umbilical cord***, which contains two arteries and one vein, connects the fetus to the placenta.

SELF CHECK

1. How long is gestation when measured from the first day of the last menstrual period?
2. What is the term for the process by which the blastocyst binds to the endometrium?
3. Which organ system is the first to function in a meaningful way in an embryo?
4. At what point in its development does the embryo become a fetus?

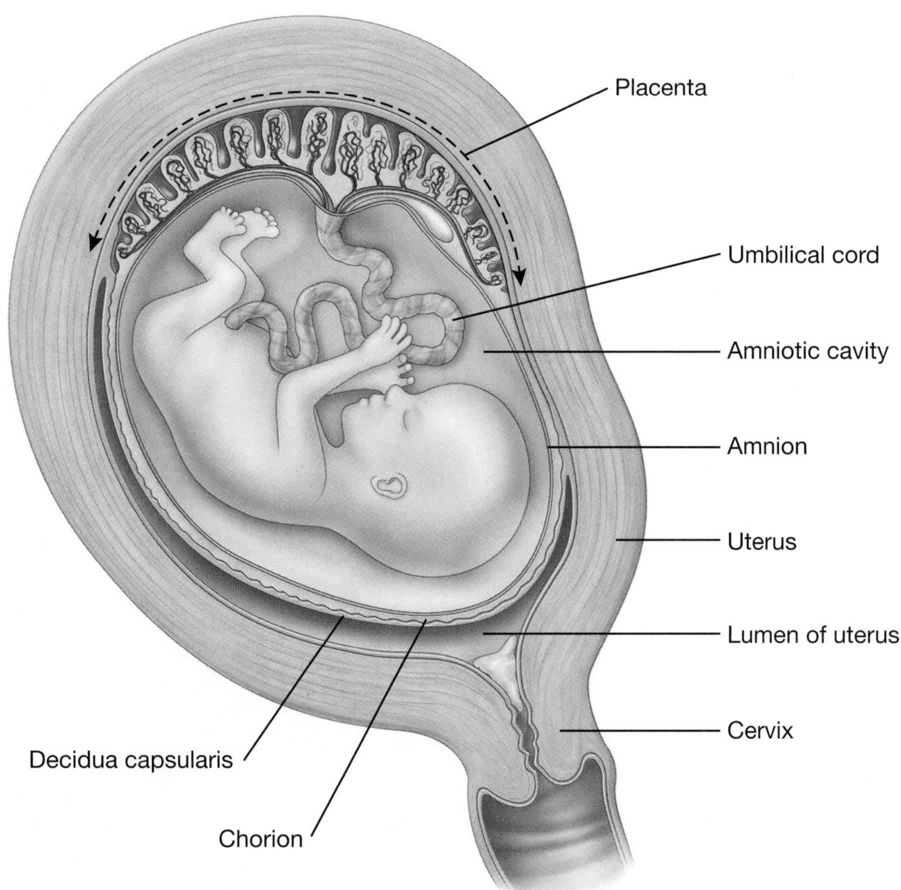

Figure 16.16 A 13-week-old fetus (end of first trimester). The fetus is about 10 centimeters long (crown to rump). The placenta is attached to the wall of the uterus. The fetus is bathed in amniotic fluid contained in a sac whose layers are (from the inside going out) the amnion, the chorion, and the decidua capsularis.

Childbirth

Childbirth, also called *parturition*, normally occurs 38 to 42 weeks after the first day of the last menstrual period. Toward the end of gestation, high levels of estrogen and progesterone cause the uterine muscle cells to become more sensitive to ***oxytocin***, a hormone that plays a key role in labor. Oxytocin is released by the pituitary glands of both the fetus and the mother.

Fetal oxytocin causes the placenta to release prostaglandins, which are lipid compounds that trigger uterine muscle contractions. Once the uterine muscle has started to contract, the baby's head is pushed into the cervical opening, causing mechanical receptors there to stretch. These receptors send messages to the brain that stimulate maternal oxytocin release, causing even more vigorous contractions of the uterine muscle and even greater stretching of the cervical receptors. This is an example of physiological positive feedback: an action triggers a response that, in turn, causes the original action to occur with greater strength and frequency.

Stages of Labor

The stages of labor are dilation, expulsion, and delivery of the placenta. When the time for birth arrives, most fetuses are in the head-down position, also called the *vertex presentation*. The vertex presentation, which causes the baby's head to exit the mother's body first, is shown in **Figure 16.17**. A rump-first position, or breech presentation, makes delivery much more difficult.

The ***dilation*** stage begins with uterine contractions and ends with a full widening of the cervical canal. In early dilation (**Figure 16.17A**), the cervix is several centimeters dilated, and the baby's head is "looking sideways" as it enters the pelvic outlet. In late dilation (**Figure 16.17B**), the cervix is fully dilated (10 centimeters), and the baby's head starts to rotate to a "looking-to-the-rear" orientation as it moves deeper into the pelvis. Dilation, which can last from 6 to 12 hours or longer, is usually the longest part of labor.

The ***expulsion*** stage (**Figure 16.17C**), the period from full dilation to delivery of the baby, lasts less than an hour in most cases. Strong contractions of

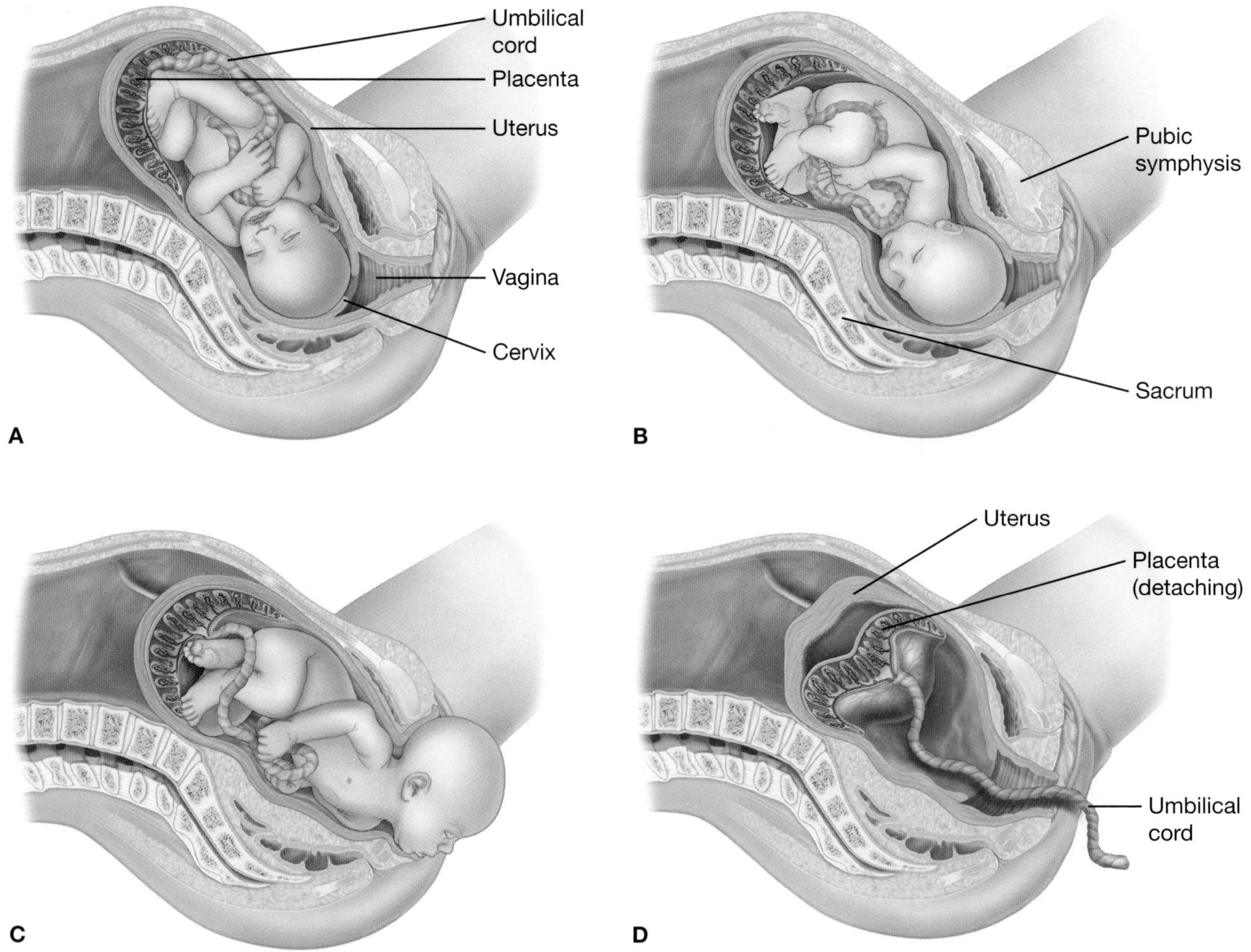

Figure 16.17 The stages of labor. A—Early dilation. B—Late dilation. C—Expulsion. D—Delivery of the placenta.

the uterus, each lasting a minute or longer, occur at two- to three-minute intervals, forcing the baby's head out. Once the head has emerged, the rest of the body usually follows quickly. The baby is still connected to the mother by the umbilical cord, which is clamped and cut.

Delivery of the placenta (**Figure 16.17D**) is the last stage of birth. During this stage, strong uterine contractions continue, causing detachment of the placenta from the uterine wall and expulsion from the mother's body.

SELF CHECK

1. What are the stages of labor?
2. Describe the difference between vertex presentation and breech presentation during the delivery of a baby.

Lactation

Lactation is the production of milk by the mother. Breast milk is a uniquely important source of nutrition for the developing infant. It contains amino acids, fats, carbohydrates, and vitamins that are well absorbed by the infant's digestive system. Breast milk also contains antibodies from the mother that help protect the infant from infection while its own immune system is immature.

Successful lactation requires activation of the normally inactive milk-producing cells of the mammary gland, as well as delivery of the milk to the baby through ducts. The two processes are regulated by two different hormones—prolactin and oxytocin.

Late in pregnancy, high levels of estrogen and progesterone stimulate the hypothalamus in the brain to produce prolactin-releasing factor, a hormone that triggers the release of ***prolactin*** from the pituitary gland. Prolactin stimulates the secretory cells of the mammary glands to produce milk.

Following birth, the infant suckling at the nipple activates receptors that trigger the release of the hormone oxytocin from the mother's pituitary. Oxytocin, which was also important for labor and delivery, causes the ***let-down reflex***—the contraction of smooth muscle cells in the mammary glands—which allows milk to be squeezed toward and out of the nipple.

Research Notes Egg Freezing as a Solution for Infertility

More women than ever are waiting until their 30s or 40s to have children. As a result, age-related infertility has become more common.

Aging can cause infertility for several reasons. A woman in her 30s or 40s has a smaller number of eggs in her ovaries, and the ovaries do not release eggs as often as they did when the woman was younger. Also, the eggs tend to be less healthy. To complicate matters, only about 25% of all fertilized eggs implant in the uterus. Miscarriage, in which the fetus is spontaneously expelled from the body, is more common in women as they age.

New technologies are available to help women who, for medical, economic, or other reasons, are postponing childbirth until later in life. One of these technologies is *oocyte cryopreservation*, more commonly known as *egg freezing*. It is less controversial than embryo cryopreservation because the oocyte is not fertilized, so it is not, by itself, a potential person.

The road to egg freezing begins when a fertility specialist—a medical doctor—prescribes drugs that stimulate a woman's ovaries to produce multiple eggs. The doctor then uses a needle, and ultrasound imaging for guidance, to harvest eggs from the ovaries. The eggs and some surrounding fluid from the pelvic cavity are extracted and placed in a flat dish. A laboratory technician identifies individual eggs through a microscope and withdraws them from the dish for freezing.

If isolated eggs were simply placed in a freezer, ice crystals would form inside them, causing irreversible damage. For this reason, various strategies have been devised to limit ice crystal formation and preserve the viability of the eggs. The two broadly used strategies are dehydration followed by slow freezing, and vitrification.

In dehydration followed by slow freezing, different chemicals are used to draw as much water as possible out of the eggs before they are slowly cooled. When the eggs reach approximately –20°F to –40°F (–30°C to –40°C), they are plunged into liquid nitrogen for long-term storage. Liquid nitrogen is simply nitrogen gas (the main component of air) that has been refrigerated to –321°F (–196°C) or cooler.

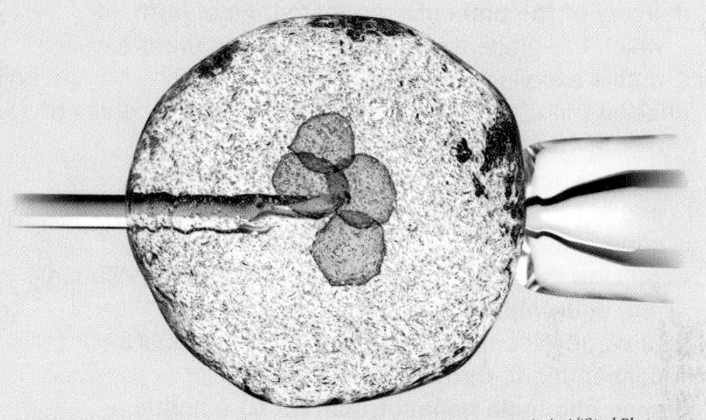

posteriori/iStockPhoto.com

A human oocyte about to be injected with sperm. This procedure, called *intracytoplasmic sperm injection*, is one type of in vitro fertilization.

In vitrification, the eggs are placed in a very small volume of chemical preservative solution for less than a minute, after which they are quickly cooled by direct exposure to liquid nitrogen. Many clinics are adopting vitrification as their standard technique for freezing eggs.

When a woman is ready to have children, the eggs are removed from the liquid nitrogen storage tank and thawed. In a procedure called *intracytoplasmic sperm injection (ICSI)*, each egg is fertilized by injection with a single sperm. When an egg has developed into an embryo, it is implanted into the uterus through a catheter, a flexible tube that is easily inserted through the vagina and the cervix.

In October 2012, the American Society of Reproductive Medicine (ASRM) reclassified oocyte cryopreservation as a proven treatment for infertility. Previously, the process was considered experimental. The ASRM based its decision on analyses of many scientific studies. The studies showed that rates of fertilization and birth, and the health outcomes of the resulting children, were just as good with eggs that had been frozen as they were with in vitro fertilization (IVF) of fresh eggs that had never been frozen.

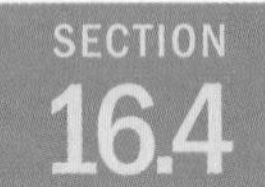

SECTION 16.4

REVIEW

Mini-Glossary

amniotic fluid a clear fluid in which the embryo, and then the fetus, is suspended

blastocyst the embryo from about four to six days after fertilization, when it includes an outer layer of cells, an inner cell mass, and a fluid-filled cavity

delivery of the placenta the last stage of birth, in which the placenta detaches from the uterine wall and is expelled

dilation the stage of labor during which the opening of the cervix dilates, or widens

embryo a developing human from the time of implantation to the end of the eighth week after conception

expulsion the stage of labor that starts at full dilation and ends when the baby is delivered

fetus a developing human from eight weeks after conception to birth

human chorionic gonadotropin (hCG) a hormone secreted by the trophoblast cells of the blastocyst that prevents deterioration of the corpus luteum and stimulates progesterone production in the placenta

implantation the binding of the blastocyst to the endometrium

lactation the secretion of milk by the mammary glands

let-down reflex the contraction of smooth muscle cells in the mammary glands that allows milk to be squeezed toward and out of the nipple

oxytocin a hormone that stimulates uterine contractions during labor and milk secretion during breast-feeding

placenta the organ that grows in the uterus to meet the nutritional needs of the embryo and fetus

prolactin a hormone that stimulates the secretory cells of the mammary glands to produce milk

umbilical cord the cord that connects the fetus to the placenta

Review Questions

1. Describe what occurs during capacitation.
2. When is the second meiotic division of the oocyte complete, and what is the result?
3. How is sperm able to penetrate the zona pellucida of the oocyte?
4. What is polyspermy and how is it prevented?
5. How is menstruation prevented once a blastocyst has successfully implanted in the endometrium?
6. What is human chorionic gonadotropin hormone, and where does it come from?
7. Which hormones are secreted by the placenta?
8. How do the embryo and, later, the fetus receive oxygen and nutrients, and how do they expel carbon dioxide and waste?
9. How is childbirth—in particular, the roles of fetal and maternal oxytocin—an example of a positive feedback system?
10. What does breast milk contain that makes it a uniquely important source of nutrition for the developing infant?
11. What is the let-down reflex?
12. You are a physician with a patient who is reluctant to breast-feed her newborn infant. What would you say to convince her of the benefits of breast-feeding?

SECTION 16.5

Disorders and Diseases of the Reproductive Systems

Objectives

- Describe common causes of male and female infertility.
- Identify common sexually transmitted infections, and describe their symptoms and treatments.
- Identify different types of cancer that affect the male and female reproductive systems.

Key Terms

adhesions
amenorrhea
chlamydia
endometriosis
genital herpes
gonorrhea
human papillomavirus (HPV)
infertility
sexually transmitted infection (STI)
syphilis

Disorders of the human reproductive system impair the ability to reproduce. Infertility is a common reproductive disorder. Because the male and female reproductive systems are open to the outside environment, they are vulnerable to infection and disease. Some reproductive system diseases, such as those that are sexually transmitted, require immediate medical attention because they can easily be spread to healthy individuals. Cancers of the reproductive system are among the most prevalent of all cancers. This section describes common disorders and diseases of the male and female reproductive systems, their signs and symptoms, and their treatments.

Infertility

Infertility is the inability to get pregnant. It is defined clinically as the inability of a couple to conceive after at least one year of unprotected intercourse. Infertility has many possible causes, and the difficulty in conceiving can arise from either the male or the female.

Male Infertility and Impotence

In males, infertility (defined above) and impotence (inability to maintain an erection) are considered to be separate conditions. Male infertility is almost always due to a semen abnormality. The volume of semen may be low, or the number of healthy sperm in the semen may be low, or both.

An insufficient quantity of healthy sperm, often called *low sperm count*, has numerous possible causes, many of which are treatable. Causes include:

- abnormal levels of the hormones that regulate sperm production (LH and FSH)
- chronic warm temperature of the testes, which need to be somewhat below normal body temperature for optimum sperm production
- smoking; heavy use of alcohol, cocaine, or marijuana
- use of anabolic steroids (performance-enhancing drugs)
- exposure to environmental toxins
- older age

If infertility is related to low sperm count, as is frequently the case, further investigation can often help determine a cause. If applicable, appropriate treatment can be given.

Low semen volume may be due to damage to the ducts that convey sperm and other components of semen. The most common cause of such damage is vasectomy (cutting of the ductus deferens to achieve permanent birth control). Other causes of damaged, blocked, or absent ducts include congenital absence of the ductus (vas) deferens (CAVD). CAVD is common in males with cystic fibrosis.

Impotence, or the inability to maintain an erection, is also called *erectile dysfunction* (ED). ED may be caused by damage to the nerves or blood vessels of erectile tissues (common in diabetes), side effects of some medications, prostate surgery, older age, stress, and psychological factors.

The drug sildenafil (better known by its trade name, Viagra) was the first oral treatment for ED to be approved by the Food and Drug Administration. Other, similar drugs are now available. These drugs work by inhibiting the enzyme that breaks down nitric oxide. As discussed earlier, nitric oxide is released from nerve endings in erectile tissues during sexual excitation, and it causes dilation of blood vessels and erection. By inhibiting the breakdown of nitric oxide, ED drugs amplify the effectiveness of the nerve activity involved in sexual excitation.

Female Infertility

Causes of female infertility include failure to ovulate, inability of the egg to reach the uterine tube and travel to the uterus, and inability of the blastocyst to implant successfully on the endometrium.

Failure to ovulate is usually accompanied by abnormal menstrual periods—either a complete absence of menstrual periods, called ***amenorrhea***, or cycles of unusual or unpredictable length. Failure to ovulate is often associated with abnormal levels of FSH or LH, or both. These abnormal levels may be a result of polycystic ovarian syndrome (PCOS), or abnormalities of the pituitary (which secretes FSH and LH) or the hypothalamus (which secretes GnRH). Failure to ovulate may also result from scarring of the ovaries, failure of the mature follicle to rupture, and premature menopause.

Inability of the oocyte to enter and make it through the uterine tube usually results from scarring and damage to the tube. Uterine tube damage can be caused by any of the following:

- diseases of the reproductive tract (usually sexually transmitted infections)
- abdominal cavity infection (appendicitis, for example)

- previous surgery, which can cause scarring or ***adhesions*** (areas where tissues stick together inappropriately)
- ectopic pregnancy
- congenital abnormalities

Failure of the blastocyst to implant on the endometrium can have multiple causes as well. These causes include scars or adhesions on the endometrium from previous infections or surgery; ***endometriosis***, the growth of endometrial cells outside the uterus (usually in the abdominal cavity), which produces inflammation and alters the balance between progesterone and estrogen; uterine fibroids—benign tumors of the muscular layer of the uterus; and abnormalities of the blastocyst itself.

Treatment for Infertility

A variety of treatments are available for male and female infertility, and they depend on the identified cause. Treatments include:

- lifestyle changes (less alcohol, drug, or tobacco use in men can help stabilize or increase sperm count, and reduced stress can be helpful for both sexes)
- drugs to induce ovulation
- surgery to correct anatomical issues

When these treatments fail, a variety of assisted reproductive technologies is available. Microsurgery to reverse tubal ligation in women and vasectomy in men is often successful. In men, if microsurgery is not feasible, it is sometimes possible to extract sperm from the testes and inject one sperm into the oocyte. In vitro fertilization (IVF) is the harvesting of one or more oocytes from the mother and combining them in a petri dish with sperm collected from the father. Fertilization occurs in the dish (*in vitro fertilization* literally means "fertilization in glass"), and the embryo is then transferred into the uterus for implantation.

SELF CHECK

1. What is the clinical definition of *infertility*?
2. What are the two most common causes of male infertility?
3. What are the three most common causes of female infertility?
4. How can male and female infertility be treated?

Sexually Transmitted Infections

A ***sexually transmitted infection (STI)*** is a condition that can be passed from one person to another through sexual intercourse or genital contact. This section discusses the most common sexually transmitted infections: AIDS, gonorrhea, chlamydia, genital herpes, syphilis, and human papillomavirus.

HIV and AIDS

Acquired immunodeficiency syndrome (AIDS) is the most lethal sexually transmitted infection. It is caused by the human immunodeficiency virus (HIV), which is shown in **Figure 16.18**. See Chapter 13 for a more detailed discussion of HIV/AIDS.

Gonorrhea

In the United States, ***gonorrhea*** infection rates have been falling for the past 35 years. However, gonorrhea is still a common infectious disease, especially among teenagers and young adults.

Gonorrhea may cause pain during urination, unusual discharge of fluid from the vagina or penis, or no symptoms at all. In women, gonorrhea can damage the endometrium and uterine tubes and can lead to infertility, even if the infection produces no symptoms. Because gonorrhea is caused by a bacterium, it can be successfully treated with antibiotics.

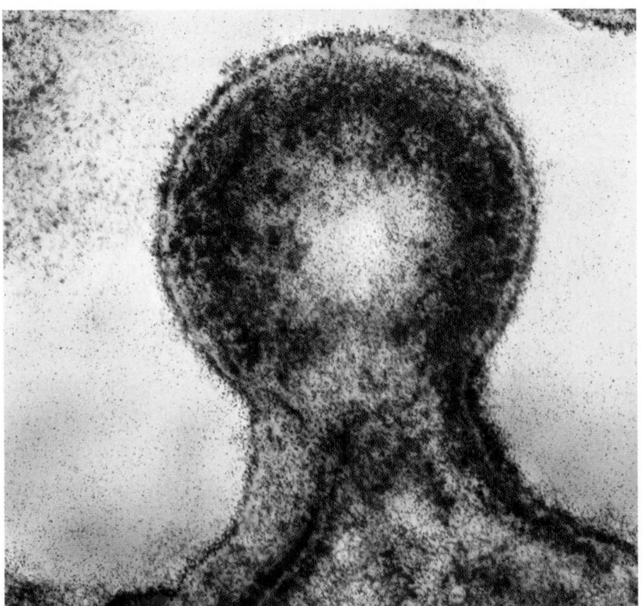

NIBSC/Science Source

Figure 16.18 A transmission electron micrograph of the HIV virus.

Chlamydia

Chlamydia is the most commonly reported STI in the United States. Its incidence has been rising.

Chlamydia often causes no symptoms, but it can damage the female reproductive tract, leading to infertility and increased risk of ectopic pregnancy. Chlamydia can be easily and successfully treated with antibiotics. The CDC recommends that all sexually active young women get an annual screening test for chlamydia.

Genital Herpes

Genital herpes is caused by herpes simplex virus type 1 (HSV-1) or herpes simplex virus type 2 (HSV-2). It is a common STI: genital HSV-2 infects about one in six Americans between 14 and 49 years of age.

Genital herpes may cause blisters or sores in the genital or anal area or near the mouth, or it may cause no symptoms. In fact, most people with genital herpes are unaware that they have it. Pregnant women who have—or have been exposed to—genital herpes need to discuss this fact with their healthcare provider. This consultation is recommended because genital herpes can spread from a pregnant woman to her unborn child with serious or fatal results. There is no cure for genital herpes, but the condition is manageable with antiviral drugs.

Syphilis

Syphilis is a highly treatable bacterial infection. If untreated, it can cause significant health problems, disability, and death, due to its cardiovascular and neurological complications. Syphilis incidence in the United States declined greatly after the widespread introduction of penicillin in the 1940s, and reached a minimum around the year 2000. Incidence has increased since then, although it is still significantly less common than chlamydia or gonorrhea. The recent increase in syphilis has led to a sharp rise in congenital syphilis, which occurs when syphilis passes from mother to baby during pregnancy. This can cause serious health problems or death to the newborn.

Human Papillomavirus

Human papillomavirus (HPV) causes genital warts and cervical cancer. The most common STI in the United States, HPV infects both men and women. Some 6 million new infections emerge each year, and one-half of all sexually active adults will be infected with HPV at some point in their lives. In most people, the immune system eliminates HPV, but it takes about two years to do so. HPV may produce no symptoms.

Pelvic Inflammatory Disease

Pelvic inflammatory disease (PID) is an inflammation of the uterus, uterine tubes, ovaries and/or other organs of the peritoneal (abdominopelvic) cavity. PID is caused by a bacterial infection. It is a potentially serious complication of chlamydia and gonorrhea in females.

The symptoms of pelvic inflammatory disease may include mild to severe pelvic pain, fever, and painful urination. When the symptoms are mild, PID often goes unrecognized. PID can be effectively treated with antibiotics. Prompt treatment is important to prevent permanent damage to the reproductive organs, including scarring of the uterine tubes. Such damage can cause infertility and increase the risk of ectopic pregnancy.

Detection and Prevention

Sexually transmitted infections can occur in any sexually active person. A person with symptoms—such as a discharge of unusual fluid from the genitals; burning during urination; or unusual sores, growths, or a rash—should stop having sex and see a healthcare provider immediately. The use of a condom during sex helps prevent the spread of most STIs. However, abstinence from sexual activity is the only foolproof method of preventing STIs.

SELF CHECK

1. How do sexually transmitted infections spread from one person to another?
2. What is the most commonly reported STI in the United States?
3. Which STI can cause infected women to develop cervical cancer?

Cancers of the Reproductive System

Cancers of the reproductive system in males and females are among the most common and among the deadliest cancers. When detected early, however, these cancers can often be successfully treated. Millions of people in the United States are cancer survivors. In discussions of cancer, you will often see the words *incidence* and *mortality*. *Incidence* refers to the number of people who get the disease; *mortality* refers to the number of people who die from it.

Prostate Cancer

After skin cancer, the cancer with the highest incidence among men in the United States is prostate cancer. Prostate cancer is also the second most frequent cause of cancer mortality among men (the first is lung cancer). Older men and men with a family history of prostate cancer are among those with an increased risk of developing prostate cancer.

Most prostate cancers, which are slow growing, originate in the gland cells that produce the fluid added to semen. Screening tests are available for prostate cancer, the most common of which is the prostate-specific antigen (PSA) test. The PSA test is valuable in the early detection and treatment of prostate cancer, and it saves lives. However, the test sometimes produces false-positive results, prompting a series of follow-up tests and treatments that have risks of their own. Furthermore, the PSA test may not distinguish between rapidly growing, malignant tumors and slow-growing tumors that might safely be left alone.

Treatment of prostate cancer includes surgery to remove cancer cells, radiation therapy, and chemotherapy. Radiation therapy is the use of X-rays to kill cancerous cells. Radiation therapy for prostate cancer is sometimes delivered to the tumor by surgically implanting radioactive "seeds"—each about the size and shape of a grain of rice—into the prostate gland. This method, known as *brachytherapy*, may have fewer unwanted side effects than other treatment options.

Cancers of the Female Reproductive Tract

The three most commonly diagnosed cancers of the female reproductive tract—and the deadliest (not including breast cancer)—are uterine, ovarian, and cervical cancers. These cancers affect about 70,000 US women annually and cause more than 20,000 deaths each year.

Uterine Cancer

Cancer of the uterus is the most frequently diagnosed cancer of the female reproductive tract. Uterine cancer almost always develops in cells of the endometrium, the inner lining of the uterus. For this reason, *endometrial cancer* is another term for uterine cancer.

Abnormal uterine bleeding often reveals the presence of uterine cancer before it spreads within the body. Surgical removal of the entire uterus (known as *hysterectomy*), uterine tubes, and ovaries is the standard initial treatment. More than 80% of uterine cancer patients survive for at least five years after diagnosis.

Ovarian Cancer

Cancer of the ovary is the fifth most common cause of cancer-related death among women in the United States. Ovarian cancer causes more deaths than any other cancer of the female reproductive tract. Unlike uterine cancer, ovarian cancer usually does not cause any symptoms until the disease has spread beyond its initial site. For this reason, the average five-year survival rate of ovarian cancer patients is about 40%.

The standard initial treatment is surgical removal of the uterus, uterine tubes, and ovaries. In most cases, surgery is followed by chemotherapy. Currently, there are no effective screening tests for ovarian cancer.

Cervical Cancer

Among cancers of the female reproductive tract, cervical cancer is the third most commonly diagnosed, and it ranks third as a cause of death among US women, after uterine and ovarian cancers. Although the cervix is part of the uterus anatomically, cervical cancer is considered a different type of cancer from uterine cancer.

The Papanicolaou test, or Pap smear, is a screening test that has significantly reduced cervical cancer mortality over the last 35 years. It is used not only to detect cervical cancer but also to detect precancerous conditions in the cervix. Cervical cancer develops slowly, and the Pap smear allows early detection and surgical treatment.

Most cervical cancers are caused by high-risk forms of human papillomavirus. HPV also causes most anal cancers and about half of all vaginal, vulvar, and penile cancers. Health professionals expect that the incidence and mortality rates of cervical cancer, and perhaps those of other reproductive system cancers, will drop over the next few years because of widespread use of vaccines that protect against HPV infection.

Research Notes Genetic Research and Cancer Treatment Breakthroughs

Cancers of the reproductive tract, like cancers of other organs and tissues, are diseases in which cells grow "out of control." Recall from Chapter 2 that cancer cells have mutations in their DNA. Often, these mutations result from damage to the genes that regulate cell division. Cells become cancerous because the mechanisms that regulate cell division—which inhibit cell division—no longer work.

Advances in technology are making it possible for scientists to decipher more information about the genetic makeup of cancer cells. Likewise, this technology is enabling scientists to identify people who, because of their genetic constitution, are more likely to develop cancer. These advances are leading to earlier detection of cancer as well as potentially significant changes in cancer care.

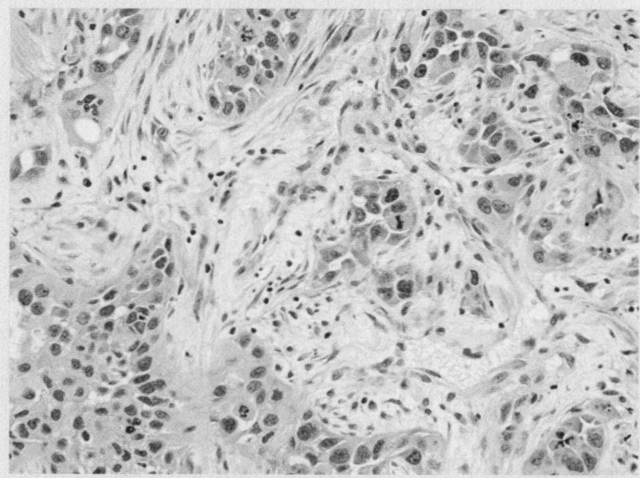

OGphoto/iStockPhoto.com

Microscopic view of ductal breast cancer cells in a tissue culture.

Genes Associated with Cancer

Researchers have found that a person's genetic makeup can make him or her more likely to develop cancer. This information can be used to detect cancer at its earliest stage, when it can be successfully treated, and to identify people at high risk of developing cancer. For example, women who inherit a mutant form of the BRCA1 or BRCA2 gene have a significantly elevated risk of developing breast or ovarian cancer. These genes, named for their association with breast cancer, provide the genetic codes for proteins that repair damaged DNA. When the BRCA1 or BRCA2 gene is damaged, cells are less able to repair the DNA damage that can occur as people grow and age. As a result, the risk of further gene mutation, and thus the risk of cancer, increases.

A woman can be tested for mutant forms of the BRCA1 and BRCA2 genes. If she has a mutation, she can undergo periodic screenings to detect precancerous changes in cells.

Women with damaged BRCA1 or BRCA2 genes account for only about 15% of breast cancer cases. In the remainder of cases, women do not have a direct hereditary cause of breast cancer, and the condition may arise from gene mutations that occur randomly throughout life.

The protein p53 is also known as the *guardian of the genome* because it suppresses tumor development by helping repair DNA. It does this by preventing cells with damaged DNA from dividing until the damage is fixed, and by causing cells whose DNA damage is unfixable to undergo *apoptosis*, or self-destruction. The gene that codes for p53 is TP53. When TP53 is damaged, tumors are much more likely to develop. TP53 is the most commonly altered gene in cancer cases. This gene is damaged or inactivated in more than half of all cancers studied.

In rare cases, a person inherits a damaged TP53 gene from a parent. However, it is much more common for mutations of TP53 to occur during the lifetime of the affected individual. These mutations often occur with no known cause, but exposure to environmental factors such as tobacco smoke and ultraviolet light can increase the odds of such mutations.

New Cancer Treatments

Besides alerting women to a potential genetic vulnerability to cancer, advances in technology are reducing the time and cost required to determine the DNA sequence of cancer cells from individual patients. These technological advances can lead to improved cancer care. For example, some tumors have a genetic mutation that makes them responsive to certain anti-cancer drugs. A doctor and patient with this knowledge can choose drug therapy accordingly.

Currently, more information is available on cancer cell mutations than there are drug therapies to effectively target and treat these mutations. Medical researchers continue their efforts to develop drugs tailored to the specific DNA mutations identified in different types of cancer cells.

Breast Cancer

Breast cancer forms in the tissues of the breast—usually in the ducts and lobules. Males can develop breast cancer, but females are more typically affected. After skin cancer, breast cancer is the most commonly diagnosed cancer among women in the United States. More women die from breast cancer than from any other cancer, with the exception of lung cancer. However, the breast cancer death rate has been declining due to early detection and more effective treatment therapies.

Factors that increase a woman's risk of developing breast cancer include advanced age, a family history of breast cancer, menarche at an early age, late onset of menopause, being overweight, and never having given birth.

Early detection of breast cancer improves the odds of successful treatment. For this reason, screening mammography is recommended. Mammography involves taking an X-ray image of the breast (a mammogram) to detect a tumor while it is still small. Different medical organizations have slightly different recommendations for when to start mammography (40, 45, or 50 years of age), and how often to do it (every year or every other year).

Why not start at a young age and do the exams frequently to be on the safe side? Simply put, there are downsides to screening tests, including mammography. The tests are designed to err on the side of caution, which means they sometimes "see tumors" that are not really tumors. This leads to follow-up tests and medical procedures that carry risks of their own. The balance between risks and benefits of screening depends on age and other risk factors. Women should consult a healthcare provider when making this decision.

Research suggests that regular clinical examination of the breast by a professional and regular breast self-examination do not improve breast cancer survival. Therefore, as of 2016, the US Preventive Services Task Force and the American Cancer Society do not recommend regular clinical breast exams or regular breast self-examination. However, women should be familiar with the normal look and feel of their breasts, and they should report any changes to their healthcare provider.

Breast cancer is treated with surgery to remove cancer cells and with radiation therapy and/or chemotherapy to kill cancer cells. Treatment options, such as what kind of surgery to have or which drugs to use, depend on the specific clinical details of each case. Surgery options range from a "lumpectomy," in which only a small region of cancer tissue is removed, to a radical mastectomy, now rarely done, in which all of the breast tissue, some underlying muscle, and nearby lymph nodes are removed.

SECTION 16.5 REVIEW

Mini-Glossary

adhesions areas in which tissues stick together inappropriately after surgery

amenorrhea complete absence of menstrual periods

chlamydia a sexually transmitted infection that often causes no symptoms but can damage the female reproductive tract, lead to infertility, and increase the risk of ectopic pregnancy

endometriosis growth of endometrial cells outside the uterus, usually in the abdominal cavity, that produces inflammation and alters the balance between progesterone and estrogen

genital herpes a sexually transmitted infection that may cause blisters or sores in the genital or anal area or near the mouth; may cause no symptoms

gonorrhea a sexually transmitted infection that may cause pain during urination, unusual discharge of fluid from the vagina or penis, or no symptoms at all; can lead to infertility

human papillomavirus (HPV) a sexually transmitted infection that causes genital warts and can cause cervical cancer

infertility the inability to get pregnant

sexually transmitted infection (STI) an infectious disease transmitted through sexual contact

syphilis a highly treatable bacterial infection; if untreated, can cause significant health problems, disability, and death due to its cardiovascular and neurological complications

Review Questions

1. What is another name for impotence?
2. Compare and contrast male and female infertility.
3. Which hormones, when present at abnormal levels, can result in failure to ovulate?
4. Name five causes of uterine tube damage.
5. What are uterine fibroids?
6. Which is the most lethal STI?
7. Which STI often causes no symptoms but can cause infertility and an increased risk of ectopic pregnancy if left untreated?
8. Which STI is the most common in the United States, affecting 50% of all sexually active adults at some point in their lives?
9. How can a sexually active lifestyle increase a person's risk of becoming infertile? What can people do to help ensure that their reproductive systems function normally when they want to have children?

(continued)

10. Explain the meanings of the words *incidence* and *mortality* as they relate to discussions of cancer.
11. How are cancer cells different from normal cells?
12. Which screening tests are used to detect cancers of the prostate, cervix, and breast respectively?
13. Which cancer of the female reproductive tract has the highest incidence among women in the United States? Which cancer has the highest mortality among women?

Medical Terminology: The Male and Female Reproductive Systems

By understanding the word parts that make up medical words, you can extend your medical vocabulary. This chapter includes many of the word parts listed below. Review these word parts to be sure you understand their meanings.

-al	pertaining to
centr/o	center
cyt/o	cell
dipl/o	double
-genesis	birth, generation
hapl/o	single, simple
inguin/o	groin
mer/o	part
metr/o	womb, uterus
o/o	egg
-ous	pertaining to
peri-	around, surrounding
-ploid	number of chromosomes in a cell
poly-	many
semin/i	semen, seed
tri-	three
-um	structure
-y	condition, process

Now use these word parts to form valid medical words that fit the following definitions. Some of the words are included in this chapter. Others are not. When you finish, use a medical dictionary to check your work.

1. cells that have two sets of chromosomes
2. central part or point of attachment
3. cells that have one set of chromosomes
4. pertaining to semen
5. pertaining to the groin
6. egg cell
7. outer layer/structure surrounding the uterus
8. generation of eggs
9. condition of having three chromosomes in a cell
10. condition of having many sperm penetrate a single egg

Chapter 16 Summary

- Of the two types of reproduction—asexual and sexual—sexual reproduction is more complicated.
- Mitosis is the cell division process that occurs in all of the body's tissues throughout life. Meiosis occurs only in the sex organs and produces gametes.
- During puberty, females experience changes such as breast growth, the growth of underarm and pubic hair, and menarche. Males experience growth of the scrotum and testes and growth of underarm, pubic, and facial hair.
- The primary organs of the male reproductive system are the testes; other organs include the penis, accessory glands, and a series of ducts.
- Sperm are produced in the testes and then delivered to the external urethral orifice through a series of ducts. Semen is ejaculated as a result of nerve impulses that cause peristaltic contractions.
- The primary organs in the female reproductive system are the ovaries; other organs include the uterine tubes, uterus, vagina, external genitalia, a series of ducts, and mammary glands.
- During the female's monthly cycle, the ovaries, uterus, and hormones undergo changes. Ovulation occurs when a follicle reaches maturity and the oocyte is released from the ovary.
- Fertilization occurs when the chromosomes of the oocyte and the sperm unite to produce a zygote.
- After fertilization, the zygote travels through the uterine tube and into the uterus, where it implants. Fetal vessels carry blood through the umbilical cord, to and from the placenta, which grows to meet the nutritional needs of the embryo/fetus.
- The stages of labor are dilation, expulsion, and delivery of the placenta.
- Lactation, the production of milk by the mother, is regulated by hormones.

- Infertility is the inability to conceive after at least one year of unprotected intercourse.
- A sexually transmitted infection (STI) is a condition that can be passed from one person to another through sexual intercourse or genital contact.
- Common sexually transmitted infections include acquired immunodeficiency syndrome (AIDS), gonorrhea, chlamydia, genital herpes, syphilis, and HPV.
- Cancers of the reproductive system are some of the most common and deadly types of cancer.

Chapter 16 Review

Understanding Key Concepts

1. *True or False?* Homologous chromosomes are the two identical chromosomes that make up one of the 23 pairs in a mother cell.
2. Which of the following helps create genetic diversity?
   A. DNA
   B. mitosis
   C. crossovers
   D. SRY genes
3. Does the presence of a Y chromosome indicate development of a male or a female?
4. Which of the following hormones is *not* involved in stimulating puberty?
   A. TSH
   B. FSH
   C. LH
   D. GnRH
5. Adolescence officially begins with the appearance of ______ and ends when ______.
6. *True or False?* By the end of puberty, mature sperm are present in semen.
7. Testes are to ovaries as sperm are to ______.
8. At which of the following temperatures would you expect sperm production to be *most* vigorous?
   A. 98.6°F
   B. 101°F
   C. 95°F
   D. 97°F
9. Identify the functions of the male reproductive system.
10. The ______ glands make the greatest contribution to the production of semen.
11. How many chromosomes does a spermatid have?
12. *True or False?* When a spermatid develops a flagellum and is released into the seminiferous tubule, it is mature.
13. What is an oocyte? Where are oocytes originally located?
14. How many ovarian follicles reach maturity each month?
15. Describe the step-by-step process that occurs during ovulation.
16. Describe where the uterus is located. What is the purpose of the uterus in reproduction?
17. Why is the pH of the vagina acidic in healthy adult women?
18. Identify the functions of the female reproductive system.
19. Which hormone stimulates milk production by the female mammary glands after childbirth?
20. After ovulation, what happens to the levels of estrogen and progesterone in the blood?
21. *True or False?* A gamete has 46 chromosomes.
22. *True or False?* After intercourse, a few thousand sperm may reach the oocyte.
23. What is the function of acrosomal enzymes in sperm?
24. Describe how pregnancy test kits work.
25. Where is the placenta located, and what is its function?
26. Which structure connects the fetus to the placenta?
27. Which stage of labor lasts the longest, and what events occur during this stage?
28. Why are the male and female reproductive systems vulnerable to infection and disease?
29. Which of the following glands secretes GnRH?
    A. hypothalamus
    B. pituitary
    C. testis
    D. ovary
30. What is erectile dysfunction, and what are some common causes of this condition?
31. What is in vitro fertilization (IVF)? Briefly describe how it is performed.
32. *True or False?* Gonorrhea and chlamydia cannot be successfully treated with antibiotics.

33. *True or False?* Genital warts are a symptom of human papillomavirus.
34. What is the most frequently diagnosed cancer of the female reproductive tract?
35. *True or False?* The breast cancer death rate has been declining slowly but steadily.
36. What is the relationship between gene mutation and cancer development?

Thinking Critically

37. Imagine that you have been asked to teach a lesson on the differences between mitosis and meiosis to an eighth-grade biology class. How would you explain the differences to the class?
38. Compare sperm cells to other cells in the human body. How are they different? How are they similar?
39. Compare and contrast the anatomy of the ovary and the testis.
40. Compare and contrast the functions of the male and female reproductive systems.
41. Explain why it is important for pregnant women to avoid drinking alcohol and taking drugs that are illegal or not prescribed.
42. Evaluate the cause and effect of the human papillomavirus on the structure and function of the female reproductive system.
43. You are a doctor who treats infertile couples. A new patient complains that she is not pregnant although she and her husband have been trying for six months. What would you tell this patient? Write a "prescription" for lifestyle changes that could help increase their chances of conceiving.

Clinical Case Study

Read again the Clinical Case Study at the beginning of this chapter. Use the information provided in the chapter to answer the questions at the end of the scenario.

44. What features of pelvic anatomy and physiology are relevant to Anika's symptoms?
45. How is Anika's family history relevant?
46. How do the laboratory test results, paired with her symptoms, help clarify the possible diagnoses?
47. What is the significance of the negative urine and blood test results for human chorionic gonadotropin?

Analyzing and Evaluating Data

The following figure shows the rate of HPV infection among surveyed females in the United States. Several factors are linked to the rate of infection among certain demographic groups. Use the chart to answer the following questions.

HPV Infection Rates Among Surveyed US Females

Factor	Demographic Group	Rate of Infection
Age	14–19	40%
	20–24	50%
	25–29	28%
	30–39	37%
	40–49	25%
	50–59	20%
Race/ Ethnicity	African-American	39%
	Caucasian	24%
	Hispanic	24%
Economic Status	Below the poverty line	38%
	At/above the poverty line	24%

48. Which race/ethnicity is most likely to become infected with HPV?
49. What is the difference in HPV infection rate between those at or above the poverty line and those below the poverty line?
50. How much more likely is a woman between 14 and 19 years of age to become infected with HPV than a woman between 50 and 59 years of age?
51. Why do you think that females 20–24 years of age are more likely to become infected with HPV than other age groups?

Investigating Further

52. Cancer screenings can detect cancer at an early stage, improving the chances of survival. Yet the value of some of these tests for people who have no symptoms and few or no risk factors has recently come into question. Research the debate surrounding either prostate or breast cancer screenings. Choose a position (yes or no) and develop an argument in response to the following question: Do the benefits of cancer screenings outweigh the risks involved?

Appendix A

English-Metric Conversion Factors

Quantity	When you know English units	Multiply by	To get Metric Units[1]
Length	inches	2.54	centimeters
	inches	0.0254	meters
	feet	30.5	centimeters
	feet	0.305	meters
Area	square inches	6.45	square centimeters
	square feet	0.929	square meters
Volume[2]	fluid ounces	29.4	milliliters
	pints	0.473	liters
	quarts	0.946	liters
Weight	ounces	28.3	grams
	ounces	0.283	kilograms
	pounds	0.454	kilograms
Pressure	pounds per square inch	51.7	millimeters of mercury
	pounds per square inch	6.89	kilopascals
Flow	gallons per minute	3.79	liters per minute
Mass	slug	0.0685	kilogram
Force	pound	0.225	newton
Torque	foot-pounds	0.738	newton-meters
Temperature[3]	Fahrenheit	$5/9 \times (F - 32)$	Celsius

[1] To convert from metric to English units, divide metric units by the number shown.
[2] For volume, note that 1 milliliter = 1 cubic centimeter.
[3] For temperature, use the formula $F = (9/5 \times C) + 32$ to convert metric to US units.

Appendix B

Anatomy and Physiology Word Elements

Many word parts that are routinely used in the study of anatomy and physiology come from Greek and Latin. The meanings of these word parts offer clues to the meanings of words used to describe structures, functions, and processes. For example, the word physiology is made up of physio- ("function") and -logy ("study of"). Thus, physiology is the study of how living things function or work. Likewise, the word anatomy comes from ana- ("apart") and -tomy ("cutting"). These word elements are appropriate when you consider that ancient anatomists gained a great deal of knowledge about the structure of tissues and organs through dissection.

The following combining forms, prefixes, and suffixes are used throughout the text. This list is not exhaustive; only commonly used forms are presented.

A

ab- away from, off (*abdominal aorta, abduction*)
abdomen/o abdomen (*abdominal, abdominopelvic cavity*)
acous/o, acoust/o hearing, sound (*external acoustic meatus*)
acr/o- extremity, highest or farthest point (*acromegaly, acromion*)
ad- to, toward, near (*adduction*)
adip/o- fat or fatty tissue (*adipocyte, adipose tissue*)
af- toward (*afferent nerves, afferent pathway*)
-agon to gather, assemble (*agonist, antagonist*)
alb/i, alb/o, albin/o white (*albinism*)
amni- fetal sac (*amnion, amniotic fluid*)
amph-, amphi/o on both sides, around (*amphiarthrosis*)
an- not, without (*anaerobic, anemia*)
ana- apart (anatomy, anaphase); up, build up (*anabolism*)
andr/o male (*androgen*)
angi/o blood vessel (*angioplasty, angiography, angiotensin*)
antero forward, from front to back (*anteroposterior*)
anti- against (*antibiotic, antidiuretic hormone*)
apo- above, away, off, separated from (*apocrine glands, aponeurosis*)
aque/o water (*aquaporins, aqueous humor*)
arteri/o artery (*arterial, arterioles*)
arthr/o joint (*synarthroses, diarthrodial*)
articul/o joint (*articular fibrocartilage, articulating bones*)
-ase enzyme (*amylase, polymerase*)
ather/o fat, plaque (*atherosclerosis*)
atri/o heart, entryway (*atrium, interatrial septum*)
audi/o, audit/o hearing (*auditory canal, audiologist*)
aur/i, aur/o, auricul/o ear, hearing (*auricle*)
aut/o self (*autoimmune disease, autonomic nervous system*)
axi/o axis, straight line (*axial skeleton, axon*)

B

bar/o pressure, weight (*baroreceptors, barometric*)
bi- two, twice, double (*bicarbonate, biceps*)
bi/o life (*biopsy, microbial*)
bil/i bile (*bilirubin*)
blast/o bud, germ, precursor (*blastocyst, osteoblast*)
brachi/o arm (*biceps brachii*)
bronch/i, bronch/o airway (*bronchus, bronchodilator*)

C

calc/o, calci/o calcium, stone (*hypercalcemia, calcitonin*)
calori- heat (*Calorie, caloric*)
carcin/o cancer (*carcinogen*)
cardi/o heart (*cardiovascular*)
carp/o wrist (*metacarpals, radiocarpal*)
centr/i, centr/o middle, center (*centromere, centriole*)
cephal/o head (*diencephalon, brachiocephalic artery*)
cerebr/o brain (*cerebrum*)
cervic/o neck, narrow part (*cervical*)
circ/um- around, about (*circumduction*)
-clast break (down), destroy (*osteoclasts*)

clavicul/o hammer, club, key (*clavicle, acromioclavicular joint*)
-cle little (*corpuscle*)
co- with, together (*cotransport*)
col-, col/o, col/ono- large intestine (*colonoscopy*)
com- with, together (*complement system, compression*)
contus/o bruise (*contusion*)
coron/o heart, crown (*coronary, corona radiata*)
corp/o, corpor/o body (*corpus luteum, corpora cavernosa*)
corti- covering (*cortical*)
cost/o rib (*intercostal nerves, sternocostal joints*)
cox/a, cox/o hip (*coxal bone*)
crani/o skull (*cranium*)
-crin/o secrete, separate (*endocrine, exocrine*)
cry/o cold (*cryotherapy, oocyte cryopreservation*)
-cule, -culus small (*molecule, canaliculus*)
cutane/o skin (*subcutaneous fascia, musculocutaneous*)
cyst/i, cyst/o bladder (*cystitis, cholecystectomy*)
-cyte, cyt/o cell (*lymphocyte, cytoplasm*)

D

de- down, away from, cessation (*dehydration, defibrillation*)
dendr/o tree, branch (*dendrites, oligodendrocytes*)
-derma, dermat/o, derm/o skin (*epidermal, dermatologist*)
-desis binding, tying together (*diapedesis*)
desm/o bond, ligament (*desmosomes, syndesmosis*)
di- two, apart, separate, through (*diuresis, antidiuretic hormone*)
dia- across, separate, through (*diaphragm, dialysis*)
dif- apart, separate (*differentiate, diffusion*)
digit- finger (*extensor digitorum*)
dilat/o widening, expanding, stretching (*dilation*)
dipl/o double (*diploid*)
dis- apart, separate (*dissect, dislocation*)
dist/o far, distant (*distal convoluted tubule*)
dors/i, dors/o back, back of body (*dorsal, latissimus dorsi*)
duc-, duct/o to lead, carry (*abduction, adduction*)
dynam/o strength, force, power, energy (*dynamic lung volume, dynamometer*)
dys- bad, abnormal, painful (*muscular dystrophy, dyspnea*)

E

e- out (*ejaculate, eversion*)
-eal pertaining to (*pineal, esophageal*)
ec-, ect/o out, outside, away (*ectopic*)
-ectomy incision, surgical removal (*cholecystectomy, mastectomy*)
-edema swelling (*lymphedema, myxedema*)
ef- out, out of (*efferent, effusion*)
-el, -elle small (*organelle, fontanel*)
electr/o electricity (*electrocardiogram, electrolytes*)
em- in, within (*embolism*)
-ema condition (*emphysema*)
-emia blood condition (*anemia, leukemia*)
en- in, into (*enzyme*)
encephal/o brain (*diencephalon*)
end/o in, inside, within (*endometrium*)
enter/o intestine (*gastroenterologist*)
epi- on, upon, above (*epidermis, epididymis*)
epitheli/o skin (*epithelium*)
erythr/o red (*erythrocyte*)
-esis action, condition, state of (*erythropoiesis, synthesis*)
estr/o female (*estrogen*)
ex-, exo- out, out of, away, away from (*exocytosis, exophthalmos*)
extra- outside (*extracellular*)

F

femor/o thigh bone (*femoral*)
fer-, -ferent to carry (*afferent, efferent*)
fibr/o fiber (*fibroblast*)
fil/a, fil/o, filament/o thread, thread-like (*microfilament, filtration*)
flex/o bend (*dorsiflexion*)
fore- before (*forearm*); in front (*forehead*)
-form, -iform having the shape or form of (*fusiform, deformed*)

G

gastr/o stomach (*gastric, gastroesophageal*)
-gen, -genic, -genesis producing, bringing about (*gluconeogenesis, oogenesis*)
germi- sprout, bud (*germinate, germinal*)

gest/o to carry (ingest); pregnancy (*gestation, progesterone*)
gingiv/o pertaining to the gums (*gingivitis*)
glauc/o having a blue or blue-gray color (*glaucoma*)
-glia glue (*neuroglia, microglia*)
globu- sphere, ball (*globulin, hemoglobin*)
gloss/o, glott/o tongue (*glossopharyngeal*)
gluc/o sugar, glucose (*glucose, glucocorticoid*)
glyc/o sugar, glucose (*glycogen, hypoglycemia, glycolysis*)
-gnosis knowledge (*diagnosis, prognosis*)
gon/o, gonad/o semen, seed, pertaining to reproduction (*spermatogonia, gonadotropic*)
gyn/o, gynec/o woman, female (*gynecology*)

H

hapl/o single, simple (*haploid*)
hema-, hemo-, hemat/o blood (*hematopoiesis, hematocrit*)
hemi- half (*hemisphere*)
-hemia blood condition (*polycythemia*)
hepat/o liver (*hepatitis*)
hist/o tissue (*histology*)
hom/o like, similar (*homologous*)
home/o unchanging, constant (*homeostasis*)
humer/o shoulder (*humerus*)
hydr/o water (*hydrophobic*)
hyper- above, above normal, excessive (*hypertrophy, hyperopia*)
hypo- under, below normal (*hypoxia, hyposecretion*)

I

-ia condition (*anemia, pneumonia*)
-iasis abnormal condition (*psoriasis*)
-iatr/o doctor, medicine (*pediatric*)
-ic, -ical pertaining to (*anatomical, biological*)
-icle, -icul small (*ossicle, canaliculus*)
-ics knowledge (*kinetics, genetics*)
-immun/o protection, safety (*autoimmune, immunotherapy*)
in- in, into, not (*inspiration*)
-in(e) protein, enzyme, chemical compound (*penicillin, creatinine*)
infra- below, beneath, inferior to (*infraspinous fossa*)
inter- between, among (*interstitial, intervertebral*)
intra- within, into (*intracellular*)
-ism process (*metabolism*); condition or disorder (*gigantism, astigmatism*)
is/o same, equal (*isometric*)
-ite little (*dendrite*)
-itis inflammation (*gingivitis*)
-ium structure, tissue (*cranium, endomysium*)

J

jaund/o yellow (*jaundice*)
jug- to join (*jugular*)
juxta- beside, next to (*juxtamedullary nephrons*)

K

kerat/o hard, horn-shaped tissue (*keratinocytes*)
kin/e, kin/o, kines/o, kinesi/o movement, motion (*kinetic, cytokinesis*)

L

lacrim/o tear (*lacrimal glands*)
lact/i, lact/o milk (*lactation*)
laryng/o voice box (*laryngeal*)
later/o side (*lateral rotation*)
-lepsy, -leptic seizure (*epilepsy, epileptic*)
-let small (*platelet*)
leuk/o white (*leukocytes, leukemia*)
lig/o to tie, bind (*ligament*)
lingu/a, lingu/o tongue (*lingual tonsil*)
lip/o fat (*lipocyte*)
lith/o stone (*lithotripsy*)
-(o)logy study of (*biology, physiology*)
-lucent, -lucid clear, light, shining (*zona pellucida, stratum lucidum*)
lumb/o lower back (*lumbar*)
lun- moon, crescent (*semilunar valves*)
lute/o yellow (*corpus luteum*)
-lymph, lymph/o lymph (*endolymph, lymphocytes*)
lys/o, lyt/o, -lyt/ic separate, break apart, break down, destroy (*lysosome, glycolysis*)

M

macro- large (*macrophage*)
mal/i bad (*malfunction, malignant*)

mamm/o breast (*mammogram*)
medi/o, mediastin/o middle (*medial, mediastinum*)
medull/o middle, deep part, marrow (*medullary canal, medulla oblongata*)
meg/a, megal/o, -megaly large, enlargement (*acromegaly, megakaryocytes*)
melan/o black color (*melanocyte, melanoma*)
men/o month, menses, menstruation (*amenorrhea, menarche*)
mening/o, meningi/o membrane (*meningitis*)
meta- after, beyond; change (*metaphase, metacarpal*)
-meter instrument or device used to measure (*spirometer, sphygmomanometer*)
metri- length, measure (*metric system*)
metri-, metr/o uterus, womb (*endometrium*)
micro- small; millionth (*microscope, microbiology*)
mon/o one, single (*monomer, monosaccharide*)
morph/o form, shape (*polymorphism*)
-mortem, mort/o death (*mortality, postmortem*)
muc/o, mucos/o mucus (*mucosal*)
multi- many (*multicellular*)
muscul/o muscle (*musculoskeletal*)
muta- change (*mutation*)
myel/o bone marrow (*myeloid*); spinal cord (*myelin*)
mysi-, my/o, myos/o muscle (*myositis, epimysium*)

N

nas/o nose (*nasolacrimal, nasopharynx*)
natr/i, natr/o sodium (*hyponatremia, natriuretic*)
neo- new (*gluconeogenesis, neonatal*)
nephr/o kidney (*nephron*)
neur/o nerve (*neuromuscular, neuroscience*)
neutr/o neutral, neither (*neutrophil, neutralization*)
nucle/o nucleus (*nuclear membrane, deoxyribonucleic acid*)
nutri/o, nutrit/o nourish (*nutrient, nutrition*)

O

obstetr/o pregnancy; birth (*obstetrician*)
ocul/o eye (*oculomotor, orbicularis oculi*)
odont/o tooth (*periodontal disease*)
-ole little, small (*arteriole, nucleolus*)
-oma tumor, mass (*carcinoma, hematoma*)
onc/o tumor (*oncologist*)
-opia vision condition (*myopia, hyperopia*)
ophthalm/o eye (*ophthalmologist, exophthalmos*)
-opsy view of (*biopsy*)
optic/o eye, vision (*optic chiasma*)
or/o mouth (*oropharynx*)
orbi- circle (*orbicularis*)
-orexia appetite (*anorexia*)
orth/o straight (*orthopedic, orthodontist*)
-ose sugar (*glucose, fructose*)
-osis process (*mitosis, apoptosis*); disease, abnormal condition (*tuberculosis, cirrhosis*)
osseo- bony (*osseous tissue, interosseous membrane*)
ossi- bone (*ossification*)
ost/e, oste/o bone (*osteoporosis*)
ov/o, ovul/o egg (*ovum, ovulation*)
ox/o oxygen (*hypoxic, oxyhemoglobin*)

P

para- near, next to, beside (*parathyroid, parasites*)
-partum birth; labor (*parturition, postpartum*)
path/o disease (*pathology*); feeling, emotion (*sympathetic*)
pector/o chest (*pectoral girdle, pectoralis major*)
ped/o child (*pediatrician*); foot (*tinea pedis*)
pelv/i, pelv/o hip (*pelvic*)
pend/o to hang (*appendix, appendicular*)
-penia deficiency (*osteopenia*)
penna- thread (*unipennate*)
penta- five, fifth (*pentapeptide, pentamer*)
peri- around (*periosteum, peritoneum*)
-phage, phag/o eat, swallow (*esophagus, phagocytosis*)
phalang/o fingers, toes (*phalanges*)
pharyng/o throat (*pharyngeal*)
phil/o loving, attracted to (*hydrophilic*)
phleb/o vein (*phlebotomist*)
-phob/o, -phobia fear (*hydrophobic*)
phon/o, -phonia voice, sound (*phonetic*)
phot/o light (*phototherapy*)
physi/o, physic/o nature, function (*physiology, physician*)
-physis growth (*diaphysis, epiphysis*)
-plasm shaped, molded (*cytoplasm, endoplasmic*)
-plasty surgical repair (*rhinoplasty*)
-plegia, -plegic paralysis (*paraplegia*)
pleur/o lung (*pleurisy*)
plex/o network of nerves (*brachial plexus*)
-pnea breath, breathing (*dyspnea*)

pneum/o, pneumon/o lung, air (*pneumonia*)
pod/o foot (*podocyte*)
-poiesis formation (*hematopoiesis, erythropoiesis*)
-poietin substance that forms (*erythropoietin, thrombopoietin*)
poly- many, much (*polymer, polysaccharide*)
-porosis condition of holes, spaces (*osteoporosis*)
post- after, behind (*postmenopausal*)
poster/o back of (the body), behind (*posterior*)
pre- before, in front of (*precursor, preganglionic*)
presby/o old age (*presbyopia*)
pro- before, in front of (*prostate*); promote (*progesterone*)
prot/o first (*protoplasm*)
proxim/o near (*proximal*)
pseudo false (*pseudopod*)
psych/o mind (*psychological*)
pulmon/o lung (*pulmonary*)
puls/o, pulsat/o to beat, vibrate, push against (*pulsation, propulsion*)
pyr/o, pyret/o, pyrex/o fire; fever (*pyrogen*)

Q

quadri- four (*quadriceps*)
quater- fourth (*quaternary structure*)

R

radiat- radiating (*corona radiata*)
radi/o X-ray; radioactive (*radiography*)
re- back, again, backward (*reabsorption, remodeling*)
-receptor, -ceptor receiver (*chemoreceptor*)
ren/o kidney (*renal cortex*)
respir/o breathe (*respiratory*)
reticul/o network (*reticular connective tissue*)
retr/o back, backward, behind (*retroperitoneal*)
rhin/o nose (*rhinoplasty*)
-rrhage, -rrhagia bursting forth of blood (*hemorrhagic stroke*)
-rrhea flow, discharge (*diarrhea, amenorrhea*)

S

sacchar/o sugar (*polysaccharide*)
sacr/o posterior section of pelvic bone (*sacroiliac joint*)
scapul/o shoulder blade (*scapulothoracic joint, subscapular*)
-scope, scop/o, -scopy see (*microscope, colonoscope*)
sect/o to cut (*dissection*)
semi- half (*semicircular canals, semilunar valves*)
semin/i semen, seed (*seminal glands, seminiferous tubules*)
-sis state of, condition (*stenosis*); process (*mitosis, glycolysis*)
son/o sound (*sonogram*)
-spasm sudden contraction of muscles (*bronchospasm*)
sperm/o, spermat/o sperm cells (*spermatid, spermatocyte*)
-sphyxia pulse (*asphyxiation*)
spir/o to breathe (*respiration, spirometer*)
stas/i, stat/i stop, remain, stay the same (*homeostasis*)
-static pertaining to stopping or controlling (*homeostatic, hydrostatic*)
sten/o narrow, constricted (*valvular stenosis*)
stern/o chest, breast (*sternum*)
steth/o chest (*stethoscope*)
strept/o twisted chains (*streptococcus*)
stri/a striped (*striated*)
sub- under, below (*subcutaneous*)
super- above, beyond (*superior, superficial*)
sym- together, with (*symphysis, symmetrical*)
syn- together, with (*synthesis, synarthroses*)
synaps/o, synapt/o to join, make contact (*synaptic*)
systol/o contraction (*systolic*)

T

tars/i, tars/o ankle, hindfoot (*metatarsal*)
tendin/o, ten/o tendon (*tendinitis*)
tens/o stretched, strained (*tensile*)
tetra- four (*tetramer, tetrad*)
therm/o heat (*hyperthermia, thermometer*)
thorac/o, -thorax chest, pleural cavity (*cardiothoracic*)
thromb/o blood clot (*thrombosis, thrombocytes*)
tom/o to cut (*splenectomy, cholecystectomy*)
tox/o, toxic/o poison (*cytotoxic*)
trans- across, through (*neurotransmitter, transverse plane*)
tri- three (*adenosine triphosphate, triglycerides*)
-tropin to act on, stimulate (*adrenocorticotropin, gonadotropin*)

U

-ul, -ule little, small (*trabecula, glomerulus*)
ultra- beyond, excessive (*ultraviolet, ultrasonic*)
-um structure, tissue, substance (*cerebrum, sodium*)
uni- one (*unipennate, unipolar*)
-uresis urination (*diuresis*)
ur/i, ur/o, -uria, urin/o urine, urination (*polyuria, urinalysis*)
-us structure, thing (*fetus, hypothalamus*)
uter/o womb (*uterus, uterine*)

V

valv/o, valvu/o valve (*valvular stenosis*)
vas/o, vascul/o vessel (*vasa recta, vascular, vas deferens*)
ven/i, ven/o vein (*venous, venule, intravenous*)
ventil/o to oxygenate (*ventilation, hyperventilation*)
ventr/o, ventricul/o belly side of body, lower part (*ventral, ventricle*)
vers/o, -verse, -version turning (*eversion, inversion*)
vertebr/o spine; backbone (*intervertebral*)
vir/o virus (*viral, virology*)
viscer/o internal organs (*visceral pleura, visceral pericardium*)
vit/a, vit/o life (*vitamin, vital signs*)
vitr/e, vitr/o glass (*vitreous humor, in vitro*)

X

xanth/o yellow (*xanthosis*)
xiph/o sword-shaped (*xiphoid process*)

Y

-y condition, process (*thermoplasty*)

Z

zo/o life (*zoology*)
zyg/o union, junction, pair (*zygote*)

Appendix C

Common Medical Abbreviations

A

ACTH adrenocorticotropin hormone
AD Alzheimer's disease
ADH antidiuretic hormone
ADP adenosine diphosphate
AED automatic external defibrillator
AIDS acquired immunodeficiency syndrome
ALL acute lymphocytic leukemia
ALS amyotrophic lateral sclerosis
AML acute myeloid leukemia
ANP atrial natriuretic peptide
ANS autonomic nervous system
APC antigen-presenting cell
ATP adenosine triphosphate
AV atrioventricular (node; valves)

B

BMI body mass index
BMR basal metabolic rate
BPM beats per minute

C

CLL chronic lymphocytic leukemia
CML chronic myeloid leukemia
CNS central nervous system
CO_2 carbon dioxide
COPD cardiopulmonary disease
CP cerebral palsy
CPR cardiopulmonary resuscitation
CT computed tomography

D

DNA deoxyribonucleic acid
DO doctor of osteopathic medicine
DOMS delayed-onset muscle soreness
DPT doctor of physical therapy

E

ECG electrocardiogram
ED erectile dysfunction
EIB exercise-induced bronchospasms
EKG electrocardiogram (*variant of* ECG)
EMD electromechanical delay
EMT emergency medical technician
EPO erythropoietin
ERV expiratory reserve volume

F

FEV_1 forced expiratory volume in one second
FEV_1/FVC forced expiratory volume in one second/forced vital capacity
fMRI functional magnetic resonance imaging
FRC functional residual capacity
FSH follicle-stimulating hormone
FT fibers fast-twitch fibers

G

GERD gastroesophageal reflux disease
GFR glomerular filtration rate
GH growth hormone
GI gastrointestinal
GnRH gonadotropin-releasing hormone

H

H_2O water
HbA1c glycosylated hemoglobin (test)
hCG human chorionic gonadotropin
HDL high-density lipoprotein
HIV human immunodeficiency virus
HPV human papillomavirus
HR heart rate
HSV-1 herpes simplex virus type 1
HSV-2 herpes simplex virus type 2

I

IRV inspiratory reserve volume
IV intravenous
IVF in vitro fertilization

L

L/min liters per minute
LBP low back pain
LDL low-density lipoprotein
LH luteinizing hormone

M

MAC membrane attack complex
MALT mucosa-associated lymphatic tissue
MAP mean arterial pressure
MD medical doctor; muscular dystrophy
mg/DL milligrams per deciliter
MHC major histocompatibility complex glycoproteins
mL/beat milliliters per beat
mmHG millimeters of mercury
MRA magnetic resonance angiography
MRI magnetic resonance imaging
mRNA messenger RNA (ribonucleic acid)
MS multiple sclerosis

N

NCV nerve conduction velocity
NK cells natural killer cells

O

O_2 oxygen
OD optometry degree

P

PA physician assistant
PACs premature atrial contractions
PCOS polycystic ovarian syndrome
PCT proximal convoluted tubule
PD Parkinson's disease
PET positron emission tomography
pH acid-base balance
PID pelvic inflammatory disease
PNS peripheral nervous system
PRO prolactin
PSA test prostate-specific antigen test
PTH parathyroid hormone
PVCs premature ventricular contractions
PVD peripheral vascular disease

Q

Q cardiac output

R

RBC red blood cell
RNA ribonucleic acid
rRNA ribosomal RNA (ribonucleic acid)
RT respiratory therapist
RV pulmonary ventilation residual volume

S

SA sinoatrial (node)
SCID severe combined immune deficiency
SNS sympathetic nervous system
ST fibers slow-twitch fibers
STI sexually transmitted infection
SV stroke volume

T

T_3 triiodothyronine
T_4 thyroxine
TB tuberculosis
TBI traumatic brain injury
TIA transient ischemic attack
TLC total lung capacity
tRNA transfer RNA (ribonucleic acid)
TSH thyroid-stimulating hormone
TV tidal volume

U

UTI urinary tract infection
UVB ultraviolet B

V

VC vital capacity

W

WBC white blood cell

Glossary

A

abdominal cavity. The open chamber that contains the stomach, digestive tract, liver, and other organs. (1)

abdominopelvic cavity. A continuous internal opening that includes the abdominal and pelvic cavities. (1)

abduction. Movement of a body segment away from the body in the frontal plane. (6)

absorption. The movement of nutrient molecules from the small intestine into the blood. (14)

acetylcholine. A neurotransmitter that stimulates skeletal muscle and inhibits activity in cardiac and smooth muscle. (6, 7)

acquired immunodeficiency syndrome (AIDS). A disease in which the immune system is greatly weakened due to infection with HIV, making a person more susceptible to rare cancers and opportunistic infections. (13)

acromegaly. A condition in which the anterior pituitary hypersecretes growth hormone (GH), causing an increase in overall body size; also known as *gigantism*. (9)

action potential. An electrical charge that travels along a nerve fiber when stimulated. (6, 7)

active immunity. A form of immunity in which the blood plasma cells in the body make antibodies as a result of previous exposure to a disease or a vaccine. (13)

active transport. Movement across a cell membrane that requires energy to move a substance against the gradient of concentration. (2)

acute bronchitis. A condition characterized by a temporary inflammation of the mucous membranes that line the trachea and bronchial passageways; causes a cough that may produce mucus. (10)

acute lymphocytic leukemia (ALL). The most common form of leukemia in children under 15 years of age characterized by overproduction of lymphocytes. (11)

acute myeloid leukemia (AML). The most common form of leukemia in adults; develops when the bone marrow produces too many myeloblasts. (11)

Addison's disease. A condition caused by hyposecretion of adrenal corticoid hormones. (9)

adduction. Movement of a body segment closer to the body in the frontal plane. (6)

adenosine triphosphate (ATP). A nucleotide composed of an adenine base, a sugar, and three phosphate groups. (2)

adrenal cortex. The outer layer of the adrenal glands, which has three sublayers that secrete steroid hormones. (9)

adrenal glands. A pair of glands that sit on top of the kidneys; consist of the adrenal cortex and adrenal medulla. (9)

adrenal medulla. The inner layer of the adrenal glands, which functions as a part of the nervous system; secretes epinephrine and norepinephrine during the fight-or-flight response. (9)

afferent nerves. Sensory transmitters that send impulses from receptors in the skin, muscles, and joints to the central nervous system. (7)

agglutination. The process by which red blood cells clump together, usually in response to an antibody. (11)

agonist. Role played by a skeletal muscle in causing a movement. (6)

agonist-antagonist pairs. Pairs of muscles that cause opposing actions at a joint. (6)

aldosterone. A steroid hormone produced in the adrenal cortex that regulates salt and water balance in the body by increasing the amount of sodium reabsorbed from urine. (15)

alimentary canal. The connected canals and cavities that run from the mouth to the anus through the pharynx, esophagus, stomach, and intestine; also known as the *gastrointestinal tract*. (14)

allergen. An antigen that causes an inappropriately strong immune system response. (13)

allergen immunotherapy. A long-term, preventive treatment for allergies; also known as *allergy shots*. (13)

all-or-none law. A rule stating that the fibers in a given motor unit always develop maximum tension when stimulated. (6)

alternative pathway. One of the primary ways in which the complement system can be activated; this pathway is triggered when the C3b complement protein binds to foreign material. (13)

alveolar capillary membrane. A structure that contains the alveoli and the capillaries surrounding the alveoli; the site where gas exchange occurs. (10)

alveoli. Air sacs that serve as the main sites of gas exchange in the lungs. (10)

Alzheimer's disease. A condition involving a progressive loss of brain function with major consequences for memory, thinking, and behavior. (7)

amenorrhea. Absence of a menstrual period in women of reproductive age. (5)

amino acid-derived hormones. Water-soluble hormones composed of proteins or protein-related substances. (9)

amino acids. The building blocks of proteins. (2)

amniotic fluid. A clear fluid in which the embryo, and then the fetus, is suspended. (16)

amphiarthrosis. A type of joint that permits only slight motion. (5)

anabolism. Process by which small molecules are assembled into larger ones. (14)

anaphylaxis. A severe and potentially life-threatening allergic reaction that may include airway obstruction and very low blood pressure. (13)
anatomical position. An erect standing position with arms at the sides and palms facing forward. (1)
anatomy. The study of the form or structure of living things, including plants, animals, and humans. (1)
anemia. A condition characterized by a decrease in the number of red blood cells or an insufficient amount of hemoglobin in the red blood cells. (11)
aneurysm. The abnormal ballooning of a blood vessel, usually an artery, due to a weakness in the wall of the vessel. (12)
angina pectoris. A condition characterized by severe, constricting pain or a sensation of pressure in the chest, often radiating to the left arm; caused by an insufficient supply of blood to the heart. (12)
angiotensin. A polypeptide hormone in the blood that constricts blood vessels and increases blood pressure. (15)
anion. A negatively charged ion. (2)
anorexia nervosa. Condition characterized by body weight 15% or more below the minimal normal weight range, extreme fear of gaining weight, an unrealistic body image, and amenorrhea. (5)
antagonist. Role played by a skeletal muscle acting to slow or stop a movement. (6)
anterior pituitary. The anterior lobe of the pituitary gland, which secretes six different hormones: growth hormone, prolactin, adrenocorticotropin hormone, thyroid-stimulating hormone, follicle-stimulating hormone, and luteinizing hormone. (9)
anterior (ventral) cavity. A continuous internal opening that includes the thoracic and abdominopelvic cavities. (1)
antibody. Immune proteins that react with the antigen that caused its synthesis. (11)
antibody-mediated immunity. A form of immunity associated with free antibodies that circulate in the blood; also known as *humoral immunity*. (13)
anticodon. A set of three bases in transfer RNA that are complementary to those in a codon on messenger RNA. (2)
antidiuretic hormone (ADH). A peptide hormone secreted by the pituitary gland that constricts blood vessels, raises blood pressure, and reduces excretion of urine; also known as *vasopressin*. (15)
antigen. A protein on the surface of RBCs that is used to identify blood type by identifying cells as "self" or "non-self" (foreign) cells. (11)
antigen-presenting cells (APCs). Cells that process protein antigens and present them on their surfaces in a form that can be recognized by lymphocytes. (13)
antihistamines. Medications that help curb the activity of histamines. (8)
aorta. A large arterial trunk that arises from the base of the left ventricle and channels blood from the heart into other arteries throughout the body. (12)
aortic arch. The curved portion of the aorta; located between the ascending and descending parts of the aorta. (12)
aortic valve. The semilunar valve between the left ventricle and the aorta that prevents blood from flowing back into the left ventricle. (12)
aplastic anemia. A rare but serious condition in which the bone marrow stem cells are incapable of making new red blood cells. (11)
aponeurosis. A flat, sheetlike fibrous tissue that connects muscle or bone to other tissues. (6)
apophysis. Site at which a tendon attaches to bone. (5)
apoptosis. A programmed process of cellular self-destruction. (13)
appendicular skeleton. Collective term for the bones of the body's appendages; the arms and legs. (5)
appositional growth. Growth accomplished by the addition of new layers to those previously formed. (5)
aqueous humor. A clear, watery substance in the anterior chamber of the eye that provides nutrients to the lens and cornea and helps maintain normal intraocular pressure. (8)
arteries. Blood vessels that carry blood away from the heart. (12)
arterioles. Microscopic arteries that connect with capillaries. (12)
arthritis. A family of more than 100 common pathologies associated with aging; characterized by joint inflammation accompanied by pain, stiffness, and sometimes swelling. (5)
articular cartilage. Dense, white connective tissue that covers the articulating surfaces of bones at joints. (5)
articular fibrocartilage. Tissue shaped like a disc or a partial disc called a *meniscus* that provides cushioning at a joint. (5)
asthma. A disease of the lungs characterized by recurring episodes of airway inflammation that causes bronchospasms and increases mucus production. (10)
atherosclerosis. Hardening of the arteries. (12)
atlas. The first cervical vertebra; specialized to provide the connection between the occipital bone of the skull and the spinal column. (5)
atom. A basic building block of matter. (1)
atomic number. The number of protons in an atom's nucleus. (2)
atrial fibrillation. A condition in which the atria contract in an uncoordinated, rapid manner (rate above 350 bpm), causing an irregular ventricular response. (12)
atrial natriuretic peptide (ANP). Peptide hormone secreted by the atria of the heart that promotes excretion of sodium and water and lowers blood pressure. (15)
atrioventricular (AV) valves. The two valves (tricuspid and mitral/bicuspid) situated between the atria and the ventricles. (12)
atrioventricular node (AV node). A small mass of tissue that transmits impulses received from the sinoatrial node to the ventricles via the bundle of His. (12)

auditory canal. A short, tubelike structure that connects the outer ear to the eardrum. (8)

auricle. The irregularly shaped outer portion of the ear; also known as the *pinna*. (8)

autoimmune disorder. A condition in which the immune system attacks the body's own tissue. (13)

autonomic nervous system. The branch of the nervous system that controls involuntary body functions. (7)

autonomic reflexes. Involuntary stimuli transmitted to cardiac and smooth muscle. (7)

axial skeleton. The central portion of the skeletal system, consisting of the skull, spinal column, and thoracic cage. (5)

axis. The second cervical vertebra; specialized with an upward projection called the *odontoid process*, on which the atlas rotates. (5)

axon. A long, tail-like projection found on a typical nerve that transmits impulses away from the cell body. (6, 7)

axon terminals. Offshoots of the axon that branch out to connect with individual muscle fibers. (6)

B

Bachmann's bundle. A tract that runs from the left atrium to the right atrium, carrying the impulse generated by the SA node; also called the *interatrial tract*. (12)

ball-and-socket joint. A synovial joint formed between one bone end shaped roughly like a ball and a receiving bone reciprocally shaped like a socket. (5)

baroreceptors. Receptors located in the atrium, aortic arch, and carotid arteries that are sensitive to changes in blood pressure. (12)

basal cell carcinoma. The most common and least malignant form of skin cancer. (4)

basal metabolic rate (BMR). The amount of energy required to sustain a person's metabolism for one day if he or she is at complete rest. (14)

base pairs. Pairs of complementary nucleic acid bases; A and T or C and G. (2)

bending. A loading pattern created by a combination of off-center forces. (1)

biopsy. Removal of a tissue sample for microscopic examination to diagnose disease. (3)

blastocyst. The embryo from about four to six days after fertilization, when it includes an outer layer of cells, an inner cell mass, and a fluid-filled cavity. (16)

B lymphocytes (B cells). Lymphatic cells that mature in the bone marrow before moving out to the blood and the rest of the body. (13)

bone marrow. Material with a rich blood supply found within the medullary cavity of long bones; yellow marrow stores fat, and red marrow is active in producing blood cells. (5)

bony labyrinth. Term that describes the winding tunnel located in the inner ear. (8)

brachial artery. The artery located at the fold of the elbow. (12)

bradycardia. A normal heart rhythm but with a rate below 60 bpm. (12)

bronchioles. The thin-walled, smallest air-conducting passageways of the bronchi. (10)

bronchospasms. Spasmodic contractions of the bronchial muscles that constrict the airways during an asthma attack. (10)

buffy coat. A thin layer of white blood cells and platelets that lies between the red blood cells and plasma in a blood specimen that has gone through a centrifuge. (11)

bulbourethral glands. Two small glands at the base of the penis that secrete mucus into the urethra. (16)

bulimia nervosa. Condition characterized by a minimum of two eating binges a week for at least three months; an associated feeling of lack of control; use of self-induced vomiting, laxatives, diuretics, strict dieting, or exercise to prevent weight gain; and an obsession with body image. (5)

bundle branches. The left and right branches that extend from the bundle of His to transport electrical impulses to the Purkinje fibers in the ventricles. (12)

bundle of His. A slender bundle of modified cardiac muscle fibers that conducts electrical impulses from the AV node, through the left and right bundle branches, to Purkinje fibers in the ventricles. (12)

bursae. Small capsules lined with synovial membranes and filled with synovial fluid that cushion the structures they separate. (5)

bursitis. Inflammation of one or more bursae. (5)

C

calcaneus. The largest of the tarsal bones; referred to as the *heel bone*. (5)

Calorie. The unit food scientists use to measure the potential energy in foods; the amount of heat required to raise the temperature of 1 kilogram of water by 1°C; also called a *kilocalorie*. (14)

capillaries. Small, thin-walled blood vessels in which oxygen and carbon dioxide gas exchange occurs. (12)

capillary bed. A network of intertwined capillaries. (12)

carcinoma. Cancer that originates in the epithelial tissue. (3)

cardiac muscle. The major muscle tissue of the heart. (3)

cardiac output. The amount of blood pumped from the heart per minute; also known as *cardiac volume*. (12)

cardiomyocytes. Cardiac muscle cells. (12)

cardiomyopathy. A disease such as an infection that weakens the myocardium and causes heart failure. (12)

cardiopulmonary system. The collective name for the respiratory and cardiovascular systems. (10)

carotid arteries. The arteries located on either side of the windpipe; where the carotid pulse is felt. (12)

carpal bones. Bones of the wrist. (5)

cartilage. A class of connective tissue that provides support and flexibility to parts of the skeleton. (3)

catabolism. Process by which large molecules are broken down into smaller ones. (14)
cation. A positively charged ion. (2)
cell body. The part of an axon that contains a nucleus and other common organelles. (7)
cell-mediated immunity. A form of immunity that arises from the activation of T lymphocytes (T cells) by antigen-presenting cells; also known as *cellular immunity*. (13)
cells. The smallest building blocks of all living beings. (1)
cellulitis. A bacterial infection characterized by a red, swollen, and painful area of skin. (4)
central nervous system (CNS). Division of the nervous system that includes the brain and spinal cord. (7)
centrioles. Short cylinders that help guide the movement and separation of chromosomes during cell division. (2)
centromere. The point on a chromosome that divides the chromosome into two arms; functions as the point of attachment for the sister chromatids; provides movement during cell division. (16)
cerebellum. The section of the brain that coordinates body movements, including balance. (7)
cerebral palsy. A group of nervous system disorders resulting from brain damage before or during birth, or in early infancy. (7)
cerebrovascular accident (CVA, stroke). A sudden blockage of blood flow, or the rupture of an artery in the brain, that causes brain cells to die from lack of oxygen. (12)
cerebrum. The largest part of the brain, consisting of the left and right hemispheres. (7)
ceruminous glands. The glands that secrete cerumen (earwax) and are located in the auditory canal. (8)
cervical region. The first seven vertebrae, comprising the neck. (5)
cervix. The narrow, lower end of the uterus that includes the opening through which a baby passes during childbirth. (16)
channel proteins. Molecules with a hollow central pore that allows water or small, charged particles of certain substances to pass into or out of cells. (2)
chelation therapy. A procedure in which excess metals, such as iron, are removed from the blood. (11)
chemical breakdown. The breakdown of large food molecules into smaller molecules by enzymes. (14)
chemoreceptors. Sensory cells that respond to chemical stimuli (10); receptors located in the aortic arch and carotid arteries that are sensitive to pH levels, decreased partial pressure of oxygen, increased partial pressure of carbon dioxide, and increased concentration of hydrogen ions. (12)
chlamydia. A sexually transmitted infection that often causes no symptoms but can damage the female reproductive tract, lead to infertility, and increase the risk of ectopic pregnancy. (16)
cholecystectomy. Surgical removal of the gallbladder. (14)
chondroblasts. Cells that secrete the extracellular matrix of cartilage. (3)
choroid. The middle layer of the wall of the eye. (8)
chromatids. Paired strands of a duplicated chromosome that become visible during cell division and are joined by a centromere. (16)
chromosome. A structure that contains the genes, or genetic code, for an individual; consists of a DNA molecule and the associated proteins that help it coil. (2, 16)
chronic bronchitis. A long-lasting respiratory condition in which the airways of the lungs become obstructed due to inflammation of the bronchi and excessive mucus production. (10)
chronic kidney disease. A condition diagnosed by evidence of kidney damage or a glomerular filtration rate less than 60 mL per minute for at least three months. (15)
chronic lymphocytic leukemia (CLL). A form of leukemia characterized by extremely high levels of lymphocytes; most often found in middle-aged adults. (11)
chronic myeloid leukemia (CML). A form of leukemia characterized by overproduction of granulocytes. (11)
chronic obstructive pulmonary disease (COPD). Any lung disorder characterized by a long-term airway obstruction that makes it difficult to breathe; the two most common forms are emphysema and chronic bronchitis. (10)
chyme. The mixture of food and digestive juices in the stomach and duodenum. (14)
cilia. Hair-like projections that actively flex back and forth to move fluid or mucus across the outside of a cell. (2)
ciliary body. The structure between the choroid and the iris that anchors the lens in place. (8)
ciliary glands. Modified sweat glands located between the eyelashes. (8)
ciliated epithelium. A cellular covering embedded with tiny, hair-like cilia that brush foreign particles upward and out of the trachea. (10)
circumduction. Rotational movement of a body segment such that the end of the segment traces a circle. (6)
classical pathway. One of the primary ways in which the complement system can be activated; this pathway is triggered when complement protein C1 recognizes an antibody bound to foreign material. (13)
clavicle. A doubly curved long bone that forms part of the shoulder girdle; also known as the *collarbone*. (5)
clitoris. A cylindrical body of erectile tissue that lies at the anterior end of the vulva. (16)
clonal selection. The repeated division of a lymphocyte that produces many exact genetic copies (clones) of itself. (13)
coagulation. The process by which the enzyme thrombin and the protein fibrinogen combine to form fibrin, a fiber that weaves around the platelet plug to form a blood clot. (11)

coccyx. The four vertebrae at the base of the spine that are fused to form the tailbone. (5)

cochlea. A snail-shaped structure in the inner ear that enables hearing. (8)

cochlear duct. The portion of the membranous labyrinth located inside the cochlea. (8)

codon. A set of three bases in DNA or RNA that codes for one amino acid. (2)

coenzyme. A molecule that is necessary for the action of an enzyme. (14)

collecting duct. A tube that collects urine from several nephrons and carries it to the renal pelvis. (15)

colon. The longest segment of the large intestine. (14)

combined loading. The simultaneous action of two or more types of forces. (1)

common warts. Warts that typically appear on the hands or fingers and disappear without treatment. (4)

complement proteins. The proteins in the blood that work with immune system cells and antibodies to defend the body against infection. (13)

complement system. A system of more than 30 proteins that circulate in the blood plasma and work together to destroy foreign substances. (13)

complete blood count (CBC). A blood test that helps detect blood disorders or diseases such as anemia, infection, abnormal blood cell counts, clotting problems, immune system disorders, and cancers of the blood. (11)

compression. A squeezing force that compresses the structure to which it is applied. (1)

compressive strength. The ability of a material to withstand compression (inward-pressing force) without buckling. (3)

concentric contraction. A type of contraction that results in shortening of a muscle. (6)

conductivity. The ability of a neuron to transmit a nerve impulse. (7)

condylar joint. A type of diarthrosis in which one articulating bone surface is an oval, convex shape, and the other is a reciprocally shaped concave surface. (5)

cones. Sensory cells in the retina that are sensitive to bright light and provide color vision. (8)

conjunctiva. A delicate external membrane that covers the exposed eyeball and lines the eyelid. (8)

connective tissue. A class of tissue that connects, supports, binds, or separates other tissues or organs. (3)

constipation. A condition characterized by difficulty in defecating. (14)

contractility. The ability to contract or shorten. (6)

control center. A system that receives and analyzes information from sensory receptors, and then sends a command stimulus to an effector to maintain homeostasis. (1)

contusion. Bruising or bleeding within a muscle as a result of an impact. (6)

cornea. A transparent tissue located over the anterior center of the eye. (8)

coronary artery disease (CAD). A condition characterized by narrowing of one or more of the coronary arteries due to a buildup of plaque. (12)

coronary sinus. The large venous channel between the left atrium and left ventricle on the posterior side of the heart that empties into the right atrium at the junction of the four chambers. (12)

cortical bone. Dense, solid bone that covers the outer surface of all bones and is the main form of bone tissue in the long bones. (5)

covalent bond. A strong connection formed between two atoms when they share a pair of electrons. (2)

cranial cavity. The open chamber inside the skull that holds the brain. (1)

cranial nerves. Twelve pairs of nerves that originate in the brain and relay impulses to and from the PNS. (7)

craniosacral division. The parasympathetic nervous system; includes nerves that originate in the brainstem or sacral region of the spinal cord. (7)

cranium. Collective term for the fused, flat bones surrounding the back of the head. (5)

creatinine. A normal by-product of muscle metabolism; produced by the body at a fairly steady rate and freely filtered by the glomerulus. (15)

Crohn's disease. A chronic inflammatory bowel disease that usually affects the small intestine or colon. (14)

cross bridges. Connections between the heads of myosin filaments and receptor sites on the actin filaments. (6)

crossovers. Connections that form between homologous chromosomes during meiosis, resulting in the swapping of portions of chromosomes. (16)

Cushing's syndrome. A disorder of the adrenal cortex caused by hypersecretion of cortisol. (9)

cutaneous membrane. Another name for skin. (4)

cyclic adenosine monophosphate (cAMP). A chemical derived from ATP that serves as a messenger to activate protein kinases, which in turn trigger a variety of responses in the cell, such as protein synthesis and glycogen breakdown. (9)

cystic fibrosis. A common inherited disease that causes exocrine gland secretions to become abnormally thick, creating buildup. (3)

cytokinesis. Division of the cytoplasm in a cell, which begins during the telophase portion of mitosis. (2)

cytoplasm. The part of a cell that contains everything inside the cell membrane except the nucleus. (2)

cytoskeleton. A network of proteins that defines the shape of a cell and gives it mechanical strength. (2)

D

data. Systematically collected and recorded observations. (1)

defecation. The discharge of feces from the anus. (14)

delayed-onset muscle soreness (DOMS). Muscle pain that follows participation in a particularly long or strenuous activity; begins 24–73 hours after activity and involves multiple, microscopic tears in the muscle tissue that cause inflammation, pain, swelling, and stiffness. (6)

delivery of the placenta. The last stage of birth, in which the placenta detaches from the uterine wall and is expelled. (16)

dementia. An organic brain disease involving loss of function in two or more areas of cognition. (7)

dendrites. Branches of a neuron that collect stimuli and transport them to the cell body of a neuron. (7)

deoxyribonucleic acid (DNA). A polymer of nucleotides with the bases adenosine, guanine, cytosine, and thymine. (2)

depolarized. A condition in which the inside of a cell membrane is more positively charged than the outside. (7, 12)

dermis. The layer of skin between the epidermis and hypodermis; includes nerve endings, glands, and hair follicles. (4)

detrusor. The smooth muscle that forms most of the bladder wall and aids in expelling urine. (15)

diabetes insipidus. A disorder caused by hyposecretion of antidiuretic hormone (ADH) by the posterior pituitary. (9)

diabetes mellitus. A disease that results from the body's inability to regulate blood glucose levels; see *type I diabetes mellitus* and *type II diabetes mellitus*. (9)

diapedesis. The passage of blood, or any of its formed elements, through the blood vessel walls into body tissues. (11)

diaphragm. A dome-shaped sheet of muscle and fibrous tissue that separates the thoracic and abdominal cavities. (6)

diaphysis. The shaft of a long bone. (5)

diarrhea. The occurrence of frequent, watery bowel movements. (14)

diarthrosis. A freely movable joint; also known as a *synovial joint*. (5)

diastole. The period of relaxation in the heart when the chambers fill with blood. (12)

diencephalon. The area of the brain that includes the epithalamus, thalamus, and hypothalamus; also known as the *interbrain*. (7)

dilation. The stage of labor during which the opening of the cervix dilates, or widens. (16)

diploid. A cell containing two sets of chromosomes, one set from the mother and one set from the father. (16)

dislocation. Injury that involves displacement of a bone from its joint socket. (5)

distal convoluted tubule. The last part of a nephron through which urine flows before reaching the collecting duct. (15)

diuresis. Urine production. (15)

DNA. See *deoxyribonucleic acid (DNA)*. (2)

dorsal ramus. The division of posterior spinal nerves that transmit motor impulses to the posterior trunk muscles and relay sensory impulses from the skin of the back. (7)

dorsiflexion. Movement of the top of the foot toward the lower leg. (6)

downregulated. Decreased. (9)

ductus arteriosus. A short, broad vessel in the fetus that connects the left pulmonary artery with the descending aorta, allowing most of the blood to bypass the infant's lungs. (12)

ductus deferens. The secretory duct of the testis, which extends from the epididymis and joins with the excretory duct of the seminal gland; also known as the *vas deferens*. (16)

dwarfism. A condition in which the pituitary gland hyposecretes growth hormone (GH), resulting in an adult height of less than four feet. (9)

dysrhythmia. An irregular heartbeat or rhythm. (12)

E

eccentric contraction. A type of contraction that results in lengthening of a muscle. (6)

ectoderm. The outermost layer of cells or tissue of an embryo in early development. (3)

eczema. A common skin condition that is characterized by unrelenting itchiness in affected areas of skin; also known as *atopic dermatitis*. (3)

effector. A unit that receives a command stimulus from the control center and causes an action to help maintain homeostasis. (1)

efferent nerves. Motor transmitters that carry impulses from the central nervous system to the muscles and glands. (7)

ejaculation. The discharge of sperm from the ejaculatory duct during the male sexual response. (16)

elastic. A response in which a structure returns to its original size and shape after the application of force. (1)

elasticity. The ability of a material to stretch when tension is applied, and spring back to its original shape when the tension is removed. (3, 6)

electron. A negatively charged fundamental particle. (2)

element. A substance composed of atoms that all have the same atomic number. (2)

embolus. A clot that has become dislodged from the wall of a blood vessel and travels through the bloodstream. (11)

embryo. A developing human from the time of implantation to the end of the eighth week after conception. (16)

emphysema. A form of COPD that leads to chronic inflammation of the lungs, which damages the alveoli and causes an accumulation of carbon dioxide in the lungs. (10)

emulsification. The breakdown of large fat particles into much smaller particles, aided by bile. (14)
endocarditis. Inflammation of the innermost lining of the heart, including the inner surfaces of the chambers and valves. (12)
endocardium. The innermost layer of the heart, which lines the interior of the heart chambers and covers the valves of the heart. (12)
endocrine gland. A gland that secretes its product into the interstitial space. (3)
endoderm. The innermost layer of cells or tissue of an embryo in early development. (3)
endolymph. A thick fluid that fills the membranous labyrinth. (8)
endomysium. A fine, protective sheath of connective tissue that surrounds a skeletal muscle fiber. (6)
endoneurium. A delicate, connective tissue that surrounds each axon, or nerve fiber, in a nerve. (7)
endoplasmic reticulum (ER). An organelle that consists of a network of membranes in the cytoplasm. (2)
endothelial cells. The cells that form the walls of lymphatic and blood capillaries, and which form the inner lining of larger blood vessels. (11, 13)
energy. The capacity of a physical system to do work. (14)
enzyme. A protein that catalyzes, or speeds up, a specific chemical reaction. (2)
epicardium. The outermost layer of the heart and the visceral layer of the serous pericardium. (12)
epidermal dendritic cells. Skin cells that initiate an immune system response to the presence of foreign bacteria or viruses. (4)
epidermis. The outer layer of skin. (4)
epididymis. A system of small ducts in the testis in which sperm mature. (16)
epiglottis. A flap of cartilaginous tissue that covers the opening to the trachea; diverts food and liquids to the esophagus during swallowing. (10)
epilepsy. A group of brain disorders characterized by repeated seizures over time. (7)
epimysium. The outermost sheath of connective tissue that surrounds a skeletal muscle. (6)
epinephrine. The chief neurohormone of the adrenal medulla; used as a heart stimulant, vasoconstrictor (narrows the blood vessels), and bronchodilator (relaxes the bronchial tubes in the lungs). (9)
epineurium. The tough outer covering of a nerve. (7)
epiphyseal plate. Growth plate near the ends of long bones where osteoblast activity increases bone length. (5)
epiphysis. The bulbous end of a long bone. (5)
epithalamus. The uppermost portion of the diencephalon, which includes the pineal gland and regulates sleep-cycle hormones. (7)
epithelial membranes. Thin sheets of tissue lining the internal and external surfaces of the body. (4)
epithelial tissue. Membranous tissue that covers internal organs and other internal surfaces of the body. (3)
erection. The condition of erectile tissue when filled with blood, which permits the penis to gain entry to the female reproductive tract. (16)
erythroblastosis fetalis. A severe hemolytic disease found in fetuses or newborns that is caused by the production of maternal antibodies against the antigens on fetal red blood cells; usually involves Rh incompatibility between the mother and fetus; also known as hemolytic disease of the newborn (HDN). (11)
erythrocytes. Red blood cells. (11)
erythropoiesis. The process by which red blood cells are produced. (11)
erythropoietin (EPO). A hormone secreted by the kidneys that stimulates the production of red blood cells. (11)
esophagus. The muscular tube that connects the pharynx and stomach. (14)
Eustachian tube. A channel that connects the middle ear to the pharynx and serves to equalize pressure on either side of the tympanic membrane. (8)
eversion. Movement in which the sole of the foot is rolled outward. (6)
exocrine gland. A gland that secretes its product to the outside world. (3)
exocytosis. A process in which the cell membranes of a vesicle and a cell fuse together and push debris from the vesicle outside of the cell. (13)
expiration. The process by which air is expelled from the lungs; also known as *exhalation*. (10)
expiratory reserve volume (ERV). The additional amount of air that can be exhaled immediately after a normal exhalation. (10)
expulsion. The stage of labor that starts at full dilation and ends when the baby is delivered. (16)
extensibility. The ability to be stretched. (6)
extension. Movement that returns a body segment to anatomical position in the sagittal plane. (6)
external respiration. The process by which gas exchange occurs between the alveoli in the lungs and the pulmonary blood capillaries. (10)
external urethral sphincter. A ring of skeletal muscle that surrounds the intermediate part of the urethra where it passes through the urogenital diaphragm; this muscle is voluntarily controlled during release of urine from the body. (15)
extracellular fluid. The liquid—consisting of mostly water—that surrounds a typical cell. (2)
extracellular matrix. The solid or gel-like substance that surrounds a typical cell in tissues. (1, 2)
extrinsic muscles. The muscles that are attached to the outer surface of the eye and are responsible for changing the eye's direction of viewing. (8)

F

facial bones. Bones of the face. (5)

false pelvis. The bony region of the pelvis that is located superior to the pelvic inlet. (5)

fascicle. A bundle of muscle fibers. (6)

fast-twitch. A type of muscle that contracts quickly. (6)

fatty acid. A molecule that consists of a hydrocarbon chain with a carboxylic acid group at one end. (2)

female athlete triad. Combination of disordered eating, amenorrhea, and osteoporosis. (5)

femur. Thigh bone. (5)

fertilization. The formation of a single cell that contains the genetic material from two gametes, one from each parent. (16)

fetus. A developing human from eight weeks after conception to birth. (16)

fever. The maintenance of body temperature at a higher-than-normal level. (13)

fibrin. A long, thread-like fiber created by the combination of thrombin and fibrinogen. (11)

fibrinolysis. The process of breaking down fibrin to dissolve a blood clot. (11)

fibrous pericardium. The tough, non-elastic outer wall of the pericardium. (12)

fibula. Bone of the lower leg that does not bear weight. (5)

first-degree burns. Burns that affect only the epidermal layer of skin. (4)

fissures. The uniformly positioned, deep grooves in the brain. (7)

flexion. Forward movement of a body segment away from anatomical position in the sagittal plane. (6)

follicle-stimulating hormone (FSH). A hormone secreted by the anterior pituitary that stimulates the production of eggs in females and sperm in males. (16)

fontanel. An opening in the infant skull through which the baby's pulse can be felt; these openings enable compression of the skull during birth and brain growth during late pregnancy and early infancy. (5)

foramen ovale. An opening in the septal wall between the atria; normally present only in the fetus. (12)

force. A push or pull acting on a structure. (1)

forced expiratory volume in one second (FEV_1). The amount of air a person can expire in one second. (10)

forced expiratory volume in one second/forced vital capacity (FEV_1/FVC). Ratio that indicates the overall expiratory power of the lungs. (10)

formed elements. The solid components of blood; includes red blood cells, white blood cells, and platelets. (11)

fourth-degree burns. Burns that involve destruction of all layers of skin, as well as nerve endings and some of the underlying tissues, such as muscle, tendon, ligament, and bone. (4)

fovea centralis. A tiny spot near the center of each retina that contains only cones and is the point of greatest visual acuity. (8)

fracture. Any break or disruption of continuity in a bone. (5)

frontal lobes. The regions of the brain located behind the forehead; include areas that control higher order intellectual functioning and speech. (7)

frontal plane. An imaginary, vertical flat surface that divides the body into front and back halves. (1)

functional residual capacity (FRC). The amount of air that remains in the lungs after a normal expiration; ERV + RV. (10)

G

gallbladder. The digestive accessory organ that stores bile and delivers it to the duodenum when needed. (14)

gallstones. Solid crystals that form from substances in the bile of the gallbladder. (14)

gametes. Mature haploid male or female cells that unite with cells of the opposite sex to form a zygote; known as *eggs* in females and *sperm* in males. (16)

ganglion. A mass of nervous tissue that is composed mostly of nerve cell bodies and acts as an enlarged junction between neurons. (7)

gastroenteritis. An inflammation of the stomach or intestine that produces some combination of nausea, vomiting, diarrhea, and abdominal pain. (14)

gastroesophageal reflux. The movement of chyme from the stomach into the lower esophagus. (14)

gastroesophageal reflux disease (GERD). Chronic inflammation of the esophagus caused by the regular upward flow of gastric juice from the stomach into the lower esophagus. (14)

gastrointestinal (GI) tract. The connected canals and cavities that run from the mouth to the anus through the pharynx, esophagus, stomach, and intestine; also known as the *alimentary canal*. (14)

genital herpes. A sexually transmitted infection that may cause blisters or sores in the genital or anal area or near the mouth; may cause no symptoms. (16)

gingiva. The soft tissue that covers the necks of the teeth, the mandible, and the maxilla; also called the *gum*. (14)

glands. Epithelial cells that are organized to produce and secrete substances. (3)

gliding joint. A type of diarthrosis that allows only sliding motion of the articulating bones. (5)

glomerular filtration. The movement of water and solutes from the capillaries into the glomerular capsular space. (15)

glomerular filtration rate (GFR). The total amount of water filtered from the glomerular capillaries into the glomerular capsule per unit of time; usually measured in milliliters per minute. (15)

glomerulus. A cluster of capillaries in a cup-like capsule at the end of a renal corpuscle. (15)

glucagon. A hormone secreted by the pancreas that causes the breakdown of glycogen stored in the liver. (9)

glucose. The main form of sugar that circulates in the blood; a monosaccharide. (2)
glycogen. A polymer of glucose that is found in animals; the stored form of glucose. (2)
glycoproteins. Proteins with carbohydrate groups attached. (2)
goiter. An enlarged thyroid gland. (9)
Golgi apparatus. An organelle that produces vesicles; consists of membranous discs. (2)
gonads. The organs that produce gametes (oocytes and sperm); the ovaries in females and the testes in males. (16)
gonorrhea. A sexually transmitted infection that may cause pain during urination, unusual discharge of fluid from the vagina or penis, or no symptoms at all; can lead to infertility. (16)
Graves' disease. An autoimmune disorder that causes an overactive thyroid gland and outward bulging of the eyes. (9)
gustatory cells. Sensory receptors located within taste buds. (8)
gustatory hairs. Tiny threads in taste buds that send nerve impulses to the brain. (8)

H

haploid. A cell containing a single set of unpaired chromosomes. (16)
Haversian canals. Major passageways running in the direction of the length of long bones, providing paths for blood vessels. (5)
Haversian system. Structural unit that includes a single Haversian canal along with its multiple canaliculi, which branch out to join with lacunae, forming a comprehensive transportation matrix for supplying nutrients and removing waste products; also known as an *osteon*. (5)
heart block. A condition in which the impulses traveling from the SA node to the ventricles are delayed, intermittently blocked, or completely blocked before they reach the ventricles. (12)
heart murmurs. Extra or unusual sounds during a heartbeat that can be heard by a stethoscope; may be harmless or indicative of a problem with one of the heart valves. (12)
hematocrit. The percentage of total blood volume that is composed of red blood cells. (11)
hematopoiesis. Process of blood cell formation. (5)
hematopoietic cells. The cells that are responsible for creating blood cells. (11)
hemodialysis. A procedure for removing metabolic waste products from the body; blood is withdrawn from an artery, pumped through a dialyzer, and then returned to the patient through a vein. (15)
hemoglobin. An essential molecule of the red blood cell that serves as the binding site for oxygen and carbon dioxide; composed of globin and heme. (11)
hemolysis. The rupture of red blood cells. (11)
hemophilia. A condition in which blood does not clot properly due to the absence of a clotting factor. (11)
hemostasis. The sequence of events that causes a blood clot to form and bleeding to stop. (11)
hepatic portal system. The circulatory system through which blood picks up nutrients for distribution throughout the body. (12)
hepatitis. A disease characterized by inflammation of and damage to the liver. (14)
Hering-Breuer reflex. An involuntary impulse that halts inspiration and initiates exhalation; triggered by stretch receptors in the bronchioles and alveoli. (10)
hernia. A balloon-like section of tissue that protrudes through a hole or weakened section of a muscle. (6)
herpes simplex virus type 1 (HSV-1). The form of herpes that generates cold sores or fever blisters around the mouth. (4)
herpes simplex virus type 2 (HSV-2). The genital form of herpes. (4)
herpes varicella (chickenpox). A highly contagious, common childhood disease that is characterized by extremely itchy, fluid-filled blisters. (4)
herpes zoster (shingles). A disease that involves a painful, blistering rash accompanied by headache, fever, and a general unwell feeling. (4)
hinge joint. A type of diarthrosis that allows only hinge-like movements in forward and backward directions. (5)
histamines. Molecules that trigger a reaction to irritation of the nasal membranes, producing nasal congestion and drainage. (8)
histology. The study of tissues. (3)
homeostasis. A state of regulated physiological balance. (1)
homeostatic imbalance. A state in which the organ systems are unable to keep the body's internal environment within normal ranges. (1)
homeostatic mechanisms. The processes that maintain homeostasis. (1)
hormonal control. The type of endocrine control in which endocrine organs are stimulated by hormones from other endocrine organs, starting with the hypothalamus. (9)
hormones. Chemical messengers secreted by the endocrine glands. (9)
human chorionic gonadotropin (hCG). A hormone secreted by the trophoblast cells of the blastocyst that prevents deterioration of the corpus luteum and stimulates progesterone production in the placenta. (16)
human genome. The complete DNA sequence of a human. (2)
human immunodeficiency virus (HIV). The virus that causes immune deficiency in humans and leads to AIDS. (13)
human papillomavirus (HPV). A sexually transmitted infection that causes genital warts and can cause cervical cancer. (16)

humerus. Major bone of the upper arm. (5)
humoral control. The type of endocrine control in which levels of various substances in body fluids are monitored for homeostatic imbalance. (9)
Huntington's disease. A genetic disease that causes degeneration of neurons in the brain, resulting in an inability to control movements, a loss of intellectual capacity, and emotional disturbance. (7)
hydrogen bond. A weak connection that forms between two molecules through an electrostatic (van der Waals) attraction. (2)
hydrostatic pressure. The pressure exerted by a liquid as a result of its potential energy. (15)
hypercalcemia. A condition characterized by increased blood calcium levels and increased calcium absorption by the kidneys; caused by the hypersecretion of parathyroid hormone (PTH). (9)
hyperextension. Backward movement of a body segment past anatomical position in the sagittal plane. (6)
hyperglycemia. A condition in which blood glucose levels are elevated. (9)
hypertension. High blood pressure; a condition that occurs when the force of blood against the arterial wall remains elevated for an extended period of time. (12)
hyperthyroidism. The condition caused by an overactive thyroid gland; characterized by a visibly enlarged thyroid gland in the neck. (9)
hyperventilation. Excessive breathing that leads to increased oxygen and expulsion of a larger amount of carbon dioxide. (10)
hypodermis. The layer of skin beneath the dermis; serves as a storage repository for fat. (4)
hypothalamic non-releasing hormones. The hormones that are produced in the hypothalamus and carried by the blood to the anterior pituitary, where they stop certain hormones from being released; also known as *hypothalamic inhibiting hormones*. (9)
hypothalamic releasing hormones. The hormones that are produced in the hypothalamus and carried by the blood to the anterior pituitary, where they stimulate the release of anterior pituitary hormones. (9)
hypothalamus. The portion of the diencephalon that regulates functions such as metabolism, heart rate, and blood pressure. (7)
hypothesis. An educated guess about the outcome of a study. (1)
hypothyroidism. The condition of an underactive thyroid gland. (9)
hypoxia. A condition of having too little oxygen in the blood. (11)

I

immune system. The cells and chemicals that contribute to the body's specific defenses against disease. (13)
immunoglobulins. Antibodies; proteins that recognize particular antigens with great specificity. (13)
immunosuppression. A reduction in the activity and sensitivity of the immune system. (13)
impetigo. A bacterial infection common in elementary school children that is characterized by pink, blister-like bumps, usually on the face. (4)
implantation. The binding of the blastocyst to the endometrium. (16)
incus. A tiny bone within the middle ear that transmits sound from the malleus to the stapes; sometimes called the *anvil* because of its shape. (8)
inferior vena cava. The largest vein in the human body, which returns deoxygenated blood to the right atrium of the heart from body regions below the diaphragm. (12)
infertility. The inability to get pregnant. (16)
inflammatory bowel disease. A condition in which the walls of the small and/or large intestine become chronically inflamed. (14)
inflammatory response. A physiological response to tissue injury or infection that is characterized by heat, redness, swelling, and pain; also called *inflammation*. (13)
influenza. A viral infection that affects the respiratory system; also known as the *flu*. (10)
ingestion. The intake of food and liquids via the mouth. (14)
insertion. The site of a muscle's attachment to a bone that tends to move when the muscle contracts. (6)
inspiration. The process by which air flows into the lungs; also known as *inhalation*. (10)
inspiratory reserve volume (IRV). The amount of air that can be inhaled immediately after a normal inhalation. (10)
insulin. A hormone that promotes glucose uptake in body tissues. (9)
insulin resistance. A condition present in type II diabetes in which the pancreas secretes insulin, but the body's insulin receptors are downregulated, causing elevated blood glucose levels. (9)
integumentary system. Term for the skin and its appendages; includes the epidermis, dermis, sudoriferous and sebaceous glands, nails, and hair. (4)
interatrial septum. The wall that separates the right and left atria in the heart. (12)
interferons. Proteins released by cells that have been infected with viruses; interfere with virus reproduction. (13)
internal respiration. The process by which gas exchange occurs between the tissues and the arterial blood. (10)

internal urethral sphincter. A layer of smooth muscle located at the inferior end of the bladder and the proximal end of the urethra; this muscle, which prohibits release of urine, is under involuntary control. (15)

interstitial fluid. The fluid located in the spaces between cells. (13)

interventricular septum. The thick wall between the two ventricles in the heart. (12)

intervertebral discs. Fibrocartilaginous cushions between vertebral bodies that allow bending of the spine and help to create the normal spinal curves. (5)

inversion. Movement in which the sole of the foot is rolled inward. (6)

ion. An atom or molecule that has a positive or negative charge. (2)

ionic bond. A connection that forms between atoms due to electric attraction. (2)

iris. The anterior portion of the choroid, which gives the eye its color. (8)

iron-deficient anemia. The most common type of anemia; caused by an insufficient dietary intake of iron, loss of iron from intestinal bleeding, or iron-level depletion during pregnancy. (11)

irritability. The ability to respond to a stimulus. (6)

ischemia. A lack of blood flow, usually due to the narrowing of a blood vessel. (12)

isometric contraction. A type of contraction that involves no change in muscle length. (6)

isotope. A form of an element that contains an equal number of protons but a different number of neutrons than other forms, or isotopes, of the element. (2)

J

jaundice. A blood disorder characterized by yellow-colored skin and whites of the eyes. (11)

K

keratin. A tough protein found in the skin, hair, and nails. (4)

keratinocytes. Cells within the epidermis that produce keratin. (4)

kidney stone. A solid crystalline mass that forms in the kidney, which may become stuck in the renal pelvis or ureter; usually made of calcium, phosphate, or uric acid. (15)

kinetics. A field of study that analyzes the actions of forces. (1)

L

labia majora. The two skin folds posterior to the mons pubis that lie parallel on either side of the vaginal opening. (16)

labia minora. A smaller set of skin folds inside the labia majora. (16)

lacrimal glands. The glands that are located above the lateral end of each eye and secrete tears. (8)

lactation. The secretion of milk by the mammary glands. (16)

lactiferous duct. The duct through which milk is secreted; opens at the nipple. (16)

large intestine. The portion of the GI tract between the small intestine and the anus; includes the cecum, colon, rectum, and anal canal. (14)

laryngitis. Inflammation of the larynx, or voice box. (10)

larynx. A triangular-shaped space inferior to the pharynx that is responsible for routing air and food into the proper passageways and producing speech; also known as the *voice box*. (10)

lateral rotation. Outward (lateral) movement of a body segment in the transverse plane. (6)

lectin pathway. One of the primary ways in which the complement system can be activated; this pathway is triggered when lectin binds to a sugar molecule present on the surfaces of bacteria. (13)

lens. A transparent, flexible structure that curves outward on both sides. (8)

let-down reflex. The contraction of smooth muscle cells in the mammary glands that allows milk to be squeezed toward and out of the nipple. (16)

leukemia. A cancer of the blood that causes the bone marrow to produce abnormal white blood cells. (3, 11)

leukocytes. White blood cells. (11)

ligament. A band of collagen and elastic fibers that connects bones to other bones. (5)

limbic system. The part of the brain responsible for emotions. (8)

linea alba. A longitudinal band of connective tissue that separates the *rectus abdominis* muscles. (6)

lingual tonsils. Two masses of lymphatic tissue that lie on either side of the base of the tongue. (13)

lipids. Fatty molecules that dissolve poorly in water but dissolve well in a nonpolar solvent; can be classified as saturated or unsaturated. (2, 14)

lobes. The regions of the brain; include the frontal, parietal, occipital, and temporal lobes. (7)

lower extremity. The hips, legs, and feet. (5)

lumbar region. Five vertebrae comprising the low back region of the spine. (5)

lumen. The hollow, inner portion of a body cavity or tube. (3)

luteinizing hormone (LH). A tropic hormone produced by the anterior pituitary that signals the egg's release from the follicle, stimulates the production of progesterone and small amounts of estrogen in women, and stimulates the interstitial cells of the testes to produce testosterone in men. (16)

lymph. A clear, transparent, sometimes faintly yellow fluid that is collected from tissues throughout the body and flows in the lymphatic vessels. (13)

lymph nodes. Small, bean-shaped structures found along the lymphatic vessels throughout the body. (13)
lymphatic nodules. Small, localized clusters of dense tissue formed by lymphocytes and macrophages. (13)
lymphatic trunks. Large lymphatic vessels that drain lymph from different parts of the body. (13)
lymphatic valves. Tissue flaps that act as one-way gates inside the lymphatic vessels. (13)
lymphatic vessels. The vessels that carry lymph. (13)
lymphedema. A buildup of extracellular fluid in the body because of disruption in lymphatic drainage. (13)
lymphocytes. The distinctive cells of the lymphatic system. (13)
lymphoma. Cancer that originates in lymph nodes and other lymphatic tissues. (3)

M

macronutrients. Substances such as carbohydrates, proteins, and fats that the body requires in relatively large quantities. (14)
macrophages. Cells that engulf and destroy foreign cells, such as bacteria and viruses. (13)
major histocompatibility complex glycoproteins (MHCs). Proteins found on the surfaces of lymphocytes and other cells; help the immune system recognize foreign antigens and ignore "self" tissues. (13)
malignant melanoma. Cancer of the melanocytes; the most serious form of skin cancer. (4)
malleus. A tiny bone in the middle ear that transmits sound from the tympanic membrane (eardrum) to the anvil; sometimes called the *hammer* because of its shape. (8)
mammary glands. The milk-producing glands in the female. (16)
mandible. Jaw bone. (5)
Marfan syndrome. An inherited connective tissue disease that causes skeletal, ocular, and cardiovascular symptoms. (3)
mass. The quantity of matter contained in an object. (1)
mast cells. Connective tissue cells that contain stores of histamine. (13)
maxillary bones. Two fused bones that form the upper jaw, house the upper teeth, and connect to all other bones of the face, with the exception of the mandible. (5)
mechanical breakdown. The breakdown of food into smaller pieces, thus increasing its surface area. (14)
mechanoreceptors. Chemical receptor cells that detect muscle contraction and force generation during exercise; they quickly increase respiration rates when exercise begins (10); receptors that are sensitive to mechanical stretch in tissues. (10, 12)
medial rotation. Inward movement of a body segment in the transverse plane. (6)
median sacral crest. Prominent elevation formed by the fused spinous processes of the upper four sacral vertebrae. (5)
mediastinum. The anatomical region between the sternum and the vertebral column, and between the lungs; houses the heart, great blood vessels, trachea, esophagus, thoracic duct, thymus gland, and other structures. (10, 12)
medulla oblongata. The lower portion of the brain stem, which regulates heart rate, blood pressure, and breathing, and controls several reflexes. (7)
medullary cavity. Central hollow area found in long bones. (5)
meiosis. A type of cell division that produces daughter cells with half the chromosomes of the parent cell; produces eggs in females and sperm in males. (16)
melanin. A pigment that protects the body against the harmful effects of ultraviolet rays from the sun. (4)
melanocytes. Specialized cells in the skin that produce melanin. (4)
membrane. Thin sheet or layer of pliable tissue. (4)
membranous labyrinth. Term that describes the membrane-covered tubes located inside the bony labyrinth. (8)
memory cells. B cells and T cells in lymphatic tissues that respond if a previously encountered antigen invades the body again. (13)
menarche. The first menstrual bleeding. (16)
meninges. The three protective membranes that surround the brain and spinal cord. (7)
meningitis. An infection-induced inflammation of the meninges surrounding the brain and spinal cord. (7)
Merkel cells. Touch receptors in the skin; also known as *Merkel-Ranvier cells*. (4)
mesenchymal cells. Stromal cells that can develop into tissues of the circulatory and lymphatic systems as well as connective tissues. (11)
mesoderm. The middle layer of an embryo in early development. (3)
messenger RNA (mRNA). A single-strand RNA molecule whose base sequence carries the information needed by a ribosome to make a protein. (2)
metabolic rate. The speed at which the body consumes energy. (1)
metabolism. All of the chemical reactions that occur within an organism to maintain life. (1, 14)
metacarpal bones. The five interior bones of the hand that connect the carpals in the wrist to the phalanges in the fingers. (5)
metastasis. The spreading of cancerous cells from their original location to another part of the body. (13)
metatarsal bones. The small bones of the ankle. (5)
metric system. International system of measurement that is used in all fields of science. (1)
micronutrients. Substances such as vitamins and minerals that are essential to the body in small amounts. (14)

microvilli. Finger-like extensions that increase the surface area of a cell. (2)
micturition. Urination. (15)
midbrain. The relay station for sensory and motor impulses; located on the superior end of the brain stem. (7)
middle ear cavities. Openings in the skull that serve as chambers for transmitting and amplifying sound. (1)
minerals. Elements that the body needs in relatively small amounts. (14)
mitochondria. Organelles in the cytoplasm that make ATP. (2)
mitosis. The division of a cell nucleus and chromosomes into two nuclei, each with its own set of identical chromosomes. (2)
mitral valve. The atrioventricular valve that closes the orifice between the left atrium and left ventricle of the heart; also known as the *bicuspid valve*. (12)
mitral valve prolapse. An incomplete closing of the mitral valve, which causes blood to flow backward into the left atrium when the left ventricle contracts. (12)
molecule. A group of two or more atoms bonded together. (1, 2)
monocytes. Leukocytes that develop into phagocytizing macrophages when they migrate out of lymphatic circulation into surrounding tissue. (13)
monounsaturated fats. One category of unsaturated fatty acids; sources include canola oil and olive oil. (14)
motor neuron. A nerve that stimulates skeletal muscle tissue. (6)
motor unit. A single motor neuron and all of the muscle fibers that it stimulates. (6)
mucosa-associated lymphatic tissue (MALT). Lymphatic tissue found in mucous membranes that line passageways open to the outside world. (13)
mucous membranes. Thin sheets of tissue lining the body cavities that open to the outside world. (4)
multiple myeloma. A cancer of the plasma cells in bone marrow. (11)
multiple sclerosis (MS). A chronic, slowly progressive disease of the central nervous system that destroys the myelin sheath of nerve cell axons. (7)
muscle cramps. Moderate to severe muscle spasms that cause pain. (6)
muscle fiber. An individual skeletal muscle cell. (6)
muscle strain. An injury that occurs when a muscle is stretched beyond the limits to which it is accustomed. (6)
muscle tissue. A type of tissue that generates force and allows the body to move. (3)
muscular dystrophy (MD). A group of similar, inherited disorders characterized by progressively worsening muscle weakness and loss of muscle tissue. (6)
myelin sheath. The fatty band of insulation surrounding an axon fiber. (7)
myocardial infarction (MI). A condition characterized by blockage of a coronary artery; also known as a *heart attack*. (12)
myocarditis. Inflammation of the middle layer of the heart, or myocardium. (12)
myocardium. The middle layer of the heart, which makes up about 95% of the heart. (12)
myositis ossificans. A condition in which a calcium mass forms within a muscle three to four weeks after a muscle injury. (6)
myxedema. A severe form of hypothyroidism that occurs when hypothyroidism goes undiagnosed or untreated. (9)

N

nares. The two openings in the nose through which air enters; also known as *nostrils*. (10)
nasal cavity. Opening within and behind the nose. (1)
nasal conchae. Three uneven, scroll-like nasal bones that extend down through the nasal cavity. (10)
nasopharyngitis. Inflammation of the nasal passages and pharynx. (10)
natural killer (NK) cells. Lymphocytes that play an important role in the nonspecific defense system by killing virus-infected cells and cancer cells. (13)
negative feedback. A mechanism that restores homeostasis by reversing a condition that has exceeded the normal homeostatic range. (1)
neonatal hypothyroidism. A form of hypothyroidism that occurs in infants and children; may develop congenitally or soon after birth. (9)
nephron. The fundamental excretory unit of the kidney. (15)
nephron loop. The U-shaped part of the nephron that is located between the proximal convoluted tubule and the distal convoluted tubule; has a descending limb and ascending limb; also known as the *loop of Henle*. (15)
nerve tissue. A type of tissue that conveys information through electric signals. (3)
net force. The single force resulting from the summation of all forces acting on a structure at a given time. (1)
neural control. The type of endocrine control in which nerve fibers stimulate endocrine organs to release hormones. (9)
neurilemma. The thin, membranous sheath enveloping a nerve fiber. (7)
neuroglia. Cells that form the interstitial or supporting elements of the CNS; also known as *glial cells*. (7)
neuromuscular junction. The link between an axon terminal and a muscle fiber. (6)
neuron. Specialized nerve cell that transmits information throughout the body in the form of electrical impulses. (3, 7)
neurotransmitter. Chemical used to pass along a message by carrying a signal from an axon to a receptor cell. (7)
neutron. A fundamental particle that has no electric charge. (2)

neutrophil. The most common type of white blood cell; can slip out of capillaries and into surrounding tissue to destroy bacteria and cellular debris. (13)

nodes of Ranvier. The uninsulated gaps in the myelin sheath of a nerve fiber, where the axon is exposed. (7)

norepinephrine. A neurotransmitter that is released by postganglionic neurons in the sympathetic nervous system and plays a role in triggering the fight-or-flight response. (7)

nucleic acids. Key information-carrying molecules in cells. (2)

nucleotides. Subunits that make up nucleic acids. (2)

nucleus. A rounded or oval mass of protoplasm within the cytoplasm of a cell that contains the cell's DNA and is bounded by a membrane. (2)

nutrients. Chemicals that the body needs for energy, growth, and maintenance. (14)

O

occipital lobes. The regions of the brain located behind the parietal lobes; responsible for vision. (7)

olfactory bulb. The thickened end of the olfactory nerve, which sends sensory impulses to the olfactory region of the brain. (8)

olfactory hairs. Tiny threads that extend from the olfactory receptor cells into the nasal cavity. (8)

olfactory nerve. A cranial nerve that sends impulses to the olfactory cortex of the brain. (8)

olfactory receptors. Sensory cells in the olfactory region that provide the sense of smell. (8, 10)

olfactory region. A dime-sized area found on top of each nasal cavity that houses the olfactory receptor cells. (8)

oocyte. An egg cell. (16)

oogenesis. The process by which oocytes are generated. (16)

opportunistic infection. An infection that rarely occurs in people with a healthy immune system but may occur in a person with a damaged immune system, such as someone with AIDS. (13)

opposition. The act of touching any of your four fingers to your thumb; this movement enables grasping of objects. (6)

opsonins. Proteins that make cells more attractive to phagocytes. (13)

optic chiasma. The point at which the optic nerves cross. (8)

optic nerve. The transmitter of visual sensory signals to the occipital lobe of the brain. (8)

optic tracts. The portion of the optic nerve fibers that extend beyond the optic chiasma. (8)

oral cavity. Opening within the mouth. (1)

orbital cavities. Openings that hold the eyes. (1)

organ. A body part organized to perform a specific function. (1)

organ of Corti. A spiral-shaped ridge of epithelium in the cochlear duct, which is lined with hair cells that serve as hearing receptors. (8)

organ system. Two or more organs working together to perform specific functions. (1)

origin. The site of a muscle's attachment to a relatively fixed structure. (6)

osmosis. The movement of water molecules from a region of low osmotic pressure to a region of high osmotic pressure. (15)

osmotic diuresis. An increase in urine production caused by high osmotic pressure of the glomerular filtrate, which "pulls" more water into the filtrate. (15)

osmotic pressure. The pressure created by the presence of dissolved substances in water. (15)

osseous tissue. Bone tissue. (3)

ossicles. The body's three smallest bones—the hammer, anvil, and stirrup; found in the middle ear. (8)

ossification. Process of bone formation. (5)

osteoarthritis. Degenerative disease of the articular cartilage; characterized by pain, swelling, range-of-motion restriction, and stiffness. (5)

osteoblasts. Specialized bone cells that build new bone tissue. (5)

osteoclasts. Specialized bone cells that resorb bone tissue. (5)

osteocytes. Mature bone cells. (5)

osteon. A Haversian system. (5)

osteopenia. Condition characterized by reduced bone mass without the presence of a fracture. (5)

osteoporosis. Condition in which bone mineralization and strength are so abnormally low that regular, daily activities can result in painful fractures. (5)

oval window. A membrane-covered opening that connects the middle ear to the inner ear. (8)

ovarian cycle. The sequence of events associated with maturation and release of an oocyte. (16)

ovaries. The female sex glands. (9)

ovulation. The release of an oocyte from the ovarian follicle. (16)

oxytocin. Hormone that stimulates uterine contractions during labor and milk secretion during breast-feeding. (16)

P

palate. A structure that consists of hard and soft components and separates the oral and nasal cavities. (10)

palatine tonsils. Two masses of lymphatic tissue that lie at the back of the mouth, on the left and right sides; the largest and most commonly infected tonsils. (13)

palpitations. Sensations of a rapid heartbeat. (12)

pancreas. A long, thin organ located posterior to the stomach; secretes insulin and glucagon as an endocrine gland; secretes digestive enzymes as an exocrine gland. (9)

pancreatitis. Inflammation of the pancreas. (14)
papillae. Tiny bumps on the tongue that house taste buds. (8)
papillary layer. The outer layer of the dermis. (4)
papillary muscle. One of the small muscular bundles attached at one end to the chordae tendineae and to the endocardial wall of the ventricles at the other; maintains tension on the chordae tendineae as the ventricle contracts. (12)
parallel fiber architecture. A muscle fiber arrangement in which fibers run mostly parallel to each other along the length of the muscle. (6)
paraplegia. A disorder characterized by loss of function in the lower trunk and legs. (7)
parathyroid glands. Four tiny glands that are located on the posterior aspect of the thyroid gland and secrete parathyroid hormone in response to low blood calcium levels. (9)
paravertebral ganglia. Mass of nerve cell bodies that lie parallel to the spinal cord. (7)
parietal lobes. The regions of the brain located behind the frontal lobes; integrate sensory information from the skin, internal organs, muscles, and joints. (7)
parietal pericardium. The parietal layer of the serous pericardium; secretes the serous fluid found in the pericardial cavity. (12)
Parkinson's disease. A chronic nervous system disease characterized by a slowly spreading tremor, muscular weakness, and rigidity. (7)
partial pressure. The individual pressure of a gas in a mixture of gases. (10)
passive immunity. A form of immunity that comes from antibodies received from an outside source, such as breast milk. (2, 13)
passive transport. Movement across a cell membrane that does not require energy because the substance is moving from an area of greater concentration to one of lower concentration. (2)
patella. Kneecap. (5)
pathogens. Disease-causing agents. (13)
pectoral girdle. The bones surrounding the shoulder, including the clavicle and scapula. (5)
pelvic cavity. Internal opening that holds the reproductive and excretory organs. (1)
pelvis. Collective term for the bones of the pelvic girdle and the coccyx at the base of the spine. (5)
penis. The reproductive organ that delivers sperm to the female reproductive tract. (16)
pennate fiber architecture. A muscle fiber arrangement in which each fiber attaches obliquely to a central tendon. (6)
peptic ulcer. A break in the lining of the stomach, duodenum, or lower esophagus. (14)
peptide bond. The chemical bond that links two amino acids by connecting the amino group of one to the acid group of another. (2)
perforating (Volkmann's) canals. Large canals that connect the Haversian canals; oriented across bones and perpendicular to Haversian canals. (5)
pericarditis. Inflammation of the pericardial sac that surrounds the heart. (12)
pericardium. The membrane that surrounds the heart. (4)
perilymph. A clear fluid that fills the bony labyrinth. (8)
perimysium. A connective tissue sheath that envelops each primary bundle of muscle fibers. (6)
perineurium. A protective sheath that surrounds a bundle of nerve fibers, or fascicle. (7)
periodontal disease. A disease that affects the supporting structure of the teeth and the gums. (14)
periosteum. Fibrous connective tissue membrane that surrounds and protects the shaft (diaphysis) of long bones. (5)
peripheral nervous system (PNS). The division of the nervous system that contains all parts of the nervous system external to the brain and spinal cord. (7)
peripheral neuropathy. A disease or degenerative state of the peripheral nerves often associated with diabetes mellitus; marked by muscle weakness and atrophy, pain, and numbness. (9)
peripheral vascular disease (PVD). A condition characterized by a narrowing of the arteries in the legs. (12)
peritoneal dialysis. A procedure for removing metabolic waste products from the body; the patient's peritoneum is used to filter fluids and dissolved substances from the blood. (15)
peritoneum. The membrane that lines the abdominal cavity. (4)
peritonitis. Inflammation of the peritoneum. (4)
pernicious anemia. A severe anemia caused by the inability of the intestines to absorb vitamin B_{12}, which is essential for the formation of red blood cells; usually develops in older adults. (11)
pH. A measure of the acidity of a solution. (2)
phagocytes. Cells that engulf and consume bacteria, foreign material, and cellular debris. (13)
phagocytosis. The process by which macrophages in the liver and spleen envelop, digest, and recycle old RBCs and other types of cells. (11, 13)
phalanges. Bones of the fingers. (5)
pharyngeal tonsil. Lymphatic tissue that lies at the back of the nasopharynx; commonly known as the *adenoid* or *adenoids*. (13)
pharyngitis. Inflammation of the pharynx, or throat. (10)
pharynx. The muscular passageway that extends from the nasal cavity to the mouth and connects to the esophagus. (10)
phlebotomy. The drawing of blood; a standard treatment for polycythemia. (11)
phospholipids. Lipids that contain phosphate groups. (2)
physiology. The study of how living things function or work. (1)

pineal gland. A pinecone-shaped gland that is located in the brain and releases the sleep-inducing hormone melatonin. (9)
pituitary gland. A pea-sized gland that activates a metabolic response in target tissues and stimulates other endocrine glands to release hormones. (9)
pivot joint. A type of diarthrosis that permits rotation around only one axis. (5)
placenta. The organ that grows in the uterus to meet the nutritional needs of the embryo and fetus. (16)
plantar flexion. Downward movement of the foot away from the lower leg. (6)
plantar warts. Warts that develop on the soles of the foot, grow inward, and can become painful. (4)
plasma. The liquid component of blood. (11)
plasma membrane. The membrane that defines the outer boundary of a cell. (2)
plastic. A response in which a structure retains some permanent deformation after a force is applied. (1)
platelet plug. A gathering of platelets that forms a small mass at the site of an injury. (11)
platelets. Cell fragments that play a vital role in blood clotting; also known as *thrombocytes*. (11)
pleura. The membrane that encases the lungs. (4)
pleural sac. The thin, double-walled serous membrane that surrounds the lungs. (10)
pleurisy. Inflammation of the pleura. (4)
plexuses. Complex interconnections of nerves. (7)
pneumonia. An infection of the lungs that causes inflammation; caused by a virus, bacterium, fungus, or—in rare cases—parasite. (10)
polarized. A condition in which the inside of a cell membrane is more negatively charged than the outside. (7)
polycythemia. A condition in which the bone marrow manufactures too many red blood cells; caused by prolonged altitude exposure and a genetic mutation. (11)
polymer. A molecule made of many similar subunits. (2)
polypeptide. A long chain of amino acids. (2)
polyunsaturated fats. One category of unsaturated fatty acids; sources include corn oil and soybean oil. (14)
pons. The section of the brain stem that plays a role in regulating breathing. (7)
pores of Kohn. Small openings in the alveolar walls that allow gases and macrophages to travel between the alveoli. (10)
positive feedback. A mechanism that restores homeostasis by further increasing a condition that has exceeded the normal homeostatic range. (1)
posterior (dorsal) cavity. Continuous internal opening located near the back of the body that includes the cranial and spinal cavities. (1)
posterior pituitary. The posterior lobe of the pituitary gland, which stores two hormones produced by the hypothalamus: antidiuretic hormone and oxytocin. (9)
postganglionic neuron. The second neuron in a series that transmits impulses from the CNS. (7)
precapillary sphincter. A band of smooth muscle fibers that encircles each capillary at the arteriole-capillary junction and controls blood flow to the tissues. (12)
precipitation. The formation of an insoluble complex, such as a clump of antigen molecules joined together by antibodies. (13)
preganglionic neuron. The first neuron in a series that transmits impulses from the CNS. (7)
premature atrial contractions (PACs). A condition in which an irritable piece of atrial heart tissue fires before the SA node, causing the atria to contract too soon. (12)
premature ventricular contractions (PVCs). A condition in which Purkinje fibers fire before the SA node, causing the ventricles to contract prematurely. (12)
pressure. The force distributed over a given area. (1)
primary bronchi. The two passageways that branch off the trachea and lead to the right and left lungs. (10)
primary immune response. The initial immune response to a foreign invader such as a virus or bacterium. (13)
primary motor cortex. The outer region of the brain in the frontal lobes that sends neural impulses to the skeletal muscles. (7)
primary somatic sensory cortex. The outer region of the brain in the parietal lobes that interprets sensory impulses received from the skin, internal organs, muscles, and joints. (7)
prolactin. A hormone that stimulates the secretory cells of the mammary glands to produce milk. (16)
pronation. Medial rotation of the forearm (palm down). (6)
propulsion. The movement of food through the GI tract; stimulated by swallowing at the pharynx and peristalsis, muscular contractions that move food through the rest of the GI tract. (14)
prostaglandins. Fatty acids involved in the control of inflammation and body temperature. (13)
prostate gland. The gland that sits directly under the bladder and surrounds the beginning of the urethra in the male; produces about one-third of the fluid volume of semen. (16)
prothrombin. A protein in the blood that is activated to form thrombin during clot formation. (11)
prothrombin activator (PTA). A protein that activates the protein fibrinogen. (11)
proton. A positively charged fundamental particle. (2)
proximal convoluted tubule (PCT). The part of the nephron between the glomerular capsule and the nephron loop; minerals, nutrients, and water are reabsorbed from the filtrate here. (15)
psoriasis. A common skin disorder that involves redness, irritation, and scales (flaky, silver-white patches) that itch, burn, crack, and sometimes bleed. (4)
pulmonary circulation. The circulation of oxygen-poor blood from the right ventricle and through the lungs, returning to the left atrium with oxygen-rich blood. (12)
pulmonary valve. The semilunar valve that lies between the right atrium and the pulmonary trunk. (12)

pulmonary ventilation. The process by which air is continuously moved in and out of the lungs. (10)
pupil. The opening through which light rays enter the eye. (8)
Purkinje fibers. Special fibers that rapidly transmit impulses throughout the ventricles, causing ventricular contraction. (12)
pyrogens. Chemicals that cause fever by increasing the set-point temperature of hypothalamic neurons. (13)

Q

quadriplegia. A disorder characterized by loss of function below the neck. (7)

R

radial artery. The artery located on the thumb side of the wrist; where the radial pulse is detected. (12)
radius. The smaller of the two bones in the forearm; rotates around the ulna. (5)
reabsorption. The movement of water and dissolved substances into the blood from the filtrate in a renal tubule. (15)
receptor. A transmitter that senses environmental changes. (1)
rectum. The short, final segment of the GI tract whose lower end is the anal canal. (14)
rectus sheath. Connective tissue that encases the *rectus abdominis* muscles. (6)
red blood cells (RBCs). Blood cells that contain hemoglobin, a protein responsible for oxygen and carbon dioxide transport; also known as *erythrocytes*. (11)
reflexes. Simple, rapid, involuntary, programmed responses to stimuli. (7)
refractory period. The time between the completion of the action potential and repolarization. (7)
remodeling. Process through which adult bone can change in density, strength, and sometimes shape. (5)
renal corpuscle. The part of a nephron that consists of a glomerulus and its surrounding glomerular capsule. (15)
renal cortex. The lighter-colored, outer layer of the kidney that contains the glomeruli and convoluted tubules. (15)
renal dialysis. The removal of wastes from the blood by artificial means. (15)
renal medulla. The darker, innermost part of the kidney. (15)
renal pelvis. A hollow, funnel-shaped cavity in the center of the kidney where urine collects before it flows into the ureter. (15)
renal tubule. The part of a nephron that leads away from a glomerulus and empties into a collecting tubule; consists of a proximal convoluted tubule, nephron loop, and distal convoluted tubule. (15)
renin. An enzyme made and secreted by the kidneys; aids in the production of angiotensin. (15)
repolarization. The reestablishment of a polarized state in a cell after depolarization. (7)
repolarize. To restore the original electrical polarity of cells that have been depolarized to their normal resting polarity, causing the heart muscle to relax. (12)
research question. The question to be answered or problem to be solved in a research study. (1)
residual volume (RV). The volume of air that never leaves the lungs, even after the most forceful expiration. (10)
respiration. Breathing; the process by which the lungs provide oxygen to body tissues and dispose of carbon dioxide. (10)
respiratory gas transport. The process by which oxygen and carbon dioxide are transported to and from the lungs and tissues. (10)
reticular layer. The inner layer of the dermis; includes blood and lymphatic vessels, sweat and oil glands, involuntary muscles, hair follicles, and nerve endings. (4)
retina. The innermost layer of the eye, which contains light-sensitive nerve endings that send impulses through the optic nerves to the brain. (8)
Rh factor. The antigen of the Rh blood group that is found on the surface of red blood cells; people with the Rh factor are Rh^+ and those lacking it are Rh^-. (11)
rheumatoid arthritis. Autoimmune disorder in which the body's own immune system attacks healthy joint tissues; the most debilitating and painful form of arthritis. (5)
RhoGAM. An immune serum that prevents an Rh^- pregnant woman's blood from becoming sensitized to her Rh^+ fetus. (11)
ribonucleic acid (RNA). A polymer of nucleotides with the bases adenine, guanine, cytosine, and uracil. (2)
ribosomes. Very large enzymes that make polypeptides. (2)
RNA. See *ribonucleic acid (RNA)*. (2)
RNA polymerase. The enzyme that makes an RNA molecule complementary to a gene on DNA. (2)
rods. Sensory cells in the retina that are activated in dim light. (8)
rotator cuff. The four muscles that attach the humerus to the scapula and their tendons. (6)
rule of nines. A method used to calculate body surface area affected by burns. (4)

S

sacral canal. Continuation of the vertebral canal in the sacral region. (5)
sacral hiatus. Prominent opening at the inferior end of the sacral canal. (5)
sacrum. Collective term for five fused vertebrae that form the posterior of the pelvic girdle. (5)

saddle joint. A type of diarthrosis in which the articulating bone surfaces are both shaped like the seat of a riding saddle. (5)
sagittal plane. An imaginary, vertical flat surface that divides the body into right and left halves. (1)
saltatory conduction. The process in which an action potential rapidly skips from node to node on myelinated neurons. (7)
sarcolemma. The delicate membrane that surrounds each striated muscle fiber. (6)
sarcoma. Cancer that originates in connective tissue. (3)
sarcomeres. Units composed of actin and myosin that contract inside the muscle fiber. (6)
scapula. Shoulder blade. (5)
science. A systematic process that creates new knowledge and organizes it into a form of testable explanations and predictions about an aspect of our universe. (1)
scientific method. A systematic process that can be used to answer questions or find solutions to problems. (1)
scientific theory. An explanation of some aspect of the natural world that is based on rigorously tested, repeatedly confirmed research. (1)
sclera. The tough, fibrous outer layer of the eye. (8)
scrotum. A sac that encases the testes. (9)
sebaceous glands. Glands that produce sebum and are located all over the body. (4)
sebum. An oily substance that helps to keep the skin and hair soft. (4)
secondary immune response. The response of the immune system to an infectious agent that it has encountered before. (13)
second-degree burns. Burns that involve damage to both the epidermis and the upper portion of the underlying dermis; characterized by blisters. (4)
secretion. The active movement of substances from the blood into the filtrate, which will become urine. (15)
semen. The fluid that contains sperm, which is delivered to the female during intercourse; also known as *penile ejaculate*. (16)
semicircular canals. Channels located in the inner ear, which contain hair cells that play an important role in balance. (8)
semilunar valves. The valves situated at the opening between the heart and the aorta, and at the opening between the heart and the pulmonary artery; prevent backflow of blood into the ventricles. (12)
seminal glands. The glands that produce up to 70% of the volume of semen; also known as *seminal vesicles*. (16)
seminiferous tubules. Small tubes in the testes in which sperm form. (16)
septum. The structure made of cartilage that divides the nose into left and right air passages. (8)
serous fluid. A thin, clear liquid that serves as a lubricant between parietal and visceral membranes. (4)
serous membranes. Thin sheets of tissue that line body cavities that are closed to the outside world. (4)
serous pericardium. The inner wall of the pericardium; divided into the parietal layer (parietal pericardium) and the visceral layer (epicardium). (12)
sexually transmitted infection. An infectious disease transmitted through sexual contact. (16)
Sharpey's fibers. Tiny connective tissue fibers that join together to firmly bind the periosteum to the underlying cortical bone. (5)
shear. A force that acts along a surface and perpendicular to the length of a structure. (1)
shin splint. Pain that is localized to the anterior lower leg. (6)
shoulder complex. All of the joints surrounding the shoulder, including the acromioclavicular, sternoclavicular, and glenohumeral joints. (5)
sickle cell anemia. A disease in which the red blood cells are shaped like a sickle, or crescent, rather than a disc; caused by irregularly shaped hemoglobin molecules in the red blood cells. (11)
simple epithelia. Epithelia that have a single layer of cells. (3)
sinoatrial node (SA node). A small mass of specialized tissue located in the right atrium that normally acts as the pacemaker of the heart, causing it to beat at a rate between 60 and 100 bpm. (12)
sinuses. The air-filled cavities that surround the nose. (10)
sinusitis. Inflammation of the sinuses. (10)
skeletal muscle. The most common type of muscle tissue; usually attached to bone and helps the body move. (3)
skull. The part of the skeleton composed of all of the bones of the head. (5)
slow-twitch. Type of muscle that contracts slowly and is resistant to fatigue. (6)
small intestine. The portion of the GI tract where most of the chemical breakdown of food, food absorption, and water absorption occurs; the longest segment of the GI tract. (14)
smooth muscle. The muscle tissue found in the walls of hollow organs. (3)
somatic nervous system. The branch of the nervous system that stimulates the skeletal muscles. (7)
somatic reflexes. Involuntary stimuli transmitted to skeletal muscles from neural arcs in the spinal cord. (7)
sperm (singular or plural). The male gamete; a haploid cell that can fertilize an egg to make a zygote. (16)
spinal cavity. The internal opening that houses the spinal cord. (1)
spinal cord. A column of nerve tissue that extends from the brain stem to the beginning of the lumbar region of the spine. (7)
spinal nerves. Thirty-one pairs of nerves that branch from the left and right sides of the spinal cord. (7)
spleen. The largest lymphatic organ in the body, located in the abdomen below the diaphragm; filters blood and activates an immune response when necessary. (13)

sprain. Injury caused by abnormal motion of the articulating bones that results in overstretching or tearing of ligaments, tendons, or other connective tissues crossing a joint. (5)

squamous cell carcinoma. A type of rapidly growing cancer that appears as a scaly, reddened patch of skin. (4)

stapes. A tiny bone in the middle ear that attaches to the anvil on one side and the oval window on the other; sometimes called the *stirrup* because of its shape. (8)

statistical inference. The practice of generalizing the findings of a research study to a large population. (1)

statistical significance. An interpretation of statistical data indicating that the results of a study can legitimately be generalized to the population represented in the study sample. (1)

sternum. Breastbone. (5)

steroid hormones. Lipid (fat-based) hormones. (9)

steroids. Lipids with a structure that is different from other lipids; includes cholesterol, testosterone, and estrogen, among others. (2)

stomach. The reservoir in which food is broken down mechanically and chemically before it enters the small intestine. (14)

stratified epithelia. Epithelia that have multiple layers of cells. (3)

stratum basale. The deepest layer of the epidermis. (4)

stratum corneum. The outer layer of the epidermis. (4)

stratum granulosum. The layer of somewhat flattened cells just superficial to the stratum spinosum and inferior to the stratum lucidum. (4)

stratum lucidum. The clear layer of thick skin found only on the palms of the hands, the fingers, the soles of the feet, and the toes. (4)

stratum spinosum. The layer of cells in the epidermis superior to the stratum basale and inferior to the stratum granulosum. (4)

stress. The force distribution inside a structure. (1)

stroke volume. The volume of blood pumped from the heart per beat. (12)

sudoriferous glands. Sweat glands that are distributed in the dermis over the entire body. (4)

superior vena cava. The second largest vein in the body, which returns deoxygenated blood to the right atrium of the heart from the upper half of the body. (12)

supination. Lateral rotation of the forearm (palm up). (6)

surfactant. A phospholipid that reduces surface tension in the alveoli and prevents them from collapsing. (10)

suspensory ligaments. Tiny structures that attach the lens of the eye to the ciliary body. (8)

sutures. Joints in which irregularly grooved, articulating bone sheets join closely and are tightly connected by fibrous tissues. (5)

symphysis. A type of amphiarthrosis in which a thin plate of hyaline cartilage separates a disc of fibrocartilage from the bones. (5)

synapse. The intersection between two neurons, or between a neuron and a muscle, gland, or sensory receptor. (7)

synaptic cleft. The microscopic gap that separates the axon terminal of a neuron from the muscle fiber. (6, 7)

synarthrosis. A fibrous joint that can absorb shock, but which permits little or no movement of the articulating bones. (5)

synchondrosis. A type of amphiarthrosis joint in which the articulating bones are held together by a thin layer of hyaline cartilage. (5)

syndesmosis. A type of synarthrosis joint at which dense, fibrous tissue binds the bones together, permitting extremely limited movement. (5)

synovial fluid. A clear liquid secreted by synovial membranes that provides cushioning for and reduces friction in synovial joints. (4)

synovial joint. A diarthrodial joint. (5)

synovial membrane. Thin sheet of tissue that lines the synovial joint cavity and produces synovial fluid. (4)

syphilis. A highly treatable bacterial infection; if untreated, can cause significant health problems, disability, and death due to its cardiovascular and neurological complications. (16)

systemic circulation. The circulation of oxygenated blood from the left ventricle, through the arteries, capillaries, and veins of the circulatory system, returning to the right atrium. (12)

systemic lupus erythematosus. An autoimmune disease in which the immune system attacks the body's own connective tissue; also known as *lupus* or *SLE*. (3)

systole. A period of contraction when the chambers pump blood out of the heart. (12)

T

tachycardia. A normal heart rhythm but with a rate above 100 bpm. (12)

tarsal bones. Bones of the ankle. (5)

tarsal glands. The glands that are located in the eyelids and secrete an oily substance. (8)

tastants. Compounds that stimulate the gustatory hairs to send nerve impulses to the brain. (8)

taste buds. The sensory receptors for taste. (8)

taste pores. Very small openings in the top of the taste buds through which gustatory hairs project. (8)

temporal lobes. The most inferior portions of the brain; responsible for speech, hearing, vision, memory, and emotion. (7)

tendinitis. Inflammation of a tendon; usually accompanied by pain and swelling. (6)

tendinosis. Degeneration of a tendon believed to be caused by microtears in the tendon's connective tissue. (6)

tendon. A band of collagen and elastic fibers that connects a muscle to a bone. (5)

tendon sheaths. Double-layered synovial structures surrounding tendons that are subject to friction because they are located so close to bones; secrete synovial fluid to promote free motion of the tendons during joint movement. (5)

tensile strength. The ability of a material to withstand tension (outward-pulling force) without tearing or breaking. (3)

tension. A pulling force on a structure. (1)

testes. The male sex glands. (9)

tetanus. A condition in which muscles are in a state of tetany, or sustained muscular contraction; a sustained, maximal level of muscle tension that occurs with high-frequency stimulation. (6)

thalamus. The largest portion of the diencephalon; communicates sensory and motor information between the body and the cerebral cortex. (7)

thalassemia. A condition that limits the body's ability to produce fully developed hemoglobin and red blood cells; also known as *Cooley's anemia.* (11)

third-degree burns. Burns that destroy the entire thickness of the skin. (4)

thoracic cage. The bony structure surrounding the heart and lungs in the thoracic cavity; composed of the ribs, sternum, and thoracic vertebrae. (5)

thoracic cavity. The internal opening that houses the heart and lungs. (1)

thoracic region. The 12 vertebrae located in the middle of the back. (5)

thoracolumbar division. The sympathetic system; includes nerves that originate from the thoracic and lumbar regions of the spine. (7)

thrombocytes. Platelets. (11)

thrombus. A clot that forms in an intact blood vessel, usually a vein. (11)

thymus. An organ that secretes thymosin; functions as both an endocrine gland and a lymphatic organ. (9)

thyroid cartilage. The largest cartilaginous plate in the larynx; commonly known as the *Adam's apple.* (10)

thyroid gland. A gland that is located below the larynx and secretes thyroid hormones (T_3 and T_4) and calcitonin. (9)

thyroiditis. Inflammation of the thyroid gland. (9)

tibia. The major weight-bearing bone of the lower leg. (5)

tidal volume (TV). The amount of air inhaled in a normal breath. (10)

tinea. A fungal infection that tends to occur in areas of the body that are moist. (4)

tissues. Organized groups of similar cells. (1)

T lymphocytes (T cells). Lymphatic cells that complete their maturation in the thymus before they move out to the blood and the rest of the body. (13)

tolerance. A reduction or elimination of the allergic response, which may occur after immunotherapy. (13)

tonsillitis. Inflammation of the tonsils. (10)

tonsils. Clusters of lymphatic tissue located in the pharynx that function as the respiratory system's first line of defense against infection. (10)

torque. The rotary effect of a force. (1)

torsion. A loading pattern that can cause a structure to twist about its length. (1)

total lung capacity (TLC). A combination of the vital capacity and the residual volume; VC + RV. (10)

trabecular bone. Interior, spongy bone with a porous, honeycomb structure. (5)

trachea. The air tube that extends from the larynx into the thorax, where it splits into the right and left bronchi; commonly known as the *windpipe.* (10)

transcription. The production of RNA from DNA. (2)

transfer RNA (tRNA). A molecule that binds to the mRNA-ribosome complex and helps assemble amino acids into polypeptides. (2)

transient ischemic attack (TIA). A temporary lack of blood flow to the brain. (12)

trans-unsaturated fats. One category of unsaturated fatty acids; artificially produced; also called *trans fats.* (14)

transverse plane. An imaginary, horizontal flat surface that divides the body into top and bottom halves. (1)

traumatic brain injury. Mild or severe trauma that can result from a violent impact to the head. (7)

tricuspid valve. The atrioventricular valve that closes the orifice between the right atrium and right ventricle of the heart; composed of three cusps. (12)

triglycerides. Compounds composed of a glycerol molecule with three fatty acids attached. (2)

trigone. The triangular region of the bladder formed by the two ureteric orifices and the internal urethral orifice. (15)

tropic hormones. Pituitary hormones that act on other endocrine glands; also known as *tropins.* (9)

true pelvis. The region of the pelvis immediately surrounding the pelvic inlet. (5)

tuberculosis (TB). A highly contagious bacterial infection caused by *Mycobacterium tuberculosis.* (10)

tunica externa. The outermost layer of a blood vessel, composed mostly of fibrous connective tissue that supports and protects the vessel. (12)

tunica intima. The innermost layer of a blood vessel, composed of a single layer of squamous epithelial cells over a sheet of connective tissue. (12)

tunica media. The thicker middle layer of a blood vessel that contains smooth muscle cells, elastic fibers, and collagen. (12)

tympanic membrane. A sheet of tissue found at the end of the auditory canal; also known as the *eardrum.* (8)

type I diabetes mellitus. An autoimmune disorder in which the immune system attacks the insulin-secreting beta cells of the pancreas, causing insulin production to decrease or stop completely. (9)

type II diabetes mellitus. A condition in which the body's insulin receptors are downregulated. (9)

U

ulcerative colitis. An inflammatory bowel disease that usually affects the colon and the mucosal layer of the intestinal wall. (14)

ulna. Larger bone of the lower arm. (5)

umbilical cord. The cord that connects the fetus to the placenta. (16)

universal donor. A person with type O blood, which has neither A nor B antigens; can donate blood for transfusion to people of all blood types. (11)

universal recipient. A person with type AB blood, which has neither A nor B antibodies; can safely receive a transfusion of any blood type. (11)

upper extremity. The shoulders, arms, and hands. (5)

upregulated. Increased. (9)

ureter. A duct through which urine travels from the kidney to the bladder. (15)

urethra. A thin tube that connects the urinary bladder to the outside environment. (15)

urinalysis. Laboratory analysis of urine to test for the presence of infection or disease. (15)

urinary bladder. A hollow, muscular organ that stores urine; also called the *bladder*. (15)

urinary system. The organs involved in the formation, storage, and excretion of urine; includes the kidneys, ureters, bladder, and urethra. (15)

urinary tract infection (UTI). An infection of the urethra, bladder, ureters, and/or kidney, usually caused by bacteria that enter the urethra at its outside opening. (15)

urine specific gravity. The density of urine divided by the density of pure water. (15)

uterine cycle. The monthly cycle of changes that the uterus undergoes; includes the menstrual, proliferative, and secretory phases. (16)

uterine tubes. The tubes in which the oocyte is fertilized; begin at the lateral end of the ovary and travel up and around the ovary to terminate at the top lateral portion of the uterus. (16)

uterus. A hollow, muscular organ located in front of the rectum and behind the bladder; also known as the *womb*. (16)

V

vagina. A thin-walled, tubular structure located below the uterus; also known as the *birth canal*. (16)

valvular stenosis. A narrowing of the heart valve due to stiff or fused valve cusps. (12)

vasa recta. Thin-walled blood vessels that begin and end near the boundary between the renal cortex and the renal medulla, and which extend deep into the renal medulla, running parallel to the nephron loops; play a role in the formation of concentrated urine. (15)

vasoconstriction. Narrowing of the blood vessels, which decreases blood flow. (12)

vasodilation. Widening of the blood vessels, which increases blood flow. (12)

veins. Blood vessels that carry blood to the heart. (12)

ventral ramus. The anterior division of spinal nerves that communicate with the muscle and skin of the anterior and lateral trunk. (7)

ventricular fibrillation. A life-threatening condition in which the heart ventricles quiver at a rate greater than 350 bpm. (12)

ventricular tachycardia. A life-threatening arrhythmia in which the ventricles, rather than the SA node, initiate the heartbeat; the heart rate is between 150 and 250 bpm, requiring swift medical attention. (12)

venules. The smallest veins; connect the capillaries with the larger systemic veins. (12)

vertebra. One of the bones making up the spinal column. (5)

vestibule. A chamber in the inner ear that contains the three semicircular canals. (8)

vestibulocochlear nerve. A cranial nerve comprising the cochlear nerve and the vestibular nerve. (8)

vital capacity (VC). The total amount of air that can be forcibly expired from the lungs after a maximum inspiration. (10)

vitamin deficiency. The long-term lack of a particular vitamin in one's diet; may result in certain health problems. (14)

vitamins. Organic chemicals needed by the body for normal functioning and good health. (14)

vitreous humor. A gel-like substance in the posterior chamber of the eye that helps maintain intraocular pressure. (8)

W

weight. The force equal to the gravitational acceleration exerted on the mass of an object. (1)

white blood cells. Blood cells that fight infection and protect the body through various mechanisms; also known as *leukocytes*. (11)

Z

zygote. A diploid cell produced by the fusion of a sperm with an egg; a fertilized egg. (16)

Index

B

C

F

I

J

K

L

N

O

Q

R

S

T

U

V

W

X

Y

Z